P9-DUD-104

Rudolph's Fundamentals of

PEDIATRICS

Second Edition

Rudolph's Fundamentals of
PEDIATRICS

Second Edition

Editors

Abraham M. Rudolph, MD
Professor of Pediatrics Emeritus and Senior Staff Member
Cardiovascular Research Institute
University of California, San Francisco
San Francisco, California

Robert K. Kamei, MD
Associate Professor of Clinical Pediatrics
Director, Residency Training Program
Department of Pediatrics
University of California, San Francisco
San Francisco, California

Assistant Editor
Paul Sagan

APPLETON & LANGE
Stamford, Connecticut

Notice: The authors and the publisher of this volume have taken care to make certain that the doses of drugs and schedules of treatment are correct and compatible with the standards generally accepted at the time of publication. Nevertheless, as new information becomes available, changes in treatment and in the use of drugs become necessary. The reader is advised to carefully consult the instruction and information material included in the package insert of each drug or therapeutic agent before administration. This advice is especially important when using, administering, or recommending new or infrequently used drugs. The authors and publisher disclaim all responsibility for any liability, loss, injury, or damage incurred as a consequence, directly or indirectly, of the use and application of any of the contents of this volume.

Copyright © 1998 by Appleton & Lange
A Simon & Schuster Company
Copyright © 1994 by Appleton & Lange

All rights reserved. This book, or any parts thereof, may not be used or reproduced in any manner without written permission. For information, address Appleton & Lange, Four Stamford Plaza, PO Box 120041, Stamford, Connecticut 06912-0041.

www.appletonlange.com

98 99 00 01 02 / 10 9 8 7 6 5 4 3 2 1

Prentice Hall International (UK) Limited, *London*
Prentice Hall of Australia Pty. Limited, *Sydney*
Prentice Hall Canada, Inc., *Toronto*
Prentice Hall Hispanoamericana, S.A., *Mexico*
Prentice Hall of India Private Limited, *New Delhi*
Prentice Hall of Japan, Inc., *Tokyo*
Simon & Schuster Asia Pte. Ltd., *Singapore*
Editora Prentice Hall do Brasil Ltda., *Rio de Janeiro*
Prentice Hall, *Upper Saddle River, New Jersey*

ISSN: 1074-7451

Acquisitions Editor: Shelley Reinhardt
Development Editor: Cara Lyn Coffey
Production Editor: Lisa M. Guidone
Art Coordinator: Maggie Darrow
Designer: Mary Skudlarek
Cover illustration: *Homage à Bleriot* by Robert Delaunay

ISBN 0-8385-8236-2

PRINTED IN THE UNITED STATES OF AMERICA

Contents

Authors

Ann Alpers, JD
Assistant Professor, University of California, San Francisco, California
Internet: ann_alpers@ucsfdgim.ucsf.edu
Ethical Issues in Pediatrics

William F. Balistreri, MD
Director, Gastroenterology and Nutrition, Children's Hospital Medical Center, Cincinnati, Ohio
Internet: W.Balistreri@chmcc.org
The Gastrointestinal Tract & Liver

Michael M. Brook, MD
Assistant Professor of Clinical Pediatrics, University of California, San Francisco, San Francisco, California
Internet: mmbrook@pedcard.ucsf.edu
Circulation

Susan Carden, MD
Fellow, Pediatric Ophthalmology, Children's Hospital Medical Center, Cincinnati, Ohio
Ophthalmology

Caroline J. Chantry, MD
Assistant Professor, Department of Pediatrics, University of Puerto Rico School of Medicine, San Juan, Puerto Rico
Internet: chantry.caroline@karloff.fstrf.org
Adolescence

John Christodoulou, MB, BS, PhD, FRACP, CGHGSA
Associate Professor, Department of Pediatrics and Child Health, University of Sydney, Sydney, NSW, Australia; Director, Western Sydney Genetics Program, Royal Alexandra Hospital for Children, Westmead, NSW, Australia
Internet: johnch@mail.usyd.edu.au
A Clinical Approach to Inborn Errors of Metabolism

Cynthia R. Curry, MD
Professor of Pediatrics, University of California, San Francisco; Director, Genetic Medicine, Valley Children's Hospital, Fresno, California
Internet: curryc@valleychildrens.org
An Approach to Clinical Genetics

Mark E. Dato, MD, PhD
Project Physician/Scientist, Procter & Gamble Pharmaceuticals, Cincinnati, Ohio
Internet: dato.me@pg.com
Respiratory Diseases

Carol A. Diamond, MD
Assistant Clinical Professor, University of California, San Francisco, San Francisco, California
Internet: Carol.Diamond@ncal.kaiperm.org
Oncology

Dennis R. Durbin, MD
Assistant Professor of Pediatrics and Epidemiology, Division of Emergency Medicine, The Children's Hospital of Philadelphia, Philadelphia, Pennsylvania
Internet: durbin@cceb.med.upenn.edu
Injuries & Emergencies

Andrew Eichenfield, MD
Assistant Professor of Pediatrics and Chief, Pediatric Rheumatology, Mount Sinai Medical Center, New York, New York
Internet: A_Eichenfield@smtplink.mssm.edu
Rheumatic Diseases

Lawrence F. Eichenfield, MD
Associate Clinical Professor, Department of Pediatrics and Medicine (Dermatology), University of California, San Diego, School of Medicine, San Diego; Chief, Division of Pediatric and Adolescent Dermatology and Laser Surgery, Children's Hospital, San Diego, California
Internet: leichenfield@ucsd.edu
Skin

Joel A. Fein, MD
Assistant Professor of Pediatrics, The University of Pennsylvania School of Medicine, Philadelphia; Attending Physician, Emergency Department, The Children's Hospital of Philadelphia, Philadelphia, Pennsylvania
Internet: fein@email.chop.edu
Injuries & Emergencies

Donna M. Ferriero, MD
Associate Professor, Neurology and Pediatrics, University of California, San Francisco; Director, Child Neurology Clinic, San Francisco General Hospital, San Francisco, California
Internet: dmf@itsa.ucsf.edu
The Nervous System

Sheila Fallon Friedlander, MD
Assistant Clinical Professor, Departments of Pediatrics and Medicine, University of California, San Diego, School of Medicine and Children's Hospital, San Diego, California
Internet: sfriedlander@chsd.org
Skin

Tina Gabby MD, MPH
Assistant Clinical Professor, Department of Pediatrics, University of California, San Francisco, San Francisco, California
Internet: tgabby@itsa.ucsf.edu
Developmental & Behavioral Pediatrics

Francesca Geertsma, MD
Assistant Clinical Professor, Department of Pediatrics,
University of California, San Francisco; Assistant Medical
Director, Infectious Diseases, Valley Children's Hospital,
Fresno, California
Infectious Diseases

Stephen E. Gitelman, MD
Associate Professor, Pediatric Endocrinology and Diabetes,
University of California, San Francisco, San Francisco,
California
Internet: sgitelma@peds.ucsf.edu
Endocrinology

William V. Good, MD
Scientist (Clinical), Smith-Kettlewell Eye Research Institute,
San Francisco, California
Internet: good@skivs.ski.org
Ophthalmology

Caroline A. Hastings, MD
Assistant Clinical Professor, Department of Pediatrics,
University of California, San Francisco; Associate
Hematologist, Children's Hospital, Oakland, California
Blood

Anna Huttenlocher, MD
Assistant Professor, Department of Pediatrics, University of
Illinois College of Medicine, Urbana, Illinois
Internet: Huttenlo@uiuc.edu
Immunologic Disorders

Donald Wayne Laney, Jr, MD
Assistant Professor of Pediatrics and Nutrition Sciences,
University of Alabama School of Medicine, Birmingham;
Medical Director, North AL Children's Specialists,
Huntsville, Alabama
Internet: wlaney@pol.net
The Gastrointestinal Tract & Liver

Allan S. Lau, MD, FRCP(C)
Associate Professor, Department of Pediatrics, University of
California, San Francisco, San Francisco, California
Internet: asylau@itsa.ucsf.edu
Infectious Diseases

Deborah Lehman, MD
Assistant Clinical Professor, University of California, Irvine;
Attending Physician, Pediatric Infectious Diseases,
Memorial Miller Children's Hospital, Long Beach,
California
Infectious Diseases

Robert H. Levin, PharmD
Professor, Clinical Pharmacy & Pediatrics, University of
California, San Francisco; Associate Director,
Pharmaceutical Services, San Francisco General Hospital,
San Francisco, California
Internet: rhl@itsa.ucsf.edu
Drug Disposition and Therapy

Bernard Lo, MD
Professor of Medicine, Director, Program in Medical Ethics,
University of California, San Francisco, San Francisco,
California
Internet: bernie@utsa.ucsf.edu
Ethical Issues in Pediatrics

Bertram H. Lubin, MD
Director of Medical Research, Children's Hospital Oakland,
Oakland, California
Internet: blubin@lanminds.com
Blood

Robert S. Mathias, MD
Assistant Professor of Pediatrics, University of California,
San Francisco, San Francisco, California
Internet: rmathias@ped.ucsf.edu
Kidneys & Electrolytes

Roderick R. McInnes MD, PhD
Professor of Pediatrics and Molecular and Medical Genetics,
University of Toronto Faculty of Medicine, The Hospital
for Sick Children, Toronto, Canada
Internet: mcinnes@sickkids.
Clinical Approach to Inborn Errors of Metabolism

Phillip Moore, MD
Assistant Clinical Professor of Pediatrics, Director, Pediatric
Catheterization Laboratory, University of California, San
Francisco, San Francisco, California
Circulation

Kim J. Overby, MD
Assistant Professor of Pediatrics, University of Iowa College
of Medicine, Iowa City, Iowa
Health Supervision

John Colin Partridge, MD, MPH
Associate Clinical Professor, Pediatrics, San Francisco
General Hospital, University of California, San Francisco,
San Francisco, California
The Perinatal Period

Anthony A. Portale, MD
Professor of Pediatrics and Medicine, Chief, Division of
Pediatric Nephrology, University of California, San
Francisco, San Francisco, California
Internet: aportale@peds.ucsf.edu
Kidneys & Electrolytes

Donald E. Potter, MD
Clinical Professor of Pediatrics, University of California, San
Francisco, San Francisco, California
Kidneys & Electrolytes

Marta R. Rogido, MD
Pediatric Resident, Cedars–Sinai Medical Center, Los
Angeles, California
Internet: mrogido@mailgate.scmc.edu
The Perinatal Period

Stephen M. Rosenthal, MD
Associate Professor of Pediatrics, University of California,
San Francisco, San Francisco, California
Internet: smr@itsa.ucsf.edu
Endocrinology

Steven M. Selbst, MD
Professor of Pediatrics, University of Pennsylvania School of
Medicine, Philadelphia, Pennsylvania
Injuries & Emergencies

Richard S. Shames, MD
Assistant Professor of Pediatrics, Stanford University School
of Medicine, Stanford, California
Internet: rshames@leland.stanford.edu
Allergy: Mechanisms & Disease Processes

John T. Smith, MD
Associate Professor, Department of Orthopedics, University
of Utah School of Medicine, Salt Lake City, Utah
Internet: john.smith@hsc.utah.edu
Orthopedic Problems

Augusto Sola, MD
Director, Division of Neonatology, Ahmason Pediatric
Center, Cedars–Sinai Medical Center; Professor of
Pediatrics, University of California, Los Angeles, Los
Angeles, California
Internet: asola@mailgate.scmc.edu
The Perinatal Period

Surachai Supattapone, MD, PhD, DPhil
Clinical Fellow in Infectious Diseases, Department of
Infectious Diseases, University of California, San
Francisco, San Francisco, California
Infectious Diseases

Diana C. Tanney, MD
Assistant Professor of Pediatrics, Stanford University,
Stanford, California
Internet: md.dct@forsythe.stanford.edu
Kidneys & Electrolytes

Alan Uba, MD
Assistant Clinical Professor of Pediatrics, University of
California, San Francisco, San Francisco, California
Internet: alan_uba@ucsfmgph.his.ucsf.edu
Infectious Diseases

George F. Van Hare, MD
Associate Professor of Pediatrics and Medicine; Director of
Pediatric Arrhythmia Service, Rainbow Babies and
Children Hospital, Cleveland, Ohio
Circulation

Diane Wara, MD
Professor of Pediatrics, Director, Pediatric
Immunology/Rheumatology, Director, Pediatric Clinical
Research Center, University of California, San Francisco,
San Francisco, California
Internet: wara@gcrc.ucsf.edu
Immunologic Disorders

William Weiss, MD
Assistant Professor of Neurology (Child Neurology), Hooper
Foundation, University of California, San Francisco, San
Francisco, California
Internet: weiss@cgl.ucsf.edu
The Nervous System

Robert W. Wilmott, MD
Professor, Department of Pediatrics, University of Cincinnati
College of Medicine, Cincinnati; The Hubert and Dorothy
Campbell Professor of Pediatric Pulmonology, Children's
Hospital Medical Center, Cincinnati, Ohio
Internet: wilmr@chmcc.org
Respiratory Diseases

Preface

In the first edition, we attempted to create a text that provided a broad information base of pediatrics and did so using a problem-oriented clinical approach. From our experience in the clinical teaching of pediatrics to medical students and residents, we recognize that traditional textbooks usually lack what is most needed: an approach that not only reviews normal and abnormal function in important areas but also provides information helpful in the analysis of common symptom complexes. Learning pediatrics by focusing on the presenting symptom complexes is important for students' understanding and in aiding their ability to remember, process, and apply information in diagnosis and treatment.

We were pleased with the positive reception of the first edition by both students and faculty. This second edition extends the goals of the first. We have added more algorithms and tables that summarize material simply, in a form that is easily assimilable. A new chapter on ethics covers issues frequently encountered by pediatric practitioners. Many sections have been rewritten and expanded for clarity and comprehensiveness. But, as with the first edition, we made particular efforts to indicate what is important—because it is common, because it is treatable, or because it is harmful if overlooked. There is still a minimum of reference citations; only selected lists are included for either historical interest or more extensive review.

As before, we greatly appreciate the contributors' efforts in responding to our comments and suggestions. We also remain grateful for the excellent editorial assistance of Paul Sagan.

Abraham M. Rudolph, MD
Robert K. Kamei, MD

San Francisco, California
February 1998

1

Health Supervision

Kim J. Overby, MD

The goal of primary care pediatrics is to facilitate optimal health and well-being for children and their families. This is accomplished through a variety of interrelated activities, including problem surveillance and management, problem prevention, health promotion, and the coordination of care for special-needs children. The traditional focus on problem diagnosis and management has been broadened to include screening for disease and its precursors in asymptomatic populations. Pediatric providers have long recognized the value of preventive programs, such as mass immunization, and continue to lead the way in this area through an emphasis on regular health supervision, anticipatory guidance, and involvement in community-based prevention strategies. Recent emphasis has also been placed on the related concept of health promotion, whereby optimal health and well-being can be positively encouraged rather than focusing only on avoiding problems. A by-product of the successes of modern medicine has been an increasing population of children with chronic illness, disability, and other special needs. The primary care provider is in a unique position to coordinate the often complex care of these children and to facilitate communication among the individuals involved in their cases. These areas form the foundation for current recommendations regarding routine child health supervision (Table 1–1), which are based largely on common sense and expert consensus. Much further research is needed to help providers determine the optimal schedule and content of the well-child visit.

Caring for children provides unique rewards and challenges. The interplay between environmental influences and factors intrinsic to the child becomes evident in many aspects of pediatric health and development. Continuity of care is based on a developmental framework that recognizes the constancy of growth and change throughout childhood. At each visit, the child's developmental level dictates both the approach to the patient and much of the visit's content. Flexibility is essential in performing the physical examination. A focus on examining the least threatening areas first and on using age-appropriate methods to minimize the child's anxiety is important. In pediatrics, the therapeutic alliance must necessarily include both children and their families; therefore, the importance of establishing a trusting long-term relationship cannot be overemphasized.

This chapter is divided into five main sections—Physical Growth, Motor and Psychological Development, Counseling and Anticipatory Guidance, Screening, and Immunizations—and is intended to provide a functional overview of the major components of pediatric health supervision as well as some issues and problems frequently encountered in each of these areas. Issues with specific relevance to adolescents are covered in more depth in Chapter 2.

PHYSICAL GROWTH

Changes in physical size and appearance are a visible manifestation of the complex morphologic, biochemical, and physiologic changes taking place during childhood. Pediatric health care providers routinely monitor weight, length, head circumference, dental development, and the appearance of secondary sexual characteristics to assess the overall adequacy of a child's growth. Common rules of thumb regarding physical growth patterns are given in Tables 1–2 and 1–3. The normal progression of secondary sexual characteristics is discussed in Chapter 2.

In the absence of an absolute definition of normality, the adequacy of a child's growth is determined by comparison with others of similar age and sex, as well as by the presence or absence of concordance between growth parameters and the consistency of growth patterns over time. Plotting a child's height, weight, and head circumference on a standard National Center for Health Statistics (NCHS) cross-sectional growth chart provides a statistical definition of normality by comparing that individual with others of similar age and sex. Although the farther a

Table 1–1. Guidelines for health supervision.[1]

	Infancy							Early Childhood				Late Childhood							Adolescence								
	New-born	By 1 mo	2 mo	4 mo	6 mo	9 mo	12 mo	15 mo	18 mo	24 mo	3 y	4 y	5 y	6 y	8 y	10 y	11 y	12 y	13 y	14 y	15 y	16 y	17 y	18 y	19 y	20 y	21 y
History: initial/interval	•	•	•	•	•	•	•	•	•	•	•	•	•	•	•	•	•	•	•	•	•	•	•	•	•	•	•
Growth parameters Height & weight	•	•	•	•	•	•	•	•	•	•	•	•	•	•	•	•	•	•	•	•	•	•	•	•	•	•	•
Head circumference	•	•	•	•	•	•	•	•	•	•																	
Tanner staging[2]															•	•	•	•	•	•	•	•	•	•	•	•	•
Physical examination	•	•	•	•	•	•	•	•	•	•	•	•	•	•	•	•	•	•	•	•	•	•	•	•	•	•	•
Developmental surveillance	•	•	•	•	•	•	•	•	•	•	•	•	•	•	•	•	•	•	•	•	•	•	•	•	•	•	•
Screening Newborn metabolic	•																										
Newborn hemoglobinopathies	•																										
Vision	S	S	S	S	S	S	S	S	S	S	S/O	O	O	S	S	O	S	O	S	S	O	S	S	O	S	S	S
Hearing[3]	S/O* →	S →	S ←	S	S	S	S	S	S	S	S/O	O	O	S	S	O	S	O	S	S	O	S	S	O	S	S	S
Blood pressure											•	•	•	•	•	•	•	•	•	•	•	•	•	•	•	•	•
Cholesterol[4]										*	*	*	*	*	*	*	*	*	*	*	*	*	*	*	*	*	*
Lead[5]							•			•																	
Hematocrit/ hemoglobin[6]						←	*	→											*	*	*	*	*	*	*	*	*
PPD[7]												*	*	*	*	*	*	*	*	*	*	*	*	*	*	*	*
STD screening[8]																	*	*	*	*	*	*	*	*	*	*	*
PAP/pelvic[9]																	*	*	*	*	*	*	←		*		→
Anticipatory guidance	•	•	•	•	•	•	•	•	•	•	•	•	•	•	•	•	•	•	•	•	•	•	•	•	•	•	•
Immunizations[10]	• →	→	•	•	•		• →	→	→			←	•	→						←	•	→					
Initial dental referral							←	←	←	←	•																

[1]Adapted from American Academy of Pediatrics (AAP) Committee on Practice and Ambulatory Medicine Recommendations 1995.
[2]Secondary sexual characteristics (see Chapter 2).
[3]Goal of universal objective hearing assessment at birth to 3 months supported by AAP. Until effective technologies/programs are in place to accomplish this, a selective screening strategy based on the presence of risk factors is recommended (see section on screening).
[4]Selective screening at 24 months based on presence of risk factors; subsequent screening interval determined by same; universal screening at 18–21 years (see section on screening).
[5]Universal screening at 12 and 24 months; earlier and more frequent screening based on presence of risk factors (see section on screening).
[6]Selective screening at 9–15 months and during adolescence based on presence of risk factors (see section on screening).
[7]Selective screening based on presence of risk factors; subsequent screening interval determined by same (see section on screening).
[8]All sexually active patients should be screened for STDs at least annually; more frequently if high risk (see Chapter 2 regarding specific tests).
[9]All sexually active females should have a pelvic examination. A pelvic examination and routine PAP smear should be offered as part of preventive health maintenance between the ages of 18 and 21 years.
[10] See section on immunizations for recommendations regarding specific vaccines and acceptable variations in shedule at administration.
• = to be performed; * = to be performed for patients at risk; S = subjective, by history; O = objective, by a standard testing method; ←•→ = range during which a service may be provided, with the dot indicating the preferred age; PAP = Papanicolaou smear; PPD = purified protein derivative; STD = sexually transmitted disease.

Table 1–2. Typical patterns of physical growth.

Weight:	Birth weight is regained by 10th–14th day. Average weight gain/day: 0–6 mo = 20 g; 6–12 mo = 15 g. Birth weight doubles at ~ 4 mo, triples at ~ 12 mo, quadruples at ~ 24 mo. During second year, average weight gain/month = ~ 0.25 kg. After age 2 y, average annual gain until adolescence = ~ 2.3 kg (5 lb).
Length/height:	By end of first year, birth length increases by 50%. Birth length doubles by 4 y, triples by 13 y. Average height gain during second year = ~12 cm (5 in). After age 2 y, average annual growth until adolescence ≥ 5 cm (2 in).
Head circumference:	Average head growth/week: 0–2 mo = ~ 0.5 cm, 2–6 mo = ~ 0.25 cm. Average total head growth from 0–3 mo = ~ 5 cm, 3–6 mo = ~ 4 cm, 6–9 mo = ~ 2 cm, 9 mo–1 y = ~ 1 cm.

Table 1–3. Chronology of tooth eruption and exfoliation.

	Eruption	
	Maxillary	**Mandible**
Primary[1]		
Central incisor	10 (8–12)	8 (6–10)
Lateral incisor	11 (9–13)	13 (10–16)
Canine	19 (16–22)	20 (17–23)
First molar	16 (13–19 boys) (14–19 girls)	16 (14–18)
Second molar	29 (25–33)	27 (23–31 boys) (24–30 girls)
Permanent[2]		
Central incisor	7–7.5	6–6.5
Lateral incisor	8–8.5	7.2–7.7
Canine	11–11.6	9.7–10.2
First premolar	10–10.3	10–10.7
Second premolar	10.7–11.2	10.7–11.5
First molar	6–6.3	6–6.2
Second molar	12.2–12.7	11.7–12
Third molar	20.5	20–20.5

	Exfoliation[3]			
			Mean Age (y/mo)	
Rank	**Mandibular Arch**	**Maxillary Arch**	**Boys**	**Girls**
First	Central incisors		6.0	5.7
Second		Central incisors	6.10	6.7
Third	Lateral incisors		7.2	6.10
Fourth		Lateral incisors	7.10	7.5
Fifth	Canines		10.5	9.7
Sixth	First molars		10.8	10.2
Seventh		First molars	10.11	10.6
Eighth		Canines	11.3	10.7
Ninth	Second molars	Second molars	11.9	11.5

[1]Mean age in months + 1 SD. Adapted and reproduced, with permission, from Lunt RC, Law DB: J Am Dent Assoc 1974;89:878.
[2]Mean age in years. Adapted and reproduced, with permission, from Burdi AR: The development and eruption of the human dentitions. Chapter 5 in: *Pediatric Dental Medicine,* Forrester DJ, Fleming J (editors). Lea & Febiger, 1981.
[3]Adapted and reproduced, with permission, from Ripa LW et al: Chronology and sequence of exfoliation of primary teeth. J Am Dent Assoc 1982;105:641.

child's growth parameters are from population norms (traditionally defined as 2 SD above and below the mean), the greater the likelihood of a growth problem, making assumptions about the adequacy of a child's growth on the basis of a single set of growth parameters can be misleading. By definition, approximately 5% of the population will be above and below the range of growth parameters statistically defined as normal. The standard NCHS growth curves were generated by measuring different groups of primarily white, middle-class children at each age, and when these data are extrapolated to those of different ethnic or racial backgrounds, may erroneously label their growth as abnormal.

Of even greater importance to the overall assessment of a child's growth is the observation of growth curves over time. Serial measurements provide the most accurate indication of whether physical growth is progressing normally for a given individual. Because most children track along a genetically determined percentile, significant deviations from a previously stable growth curve should provoke concern. However, downward crossing of percentiles during the first 2 years of life can also result from several normal growth variants.

A third aspect of growth assessment involves observing the relationship between growth parameters in a given child. For most individuals, general concordance is observed between percentiles for height, weight, and head circumference. Major discrepancies between or disproportionate fall-off in growth parameters may suggest a variety of specific growth problems.

Routine surveillance of a child's growth provides a framework for periodic discussions regarding normal growth patterns, nutritional needs, and developmental feeding behaviors of infants and children. The primary care provider is also in a unique position to detect and orchestrate subsequent evaluation and management of a variety of growth problems. Knowledge of both normal and pathologic growth patterns is essential to this process. The following section focuses on several of the most common growth concerns pediatricians must confront, including failure to thrive, obesity, and variations in head size. The approach to short stature and variations in pubertal development are discussed in Chapter 19.

COMMON GROWTH CONCERNS

Failure to Thrive

The term **failure to thrive,** first used to describe the malnourished and depressed condition of many institutionalized infants in the early 1900s, remains a descriptive rather than a diagnostic label. It is generally applied to children whose attained weight or rate of weight gain is significantly below that of other children of similar age and sex. Depending on the length and severity of malnourishment, linear growth and head circumference may also be affected. Although the adverse acute and long-term consequences of childhood malnutrition are well established, the point at which deviations from age-related norms exceed normal growth variation and place the child at risk is less certain. Lack of consensus regarding specific anthropomorphic criteria for identifying the child who is failing to thrive is reflected in the number of commonly used definitions (Table 1–4).

Growth failure in infancy and childhood can result from a wide range of factors, including serious medical disease, dysfunctional child-caregiver interactions, poverty, parental misinformation, and child abuse (Table 1–5). In most cases, an underlying organic etiology is not found; when one is identified, it rarely presents with growth failure as its only manifestation. On the other hand, psychosocial problems resulting in growth failure are common and should no longer be perceived as diagnoses of exclusion. Whether primarily organic or psychosocial in origin, all children who fail to thrive suffer the physical and psychological consequences of malnutrition and are at significant risk for long-term physical and psycho-developmental sequelae. In recognition of this fact and that biologic and psychosocial problems frequently coexist, the approach to the child with apparent growth failure has shifted away from attempts to define a purely organic or nonorganic etiology to focus instead on assessing both physical and psychosocial risk factors, the degree of malnourishment present, and the resultant physiological and psychodevelopmental consequences for that child. Key aspects of the evaluation include a review of past and present growth data, a thorough history and physical examination, a developmental and behavioral assessment, observation of a feeding, assessment of both situation-specific and global child-parent interaction, and selected laboratory studies based on concerns raised by the evaluation (see Table 1–6).

Table 1–4. Definitions of failure to thrive.

Attained growth
Weight < 3rd percentile on NCHS growth chart
Weight for height < 5th percentile on NCHS growth chart
Weight 20% or more below ideal weight for height
Triceps skin fold thickness ≤ 5 mm
Rate of growth
Depressed rate of weight gain
< 20 g/d from 0–3 mo of age
< 15 g/d from 3–6 mo of age
Falloff from previously established growth curve:
downward crossing of ≥ 2 major percentiles on NCHS growth charts
Documented weight loss

NCHS = National Center for Health Statistics.

Table 1–5. Causes of inadequate weight gain.

Inadequate intake
Poverty
Misperceptions about diet and feeding practices
Inadequate breast milk production
Errors in formula reconstitution
Dysfunctional parent-child interaction:
Behavioral feeding problem
Neglect
Child abuse
Mechanical problems with sucking, swallowing, and feeding
Primary neurologic disease
Chromosomal abnormality
Prenatal insult
Systemic disease resulting in anorexia/food refusal
Calorie wasting
Persistent vomiting
Gastroesophageal reflux
Gastrointestinal obstruction
Rumination
Metabolic problems
Increased intracranial pressure
Malabsorption/chronic diarrhea
Primary gastrointestinal diseases
Cystic fibrosis
Infections
Endocrinopathies
Structural problems
Renal losses
Diabetes
Renal tubular acidosis
Increased caloric requirements
Congenital heart disease
Chronic respiratory disease
Neoplasm
Hyperthyroidism
Chronic or recurrent infection
Altered growth potential/regulation
Prenatal insult
Chromosomal abnormality
Endocrinopathies

Because many parents occasionally worry about their child's growth, and because several normal variants can be confused with growth failure, the first issue that must be addressed is whether the child is truly failing to thrive. This question can best be answered by reviewing the child's past and present growth data for deviations from population norms, consistency over time, and concordance between growth parameters. As previously mentioned, care must be taken when applying NCHS growth norms, which were derived primarily from a white, middle-class population, to children of different ethnic or racial backgrounds. Children who are genetically short or small tend to be small at birth, and their growth parameters are consistent with parental size. They have a normal weight for height (both equally below the 3rd percentile), growth curves that fall below but parallel to NCHS curves, a normal skinfold thickness, and a bone age consistent with chronologic age.

The shape and placement of growth curves over time

provide important information (Figure 1–1). Children who are growing normally parallel their genetically determined percentile on the standard NCHS growth curves. Children who are genetically small parallel the standard curves at the low end of, or just below, the statistically defined normal range of heights and weights in the population. Children who have suffered a significant prenatal event leading to growth failure typically are proportionately small for gestational age at birth and, with time, continue to fall farther away from population means on all parameters. The postnatal onset of a growth problem is manifest by a downward trend in a previously stable growth curve. While the downward crossing of percentiles should always provoke concern, during the first 2 years of life this pattern can also result from two normal growth variants that may be difficult to differentiate from growth failure. A baby's size at birth is significantly influenced by maternal intrauterine conditions, and some downward shifting may occur as the percentile representing the child's true genetic growth potential is achieved. Such shifting generally occurs between 6 and 12 months of age and is associated with a steady, although decreased, rate of weight gain. Downward percentile shifting can also occur owing to normal variations in the rate and timing of growth spurts. Because NCHS growth curves were constructed by using different samples of children at each age rather than by observing the same cohort over time, they cannot differentiate normal variations in the rate of growth from early pathologic growth. In constitutional growth delay, a child's height and weight are normal at birth, drop off proportionately during the first 2 years of life, eventually parallel the NCHS growth curves at or just below the 5th

percentile for most of middle childhood, and then cross percentiles upward to achieve a final normal adult size. Bone age is delayed for the child's chronologic age but is consistent with height age (the age at which the child's height is at the 50th percentile). Although delays in early growth spurts may raise concerns regarding growth failure, constitutional growth delay is often first recognized when the shifted adolescent growth spurt results in the delayed appearance of secondary sexual characteristics. Like genetic short stature, constitutional growth delay is familial, and parents frequently report delayed adolescent development themselves ("late bloomer") or similar growth patterns in other offspring. The recent availability of longitudinal growth charts, which provide normative data for early-, average-, and late-developing children, allows the physician to identify more readily these constitutional growth variants as normal.

Major discrepancies between growth parameters may also indicate a variety of problems. Several characteristic patterns have been described (Figure 1–2). Weight, height, and head circumference that are all significantly below that expected for the child's chronologic age suggest the possibility of an intrauterine insult or genetic abnormality. Relative sparing of the head circumference in relation to weight and height that are significantly below that predicted for chronologic age is more characteristic of the normal variants of constitutional growth delay and genetic short stature, as well as structural dystrophies and endocrine causes of growth failure. Caloric insufficiency from inadequate intake, increased loss, or a hypermetabolic state is suggested when weight is significantly below that expected for chronologic age, with relative sparing of both head circumference and height.

When review of growth data reveals inadequate growth, the physician must ascertain whether this is due primarily to inadequate caloric intake, calorie wasting, an increased caloric requirement, or alteration in growth potential (Table 1–6). Evidence should be elicited to support a specific situational, behavioral, interactional, or medical problem. In addition to detailed medical information, a thorough dietary, feeding, social, behavioral, and developmental history is essential. Most cases of failure to thrive result from inadequate consumption of appropriate amounts or kinds of food. Inadequate caloric intake is most often due to psychosocial problems, including lack of access to food, parental ignorance and misperceptions regarding appropriate feeding, dysfunctional feeding environment or interaction, or more global problems within the parent-child relationship. However, inadequate intake also can be due to oromotor or other feeding dysfunction or to medical problems that result in secondary anorexia or food refusal. When caloric intake appears to be adequate, evidence must be sought to suggest a condition associated with calorie wasting, an increased caloric requirement, or an alteration in growth potential. Excessive caloric losses occur primarily with several gastrointestinal and renal disorders. Children with cardiopulmonary problems, malignant tumors, hyperthyroidism, and chronic or

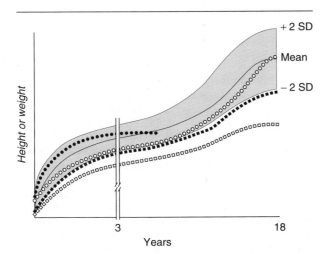

Figure 1–1. Growth curve patterns for children with postnatal-onset pathologic growth (closed circles), prenatal-onset pathologic growth (open squares), constitutional growth delay (open circles), genetic short stature (closed squares). Shaded area represents mean growth curve ± 2 SD.

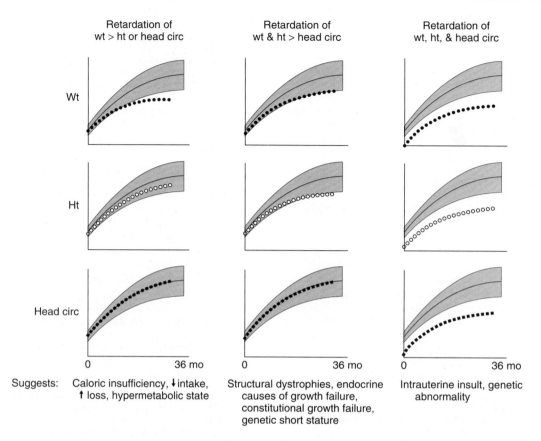

Retardation of wt > ht or head circ   Retardation of wt & ht > head circ   Retardation of wt, ht, & head circ

Wt

Ht

Head circ

0   36 mo   0   36 mo   0   36 mo

Suggests: Caloric insufficiency, ↓intake, ↑ loss, hypermetabolic state   Structural dystrophies, endocrine causes of growth failure, constitutional growth failure, genetic short stature   Intrauterine insult, genetic abnormality

Figure 1–2. Relationships between growth parameters (weight, height, and head circumference) and suggested causes.

recurrent infections may have increased caloric needs. A variety of prenatal insults, genetic abnormalities, and endocrinopathies may lead to alterations in the child's growth rate and potential.

Physical examination of a child who is growing poorly should focus on identifying signs of underlying organic disease, severity of malnutrition, and important concomitant findings, such as evidence of physical abuse or neglect and the presence of deprivational behaviors. Observation of the parent-child interaction should occur throughout the visit. Watching a feeding session is an excellent way to identify specific behavioral and interactional problems occurring during the feeding situation. A psychomotor developmental assessment should also be obtained. Children with severe psychosocial failure to thrive may manifest a variety of gaze disturbances, ranging from hyperalert, wary watchfulness to total avoidance of eye contact and apathetic withdrawal. Infants may resist cuddling and prefer interactions with inanimate objects, whereas toddlers may demonstrate indiscriminate affection-seeking behaviors. Many of these children also manifest developmental delays, especially in the areas of language and social adaptive behavior, which are most dependent on environmental stimulation.

The diagnostic laboratory evaluation should be guided by concerns raised in the history, physical examination, and review of growth data. Organic disease presenting only with growth failure is extremely uncommon. An undirected laboratory evaluation is rarely productive of an unsuspected diagnosis and is potentially harmful. Depending on the length and severity of the growth failure, additional laboratory studies may be useful to help assess nutritional status and the presence of concomitant problems, such as iron deficiency anemia. Most children with failure to thrive should receive a complete blood count, serum electrolytes, serum creatinine, total protein:albumin, urinalysis, urine culture, and determination of bone age (if height growth is also poor) as part of their evaluation.

Most children with growth failure can be evaluated and managed as outpatients, but some will require hospitalization. Among these are children with psychosocial failure to thrive who manifest evidence of, or are at high risk for, physical abuse or severe neglect, who are severely malnourished or medically unstable, or who have failed a trial of outpatient management. The approach to a child with failure to thrive requires both time and sensitivity. To facilitate subsequent communication and management, it is important to understand the parents' perspective regarding

Table 1–6. Evaluating the child with failure to thrive.

Growth data
Key issues
Is the child failing to thrive or does growth represent a normal variant?
Do growth parameters and curves suggest a specific etiology?
Components
Current growth parameters
Growth curves over time
Relationship of growth parameters to each other

History
Key issues
Do caretakers perceive growth to be a problem?
Is growth failure due to inadequate caloric intake, calorie wasting, increased caloric requirements, or altered growth potential?
Does the history suggest a specific situational, behavioral, interactional, or medical problem?
Components
Problem context
Parents' perception of child's growth and overall health
When growth problems first became a concern
Previous interventions attempted
Medical
Prenatal care and complications (infection, maternal, nutrition, drug exposure)
Gestational age and growth parameters at birth (small for gestational age, prematurity)
Perinatal complications (infections, central nervous system insults, anomalies)
Previous hospitalizations, illnesses, and surgery
Current medications
Review of systems (vomiting, stooling patterns, mechanics of feeding/swallowing, anorexia, distress/tiring with feedings)
Nutritional feeding
Caloric intake
Breast fed: schedule and length of feedings; maternal cues to prefeeding engorgement, milk let-down, and drainage; postfeeding; maternal diet, rest, stress, and medications
Formula fed: type, method of preparation, feeding schedule, and amount offered and consumed
Mixed diet: 3-day diet history (food/beverage type, method of preparation, quantity consumed)
Schedule and length of feedings
Cues to infant's/child's hunger and satiety
Daily feeding/ mealtime environment
Location/positioning during feedings
Perceptions of sucking, swallowing, and grasping of nipple
Caregivers involved with feedings
Amount and type of mealtime supervision
Behavior during feedings
History of progression to solid/table foods
Favorite/disliked foods
Parental knowledge/beliefs regarding child/infant feeding
Family eating practices and beliefs
Financial constraints affecting food availability
Psychosocial
Caregiving environment
Family support systems
Family finances
Stability of parents and their relationship
Family/household composition
Parent-child relationship
Attitudes toward parenting

Content/structure of typical day for the child
Parents' perceptions of child's needs
Developmental/behavioral
Age-related behavior problems (eg, attachment, autonomy)
Developmental milestones: gross/fine motor, language, social/emotional, cognition
Parents' perception of child's temperament/behavior

Physical examination
Key issues
Is there evidence to suggest an underlying organic etiology?
Is there evidence of severe malnutrition and/or nutritional deficiency?
Is there evidence of a disturbed parent-child relationship, including the presence of deprivational behaviors and/or signs of physical abuse/neglect?
Components
Physician-child interaction
Skinfold measurements
Complete physical examination

Developmental and behavioral assessment
Key issue
Is there global or asymmetric developmental delay?
Component
Neurodevelopmental assessment of gross/fine motor, language, socio-emotional, cognitive skills

Observation of a feeding
Key issue
Is there a specific situational, behavioral, interactional, and/or medical problem observed?
Components
Feeding environment (home observation)
Type and amount of food offered
Pace and duration of feeding
Child's oral-motor and fine motor skills
Child's cues to and prenatal response regarding readiness to eat and satiation
Parents' use of opportunities for positive reinforcement and social interaction
Parents' awareness and use of child's developmental abilities
Overall parent-child interaction

Laboratory studies
Key issues
Are any specific diagnostic studies indicated?
Does the extent of malnutrition warrant further laboratory studies?
Components
Diagnostic tests directed by positive findings on history, physical, and review of growth data
Consider: complete blood count, serum electrolytes, serum creatinine, urinalysis (± culture), total protein:albumin, bone age (if height growth is also poor)

Disposition
Key issue
Is inpatient evaluation warranted?
Hospitalize if
Evidence of physical abuse or severe neglect
High risk of abuse or neglect due to very disturbed parent-child interaction, poor parent functioning, or an extremely stressful environment
Severe malnutrition or medical instability
Outpatient management failure

their child's growth and health as well as to be cognizant of previous efforts to intervene when concerns have been present. Many parents of children who are failing to thrive experience feelings of guilt, inadequacy, and anger when psychosocial problems are uncovered; subsequent efforts to intercede are often perceived as being critical of their parental abilities. Focusing concern on the child's health and well-being, as well as the positive goal of enhancing the parent-child relationship, may help to defuse some of these feelings. Ultimately, the success of treatment often depends on establishing a positive and caring long-term alliance with children and their caretakers. Management of the child with psychosocial failure to thrive must be individualized to the specific needs of the child and family. In addition to nutritional rehabilitation, efforts are focused on correcting any dysfunctional child-parent interactions by addressing areas of parental misinformation, providing and helping to implement specific feeding guidance, and addressing the larger psychosocial needs of the family. A multidisciplinary team approach involving the primary care provider, nutritionist, social worker, child behavior specialist, and community-based outreach services is often the most beneficial.

Obesity

Childhood obesity is one of the most frequent as well as challenging growth problems faced by the pediatric health care provider. It is estimated that as many as 25% of children in the United States are significantly overweight. Concern for their well-being has focused on several immediate and future issues. Obesity in both children and adults has been associated with increased risk of hypertension, diabetes, and hyperlipidemia. The longer children remain obese, the more likely they will continue to be overweight as adults and to suffer the long-term cardiovascular consequences. Excessive weight may also predispose some children to orthopedic problems, such as Blount disease and slipped femoral capital epiphyses. Of equal importance to these medical concerns are the psychological consequences of obesity. Despite secular trends in food consumption and physical activity that have encouraged the rising prevalence of childhood obesity, our society puts a high premium on thinness. Children who are overweight are frequently subjected to conscious and unconscious stereotyping and discrimination by both adults and other children. They are often less popular with their peers than normal-weight individuals and may find themselves socially ostracized or isolated. Despite the complex causal relationship between biologic, environmental, and psychological factors, many individuals, including parents, simply blame these children for their weight problems, assuming them to be slovenly and lacking in self-control. Several investigators have described a higher incidence of poor self-concept and personality disturbances among obese as compared with normal-weight children. However, it should also be remembered that many overweight children suffer no psychological problems as a result of their obesity.

Childhood obesity is defined in most settings by comparison of indirect measures of body composition and fat distribution with population norms (Table 1–7). Unfortunately, these statistical definitions do not identify the point at which a given child is at risk for present or future morbidity. The simplest way to assess children's body fatness is to compare their weight with that of other children of similar age and sex. However, weight alone is a poor indicator of body fatness because it fails to take into account differences in body size and lean body mass. Measure-

Table 1–7. Commonly used measures and definitions of obesity.

Measure	Definition of Obesity	Comments/Limitations
Weight[a]	> 95th percentile for age/sex norms	Easy to obtain, reliable, does not take into account variations in frame size (height) and body composition (lean versus fat mass).
% Overweight	20% or more above ideal body weight[b] for age/sex norms	Reliable, easy to obtain. Corrects for variations in frame size (height) but still does not take into account variations in body composition (lean body versus fat mass).
Weight for height[a] Body mass index (weight/height^2)	> 95th percentile for age/sex norms > 85th percentile for age/sex norms	
Subcutaneous fat thickness (skinfolds)	> 85th percentile for age/sex norms	Best office-based, noninvasive method to directly assess degree of adiposity. Independent of above anthropometric measures.
Densitometry: Air versus hydrostatic (underwater) weighing Radioisotope distribution (K 40 space)		Gold standard for assessing adiposity and body fat. Not practical for use in office setting.

[a]Using National Center for Health Statistics growth charts.
[b]Ideal body weight = weight at the percentile that corresponds to the patient's height percentile on National Center for Health Statistics growth charts.

ments that incorporate weight and height, such as the body mass index (weight in kilograms divided by the height squared), are an improvement, in that they allow correction for body size (height), but they still do not differentiate differences in body composition (adiposity versus lean body mass). Skinfold measurements, obtained by gently compressing and measuring with calipers the skin and subcutaneous tissue in the triceps and subscapular areas, are a practical way to assess body adiposity and thereby differentiate the child who is overweight because of excess fat versus lean body mass.

Excess body fat results from energy intake that is in excess of energy expenditure. Although parents are frequently concerned about an underlying organic etiology, this occurs in fewer than 5% of children with excessive weight gain (Table 1–8). Most cases of childhood obesity are caused by a complex interaction between genetic and environmental factors affecting food consumption, activity level, and metabolic rate. The obese child is often the visible result of much broader family patterns of food intake, eating behavior, and physical activity, making intervention extremely challenging. Components of the evaluation of an obese child and their family are given in Table 1–9.

By reviewing past and present growth data and performing skinfold measurements, the physician can assess the extent to which the child's weight exceeds predicted norms based on height and represents an excess of adiposity as opposed to lean body mass. Knowledge of birth weight and growth curves over time can assist the physician in identifying and exploring events surrounding changes in a previously stable growth pattern. It is also important to assess the adequacy of the child's linear

growth. With the exception of hyperinsulinemia, most of the endocrinopathies and congenital syndromes causing secondary obesity are associated with poor height growth. Children with endogenous obesity are typically average or above average in height.

When the child's weight gain or adiposity are found to be excessive, the physician must seek to understand both the child's and parents' perspectives on the weight issue, how this problem fits into the larger family dynamic, and previous interventions that have been attempted. In addition to exploring these issues, the history should focus on documenting the amount and type of foods consumed, physical activity, individual and environmental factors influencing food consumption and activity level, the presence of or risk for medical or psychological morbidity, and evidence of an underlying disease process. Blood pressure assessment is an important aspect of the evaluation. Hypertension is a frequent complication of obesity and, when present, underlines the need for intervention. The physical examination may provide important clues to the rare presence of an underlying disease process. The presence of a centrifugal fat distribution, abdominal striae, skin and hair changes, dysmorphic features, and advanced or delayed pubertal development should be noted. Because of secondary endocrinologic effects, obese children tend to experience the physical changes of adrenarche and pubarche at an earlier age than their lean age-matched peers. Obesity in conjunction with delayed pubertal development should suggest a potential hypothalamic abnormality. Because the obese child's level of physical activity is an important part of both the problem and the solution, assessment of the child's overall cardiorespiratory fitness can be helpful. Laboratory evaluation of the obese child should be directed at confirming diagnostic concerns raised by the history and physical examination. Depending on the severity of obesity and family history, screening for concurrent morbidity and cardiovascular risk factors should also be done. A lower threshold for obtaining thyroid screening tests may be warranted, because infants and children with obesity secondary to hypothyroidism may not present with the classic findings.

Once a child's adiposity is identified as a problem, making significant and sustained changes is a difficult but not an impossible task. For this to occur, however, it is imperative that both the child (if age-appropriate) and parents perceive the obesity as a problem and recognize the importance of intervention. Treatment efforts that tailor suggestions to individual children and their environment, address controlling factors for both food intake and energy expenditure, and focus assessment and management at the family rather than the individual level have the greatest chance of success (Table 1–10). Older children, in particular, may also benefit from the mutual support and camaraderie provided by group activities with others who are also overweight. Because of the potential adverse effects of therapeutic dieting on brain and linear growth in children, caloric restriction is rarely encouraged. Rather than weight loss, the goal is to slow the rate of fat deposi-

Table 1–8. Causes of secondary obesity.[1]

Central nervous system damage
Trauma
Tumor
Postinfection
Endocrinopathies
Hypothyroidism
Insulinoma
Cushing syndrome
Exogenous corticosteroids
Mauriac syndrome (diabetes with excess insulin administration, characterized by short stature and hepatomegaly)
Congenital syndromes
Prader-Willi
Laurence-Moon-Biedl (mental retardation, short stature, polydactyly, hypogonadism, retinitis pigmentosa, deafness)
Alström syndrome (deafness, diabetes mellitus, retinitis pigmentosa, short stature, hypogonadism)
Vasquez syndrome (males with X-linked short stature, mental retardation, hypogonadism, gynecomastia)
X-Chromosome disorders
Pseudohypoparathyroidism
Pseudopseudohypoparathyroidism

[1]Reproduced, with permission, from Merritt RJ: Obesity. Curr Prob Pediatr 1982;12(11):1–58.

Table 1–9. Evaluating the obese child.

Growth data
  Key issues
    Is the child's weight growth and adiposity excessive?
    Is height growth normal, advanced, or stunted?
  Components
    Current growth parameters
    Growth curves over time
    Relationship of growth parameters to each other: body
      mass index, pattern of height growth
    Skinfold measurements

History
  Key issues
    Do caretakers or child perceive weight to be a problem?
    Does the history suggest an underlying disease process or
      syndrome?
    Are there identifiable individual and environmental factors
      encouraging excessive caloric intake or inadequate
      physical activity?
    Does the history suggest current or future high risk for
      medical/psychological morbidity?
  Components
    Problem context
      Parents'/child's perceptions of weight/size
      When excess weight first became a concern
      Previous interventions attempted
    Medical
      Prenatal care and complications
      Growth parameters at birth
      Perinatal complications: infections, central nervous
        system insults, anomalies
      Previous hospitalizations, illnesses, and surgery
      Current medications
      Review of systems: cold intolerance, constipation,
        fatigue (hypothyroidism), hypoglycemia, hyperphagia
        (primary hyperinsulinemia), pubertal delay (hypothala-
        mic problem)
    Family history
      Weight problems
      Endocrinopathies
      Cardiovascular risk factors and disease
    Nutritional/eating
      Three-day diet history: food/beverages consumed,
        method of preparation, quantity consumed
      Feeding/mealtime context:
        Schedule and length of feedings/meals
        Cues to infant's/child's hunger and satiety
        Daily feeding/mealtime environment
        Location/positioning during feedings
        Caregivers involved with feedings
        Amount and type of mealtime supervision
        Behavior during feeding/mealtime
      Factors affecting eating behavior:
        Availability of foods at home and school and in neigh-
          borhood
        Parents' knowledge, attitudes, and feelings regarding
          food, eating, and overeating
        Family eating behavior
        Eating environment (eg, television)
        Non-appetite–driven cues to eat
        Parental reinforcement/mixed messages
    Activity level
      Diary of type and amount of daily physical activity (espe-
        cially aerobic)
      Factors affecting exercise behavior and activity level
        Competing daily activities
        Availability of exercise facilities/equipment and role
          models
        Family exercise behavior patterns
        Peer exercise behavior
        Parents' knowledge and attitudes about exercise

        Child's knowledge and attitudes about exercise
        Environmental cues and reinforcers
        Perceived energy level, physical abilities
        Perceived reward value of exercise compared with
          sedentary activities (eg, television)
        Past experience with exercise
    Psychosocial
      Family/household composition
      Parent-child relationship
      Relationships between other family members
      Family stressors
      Role of child's obesity in family dynamics
      Peer relationships
      Child's self-esteem/self-concept
      Content/structure of typical day for child
    Developmental/behavioral
      Age-related behavior problems (eg, attachment,
        autonomy)
      Developmental milestones: gross/fine motor, language,
        social/emotional, cognition
      Parents' perception of child's temperament/behavior

Physical examination
  Key issues
    Is there evidence of an underlying disease process or syn-
      drome?
    Is there evidence of current or high risk of subsequent,
      medical/psychological morbidity?
  Components
    Observation of parent-child interaction
    Assessment of child's interaction with physician
    Blood pressure measurements
    Skinfold measurements
    Complete physical examination with emphasis on fat distri-
      bution (central distribution may suggest Cushing syn-
      drome), presence of dysmorphism (syndromes),
      neurologic examination (primary hypothalamic prob-
      lems), presence of striae (Cushing syndrome), presence
      of dry/coarse skin or hair (hypothyroidism), secondary
      sexual characteristics (delay may suggest hypothalamic
      problem)

Developmental/behavioral assessment
  Key issue
    Is there developmental delay/mental retardation?
  Component
    Neurodevelopmental assessment of gross/fine motor, lan-
      guage, socio-emotional, cognitive skills (delay/retarda-
      tion may suggest syndrome)

Assessment of cardiorespiratory fitness
  Key issue
    What is the child's current fitness level?
  Components
    Submaximal step test
    Submaximal bicycle ergometer test
    Twelve-minute run-walk test
    Steady-state run test

Laboratory studies
  Key issues
    On the basis of history and physical examination, are diag-
      nostic laboratory tests indicated?
    Does the severity of obesity and family history warrant
      screening for additional morbidity and cardiovascular
      risk factors?
  Components
    Diagnostic tests directed by concerns raised in history and
      physical examination
    Consider thyroid screening (classic physical findings of hy-
      pothyroidism may be absent)
    Depending on severity of obesity and family history: cho-
      lesterol and lipid screening, glucose tolerance testing

Table 1–10. Treating the child with endogenous obesity.

Develop an alliance with the child and family regarding the issues involved and the importance of therapy.

Focus assessment and management at the family rather than individual level (eg, How can the whole family develop healthier eating habits?).

Tailor suggestions to the specific child and his or her unique family circumstances/environment.

Dispel misperceptions and provide accurate factual information regarding the child's nutritional needs.

Encourage dietary and activity changes that can be maintained long-term.

Address specific controlling factors regarding the type and quantity of food ingested and energy expenditure:
- Inappropriate behavioral dynamics, such as use of food as a reward
- Vulnerable times, such as after school or before bed
- Situational/environmental cues, such as watching television or feeling stress, that encourage unhealthy eating habits

Emphasize qualitative changes in diet rather than calorie restriction (dieting), which will slow rate of fat deposition and allow the child to grow into his or her weight:
- Decrease fat content
- Remove unhealthy foods from house
- Identify and substitute preferred healthy foods for preferred unhealthy foods

Encourage participation in aerobic activities to increase energy expenditure, increase cardiovascular fitness, and improve self-esteem.

Limit television watching.

Use specific behavioral techniques:
- Self-monitoring
- Contingency training
- Positive reinforcement

Use "groups" if available, especially for older children.

Use a team approach (physician, psychologist, nutritionist, case-manager/social worker) for children with significant obesity; may be most beneficial.

Provide long-term encouragement and follow-up.

---

tion, to allow children to "grow into" their weight. Emphasis is placed on making qualitative changes in diet, such as reductions in fat content, and encouraging participation in aerobic activities, which serve to increase energy utilization, cardiovascular fitness, and self-esteem. With significantly obese children, a team approach involving a primary care provider, nutritionist, behavior therapist, and family or child counselor may be the most beneficial. Long-term encouragement and follow-up is important, as many children and their families return to old behavior patterns once the intense period of treatment is completed. Despite our inability to document long-term success in dealing with many obese children, the potential benefits of establishing more healthful eating and activity patterns warrant our continued efforts to intervene early on as well as to develop more effective therapies.

Variations in Head Growth

Head size is obtained by measuring the greatest occipitofrontal circumference and reflects the volume of intracranial contents, including brain, cerebrospinal fluid, and blood, as well as the thickness of the skull and scalp. Macrocephaly and microcephaly are statistically defined as a head circumference greater than 2 SD above and below the mean for children of similar age. According to this definition, approximately 5% of the population is labeled as either macrocephalic or microcephalic. As with other growth parameters, the significance of a given measurement is best defined within the context of a knowledge of normal variations, the pattern of past head growth, the relationship of head size to other growth parameters, and the presence or absence of associated historical or physical findings.

Unrelated to intracranial volume, the presence of scalp edema or a cephalhematoma may significantly increase the head circumference. The effect of head shape on circumference should also be kept in mind. For the same intracranial volume, a round head has a smaller head circumference than a more oval-shaped one. Gestational rather than chronologic age should be used when plotting the head circumference of preterm infants. As a result of catch-up growth, these infants also exhibit an accelerated rate of head growth compared with that of full-term babies, initially exceeding gains in weight and height. The disproportionately enlarging head may raise concerns regarding hydrocephalus. The fact that many premature infants are also at increased risk for this complication emphasizes the need for close observation.

When a child's head size or rate of head growth provokes concern, a thorough history, physical examination, and review of growth curves should be obtained. Knowledge of head size at birth and the pattern of prior head growth is important. A child whose head circumference consistently falls within the same percentile is more likely to be normal than the child whose growth channel is shifting upward or downward across percentiles. Head size must also be assessed within the context of the child's overall body size. General concordance exists between growth parameters in a given individual, and significant discrepancies between head circumference and body size (height and weight) increase the likelihood of pathology. The influence of benign familial factors as well as specific syndromes and problems often can be identified by evaluating the head circumference of the child's parents and siblings. The history and physical examination should seek to identify signs and symptoms of causal or concomitant problems, including developmental disabilities; mental retardation; neurologic abnormalities, such as cerebral palsy, seizures, and focal deficits; dysmorphology; abnormal fontanelles and sutures; and skin findings suggestive of a neurocutaneous disorder. A history of prenatal, perinatal, and postnatal factors with potential import to subsequent central nervous system growth and development should be elicited, including poor prenatal care, maternal drug use or infection during pregnancy, prematurity, perinatal asphyxia, hypoglycemia, hypotension, and central nervous system infection.

Macrocephaly can result from excess cerebral spinal fluid (**hydrocephalus**), excess brain tissue (**megalen-**

cephaly), thickening of the skull, or hemorrhage into the subdural or epidural spaces. Each of these problems, in turn, may be secondary to a variety of inborn and acquired disorders, which rarely present exclusively with head growth abnormalities. Hydrocephalus may result from conditions causing increased production, decreased absorption, or obstruction to flow of the cerebral spinal fluid and, among potential causes of macrocephaly at birth, is the only one associated with increased intracranial pressure. Megalencephaly refers to the presence of excess brain tissue secondary to an increased size or number of brain cells. This may be a primary anatomic condition with or without concomitant syndromic or neurologic abnormalities, or may be due to a variety of metabolic disorders that are associated with cerebral edema or brain cell storage of accumulated substances. Infants with anatomic megalocephaly generally are born with large heads, whereas those with metabolic causes of megalocephaly typically have normal head size at birth with subsequent enlargement during the neonatal period. Metabolic megalencephaly is frequently accompanied by developmental regression or delay, signs of increased intracranial pressure, and concomitant neurologic problems, such as seizures.

The widespread availability and use of the computed tomography (CT) scanner has also resulted in the identification of several benign conditions associated with macrocephaly. Benign enlargement of the subarachnoid space is a relatively common cause of macrocephaly in an otherwise normal infant. These children typically have large but normal-sized heads at birth and provoke concern during infancy when their head circumference subsequently crosses percentiles upward to exceed and then parallel the 98th percentile for children of similar age and sex. A head CT, if obtained, demonstrates an enlarged subarachnoid space, normal to slightly increased ventricular size, and widened sulci and sylvian fissure. A genetic etiology is suspected because of the observed male predominance of this condition and the frequent concomitant finding of macrocephaly in the identified child's father. Aside from the head growth abnormalities, these children are neurologically and intellectually normal. Genetic megalencephaly (large brain), another common normal variant causing macrocephaly, may be indistinguishable from the previously described condition unless a head CT is performed. These children may or may not have large heads at birth but subsequently cross percentiles upward to parallel the curve above the 98th percentile. A head CT, if obtained, is normal. The family history is usually positive for megalencephaly and, as with children identified with benign enlargement of the subarachnoid space, neurologic and mental function are normal. A child identified as having one of these two benign conditions does not require further evaluation unless head growth subsequently deviates further from the normal curve, or a neurologic abnormality or developmental delay is detected.

Microcephaly is indicative of a small-sized brain and is typically the result of a primary or secondary defect in brain development. It is frequently associated with mental retardation, although normal intelligence can occur. **Primary microcephaly** refers to the presence of a genetic or chromosomal condition in which bulk or structural brain growth is intrinsically flawed. In **secondary microcephaly,** previously normal brain development is impaired by a variety of prenatal and postnatal infections, toxins, and central nervous system injuries. Because brain expansion dictates skull growth, inadequate brain growth may result in premature fusion of the cranial bones. This cause of premature suture closure can usually be differentiated from primary craniosynostosis by the absence of both an abnormally shaped skull and palpably thickened suture lines.

The presence of microcephaly at birth establishes the antenatal timing of impaired brain growth but does not differentiate primary from secondary etiologies. With the exception of some chromosomal disorders, a normal-sized head at birth with subsequent development of growth failure strongly suggests a secondary etiology for the microcephaly. Perinatal insults to the central nervous system rarely result in recognizably impaired head growth before the ages of 3–6 months. When such insults cause microcephaly and mental retardation, they are also associated with motor deficits (cerebral palsy) and frequently with seizures. Cranial CT scans of children with primary microcephaly typically either are normal or reveal dysmorphology characteristic of the specific etiology, whereas CT scans of those with secondary microcephaly are usually abnormal, showing a combination of nonspecific findings such as ventricular enlargement and cerebral atrophy.

MOTOR & PSYCHOLOGICAL DEVELOPMENT

To assess their patients' overall developmental progress and functioning and to counsel parents regarding a variety of developmentally based issues, physicians must have a firm understanding of both normal patterns and common variations in the developmental process. Knowing the average ages at which children achieve certain neurodevelopmental milestones and encounter specific developmental tasks helps to provide a conceptual framework for normative child development. However, developmental normality cannot be defined in absolute terms. Whereas the sequence of development is similar for all children, the rate of progress may vary from child to child, and "dissociation" of performance between developmental fields can often be normal. By comparing a child's performance with others, one can say only that the further a child is from "average," the less likely he or she will be "normal." It is important to remember that a child's developmental level and progress are the result of a variety of factors, many unrelated to the child's genetic mental endowment, such as the presence of acute or chronic illness, physical or sensory handicaps, and the quality of the nurturing environment. Current developmental thinking emphasizes the interactional contributions of both "nature" and "nurture" to the child's overall functioning. Developmental assessment should emphasize their shared importance by addressing the child's medical history, physical examination, and psychosocial history, in addition to eliciting specific developmental skills and information. A longitudinal and multidimensional approach to developmental monitoring should be encouraged, and overreliance on isolated developmental scales and tests avoided.

Table 1–11 outlines general areas of developmental observation and the average ages at which common milestones occur. Motor development tends to parallel central nervous system maturation, progressing in a cephalocaudal and proximal-to-distal direction. The disappearance of primitive reflexes must precede the appearance of volitional movements, and generalized mass activity is replaced by specific responses. Controlled use of the upper extremities precedes that of the lower extremities, and truncal coordination occurs before mastery of the extremities. In general, there is greater variation in the timing of gross motor development than in the acquisition of fine motor skills. It must be remembered that some of the most important aspects of developmental assessment, such as alertness, responsiveness, persistence, and concentration, defy objective scoring, whereas some of the most easily scored items, such as gross motor development in infancy, are the least reliable indicators of overall mental ability. Among objective areas of assessment, speech and language development is the best predictor of subsequent cognitive performance. However, problems in this area may also be related to a variety of factors unrelated to mental endowment.

An important aspect of the pediatric health supervision visit is the opportunity for periodic assessment of a child's overall developmental functioning. For this purpose, standardized developmental screening instruments, such as the Denver II, are frequently used. Developmental screening implies the detection of children at high risk for otherwise unsuspected developmental problems. Screening tests by definition are not diagnostic and, when findings are abnormal, must be followed by a thorough diagnostic evaluation. The value of a screening test lies in its ability to decrease morbidity through early detection and treatment. Definitive diagnostic strategies and effective treatment programs must exist and be supported to achieve this goal. A screening test of sufficient sensitivity, specificity, and predictive value for the population in which it is to be used must be available to minimize the psychological and financial costs of identifying false-positive cases and missing true cases. Each of these areas has provoked considerable controversy with regard to developmental screening. Most moderate to significant disabilities, rather than being identified during routine developmental screening, are suspected and identified because of concerns raised by a parent, teacher, or physician in the context of an ongoing relationship with the child. Information regarding the efficacy of intervention programs for children with a variety of developmental disabilities remains incomplete, and in many communities, the availability of subsequent comprehensive diagnostic and treatment programs is limited. Much discussion has focused on the strengths and weaknesses of specific developmental screening tests. Such tests are designed to assess the likelihood of a developmental problem at one point in time. Given the dynamic and multifactorial nature of the developmental process, it is not surprising that developmental screening tests are only weakly predictive of later developmental performance and correlate poorly with subsequent school problems or failure. The sensitivity, specificity, and predictive value of a test varies with the population to which it is applied. Considerable problems in interpretation and validity arise when a test is administered to individuals in populations significantly different from those in which the instrument was standardized. Concern has arisen especially with respect to cross-cultural applications and the screening of developmentally "high-risk" populations, such as premature infants, not originally included in the population used to validate the screening instruments.

Despite the concerns and uncertainties, developmental screening instruments provide a measure of normative development within a given population and a useful framework on which to structure developmental observation and discussion during the health supervision visit. If a screening tool is used, one should be familiar with the specific strengths and weaknesses of the instrument chosen and consider whether its use is appropriate in the intended patient population. When evaluating developmental performance in the office, it is important to allow children to demonstrate their best effort and ability. Testing should not occur when the child is sick or frightened. Care must be taken to avoid prognosticating or labeling a child on the basis of a screening test.

The information obtained through screening tests should enhance rather than supplant broader ongoing developmental monitoring in the context of a primary care relationship with the parents and family. Given the limitations of developmental screening tests, the much broader, time-honored concept of developmental surveillance is receiving renewed attention and growing support. Surveillance, while requiring no less thorough a knowledge of normal and deviant patterns of development, relies less on developmental testing and more on continual monitoring of developmental functioning and well-being by paying attention to parental concerns and making longitudinal observations during all encounters with children and their families.

In the context of such a relationship, pediatric primary care providers frequently face concerns regarding a child's global or selective developmental abilities. The re-

Table 1–11. Aspects of developmental assessment and common developmental milestones.[1,2]

Perceptions/concerns of others: Parents, teachers, and other caregivers	
General responsiveness and alertness	
Symmetry of movement	
Use of eyes and ears	
Follows dangling object from midline through a range of < 45 degrees:	0–1 mo
Follows dangling object from midline through a range of 90 degrees:	1 mo
Follows dangling object from midline through a range of 180 degrees:	3 mo
Consistent conjugate gaze (binocular vision):	4 mo
Alerts or quiets to sound:	0–2 mo
Lateralizes sound (turns head to sound made on level with ear):	3 mo
Localizes sound well in all directions:	7–10 mo

Tone: posture, resistance to passive movement, clonus, deep tendon reflexes, head and truncal control
Primitive and postural reflexes

	Present by	Absent by
Moro:		3–4 mo
Palmar grasp:		2–3 mo
Asymmetrical tonic neck:		2–3 mo
Placing/stepping:		1.5–2 mo
Landau:	3 mo	1 y
Parachute:	6–9 mo	

Head control: prone, ventral suspension, pull to sitting

Prone	
Head rests on table turned to one side:	1 mo
Lifts head momentarily:	1 mo
Head up 45 degrees:	2 mo
Head up 90 degrees:	3–4 mo
Weight on forearms:	3–5 mo
Weight on hands with arms extended:	5–6 mo
Ventral suspension	
Head hangs completely down:	newborn
Momentarily holds head in plane of body:	6 wk
Head sustained in plane of body:	2 mo
Maintains head beyond plane of body:	3 mo
Pull to sitting	
Complete head lag, back uniformly rounded:	newborn
Slight head lag:	3 mo
No head lag, back straightening:	5 mo
Lifts head off table when about to be pulled up:	6 mo
Raises head spontaneously from supine:	7 mo

Rolling

Rolls front-to-back:	4–5 mo
Rolls back-to-front:	5–6 mo

Sitting

Back uniformly rounded, cannot sit unsupported:	newborn
Back straightening, sits with propping:	5–6 mo
Back straight, sits with arms forward for support:	6–7 mo
Sits with no support:	7 mo

Fine motor/manipulation

Hands predominantly closed:	1 mo
Hands predominantly open:	3 mo
Hand regard:	3–5 mo
Hands come together:	4 mo
Foot play:	5 mo
Voluntary grasp (no release):	5 mo
Transfers objects from hand to hand:	6 mo
Ulnar grasp of cube:	5–6 mo
Grasps cube against thenar eminence:	6–8 mo
Grasps cube against lower thumb:	8–10 mo
Mature cube grasp—finger tips and distal thumb:	10–12 mo
Index finger approach to small objects and finger-thumb opposition:	10 mo
Voluntary release of objects:	10 mo
Plays pat-a-cake:	9–10 mo
Enjoys putting objects in and out of box:	≥ 11 mo
Casting objects:	10–13 mo
Tower of 2 cubes:	13–15 mo
Tower of 4 cubes:	18 mo
Tower of 6–7 cubes:	2 y
Tower of 10 cubes:	3 y
Good use of cup and spoon:	15–18 mo

Weight-bearing and walking

Some weight-bearing:	3 mo
Supports most weight:	6 mo
Pulls to stand:	9 mo
Walks holding onto furniture (cruising):	11 mo
Walks with one hand held:	12 mo
Walks without help:	13 mo
Walks well:	15 mo
Runs well:	2 y
Up and down stairs, two feet each step:	2 y
Up and down stairs, one foot per step down, two feet per step up:	3 y
Up and down stairs, one foot per step:	4 y
Jumps off ground with two feet:	2.5 y
Hops on one foot:	4 y
Skips:	5–6 y
Balance on one foot 2–3 s:	3 y
Balance on one foot 6–10 s:	4 y

Personal/social and cognitive

Social smile:	1–2 mo
Smiles at image in mirror:	5 mo
Looks after dropped toy—beginning of object permanence:	6 mo
Separation anxiety/stranger awareness:	6–12 mo
Interactive games: peek-a-boo and pat-a-cake:	9–12 mo
Waves "bye-bye":	10 mo
Rolls ball to examiner:	12 mo
Feeds self with cup and spoon:	15–18 mo
Dresses self, except for buttons in back:	3 y
Ties shoe laces:	5 y
Autonomy and independence issues often begin:	18 mo–2 y
Parallel play:	1–2 y
Cooperative play:	3–4 y
Magical thinking and symbolic (pretend) play:	18 mo–5 y
Able to distinguish fantasy from reality:	5 y

Speech and language

Cooing:	2–4 mo
Babbles with labial consonants ("ba, ma, ga"):	5–8 mo
Imitates sounds made by others:	9–12 mo
First words (~ 4–6, including "mama," "dada"):	9–12 mo
Understanding one-step command (without gesture):	15 mo
Jargon (ie, expressive, unintelligible language) Recognizable words increase with age:	15–24 mo
Vocabulary of 10–50 words:	13–18 mo
Vocabulary of 50–75 words:	18–24 mo
Vocabulary of 250 words:	3 y
Two-word sentences:	18–24 mo
Three-word sentences:	2–3 y
Four-word sentences:	3–4 y
Five-word sentences:	4–5 y

[1]Modified and reproduced, with permission, from Illingworth RS: *The Development of the Infant and Young Child: Normal and Abnormal,* 9th ed. Williams & Wilkins, 1980, 1987.
[2]Ages are averages based primarily on data of Arnold Gesell.

mainder of this section addresses the initial evaluation and management of children with suspected developmental delay and speech or language problems. The approach to the child with school failure and learning disabilities is discussed in Chapter 3.

COMMON ISSUES & CONCERNS

Suspected Developmental Delay

Because parents more commonly overestimate than underestimate their child's abilities, developmental concerns, when such concerns are expressed, should be taken seriously. Although parents of children with suspected developmental delays most often worry about the possibility of mental retardation, many factors besides inherent mental ability can affect a child's apparent developmental level. Performance can be artificially lowered if testing occurs when a child is sick, frightened, or uncooperative, or if screening instruments are indiscriminately applied as previously noted. Otherwise normal premature infants may manifest slight differences in their patterns of development, particularly with respect to gross motor skills, and may be labeled erroneously as abnormal when compared with the performance of full-term babies. Furthermore, an age correction for the extent of prematurity should be made until the child is 18–24 months old. Developmental disabilities, frequently unrelated to intellectual endowment, may result from cerebral palsy; major sensory deficits, such as hearing or vision loss; specific speech or language problems; and emotional or behavioral disturbances, such as autism, specific learning disabilities, a neglectful or abusive environment, or chronic illness. Many of these conditions interfere with a child's developmental performance and may present initially as developmental delay. The therapeutic and prognostic implications of differentiating these conditions are great.

When a developmental problem is suspected, a definitive diagnostic evaluation should be undertaken to determine whether a delay is truly present and, if so, whether a specific etiology can be identified with implications for prognosis, therapy, and subsequent offspring (Table 1–12). A comprehensive developmental assessment, using a standard age-appropriate instrument, should be obtained by trained personnel. If a developmental problem is confirmed, it is important to ascertain whether the delay is global or selective. For example, a problem primarily with language may suggest a hearing problem, inadequate environmental stimulation, or autism. An isolated motor problem may occur with neuromuscular disease, hemiplegia or paraplegia, and cerebral palsy. With confirmation of a delay, a complete history and physical examination, as well as formal evaluation of hearing and vision, are essential. It is important to ascertain from the parents whether their child's developmental problems had a distinct age of onset, suggesting specific causal factors, and whether any developmental regression has been noted. Slow developmental progress may be indicative of either a static or a progressive process. However, developmental regression, as manifest by loss of previously achieved developmental milestones, should always suggest a progressive neurologic disorder. The presence of prenatal, perinatal, and postnatal risk factors for subsequent developmental problems, as well as a positive family history for similar problems, should be elicited. A thorough psychosocial and behavioral assessment should also be obtained with an emphasis on exploring the care-taking environment and any concomitant behavioral problems. Nonwillful problems, such as hyperactivity, impulsivity, distractibility, and poor social interactions, should be differentiated from willful behavioral problems, such as tantrums, hitting, and disobedience, which may be indicative of a specific underlying behavioral problem. Overall patterns of growth with special emphasis on head circumference should be noted. A complete physical examination should be performed with a focus on detecting the presence of neurologic problems, dysmorphic features, congenital anomalies, and skin pigment abnormalities suggestive of neurocutaneous disorders. When congenital anomalies or dysmorphic features are identified, evaluation by a dysmorphologist skilled in the identification of specific syndromes is warranted. During the examination, the child's general alertness, curiosity, persistence, and interpersonal interactions can also be assessed. Perhaps parents' greatest concern during such an evaluation is that their child will be discovered to be mentally retarded. **Mental retardation** is defined as subnormal intellectual functioning statistically represented by an IQ less than 2 SD below the population mean on standardized intelligence testing and associated with coexisting delays in adaptive skills, such as self-care, home living, communication, and social interactions. This corresponds to an IQ of approximately 70–75 on both the Stanford-Binet and Wechsler intelligence tests. **Mild mental retardation** is generally defined as an IQ of 50–70, and **moderate to severe retardation,** as an IQ less than 50. In more recent definitions, an effort has been made to avoid categorization on the basis of IQ levels and to place greater emphasis on descriptions of functional deficits in a variety of adaptive skill areas. Mild mental retardation occurs with an incidence of 20–30:1000 individuals, is often familial or polygenic, and is more frequently noted in boys and in groups of lower socioeconomic status. Identifiable chromosomal abnormalities account for only 4–8%. Although the majority of these abnormalities are believed to be idiopathic, a variety of insults and pathogenic processes, such as prenatal substance exposure and postnatal lead toxicity, may be causal. By contrast, severe mental retardation occurs with an incidence of 3–4:1000 individuals, is typically sporadic, and although still more common in boys, shows no socioeconomic predilection. An etiology can be determined in approximately 60–70% of cases. Chromosomal abnormalities are the single largest group of etiologies detected (30%), and among these, Down syndrome, or trisomy 21, is the most frequent disorder identified. Because of the recent availability of specific molecular and

Table 1–12. Evaluating the child with suspected developmental delay.

Developmental assessment
Key issues
Is a developmental delay present?
Is delay global or selective?
Components
Developmental screening/surveillance
Definitive developmental test using standardized instrument (eg, Bayley Scales of Infant Development)

History
Key issues
Do caretakers perceive development to be a problem?
Was there a distinct onset to the developmental problems?
Has developmental regression been noted?
Does the history suggest a potential etiology?
Components
Problem context
Parental concerns/problem perceptions
Parental expectations
Developmental history
Parental recollection of milestones, problem onset
Family history
Family history of developmental problems/syndromes
Medical history
Prenatal care and complications: infections, toxin/drug exposure
Perinatal complications: problems with delivery, asphyxia, infection, central nervous system insults, anomalies, postpartum problems
Gestational age and growth parameters at birth: prematurity, small for gestational age, microcephaly
Previous hospitalizations, illnesses, and surgery
Current medications
Review of systems:
Complete review of systems with emphasis on detecting symptoms of neurologic disorders (eg, seizures) and chronic illness

Psychosocial and behavioral assessment
Key issues
What is the nature of the care-giving environment?
Are significant emotional/behavioral problems present?

Components
Care-giving environment
Parent-child relationship
Family stressors
Behavioral problems: "willful" (eg, tantrums, hitting, disobedience); "nonwillful" (eg, hyperactivity, impulsivity, distractibility, problems with interpersonal relationships)

Physical examination
Key issues
Is there physical evidence of a potential etiology?
Is growth retardation or microcephaly present?
Components
Growth parameters (especially head circumference)
Observations of child's interpersonal interactions, alertness, curiosity, and persistence
Complete physical examination with emphasis on detecting neurologic abnormalities, dysmorphic features, congenital anomalies, skin pigment abnormalities

Sensory evaluation
Key issue
Is a sensory deficit present?
Components
Hearing test
Vision test

Laboratory studies
Key issue
Are specific diagnostic tests warranted?
Components
Diagnostic tests directed by concerns raised in history and physical examination
Newborn/infant: follow-up of state metabolic screening
Idiopathic mental retardation: determined on the basis of clinical presentation and philosophy (see Table 1–13)
Chromosomal testing (cytogenetic testing for fragile X syndrome must be specifically requested)
Magnetic resonance imaging
Metabolic screening
Serum lead level

cytogenetic techniques, a syndrome called **fragile X** has increasingly been identified as a cause of mental retardation. This X-linked–inherited disorder typically affects males (although approximately one third of female carriers are also affected) and is classically characterized by mental retardation, facial dysmorphism, and macroorchidism. A history of central nervous system injury secondary to teratogens, infection, and prenatal, perinatal, and postnatal insults can be found in 15–20% of cases of severe mental retardation in children. Neuroradiologic imaging studies can identify another 10–15% as having significant cerebral dysgenesis. When found in the absence of other anomalies or the stigmata of a specific syndrome, this usually indicates a sporadic and nonprogressive process. Children with multiple congenital anomalies and an identifiable syndrome constitute only 4–5% of cases of severe mental retardation. However, it is important to identify these conditions through a thorough assessment of dysmorphology and family history, because many represent single-gene disorders with important im-

plications for parents' subsequent childbearing. Endocrine and metabolic causes of severe mental retardation account for 3–5% of cases.

Laboratory evaluation of a child with a confirmed developmental delay in general should be guided by the history and physical examination (Table 1–13). Given our growing awareness of the deleterious effects of relatively low levels of ingested lead and its pervasive presence in our environment, children with unexplained developmental delay should be screened for lead toxicity. A child with significant unexplained mental retardation should also have chromosomal studies performed, including specific cytogenetic testing for fragile X syndrome. The routine use of neuroimaging in the evaluation of idiopathic mental retardation is controversial. The recent availability of high-resolution magnetic resonance imaging has increased our ability to detect varying degrees of cerebral dysgenesis and to provide parents with at least a partial explanation for their child's disability, although it may not necessarily be the primary etiology. The desire to identify

Table 1–13. Suggested indications for diagnostic or screening tests recommended in children with unexplained mental retardation and specific findings.[1]

Magnetic resonance imaging of the brain
Cerebral palsy or motor asymmetry
Abnormal head size or shape
Craniofacial malformation
Loss or plateau of developmental skills
Multiple somatic anomalies
Neurocutaneous findings
Seizures
IQ < 50
Cytogenetic studies[2]
Microcephaly
Multiple (even minor) somatic anomalies
Family history of mental retardation
Family history of fetal loss
IQ < 50
Skin pigmentary anomalies (mosaicism)
Suspected contiguous gene syndromes (eg, Prader-Willi, Angelman, Smith-Magenis)
Metabolic studies[3]
Episodic vomiting or lethargy
Poor growth
Seizures
Unusual odors
Somatic evidence of storage
Loss or plateau of developmental skills
Movement disorder (choreoathetosis, dystonia, ataxia)
Sensory loss (especially retinal abnormality)
Acquired cutaneous disorders

[1]Reproduced, with permission, from Palmer FB, Capute AJ: Mental retardation. Pediatr Rev 1994;15:473.

[2]Because of high prevalence, lack of specific clinical features, and variable developmental manifestations, some experts suggest specific cytogenetic testing for fragile X syndrome in both males and females with otherwise unexplained mental retardation.

[3]Basic laboratory screen: fasting plasma amino acids, blood lactate, ammonia, very–long-chain fatty acids, urinary oligosaccharides/mucopolysaccharides. Further metabolic evaluation is usually directed best by a specialist.

a specific etiology, however, must also be weighed against the cost of the test and the low likelihood of identifying specific findings with relevance to the child's subsequent treatment and prognosis. Routine screening for metabolic disorders in otherwise asymptomatic children with idiopathic mental retardation is usually nonproductive. Most of these conditions present with additional findings, such as seizures, failure to thrive, lethargy, hypoglycemia, acidosis, vomiting, and a plateau or progressive loss of developmental skills. When the clinical situation is suggestive, however, appropriate metabolic screening tests should be obtained. In addition, results of state-mandated newborn metabolic screening should always be followed up in the newborn period. While a developmental evaluation is ongoing, it is important to avoid labeling the child with terms such as **developmentally delayed, disabled,** or **mentally retarded.** If an otherwise unexplained problem is confirmed by definitive testing, it should be pointed out to parents that the delay observed relates to the child's current performance. Although the likelihood of a child's ability being normal decreases the farther their performance is from expected norms, present developmental tests are poor predictors of future performance, particularly those used during infancy and toddlerhood.

Many physicians, as well as parents, may delay evaluation of a child for whom they have developmental concerns because of the perception that effective interventions are lacking. However, given the many factors that can affect developmental performance, a variety of specific treatable conditions can be detected. The physician may also identify conditions with important implications for parents' future childbearing. Furthermore, although the field of developmental intervention is relatively new and many questions remain, a growing body of data suggests that long-term, comprehensive programs that combine child-focused services with parental education and family support can effectively enhance the developmental abilities of many children with established disabilities and help families to cope better with the varying demands of having a child who is developmentally disabled. Helping parents adjust to the realization that their child has a developmental disability can be difficult. Feelings of denial, guilt, anger, and sadness are often exacerbated by the frequent underlying uncertainty regarding cause, subsequent prognosis, and recurrence risk. Pediatric primary care providers can provide the long-term support and coordination of care so important to these families and are also in a unique position to advocate effectively for the needs of these children and their families with schools and other outside agencies.

Suspected Speech & Language Delay

Although speech and language problems frequently coexist with more global developmental delays, pediatricians are often faced with specific concerns regarding a child's progress in this area. Approximately 50% of children with delayed language development have delays in other areas. Particularly when more global problems are present, a child's language ability is highly correlated with subsequent cognitive performance. However, problems in this area can be indicative of a variety of primary language disorders and additional factors that are independent of intellectual endowment.

The most frequent causes of inadequate language development are given in Table 1–14. Both sensorineural

Table 1–14. Causes of inadequate language development.

Hearing problem
Mental retardation
Dysphasia (developmental language disorder)
Autistic spectrum disorder
Dysarthria
Structural problems of the oropharynx and upper respiratory tract
Elective mutism
Child abuse and neglect

and recurrent conductive hearing loss can result in abnormal language development. Although deaf infants produce vowel sounds (cooing), progression beyond this point is usually impaired. Formal hearing assessment is essential, as parental impressions and crude office testing are notoriously inaccurate. **Autism, or autistic spectrum disorder,** is an organic brain disorder of unknown and probably multifactorial etiology, characterized by a behavioral symptom complex consisting of abnormalities in socialization and interpersonal interactions (eg, prefer inanimate objects to people, little affection with caretakers), affect modulation (eg, mood swings), communication (usually both receptive and expressive aspects of language affected), and play (eg, narrow focus of interest, little interactive or pretend play). It is also frequently associated with cognitive abnormalities, stereotypic motor behaviors (eg, toe walking, hand flapping, rocking, twirling), sensory abnormalities (eg, relative pain insensitivity, increased or decreased response to sensory stimuli), and a variety of nonspecific behavioral problems (eg, attention problems, sleep problems). **Developmental language disorders,** or **dysphasic syndromes,** are disorders of higher cerebral functioning resulting in impaired language development. Dysphasia is typically classified into multiple subtypes based on whether primarily expressive, receptive, or a combination of both types of language deficits are present and whether higher-order language processing is impaired (semantics, syntax). **Dysarthria** (neuromotor abnormalities of the orofacial muscles) and anatomic problems of the oropharynx and larynx can also impair speech. Children who grow up in neglectful or overtly abusive environments frequently manifest language as well as other developmental delays. **Elective mutism** refers to a child who uses language in some environments but not in others and can be indicative of an underlying language disorder or a significant emotional disturbance.

Because of the influence of individual temperament, social or cultural factors, and the child's verbal and language environment, children manifest greater variability in the acquisition of language than in other developmental areas. This is especially true with respect to expressive verbal skills. Furthermore, the pace of observable development is not constant. Parents frequently become concerned during the beginning of their child's second year of life when the acquisition and use of new words occurs rather slowly, only to be amazed by the veritable explosion in vocabulary and comprehension during the second half of the same year. A transient and relative delay in the emergence of expressive language skills of later-born compared with first-born children is often noted and may reflect differences in the kinds and extent of opportunities for verbal interaction encountered by children in families with one compared with multiple children. Children from bilingual families may also manifest transient delays in their expressive language and frequently combine elements of both languages in their early verbalizations. By 2–3 years of age, however, most of these children are able to separate the languages appropriately and use them in their respective contexts. No long-term language problems have been associated with multilanguage exposure, and there is some evidence to suggest that subsequent language development may actually be facilitated by this experience. As children learn the patterns of their language, rules are often overgeneralized, leading to common developmental "mistakes" (eg, "sheeps" instead of "sheep," "goed" instead of "went"), which must be differentiated from deviant language development. In general, screening instruments rely heavily on the assessment of expressive language abilities. Because of normal variability in this area and because of the frequently encountered difficulties with obtaining an accurate expressive performance in an office setting, many children may be erroneously labeled as language delayed. A longitudinal perspective regarding the child's language and overall development can help to put concerns into perspective. While care must be taken to avoid mislabeling normal children, the availability of effective treatments for a variety of conditions with primary or secondary effects on speech and language development makes prompt evaluation of significant or persistent concerns important.

Initial evaluation of a child with a suspected language delay should include direct assessment of the child's language abilities through the use of informal observation and specific language screening instruments; a thorough developmental history and assessment; formal hearing evaluation; a complete medical, family, psychosocial, and behavioral history; and a thorough physical examination. Table 1–15 lists important expressive and receptive developmental language milestones as well as specific indications for further evaluation and referral. Key findings that should prompt concern include the absence of apparent response to sound in an infant, the absence of babbling by 9–12 months of age, the absence of any words by 18 months, the absence of meaningful phrases by 24 months, speech that is largely unintelligible to strangers at 3 years, an inability to use language communicatively, and apparent difficulties with language comprehension. To optimize the likelihood of an accurate assessment, attempts to evaluate a child's language ability should take place in a quiet, nonthreatening environment when the child is otherwise well and before other more distressing aspects of the visit are performed. While observation of children's verbal interaction with their parents and the use of simple toys and picture books to engage them in casual conversation can be very useful, a variety of specific language screening instruments, such as the Early Language Milestone (ELM) scale and Clinical Linguistic Assessment Measurement, are available for use in the office setting. These scales are designed to differentiate receptive, expressive, and mixed language disorders. It is also important to ascertain, through a thorough developmental assessment, whether the language delay is an isolated problem or part of more global developmental concerns. A formal hearing assessment using behavioral or brain stem–evoked response audiometry should always be performed on a child with

Table 1–15. Clinical evaluation of language skills.[1]

Age	Receptive Skills	Expressive Skills	Specific Indication for Referral
0–1 mo	Recognizes sound with startle; turns to sound and looks for source; quiets motor activity to sound; "prefers" human speech with high inflection.	Differentiated crying; body language of positive and negative response.	No response to pleasing sound when alert; neonatal sepsis; meningitis; neonatal asphyxia; prematurity; congenital infection; familial deafness; renal abnormalities; aminoglycoside therapy.
2–4 mo	Prolonged attention to sounds; responds to familiar voice; watches the speaking mouth; enjoys rattle; attempts to repeat pleasing sound with objects; shifts gaze back and forth between sounds.	"Ee, ih, uh" (hindmouth vowels); cooing, blows bubbles; enjoys using tongue and lips; reciprocal cooing; play dialogues; loudness varies.	No response to pleasing sounds; does not attend to voices.
5–8 mo	Seeks out speaker; localizes sounds; understands own name, familiar words; associates word to activity (eg, bath, car).	Pitch varies; babbles with labial consonants ("ba, ma, ga"); uses sounds to get attention, express feeling; sounds directed at object.	Decrease or absence of vocalizations.
9–12 mo	Responds to simple commands: "point to your nose," "say bye-bye"; knows names of family members; responds to a few words (ie, words associated with specific objects).	First words, five to six: "mama, dada"; inflected vocal play; repeats sounds and words made by others; "oo, ee" (foremouth vowels).	No babbling with consonant sounds; no response to music.
13–18 mo	Some understanding of words; single-element commands; identifies familiar objects.	Points to objects with vocalization; vocabulary of 10–50 words, pivot and open class words, rate and content varies; jargon with proper stress and intonation, monologues and dual monologues.	No comprehension of words; does not understand simple requests.
18–24 mo	Recognizes many nouns; understands simple questions.	Telegraphic speech; vocabulary of 50–75 words; two-word sentences, phrases; stuttering very common.	Vowel sounds but no consonants.
24–36 mo	Understands prepositions; can follow story with pictures.	Vocabulary of 200 words; dependent on phrases, two-word sentences; uses words for expressive needs; pronouns; uses action verbs.	No words; does not follow simple directions.
30–36 mo	Understands some syntax (difference between car hit train and train hit car); understands opposites; understands action in pictures.	Sentences of four to five words, three elements; tells stories; uses questions: what, where; uses negation; uses progressive and past tense, all regular form; uses plurals, regular form.	Speech largely unintelligible to stranger; dropout of initial sonants; no sentences.
3–4 y	Understands three-element commands.	Grammar by own rules; vocabulary 40–1500 words; speech intelligible to strangers; "why" questions; commands; uses past and present tense; spontaneous speech; nursery rhymes; colors, one to four numbers up to five; tells sex, full name; articulation; "m, n, p, h, w"; four-word sentences.	Speech not comprehended by strangers; still dependent upon gestures; consistently holds hands over ears; speech without modulation.
4–5 y	Understands four-element commands; links past and present events.	2700-word vocabulary; defines simple words; auxiliary verbs: "has, had"; conversationally mature; "how" and "why" questions in response to others; articulation: "b, k, g, f"; five-word sentences; "normalizes" irregular verbs and nouns.	Stuttering; consistently avoids loud places.
5–6 y	Understands five-element commands; can follow a story without pictures; enjoys jokes and riddles; can comprehend two meanings of word.	Correct use of all parts of speech; vocabulary 5000 words; articulation: "y, ng, d"; six-word sentences; corrects own errors in speech; can use logic in recounting story plots.	Word endings dropped; faulty sentence structure; abnormal rate, rhythm, or inflection.
6–7 y	Asks for motivation and explanation of events; understands time intervals (months, seasons); right and left differences.	Articulation: "l, r, t, sh, ch, dr, cl, bl, gl, cr"; has formal (adult) speech patterns.	Poor voice quality, articulation.
7–8 y	Can use language alone to tell a story sequentially; reasons using language.	Articulation: "v, th, j, s, z, tr, st, sl, sw, sp."	
8–9 y		Articulation: "th, sc, sh."	

[1]Reproduced, with permission, from Dixon SD, Stein MT: Page 241 in: *Encounters with Children: Pediatric Behavior and Development.* Year Book Publishers, 1987.

suspected speech and language problems. Medical and familial risk factors for hearing or speech and language problems, such as prematurity, perinatal asphyxia, prolonged aminoglycoside use, known central nervous system insults, and a family history of prior syndromes or hearing and language problems, should be elicited. A thorough behavioral assessment is essential, with special emphasis on detecting behaviors suggestive of autism. The nature and quality of the child's psychosocial environment should also be evaluated. Children exposed to neglectful or abusive environments frequently manifest delays in language and personal social skills disproportionate to their motor abilities. The physical examination should focus on identifying abnormal growth patterns (especially microcephaly), congenital anomalies and dysmorphism suggestive of an underlying syndrome or prenatal insult, neurologic abnormalities, ear pathology, and abnormalities of the oropharynx.

Specific therapies are available for a variety of conditions resulting in inadequate speech and language development. Success in treating primary developmental language disorders depends on the type and severity of dysphagia; the age of diagnosis; and the presence of concomitant developmental, behavioral, psychosocial, and other medical disorders.

COUNSELING & ANTICIPATORY GUIDANCE

An integral part of child health supervision is the provision of information, support, and anticipatory guidance to parents and children regarding a variety of age-related topics important to the health and well-being of the growing child. Parents increasingly turn to their pediatrician for the advice and support once provided by extended family. The physician, by developing a strong long-term relationship with patients and their families, is in a unique position to respond to specific problems and concerns as they arise, as well as to facilitate health promotion and disease prevention by providing and personalizing information and support.

The pediatric health supervision visit allows for discussion of age-appropriate topics related to nutrition, daily care, behavior and development, injury prevention, family functioning, and the management of minor medical problems. While prevention of specific problems is an important aspect of anticipatory guidance, an equally important goal is the promotion of health and development by optimizing the parent-child relationship and encouraging positive health behaviors. Helping parents to understand the impact of their child's temperament and environment on growth and development, and to anticipate abilities, behaviors, and issues that typically emerge at different ages, encourages an understanding of how the child is both similar to and different from other children.

Despite the potential for benefit, limited and conflicting data exist regarding the optimal content, technique, and overall effectiveness of anticipatory guidance. Further research is needed to help define the most effective use of the clinician's limited time during the well-child visit. Several general principles, however, should be kept in mind when incorporating anticipatory guidance into child health supervision.

- The perceived need to cover a predetermined list of topics at each visit should not overshadow the importance of establishing a strong doctor-parent-child relationship. Advice given within the context of such a relationship can have a powerful effect on health behavior choices.

- Discussion, using appropriate language and explanations, should be encouraged and advice personalized to the resources and experience of the child and family.

- Emphasizing the developmental basis for age-appropriate issues, although enjoyable for some parents, is not essential to providing meaningful information and discussion.

- More is not always better. It is important to prioritize the information one wishes to convey and not to try to cover too much at each visit.

- It is also wise to recognize when scientific evidence regarding a particular approach or issue is unclear and therefore to avoid being overly dogmatic or judgmental when giving advice. Making an issue over a relatively minor point may, in the long run, diminish your chances of influencing the parents on matters of importance where data are well established.

- Given the time constraints of the health supervision visit, clinicians should make use of "natural" counseling moments as they occur, such as when reviewing the child's growth chart with the parents, when performing the physical examination, or when observing a particular behavior in the office.

- Important information should be repeated several times during the visit.

- Both children and adults respond best to positive rather than negative reinforcement. It is always important to recognize and acknowledge good parenting and child-parent interactions when observed.

On the basis of primarily expert consensus, the National Center for Education in Maternal and Child Health and the American Academy of Pediatrics have issued guidelines regarding recommended anticipatory guidance content for child health supervision visits. The *Guidelines for Adolescent Preventive Services* expand on issues relevant to the preventive health care needs of adolescents. These areas are addressed further in Chapter 2. A condensation of suggested topics for discussion at different ages is given in Table 1–16. The following section focuses on common issues addressed during the health supervision visit, including nutrition/feeding, sleep, crying and fussiness, discipline, and safety/accident prevention. Specific sleep problems and colic are discussed in Chapter 3.

COMMON ISSUES IN NUTRITION & FEEDING

Breast-feeding

Infant feeding practices, influenced by a variety of social, cultural, scientific, and commercial factors, have varied widely over the last half century. The availability of nutritionally sound infant formulas has given parents more flexibility and options in the feeding of their infant. However, the nutritional, immunologic, and psychological advantages of breast-feeding remain compelling. The decision to breast-feed or bottle-feed an infant usually is made before the baby is born and, therefore, is an important topic for discussion during the prenatal visit. Physicians should promote the benefits of breast-feeding by providing information, dispelling misconceptions, and helping parents to clarify their own feelings and attitudes about infant feeding. Once a decision is made, however, it is important to be supportive and nonjudgmental.

Most breast-feeding mothers who wean their infants in the first several weeks postpartum do so because of a lack of information regarding breast-feeding norms and supportive guidance in dealing with a variety of common problems. Postpartum counseling should encourage maternal confidence by providing training in correct nursing technique, as well as anticipatory guidance regarding breast-feeding physiology, norms, and common problems. Because questions commonly arise, it is especially important to offer early follow-up counseling to parents who elect to breast-feed their infants.

The suckling newborn stimulates the mother's pituitary to release prolactin and oxytocin, which in turn stimulate the production and "let-down" of breast milk. During the first several days postpartum, the infant receives antibody-rich colostrum. Suboptimal feeding routines during this time rarely interfere with ultimate breast-feeding success. However, once the mother's milk has "come in," usually 2–5 days after delivery, and she begins to produce a significant volume, suboptimal breast emptying or other factors that interfere with the complex hormonal balance may jeopardize the success of continued lactation. Parents who wish to supplement breast-feeding with an occasional bottle are advised to wait several weeks until the breast-feeding pattern is well established. The mouth and tongue movements used in breast-feeding are different from, and generally more effort-intensive than, those used with an artificial nipple. Some infants may have difficulty switching back and forth or may prefer the artificial nipple once exposed.

Most women find the optimal position for nursing to be one where the infant is cradled at the level of the breast in front of and completely facing the mother. In this position the mother's other hand is used to squeeze the nipple gently, making it more protractile and therefore easier for the infant to latch onto as much of the areola as possible. Stroking the infant's lips with the nipple to stimulate mouth opening and waiting until the mouth is opened wide enough to cover as much of the areola as possible help to optimize placement at the breast. Mothers should be encouraged to note the occurrence of symptoms of milk let-down (breast/nipple tingling, milk dripping) and to listen for audible infant swallowing. When removing the infant from the breast, the mother should gently insert a finger between the infant's mouth and the breast to break the suction and minimize nipple trauma. Current breast-feeding philosophy discourages rigid schedules for feeding duration and timing. Nipple soreness, once thought to be due to early prolonged suckling, is now believed to be primarily related to poor positioning of the infant and trauma when the infant is removed without breaking suction. Most women work up to feedings of 10–20 minutes or more at each breast with each feeding over the first several days postpartum. In general, the infant will determine when the feeding is over, and parents should be helped to recognize the signs of satiety. To facilitate optimal breast drainage and milk production, it is important that the infant take milk from both breasts at each feeding. Alternating the breast offered first is encouraged for the same reason. Intervals between demand feedings vary, but average every 1½–3 hours in the first several weeks (8–12 times per day). Newborns should not be allowed to go longer than 4–5 hours between feedings. In most infants, one or more of the middle-of-the-night feedings is given up by 2 months of age.

Sore nipples, engorgement, and maternal fatigue are common problems that may undermine successful breast-feeding. Nipple soreness is a frequent and almost always a self-limited condition that diminishes as nipples become conditioned. However, it can be exacerbated by improper nursing technique or factors that interfere with successful milk let-down and flow. Problems with technique most frequently observed include not using the ventral-to-ventral position, so that the infant ineffectively grasps and puts tension on the nipple, not getting enough of the areola in the baby's mouth, and forgetting to break suction before removing the baby from the breast. A warm shower or heating pad may help enhance milk let-down and flow. Spreading a thin layer of breast milk on nipples and allowing them to air-dry with the help of a warm lamp facilitates healing and conditioning. Application and removal of creams and ointments with each feed may actually increase trauma and abrasion, and therefore are generally discouraged. Trying different nursing positions to vary the pressure points during suckling may also be helpful. Other suggestions to reduce nipple soreness include initiating the feeding and milk let-down on the less sore side then switching to the sore nipple and manually

Table 1–16. Anticipatory guidance—suggested topics at each visit.[1]

Prenatal	
Injury prevention:	Safe baby furniture; car safety restraints; smoke detector; water thermostat set < 120 °F.
Feeding/nutrition:	Breast vs. bottle.
Medical:	Circumcision; what to expect at delivery; schedule of health supervision visits.
Other:	Maternal health issues; social supports; siblings.
Newborn	
Injury prevention:	Review above. Emphasize: never leave infant unattended, use car restraints.
Feeding/nutrition:	Issues with breast-feeding or bottle feeding: norms, common problems.
Daily care/activities:	Crying, sleeping, sleep position and SIDS, stooling patterns; bathing and skin care; hiccups, sneezing, "wet burps."
Developmental/ behavioral issues:	Normal reflexes (startle); individuality of infant; importance of close interaction and responding to infant's needs (cannot spoil).
Medical:	Care of umbilical cord and circumcision; jaundice; how to take a baby's temperature; when and how to call the doctor: fever, vomiting, diarrhea, decreased feeding; review schedule of health supervision visits.
Other:	Postpartum adjustment; change in parent and family relationships; sibling reactions.
2–4 wk	
Injury prevention:	Review above; bath safety; sun exposure/protection.
Feeding/nutrition:	Issues with breast-feeding vs. bottle feeding; fluoride supplementation, if indicated.
Daily care/activities:	Sleep patterns; crying and "colic"; bladder and bowel habits.
Developmental/ behavioral issues:	Emphasize infant's abilities; enjoy holding, cuddling, talking to baby (cannot spoil).
Medical:	Reinforce when to call the doctor.
Other:	Time to themselves for parents: baby sitters; spending time with siblings; plans for substitute care if mother works outside home.
2 mo	
Injury prevention:	Review above. Emphasize: use car restraints, protect from falls, rolling; do not leave unattended on bed or table; caution about hot liquids, burns; advise against infant walkers.
Feeding/nutrition:	As above; waiting to introduce solids at 4–6 mo.
Daily care/activities:	Sleep, crying, and bowel patterns.
Developmental/ behavioral issues:	As above.
Medical:	Immunizations; URI management: bulb syringe, saline nose drops.
Other:	As above; child care arrangements and support.
4 mo	
Injury prevention:	Review above. Emphasize: keep small objects out of reach.
Feeding/nutrition:	Introducing solid foods: iron-fortified cereal, fruits and vegetables.
Daily care/activities:	Sleep: night awakening; teething/drooling.

Developmental/ behavioral issues:	As above; talk to baby: respond to vocalizations.
Medical:	Immunizations; management of mild gastroenteritis.
Other:	Parent and family functioning; child care arrangements and support.
6 mo	
Injury prevention:	"Child-proofing" house in preparation for mobility; syrup of ipecac/Poison Control Center number; car safety; walkers and stair gates; window-guards; bathtub safety; electrical cords and outlets; burn risks.
Feeding/nutrition:	Issues with feeding solids; norms regarding caloric needs (volumes); introducing finger foods (7–9 mo); begin practice with cup; discourage milk or juice as pacifier or bottle to bed; discuss when to introduce cow's milk (end of first year, if possible).
Daily care/activities:	Resistance to sleep: suggest favorite toy or possession (transitional objects); teething/dental care; shoes (soft, flexible).
Developmental/ behavioral issues:	Separation and stranger anxiety.
Medical:	Immunizations.
Other:	As above.
9 mo	
Injury prevention:	Review above. Emphasize: toddler car restraint when ≥ 20 lb; ingestants (eg, small objects, peanuts, grapes, hot dogs; burns).
Feeding/nutrition:	Finger/table foods; self-feeding: cup and spoon practice; begin to wean from bottle; anticipate decreased food intake; introducing cow's milk.
Daily care/activities:	Sleep: night awakening, favorite toy or possession; shoes; dental care.
Developmental/ behavioral issues:	Separation and stranger anxiety; vocalization, communication, imitation; social games; anticipate autonomy issues of toddler period; discipline: limit-setting, consistency, distraction.
Other:	Parent and family functioning; child care arrangements and support.
12 mo	
Injury prevention:	Reinforce: syrup of ipecac/Poison Control Center number; tap water at maximum of 120 °F; kitchen, stair, water, and car safety; fences, gates, and latches; burn risks.
Feeding/nutrition:	Table foods, weaning from bottle; decreased food intake; introducing cow's milk.
Daily care/activities:	As above.
Developmental/ behavioral issues:	Speech development; talk to baby; discuss autonomy, limit-setting, discipline; praise desired behavior (positive reinforcement); prohibitions: few but firm.
Other:	As above.
15 mo	
Injury prevention:	Review above.
Feeding/nutrition:	Self-feeding, eats meals with family; phase out bottle use, advise against bottle in bed.

(continued)

Table 1–16 (cont'd). Anticipatory guidance—suggested topics at each visit.[1]

Daily care/activities:	As above.
Developmental/ behavioral issues:	Review indicators of toilet training readiness; discipline/temper tantrums: remove from temptation, consistency between parents, time-out, substitution, avoid reinforcing tantrum behavior, praise good behavior; read books together.
Medical:	Immunizations.
Other:	Parent and family functioning; child care arrangements and support; sibling rivalry.

18 mo

Injury prevention:	Review above. Emphasize: supervised play near street, in driveway; yard, pedestrian, and playground safety; dangers of climbing; never leave unattended in car or in house; unsafe toys, plastic bags and balloons.
Feeding/nutrition:	Wean from bottles; good use of spoon and cup in self-feeding.
Daily care/activities:	Sleep: short ritual before regular bedtime, night fears, night awakening; self-comforting behaviors: thumb sucking, masturbation, favorite toy or possession.
Developmental/ behavioral issues:	Discipline; need for autonomy and independence; "rapprochement"—transient return to clinging behavior; may show toilet training readiness at 18–24 mo; play games: praise, show affection; read simple stories to child regularly.
Medical:	Immunizations.
Other:	As above.

24 mo

Injury prevention:	Review above.
Feeding/nutrition:	Avoid struggles about eating; discourage non-nutritious snacks; encourage social/family aspects of meals.
Daily care/activities:	Sleep: discuss a move to regular bed; reassure that day napping varies; use of toothbrush.
Developmental/ behavioral issues:	Autonomy: do not hurry, consistent limits, present choices. Toilet learning: does child show interest and readiness, understand expectations? Curiosity about body parts; provide for play and peer contacts; imaginary friends.
Other:	Parent and family functioning; child care arrangements and support; sibling rivalry.

3 y

Injury prevention:	Review above. Emphasize: car safety restraints; street and water safety; animals and pets; teach full name, emergency number, and address.
Feeding/nutrition:	Balanced diet, avoidance of junk foods.
Daily care/activities:	First dental appointment; sleep: regular bedtime and routine, napping variability.

Developmental/ behavioral issues:	Discipline; toilet training; nursery school, day care, baby sitters: encourage out-of-home experiences, peer interactions; allow to explore, show initiative, and communicate; talk about activities with child; reserve time alone with child; limit television viewing; watch children's programs with child; masturbation; satisfy curiosity about babies, sex differences.
Other:	Family functioning.

4 y

Injury prevention:	Review above. Emphasize: bicycle and pedestrian safety; water safety; car seat, booster, or seat belt; refusal of food or rides from strangers; electrical tools, firearms, matches, and poisons; know emergency number and address; home fire safety drills.
Feeding/nutrition:	Balanced diet, social aspects of meals.
Daily care/activities:	Dental care, sleep.
Developmental/ behavioral issues:	Toilet training; discipline; provide interactions with other children; assign chores; limit television viewing; sexual curiosity, masturbation; nursery school, day care; issues around school, readiness assessment.
Other:	Family functioning.

5 y

Injury prevention:	Review above.
Feeding/nutrition:	Balanced diet.
Daily care/activities:	Dental care, sleep.
Developmental/ behavioral issues:	School readiness; plays well with other children, normal development, endures half-day separation from home; promote interactions with other children; assign chores; discipline; sexual curiosity, masturbation.
Medical:	Immunizations.
Other:	Family functioning.

6 and 8 y

Injury prevention:	Bicycle safety; seat belts; learn to swim; child supervision when away.
Feeding/nutrition:	Avoid junk food, maintain appropriate weight; encourage social aspects of mealtime.
Daily care/activities:	Exercise regularly; brush teeth; get adequate sleep; school and academic activities; peer interactions; family interactions.
Developmental/ behavioral issues:	Establish rules, act as role model; provide allowance; spend time with child; show interest in school; praise, encourage, show affection; limit television viewing.
Other:	Library card.

10 y

Injury prevention:	Review above. Emphasize: skateboard and bicycle safety; drugs, alcohol, and tobacco; supervise potentially hazardous activities; sport safety.
Feeding/Nutrition:	As above.
Daily care/activities:	As above.

(continued)

Table 1–16 (cont'd). Anticipatory guidance—suggested topics at each visit.[1]

Developmental/ behavioral issues:	As above; social interactions: peers, hobbies, social skills; sex education at home, school; discuss pubertal changes; academic activities; family communications: method of resolution, limit setting, sense of responsibility.	Feeding/nutrition:	As above.
		Daily care/activities:	As above.
		Developmental/ behavioral issues:	Review above. Emphasize: dating, peer pressure; sexuality.
12 y		**16–20 y**	
Injury prevention:	Review above.	Injury prevention:	Review above. Emphasize: responsibility for health; driving safety; substance abuse; CPR training.
Feeding/nutrition:	Avoid junk food, maintain appropriate weight; encourage social aspects of mealtime.	Feeding/nutrition:	Healthy diet, maintaining appropriate weight.
Daily care/activities:	Exercise regularly, brush teeth, get adequate sleep; school and academic activities; sports, hobbies, and weekend jobs; peer and family interactions.	Daily care/activities:	School and academic activities; sports, hobbies, jobs; regular physical exercise; peer and family interactions.
Developmental/ behavioral issues:	Discuss: rapid physical growth and sexual development, body image; sex education; establish rules, communicate with child; respect privacy, allow decision making.	Developmental/ behavioral issues:	Goals and values clarification, future plans; fair rules, allow decision-making; family and peer communication; expect periods of estrangement; respect privacy; encourage independence; serve as role model; sexuality and activity, contraception and prevention of sexually transmitted diseases.
14 y			
Injury prevention:	Review above. Emphasize: risk-taking behaviors; encourage responsibility for health and health behavior choices.		

[1]Modified and reproduced, with permission, from: *Guidelines for Health Supervision II,* 2nd ed. American Academy of Pediatrics, Committee on Psychosocial Aspects of Child and Family Health, 1985–88, 1988.

CPR = cardiopulmonary resuscitation; SIDS = sudden infant death syndrome; URI = upper respiratory infection.

expressing enough milk to initiate milk let-down so that the most vigorous period of sucking is avoided. It is, however, very important that the nursing mother not decrease feeding because of sore nipples as this may lead, through inadequate breast drainage, to engorgement.

Engorgement refers to the uncomfortable swelling of the breasts that occurs when regular effective breast emptying does not take place. Feedings on an engorged breast may be both painful and difficult because of decreased nipple protractility. A cycle of decreased feeding leading to increasing engorgement, involution of the milk supply, and possible mastitis can result if adequate drainage does not occur. Engorgement can be avoided with regular, frequent nursing. If it occurs, it is important to counsel mothers that increasing rather than decreasing feedings on the affected side will hasten relief. This may be initially facilitated by manually expressing some milk or using a hand pump until it is easier and less painful for the infant to suckle. Warm compresses to facilitate milk let-down during feedings and cool compresses between feedings may be helpful.

Maternal pain, stress, fatigue, and anxiety can have a significant impact on the hormonal milieu necessary for effective lactation. It is important to encourage the lactating mother to get as much rest as possible and to enlist the assistance of the baby's father or other support persons in this regard. Her diet should be nutritious and include plenty of fluids. Suggestions to help facilitate milk let-down during feedings include nursing in a quiet, comfortable place; nursing while lying down; and taking a hot shower or bath just before a feeding.

Breast-feeding mothers frequently worry about whether their milk supply is adequate and whether the infant is getting enough. Not all women experience fullness or the sensation of milk let-down despite successful breast-feeding. Parents should be counseled on ways to assess indirectly whether intake is adequate, such as weight gain, signs of hydration, and satiety behavior (Table 1–17). Breast-fed infants may lose up to 10% of their birth weight before regaining it by 10–14 days of age. Greater or more prolonged weight loss may be a sign of feeding difficulty. During growth spurts (typically at 3, 6, and 12 weeks), the infant may transiently decrease the interval between feedings to stimulate more milk production. It is important to inform parents of this normal phenomenon,

Table 1–17. Cues to assessing adequacy of breast-feeding.

- Nursing frequency no greater than 8 feeds per day
- Presence of fullness before feeding and relief of fullness after feeding
- Presence of symptomatic milk ejection reflex
- Audible swallowing by infant
- Signs of satiation in infant after feeding
- At least 6 wet diapers/day (normally 6–8/d)
- At least 4 stools per day (normally 6–10)
- Birth weight loss less than 10% (birth weight regained by 2 weeks of age)

so that the change is not perceived as a sign of inadequate milk supply. The use of vitamin and fluoride supplements and the introduction of solid foods in conjunction with breast-feeding are discussed below.

The decision about when to begin weaning should take into account the needs and realities of both the infant and the mother. Weaning ideally is a gradual process whereby nutritive and psychological needs are increasingly provided by other sources and activities. One can begin by substituting a cup or bottle for the least favorite breast-feeding session at the same time each day. The last feeding to be eliminated should be the one to which the child is most attached. Cuddling and holding without nursing should also be encouraged. In the somewhat older child, periods of separation from the mother and the use of distraction techniques may be helpful. A supportive bra increases the comfort of the mother during the weaning process, and maternal fluid intake should be decreased accordingly.

Formula Feeding

For parents who elect not to breast-feed, various manufactured formulas are available. Parents should be informed regarding similarities and differences between formulas, their appropriate preparation and storage, and what to expect in terms of frequency and volume of feedings.

Most of the common commercial formulas designed for healthy, full-term infants are cow's milk–based and are composed of reconstituted skim milk or skim milk with added whey protein. The source of carbohydrate is lactose, and the fat content consists of a mixture of vegetable oils that are better digested and absorbed than butter fat. The composition of these formulas is thought to provide an adequate nutritional alternative to breast milk. Differences within this group are relatively small, and in choosing among them, weight should be given to relative cost and the taste preference of the infant. Soy-protein formulas, introduced in the 1920s as hypoallergenic alternatives to cow's milk–based preparations, were initially deficient in several important nutrients. Since then they have undergone a series of refinements and are now considered a nutritionally sound alternative to the milk-based formulas for full-term infants. They are, however, of limited value as hypoallergenic preparations because of the high incidence of cross-reactivity to soy protein among infants with cow's-milk protein allergy and to the development of protein hydrolysate formulas. The fat composition of soy formulas is similar to that of the cow's milk group. Because the source of carbohydrate is sucrose or corn syrup solids, soy protein formulas may also be useful as a transitional formula for the infant with transient lactase deficiency that follows significant diarrheal illness. Formula switching for vague constitutional and gastrointestinal symptoms or for mild viral gastroenteritis risks inappropriately labeling the child as allergy-prone or having gastrointestinal problems and should be discouraged. The lack of gastrointestinal symptoms from the concentration

of iron in both cow's-milk and soy-based formulas should be discussed with parents and is addressed further below. Recently, weaning formulas designed for infants older than 6 months have been introduced into the market. Although these formulas provide satisfactory nutrient content, they offer no advantage over the currently recommended combinations of breast-feeding, infant formula, and iron- or vitamin-containing solids for children of this age.

Most formulas may be purchased in a powdered, concentrate, or ready-to-eat form. While powdered and concentrate preparations are the least expensive, they require care in reconstituting to the appropriate concentration. Unless the family lives in an area where the water supply is potentially unsafe, sterilization of both bottle and formula is no longer necessary. Between use, bottles and nipples should be cleaned with warm, soapy water. Once opened, a can of concentrate or ready-to-eat formula should be refrigerated and used within 48 hours.

As with breast-feeding, an on-demand feeding schedule should be encouraged. Most newborns will feed 2–3 oz every 2–3 hours and should not be allowed to go longer than 5 hours between feedings. Formula-fed infants usually lose less than 8% of their birth weight and regain this weight by 7–10 days after birth. After the first week, most infants take 2–4 oz every 2–4 hours or average approximately 2–3 oz/lb/d. By 2 months of age, the middle-of-the-night feeding usually drops out. During the second half of the first year, the infant generally should be taking less than 30 oz of formula per day in combination with solids, and calories from formula should not exceed 65% of the total daily intake. Especially with bottle-fed infants, it is important to encourage parents to learn to distinguish crying due to hunger from that due to other causes and to recognize the signs of satiety to avoid the common problem of overfeeding. Putting the older infant to sleep with a bottle should be discouraged because of the risk of nursing-bottle caries and the likely exacerbation of subsequent problems with discontinuing its use. Most parents begin weaning the infant from the bottle at 9–12 months of age. Allowing a toddler or preschool child to "roam" with a bottle on demand will make eventual discontinuation much more difficult and can lead to a variety of feeding problems, such as inadequate intake and restricted acceptance of solid foods.

Vitamin, Iron, & Fluoride Supplementation

Commercial formulas are fortified with vitamins and minerals. Formula-fed full-term infants require no additional supplementation. Although quantitative levels of vitamin D are low in breast milk, clinical rickets is uncommon in full-term breast-fed infants when maternal vitamin D intake during pregnancy and lactation is adequate and when mother and child receive normal amounts of sunlight exposure. Although some pediatricians advocate vitamin D supplementation for all breast-fed infants, most recommend selective supplementation (400 IU/d) of those breast-fed infants thought to be at greatest risk for deficiency, including infants of mothers with inadequate prenatal or postnatal dietary vitamin D intake; infants with little sunlight absorption because of factors related to climate, skin pigmentation, and cultural clothing practices; and older infants whose diets consist exclusively of breast milk. Vitamin B_{12} deficiency may also occur in breast-fed infants of mothers who are strict vegetarians. There is no evidence to suggest that breast-fed infants need routine supplementation with vitamin A, C, or E.

If dietary iron is not provided, full-term infants begin to deplete their iron stores by 4 months of age. For all but exclusively breast-fed infants, iron supplementation from one or more sources, such as formula, iron-fortified cereal, or ferrous sulfate drops, should begin at 4–6 months of age in the full-term infant and 2 months of age in the preterm infant. Although the iron content of breast milk is lower than that of formula, exclusively breast-fed infants require no extra source of iron because of its greater bioavailability. However, when solids are started and breast-milk intake is decreased, as with formula-fed children, iron-rich foods are indicated. Early introduction of whole cow's milk can cause iron deficiency anemia because of its low iron content and potential for causing occult gastrointestinal blood loss and should be discouraged before 1 year of age. Contrary to popular belief, ample evidence now supports the statement that iron-containing formulas do not cause an increase in gastrointestinal symptoms, such as constipation or gas, in most children. It is wise to discuss this with parents and to explain why iron is important to their child's diet.

The topical and systemic use of fluoride has dramatically decreased the incidence of dental caries. Excess fluoride, however, can cause fluorosis of the enamel, a cosmetically disfiguring condition. Current recommendations regarding the need for supplementation are based on the concentration of fluoride in the local water supply. When this is inadequate, the American Academy of Pediatrics (AAP) and the American Dental Association Council on Dental Therapeutics recommend beginning fluoride supplementation at 6 months of age. The dose given depends on the age of the child and the fluoride content of the local water supply (Table 1–18). Levels of fluoride in breast milk are low and only slightly related to the

mother's intake. However, the incidence of caries in exclusively breast-fed infants whose mothers drink fluoridated water is similar to that of formula-fed infants living in the same area; therefore, whether breast-fed infants living in areas with adequately fluoridated water need additional fluoride supplementation is debatable. It is important to remember to supplement the formula of the rare infant who is ingesting only ready-to-eat formula, because these are manufactured with nonfluoridated water. When assisting the toddler in brushing primary teeth, it is important to use only a small amount of fluoridated toothpaste as much of it is swallowed and can lead to excess fluoride intake with subsequent enamel fluorosis.

Advancing to Solids, Cow's Milk, Self-feeding, & a Prudent Diet

Current recommendations regarding the introduction of solid foods are based on considerations of developmental readiness, nutrient needs, and the potential for adverse reactions. In the first 4 months of life, breast milk or infant formula provides optimal nutrition for the baby, and the use of solid foods should be discouraged. Although they can be force-fed, babies younger than 4 months of age have a strong tongue-protrusion reflex and have not yet developed the mouth and tongue movements necessary for coordinated swallowing of solid foods. By 4–6 months, the infant's head and oromotor control are sufficiently developed to begin to participate actively in exploring the different tastes and textures of solid food. Initially, the volume of food consumed is less important than the experience. Parents should be prepared for some fun and mess. Many begin by offering solid foods at one or two feedings a day and then advance to a schedule that gradually approaches the family mealtimes. The order in which foods are introduced is, to a large extent, dictated by tradition. However, because of concerns about the impact of gastrointestinal immaturity on the development of food allergy, it is generally recommended that substances frequently associated with allergic symptomatology, such as egg white, wheat, and fish, be introduced later. Most parents begin with iron-fortified infant cereals and advance to strained or pureed vegetables, fruits, and meats. It is important to remind parents to introduce one new food at a time and to wait 3–5 days before adding another to appreciate any adverse effects. When purchasing baby food, one-item foods are preferable to combination dinners. Infant preparations can also be easily and cheaply made at home by cooking foods until tender and then pureeing them with a blender, food mill, or kitchen strainer. Food can be prepared in advance and stored in meal-sized portions by freezing the puree in ice cube trays. Babies appear to be born with a preference for sweetness. An innate preference for saltiness appears later in the first year of life. However, both sweet and salty taste preferences can be exaggerated by dietary exposure. Parents should avoid adding salt or processed sugar to their infant's food.

As previously mentioned, the early introduction of

Table 1–18. Fluoride supplementation.[1,2]

Age	Water Fluoride Content (ppm)		
	< 0.3	0.3–0.6	> 0.6
Birth to 6 mo	0	0	0
6 mo to 3 y	0.25	0	0
3–6 y	0.50	0.25	0
6–16 y	1.00	0.50	0

[1]Reproduced, with permission, from: Committee on Nutrition, American Association of Pediatrics, Fluoride Supplementation for Children: Interim policy recommendations. Pediatrics 1995;95: 777.
[2]Fluoride daily doses are given in milligrams.

whole cow's milk has been associated with occult gastrointestinal blood loss and iron deficiency in young infants. This should be delayed until the end of the first year of life. As discussed below, whole or 2% fat milk rather than skimmed milk is recommended in the first 2 years of life.

By 6–8 months of age, most infants can sit, bring objects to their mouth, and begin holding a cup and spoon. With practice, relatively controlled use of the cup and spoon usually occurs between 15 and 18 months of age. Most infants are ready to enjoy finger foods by 7–9 months. Mature chewing skills are usually present by 18 months. In choosing what to offer, it is important to avoid large, hard, spheric, or coin-shaped items that could cause airway obstruction if aspirated. These include foods such as raw carrots, large pieces of raw apple, whole hot dogs or hot dog coins, whole grapes, large cookies, peanuts, and hard candy. Infants and toddlers should always be observed by an adult when eating.

Ample evidence now exists that atherosclerotic disease begins in childhood. Prudent dietary and other life-style practices that are begun early may prevent or decrease atherosclerotic morbidity in later life. However, excessive dietary fat restriction may lead to impaired growth and nutrition in the developing child. Many expert panels and groups, including the National Cholesterol Education Program (NCEP), the AAP, and the American Heart Association, have issued recommendations regarding a prudent diet for children. These guidelines all emphasize the need to eat a varied and nutritionally balanced diet, maintain ideal body weight, decrease total fat intake, increase polyunsaturated fats at the expense of saturated fats and cholesterol, and avoid excessive salt. Children younger than 1–2 years of age need adequate amounts of dietary fat (30–50% of daily calorie intake) for optimal growth and development. During this time, dietary fat and cholesterol should not be restricted, and whole milk, rather than skim or 2% fat-free milk, should be used. After age 2 years, the child should gradually make the transition to a prudent diet consisting of approximately 30% of daily calories from fat, less than 10% from saturated fats, and less than 300 mg/d of cholesterol.

Common Toddler Feeding Issues

Parents of toddlers often become concerned about their child's dietary intake and eating habits. Worry frequently centers around the volume and variety of food consumed. It is important to inform parents that the child's rate of growth slows considerably after the first year of life, and caloric needs per pound decrease even as activity increases. Reviewing the growth chart with parents can be very reassuring. It is also important to point out that otherwise healthy (physically/psychosocially) children will not willfully starve themselves. Parents should be advised to evaluate success at meeting nutritional needs, such as sufficient intake from various food groups, over the course of a week rather than at each meal.

Issues of autonomy and self-assertion also frequently

present themselves around mealtime at this age. Suggestions to help prevent common toddler feeding and mealtime behavior problems are given in Table 1–19. Long, drawn-out battles are rarely productive. Parents should also resist the temptation to prepare a separate meal of limited, preferred foods for the child and should continue to offer previously refused foods at periodic intervals. The social aspects of mealtime should be emphasized by having the family sit down together and avoiding other distracting activities, such as watching television and reading, during the meal. Finally, because children learn by observation, parents should model the same good eating behaviors that they wish their child to exhibit.

NORMAL AGE-RELATED SLEEP PATTERNS & COMMON PROBLEMS

The character and patterns of sleep undergo a normal transition from infancy to adulthood that is influenced not only by neuromaturational factors but also by the child's temperament and care-taking environment. Sleep comprises two distinct states: active or REM sleep, characterized by rapid eye movements, motor movements, vocalizations, dreaming, and easy awakening; and the deeper quiet or non-REM sleep. Fifty percent of an infant's sleeptime is spent in the REM state with non-REM intervals of 50–60 minutes between active phases, whereas only 20% of the adult sleep cycle consists of REM sleep interspersed with 90–100 minute intervals of quiet sleep.

Table 1–19. Preventing common toddler feeding/mealtime behavior problems.

- Don't make mealtimes a battle ground; should be pleasant
- Establish mealtime routine and rules
- Eat as a family and encourage social aspects
- Avoid other concurrent activities (television, reading)
- Don't carry on conversations with another adult for longer than a few minutes; include child in table talk
- Find opportunities to praise your child for appropriate mealtime/daytime behaviors
- Provide opportunities for mealtime choice while regaining control over important issues
- Provide variety: praise trying (taste test); offer previously refused types of foods at periodic intervals
- Allow and encourage self-feeding (even if messy)
- Portion control: give realistic (small) portions, seconds if child finishes
- Mealtimes should be of a finite/realistic duration (15–30 min)
- When food refused, avoid routinely preparing a "special" meal for child
- Don't make leaving table contingent on cleaning plate
- Remove food not finished after the prediscussed time period and, except for routine snacks, avoid additional feedings until next meal
- Avoid excessive intake of liquids (juice, milk) and continual "grazing" between meals
- Provide nutritious between meal snacks; avoid excessive snacking
- Model good eating behavior as parents

Newborns sleep approximately 18 hours per day, with sleep time distributed evenly over the day and night hours. However, sleep-wake patterns quickly become entrained to a day-night cycle because of inherent circadian rhythms and parental care-giving schedules. Between 6 and 15 months of age, most children sleep approximately 10–12 hours at night and take two daytime naps, each lasting more than an hour, in the midmorning and afternoon. After 15 months of age, children usually take only one nap during the day, and by 4 years of age have discontinued napping altogether. Although individual differences are significant, the 5 year old requires approximately 11 hours, and the 10 year old, 9½ hours of sleep per night. Most adolescents need 8–9 hours of sleep each night.

By inquiring about sleep habits or problems and providing information and anticipatory guidance, pediatric primary care providers are in a unique position to diagnose and manage, as well as prevent, many common age-related sleep problems. Several excellent suggestions to help parents facilitate optimal sleep habits and prevent subsequent sleep problems in their infant and young toddler are given in Table 1–20. Parents may inadvertently slow their early infant's adaptation to a day-night sleep schedule by prolonged or frequent periods of nocturnal feeding and attention. Spontaneous awakenings are normal and occur often during periods of REM sleep. The ability of infants to use internal mechanisms to return themselves to sleep usually develops around 3–4 months

Table 1–20. Strategies to encourage night settling.[1]

Early infancy (birth to 4 mo)
  During the day, limit the duration of sleep to 3–4 consecutive hours
  Place baby to sleep in crib in own room, if feasible
  Place baby in crib sleepy, but awake
  Allow baby to fall asleep alone (eg, without rocking, feeding, or pacifier)
  Allow baby to self-calm (eg, find his or her own thumb)
  Make middle-of-the-night feedings "brief and boring"
  Do not respond to normal sounds made during sleep by picking up the baby

Middle infancy (4–6 mo)
  Delay response to fussing for several minutes to allow infant opportunity to fall back asleep
  Gradually reduce duration and amount of nighttime feeding
  Avoid unnecessary stimulation (eg, picking up) when checking on fussy infant

Later infancy (6–12 mo)
  For separation anxiety: Provide a transitional object (eg, blanket, toy) or night light; leave door to bedroom open
  Provide extra reassurances and cuddling during day
  Make bedtime routine pleasant, predictable, and quiet
  Set firm limits after infant is put to bed (eg, "once in bed, stay in bed")
  Further delay response in infant fussing and avoid physical contact and extra stimulation
  Promptly respond to nightmares and bedtime fears
  Promptly reinstitute strategies after recovery from illness

---

[1]Reproduced, with permission, from: Algranati PS, Dworkin PH: Infancy problem behaviors. Pediatr Rev 1992;13:16.

of age and is referred to as "settling." At this time an infant begins to sleep for 6–8 uninterrupted hours during the night. Although the vast majority of infants "settle" by 6 months of age, some children continue to have frequent and prolonged nighttime awakening. Aside from inherent temperamental differences, several environmental factors may be involved. First, parents may misperceive the movements, vocalizations, and brief awakenings of REM sleep as indicating a need for intervention and, in attending to the infant, may inadvertently cause the child to arouse further. Frequent feedings and prolonged attention at night may also encourage this pattern. Infants who always fall asleep while being rocked, fed, or otherwise soothed may be unable to return themselves to sleep when normal nighttime awakening occurs and the same conditions are not present. To avoid this problem, parents should be encouraged to allow infants to fall asleep in their cribs.

Normal separation issues may make going to sleep difficult for the 9- to 18-month-old child. Use of a transitional object, such as a favorite blanket or stuffed animal, that the child can take to bed may make falling and staying asleep easier. The older toddler frequently resists going to bed. A passion for experience and the desire for autonomy and control contribute to this behavior. At this age, it is especially important to have established consistent bedtime routines and rituals that allow the child to "wind down" from more stimulating activities and, at the same time, to take charge of certain aspects of the bedtime process.

During the preschool and school-age years, nighttime fears are frequent and usually transient. Nightmares are also common during this period. These occur during REM sleep and frequently cause spontaneous wakening with vivid recall. Nightmares are usually easily distinguished from night terrors, which affect approximately 5% of young children and occur during deepest non-REM sleep. During a night terror the child appears extremely frightened and agitated and, although seemingly awake, is actually in deep sleep and difficult to arouse. Upon awakening, the child has no apparent memory of the event. Although frightening to parents, night terrors are believed to be self-limited and benign. A more detailed discussion regarding the diagnosis and management of common sleep problems encountered during infancy and childhood is provided in Chapter 3.

CRYING & FUSSINESS

Crying is a normal physiologic response to distress or discomfort and serves to alert the caretaker to the baby's needs. The quality and duration of an infant's crying may vary with the cause of distress, the temperament of the child, and the caretaking response that it elicits. The results of Brazelton's study of 80 otherwise healthy middle-class infants indicated that a 2-week-old infant cries approximately 2 hours per day. Crying tends to increase to an average of 3 hours per day at 6 weeks and then decrease to 1 hour per day by 3 months of age. Most crying occurs during the evening hours. All parents worry about how best to manage their infant's fussy periods; caretakers should be encouraged to develop a consistent set of responses to the crying episodes (Table 1–21).

Many parents become concerned about what they perceive to be excessive crying. Parents' perceptions of their baby's crying may be affected by prior expectations about what is normal, the duration or character of the crying, the baby's responsiveness to attempts at consoling, and parental functioning in the face of various environmental stresses. Evaluation of such a complaint should involve a thorough history, including a description of the character and pattern of crying, past and current attempts at management, specific parental concerns, environmental stresses, and overall parental coping. A physical examination is important to rule out underlying medical problems and to reassure the parents. The approach used for the otherwise well-nourished, healthy infant with excessive, unexplained paroxysms of crying (colic) is discussed in Chapter 3.

DISCIPLINE

Parents frequently consult pediatricians for advice regarding discipline. The health supervision visit provides an excellent opportunity to discuss age-appropriate guidelines, as well as to help parents understand how normal developmental pressures, parental styles, environmental factors, and individual temperamental differences interact to affect a child's behavior and socialization. Although frequently used to refer to punishment, **discipline** is derived from the word "disciple," meaning to teach, and, in its broadest definition, is the structure provided by parents that helps to foster a child's sense of being a lovable and capable human being. Parents who make an effort to listen to and get to know their child, and who spend even a short period of uninterrupted "special" time with their child each day, are conveying the powerful message that the child is loved and important. By showing interest and caring, complimenting good behavior, providing consistent appropriate limits, and setting a good example, parents can best shape their child's behavior and conscience according to their own values and practices. Punishment, when necessary, should be age-appropriate and close in time to the misbehavior and should not be physically or psychologically destructive. Corporal punishment is less effective than positive reinforcement, is potentially harmful, and teaches children that physical aggression is an acceptable means of dealing with anger.

Contrary to common belief, infants younger than 4 months cannot be "spoiled," and parents should be encouraged to respond to their child's needs with unrestricted nurturing and care. By age 4–6 months, infants can begin to use crying in manipulative ways, and behavior modification techniques may be helpful. As discussed in the sections on sleep and crying, care must be taken not to inadvertently reinforce behaviors such as frequent nocturnal awakening or feeding by providing excessive nighttime attention. Limit setting becomes important for the older infant and beyond, and the expression of verbal or nonverbal disapproval is an effective form of punishment for this and older age groups. At all ages, verbal disapproval is most effective when combined with positive instruction regarding appropriate behavioral alternatives and should be focused on the misbehavior rather than on personally belittling the child. The older infant and early toddler may respond to constructive distraction or redirecting, techniques that have the added advantage of being useful preventively. As the naturally curious child develops mobility, the parent must take responsibility for structuring an environment that not only is safe but also minimizes temptations for misadventure. Parents who accommodate their playing toddler's need for frequent, brief, verbal and nonverbal contact may prevent an escalation of negative attention-seeking behavior, which can occur when a parent is otherwise preoccupied. Toddlers often have difficulty with shifts in their routine and abrupt transitions from one activity to the next and, when possible, should be given advance warning of such changes. Providing toddlers with the opportunity to make choices among acceptable options (eg, clothing, food) allows them to express positively their growing need for control and independence. Negativism and temper tantrums are common expressions of the toddler's struggle for autonomy and self-control. Harmless behaviors, such as tantrums, sulking, and whining, can frequently be averted by redirecting the child or avoiding excessive fatigue and hunger, and are most effectively extinguished by ignoring them. Children who are engaging in harmful or potentially harmful behavior may

Table 1–21. Strategies to manage fussy periods during early infancy.[1]

To diminish the amount of crying and fussing
Carry and cuddle frequently during both fussy and nonfussy periods
Respond promptly to baby's cry, and do not worry about "spoiling" infant
Help baby to become a self-soother (eg, help baby to find own thumb or a comfortable body position)
Develop a routine series of responses to soothe baby
Pick up baby
Change diaper if soiled
Cuddle
Offer feeding if last feeding was more than 2 h ago
Burp
Offer a pacifier
Check to see that baby is neither too hot nor too cold and that clothing or diaper is not constricting
Place baby in a swing or crib rocker or carry in a front pack
Turn on music or heartbeat simulator
Go for a walk or ride in the car
Put baby in crib and allow to cry and fuss
Repeat routine

[1]Reproduced, with permission, from: Algranati PS, Dworkin PH: Infancy problem behaviors. Pediatr Rev 1992;13:16.

need to be manually removed from the situation. The technique of "time-out," described below, is an effective method for dealing with harmful or disruptive behavior and can be implemented successfully as early as 9–12 months of age. From an early age, it is also important to help children recognize and verbalize their feelings rather than act them out physically. The preschooler and older child often respond to natural and logical consequences whereby, within the bounds of safety, they learn by experiencing the negative natural or social consequences of their actions. For example, the child who is late for dinner is confronted by a plate of cold food, toys that are mishandled are removed, and the child who spills juice helps to clean it up. Family conferences that permit the child to participate in discussion and negotiation are important when establishing rules for older school-aged children. Delaying privileges until other less pleasurable tasks are completed is also frequently effective.

Time-out is an effective method for extinguishing harmful or disruptive behavior and works by temporarily withdrawing social interaction. It may be used as early as 8 months of age and should begin being phased out by 5–6 years. A time-out location, such as a chair in the corner of the room, that is devoid of interesting distractions but not frightening to the child, should be chosen in advance. For young children, this should always be an area in which they can be easily observed by an adult. When a pre-agreed behavior warranting time-out occurs, parents should give one warning and then ask the child to go to the time-out location if the behavior persists. The child who does not go voluntarily may need to be manually guided there. Parents should attempt to maintain a perspective of calm control and avoid engaging in angry lecturing or negotiations when applying time-out. Out-of-control behavior may initially be exacerbated by attempts to establish control. However, consistency and persistence are essential to the success of this technique. The length of time-out should be brief, approximately 1 minute for every year of life up to a maximum of 5 minutes. Use of a kitchen timer may be helpful. Children who leave the time-out location prematurely should be calmly returned, and the clock restarted. It is not important that the child be quiet, only that he or she stay in time-out. Occasionally it may be necessary to gently hold the child in the chair for the prescribed duration while minimizing conversation and interaction. When the time period is over, the child should be verbally released from time-out and welcomed back into the social setting without further mention of the previous infraction. After time-out, it is important to help the child learn socially acceptable alternative behaviors and, as soon as is possible, to recognize and compliment positive behavior.

SAFETY & ACCIDENT PREVENTION

Injuries, both unintentional and intentional, are responsible for more childhood morbidity and mortality than all other diseases and conditions combined. Perhaps not surprisingly, toddlers and adolescents are at highest risk for injury-related morbidity and mortality. Three quarters of all injury-related deaths among infants result from homicide (22%), suffocation (15%), choking (13%), motor-vehicle accidents (12%), and fires and burns (11%). Among preschoolers, fire (20%), drowning (19%), motor-vehicle accidents (15%), and pedestrian injuries (14%) account for two thirds of such deaths. Causes of injury-related death in school-aged children are similar to those in preschoolers, with a notable increase in pedestrian injuries (23%). Among adolescents, motor-vehicle accidents (44%), suicide (15%), and homicide (14%) account for three quarters of all injury-related deaths. Such mortality statistics underestimate the frequency of injuries that less often result in death. Common nonfatal injuries include falls, cuts, being struck by objects, burns, poisonings, animal bites, solitary (eg, bicycling or skating) and team sports injuries, and motor-vehicle accidents. Many people believe that injuries are random, unavoidable events and that children who incur them are simply "accident-prone." However, an increasing body of data suggests that, with appropriate personal, community, and legislative action, many injuries can be either prevented or diminished in severity. Furthermore, while certain behavioral and environmental characteristics may be associated with higher rates of injury, most injuries occur to children without such risk factors.

Recent years have also witnessed an alarming increase in intentional injury and violence within the pediatric population. Homicide is currently the second leading cause of death among adolescents, and suicide is a close third. Children and teens are increasingly confronted with violence in their homes, schools, communities, and larger society. The causes of these trends are complex and multifactorial. However, disintegration of traditional social networks and institutions, socioeconomic inequities, lack of appropriate adult role models or guidance regarding nonviolent conflict resolution and tolerance of differences, media glorification of violence as entertainment, and the availability of handguns and other weapons all contribute to the growing problem with violence.

The pediatrician is in a unique position to become involved in the area of injury and violence prevention as an advocate for safety legislation and as a resource and counselor for prevention strategies in which both individual families and communities can engage. Getting parents to translate the information provided into actual preventive action and changes in behavior provides a key challenge for the primary care provider. Individuals are much more likely to engage in preventive behaviors if they feel personally susceptible to a given problem and believe that they can favorably alter their risk by modifying behavior. It is easier to get people to take onetime actions, such as buying a car seat, installing a smoke detector, or turning down the temperature on the hot-water heater, than to engage in behaviors that require regular or frequent action, such as consistent, appropriate use of car restraints. The amount of effort, decrease in comfort, and cost associated with a particular prevention strategy also affect how widely it is adopted. At the health supervision visit, providing an all-inclusive list of potential safety hazards to parents is less important than focusing on the most prevalent problems at each age and attempting to facilitate preventive action by personalizing the information provided. An integrated approach to accident prevention involving both individual counseling and community-based action

has a greater chance of success than either approach alone.

The AAP recommends that all parents be counseled regarding the safety measures outlined in Table 1–22, which focus on the major causes of accidental death and injury in childhood. In addition to these specific topics, the AAP suggests regular discussion during the health supervision visit of age-, season-, and locality-appropriate safety issues and corresponding prevention strategies. Suggested

Table 1–22. Office-based counseling for injury prevention.[1]

All children should grow up in a safe environment.

Anticipatory guidance for injury prevention should be an integral part of the medical care provided for all infants and children.

In addition to below, all physicians caring for children should counsel parents in age-appropriate, season-appropriate, and locality-appropriate prevention strategies that reduce common serious injuries. Medical records should reflect this counsel.

Infants and preschoolers

Physicians caring for infants and preschool children should advise parents about the following issues:

- Traffic safety: appropriate use of currently approved child safety restraints (car seats); parental use of their own seat belts.
- Burn prevention: installation and maintenance of smoke detectors in home; setting of hot-water heater temperature between 120 and 130 °F, or lower.
- Fall prevention: use of window and stairway guards/gates in place; use of infant walkers discouraged.
- Poison prevention: storage of medicines/household products out of sight and reach and in original childproof containers; storage of 1 oz bottle of syrup of ipecac at home for use as advised by pediatrician.
- Choking prevention: provision of age-appropriate foods; avoidance of running/playing during eating; supervision of mealtime; use of age-appropriate toys.
- Drowning prevention: supervision of infant/young child in bathtub or wading pool; emptying of all buckets, tubs, wading pools immediately after use; installation of appropriate fencing/safety guards with swimming pools; supervision of preschool-aged child while swimming (irrespective of child's swimming ability).
- Cardiopulmonary resuscitation (CPR) training: training of parents in CPR; knowledge of how to access local emergency care system.

School-aged children

Physician advice to parents of elementary school–aged children begins to be more focused on the child's behavior. The child is included in this process as well, while the parents are reminded of their need to model safe behaviors.

- Traffic safety: use of seat belts/booster seats; knowledge of safe pedestrian practices; use of approved bicycle helmets when cycling and protective equipment for in-line skating/skate boarding.
- Water safety: provision of swimming instruction for children older than 5 years of age; knowledge of appropriate rules for water play; supervision of swimming; use of personal flotation devices with boating activities.
- Sports safety for adults who supervise children participating in organized sports: importance of appropriate safety equipment and physical conditioning.
- Firearm safety: removal of any handguns in the home. (If parents choose to keep a firearm, gun must be unloaded and both gun and ammunition must be kept in separate locked cabinets.)

Adolescents

Injury prevention advice to adolescents should be included in a broader discussion of healthy life-style choices (eg, alcohol/drug use, sexual activity, diet/physical activity). Specific areas of injury prevention guidance should include the following:

- Traffic safety: use of seat belts; role of alcohol in teenage motor vehicle accidents; use of motorcycle/bicycle helmets; use of protective equipment for in-line skating and skateboarding.
- Water safety: alcohol use in water-related activities; use of approved personal flotation devices when boating.
- Sports safety: importance of proper safety equipment and physical conditioning for adolescents participating in organized sports programs.
- Firearm safety: knowledge of unique dangers of in-home firearms during adolescence—risk of impulsive, unplanned use resulting in suicide, homicide, or other serious injuries. (If parents choose to keep a firearm, unloaded gun and ammunition must be kept in separate locked cabinets.)

[1]Modified and reproduced, with permission, from: Committee on Injury and Poison Prevention, American Academy of Pediatrics: Pediatrics 1994;94:566.

safety topics to cover at each visit are given in Table 1–16.

A developmental approach to counseling allows the pediatrician to emphasize the normal age-related variations in cognitive, motor, and perceptual skills that significantly affect the frequency and kinds of problems children encounter. Not surprisingly, infants 1–2 years of age have the highest rates of accidental injury. At this age, an insatiable desire for experience and autonomy, coupled with difficult impulse control, may outstrip cognitive and motor abilities, leading to unfortunate consequences. Recently acquired mobility, a pincer grasp, and an enjoyment of oral exploration also put children of this age at increased risk. With the achievement of object permanence, the infant and toddler actively search for objects and, as they begin to learn about cause and effect, may engage in dangerous behavior in an attempt to re-create a particularly fascinating event. Children at this age cannot understand or foresee the consequences of their actions and require parents to provide a safe environment, firm limit-setting, and appropriate supervision. This continues to be important for preschoolers, who, immersed in magical and egocentric prelogical thinking, have difficulty understanding that cause and effect is not a function of their own desires and intentions. Three-year-olds may believe that just by not intending or wanting something to happen, an undesirable outcome of their actions can be avoided. At this age, fantasy and reality may sometimes be confused. Preschoolers are, in general, unable to empathize with others who might be hurt by their actions. An inability to generalize or learn from past experiences is also common during this period.

To the school-aged child, peer group identification and acceptance becomes increasingly important. Dangerous or irresponsible behavior may arise out of a desire to be accepted by or not to "lose face" within a peer group. In challenging themselves to do things on their own, children at this age may overestimate their skills and competence. During this period, children develop the capacity for concrete operational thinking. Although they understand the concept of rules, they may often challenge them, believing that they know more than their parents. It is important to allow school-aged children to be involved in the rule-making process and, within the constraints of safety, to learn from experience and gradually increasing responsibility. Parents should also be encouraged to help their child develop empathy and problem-solving and conflict-resolution skills by providing opportunities for family discussion, as well as role-modeling tolerance of differences and nonviolent means of resolving disagreements.

After toddlers, adolescents have the highest rate of accidental death during childhood. Motor-vehicle accidents are the most common cause of injury and death among teenagers and often involve the concomitant use of alcohol or other mind-altering substances. Homicide, suicide, and violent trauma are the next most common causes of death in this age group. Feelings of invulnerability, susceptibility to peer pressure, a need to establish independence, and high rates of substance use and experimentation all contribute to these problems. One cannot overemphasize the importance of providing teens with specific situational skills to avoid uncomfortable or potentially dangerous situations with their peer group and to resolve conflicts nonviolently when they arise.

Adolescent risk-taking behavior is discussed in more depth in Chapter 2.

SCREENING

Much of the history and physical examination findings obtained at each health supervision visit are directed toward identification of undetected problems and their risk factors. Pediatricians need to be aware of not only current recommendations regarding screening and the specific tests available, but also the basic principles and concepts behind screening to evaluate whether a given program does more good than harm for their patients and community. Screening implies the presumptive identification of disease or its precursors in an otherwise asymptomatic individual or population and is, by definition, not diagnostic. It assumes that persons so identified will undergo definitive diagnostic testing and will subsequently benefit by the earlier implementation of treatment or prevention programs. The effectiveness of a given screening program can be demonstrated by performing a randomized clinical trial in which all pertinent outcomes are evaluated. Unfortunately, such data are often lacking and difficult to obtain. In the absence of such studies, the value of a given screening program must be defined in relation to certain characteristics of the condition being screened for, the test being used, the population being evaluated, and the larger social context in which decisions regarding the value of detection and the allocation of resources are being made.

When deciding what conditions are worth screening for, one must consider both the burden of suffering caused by a particular condition, as defined by its prevalence and severity, and the availability of a specific treatment or prevention strategy that, when implemented early, results in a longer or greater benefit to the individual than would have occurred with diagnosis at the onset of symptoms. The identification of conditions for which no treatment exists, or for which the benefit of existing therapy is unproved, is of questionable value and potentially harmful. Even when effective interventions do exist, one must weigh the potential risks and benefits of the treatment itself with those of the identified condition and consider the impact of public acceptance on compliance with screening and treatment recommendations.

The value of screening also depends on the existence of a good screening test. The accuracy of a test is defined by its sensitivity and specificity when compared with gold-standard measures of the presence or absence of disease, and its positive and negative predictive value within a population with a given disease prevalence. It is important to understand how these test characteristics affect the overall value of and implementation strategies for screening programs.

The sensitivity of a test refers to the proportion of individuals with a condition who have an abnormal test result. Thus, a highly sensitive test misses few true cases, because a high proportion of individuals with the disease have an abnormal test. The specificity of a test refers to the proportion of individuals without disease who have a normal test result. A highly specific test identifies few false-positive results because most individuals without the disease have a normal test. The sensitivity and specificity acceptable in a screening test reflect a relative weighing of the risk of missing true cases (sensitivity) compared with the risk of identifying false-positive results (specificity).

The predictive value of a test is the probability of the presence or absence of disease given an abnormal or normal test result. Positive predictive value refers to the probability that, given an abnormal result, an individual actually has the condition. Negative predictive value indicates the probability of the absence of the condition in an individual whose test result is normal. Predictive value depends on the sensitivity and specificity of the screening test being used, as well as on the prevalence of the disorder in the population being screened. The greater the sensitivity of a test, the greater its negative predictive value, and the greater the specificity of a test, the greater its positive predictive value. Independent of the screening test's sensitivity and specificity, decreasing the population prevalence of the condition being sought diminishes the positive predictive value of the test by changing the proportion of true-to-false positive results. One should be aware of the population on which the test was standardized and whether the group you wish to screen is sufficiently similar that measures of predictive ability are comparable and application of the instrument is appropriate. For most screening situations, it is important to know the predictive ability of the test in a population with low disease prevalence because this is generally how screening tests are used. In many cases, selective testing of high-risk subgroups may make more sense than mass screening.

The costs associated with a screening program must be broadly defined. These include not only the screening itself but also the subsequent diagnostic, therapeutic, and supportive services required. The psychological impact on individuals identified as false-positives and the costs involved in definitive evaluation of these individuals may be significant. Early identification through screening does not always imply a better outcome. One must question the ultimate value of the screening program if the health care system or community are unable to provide the subsequent necessary diagnostic and therapeutic services. If persons who are at greatest risk do not avail themselves of the screening program or individuals with abnormal screening tests do not follow through with subsequent diagnostic and therapeutic recommendations, the screening program will fail to achieve the benefits intended.

Current recommendations regarding screening during routine health supervision visits (see Table 1–1) reflect an increasing awareness of the importance of these issues when deciding the value of specific screening programs. They also recognize that different strategies may be appropriate for different populations. The following section addresses specific aspects of screening during the health supervision visit. Recommendations regarding additional screening for the sexually active adolescent are discussed in Chapter 2.

SPECIFIC SCREENING AREAS

Newborn Screening for Metabolic Diseases

The number of metabolic diseases that can be diagnosed and treated in the newborn period, before the onset of symptoms or morbidity, is rapidly increasing. While all states in the United States have initiated neonatal metabolic screening programs, because of the absence of federal guidelines, considerable state-to-state variability exists. Currently, all states screen for congenital hypothyroidism and phenylketonuria (PKU). Two thirds also screen for galactosemia. All these disorders are treatable and, if not diagnosed early, lead to irreversible brain damage. A blood sample should be obtained from all full-term neonates just before hospital discharge. Special testing arrangements must be made if birth takes place in a nontraditional setting. Identification of some disorders, such as PKU, requires sufficient build-up of metabolites to be detected. If, because of early discharge, blood was drawn before the infant was 24 hours old, a second sample should be obtained when the child is 1–2 weeks of age. Blood transfusions and dialysis, which introduce foreign blood cells and reduce concentrations of circulating metabolites, may result in both false-negative and false-positive results when screening newborns for metabolic disorders and hemoglobinopathies. When feasible, samples should be obtained before these procedures are done. Preterm and sick infants should be screened by 1 week of age regardless of the presence of these or other factors (eg, parenteral feeding, antibiotic use, or prematurity) that may interfere with specific assays or the interpretation of test results. When such concerns exist, a repeat sample should be obtained at a time interval appropriate to resolution of the confounding factors.

Newborn Screening for Hemoglobinopathies

Hemoglobinopathies occur with significant frequency and are a major cause of illness and death in this country. Sickle cell disease alone (SS, SC, and SB-thalassemia) affects approximately 1 of every 400 African-American newborns, as well as newborns from a variety of other ethnic and racial groups. Although the technology has existed for some time, compelling support for hemoglobinopathy screening in the newborn period was provided when a significant decrease in morbidity and mortality was demonstrated for children with sickle cell disease when diagnosis and initiation of a comprehensive treatment program, including prophylactic penicillin, occurred before symptomatic presentation.

In 1987, a National Institutes of Health Consensus Conference on this subject recommended that universal newborn screening for hemoglobinopathies be provided by each state. Debate continues as to the need for universal versus selective screening and the optimal screening procedure. Concern has also been raised over variability in laboratory accuracy and the adequacy of subsequent diagnostic and counseling services for individuals identified as either heterozygotes or homozygotes for these conditions. Current screening policies vary widely from state to state. Both heel-stick and cord blood samples may be used. Specimens are usually examined using electrophoresis at an alkaline pH, and abnormal samples are further evaluated using acid electrophoresis.

Physical Examination

During routine health supervision visits, a physical examination is performed for diagnostic or case-finding (screening) purposes. In addition, it provides a useful framework for parent-child education and reassurance. Although the importance of the latter function should not be overlooked, the case-finding value of routine physical examinations, when pathology is otherwise unsuspected, is limited and may not be the most effective use of the time available during the well-child visit. Except in the newborn period, among high-risk populations, or in the absence of adequate history, the primary aim of the well-visit physical examination should be to rule in or out pathology suspected by history or observation and to provide reassurance and guidance to families.

Developmental Screening

See section on development earlier in this chapter (Motor & Psychological Development).

Vision Screening

Routine vision screening is an effective way to identify otherwise unsuspected problems that are amenable to correction. Because normal visual development depends on the brain's receipt of clear binocular visual stimulation and because the plasticity of the developing visual system is time-limited (first 6 years of life), early detection and treatment of various problems that impair vision are essential to prevent permanent and irreversible visual deficits. Routine age-appropriate assessments should be incorporated into each health-supervision visit, beginning with the newborn examination. In the infant, assessment should include gross eye inspection and evaluation of the red reflex and fundi, pupillary light reflex, ability to track or follow an object, and the position and symmetry of the corneal light reflex. Ocular alignment should be consistently present by 4 months of age. In the toddler and preschooler, this is assessed by evaluation of the corneal light reflex, extraocular muscle movements, and fixation preference tests (cover-uncover and alternate cover tests). At approximately 3 years of age, visual acuity testing generally can be accomplished by using a standard Snelling alphabet chart, Allen picture cards, or instrumented screening equipment. Stereoscopic screening machines also allow assessment of binocular vision. School-aged children should have their visual acuity checked on a yearly basis. Preschoolers should be referred for further testing if the acuity in either eye is 20/40 or worse. In children 5 or 6 years of age, an inability to read the majority of the 20/30 line warrants referral. At all ages, a difference in the acuity measurements between eyes of more than one line necessitates further evaluation.

Hearing Screening

Approximately 1 of every 1000 infants is born deaf, and in many children sensorineural hearing deficits develop during childhood. Timely detection of these problems allows for earlier initiation of interventions aimed at enhancing the communication, social, and educational skills of these children. Controversy has recently centered around the value of selective versus universal audiologic screening during infancy. Only half the infants with significant hearing impairment are identified with the use of a selective screening strategy based on the presence or absence of risk factors for hearing impairment. However, both the limitations in screening technologies, which lead to inconsistencies in interpretation and high rates of false-positive results, and the logistical problems with availability and implementation raise concerns about the larger implications of a universal screening policy. In 1995, after reviewing these issues, the AAP affirmed the principle of universal hearing screening during infancy with the goal of identifying all infants with significant hearing impairment by 3 months of age so that intervention could be initiated by 6 months of age. Infants younger than 6 months of age have traditionally been screened with the use of brainstem response testing. A newer physiologic measure, otoacoustic emissions testing, holds promise as a simpler screening technique. However, problems with specificity (overreferral) and logistical issues with consistent use and interpretation have raised questions regarding the implementation of this method for universal screening. Children older than 6 months of age may be screened by using behavioral, auditory brainstem response, or otoacoustic emissions testing. Regardless of the technique used, screening programs must be able to detect a hearing loss of 30 dB or greater in the 500–4000 Hz region (speech frequencies), the level of deficit at which normal development of speech and language may begin to be impaired. If a hearing deficit is identified, the child should be referred in a timely manner for further evaluation and early intervention services.

Until optimal universal screening procedures and programs can be developed, the AAP recommends continuation of the selective screening strategy currently in place, which is based on the presence of specific hearing concerns and risk factors for sensorineural hearing loss. Risk factors for neonates (birth to 1 month) include family history of childhood hearing abnormalities; history of congenital infection; anatomic malformations of the head, neck, or ears; birth weight of less than 1500 g; a history of hyperbilirubinemia exceeding exchange levels; an APGAR score of 0–4 at 1 minute or 0–6 at 5 minutes; history of bacterial meningitis; significant exposure to ototoxic medications; prolonged mechanical ventilation; and presence of a syndrome or its stigmata associated with sensorineural hearing loss. Infants with one or more of these factors should receive audiologic screening by 3 months of age with the use of brainstem response testing. Risk factors warranting screening in older infants and children (1 month to 2 years) include parental concerns regarding hearing and language or developmental delay; history of bacterial meningitis or other infection known to be associated with hearing loss (eg, mumps, measles); history of significant head trauma, especially involving loss of conscientiousness or skull fracture; presence of a syndrome associated with sensorineural hearing loss; significant exposure to ototoxic medications; and presence of chronic middle-ear effusions (lasting at least 3 months). Periodic screening or rescreening of children aged 1 month to 3 years is recommended for individuals with a history of risk factors associated with delayed-onset and progressive sensorineural or conductive hearing loss. Such factors include family history of childhood hearing loss, history of congenital infection, neurofibromatosis type II, neurodegenerative disorders, anatomic abnormalities of the head and neck associated with eustachian tube dysfunction, and recurrent or chronic otitis media with effusion.

Because a variety of transient conditions, such as middle-ear effusion, as well as testing problems, can affect the hearing evaluation of older otherwise healthy children, the results of audiologic screening must be interpreted within the context of the child's history of ear disease and the results of physical examination.

Blood Pressure

Routine blood pressure screening during the well-child visit allows identification and potential treatment of children with persistently elevated blood pressure who are at increased risk for hypertension and its subsequent complications as adults. In a minority of patients, an underlying medical etiology may be found. Screening also provides an opportunity to evaluate and potentially modify additional cardiovascular risk factors and to provide education regarding prudent dietary and life-style choices.

In 1987, the Task Force on Blood Pressure Control in Children issued updated guidelines for pediatric blood pressure screening, evaluation, and treatment. In addition, age- and gender-specific standards, which acknowledge the independent influence of body size (as reflected by height) on normal blood pressure, have been recently published. Routine blood pressure screening is recommended for all otherwise healthy children aged 3 years and older at least once a year. Blood pressure measurements should also be taken in ill and potentially symptomatic children as well as in children younger than 3 years who are believed to be at increased risk for hypertension due to coexisting medical conditions.

In the child, blood pressure should be measured in the sitting position with the arm held at heart level. The bladder of the blood pressure cuff must completely encircle the circumference of the arm with or without overlap and be wide enough to cover 75% of the upper arm, from the top of the shoulder to the olecranon, to avoid an artificially elevated reading. The cuff is inflated to approximately 20 mm Hg above the point at which the radial pulse disappears and deflated 2–3 mm Hg/s while listening over the brachial artery. The level at which the first tapping sound is heard (Korotkoff sound 1 or K1) is recorded as the systolic blood pressure. In adults and children older than 12 years, the level at which all sounds disappear (K5) represents the diastolic pressure. Depending on the normative standards being used, the diastolic blood pressure in children younger than 13 years of age may be represented by either K5 or K4 (the point at which the sound becomes muffled and low-pitched). Care must be taken to use the Korotkoff sound appropriate to the standards in use. Normal blood pressure is defined as systolic and diastolic readings less than the 90th percentile for age and sex. High-normal and high blood pressure are defined, respectively, as readings between the 90th and 95th percentile and greater than or equal to the 95th percentile for age and sex, found on at least three separate occasions. Children with persistently elevated blood pressure readings (> 90th percentile) warrant a thorough history and physical examination to identify underlying causal factors, end-organ damage, and concomitant cardiovascular risk factors, as well as a long-term surveillance and treatment plan.

Cholesterol & Lipids

Epidemiologic data support the hypothesis that atherosclerosis and coronary heart disease have their precursors in childhood and that identifiable risk factors, such as hypertension, obesity, and hypercholesterolemia, are associated with an increased incidence of atherosclerotic disease. Serum cholesterol as well as other cardiovascular risk factors can be significantly influenced by dietary and life-style choices. Although long-term pediatric data are lacking regarding the risks and benefits of following prudent life-style recommendations during childhood, until more definitive information is available, it seems reasonable that pediatricians should provide preventive counseling to all their patients and families in these areas.

Controversy has centered around the value of selective versus universal cholesterol and lipid screening strategies for children as a part of routine pediatric health supervision. The AAP, the American Heart Association, and the recent National Cholesterol Education Program (NCEP) report endorse a selective screening strategy for children based on the presence of a high-risk family history and, when this is unknown, the presence of additional risk factors for atherosclerotic disease. Given the current paucity of information regarding the risks and benefits of treatment for hyperlipidemia in childhood, the costs and limitations of available screening tests, and the potential benefit of promoting healthful life-style and dietary choices to all families, these groups do not support universal cholesterol screening for children. On the basis of the recent NCEP report, the AAP recommends that children older than 2 years whose parents or grandparents have a history of early atherosclerotic disease (eg, a myocardial infarction, positive coronary arteriogram, or cerebrovascular or peripheral vascular disease before age 55), should be screened with a fasting (12-hour) serum lipid profile (total cholesterol, high-density lipoprotein cholesterol, triglycerides, and low-density lipoprotein cholesterol). In children whose parents have a significantly elevated blood cholesterol level (≥ 240), a nonfasting total serum cholesterol level should be obtained followed by the fasting lipid panel if this is significantly elevated. When family history is unclear or unknown, screening with a nonfasting total serum cholesterol may also be appropriate if a child presents with additional cardiovascular risk factors, such as obesity, smoking, hypertension, physical inactivity, or diabetes. The paradigm recommended by the AAP for selective screening and subsequent follow-up of children with elevated cholesterol levels is given in Figures 1–3 and 1–4.

Iron Deficiency Anemia

The recent decline in the prevalence of iron deficiency anemia in the United States has caused a reevaluation of the standard policy of obtaining screening hematocrits or hemoglobins for all children at ages 9–15 months and 4–6 years and during adolescence. Current thinking favors a

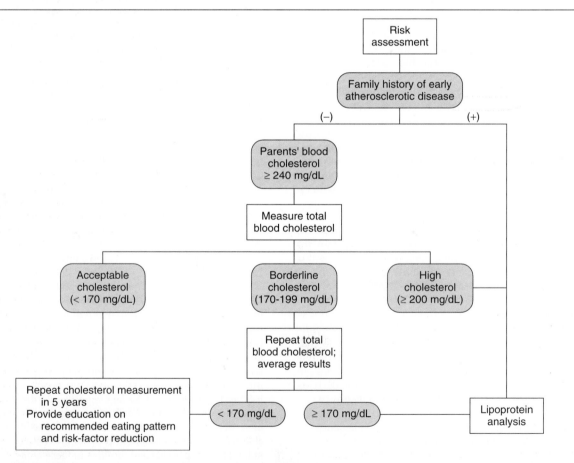

Figure 1–3. Risk assessment for elevated cholesterol and low-density lipoprotein cholesterol. (Reproduced, with permission, from National Cholesterol Education Program. Report of the Expert Panel on Blood Cholesterol Levels in Children and Adolescents. Pediatrics 1992;89[Suppl, part 2]:548.)

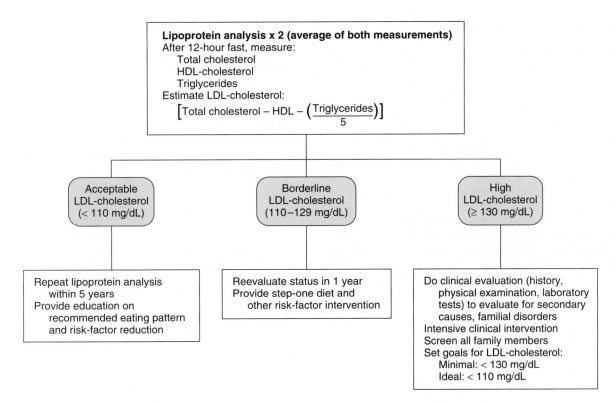

Figure 1–4. Classification, education, and follow-up based on low-density lipoprotein (LDL) cholesterol. HDL = high-density lipoprotein. (Reproduced, with permission, from National Cholesterol Education Program. Report of the Expert Panel on Blood Cholesterol Levels in Children and Adolescents. Pediatrics 1992;89[Suppl, part 2]:549.)

selective screening approach including infants (at 9–15 months) and adolescents (at health supervision visits) who belong to groups at increased risk for iron deficiency, as well as any children in whom anemia is suspected by history or examination. Risk factors for iron deficiency during infancy include prematurity, low birth weight, introduction of cow's milk before age 12 months, insufficient dietary iron intake, and low socioeconomic status. At increased risk for iron deficiency are menstruating female adolescents and both male and female athletes. Because of the frequent occurrence of mild transient anemia with acute illness, hemoglobin screening should not be done while a child is ill or within several weeks of a fever or infection. Hemoglobin measurements obtained by venipuncture are more accurate and reproducible than capillary hematocrits obtained by skin puncture. Abnormally low values are defined as being more than 2 SD below the mean for children of similar age and sex.

Lead Screening

The United States has made significant progress toward eliminating ongoing sources of environmental lead contamination. However, lead poisoning remains a significant health problem for children in this country. Although the use of lead-containing paint was effectively banned in the 1970s, ingestion of lead-containing paint chips and dust created by the deterioration or renovation of older homes remains the primary source of lead contamination in children. Considerable attention has recently been focused on this issue because of a growing body of evidence that suggests an association between subtle neurobehavioral effects and blood lead levels previously believed to be innocuous. Although controversial, these studies, in combination with initial national data demonstrating a significant prevalence of low but potentially clinically significant lead levels among children in the United States, prompted the Centers for Disease Control and Prevention (CDC) in 1991 to recommend universal blood lead screening for all children aged 6–72 months and to lower the intervention threshold to levels greater than 10 μg/dL. These CDC recommendations have provoked ongoing debate regarding the risks and benefits of universal versus selective lead screening because of the following concerns: the significance of low-level lead exposure, the value of intervention at these levels, the limitations of current testing technologies, and the availability of resources for subsequent follow-up, treatment, and lead abatement. On the basis of more recent national prevalence data regarding lead exposure in each area, the CDC is currently in the process of revising their recommendations and likely will endorse a regional policy of selective or universal screening that takes into account these findings. Such recommendations would be issued and monitored at the state and local levels.

Until such changes are made, however, the current CDC recommendations for the timing and frequency of routine screening, as well as subsequent interventions, depend on both the presence or absence of identified risk factors for lead exposure (Table 1–23) and the blood levels obtained (Table 1–24). Risk factors identified by the CDC include children aged 6–72 months who (1) live in housing built before 1960 that is either deteriorating or undergoing renovation; (2) have siblings, housemates, or playmates with known lead poisoning; (3) have family members who participate in a lead-related occupation or hobby; or (4) live near active lead smelters, battery recycling plants, or other industries that release atmospheric lead. If one uses the 1991 CDC paradigm, otherwise asymptomatic children at low risk for lead exposure (as defined by the absence of any of the above risk factors) should be routinely screened at 12 and 24 months of age. Asymptomatic children who have at least one identified risk factor should be screened initially at 6 months and again at 12 months. If the levels at both screenings are normal, the testing frequency is decreased to once a year. Because of an increased potential for contamination from environmental sources, venous blood specimens are preferred over capillary (finger-stick) samples. Elevated values obtained from capillary specimens should be confirmed with the use of venous blood testing. Regardless of age or risk factors, children who exhibit pica or excessive hand-to-mouth activity or have unexplained seizures or neurologic symptoms consistent with lead poisoning should also have their blood lead level tested.

Urinalyses & Urine Cultures

In the absence of clinical concerns or risk factors, routine surveillance urinalyses and urine cultures are not cost-effective. The relatively frequent occurrence of minor abnormalities, such as microscopic proteinuria, is of questionable significance yet, along with contaminated culture specimens, necessitate costly and inconvenient repeated urine studies. Routine screening rarely leads to the detection of significant asymptomatic renal disease, and, when it does, one must ask whether early detection results in benefit to the patient over diagnosis with the onset of symptoms. Urine studies should be obtained when disease is suspected or when the child is at increased risk for specific renal problems.

Tuberculosis

Yearly tuberculin testing is no longer recommended for all children. Although the number of cases of tuberculosis in the United States has increased in recent years, these cases continue to occur primarily within the previously identified high-risk groups. In populations with a low prevalence of tuberculosis, most reactive tests reflect false-positive results, often due to cross-reactivity with nontubercular mycobacterium leading to unnecessary treatment with isoniazid. The AAP, the American Thoracic Society, and the CDC currently endorse a selective screening strategy based on the presence of risk factors and residence in a community with a high prevalence of tuberculosis (Table 1–25). Routine tuberculin testing is no longer recommended for low-risk, asymptomatic children who live in areas of low disease prevalence. Children with one or more risk factors should be screened on a regular basis; the frequency is determined by the degree of risk present. Children who do not have risk factors but reside in high-prevalence communities and those whose history regarding risk status is unknown or incomplete may be screened on a periodic basis at 4–6 and 11–16 years of age. In all screening situations, intradermal Mantoux testing should replace multipuncture testing, and the results should be read by qualified medical personnel. Prior bacillus Calmette-Guérin vaccination is not a contraindication to placement of a purified protein derivative (PPD). Individuals who have received this vaccine can still acquire tuberculosis. Although some previously vaccinated individuals have a positive tuberculin skin test result, there is no reliable way to differentiate this reaction from that resulting from a natural infection with *Mycobacterium tuberculosis*; recommendations regarding screening, test interpretation, and subsequent evaluation and treatment remain the same.

Tuberculin testing relies on the presence of skin hypersensitivity to indicate subclinical or clinical infection. Reactivity usually develops within 2–12 weeks of infection. Two forms of tuberculin are currently available: Old Tuberculin, used in the Tine and Mono-Vacc tests, and the less expensive and more commonly used PPD. Multiple puncture tests, such as the Tine and Mono-Vacc, have the advantage of easy administration but lack consistency in the amount of tuberculin to be delivered. Reactions cannot be quantified accurately, and the numbers of false-positive and false-negative results are significant. All positive multiple puncture test results must be confirmed by subsequent Mantoux testing. However, some individuals may experience a booster effect when retesting occurs within 10 days to 12 months of the previous tuberculin exposure, thereby falsely enhancing the degree of reactivity. Be-

Table 1–23. Priority groups for lead screening based on risk factors for exposure in children aged 6–72 months.[1]

Those who live in or are frequent visitors to deteriorated housing built before 1960.
Those who live in housing built before 1960 with recent, ongoing, or planned renovation or remodeling.
Those who are siblings, housemates, or playmates of children with known lead poisoning.
Those whose parents or other household members participate in a lead-related occupation or hobby.
Those who live near active lead smelters, battery recycling plants, or other industries likely to result in atmospheric lead release.

[1]Reproduced, with permission, from: 1991 Centers for Disease Control Lead Poisoning Guidelines.

Table 1–24. Centers for Disease Control and Prevention recommendations for lead screening.[1]

Low Risk for Lead Exposure[2] Initial Screen at 12 Months			
< 10 µg/dL	10–14 µg/dL	15–19 µg/dL	> 20 µg/dL
Rescreen at 24 mo	Rescreen every 3–4 mo If two consecutive levels < 10 µg/dL or three < 15 µg/dL, rescreen in 1 y	Rescreen every 3–4 mo Education/nutritional counseling Environmental survey and abatement if two consecutive levels in same range	Repeat for confirmation Medical evaluation, treatment, and follow-up dependent on level
High Risk for Lead Exposure[2] Initial Screen at 6 Months			
< 10 µg/dL	10–14 µg/dL	15–19 µg/dL	> 20 µg/dL
Rescreen every 6 mo If two consecutive levels < 10 µg/dL or three < 15 µg/dL, rescreen once a year	Rescreen every 3–4 mo If two consecutive levels < 10 µg/dL or three < 15 µg/dL, rescreen once a year	Rescreen every 3–4 mo Education/nutritional counseling Environmental survey and abatement if two consecutive levels in same range	Repeat for confirmation Medical evaluation, prescription, and follow-up dependent on level

[1]Reproduced, with permission, from: 1991 CDC Lead Poisoning Guidelines.
[2]Based on presence of identified risk factors—see Table 1–23.

cause of these problems, the intracutaneous test (Mantoux) should be used preferentially in tuberculosis screening, when the disease is clinically suspected, and in the evaluation of persons known to have been exposed to tuberculosis. In the Mantoux test, a standardized dose of tuberculin (5 tuberculin units in 0.1 mL solution) is delivered intradermally using a 26-gauge needle and has the advantage of allowing quantification of the subsequent response. The Mantoux test should be read at 48–72 hours by tactile measurement of the margins of induration. Erythema alone does not signify a positive reaction. Test interpretation is based on the size of induration, reason for testing, and the presence or absence of other risk factors. Guidelines for interpreting test findings have been defined by the AAP, the American Thoracic Society, and the CDC (Table 1–26). This classification presumes the physician's knowledge of the child's and family's risk factors, as well as the background prevalence of tuberculosis in the community. It should be remembered that skin testing results may be negative early in the course of the disease or in the presence of anergy. A positive Mantoux test result necessitates obtaining a posteroanterior and lateral chest radiograph and investigating contacts for disease. Decisions regarding the need for prophylactic or therapeutic treatment are based on the subsequent evaluation.

IMMUNIZATIONS

Routine immunization has dramatically decreased the morbidity and mortality from a variety of infectious diseases and has become an important aspect of preventive well-child care. While the value of such programs is well established, the field is dynamic and rapidly changing. Currently, children are routinely immunized against 10 infectious diseases (Table 1–27). All are examples of active immunization, whereby live-attenuated or inactivated organisms, their components, or their products are administered to the recipient in order to stimulate a protective immunologic response. The Committee on Infectious Diseases of the AAP (Red Book) and the Advisory Committee on Immunization Practices (ACIP) of the US Public Health Service (MMWR) both regularly publish updated recommendations, which differ only in minor ways, regarding the administration and schedule of routine immunizations. These guidelines offer a current standard of care, which is subject to change as our knowledge continues to evolve (Table 1–28).

To maximize efficacy and minimize toxicity, recommendations regarding schedule, dose, route, and site of administration should be followed for each immunization. Subcutaneous and intramuscular injections are usually given in the anterolateral upper thigh in infants and, when muscle mass is sufficient, in the deltoid area in children and adults. The buttock should be avoided as a site of injection because of the potential for sciatic nerve damage and inconsistent intramuscular deposition. For intramuscular injections in infants and children, a 20- or 22-gauge ⅝–1¼-inch needle is used, whereas in adults, the standard needle length is 1½-inch. Subcutaneous injections are administered using a 25-gauge ⅝–¾-inch needle for all ages. To avoid accidental intravascular injection, it is important to pull the syringe plunger back and observe for blood return before injecting any substance.

The value of and need for a given vaccine depend on the prevalence and severity of the disease targeted, its ability to prevent or ameliorate this disease, and the inci-

Table 1–25. Revised tuberculin skin test recommendations.[1,2]

Children for whom immediate skin testing is indicated
Contacts of persons with confirmed or suspected infectious tuberculosis (contact investigation); this includes children identified as contacts of family members or associates in jail or prison in the last 5 y
Children with radiographic or clinical findings suggesting tuberculosis
Children immigrating from endemic countries (eg, Asia, Middle East, Africa, Latin America)
Children with travel histories to endemic countries and/or significant contact with indigenous persons from such countries

Children who should be tested annually for tuberculosis[3]
Children infected with HIV
Incarcerated adolescents

Children who should be tested every 2–3 y[3]
Children exposed to the following individuals: HIV infected or homeless individuals, residents of nursing homes, institutionalized adolescents or adults, users of illicit drugs, incarcerated adolescents or adults and migrant farm workers; this would include foster children with exposure to adults in the above high-risk groups

Children who should be considered for tuberculin skin testing at ages 4–6 and 11–16 y
Children whose parents immigrated (with unknown tuberculin skin test status) from regions of the world with high prevalence of tuberculosis; continued potential exposure by travel to the endemic areas and/or household contact with persons from the endemic areas (with unknown tuberculin skin test status) should be an indication for repeat tuberculin skin testing
Children without specific risk factors who reside in high-prevalence areas; in general, a high-risk neighborhood or community does not mean an entire city is at high risk; it is recognized that rates in any area of the city may vary by neighborhood, or even from block to block; physicians should be aware of these patterns in determining the likelihood of exposure; public health officials or local tuberculosis experts should help clinicians identify areas that have appreciable tuberculosis rates

Risk for progression to disease
Children with other medical risk factors, including diabetes mellitus, chronic renal failure, malnutrition, and congenital or acquired immunodeficiencies deserve special consideration; without recent exposure, these persons are not at increased risk of acquiring tuberculous infection; underlying immune deficiencies associated with these conditions theoretically would enhance the possibility for progression to severe disease; initial histories of potential exposure to tuberculosis should be included on all of these patients; if these histories or local epidemiologic factors suggest a possibility of exposure, immediate and periodic tuberculin skin testing should be considered in these patients; an initial Mantoux tuberculin skin test should be performed before initiation of immunosuppressive therapy in any child with an underlying condition that necessitates immunosuppressive therapy.

[1]Reproduced, with permission, from: Committee on Infectious Diseases, American Academy of Pediatrics: Update on tuberculosis skin testing of children. Pediatrics 1996;97:282.
[2]Bacillus Calmette-Guérin immunization is not a contraindication to tuberculin skin testing.
[3]Initial tuberculin skin testing initiated at the time of diagnosis or circumstance.

Table 1–26. Definition of a positive Mantoux skin test result (five tuberculin units of purified protein derivative) in children.[1,2]

Reaction ≥ 5 mm
Children in close contact with known or suspected infectious cases of tuberculosis
Households with active or previously active cases if treatment cannot be verified as adequate before exposure, treatment was initiated after the child's contact, or reactivation is suspected
Children suspected to have tuberculous disease
Chest roentgenogram consistent with active or previously active tuberculosis
Clinical evidence of tuberculosis[3]
Children receiving immunosuppressive therapy[4] or with immunosuppressive conditions, including HIV infection

Reaction ≥ 10 mm
Children at increased risk of dissemination
Young age (< 4 y)
Other medical risk factors, including diabetes mellitus, chronic renal failure, or malnutrition
Children with increased environmental exposure
Born, or whose parents were born, in high-prevalence regions of the world
Frequently exposed to adults who are HIV infected, homeless, users of illicit drugs, medically indigent city dwellers, residents of nursing homes, incarcerated or institutionalized persons, and migrant farm workers
Travel and exposure to high-prevalence regions of the world

Reaction ≥ 15 mm
Children ≥ 4 y of age without any risk factors

[1]Reproduced, with permission, from: Committee on Infectious Diseases, American Academy of Pediatrics: Update on tuberculosis skin testing of children. Pediatrics 1996;97:282.
[2]The recommendations should be considered regardless of previous Bacillus Calmette-Guérin administration.
[3]Evidence on physical examination or laboratory assessment that would include tuberculosis in the working diagnosis (ie, meningitis).
[4]Including immunosuppressive doses of corticosteroids.

dence and severity of vaccine-related morbidity. With the dramatic decrease in morbidity and mortality brought about by our current immunization practices, attention has focused increasingly on the potential adverse effects of the vaccines themselves.

In addition to the active-immunizing antigen(s), vaccines contain a variety of other materials, including suspending fluids such as saline or complex tissue culture, preservatives, stabilizers, antibiotics to prevent bacterial overgrowth, and adjuvants to enhance immunogenicity. All of these components may contribute to local and systemic side effects attributed to the vaccine. Although rare, anaphylactic allergic reactions are most frequently due to egg antigens in the suspending fluid of vaccines prepared in embryonated egg or chick embryo tissue culture (influenza, yellow fever, measles, mumps) and to antibiotics used to prevent bacterial overgrowth (neomycin in measles, mumps, rubella [MMR] vaccine, varicella vaccine, and oral poliovirus vaccine [OPV] and streptomycin in OPV and inactivated poliovirus vaccine [IPV]). Indi-

Table 1–27. Routine childhood vaccines: route and dose.[1]

Vaccine	Type	Route	Dose
DTP/DT/Td 　D = diphtheria 　d = reduced amount toxoid 　T = tetanus 　P = whole cell pertussis 　aP = acellular pertussis	Toxoids (D&T) Inactivated bacteria (P) Bacterial components (aP)	Intramuscular	0.5 mL
Hib 　*Haemophilus influenzae* b 　　conjugate vaccine	Bacterial polysaccharide 　conjugated to protein	Intramuscular	0.5 mL
Poliovirus vaccines 　OPV = oral 　e-IPV = inactivated	Live viruses of all three 　serotypes Inactivated viruses of all 　three serotypes	Oral Subcutaneous	Unit dose 0.5 mL
MMR 　M = measles 　M = mumps 　R = rubella	Live viruses	Subcutaneous	0.5 mL
Hep B 　Hepatitis B vaccine	Plasmid-derived viral 　antigen	Intramuscular	Varies with 　preparation and 　child's age
Var 　Varicella zoster virus vaccine	Live virus	Subcutaneous	0.5 mL

[1]Modified and reproduced, with permission, from Rudolph AM (editor): *Rudolph's Pediatrics,* 20th ed. Appleton & Lange, 1996, p. 30.

viduals with a history suggestive of an anaphylactic reaction to egg or the above antibiotics should undergo skin testing to determine the safety of subsequent immunization with these vaccines.

Many side effects, such as local tenderness, low-grade fever, and allergic reactions, can be attributed directly to the vaccine owing to their temporal relationship, frequency, and unique presentations. These adverse reactions, whether common or rare, are predictable and unavoidable. The relationship between vaccination and other uncommon but naturally occurring events, such as seizures, mental retardation, and encephalopathy, is much less well established. Such outcomes, if sometimes vaccine-related, occur against a background of indistinguishable idiopathic events, making differentiation between a temporal and a causal relationship difficult. Issues pertaining to specific immunizations are addressed below. Current standards regarding valid and nonvalid contraindications to specific vaccines are given in Table 1–29.

In recognition that some persons may be adversely affected by their participation in mass immunization programs and in order to provide some stability to vaccine supply and cost in the face of escalating liability litigation, Congress passed the National Childhood Vaccine Injury Compensation Act in 1986. This act, which was amended in 1987 and became effective in 1988, establishes an optional no-fault system of compensation with mandatory initial approach for a predefined list of possible vaccine-related reactions. The act also requires that all physicians and health care workers who administer vaccines comply with new guidelines regarding record keeping, centralized reporting of potential vaccine reactions, and distribution of standardized pamphlets describing risk-benefit information to vaccine recipients and their parents. The Red Book should be consulted for more detailed information.

SPECIFIC VACCINES

Diphtheria, Tetanus, Pertussis & Diphtheria, Tetanus, Acellular Pertussis

The diphtheria, tetanus, pertussis (DTP) vaccine is composed of diphtheria toxoid, tetanus toxoid, and inactivated whole *Bordetella pertussis* cells. Since 1991, a preparation substituting acellular for whole-cell pertussis vaccine (DTaP) has also been available for booster use in children aged 15 months to 7 years. Licensure of this product for primary vaccination of young infants is expected in the near future. Single-antigen products, combinations of diphtheria and tetanus toxoids, and, since 1993, a combined DTP/*Haemophilus influenzae* type b conjugate vaccine, are also available. Adults and children older than 7 years are not given pertussis vaccine as potential morbidity from wild-type disease is greatly diminished by this age. Because of enhanced local reactivity, these individuals receive a booster vaccine containing 1/10 the concentration of diphtheria toxoid (dT) given to younger

Table 1–28. Recommended childhood immunization schedule: United States, January–June 1996.[1]

Vaccine	Age										
	Birth	1 mo	2 mo	4 mo	6 mo	12 mo	15 mo	18 mo	4–6 y	11–12 y	14–16 y
Hepatitis B[2,3]	Hep B-1										
			Hep B-2			Hep B-3				Hep B[3]	
Diphtheria, tetanus, pertussis[4]			DTP or DTaP	DTP or DTaP	DTP or DTaP	DTP[4] (DTaP at ≥ 15 + mo)			DTP or DTaP	Td	
Haemophilus influenzae type b[5]			Hib	Hib	Hib[5]	Hib[5]					
Polio[6]			OPV[6]	OPV	OPV				OPV		
Measles, mumps, rubella (MMR)[7]						MMR			MMR[7] or MMR[7]		
Varicella zoster virus vaccine[8]						Var				Var[8]	

[1]Approved by the Advisory Committee on Immunization Practices (ACIP), the American Academy of Pediatrics (AAP), and the American Academy of Family Physicians (AAFP). Vaccines are listed under the routinely recommended ages. Bars = range of acceptable ages for vaccination. Shaded bars = catch-up vaccination: at 11–12 years of age, hepatitis B vaccine should be administered to children not previously vaccinated, and varicella zoster virus vaccine should be administered to children not previously vaccinated who lack a reliable history of chickenpox.

[2]Infants born to HBsAg-negative mothers should receive 2.5 μg of Merck vaccine (Recombivax HB) or 10 μg of SmithKline Beecham (SB) vaccine (Engerix-B). The second dose should be administered ≥ 1 month after the first dose. Infants born to HBsAg-positive mothers should receive 0.5 mL hepatitis B immune globulin (HBIG) within 12 hours of birth and either 5 μg of Merck vaccine (Recombivax HB) or 10 μg of SB vaccine (Engerix-B) at a separate site. The second dose is recommended at 1–2 months of age and the third dose at 6 months of age. Infants born to mothers whose HBsAg status is unknown should receive either 5 μg of Merck vaccine (Recombivax HB) or 10 μg of SB vaccine (Engerix-B) within 12 hours of birth. The second dose of vaccine is recommended at 1 month of age and the third dose at 6 months of age.

[3]Adolescents who have not previously received three doses of hepatitis B vaccine should initiate or complete the series at the 11–12-year-old visit. The second dose should be administered at least 1 month after the first dose, and the third dose should be administered at least 4 months after the first dose and at least 2 months after the second dose.

[4]DTP4 may be administered at 12 months of age, if at least 6 months have elapsed since DTP3. DTaP (diphtheria and tetanus toxoids and acellular pertussis vaccine) is licensed for the fourth and/or fifth vaccine dose(s) for children aged ≥ 15 months and may be preferred for these doses in this age group. Td (tetanus and diphtheria toxoids, adsorbed, for adult use) is recommended at 11–12 years of age if at least 5 years have elapsed since the last dose of DTP, DTaP, or DT.

[5]Three H influenzae type b (Hib) conjugate vaccines are licensed for infant use. If PRP-OMP (PedvaxHIB [Merck]) is administered at 2 and 4 months of age, a dose at 6 months is not required. After completing the primary series, any Hib conjugate vaccine may be used as a booster.

[6]Oral poliovirus vaccine (OPV) is recommended for routine infant vaccination. Inactivated poliovirus vaccine (IPV) is recommended for persons with a congenital or acquired immune deficiency disease or an altered immune status as a result of disease or immunosuppressive therapy, as well as their household contacts, and is an acceptable alternative for other persons. The primary three-dose series for IPV should be given with a minimum interval of 4 weeks between the first and second doses and 6 months between the second and third doses.

[7]The second dose of MMR is routinely recommended at 4–6 years of age or at 11–12 years of age, but may be administered at any visit, provided at least 1 month has elapsed since receipt of the first dose.

[8]Varicella zoster virus vaccine (Var) can be administered to susceptible children any time after 12 months of age. Unvaccinated children who lack a reliable history of chickenpox should be vaccinated at the 11–12-year-old visit.

children. At all ages, a dose of 0.5 mL is delivered intramuscularly using needle sizes and sites as described above. The recommended DTP, DTaP, and dT immunization schedule for children vaccinated at standard ages is given in Table 1–28. Studies of the immunologic response to DTP vaccination and side effects in premature infants support the approach of ignoring gestational age and beginning immunization at the usual chronologic age. The DTP or DTaP vaccine can be given concurrently (different sites) with the MMR vaccine, H influenzae type b conjugate vaccine (HbCV), hepatitis B vaccine, IPV, and

OPV without diminishing antibody responses. Concurrent administration with varicella vaccine is also believed to be effective, although data are currently limited.

Common side effects of the DTP vaccine, which are attributed primarily to the whole-cell pertussis component, include local redness, swelling, pain at the site of injection, and systemic reactions such as low to moderate fever, fretfulness, drowsiness, vomiting, and anorexia. The incidence of local reactions and fever appear to increase with the number of doses given, whereas the likelihood of other minor systemic reactions decreases.

Table 1–29. Overview of valid and nonvalid contraindications to vaccination.[1,2]

True Contraindications and Precautions	Not True (Vaccines May Be Administered)
General for All Vaccines (DTP/DTaP, OPV, IPV, MMR, Hib, HBV)	
Contraindications Anaphylactic reaction to a vaccine contraindicates further doses of that vaccine Anaphylactic reaction to a vaccine constituent contraindicates the use of vaccines containing that substance Moderate or severe illnesses with or without a fever	Mild to moderate local reaction (soreness, redness, swelling) after a dose of an injectable antigen Mild acute illness with or without low-grade fever Current antimicrobial therapy Convalescent phase of illnesses Prematurity (same dosage and indications as for normal, full-term infants) Recent exposure to an infectious disease History of penicillin or other nonspecific allergies or family history of such
DTP/DTaP	
Contraindication Encephalopathy within 7 days of administration of previous dose of DTP **Precautions[3]** Temperature of $\geq 40.5\,°C$ (105 °F) within 48 h after vaccination with a prior dose of DTP Collapse or shocklike state (hypotonic-hyporesponsive episode) within 48 h of receiving a prior dose of DTP Seizures within 3 days of receiving a prior dose of DTP[4] Persistent, inconsolable crying lasting ≥ 3 h within 48 h of receiving a prior dose of DTP	Temperature of $< 40.5\,°C$ (105 °F) after a previous dose of DTP Family history of convulsions[4] Family history of sudden infant death syndrome Family history of an adverse event after DTP administration
OPV[5]	
Contraindications Infection with HIV or a household contact with HIV Known altered immunodeficiency (hematologic and solid tumors; congenital immunodeficiency; and long-term immunosuppressive therapy) Immunodeficient household contact **Precaution[3]** Pregnancy	Breast-feeding Current antimicrobial therapy Diarrhea
IPV	
Contraindication Anaphylactic reaction to neomycin or streptomycin **Precaution[3]** Pregnancy	
MMR[5]	
Contraindications Anaphylactic reactions to egg ingestion and to neomycin[6] Pregnancy Known altered immunodeficiency (hematologic and solid tumors; congenital immunodeficiency; and long-term immunosuppressive therapy) *Except kids w/HIV, They SHOULD receive MMR* **Precaution[3]** Recent (within 3 mo) immune globulin administration	Tuberculosis or positive skin test Simultaneous tuberculin skin testing[7] Breast-feeding Pregnancy of mother of recipient Immunodeficient family member or household contact Infection with HIV Nonanaphylactic reactions to eggs or neomycin
Hib	
None identified	
HBV	
None identified	Pregnancy

(*continued*)

Table 1–29 (cont'd). Overview of valid and nonvalid contraindications to vaccination.[1,2]

True Contraindications and Precautions	Not True (Vaccines May Be Administered)
Var	
Contraindications	
Known immunodeficiency and long-term immunosuppressive therapy	Pregnant family member or household contact
	Immunodeficient family member or household contact
Pregnancy	Nonanaphylactic reaction to neomycin
Anaphylactic reaction to neomycin	
Precautions	Breast-feeding
Recent administration of immune globulin	
Children receiving long-term salicylate therapy	

[1]Reproduced, with permission, from: National Vaccine Advisory Committee: Standards for pediatric immunization practices. MMWR 42, 1993;RR-5:1.

[2]This information is based on the recommendations of the Advisory Committee on Immunization Practices (ACIP) and those of the Committee on Infectious Diseases (Red Book Committee) of the American Academy of Pediatrics (AAP) as of October 1992. Varicella vaccine information from the Committee on Infectious Diseases Statement, AAP: Pediatrics 1995;95:791. Sometimes these recommendations vary from those contained in the manufacturer's package inserts. For more detailed information, providers should consult the published recommendations of the ACIP, AAP, American Association of Family Practice Physicians, and the manufacturer's package inserts.

[3]The events or conditions listed as precautions, although not contraindications, should be carefully reviewed. The benefits and risks of administering a specific vaccine to an individual under the circumstances should be considered. If the risks are believed to outweigh the benefits, the vaccination should be withheld; if the benefits are believed to outweigh the risks (eg, during an outbreak or foreign travel), the vaccination should be administered. Whether and when to administer DTP to children with proven or suspected underlying neurologic disorders should be decided on an individual basis. It is prudent on theoretical grounds to avoid vaccinating pregnant women. However, if immediate protection against poliomyelitis is needed, OPV, not IPV, is recommended.

[4]For children with a personal or family (siblings or parents) history of convulsions, acetaminophen should be considered before DTP is administered and thereafter every 4 hours for 24 hours.

[5]There is a theoretical risk that the administration of multiple live-virus vaccines (OPV and MMR) within 30 days of one another if not administered on the same day will result in a suboptimal immune response. There are no data to substantiate this lack of response.

[6]Persons with a history of anaphylactic reactions after egg ingestion should be vaccinated only with extreme caution. Protocols that have been developed for vaccinating such persons should be consulted (J Pediatr 1983;102:196, J Pediatr 1988;113:504).

[7]Measles vaccination may temporarily suppress tuberculin reactivity. If testing cannot be done the day of MMR vaccination, the test should be postponed for 4–6 weeks. DTP = diphtheria-tetanus toxoid and pertussis vaccine; DTaP = diphtheria and tetanus toxoids and acellular pertussis vaccine; OPV = oral poliovirus vaccine; IPV = inactivated poliovirus vaccine; MMR = measles-mumps-rubella vaccine; Hib = *Haemophilus influenzae* type b vaccine; HBV = hepatitis B vaccine.

However, for any given child, the risk of a mild systemic reaction is greater with subsequent doses if it occurred with the first dose. Splitting or halving the dose in the hope of diminishing local reactions and fever is not recommended by either the AAP or the ACIP, as some evidence suggests that this practice may lead to inadequate protection, particularly against pertussis. Switching needles between drawing up and administering the vaccine is unnecessary as it does not appear to diminish the incidence of local reactions. Giving prophylactic acetaminophen (15 mg/kg) at the time of DTP administration and during the ensuing 24 hours at appropriate intervals has been shown to decrease the incidence and severity of local reactions and fever. Use of the acellular pertussis vaccine for booster doses results in significantly lower rates of minor local and systemic reactions, such as tenderness and fever, than the whole cell-containing product.

More serious but less frequent systemic events have also been reported in relation to the DTP vaccine, including persistent inconsolable crying for more than 3 hours, a high-pitched cephalic cry, temperature greater than 40.5 °C, hypotonic-hyporesponsive episodes, convulsions with or without fever, encephalopathy, and a variety of permanent neurologic deficits, including mental retardation and cerebral palsy. Considerable controversy has surrounded the relationship between pertussis vaccine and several serious neurologic conditions that, although indistinguishable from otherwise naturally occurring idiopathic events, have at times appeared temporally related. Several recent studies using sophisticated statistical and experimental techniques have found no evidence to support a causal relationship between pertussis vaccination and some alleged reactions (eg, sudden infant death syndrome) and, with respect to others, have suggested that vaccination may bring forward in time events otherwise destined to occur in a given individual (eg, seizures). While an increased incidence of seizures after DTP administration has been consistently observed, most are associated with fever and have the clinical characteristics of benign febrile seizures. There is no evidence that convulsions after DTP administration cause neurologic damage or epilepsy. As an outgrowth of the National Childhood Vaccine Injury Act, the National Academy of Science's Institute of Medicine recently undertook an extensive analysis of all existing scientific data pertaining to potential adverse effects of the pertussis vaccine. It found that evidence was consistent with a causal relationship between DTP vaccination and several rare events, including acute encephalopathy, hypotonic–hyporesponsive shock-like episodes, anaphylaxis, and prolonged inconsolable crying. It also found that children experiencing a severe acute neurologic illness (eg, encephalopathy) within 7 days after DTP vaccination were at increased risk for chronic neurologic dysfunction at levels similar to those in children experiencing acute neurologic illness unrelated in time to DTP vaccination. In these children, the committee believed that evidence was consistent with, but did not prove, a causal relationship between DTP vaccination and chronic neurologic dysfunction. The committee's conclusions have been used to modify our current guidelines regarding vaccine contraindications and conditions covered by the National Vaccine Injury Compensation Program. Current contraindications to vaccination with DTP/DTaP are given in Table 1–29. Although minor adverse effects occur less frequently with the acellular than with the whole-cell pertussis vaccine, data regarding the relative incidence of more serious reactions are limited, and contraindications are similar.

Poliovirus

Two forms of trivalent poliovirus vaccine are available for use—the enhanced-potency inactivated injectable (introduced at original potency by Salk in 1954) and Sabin's live-attenuated oral vaccine. In addition to the immunizing agents, the inactivated injectable vaccine also contains a small amount of neomycin and streptomycin to prevent bacterial outgrowth. The OPV is currently the vaccine of choice for routine immunization in the United States, although recent improvements in the immunogenicity of the injectable form (e-IPV), coupled with its inability to cause paralytic disease, have raised new questions regarding the continued advantage of this policy.

For a heterogeneous, mobile society, which receives many immigrants from polio endemic areas and in which universal health care cannot be assured, OPV offers several advantages. First, oral vaccination with attenuated-live virus is believed to induce lifelong immunity in much the same way as a natural infection, thus eliminating the need for periodic boosters. Second, because of the induction of local gut as well as systemic immunity, the transmission of wild-type virus in the population is interrupted. Third, because of fecal shedding of the vaccine viruses for several weeks after vaccination, indirect immunization or boosting of immunity in contacts is also achieved. The disadvantage to the use of OPV is its ability to induce paralytic disease in both recipients and their contacts. Only 10–15% of vaccine-induced paralytic disease is found in individuals with an underlying immunodeficiency. However, immunodeficient individuals are at increased risk of vaccine-induced disease; therefore, they and their family members should not be immunized with live-virus vaccine. Household contacts are at higher risk of disease than community contacts, and the risk for both recipients and contacts is highest after exposure to a first dose.

The inactivated injectable poliovirus vaccine offers the advantage of being unable to induce paralytic disease; however, at its original potency, it provides minimal gut immunity and requires booster doses every 4–5 years. The current enhanced-potency inactivated vaccine, while still providing minimal gut and therefore "herd" immunity, appears to induce significantly prolonged and possibly lifelong protection, thereby decreasing or perhaps eliminating the need for subsequent periodic boosters. This improvement has rekindled the debate regarding the optimal poliovirus vaccine for routine vaccination in this country. The use of a combination of e-IPV followed by OPV for the primary immunization series against polio is currently being considered.

The current recommended schedule of immunization with OPV is given in Table 1–28. Valid and nonvalid contraindications to vaccination are listed in Table 1–29. OPV can be administered on the same day as other live-virus vaccines. However, if not given on the same visit, live-virus vaccines should be spaced by 4 or more weeks owing to the potential for interference with immunologic response. In children, e-IPV is used primarily to vaccinate individuals who are immunodeficient or who live in households with an immunodeficient individual. The primary series for e-IPV consists of two doses (0.5 mL, subcutaneous) given 4–8 weeks apart starting at 2 months of age; a third dose is given 6–12 months later. A booster injection is administered at school entry (4–6 years of age). Additional periodic booster doses may be recommended as experience with the enhanced potency injectable vaccine is gained. Because of the relatively low incidence of wild-type poliovirus in this country and the increased risk of acquiring vaccine-induced disease among adults receiving the live-virus vaccine, previously unimmunized individuals older than 18 years are not routinely vaccinated. Because vaccine-induced poliovirus can occur among household contacts of oral vaccine recipients, controversy remains as to whether immunization of an infant with OPV should be delayed until unimmunized adults in the household have received a series of IPV.

Measles, Mumps, Rubella

The MMR vaccine combines three attenuated live viruses. Single-agent preparations are also available. Vaccine strains of measles and mumps are grown in chick-embryo tissue culture, whereas rubella is grown in human diploid-cell culture. All of these vaccines contain minute quantities of neomycin to prevent bacterial overgrowth. A 0.5-mL dose is administered subcutaneously using the needle size and sites described previously. The MMR vaccine can be administered concurrently (different sites) with HbCV, DTP vaccine, hepatitis B vaccine, varicella vaccine, and OPV without diminishing antibody response. However, it is recommended that live-virus vaccines, if not given on the same day, should be spaced 4 or more weeks apart. Measles vaccination may temporarily suppress tuberculin reactivity for 4–6 weeks after immunization but will not interfere with the accuracy of the test placed on the same day.

Recommendations regarding optimal timing and frequency of immunization against measles, mumps, and rubella (Table 1–28) reflect a balance between several factors, including the duration of maternal antibody protection, the seroresponse to vaccine at different ages, the rate of primary vaccine failure, the duration of immunity achieved without booster doses, and the overall level of vaccination achieved in the population. As a result of epidemic increases in the number of measles cases reported in the mid to late 1980s, significant changes recently have been made in our MMR immunization policy. Cases during these outbreaks were noted to have occurred in primarily three populations: unvaccinated preschool children younger than 15 months of age (the recommended age for vaccination at that time), unvaccinated preschool children who had not received the MMR vaccine at the recommended age, and previously vaccinated school-aged children. Cases occurring in children younger than 15 months of age were believed to result in part from an earlier decline in levels of maternal antibody among infants born to women who themselves had received measles vaccine rather than experienced a natural infection. A 2–10% primary vaccine failure rate was believed to be the primary cause of cases occurring in previously vaccinated school-aged children, although waning immunity was also a potentially important factor. Outbreaks among unvaccinated children who had not received the MMR vaccine at the recommended age represented a failure of the vaccine delivery system to maximize access, catchment, and public acceptance.

These changes in measles incidence and patterns of susceptibility prompted both the AAP and the ACIP of the US Public Health Service to recommend a two-dose MMR vaccination schedule, with the first dose to be given routinely at 12 months of age. Currently, the AAP suggests that the second (booster) dose be given at the time of entrance to middle or junior high school (ages 11–12 years), whereas the ACIP recommends giving this dose at the time of school entrance (ages 5–6 years).

A recent increase in the number of mumps cases among adolescents and young adults has also been observed and is believed to be due primarily to the existence of a relatively underimmunized cohort of children, born between 1967 and 1977 when mumps vaccine was available but not routinely recommended. Individuals who were not immunized with live mumps-virus vaccine on or after their first birthday, or who have not experienced a natural infection as diagnosed by a physician or documented by the presence of serum antibody, should be vaccinated against mumps. Most people born before 1957 are likely to have been infected naturally and generally can be considered immune even if they do not remember having had a symptomatic case. Unlike the characteristic presentation of mumps, a clinical diagnosis of rubella is notoriously unreliable. Individuals should not be considered immune to rubella unless they have been immunized with live-virus vaccine on or after their first birthday or have evidence of serum antibody present.

There is no evidence to suggest that it is harmful to immunize someone against mumps or rubella who has previously received vaccine or had a natural infection.

Contraindications to receiving the MMR vaccine are given in Table 1–29. A history of anaphylactic allergy to egg or neomycin warrants withholding this vaccine until skin testing can be obtained. Lesser degrees of allergy to antibiotics, chicken, or chicken feathers are not contraindications to vaccination.

In general, live-virus vaccines should not be given to individuals who are known to be or are suspected of being immunodeficient. An exception to this rule, however, is the recommendation that asymptomatic and probably symptomatic HIV-infected children should receive the MMR vaccine because of their significantly increased risk of morbidity and mortality if they acquire these wild-type infections.

Concerns about immunization during pregnancy apply to all live-virus vaccines, although the greatest concern has centered on rubella. The CDC reporting registry shows no evidence of defects consistent with wild-type congenital rubella syndrome among the live-born infants or aborted fetuses of women inadvertently vaccinated against rubella during or just before pregnancy. However, vaccine virus has been isolated from aborted products of conception, proving that the attenuated virus can cross the placenta. Although it is to be avoided, rubella vaccination just before or during pregnancy is not by itself a reason to interrupt pregnancy.

Side effects of measles vaccination include frequent local tenderness and swelling, fever appearing 5–7 days after immunization (5–15%), and a morbilliform rash after the same time course (5%). Recipients of the killed measles vaccine, available between 1963–1967, have a higher incidence of local reactions when revaccinated with the live-virus vaccine. However, because of a greater risk of having serious atypical measles if exposed to wild-type virus, these individuals should be revaccinated. Encephalitis and encephalopathy have occasionally been reported to follow measles and mumps vaccination, but at an incidence lower than the "background" frequency of encephalitis from unknown etiology, suggesting a temporal relationship only. Although subacute sclerosing panencephalitis, a late complication of wild-type measles infection, has been reported to occur after measles vaccination in the absence of a known natural infection, the incidence of this devastating disease has been dramatically reduced by mass immunization. Side effects of the mumps vaccine include local tenderness, low-grade fever, and, rarely, a mild orchitis or parotitis. In addition to local tenderness and a rubella-like syndrome consisting of rash, fever, and lymphadenopathy, rubella vaccination is associated with transient arthritis and arthralgias occurring 1–3 weeks after vaccination, most commonly among postpubertal women (10–15%). In a recent review of all scientific data pertaining to potential adverse effects of the rubella vaccine conducted by the National Academy of Science's Institute of Medicine, a possible causal relationship between this vaccine and chronic arthritis could not be ruled out. This review yielded insufficient evidence, however, to support a causal relationship between rubella vaccination and reports of subsequent neuropathies and thrombocytopenic purpura.

H influenzae Type b Conjugate Vaccine

Vaccines against invasive *H influenzae* type b infections have undergone a dramatic evolution since their initial licensure in 1985. Currently, three conjugate *H influenzae* type b vaccines are available for use. The *H influenzae* type b oral conjugate vaccine (HbOC) consists of purified type b capsular oligosaccharide linked to a nontoxic mutant diphtheria toxin protein. A vaccine combining HbOC with DTP has also been available since March 1993. The PRP-OMP consists of purified type b capsular polysaccharide complexed with membrane proteins of *Neisseria meningitidis.* Most recently, a tetanus toxoid conjugate vaccine (PRP-T) has become available for use. Conjugate vaccines offer a significant advantage over the original unconjugated vaccine in their ability to elicit a protective antibody response in young infants when the incidence of invasive *H influenzae* disease is greatest. As with the original vaccine licensed in 1985, the conjugate *H influenzae* vaccines do not protect against nontypable strains of *H influenzae,* which are responsible for many recurrent upper respiratory diseases, such as otitis media. Conjugate vaccine should also not be considered a protective immunizing agent against diphtheria, *N meningitidis,* or tetanus.

Current recommendations regarding the routine schedule of administration are given in Table 1–28. For children aged 2–6 months in whom vaccination is not initiated at the recommended age, a primary series of three HbOC or PRP-T (or two PRP-OMP) vaccines, each separated by at least 2 months, and a booster dose at 12–15 months of age, should be given. Unvaccinated children 7–11 months of age require two primary doses using any of the three preparations available, separated by at least 2 months, and a booster dose (at least 2 months from the last) at 12–18 months of age. Children aged 12–14 months should receive a total of two doses of vaccine (given 2 months apart). Unvaccinated children 15–60 months of age require only one dose using any of the conjugate vaccines available. Irrespective of age, children who are believed to be at increased risk for invasive *H influenzae* disease, such as individuals with functional or anatomic asplenia, should also receive conjugate vaccine. For all products, a dose of 0.5 mL is given intramuscularly using needle sizes and sites described previously. HbCV, OPV, DTP vaccine, DTaP vaccine, hepatitis B vaccine, and the MMR vaccine can be given simultaneously at different sites without diminishing immunologic response. Concurrent administration with varicella vaccine is also believed to be effective, although data are currently limited. Side effects attributed to the conjugate *H influenzae* vaccines are minimal and include primarily local tenderness and low-grade fever in a minority of recipients.

Hepatitis B Vaccine

Acute hepatitis B and its chronic sequelae are the cause of significant morbidity and mortality in this country. A plasma-derived hepatitis B vaccine, licensed in 1982, has since been replaced by two recombinant vaccines (Recombivax and Engerix B) that use synthetic hepatitis B surface antigen (HBsAg) produced in yeast by plasmid gene insertion. These vaccines are highly immunogenic, conferring protection against hepatitis B infections in greater than 90% of recipients, including infants. Failure of control strategies using selective immunization of high-risk groups and HBsAg screening of pregnant women has led both the AAP and ACIP to recommend universal hepatitis B immunization during infancy. Although many questions remain, such as the duration of immunity conferred and the optimal immunization schedule for infants, these groups believe that from both a risk-benefit and cost perspective, this approach is warranted. Current recommendations regarding the schedule, dose, and volume of vaccination vary with the preparation used, the age of the child being vaccinated, the mother's HBsAg serologic status, and the presence of relevant underlying disease (Table 1–30). The vaccine is administered intramuscularly and can be given simultaneously at different sites with the DTP vaccine, HbCV, OPV, IPV, varicella vaccine, and MMR vaccine. Both the AAP and ACIP advocate giving healthy infants born to HBsAg-negative mothers their first immunization before discharge from the nursery, the second when the child is 1–2 months old, and a third at 6–18 months (see Table 1–28). An acceptable alternative schedule for the first two doses would be to use the 2- and 4-month visits. Infants born to HBsAg-positive mothers should receive hepatitis B immune globulin (HBIG) and their first immunization at birth. For these infants, the second and third doses are currently recommended to be given at 1 and 6 months of age. Although routine testing for postimmunization antibody response is not recommended for all infants, babies born to HBsAg-positive women should be tested for HBsAg and anti-HBs at 9 months of age and revaccinated if measured antibody titers are below 10 mIU/mL. When the HBsAg status of the mother is unknown, the infant should receive the first immunization at birth and HBIG should be given as close to this as possible (within 1 week) if the mother subsequently is found to be HBsAg-positive. Because of concerns regarding diminished antibody responsiveness in small preterm infants immunized at birth, such infants who are born to HBsAg-negative women should not receive their first hepatitis B vaccination until they are 2 months of age or weigh at least 2000 g. Preterm infants born to HBsAg-positive women should receive HBIG and immunization at birth, as previously described. In addition to universal immunization of infants, both the AAP and the ACIP recommend vaccination of older children, adolescents, and adults at high risk for hepatitis B exposure (Table 1–31). The recommended schedule for these individuals is 0, 1, and 6 months. Given the current prevalence of sexual activity among adolescents and the frequent difficulty with eliciting information regarding risk status in this population, universal immunization of

Table 1–30. Recommended doses of licensed hepatitis B vaccines.[1,2]

	Vaccine[3]			
	Recombivax HB (MSD[4])		Engerix-B[5] (SK[6])	
	μg	(mL)	μg	(mL)
Infants of hepatitis B surface antigen (HBsAg)-negative mothers and children < 11 y	2.5	(0.25)	10	(0.5)
Infants of HBsAg-positive mothers (HBIG [0.5 mL] should also be given)	5	(0.5)	10	(0.5)
Children and adolescents 11–19 y	5	(0.5)	10	(0.5)
Adults ≥ 20 y	10	(1.0)	20	(1.0)
Dialysis patients and other immunosuppressed persons	40	(1.0)[7]	40	(2.0)[8]

[1]Reproduced, with permission, from Committee on Infectious Diseases, American Academy of Pediatrics: Universal hepatitis B immunization. Pediatrics 1992;89:795; and Report of the Committee on Infectious Diseases, American Academy of Pediatrics: (Red Book), 1994.
[2]Hepatavax B (MSD), a plasma-derived vaccine, is also licensed, but no longer produced in the United States.
[3]Vaccines should be stored at 2–8 °C. Freezing destroys effectiveness.
[4]Merck, Sharp & Dohme.
[5]The Food and Drug Administration has approved this vaccine for use in an optional schedule: four doses at 0, 1, 2, and 12 months (see 1991 Report of the Committee on Infectious Diseases).
[6]SmithKline Biologicals.
[7]Special formulation for dialysis patients.
[8]Four-dose schedule recommended at 0, 1, 2, and 12 months.

all adolescents should also be encouraged. Adverse effects associated with hepatitis B vaccination are minimal and limited primarily to local tenderness, although several rare hypersensitivity reactions to yeast and vaccine preservative have been reported.

Table 1–31. High-risk groups who should receive hepatitis B immunization regardless of age.[1]

- Hemophiliac patients and other recipients of certain blood products
- Intravenous drug users
- Heterosexual persons who have had more than one sex partner in the previous 6 mo and all persons with a recent episode of a sexually transmitted disease
- Sexually active homosexual or bisexual men
- Household and sexual contacts of hepatitis B virus (HBV) carriers
- Members of households with adoptees from HBV-endemic, high-risk countries who are hepatitis B surface antigen–positive
- Children and other household contacts in populations of high HBV endemicity
- Staff and residents of institutions for the developmentally disabled
- Staff of nonresidential day-care and school programs for developmentally disabled if attended by known HBV carrier; other attendees in certain circumstances
- Hemodialysis patients
- Health care workers and others with occupational risk
- International travelers who will live for more than 6 mo in areas of high HBV endemicity and who otherwise will be at risk
- Inmates of long-term correctional facilities

[1]Reproduced, with permission, from Committee on Infectious Diseases, American Academy of Pediatrics: Universal hepatitis B immunization. Pediatrics 1992;89:798; and the Report of the Committee on Infectious Diseases, American Academy of Pediatrics: (Red Book), 1994.

Varicella Vaccine

Although most of the 3.9 million cases of chickenpox reported annually in this country are self-limited and do not lead to serious medical complications, approximately 90 fatal cases are reported each year. In addition, many more children have significant morbidity, such as bacterial superinfection, pneumonitis, encephalitis, glomerulonephritis, and arthritis. Furthermore, the economic and social costs of this infection, which necessitates prolonged home care by a parent or other caregiver, are great. After weighing these issues and the potential risks and benefits of the current vaccine (licensed in March 1995), the AAP and ACIP have recommended routine varicella vaccination for all children who have not had the clinical disease. Varicella vaccine is composed of a live attenuated virus and minute quantities of neomycin. A dose of 0.5 mL is delivered subcutaneously using needle sizes and sites as described above. Routine vaccination is recommended at 12–18 months of age (Table 1–28). Children younger than 18 years of age who lack a history of natural infection should also be vaccinated. Because adults who do not recall an episode of varicella often will have antibody evidence of prior infection, it is recommended that individuals older than 18 years of age have their immune status tested before receiving the vaccination. There are no problems, however, if an individual who has already had natural varicella also receives the vaccine. Ninety-five percent of children 12 years of age or younger will seroconvert after one dose of vaccine. However, a diminished antibody response is observed in adolescents and adults. It is therefore recommended that individuals 13 years of age or older be given a two-dose regimen separated by 4–8 weeks. Varicella vaccine may be given concurrently with MMR, using separate sites and syringes. If not given on the same day, however, these live-virus vaccines should be administered at least 1 month apart. Although data currently are limited, there is no reason to suspect that varicella vaccine cannot be effectively administered simultaneously with DTP, DTaP, hepatitis B, *H influenzae,* OPV, or e-IPV. On the basis of follow-up studies to date, serologic evidence of immunity appears to be long-lasting. However, the need for subsequent booster doses at some point cannot be ruled out. A small number of vaccine recipients may experience an attenuated clinical infection when subsequently exposed to the wild-type virus. Even in these situations, however, the vaccine appears to be highly protective against severe disease. Side effects of varicella vaccination are minimal. Approximately 20–35% of recipients will experience transient pain and tenderness at the site of injection. Of greater significance, a mild varicelliform skin eruption will develop in approximately 7% of children within 1 month of receiving the immunization. Because the vaccine virus has rarely been recovered from these lesions, a very small risk exists for exposing others to the attenuated virus. Relevant precautions are given below. A mild zoster-like disease also has been reported to occur in some vaccine recipients. This appears to be less severe and occurs at no greater frequency than that observed with reactivation of the wild-type virus. Valid and nonvalid contraindications to varicella vaccination are given in Table 1–29. With the exception of some children with acute lymphocytic leukemia under study conditions, immunocompromised individuals should not receive this vaccine. However, children living in households with other immunodeficient individuals can and should receive it. If a vaccine-related skin rash develops, contact between the recipient and the immunocompromised individual should be avoided until the rash resolves. Varicella vaccine should not be given to a pregnant woman, and pregnancy should be avoided for at least 1 month after receiving the vaccine because of the potential risk to the fetus. However, the presence of a pregnant woman is not a contraindication to vaccinating a child living in the same household. The varicella vaccine should also not be administered to individuals with a history of an anaphylactic reaction to neomycin. Although no cases of Reye syndrome have been reported in association with the varicella vaccine, it is recommended that salicylates be avoided for 6 weeks after administration of the vaccine because of the well-established relationship between Reye syndrome and the use of salicylates during wild-type infection.

REFERENCES

American Academy of Pediatrics: *Policy Reference Guide, A Comprehensive Guide to AAP Policy Statements Published through December 1995,* 8th ed. American Academy of Pediatrics, 1996.

Committee on Infectious Diseases, American Academy of Pediatrics: *Report of the Committee on Infectious Diseases (Red Book).* American Academy of Pediatrics, 1994.

Committee on Psychosocial Aspects of Child and Family Health 1985–1988, American Academy of Pediatrics: *Guidelines for Health Supervision II.* American Academy of Pediatrics, 1988.

Dixon SD, Stein MT: *Encounters with Children: Pediatric Behavior and Development,* 2nd ed. Mosby–Year Book, 1992.

Elster AB, Kuznets NJ (editors): *AMA Guidelines for Adolescent Preventive Services (GAPS).* Williams & Wilkins, 1994.

Fletcher RH et al: *Clinical Epidemiology—The Essentials.* Williams & Wilkins, 1996.

Green M (editor): *Bright Futures: Guidelines for Health Supervision of Infants, Children, and Adolescents.* National Center for Education in Maternal and Child Health, 1994.

Illingworth RS: *The Development of the Infant and Young Child: Normal and Abnormal,* 9th ed. Churchill Livingstone, 1987.

Sackett DL et al: *Clinical Epidemiology: A Basic Science for Clinical Medicine,* 2nd ed. Little Brown, 1991.

2

Adolescence

Caroline J. Chantry, MD

Adolescence is the period that bridges childhood and adulthood. Varied factors, including dramatic biologic, psychological, social, and environmental changes, determine the age of onset. Usually the onset of puberty is used to define the beginning of adolescence; alternatively, a chronologic definition of 10–21 years of age may be used.

GROWTH & DEVELOPMENT

SOMATIC GROWTH & DEVELOPMENT

The major biologic changes occurring during puberty involve body composition, skeletal growth, cardiovascular changes, neuroendocrine development, and reproductive maturity. Because chronologic age correlates poorly with many of these developmental processes, the sexual maturity rating (SMR) scale of Marshall and Tanner, also known as Tanner stages, better measures the stage of biologic development.

The SMRs for secondary sexual development characterize genital development and pubic hair growth in boys and breast development and pubic hair growth in girls. On all scales, preadolescent sexual development is Tanner stage 1, and adult sexual development is usually stage 5. For male genital development, stage 2 is defined by the onset of testicular and scrotal enlargement. In stage 3, testicular and scrotal growth continue, and penile enlargement, primarily in length, begins. Further testicular and scrotal growth and penile growth in breadth constitute stage 4.

Stages of pubic hair development are the same for men and women. The first appearance of straight, slightly pigmented hair is in stage 2. Stage 3 is characterized by sparse growth of coarser, curly, pigmented hair, and stage

4 by adult-type hair that has not yet spread to the medial thigh surface. Adult-type and quantity of hair that spreads to the medial thigh surface appears in stage 5.

Tanner stage 2 of female breast development is defined by the presence of a breast bud with areolar widening. In stage 3, further breast and areolar enlargement without separation of their contours are seen. Stage 4 is reached with the presence of a secondary areolar mound, distinct from the configuration of the breast. This mound persists in some adult women, whereas in others, breast development progresses directly from stage 3 to stage 5, in which the areola recedes to the level of the breast with disappearance of the mound. Tanner stages are depicted in Figures 2–1 and 2–2.

In 98% of boys, puberty begins between 9.5 and 13.8 years of age, with a mean of 11.5 years. Testicular enlargement is usually the first sign of puberty. Discordance of more than one stage between genital and pubic hair development is rare (< 1% of white boys in the United States). Pubic hair usually follows testicular enlargement within 6 months, penile growth follows within 12–18 months, and the skeletal growth spurt peaks within 2–2½ years (at Tanner stage 4). Axillary hair usually follows pubic hair growth by 2 years. While growth of facial hair is highly variable, it most often occurs at the same time or shortly after axillary hair. Sperm are usually present in ejaculate by stage 3, and fertility is usually established by stage 4. Acne is a midpubertal event that usually occurs at Tanner stage 3. Most boys (95%) complete genital development within 4.5 years of pubertal onset, with a mean duration of puberty of 3.5 years. This sequence is depicted in Figure 2–3.

Breast development is the first secondary sex characteristic to appear in 85% of girls in the United States, with pubic hair developing first in the remainder. This occurs at a mean age of 10.5 years but can occur anywhere between 8 and 13 years of age. As with boys, it is unusual for girls (< 3% in the United States) to have discordance of more than one stage between breast and pubic hair development. Also, as with boys, axillary hair growth in girls usually follows pubic hair growth by about 2 years. However, the

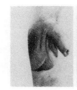

Figure 2–1. Stages of genital development in boys. (Reproduced, with permission, from Van Wieringen JD et al: *Growth Diagrams 1965,* Wolters-Noordhoff, 1971.)

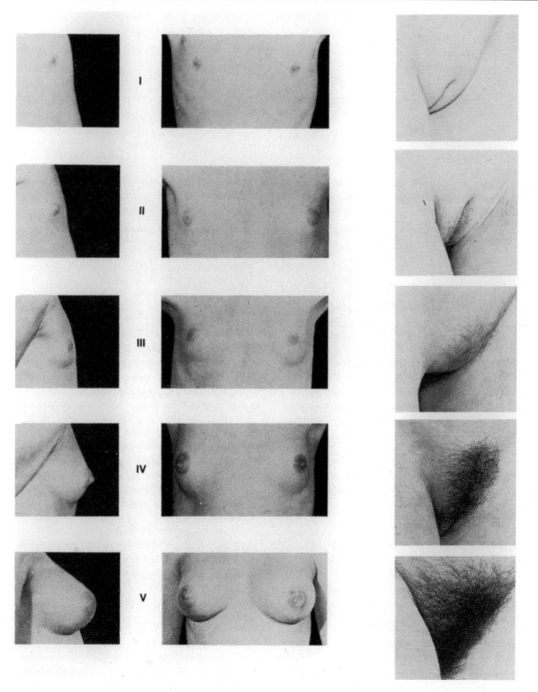

Figure 2–2. Stages in breast development and the appearance of pubic and labial hair in girls. (Reproduced, with permission, from Van Wieringen JD et al: *Growth Diagrams 1965,* Wolters-Noordhoff, 1971.)

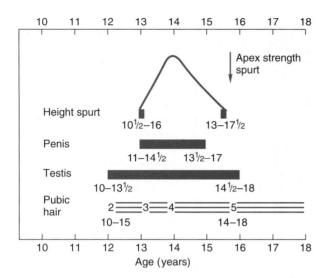

Figure 2–3. Diagram of sequence of events at adolescence in boys. The range of age of each event is indicated. (Reproduced, with permission, from Tanner JM: *Growth at Adolescence,* Blackwell, 1962.)

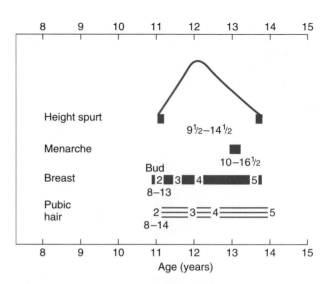

Figure 2–4. Diagram of sequence of events at adolescence in girls. The range of age of each event is indicated. (Reproduced, with permission, from Tanner JM: *Growth at Adolescence,* Blackwell, 1962.)

growth spurt occurs comparatively earlier in girls' than in boys' puberty, beginning with the onset of puberty and peaking at Tanner stage 3. Acne also occurs earlier in girls than in boys, usually at Tanner stage 2. Menarche is a late event, typically occurring 2 years after breasts bud at stage 3 or, more commonly, during stage 4 breast development, which occurs at a mean age of 12.8 years. The majority of menstrual cycles during the first 2 postmenarchal years are anovulatory; by 21 years of age, 60–80% of cycles are ovulatory. The rate of sexual maturity in girls is highly variable, ranging from 1.5 to 8 years to complete the process, with an average of 4.2 years. The sequence of female pubertal events is shown in Figure 2–4. Although the normal timing of onset, sequence, and rate of pubertal changes are variable, it is essential to understand these factors in order to detect the occasional abnormal individual. Premature or delayed developers, or those with abnormal patterns of development, may have underlying pathology and require further evaluation. See Chapter 20 for discussion of abnormal pubertal development.

Changes in body composition also occur during puberty. Muscle mass increases during early puberty in both boys and girls. In girls, muscle mass peaks at menarche and then decreases; in boys, it continues to increase throughout puberty. This increased muscle mass, together with increasing testosterone levels, accounts for the marked increase in strength found in pubertal boys. Mean body fat increases from 16% in prepubertal girls to 27% in pubertal girls and decreases from 14% to 11% in boys. Adipose tissue is also distributed differently; girls have

more in the areas of the breast, pelvis, upper arm, and back. Skeletal changes include the obvious growth spurt, as well as widening of the hips in girls and of the shoulders in both sexes, but especially in boys.

Cardiovascular development results in doubling of the heart size; systolic blood pressure continues to increase in boys but plateaus in girls. Related changes include increased lung size with decreasing respiratory rates. Although hematocrit and blood volume both increase in boys, they plateau in girls.

Neuroendocrine maturation is incompletely understood but involves maturation of the hypothalamic-pituitary-gonadal axis, the primary modulator of pubertal development. Puberty is characterized by a diminished sensitivity of the hypothalamic-pituitary-gonadal axis to negative feedback of the sex steroids estrogen and testosterone. This allows nocturnal pulses of gonadotropin-releasing hormone (GnRH) to be released from the hypothalamus, effecting release of the gonadotropins luteinizing hormone (LH) and follicle-stimulating hormone (FSH), which in turn stimulate increased release of the sex steroids. In addition, there is a more marked pubertal response to GnRH, resulting in higher levels of LH release in particular. Late puberty involves development of a positive feedback of estrogen to induce the LH surge necessary for ovulation. The gonadotropins effect release of estrogen and testosterone from the gonads; these hormones, in addition to adrenal androgens, are responsible for development of the secondary sex characteristics. For further discussion of the endocrinologic bases of puberty, see Chapter 20.

PSYCHOSOCIAL DEVELOPMENT

NORMAL PSYCHOSOCIAL DEVELOPMENT

Adolescence entails the successful completion of three primary psychosocial tasks. The first task is separation and individuation, which involves developing psychological, social, and physical independence from the family. As the family becomes less prominent in the adolescent's life, the peer group becomes more important. The second task involves establishing competence in relationship skills and developing the capacity for intimacy. The third task is achieving a new sense of self, which requires the integration of a growing and reproductively mature body with qualitatively changing cognitive skills. Cognitively, adolescents are in transition from the concrete operational logic of late childhood to formal operational logic, which characterizes adolescence and adulthood. This level of cognitive development allows adolescents to understand consequences and modulate the impulsive behavior that characterizes early adolescence. A sexual identity must be formed as part of the adolescent's evolving self-image; the older adolescent begins to plan a future societal role. More detailed information on psychosocial development is presented in Table 2–1.

Teenagers need a gradual increase in their responsibili-

Table 2–1. Biopsychosocial development during adolescence.[1]

Early Adolescence (Ages 10–13 Years)	
Characteristics	Impact
Onset of puberty, becomes concerned with developing body.	Adolescent has major questions concerning normalcy of physical maturation; often concerned about stages of sexual development and how his or her process relates to peers of same gender. Occasional masturbation.
Begins to expand social radius beyond family and concentrate on relationships with peers.	Can begin to encourage some external responsibilities alone in consultation with parents (ie, visit with health care provider, contacts with school counselors).
Cognition is usually concrete.	Concrete thinking necessitates dealing with most health situations in a simple, explicit manner using visual as well as verbal cues.
Middle Adolescence (Ages 14–16 Years)	
Characteristics	Impact
Pubertal development usually complete, and sexual drives emerge.	Explores ability to attract opposites. Sexual behavior and experimentation (same and opposite sex) begin. Masturbation increases.
Peer group sets behavioral standards, although family values usually persist.	Peer group will often have an effect on compliance; peers rather than parents may offer key support for such activities as visits to health care providers.
Conflicts over independence.	Increased assumption of independent action, together with continued need for parental support and guidance; able to discuss and negotiate changes in rules. Ambivalence on part of adolescent in discussion and negotiation.
Cognition begins to be abstract.	Begins to consider full range of possibilities with poor ability to integrate into real life because ego identity not fully formed and cognitive growth not complete.
Late Adolescence (Ages 17–21 Years)	
Characteristics	Impact
Physical maturation complete. Body image and gender role definition is secured.	The adolescent begins to feel comfortable with relationships and decisions regarding sexuality and preference. Movement to individual relationships being more important than peer group.
Relationships are no longer narcissistic; there is a process of giving and sharing.	Adolescent more open to specific questioning regarding behavior.
Idealistic.	Idealism may lead to conflicts with family.
Emancipation is nearly secured.	With emancipation, the young person begins to more fully recognize the consequences of his or her actions.
Cognitive development is complete.	Most are capable of understanding a full range of options for health issues.
Functional role begins to be defined.	Often interested in significant discussion of life goals because this is the primary function of this stage.

[1]Reproduced, with permission, from Irwin CE Jr et al: The adolescent patient. Page 39 in: Rudolph AM et al (editors): *Rudolph's Pediatrics,* 20th ed. Appleton & Lange, 1996.

ties and support for moves toward independence in this stressful period of identity formation. A supportive context may also enhance the development of their reasoning skills. Available information suggests that most elements of competent decision making are achieved by early to middle adolescence, but stress may reduce available cognitive resources, resulting in the use of less rational skills in decision making. Experimentation also serves to improve decision-making skills; hence, some risk-taking can be seen as a normal, transitional behavior of adolescence, filling a role in the developmental tasks of identity formation, establishment of relationships, and separation from the family.

RISK-TAKING BEHAVIORS

Risk-taking refers to engaging in potentially destructive behavior whether or not one understands the immediate or long-term consequences. These behaviors account for the majority of injuries and death within this age group. Specifically, substance use, premature sexual activity, and unintentional injuries account for greater than 50% of morbidity during adolescence. Although some risk-taking is a normal part of psychosocial maturation, some adolescents are predisposed to place themselves at very high risk. Table 2–2 presents factors associated with increased likelihood of taking risks, which can aid in identifying individuals at whom to aim preventive strategies.

Substance Use

The vast majority of teens have at least tried alcohol and cigarettes; in 1995, the lifetime prevalence among 12th graders was 81% and 64%, respectively. More troubling, almost 30% of high-school seniors interviewed reported an episode of heavy drinking within the previous 2 weeks, and almost 22% reported daily tobacco use, the latter an increase of almost one third in the past 4 years. Even among 8th graders, lifetime prevalence of alcohol and cigarette use was 54% and 46%, with more than 9% smoking daily. The mean age of onset is 12.6 years for use of alcohol and 12 years for cigarettes. The corresponding percentage of 12th graders who had a lifetime history of marijuana use in 1995 was 42%, and the percentage who used cocaine, 6%. More than half reported having used an illicit drug at some time. Although use of most drugs remains below the peak rates observed in the 1970s (except for inhalants), most of these rates have increased over the past few years, particularly that of marijuana; among younger adolescents in particular, the rates of use of alcohol and illicit drugs in general are increasing. In 1995, the proportion of 8th graders taking any illicit drug in the past year was almost doubled since 1991 and is now 21%. Inhalant use is especially prominent and continues to increase dramatically in young adolescents; 12.8% report such use within the past year—more than among the older age groups. Other drugs used by adolescents include amphetamines; hallucinogens, such as lysergic acid diethylamide (LSD) and phencyclidine (PCP); inhalants; and opiates, such as heroin. In addition, approximately 4% of male adolescents report current or past use of anabolic steroids; again, this usually is initiated at a young age, 16 years or younger. For treatment of acute intoxications, the reader is referred to Chapter 10.

It is important, but difficult, to distinguish the occasional from the habitual user. The transition from occasional to habitual user follows a predictable sequence, in which the individual initially uses tobacco and alcohol and may then follow these with marijuana, then other illicit drugs, and finally prescription psychoactive drugs. Cigarettes are a particularly notorious gateway drug for adolescent girls. Determining where individuals are in this sequence may help to establish habituality of use. Disclosure of such information is more likely to occur within the context of a therapeutic relationship, in which confidentiality is ensured as much as possible (see this chapter, Legal Issues).

Other signs of problem use may include lack of motivation or poor school performance, changes in personal appearance, legal problems, difficulties with family or peer relationships, or medical complications. Psychological dependence is more common during adolescence than is physical dependence, which carries a worse prognosis. Incorporation of drug use and drug-seeking behavior into daily activities suggests psychological dependence; often these adolescents use drugs to cope with stress, anxiety, or conflict or as a means of acceptance to a peer group. There is increasing recognition that many adolescents who develop problematic substance use have primary psychiatric diagnoses that contribute to drug use. A high index of suspicion for such comorbidity should be maintained, particularly in adolescents who do not respond to therapy.

Management involves prevention. A national health objective is to delay the first use of alcohol and marijuana by at least 1 year, a delay that may result in less serious drug problems for young adults. The most successful programs involve teaching coping skills to resist social pressures in combination with problem-solving, decision-making, and self-esteem enhancement skills. Self-help groups and family involvement may be adequate when use is already regularly established but dependency does not yet exist.

Table 2–2. Risk factors for onset of risk-taking behaviors.[1]

Asynchrony of biologic/psychosocial development
Male gender
Attitudes and beliefs that demonstrate a lack of awareness
Peer group that considers behavior normative
Multiple school transitions
Permissive or authoritarian family
Chronic family conflict
Familial engagement in risk behavior
Lack of skills to resist engagement
Sensation-seeking personality
Depression, anxiety, or poor self-esteem
Aggressiveness

[1]Adapted and reproduced, with permission, from Irwin CE: Risk taking behaviors in the adolescent patient: Are they impulsive? Pediatr Ann 1989;18:128.

Successful treatment is geared to the adolescent's developmental rather than chronologic age, in recognition of the fact that regular users often have arrested developmentally. A more comprehensive treatment program is indicated for those with psychological or physical dependency; appropriate referrals should be made.

Sexual Activity

Teenagers in the United States today initiate sexual activity earlier than did their predecessors: 76% of 12th-grade boys and 67% of 12th-grade girls have experienced intercourse. The corresponding numbers for 9th-grade students are 49% and 32%. Blacks are more likely than whites or Hispanics to have had intercourse. Adolescents do not protect themselves well against the risks of unintended pregnancy and sexually transmitted diseases (STDs), including HIV, imposed by this early sexual activity. Although 78% of teens report using some form of contraception at last intercourse, only 59% of male adolescents and 46% of female adolescents reported in 1993 that they or their partner used a condom to protect against STDs at last intercourse. Furthermore, studies reveal that fewer than half of those who have used condoms recently do so all the time. STD rates are higher in sexually active teens than in any other age group. More than one third of sexually active adolescents report multiple partners, further compounding the unsafe sex practices prevalent in this population.

Unintentional Injury

Unintentional injuries are the single most common cause of both injury (as measured by days of hospitalization) and death in the adolescent population. This is no surprise when one considers the sheer number and variety of risks taken by this group: a survey of young adolescents reveals that two thirds of them acknowledge taking chances on bicycles or skateboards, more than one half use seat belts inconsistently or not at all, and one third have ridden with a driver who is under the influence of alcohol or other drugs. In the United States, these unintentional injuries account for 46% of deaths in young adolescents and 80% of deaths in the 15–19-year-old age group. Motor vehicle accidents account for half of these fatalities.

Violence

Violence, defined here as intentional injuries, includes both fatal and nonfatal intentional injuries: homicides, suicides, assaults, rapes, physical fights, and domestic violence. Homicide is currently the second leading cause of death in adolescents as a whole and the leading killer of black teens. Gunshot wounds account for 75% of teen homicides. Fighting is a prominent cause of injury in adolescents and often precedes homicide. Suicide, the third leading cause of adolescent death, is usually accomplished by guns. Moreover, for every fatality due to violent crime, 41 teens are hospitalized and 1100 are treated in emergency departments. One teen in 15 is the victim of a violent crime.

Both internal and external factors predispose adolescents to violence, and many of the factors that predispose

to risk-taking also predispose to violence: male gender, asynchronous puberty (eg, late or early developing male), feelings of invulnerability, a need for peer acceptance, and lack of a sense of future. Of the environmental factors predisposing to violence, poverty is probably the most potent. There is also good evidence that children exposed to violence on television behave with more physical aggression and violence. Access to guns and alcohol or drug use are common precipitants.

Prevention must involve multilevel interventions. Primary prevention includes limiting exposures to situations that promote violence, such as poverty and family dysfunction. One can also reduce the exposure of children and adolescents to violence in the media. The American Academy of Pediatrics recommends that parents limit television viewing to 1–2 hours daily. Many experts recommend that schools teach nonviolent conflict-resolution skills as a means of prevention. There is also good evidence that stricter gun control would lessen violence. These are complex tasks, but nonetheless vitally important ones, because early identification and treatment of high-risk individuals and victims may limit the spread of this epidemic.

INTERRELATIONSHIP OF HIGH-RISK BEHAVIORS

Evidence is growing that many adolescent problem behaviors are interrelated. Substance use, in particular, tends to be associated with other high-risk behaviors. Alcohol is associated with many different kinds of injuries, both vehicular and nonvehicular; marijuana has been shown to be associated with vehicular injuries as well. Substance use has also been shown to correlate with earlier initiation of sexual activity and less safe sexual practices. Whereas some of these associations might be ascribed to effects of alcohol on coordination or inhibition, other examples, such as the association of cigarette smoking with high-risk sexual behavior, suggest that those predisposed to take risks often do so in varied form. Another such example is that frequency of drug use, smoking status, and frequency of driving under the influence of alcohol are all correlated to the frequency of not using a seat belt. Apparently, the proclivity to one risk-taking behavior increases the likelihood of undertaking another.

COMMON MENTAL HEALTH PROBLEMS

DEPRESSION

An individual is depressed when sadness, flatness, or emptiness pervades perception, thinking, and behavior. If depression occurs in the absence of a loss and interferes with life and relationships, it may indicate a depressive disorder. The prevalence of depression in adolescents aged 14–18 years is approximately 3–5%, with a female-to-male preponderance that approaches that seen in adults (2:1). Depressed adolescents can manifest with one or more of the following symptoms: eating and sleep disturbances, dysphoria, low self-esteem, somatic complaints, substance abuse, deteriorating school performance, problems with the law, and family conflict. Whereas transient symptoms may be considered developmentally normal, persistent symptoms should be considered clinically significant. For a more thorough discussion of depression, please see Chapter 3.

SUICIDAL BEHAVIOR

Epidemiology

Suicidal behavior encompasses two distinct but overlapping phenomena: suicide attempts and completed suicides. Suicide, while uncommon, is the third leading cause of death among older adolescents (15–19 years old) in the United States today, with a rate in 1992 of 10.9 per 100,000 population, and the fourth leading cause of death among young adolescents (10–14 years old), with a rate of 1.7 per 100,000. Male suicides far outnumber female suicides by as much as fivefold. Suicide is more common among whites, Latinos, and Native Americans than among blacks, although this gap is closing. These rates are underestimated because of underrecognition and underreporting; nevertheless, they have increased dramatically over the past 30 years. Firearms are the most commonly used method for completed suicides, followed by hanging and poisoning. Suicide attempts are far more common; the ratio of attempts to completion ranges from 60:1 for older male teens to 600:1 for younger female teens. National samples indicate slightly more than 8% of adolescents have made prior suicide attempts.

Risk Factors

Multiple risk factors for suicidal behavior have been identified that are reasonably sensitive but have low specificity. The most common risk factor is depression. Other factors include interpersonal loss, family conflict, alcohol or drug abuse, homosexuality and sexual orientation conflicts, personality characteristics (particularly those resulting in feelings of hopelessness and helplessness), other psychiatric disorders such as psychosis, and a family history of depression or suicide. There may be biologic markers involving serotonin metabolism in the central nervous system (CNS), but this has yet to be studied in adolescents. In addition, there are often acute precipitants, such as a disciplinary crisis with a parent, a fight with a peer, a romantic dispute or break-up, or interaction with a psychotic parent. Behaviors that increase suicide risk include a prior suicide attempt, suicidal ideation or threats,

deteriorating school performance, antisocial behavior, social isolation, and running away.

Prevention & Management

Prevention entails identifying high-risk individuals by means of a thorough patient interview. The concurrence of multiple risk factors in particular should raise concern. Any adolescent who is considered at risk should be questioned about suicidal ideation, planned method, and past suicide attempts. The lethality of the intended method should be assessed. Whether or not the adolescent is actively suicidal, the home environment should be made safe, including removal of firearms in particular. The acute goals are to ensure the safety of suicidal individuals and to guide them into long-term therapy. A no-suicide agreement should be reached, and very high-risk individuals, such as those who have recently attempted suicide, should be hospitalized until the crisis has passed. Others should begin outpatient mental health treatment so that alternative methods of dealing with stressors and resolving conflict can be identified and practiced. In all cases, long-term noncrisis therapy should follow and address underlying psychopathology. Whether primary care physicians elect to manage or refer these patients depends on their training and the individual case involved; compliance with referrals improves when an appointment is made for the patient. In any case, the primary care physician should see the patient in follow-up.

EATING DISORDERS

Eating disorders are common in female adolescents. Because significant physical and psychological illness and death can result from these disorders, the primary care physician's role is prevention and early recognition. Management should be aggressive and include treatment of any existing medical complications and referral for psychological treatment.

Anorexia Nervosa

Anorexia nervosa usually begins during adolescence and has an overall prevalence in girls of approximately 1%; subthreshold criteria are encountered more often. The incidence has doubled over the past 20 years, presumably because of our societal emphasis on thinness as a manifestation of success. Female adolescents are affected 10–20 times more often than male adolescents. Anorexia is a syndrome characterized by significant weight loss, usually more than 15% below normal, as well as disturbed body image, marked fear of fatness, and amenorrhea (see Table 2–3). Other physical symptoms can include hyperactivity (in an attempt to burn calories) and sleep disturbances. Mental disturbances often include denial of illness and bizarre attitudes and behaviors toward food. One must exclude other illnesses, physical or psychiatric, that could account for anorexia or weight loss (Table 2–4). Specifically, affective disorders and schizophrenia may masquer-

Table 2–3. Diagnostic criteria for eating disorders.[1]

Anorexia nervosa
Refusal to maintain body weight at or above a minimal normal weight for age and height, eg, weight loss leading to maintenance of body weight 15% below that expected, or failure to make expected weight gain during period of growth, leading to body weight 15% below that expected.
Intense fear of gaining weight or becoming fat, even though underweight.
Disturbance in the way in which body weight, size, or even shape is experienced, eg, the person claims to "feel fat" even when emaciated, believes one area of the body is "too fat" even when obviously underweight; undue influence of body weight or shape on self-evaluation or denial of the seriousness of the current low body weight.
In females, absence of at least three consecutive menstrual cycles when otherwise expected to occur (primary or secondary amenorrhea).

Bulimia nervosa
Recurrent episodes of binge eating (rapid consumption of a large amount of food in a discrete period of time), with a minimum average frequency of two episodes per week for 3 or more months.
During the eating binges, a feeling of lack of control over eating behavior.
Recurrent, inappropriate compensatory behavior to prevent weight gain, eg, self-induced vomiting, use of laxatives or diuretics, strict dieting or fasting, or vigorous exercise.
Persistent overconcern with body shape and weight.

[1]Adapted and reproduced, with permission, from Pages 544–550 in: *Diagnostic and Statistical Manual of Mental Disorders (DSM-IV)*, 4th ed. American Psychiatric Association, 1994.

ade as anorexia nervosa. However, the characteristic pattern of mental and physical findings typically precludes the need for extensive diagnostic testing.

Myriad physical findings may be encountered in these patients, particularly when their disease has progressed to the point of cachexia. These findings include hypothermia, bradycardia, and postural hypotension. There may be mottled skin, loss of scalp hair, and appearance of lanugo hair over the trunk. Other signs of malnutrition may occur, such as pretibial or ankle edema or constipation. If there is

Table 2–4. Differential diagnosis of anorexia nervosa.[1]

Organic disease	Psychiatric disease
Endocrine	Depression
Diabetes mellitus	Thought disorder
Hyperthyroidism	Substance abuse
Neurologic	
Central nervous system neoplasm	
Gastrointestinal	
Inflammatory bowel disease	
Achalasia	
Neoplastic	
Any malignancy	
Gynecologic	
Pregnancy	
Immunologic	
Lupus erythematosus	

[1]Reproduced, with permission, from Litt IF: Page 130 in: *Evaluation of the Adolescent Patient*. Hanley & Belfus, 1990.

purging, one may see abrasions of the palate or buccal mucosa and etching of tooth enamel consistent with self-induced vomiting. Complications of malnutrition are not uncommon and may include hypoglycemia, leukopenia, cardiac arrhythmias, hypothalamic or pituitary abnormalities, pain, and vomiting secondary to duodenal obstruction by the superior mesenteric artery after loss of mesenteric fat.

These patients often present a therapeutic challenge because of denial; the first principle of management therefore involves establishment of trust. One aims for an early restoration of a normal nutritional and physiologic status. An outpatient trial may be appropriate if food restriction and weight loss are of recent onset (< 3–4 months), binge eating or purging are absent, the family is reasonably functional, and one can anticipate cooperation from both patient and family. Often hospital admission is required because of either medical or psychologic instability. Long-term therapy requires a team approach involving both the patient and the family.

Prognosis for all of these patients is guarded because eating problems persist in more than half of these patients and often coexist with depression and obsessional behavior. Therefore, follow-up needs to continue for years, with assessment of nutritional and mental status, menstruation, eating behaviors, and psychosocial and psychosexual development. After 5 years, approximately one third of patients with anorexia nervosa or bulimia recover, one third improve but continue to have symptoms, and one third will be severely affected. Depending on the duration of illness, time of intervention, and any associated bulimia, purging, or depression, the mortality rate ranges from 5% to 18%. Death is secondary to fluid and electrolyte disturbances, starvation and its complications, or suicide. Because the mortality rate is significantly reduced by early intervention, emphasis must be placed on early diagnosis. Therefore, strict criteria for weight loss (eg, 15%) should not be enforced if other criteria for diagnosis are met.

Bulimia & Bulimia Nervosa

Bulimia is episodic binge eating, which may occur with or without purging behavior (vomiting, fasting, or laxative or diuretic abuse). Binge eating is common and may be considered normative behavior, but it constitutes the disorder of bulimia if frequent or severe. Evaluation must occur if there is unexplained weight loss, persistent binge-purge cycles, fatigue, depression, poor self-esteem, amenorrhea, delayed or arrested puberty, or parental concern regarding eating behaviors. From 10 to 50% of patients with anorexia nervosa engage in bulimia.

Bulimia nervosa is a distinct syndrome characterized by bingeing and purging that is recognized by the patient as abnormal with a fear of loss of control over eating behavior. There is also a nonpurging variant that involves the use of other compensatory mechanisms, such as fasting or excessive exercise. There is bodily dissatisfaction, particularly after a binge, and often associated depressive symptoms. Bulimia nervosa has a prevalence in adolescent and young adult women of 1–3%; the occurrence rate in males is approximately one tenth of that in females. The prognosis is guarded, similar to anorexia, but patients are more likely to have medical complications secondary to fluid and electrolyte abnormalities. Death, when it occurs, is more likely to be secondary to either severe fluid and electrolyte disturbances or suicide.

REPRODUCTIVE HEALTH ISSUES

MALE ADOLESCENTS

BREAST DISORDERS

Gynecomastia, glandular enlargement of male breast tissue, occurs in the majority of pubertal boys, usually between Tanner stages 2 and 4. It can be either unilateral or bilateral and either subareolar (type I) or generalized (type II). It often produces breast tenderness and therefore may come to the physician's attention when it is palpable but not visible. There are pathologic as well as physiologic causes of type II gynecomastia, which can be differentiated on the basis of history and physical examination. The pathologic causes of type II gynecomastia are summarized in Table 2–5. In particular, drugs, both prescription and recreational, are a common cause of pathologic gynecomastia. When the condition is physiologic, it usually resolves within 1–2 years; therefore, reassurance is indicated. Marked enlargement, or pendulous breasts, can have a devastating effect on the teenager's developing sense of masculinity, occasionally indicating the need for counseling and either medical or surgical treatment. There has been some recent success with hormonal therapies, primarily antiestrogens such as tamoxifen or the aromatase inhibitor testolactone, to decrease the estrogen-androgen ratio.

SCROTAL MASSES

Scrotal masses are best approached by first considering whether the mass is painful. Painful masses include torsion of the spermatic cord, torsion of the testicular appendix, epididymitis, orchitis, and hematoceles. Painless masses include neoplasms, hernias, hydroceles, spermatoceles, and varicoceles.

Painful Masses

Testicular Torsion. The most common cause of an acute, painful scrotal swelling in adolescents is torsion of the spermatic cord, also called testicular torsion. It is usu-

Table 2–5. Pathologic causes of type II gynecomastia.[1]

Idiopathic
Familial
    Associated with anosmia and testicular atrophy
    Reifenstein syndrome
    Associated with hypogonadism and a small penis
    Friedreich ataxia
    Others
Klinefelter syndrome
Male pseudohermaphroditism or true hermaphroditism
Testicular feminization syndrome
Hypogonadism, primary or secondary
Excessive extraglandular aromatase
Tumors producing steroids, human chorionic gonadotropin or aromatase (adrenal, testis, others)
Leukemia
Hemophilia
Leprosy
Thyroid dysfunction (hyperthyroidism and hypothyroidism)
Cirrhosis of the liver
Traumatic paraplegia
Chronic glomerulonephritis or other renal failure
Starvation (on refeeding)
Herpes zoster
HIV infection
Chest wall trauma
Psychological stress
Drugs
    Drug classes
        Estrogens
        Gonadotropins
        Androgens (aromatizable)
        Anti-androgens (cyproterone, flutamide)
        Corticosteroids
        Cancer chemotherapeutic agents (especially alkylators)
        Calcium channel blockers
        Angiotensin-converting enzyme inhibitors
        Antihypertensives (methyldopa, reserpine)
        Digitalis preparations
        Dopamine blockers
        Central nervous system agents (tricyclics, diazepam, phenytoin)
        Drugs of abuse (marijuana, heroin, methadone, amphetamines)
        Antituberculous agents (isoniazid and others)
    Individual drugs
        Cimetidine
        Spironolactone
        Ketoconazole
        Insulin
        Clomiphene
        Metronidazole
        Theophylline
        Others

[1]Adapted and reproduced, with permission, from Greydanus DE et al: Breast disorders in children and adolescents. Pediatr Clin North Am 1989;36:601; and Glass AR: Gynecomastia. Endocr Metab Clin North Am 1994;23:825.

ally caused by anomalies of testicular suspension or descent and occurs most commonly in boys aged 12–14 years. Presentation is usually acute onset of pain in the scrotum, inguinal canal, or lower abdomen, often associated with nausea and vomiting. Physical examination reveals a diffusely swollen and tender testicle; there can be secondary scrotal edema and hydrocele. Although the cremasteric reflex is usually absent, this is of limited diagnostic utility as its absence can be a normal variant. The abnormal axis of the other testis supports the diagnosis because the abnormal suspension, which predisposes to torsion, affects both sides. If reasonable suspicion exists, emergent surgery should be performed, because survival of the testis is directly correlated with time from torsion to detorsion. Radionuclide scan demonstrating decreased testicular uptake and Doppler ultrasound findings of absent pulsation should be sought only when there is a low index of suspicion. Otherwise, surgery should not be delayed to perform these confirmatory tests.

The differential diagnosis includes torsion of the testicular appendage, epididymitis, orchitis, and hematoceles. Torsion of the testicular appendix presents similarly to testicular torsion, although the pain can be less severe, begins more gradually, and is localized to the upper pole of the testis. Physical examination done early in the course of the illness may reveal a tender, pea-sized swelling at the upper pole, and the cyanotic appendix may be visible through the scrotal skin, the so-called blue dot sign. Later, generalized erythema and a reactive hydrocele may make diagnosis more difficult. If the diagnosis is confirmed by a urologist or radiologic studies, surgery may be deferred. Treatment includes analgesics and anti-inflammatory agents. Pain usually resolves within 2–12 days, but if it is severe or persistent, surgery is indicated.

Epididymitis. Inflammation of the epididymis can be secondary to infection or trauma. It usually occurs in sexually active male teens but can occur in those with urinary tract pathology or secondary to instrumentation in the absence of sexual activity. It also presents with acute onset of scrotal pain and swelling but may be associated with urinary symptoms of frequency and dysuria as well as urethral discharge. Early in the course, the epididymitis is distinct from the testis; with time, the inflammatory process generalizes, and epididymo-orchitis results. If testicular torsion is a concern, radiologic studies can be used to verify the diagnosis. The common pathogens in a sexually active teen are *Chlamydia trachomatis* or *Neisseria gonorrhoeae*. If anal intercourse has occurred, the spectrum of pathogens is broader. As with urethritis, STDs should be evaluated and treated, and urinary tract infection should also be ruled out. Adjunctive therapy includes analgesia, bed rest, and cold compresses. Partners of sexually active individuals should be examined and treated as with other STDs.

Orchitis. This inflammation of the testis presents with mild to severe scrotal pain and swelling; nausea and vomiting may be associated. It is usually a viral process but can be secondary to bacterial or tubercular epididymitis. It is most commonly caused by mumps, but it can also be caused by Epstein-Barr, influenza, and varicella viruses, as well as by coxsackieviruses. Treatment is analgesia, bed rest, and scrotal support. Post-traumatic hematoceles are another cause of scrotal pain and swelling. Usually the diagnosis is made clinically but can be confirmed by ultrasound when in doubt. Treatment is elevation, ice, and analgesia, unless bleeding continues, which is an indication for surgical drainage.

Painless Masses

The differential diagnosis of painless scrotal masses includes testicular neoplasms, inguinal hernias, hydroceles, spermatoceles, and varicoceles. The incidence of testicular neoplasms—95% of which are germ cell tumors—is on the rise, and these neoplasms represent the third most common malignancy in the 15–19-year-old age group. (Lymphoma and leukemia are most common.) They typically present as firm, painless swellings discovered on routine examination, and they gradually increase in size. The mass may become painful if necrosis or hemorrhage occurs, resulting in misdiagnosis of infection or inflammation. Ultrasound examination can further characterize the mass. Urologic referral should be immediate if a tumor is found. The tumor markers human chorionic gonadotropin (hCG) and α-fetoprotein, when present, can be used to follow the disease during treatment, which varies according to age, histology, and stage of disease. The overall 5-year survival rate is 92%; the rate is even higher when diagnosis occurs before the tumor spreads beyond the testis, emphasizing the importance of early diagnosis.

The differential diagnosis includes both indirect and direct inguinal hernias, indirect hernias being much more common in adolescents than direct hernias. This type of hernia allows the intestine to protrude through the internal inguinal ring (Figure 2–5). This is caused by failure of the processus vaginalis to obliterate after testicular descent. The Valsalva maneuver may push the bowel down the inguinal canal, or less commonly, the bowel extends into the scrotum at rest. Pain or erythema suggests bowel incarceration, a surgical emergency. Referral should be made for elective repair of all other hernias to avoid potential incarceration.

Hydroceles. The presence of fluid within the tunica vaginalis is another cause of painless masses (Figure 2–5). Hydroceles may be noncommunicating, when the mass is confined to the scrotum, or communicating, when there is continuity from the tunica vaginalis to the peritoneum and between their respective cavities. Because of this continuity, communicating hydroceles increase in size with standing and decrease with lying down. Physical examination reveals a transilluminating mass that interferes with palpation of the other scrotal contents. As hydroceles can be secondary to other pathology, including tumors, infection, or lymphatic obstruction, referral to a urologist is indicated. Ultrasound may help rule out associated pathology. Surgery is indicated only with large, painful, or communicating lesions.

Spermatoceles. These painless cysts develop in the spermatic cord. On physical examination, they are transilluminating cystic nodules found above and posterior to the testicle. They may be bilateral and multiple. As with hydroceles, surgery is indicated only for very large or painful lesions.

Varicoceles. These dilated tortuous veins in the ve-

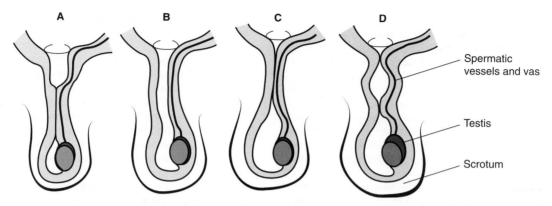

A B C D

Spermatic vessels and vas

Testis

Scrotum

Figure 2–5. Painless scrotal masses. **A:** Inguinal hernia with partial opening of process vaginalis. **B:** Complete inguinal hernia. **C:** Hydrocele of scrotum. **D:** Communicating hydrocele. (Modified and reproduced, with permission, from Schwartz MW [editor]: In: *Principles and Practice of Clinical Pediatrics*. Year Book Medical Publishers, 1987.)

nous plexus of the scrotum are found in 15–20% of male adolescents. Although they are usually asymptomatic, engorgement caused by prolonged standing can cause pain. They are usually either left-sided or bilateral; right-sided lesions should prompt investigation for associated venous obstruction. Palpation along the spermatic cord reveals the typical "bag of worms" mass superior to the testis. The size of the varicocele decreases with lying down and increases with the Valsalva maneuver. Referral is indicated for unilateral, right-sided lesions or for associated testes that are either small or not growing normally at puberty. Fertility is usually intact for an estimated 75% of men with varicoceles.

FEMALE ADOLESCENTS

BREAST DISORDERS

Serious breast disorders are uncommon in adolescents, but a variety of processes may cause concern. Questions may arise regarding the timing of development, which normally occurs between the ages of 8 and 13 years. Often one breast develops before the other; therefore, unilateral subareolar swelling in a girl of this age should be considered a normal variant unless proved otherwise by careful examination and close follow-up. Breast asymmetry frequently persists with one breast growing more rapidly, most commonly between Tanner stages 2 and 4. Symmetry usually occurs by late adolescence, but 25% of adult women continue to have visible asymmetry.

Physiologic, cyclic changes of swelling and tenderness of the breast can occur premenstrually, accounting for as much as a 50% increase in breast volume. There can be an associated cyclic lumpiness on examination. It is important to recognize these physiologic changes and reassure

the patient. The accompanying mastalgia is usually mild, and all that is required is firm brassiere support and mild analgesics.

Congenital Anomalies. These may first present during adolescence and include polythelia (extra nipples anywhere along the embryonic milk line), occurring in 2% of the population, and less commonly, polymastia. Athelia and amastia occur rarely and often as part of a more extensive chest wall deformity. Inverted nipples can also be congenital.

Breast Atrophy. This can occur in adolescence, usually secondary to severe dieting, as seen in anorexia nervosa, but can also be associated with wasting due to any chronic illness or premature ovarian failure. Hypoplastic breasts can be unilateral or bilateral and can be caused by failure of the breasts to respond to estrogen or possibly by ovarian dysfunction. Hyperplastic, or massively enlarged breasts in adolescence, a condition termed **virginal** or **juvenile hypertrophy,** can be unilateral or bilateral. This condition is sometimes familial and is presumed to be secondary to increased hormonal sensitivity or increased local production of hormones. Treatment is surgical reduction once physiologic breast development is complete.

Breast Masses. These masses often alarm the adolescent who is aware of the high rate of breast cancer in adult women. However, breast cancer is exceedingly rare in teens, with an average annual incidence of 0.1:100,000 among adolescents aged 15–19 years. Although the differential diagnosis is quite broad, there are only a few common lesions. The most common mass in this age group is a solitary cyst, which usually is fluctuant but can be tense or hard and usually resolves over 2 or 3 months. Most masses in teens undergoing biopsy are fibroadenomas (75–90%); these occur most frequently during late adolescence. Clinically, these are rubbery, nontender masses that enlarge slowly over weeks to months to a maximal size of 10–15 cm with occasional associated skin changes overlying the lesion. Most often these are unilateral, but they can be bilateral or multiple. They may have a cyclic component with premenstrual exacerbation and some regression thereafter. Although fibroadenomas may regress altogether, they usually persist. These are histologically varied and have no malignant potential. The juvenile fibroadenoma is similar but occurs more frequently in young adolescents, has less well-defined edges, and grows more rapidly to larger sizes than does the classic fibroadenoma.

Clinically, it is difficult to distinguish fibroadenomas from the rare cystosarcoma phylloides. Usually benign in adolescents, but with a small potential for malignancy, this tumor accounts for most adolescent breast cancers. It presents as a slowly growing, painless mass, often 8–10 cm at presentation. Associated skin changes, nipple discharge, and axillary adenopathy from necrosis and infection may occur. Trauma can cause a firm, tender breast mass, which may take months to resolve or may develop into fat necrosis, itself a firm, mobile, nontender mass.

Evaluation of the breast mass includes questioning for a history of cyclic pain or other symptoms, trauma, fever, weight loss, nipple discharge, medications or street drugs, and previous lesions. The physical examination is directed at determining the Tanner stage (to delineate potentially normal breast buds, on which biopsy should never be performed), size, location, and characteristics of the mass. Any lesion that is hard or nonmobile, or has associated skin changes or nipple discharge, should be referred for biopsy to evaluate for cancer. Apparently benign lesions may be observed for 2–3 months, and changes occurring with the menstrual cycle noted. Cystic or solid (probable fibroadenomas) lesions that improve over this time may continue to be observed. For masses that persist unchanged or increase in size, fine-needle aspiration (cystic) or biopsy (solid) should be performed. When necessary, ultrasound is useful in differentiating cystic from solid lesions.

Mastitis. This is an infection of the breast presenting with swelling, tenderness, erythema, and heat. It is seen almost exclusively during lactation. Treatment is heat, antibiotics, and analgesia, unless it proceeds to abscess, when incision and drainage are indicated. Nipple trauma can predispose to nonlactational mastitis, although this is rare. Trauma may simulate infection.

Fibrocystic Breast Disease. This is a vague term that some authors favor abandoning. It usually is used to refer to diffuse, firm nodularity of the breast, which may become tender premenstrually. On physical examination, these breasts have bilateral, cordlike thickening and cysts that may enlarge or collapse from month to month. The incidence in adolescents is unknown. Treatment with oral contraceptive pills and restriction of methylxanthines is controversial; rarely, other medications are used.

Galactorrhea. This refers to a persistent, bilateral milky discharge in an individual who is not pregnant or lactating. The list of potential causes is extensive; the major causes in adolescents are prolactinomas, hypothyroidism, drugs, and psychological factors, such as stress, anxiety, or depression.

MENSTRUAL PROBLEMS

Menstrual disorders are common, particularly in the younger adolescent, aged 9–15 years. Fortunately, most of these disorders are minor and can be treated with education and reassurance, although occasionally investigation or treatment are indicated. Every female adolescent should be questioned regarding her menstrual history, including age at menarche, usual cycle length, number of menstrual days per cycle, amount of flow, date of the last two menstrual periods, and any associated symptoms. Commonly, adolescents do not have information regarding their last menstrual periods and may be encouraged to keep menstrual calendars.

A clear understanding of normal menstrual physiology is required to understand the pathophysiology of these disorders. The average age of menarche in the United States is 12.8 years (normal range, 10–16 years), with anovulatory cycles and irregular, estrogen-withdrawal bleeding for a variable amount of time thereafter. A normal, ovulatory menstrual cycle requires a mature hypothalamus-pituitary-gonadal axis, wherein the hypothalamus releases GnRH, the pituitary releases FSH and LH, and the ovary produces estrogens and progesterones. During the first half of the cycle, FSH stimulates the ovary to produce estrogen, which in turn stimulates the endometrium to proliferate. There is a midcycle LH surge resulting in ovulation, after which the corpus luteum secretes progesterone, which matures the endometrium in combination with estrogen. If fertilization does not occur, the corpus luteum atrophies, estrogen and progesterone levels decrease, and the endometrium sloughs. This cycle is extremely sensitive to psychological and physiologic stressors, such that minor changes can result in altered or absent menses.

Amenorrhea

Primary amenorrhea is defined as the absence of menarche by the age of 14 years (or a bone age of 14.5 years) in the absence of secondary sexual characteristics, by age 16 regardless of the presence of secondary sexual characteristics, or by 5 years after the onset of secondary sexual characteristics. **Secondary amenorrhea,** the absence of cyclic bleeding after menarche, is very common in adolescents. The duration of amenorrhea considered clinically significant varies from 3 to 6 months.

The differential diagnosis of amenorrhea is extensive; the etiologies may be divided by organ level into hypothalamic, anterior pituitary, gonadal, and end-organ (uterine, cervical, or vaginal) causes. Primary amenorrhea may be caused by congenital or chromosomal anomalies in addition to the causes of secondary amenorrhea. Foremost, pregnancy should always be considered, even with primary amenorrhea or despite a negative history of sexual activity.

Hypothalamic Causes. These causes of amenorrhea act via the hypothalamus effecting partial or complete inhibition of GnRH release. The pathology thus affecting the hypothalamus can be quite diverse and includes local processes such as abscess, tumor, granulomatous disease, and irradiation effects, as well as systemic processes such as malnutrition, emotional or physical stress, strenuous exercise, drugs (most notably hormones, chemotherapy, and drugs of abuse, including marijuana, cocaine, heroin, and methadone), and endocrinopathies, particularly thyroid or adrenal disease. Notably, the amenorrhea associated with anorexia nervosa may actually represent a hypothalamic dysfunction inherent to the disease rather than to malnutrition per se, as the amenorrhea precedes the weight loss by several months. There can also be congenital deficiency of GnRH; when associated with impaired smell, this is known as Kallman syndrome.

Anterior Pituitary Causes. Pituitary lesions, such as infarct, tumor, or granulomatous disease, can present with amenorrhea; prolactin-secreting tumors are the most common pituitary cause of amenorrhea. Isolated gonadotropin deficiencies are rare but are part of the more common panhypopituitarism. Endocrinopathies such as hypothyroidism are thought to effect amenorrhea via thyroid-stimulating hormone (TSH) inhibition of gonadotropin release at the level of the pituitary.

Gonadal Causes. The most common cause of amenorrhea, either primary or secondary, in patients who have completed their sexual development is polycystic ovary syndrome (PCO). This complex disorder involves inappropriate gonadotropin secretion, a spectrum of ovarian pathology, which includes hyperthecosis; less commonly, polycystic ovaries; and excessive levels of androgens. These androgens may result in clinical stigmata of obesity and hirsutism. A useful laboratory definition of PCO is an increased LH:FSH ratio of greater than 2.5:1.0, but not all affected women have this finding. Gonadal causes include gonadal dysgenesis, which can cause primary or secondary amenorrhea. Although many patients with gonadal dysgenesis either have Turner syndrome or are mosaics, they may be chromosomally normal. Other ovarian causes of amenorrhea include hemorrhage, ischemia, prior radiation and chemotherapy, autoimmune disease, and premature ovarian failure.

End-organ Causes. Finally, end-organ causes of amenorrhea include obstructive müllerian anomalies, such as imperforate hymen and cervical stenosis (which may present with cyclic pain with or without an abdominal mass); complete or partial müllerian agenesis; testicular feminization; and other hormone receptor (gonadotropin) or synthetic (estrogen) defects. Endometrial hypoplasia and scarring (Asherman syndrome) from infection, radiation, or curettage also result in amenorrhea.

Clinical Approach. In general, the clinical approach to primary and secondary amenorrhea is similar. It begins with a history and physical examination to sort out any of the known causes. Important historical points include a thorough pubertal, menstrual, sexual, contraceptive, and obstetric history, as well as a family history of menarchal patterns. General physical, nutritional, and psychosocial health status and exercise pattern must be determined, as well as any associated symptoms of pregnancy; CNS or pituitary tumor (headache, visual disturbance, galactorrhea); or endocrinopathies (thyroid, androgen excess). The physical examination is similarly focused:

- Evaluation of general appearance and mental status (flat affect may denote depression, drugs, or both); height, weight, and nutritional status; signs of chronic illness; or stigmata of Turner syndrome

- Staging of secondary sexual characteristics for both breast and pubic hair development

- Neurologic examination for assessment of visual fields and cranial nerves, including tests for anosmia (Kallman syndrome), and evidence of increased intracranial pressure

- Evaluation of evidence of abnormal hormonal effects, particularly thyroid, androgens (hirsutism, acne), or prolactin (galactorrhea)

- Pelvic examination for assessment of normalcy of external anatomy, presence of a uterus, evidence of estrogen effect on the vaginal mucosa, and presence of masses, either midline or unilateral or possible pregnancy. Palpation can be done rectovaginally if the patient is not sexually active; if in doubt, an ultrasound can confirm normal internal anatomy.

If history and physical examination do not reveal a likely cause, they should be followed by laboratory evaluation. A pregnancy test must be included in every evaluation of primary or secondary amenorrhea, as should TSH and prolactin assays. General screening tests should also be considered: complete blood count (CBC), erythrocyte sedimentation rate, and T_4. A staged approach is used to determine which organ is affected; one such approach is presented in Figure 2–6. The progestational challenge is a simple test using a 5- to 7-day course of oral progesterone. Withdrawal bleeding is normally expected 2–7 days after completing the course of progesterone. This test is helpful to assess endogenous estrogen levels as well as competence of the outflow tract, which is not yet established in the case of primary amenorrhea.

Dysmenorrhea

Dysmenorrhea, defined as crampy lower abdominal or back pain occurring with menses, is the most common gynecologic complaint of female adolescents. It may be accompanied by systemic symptoms, including nausea, diarrhea, and headache. The incidence increases with increasing age because of its association with ovulatory cycles; it occurs in approximately 40% of 12-year-old girls and in more than 70% of 17-year-old girls. More than half of those affected complain of moderate to severe pain. It is the most common cause of school absenteeism in these young women, yet few seek medical attention.

Dysmenorrhea can be divided into primary and secondary types. Either can be mild, moderate, or severe.

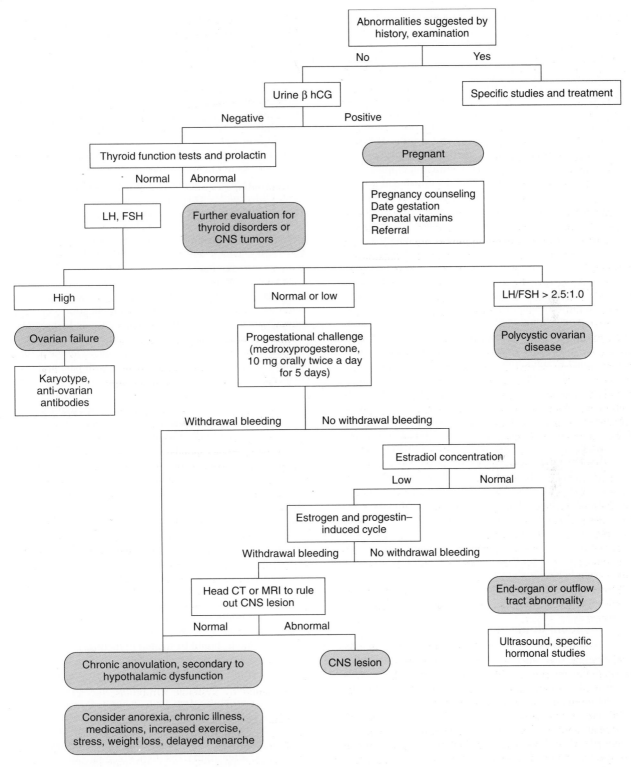

Figure 2–6. Diagnostic approach to amenorrhea. CNS = central nervous system; CT = computed tomography; FSH = follicle-stimulating hormone; hCG = human chorionic gonadotropin; LH = luteinizing hormone; MRI = magnetic resonance imaging; TSH = thyroid-stimulating hormone.

Eighty percent of adolescents with dysmenorrhea have primary dysmenorrhea, which is related to the increased amounts of prostaglandin E_2 and prostaglandin F_2 produced in these patients, causing increased uterine tone and resulting in painful ischemia. The prostaglandins also account for associated systemic symptomatology, when present. There is a familial predisposition to this disorder.

Secondary dysmenorrhea, most often due to STD, endometriosis, congenital anomalies, or complications of pregnancy, often can be suspected on the basis of history. An isolated, atypical painful menses suggests an acute pathologic process, such as endometritis or salpingitis, or a complication of pregnancy, such as threatened abortion or an ectopic pregnancy. A chronic history of progressive pain in an older adolescent suggests endometriosis, particularly when the pain is severe and occurs before menses. Congenital malformations typically cause pain by obstruction of flow or adhesions and often present with the onset of pain at menarche; flow also may be scant. Other possible causes of secondary dysmenorrhea include intrauterine devices, neoplasms, cysts, or severe psychosocial disease, which can lower pain tolerance.

Assessment should include a thorough menstrual, sexual, and pain history to find a pattern suggestive of either primary or secondary disease. An external genital and rectoabdominal examination should be done on patients suspected of having primary disease who are not sexually active, whereas a full pelvic examination should be done on patients who are sexually active and on those who are suspected of having secondary disease. Treatment of primary dysmenorrhea typically involves nonsteroidal anti-inflammatory drugs (NSAIDs), which provide relief in 70–80% of adolescents. Alternatively, low-dose oral contraceptive pills can be used as first-line therapy in sexually active teens. Because ovulation is suppressed, the endometrium is hypoplastic and prostaglandin concentrations are decreased, an effect that may take 2–3 months to achieve. If relief is not obtained with NSAIDs or oral contraceptives, one should suspect secondary disease and consider laparoscopy if other treatable causes have been ruled out. Underlying disease should be treated, when present, but symptomatic treatment with the above agents is also appropriate.

Dysfunctional Uterine Bleeding

Normal menses occurs an average of every 28 days (normal range, 21–45 days) and have a mean duration of flow of 5 days (normal range, 2–8 days). Blood loss is typically 20–80 mL. Any deviation from this is abnormal uterine bleeding. Dysfunctional uterine bleeding (DUB) is abnormal bleeding for which no organic lesion can be demonstrated. It is therefore a diagnosis of exclusion. Clinically, it is irregular bleeding that typically is excessive, prolonged, and painless. It can be difficult to quantify blood loss; practically, clots for more than 5 days or soaking more than 6 pads per day can be considered excessive.

Pathophysiologically, DUB is associated with anovulation or oligo-ovulation caused by an immature hypothalamic-pituitary-ovarian axis wherein estrogen feedback mechanisms are not yet fully developed. This results in failure of the midcycle LH surge, chronic anovulation, and tonic estrogen production, unopposed by corpus luteal secretion of progesterone. The endometrium remains proliferative until the follicle eventually involutes, causing withdrawal bleeding, an incomplete shedding that is painless and excessive, irregular, or prolonged. At least 50% of cycles in girls aged 9–13 years are anovulatory, only a minority of which cause clinically significant abnormal bleeding. Anovulatory cycles that are relatively regular are not considered abnormal in a perimenarchal adolescent. Older adolescents can also have anovulatory cycles, particularly in times of stress or illness.

As DUB is a diagnosis of exclusion, other causes of abnormal uterine bleeding must be considered. These potential causes, which will be found in approximately 5% of patients, are summarized in Table 2–6. The major causes of heavy bleeding aside from DUB are complications of pregnancy, trauma, bleeding disorders, medications, infections, and endocrinopathies. Complications of pregnancy, including ectopic pregnancies and threatened abortions, can present similarly, although usually with pain or cramping whereas DUB is painless. Pelvic inflammatory disease (PID) usually presents with pain and minimal bleeding, but bleeding can be more prominent. Endocrine disorders that can cause abnormal uterine bleeding include hyperprolactinemia, hyperthyroidism, or more commonly, hypothyroidism, which may present with abnormal bleeding as the first symptom. PCO can cause heavy bleeding. Classically, these patients have infrequent, irregular menses more than 2 years beyond menarche; they may be hirsute and obese. Ovarian cysts and tumors usually present with minimal bleeding but should be considered. Oral contraceptive use, and especially misuse, can cause excessive, irregular bleeding. Finally, anticoagulant use, including aspirin, and coagulopathies, both congenital and acquired, can present this way. von Willebrand disease, the most common congenital coagulopathy, often presents for the first time with excessive bleeding at menarche.

Assessment should first be directed at determining the degree of blood loss by history and physical examination. Orthostatic vital signs should be taken to assess for hypovolemia, which should be treated immediately. Thereafter, the history should be directed at determining the etiology of the bleeding by reviewing past and present menstrual history; amount, duration, and timing of flow; associated signs and symptoms (eg, pain, nausea, bruising, or petechiae); sexual activity; contraception; history of excessive bleeding from any site; endocrine review of systems; and any medication use (including aspirin). Physical examination, after ruling out hypovolemia, should be directed toward detecting secondary causes; one should assess for bleeding disorders (petechiae, purpura), endocrinopathies (thyroid palpation, skin and hair changes, reflexes, hirsutism), tumors (lymphadenopathy, hepato-

Table 2–6. Causes of abnormal uterine bleeding in adolescents.[1]

Dysfunctional uterine bleeding (anovulation)
Complications of pregnancy
  Ectopic or molar pregnancy
  Threatened or incomplete abortion
  Spontaneous abortion
  Placental polyp
Bleeding disorders
  von Willebrand disease
  Other hemophilias including factor VIII and IX deficiencies
  Thrombocytopenia—congenital or acquired (including idio-
    pathic thrombocytopenic purpura)
  Platelet dysfunctions—congenital or acquired
Infections
  Endometritis
  Cervicitis
  Pelvic inflammatory disease
Endocrine disorders
  Hypothyroidism or hyperthyroidism
  Adrenal dysfunction (Addison or Cushing disease), congenital
    adrenal hyperplasia
  Polycystic ovary syndrome
  Hyperprolactinemia
  Premature ovarian failure
Local pathology
  Endometriosis
  Uterine polyp or myoma
  Trauma
  Foreign body
  Tumors—ovarian, uterine, vaginal
  Ovarian cysts
Systemic illnesses
  Systemic lupus erythematosus
  Inflammatory bowel disease
  Chronic renal failure
  Severe liver disease
  Malignancies
Medications
  Oral contraceptives
  Aspirin
  Anabolic steroids
  Others

[1]Reproduced, with permission, from Neinstein LS: Menstrual problems in adolescents. Med Clin North Am 1990;74:1190; and Blythe M: Common menstrual problems: Part 3: Abnormal uterine bleeding. Adolescent Health Update 1992;4:2.

splenomegaly), and pain or masses on abdominal examination (tumor, infection, pregnancy).

A pregnancy test, CBC, and reticulocyte count should be obtained in all patients. Other laboratory studies should be individualized. For recurrent or severe bleeding, coagulation tests (bleeding time, prothrombin and partial thromboplastin times, and, if these are normal, tests for von Willebrand disease), as well as tests of thyroid and synthetic liver function, are indicated. If irregular cycles are chronic, prolactin and LH:FSH levels and thyroid studies should be considered. Hirsutism should be evaluated appropriately. When ectopic pregnancy is a concern, pelvic sonogram and quantitative serum β-hCG levels are required, as well as urgent referral to a specialist.

Treatment for mild or moderate DUB is directed at preventing or correcting anemia by iron supplementation and controlling the blood flow until the axis matures. More severe DUB may require restoration of hemodynamic stability in addition to the above; these treatments are summarized in Table 2–7. In addition, any cause of secondary bleeding needs to be treated as hormonal regulation of the menstrual cycle can camouflage underlying disease.

CONTRACEPTION

The majority of teenage girls in the United States are sexually active by the age of 18. Typically, contraception is not practiced for the first 6–12 months after first sexual intercourse; often contraceptive advice is first sought when the teenager believes she may be pregnant. Indeed, nearly half of teen pregnancies annually occur within the first 6 months of sexual activity. Accordingly, frank discussions of sexuality, reproduction, and contraception should be part of health supervision visits for all adolescents. Opportunities for these discussions should also be made during acute visits or sports physical examinations for those who are not otherwise seen, as is often the case for male adolescents.

Table 2–7. Management of dysfunctional uterine bleeding (DUB).[1]

Mild DUB (Hb > 11 g/dL)	Moderate DUB (Hb ≥ 9–11 g/dL)	Severe DUB (Hb ≤ 8 g/dL +/or Hypovolemia)
Reassurance Iron Follow-up in 2 mo	OCP: up to 4 pills/d until bleeding has stopped for 24 h; then taper by 1 pill/d every week until off Withdrawal bleeding in next 7 days OCP: cycle for 3–6 mo Iron Follow-up: weekly, then monthly	Treatment of hemodynamic instability Premarin, 20–40 mg IV q 2–4 h (maximum: 6 doses) and Enovid, 5 mg, or norethindrone acetate, 5 mg—4 pills/d tapering to 1 pill/d for 21 days Withdrawal bleeding in next 7 days OCP: cycle for 6–12 mo Iron Follow-up: daily, then weekly, then monthly

[1]Adapted and reproduced, with permission, from Coupey SM, Ahlstrom P: Common menstrual disorders. Pediatr Clin North Am 1989;36:563.
Hb = hemoglobin; OCP = oral contraceptive pill.

Adolescents' cognitive ability, need for protection from both pregnancy and STDs, comfort with touching their own bodies, and self-acknowledgment regarding sexual activity all change over time; consequently, so may the contraceptive method of choice. A summary of the available methods, their effectiveness, and advantages and disadvantages is presented in Table 2–8. The following discussion highlights more commonly used methods. Because adolescents' contraceptive behavior does not always follow their knowledge, it is critical to consider compliance-dependent effectiveness as opposed to theoretic effectiveness. Compliance has been demonstrated to increase with extreme ease of availability; instructions should also be simple, clear, and frequently reinforced.

NONHORMONAL METHODS

Abstinence from intercourse should always be acknowledged as a healthy and positive choice that does not necessarily preclude sexual activity. A discussion regarding sex that is safe from both disease and pregnancy can include myriad noncoital alternatives, such as hugging, kissing, sexual massage, mutual masturbation, and body rubbing.

Mechanical and chemical barrier methods have become a more popular choice with increasing concern since the 1980s regarding STDs, particularly HIV, as these methods have been shown to have some protective effect against most STDs. Protection is improved by using mechanical and chemical barriers together, such as a condom, diaphragm, or cervical cap with a spermicide. The female condom was approved by the Food and Drug Administration in 1993 and is available over the counter. It is made of polyurethane, lines the vagina entirely, and partially shields the perineum. It is an important addition to the contraception armamentarium in that its use can be independent of the male partner. Of the barrier methods, the latex male condom, when used properly and in combination with spermicide containing nonoxynol-9, provides optimal protection against most types of infection; the condom prevents exchange of bodily fluids, and nonoxynol-9 has both a bactericidal and virucidal effect. The relationship between nonoxynol-9 and HIV transmission, however, remains unclear. Although nonoxynol-9 is lethal to HIV in vitro and reduces the risk of transmission of gonorrhea and chlamydia, themselves a risk for HIV transmission, it can have an irritating effect on the vagina, particularly with high exposure. At least one study has documented an increased seroconversion rate in prostitutes using nonoxynol-9 compared with placebo, although other studies have documented a positive effect. A threshold effect is postulated. Natural membrane condoms should not be considered protective against viral STDs. This condom and spermicide combination is often a good contraceptive choice for adolescents who only have very intermittent activity. In addition, barrier methods should be recommended for all sexually active adolescents for disease prevention.

The diaphragm can be considered for mature, educated, motivated adolescents who are comfortable with insertion and removal. The cervical cap can be considered in the same population when available, with the additional concern that it is associated with an increased incidence of cervical abnormalities on Papanicolaou (Pap) smear. Therefore, it should be used only in individuals with normal Pap smears, which should be repeated after 3 months. There is particular concern that adolescents may be more susceptible to these abnormalities because of their external cervical transformation zone.

Other nonhormonal methods include intrauterine devices (IUDs) and periodic abstinence (fertility awareness). These are rarely indicated in the adolescent population. Coitus interruptus and sterilization are also not indicated in adolescents.

HORMONAL METHODS

Hormonal methods include oral contraceptive pills (OCPs), both combined and progestin-only (mini-pills), and various forms of long-acting progestins, including implants (eg, levonorgestrel and Norplant), which confer protection for up to 5 years; injections (eg, depomedroxyprogesterone [DMPA] and Depo-Provera), which provide protection for 3 months; and progestin-containing intrauterine devices (IUDs). OCPs are the most popular contraceptive among adolescents, because their use is independent from sexual activity and because of their high rate of effectiveness. Unfortunately, they provide no protection against STDs; therefore, the adolescent should be advised to use condoms and spermicide in addition to OCPs.

The most frequently prescribed OCPs are the fixed low-dose or triphasic combination pills containing estrogen and progesterone. These principally work by the inhibition of ovulation and implantation if fertilization occurs. Despite an effectiveness over time among experienced users of greater than 99.6%, first-year failure rates in adolescents approach 5%. There is also a high attrition rate; 25–50% of teen users discontinue the pill during the first year even in the absence of major side effects or complications, often because of minor side effects such as nausea or spotting. The clinician should therefore observe the patient and follow her status closely and attempt to minimize side effects whenever possible. Adolescents also benefit from a frank discussion of the risks and benefits of OCPs. Some of the noncontraceptive benefits include a lesser frequency of anemia, dysmenorrhea, premenstrual syndrome, benign breast tumors, recurrent ovarian cysts, and mittelschmerz, as well as a protective effect against both ovarian and endometrial cancers.

All health care providers should be familiar with both the absolute and the relative contraindications to OCP use (Table 2–9). Relative contraindications need to be individ-

Table 2–8. Methods of contraception.[1,2]

Method	Mechanism of Action	Efficacy: Rate of Pregnancy First Year of Use[3]		Coital Dependence	Prescription Required	Protection from STDs/HIV	Complications	Comments
		Theoretical	Actual					
Abstinence	No intercourse	0%	0%	No	No	Yes	None	Can encourage
Implants: Norplant (L-norgestrel)	Inhibits ovulation, prevents implantation	0.09%	0.09%	No	Yes	No	Infection at implant site	Menstrual changes
Injections: Depo Provera (medroxy-progesterone)	Inhibits ovulation, prevents implantation	0.3%	0.3%	No	Yes	No	Possible increase in osteoporosis with long-term use	Menstrual changes, delayed fertility return
Oral contraceptive pill	Inhibits ovulation Alters cervical mucus and endometrium	0.1–0.5%	3%[4]	No	Yes	Some protection against PID	Side effects, STDs (see text)	See text
Intrauterine device	Probably prevents implantation	1–2%	3%	No	Yes	No	Bleeding, cramping, pain, expulsion, increased risk of PID, ectopic pregnancy	Not recommended for teenagers
Condom Female (Reality)	Barrier	5%	21%	Yes	No	Yes	Rare	Does not depend on male partner
Male	Barrier	3%	12%	Yes	No	Yes	Reaction to latex	Some dislike
Vaginal spermicides (foam, jelly, suppositories)	Spermicidal agent	3%	21%	Yes	No	Yes	Reaction to spermicide	Some describe as "messy" to use
Condom and foam[5]	Barrier with spermicidal agent	0.01%	12%	Yes	No	Yes	Reaction to latex or spermicide	Requires using two methods
Diaphragm with spermicide	Barrier with spermicidal agent	6%	18%	Can be inserted up to 6 hours before intercourse	Yes	Some	Reaction to spermicide, pelvic discomfort, recurrent UTIs ↑Risk of toxic shock syndrome	Requires comfort with body
Coitus interruptus	Withdrawal prior to ejaculation	4%	18%	Yes	No	No	None	Requires self-control Preejaculatory semen contains sperm
Cervical cap with spermicide	Barrier with spermicidal agent	6%	18%	Can remain in place 2–3 days	Yes	?	Recurrent UTI, ↑ risk of cervical dysplasia and toxic shock syndrome	Difficult to insert/ remove
Periodic abstinence	Abstinence during times of peak fertility	1–9%	20%	No	No	No	None	Requires monitoring menstrual cycle
Chance	Chance	85%	85%	Yes	No	No	Pregnancy	Can intervene

[1]Adapted and reproduced, with permission, from Page 70 in Rudolph AM et al (editors): *Rudolph's Pediatrics*. 20th ed. Appleton & Lange, 1996.

[2]In approximate order of decreasing theoretical efficacy.

[3]Reproduced and adapted, with permission, from Hatcher RA et al: *Contraceptive Technology, 1990–1992*, 15th ed. Irvington, 1990: *Theoretical efficacy* is defined as the best *estimate* of the accidental pregnancy rate during the first year of use among couples who initiated the use of a method (not necessarily for the first time) and who used it consistently and correctly. Actual efficacy is defined as a measure of the accidental pregnancy rate during the first year among "typical couples" who initiated the use of a method (not necessarily for the first time) if they did not stop use for any other reason.

[4]All ages; 4–7% in adolescents.

[5]Efficacy rates based on use of condom *without* addition of spermicide.

STD = sexually transmitted disease; PID = pelvic inflammatory disease; UTI = urinary tract infection.

Table 2–9. Contraindications to oral contraceptive pill (OCP) use by adolescents.[1]

Absolute contraindications
Thrombophlebitis or thromboembolic disorder (or history thereof)
Cerebrovascular or coronary artery disease (or history thereof)
Known or suspected breast cancer or estrogen-dependent neoplasia (or history thereof)
Pregnancy (or strong suspicion thereof)
Benign or malignant liver tumor (or history thereof)
Known, current liver dysfunction
Undiagnosed, abnormal vaginal bleeding
Strong relative contraindications
Severe headaches, particularly vascular, which begin or worsen with OCP use
Hypertension
Hyperlipidemia
Mononucleosis, acute
Elective major surgery or surgery requiring immobilization within next 4 weeks
Long leg cast or major injury to lower leg
Exercise caution
Immature hpg axis (lack of regular menses for 12–18 mo postmenarche)
Depression
Diabetes, prediabetes, or a strong family history of diabetes
Sickle cell or sickle C disease
Active gallbladder disease or congenital hyperbilirubinemia
Completion of term pregnancy within 10–14 days[2]
Lactation[2]
Weight gain > 10 lb with OCP[2]
Cardiac or renal disease (or history thereof)[2]
Family history of myocardial infarction before age 50, particularly in a mother or sister (indicates lipid evaluation)
Family history of hyperlipidemia
Concurrent use of rifampin or other interfering drugs
Conditions likely to make patient unreliable at following OCP instructions (mental retardation, major psychiatric illness, substance abuse, history of poor compliance)
Others

[1]Adapted and reproduced, with permission, from Hatcher RA et al: Page 247 in: *Contraceptive Technology, 1990–1992,* 15th ed. Irvington, 1990.
[2]May be less of a contraindication to progesterone-only pills than combined pills.
hpg = hypothalamic-pituitary-adrenal axis.

ualized. In the absence of contraindications, any adolescent requesting maximal protection is an appropriate candidate, regardless of frequency of sexual activity.

Patients at the first visit should have a thorough medical and sexual history and physical examination, including weight, a pelvic examination, Pap smear, and STD screening. Other laboratory examinations to consider include a CBC, urinalysis, pregnancy test, and cholesterol and triglyceride screen, particularly if there are other risk factors for cardiovascular disease. Minimally, the first-year follow-up should include visits at 1, 3, 6, 9, and 12 months to check compliance, weight, and blood pressure and to review possible side effects, instructions, and danger signs (ACHES: abdominal pain, chest pain, headaches, eye problems, severe leg pain). In addition, condoms with the sper-

micide nonoxynol-9 should be recommended for protection against STDs, as back-up contraception for the first month, and as a second method of birth control should she discontinue OCPs.

Table 2–10 lists symptoms that can be attributed to the estrogenic, progestogenic, or androgenic effects. In choosing which pill to prescribe, any of the low-dose (sub-50 µg) pills may be used by most teens. Dose of hormone(s), particularly estrogen, price, and experience of the clinician or user with a particular pill all may be considered. For many new contraceptive users, the new progestins may be appropriate with several potential advantages, including improved lipid profiles, reduced amenorrhea, and lower free testosterone. Additional considerations are presented in Table 2–11.

The most common side effects of OCP include nausea, breast tenderness, weight gain, and breakthrough bleeding, particularly common during the first 3 months of therapy. In most cases, the patient can be reassured that these symptoms will disappear. If these or other symptoms persist, switching to a pill with a different estrogen-progesterone ratio often will lessen the symptoms. Clinicians should be thoroughly familiar with how to recognize the danger signs of OCP side effects, as well as how to manage specific symptoms, as compliance can be greatly affected.

Table 2–10. Hormonal side effects.[1]

Estrogenic effects
Nausea
Increased breast size (ductal and fatty tissue)
Stimulation of breast neoplasia
Fluid retention
Cyclic weight gain due to fluid retention
Leukorrhea
Cervical erosion or ectopia
Thromboembolic complications (pulmonary emboli, cerebrovascular accidents)
Hepatocellular adenomas and cancer
Increased cholesterol concentration in gallbladder bile
Growth of leiomyomata
Telangiectasia
Progestogenic effects (progestin and/or estrogen related)
Breast tenderness
Headaches
Hypertension
Myocardial infarction
Androgenic effects (caused by some progestins, minimized with new progestins)
Increased appetite and weight gain
Depression, fatigue, and tiredness
Decreased libido and enjoyment of intercourse
Acne, oily skin
Increased breast size (alveolar tissue)
Increased low-density lipoprotein cholesterol levels
Decreased high-density lipoprotein cholesterol levels
Diabetogenic effect
Pruritus
Decreased carbohydrate tolerance

[1]Adapted and reproduced, with permission, from Hatcher RA et al: *Contraceptive Technology, 1994–1996,* 16th ed. Irvington, 1994.

Table 2–11. Additional clinical considerations in oral contraceptive pill (OCP) choice.

To minimize nausea, breast tenderness, vascular headaches, and estrogen-mediated side effects, prescribe:
- Loestrin 1/20

Or a 30-µg pill, such as:
- Desogen
- Levlen
- Loestrin 1.5–30
- Lo/Ovral
- Nordette
- Ortho-Cept

To minimize spotting and/or breakthrough bleeding, prescribe:
- Lo/Ovral, Nordette, or Levlen
- A new progestin pill: Desogen, Ortho-Cept, Ortho-Cyclen, or Ortho Tri-Cyclen

To minimize androgen effects such as acne, hirsutism, oily skin, sebaceous cysts, pilonidal cysts, or weight gain, prescribe:
- Desogen, Ortho-Cept
- Ortho Tri-Cyclen
- Ortho-Cyclen
- Ovcon-35, Brevicon, or Modicon (norethindrone pills)
- Demulen-35 (ethnodiol diacetate pills)

To produce the most favorable lipid profile, prescribe:
- Ortho-Cyclen or Ortho Tri-Cyclen
- Desogen or Ortho-Cept
- Ovcon-35, Brevicon, or Modicon (norethindrone pills)

Adapted and reproduced, with permission, from Page 253 in: Hatcher RA et al: *Contraceptive Technology, 1994–1996,* 16th ed. Irvington, 1994.

Brief Management Guidelines

Acne. In general, acne improves with use of the pill. Management is directed at decreasing androgens by providing a low-androgen pill that suppresses ovarian androgen production but provides little exogenous androgen. Increasing the estrogen in the OCP may also help via increased serum hormone binding globulin (SHBG) and subsequently decreased free testosterone levels. Customary acne treatments, including dermatologic referral if necessary, may be indicated if acne persists.

Amenorrhea. Missed periods are more common with low-dose pills, as the build-up of the uterine lining is almost always less during their use than during a normal ovulatory cycle. The primary differential diagnosis is between pregnancy and inadequate endometrial build-up.

Amenorrhea may be reduced by providing a pill with higher progestin potency or one of the new progestin preparations (norgestimate or desogestrel; gestodene is not yet available in the United States).

Breakthrough Bleeding and Spotting. The differential diagnosis of breakthrough bleeding (BTB) associated with OCPs includes inadequate estrogenic or progestogenic effect on the endometrium, missed pills or altered pill schedule, ectopic pregnancy, threatened or spontaneous abortion, cervical inflammation, condylomata, polyp or cancer, pelvic inflammatory disease (PID), and endometriosis.

Accordingly, pregnancy, cervicitis, PID, and other gynecologic causes of bleeding should be ruled out, and a

hematocrit obtained if bleeding is significant. The user should be reassured and informed that BTB usually decreases markedly during the first 4 months of OCP use. Thereafter, the progestin potency may be increased or, if unsuccessful, a pill with more estrogen may be used.

Breast-feeding. As combined OCPs slightly decrease both the volume and protein content of breast milk, it is preferable to use alternative contraceptives, such as progestin-only OCPs or other progestin contraceptives, while lactating. If prescribing combined OCPs to a woman who is breast-feeding, do not initiate use until the breast-milk supply is well established, usually by 6 weeks postpartum. Before this, a woman who is exclusively breast-feeding and amenorrheic is reasonably well protected via the lactational-amenorrhea method (LAM).

Breast Tenderness (Mastalgia). The differential diagnosis of breast tenderness generally includes actual growth of breast tissue, cyclic edema from either estrogen or progestin, pregnancy, benign breast disease, cancer, or elevated prolactin levels. After pregnancy and cancer have been ruled out, an OCP with less estrogen or progestin may be tried, eg, the 20-µg pill or a progestin-only preparation. Management as for fibrocystic breast disease may be helpful.

Depression. In general, premenstrual symptoms, such as irritability and depression, are less in teens who are taking low-dose pills, but OCPs can exacerbate premenstrual symptoms or cause depression. Pills may induce depression via direct progestin effects, causing depression, fatigue, and lethargy; by decreasing pyridoxine (B6) levels; or via cyclic fluid retention caused by estrogen or progestin or drug interaction with diazepam.

One approach is to discontinue pills completely for 3–6 months and reassess the patient's status. As OCP-induced depression is most likely caused by progestin excess, reducing the progestin may have a beneficial effect, as may reducing the estrogen or both hormones. Pyridoxine supplements also may be helpful. Moderate or severe symptoms indicate referral to a mental health professional.

Galactorrhea. Galactorrhea in teens using OCPs may be caused by suppression of prolactin-inhibiting factor, a prolactin-secreting tumor, or breast stimulation. Galactorrhea related to excess estrogen in OCPs is uncommon with the use of low-dose pills and is most marked during the pill-free week. If problematic, the pill may be discontinued, in which case OCP-induced galactorrhea will disappear within 3–6 months.

Nausea. Nausea is less a problem with low-dose pills and, when it does occur, most often does so only during the first one or few cycles or the first few pills of each cycle. If nausea occurs at other times, signs of pregnancy, acute viral infection, or gallbladder disease should be sought.

Management involves taking pills with food or at bedtime or changing to a pill with less estrogen, eg, a 20-µg or progestin-only pill. Catch-up pills should be taken at 12-hour intervals, rather than two at a time, to minimize nausea.

Pregnancy. Although rare, pregnancy can occur even if pills have been taken perfectly. If a diagnosis of pregnancy is made, OCPs should be discontinued. Althuogh there is little, if any, increased risk of birth defects as a result of pill use during pregnancy, pills should be discontinued if the patient would not want an abortion and an early pregnancy cannot be reasonable ruled out. Alternative contraceptive methods, such as barriers, should be offered.

Visual Changes. OCP-related visual changes may occur through various mechanisms: retinal artery or vein thrombosis, corneal edema from fluid retention, transient ischemia with headaches, or, rarely, optic nerve inflammation with loss of vision, double vision, swelling, or unilateral or bilateral pain. Corneal edema may lead to discomfort or corneal damage with use of contact lenses.

Worsening of visual symptoms accompanying migraine headaches indicates immediate discontinuation of OCPs. Other transient, total, or partial loss of vision also indicates immediate discontinuation and neurologic referral.

Weight Changes. Weight change is usually minimal and unrelated to pill use; as many women lose weight as gain weight while taking OCPs. Some women, however, may experience weight gain definitively related to pill use caused by one of the following mechanisms: fluid retention due to either the progestin or the estrogen, usually during the first month of pill use; estrogen-induced weight gain due to increased subcutaneous fat, particularly in the hips, thighs, and breasts, usually after several months of pill use; increased appetite and food intake, an anabolic effect that occurs over several years; or depression associated with hyperphagia.

Depending on the pattern of weight gain, the pill may be changed to one with less androgenic activity (anabolic effect over years); less estrogen, progestin, or both (cyclic weight changes); or less estrogen (breast and subcutaneous thigh and hip fat). In addition, management may involve usual weight-control techniques, including increasing exercise and decreasing caloric intake.

Other Hormonal Methods

Other hormonal methods include the long-acting progestins: implants (eg, levonorgestrel and Norplant), which can last up to 5 years; injections (eg, DMPA and Depo-Provera), which provide protection for 3 months; and progestin-containing IUDs. Progestins provide contraception by inhibiting ovulation, thickening the cervical mucus so that sperm cannot penetrate (also protecting against PID), and creating an atrophic endometrial lining. Implants have the advantage of being highly effective, safe, and reversible; moreover, compliance is not an issue. There has been surprising interest in this method among adolescents. Implants are contraindicated only with undiagnosed vaginal bleeding, liver dysfunction, coagulopathies, and hormone-sensitive tumors; many anticonvulsants decrease their effectiveness, indicating a back-up method. The most common side effects are menstrual irregularity, which may include more prolonged bleeding initially, spotting

between periods, amenorrhea, or a combination thereof. These effects usually diminish with time; management may include NSAIDs or supplemental estrogen for 1–3 months.

Injectable progestin (Depo-Provera) has been rapidly accepted by teens since its approval by the FDA in 1992. This method is highly effective, convenient, and confidential. There is an incidental decrease in seizure frequency, making this the preferred contraceptive method for patients with seizure disorders. Menstrual patterns are disrupted, and amenorrhea develops in most women within 1 year of use. Moderate weight gain is also typical. Fertility eventually returns to normal, although ovulation may not resume until 1 year after the last dose.

PREGNANCY

EPIDEMIOLOGY & PREVENTION

Pregnancy rates are higher among US teens than teens in any other developed country for which data exist; similarly, adolescent birth rates are higher than for all but a handful of developed countries. At least 1 in 10 adolescents aged 15–19 years get pregnant each year; 40% will experience a pregnancy by the time they are 20 years old. There are approximately 1 million teen pregnancies each year, 40% of which terminate by therapeutic abortion, 13% by miscarriage, and 47% with live births. Most of these pregnancies are resolved outside of marriage. Of teens who give birth at term, 96% choose to raise their child even though more than half are both poor and unmarried; placing infants for adoption by this population is becoming less common. Black teens have nearly double the pregnancy rate of white teens and are less likely to abort, yielding a birth rate more than double that of whites; Hispanics have 80% the birth rate of blacks. Much of this difference is accounted for by the lower standard of living among nonwhites in this country, as birth rates are higher among the poor of any ethnicity.

In general, higher pregnancy rates in the United States are not associated with more prevalent sexual experience, but rather with less effective contraceptive use. Lack of knowledge, as well as less available and more expensive contraceptive supplies and services, contributes to this situation. Although only an estimated 5–16% of these pregnancies are intentional, the strength of the desire not to become pregnant varies with perception of the benefit of deferring parenthood; environmental factors, such as poverty and substance abuse, may make parenthood look attractive.

The estimated teen pregnancy rates for 1992 show a slight decrease from 1991, reflected in both abortion and birth rates, possibly because of increasing percentages of experienced teens who used condoms during the period 1990–1993. School-based programs that focus on risks of unprotected sexual intercourse and aid in the development of appropriate values, self-efficacy, and negotiation skills, have demonstrated effectiveness in postponing initiation of sexual intercourse and decreasing rates of unprotected intercourse.

IMPACT

Teen parenthood has both health and socioeconomic consequences. The complications of pregnancy found in adolescent mothers (eg, anemia, hypertension, and prematurity) can be eliminated with adequate prenatal care with outcomes that should be, but are not, the same or better as for older women. Even with good prenatal care, these children have more medical, emotional, and behavioral problems and lower cognitive abilities and academic achievement than do children of older mothers. The socioeconomic consequences are tremendous: teen mothers are more likely to bear subsequent children more rapidly, have more unwanted and out-of-wedlock births, experience greater marital instability, be more poorly educated, have fewer assets and lower incomes later in life, and be less satisfied with their vocational achievements than their counterparts. Short-term social programs for adolescent mothers can decrease this economic impact and improve child-raising abilities.

INTRAUTERINE PREGNANCY

The diagnosis of intrauterine pregnancy (IUP) should be considered whenever there is a history of unprotected intercourse with or without associated amenorrhea or abnormal vaginal bleeding. A menstrual history should be elicited whenever evaluating a female adolescent. As many teens are reluctant to disclose their sexual history, a negative history does not rule out pregnancy. Typical symptoms, such as amenorrhea, nausea, vomiting, breast tenderness, spotting, weight gain, urinary frequency, and fatigue, may be present or absent. If the diagnosis of pregnancy is considered, a pregnancy test and pelvic examination should be performed. Serum or urine tests for β-hCG usually are sufficient, unless quantitative levels to rule out ectopic or molar pregnancy indicate serial serum tests. Urine tests are easy to perform, inexpensive, and quite sensitive; they are positive 1 week after implantation, which is several days before a missed menses.

Once the presence of an IUP is established, counseling of the adolescent regarding her options needs to occur with a support person, her partner, or one or both of her parents, when appropriate. The adolescent, as well as her family, may be in crisis at this time. Referral sources for all options should be available, as well as legal counsel. If the adolescent chooses to remain pregnant, prenatal vitamins should be prescribed, and follow-up should ensure that prenatal care has begun as the level of denial is often high. Social-work referrals should also be made as neces-

sary to ensure that the pregnant teen has access to such necessities as housing, education, parenting classes, insurance coverage for pregnancy-related services, and entitlement benefits such as WIC. Counseling regarding her options should continue throughout the pregnancy.

ECTOPIC PREGNANCY

Ectopic pregnancy is an increasing problem. Although women aged 15–24 years have the lowest incidence of ectopic pregnancies, they have the highest related death rate. The most common predisposing factor is chlamydial salpingitis, but adhesions, endometriosis, IUDs, endometritis after therapeutic abortions, and congenital anomalies also can cause ectopic pregnancy. The condition is life-threatening as tubal rupture can occur, causing hemorrhage into the peritoneum, hypovolemia, and shock. Tubal abortions can also occur.

The diagnosis should be considered when patients present with lower abdominal pain or tenderness, amenorrhea or spotting, adnexal mass, or uterine enlargement mimicking early changes of an IUP. When suspected, diagnosis can be confirmed by a combination of serial quantitative hCG measurements, where the increase in hCG is usually less than that with an IUP; pelvic ultrasound; and, when necessary, culdocentesis and laparoscopy. The differential diagnosis includes other conditions that cause acute lower abdominal pain, such as acute salpingitis, torsion or rupture of an ovarian cyst, appendicitis, or acute gastroenteritis (see Table 2–12). When the predominant clinical presentation is bleeding rather than pain, threatened or incomplete abortion should also be considered. Treatment is

Table 2–12. Differential diagnosis of acute lower abdominal pain in the adolescent female by organ system.[1]

Urinary	Reproductive
Cystitis	Acute or chronic pelvic inflammatory disease
Pyelonephritis	
Urethritis	Cervicitis
Other	Dysmenorrhea (primary/secondary)
Gastrointestinal	Ectopic pregnancy
Acute cholecystitis	Endometriosis
Appendicitis	Endometritis
Constipation	Mittelschmerz
Diverticulitis	Ovarian cyst (torsion/rupture)
Gastroenteritis	Pregnancy (intrauterine, ectopic)
Inflammatory bowel disease	Ruptured follicle
Irritable bowel syndrome	Septic abortion
Mesenteric lymphadenitis	Threatened or incomplete abortion
Other	Torsion of the adnexa
	Tubo-ovarian abscess

[1]Adapted and reproduced, with permission, from Shafer MA, Sweet RL: Pelvic inflammatory disease in adolescent females: Epidemiology, pathogenesis, diagnosis, treatment, and sequelae. Pediatr Clin North Am 1989;36:513.

emergent surgical intervention (salpingostomy or, if rupture has occurred, salpingectomy), although medical treatment with methotrexate has been used successfully in selected cases recently. Fertility in these patients is reduced, although with improved methods of early diagnosis and conservative treatment, most (approximately 60%) are subsequently able to conceive and bear term infants.

SEXUALLY TRANSMITTED DISEASES

Sexually transmitted diseases, the most common infections in adolescents, account for much of the morbidity of this age group. The sequelae can be quite serious, and for female adolescents include complications of PID such as ectopic pregnancy, infertility, and chronic pelvic pain, as well as anogenital cancers and HIV. The outcomes for male adolescents can also include infertility, anogenital cancers, and HIV, as well as myriad other sequelae.

EPIDEMIOLOGY

Sexually active adolescents have the highest incidence of STDs of any age group; more than half of the 20 million cases reported annually occur in individuals younger than 25 years of age. Multiple factors contribute. The age of first sexual intercourse has become increasingly younger over the past 2 decades, resulting in an increase in STDs in this age group by virtue of there being more adolescents at risk. Adolescents are also often at higher risk than their adult counterparts owing to multiple sexual partners and inconsistent or no condom use. Fortunately, the percentage of high-school students reporting condom use at last sexual intercourse has increased in 1993 to 52.8% (from 46.2% in 1991). Presumably this reflects development and implementation of HIV prevention programs, also reflected in decreasing rates of some STDs, eg, gonorrhea. Although encouraging, these numbers demonstrate great room for improvement. Physiologically, the immature adolescent cervix may be more prone to infection as well.

Four percent of all high-school students report a history of STD. Actual rates are much higher, as many infections are subclinical. The most common bacterial STD is *C trachomatis*; it is at least twice as common as *N gonorrhoeae*. The prevalence of syphilis in this population, although only 0–3%, is increasing, particularly among ethnic minorities. The most common viral STD is human papillomavirus (HPV). Seroconversion to herpes simplex virus (HSV) type 2 occurs in 4% of whites and 17% of blacks by the end of their teenage years. HIV seroprevalence rates in adolescents vary widely by population tested. Up to 5.3:1000 military applicants had positive test results, depending on locale, as early as 1989 and from 0 to 4.6% (median, 0.5%) had positive results in STD clinic surveys. Although adolescents represent fewer than 1% of

the actual AIDS cases, nearly 20% of the total AIDS cases (more than half a million in the United States by December 1995) occur in the 20–29-year-old age group; many of these young adults contracted the virus during adolescence. Increasingly, transmission of this virus in adolescents is occurring by heterosexual contact; this mode now accounts for most HIV infections in female adolescents.

Ethnicity is correlated with risk for acquiring STDs, with black teens having much higher rates of gonorrhea, chlamydia, syphilis, and HIV infection and PID than their white counterparts. Gender influences infection rates as well, with female adolescents having higher reported rates than male adolescents. This may be secondary in part to the adolescent cervix being particularly susceptible to infection at the area of ectopy, and in part to higher utilization of health care services by females seeking contraception or prenatal care. Contraceptive method influences risk; mechanical barriers exert a protective effect, as does the spermicide nonoxynol-9. The effect of oral contraceptives is organism dependent; there is increased risk of chlamydial cervicitis and decreased risk of gonorrheal cervicitis. Their effect on PID is controversial but probably also organism dependent. Substance use may place the individual at higher risk via disinhibition; lack of condom use; trading sex for drugs, particularly crack; or contact with infected individuals through intercourse or shared intravenous equipment.

PREVENTION

As with any other preventable illness, the goal of the pediatrician with regard to STDs should be prevention. Primary prevention involves delaying initiation of sexual intercourse. Skill-building educational curricula focusing on behaviors, such as resisting peer and social pressures, have been successful. Clinicians also need to include sexuality issues routinely in their patient encounters. Secondary prevention entails preventing STDs in teens who are already sexually active, as well as providing early diagnosis and treatment for those who may already have acquired infection. This can be achieved by encouraging consistent condom use in conjunction with the spermicide nonoxynol-9, periodically screening those who have not used condoms consistently, ensuring access to care for those who have symptoms, and being vigilant in evaluating and treating partners of infected individuals. Tertiary prevention uses these same strategies but focuses particularly on individuals who have already experienced one or more negative outcomes. A thorough medical and psychosocial evaluation needs to be performed to delineate risk factors that may be modified.

CLINICAL SYNDROMES

The adolescent with an STD often will present with a symptom complex. The more common syndromes are discussed below with the associated etiologic agents. For further information about specific organisms, the reader is referred to Chapter 9.

Genital Lesions. These include both ulcerative diseases and venereal warts. There are several ulcerative diseases, the most common being HSV and syphilis. Less common are chancroid and lymphogranuloma venereum. In addition to the morbidity caused by these diseases, the ulcers may serve as a portal of entry for HIV. Although any of these ulcers may be asymptomatic, the lesions of HSV are classically painful, grouped vesicles, papules, or ulcers with associated tender inguinal adenopathy. Both type 1 and type 2 virus may be causative; the latter is more commonly associated with genital disease. Associated symptoms may include dysuria, vaginal or urethral discharge, pruritus, and dyspareunia. The classic chancre of primary syphilis, caused by *Treponema pallidum,* is sharply demarcated, solitary, superficial, and painless. Because it often goes unnoticed and is increasing in frequency, screening should be considered for any adolescent presenting with an STD with a serologic test for syphilis, particularly in endemic areas. Venereal warts or condyloma acuminatum are caused by HPV. Usually they are either asymptomatic or a papule is noticed, but there may be associated pain, pruritus, or dyspareunia. Their primary significance lies in their associated increased risk for anogenital cancers.

Urethritis. In adolescents, this is almost exclusively an STD. It occurs in male adolescents with much greater frequency than in female adolescents. Urethritis may be asymptomatic or symptomatic, with common symptoms including urinary complaints of dysuria, frequency, or urgency, as well as urethral discharge and edema or erythema at the urethral meatus. It is typically categorized into gonococcal or nongonococcal, the primary etiologies for the latter being *C trachomatis* and *Ureaplasma urealyticum.* Gram's stain of urethral discharge may reveal gram-negative intracellular diplococci if gonorrhea is the causative organism. Nongonococcal urethritis (NGU) is more common than gonococcal urethritis (GU) and frequently coexists; therefore, treatment for GU should include treatment for NGU. Epididymitis, discussed earlier in this chapter under painful scrotal masses, is often a manifestation of an STD as well.

Vaginitis. Vaginitis, or inflammation of the vaginal mucosa, may be asymptomatic or have abnormal quantity or quality of vaginal discharge as the primary symptom. There also may be associated perineal pruritus or rash, as well as urinary complaints. The most common etiologies include *Trichomonas vaginalis, Candida albicans* and other fungi (which may be, but are not necessarily, sexually transmitted), and bacterial vaginosis. The latter, not truly a vaginitis because of limited inflammatory changes, is caused by interaction of multiple bacteria normally present, including *Gardnerella vaginalis,* anaerobes, and others.

Mucopurulent Cervicitis (MPC). This inflammation of the endocervix caused by infection is most commonly

caused by *C trachomatis, N gonorrhoeae,* or HSV. Again, it is often asymptomatic but may cause the symptoms associated with vaginitis as well as irregular or painful vaginal bleeding and abdominal or pelvic pain. Because cervicitis can progress, it is important to rule out PID when pain, fever, or bleeding is present. Diagnosis of MPC can be made clinically when mucopurulent endocervical secretions are visible or demonstrated microscopically (> 10 polymorphonuclear leukocytes per high-power field of gram-stained os secretions). The cervix is often friable as well. Specific organisms should be sought once the clinical diagnosis of cervicitis has been made, as well as in asymptomatic high-risk individuals. However, empiric treatment is often indicated before definitive results are available, particularly in an individual who is unlikely to return for treatment.

Cervical Intraepithelial Neoplasia (CIN). This term refers to a precancerous or cancerous change of the cervical epithelial cells. This condition is relatively common in adolescents, occurring in 5–10% of sexually active teen girls. It begins in the transformation zone of the cervix, where columnar cells are undergoing metaplastic change to squamous epithelium under the influence of pubertal hormones, also known as the **area of ectopy.** This transition zone extends into the vagina during adolescence and regresses into the endocervical canal with age. This cervical immaturity is an important risk factor for the development of CIN. CIN is associated with sexual activity, apparently by transmission of one or more oncogenic agents. It has been associated with HPV in particular but also with a history of HSV or chlamydial infection. Other associations include smoking, earlier onset of sexual activity, later onset of menarche, and more lifetime sexual partners. Long-term OCP use may increase the risk of disease, whereas barrier contraception exerts a slight protective effect. Possibly some of these factors work by increasing cervical vulnerability.

CIN is often asymptomatic but may present with abnormal vaginal bleeding or spotting. The most cost-effective method of diagnosis, although not as sensitive as colposcopy and biopsy, remains the Pap smear, which can sometimes also detect subclinical HPV infection. CIN I, II, and III refer to mild, moderate, and severe dysplasia, now also referred to as low-grade (CIN I) or high-grade (CIN II, III) squamous intraepithelial lesions. Abnormal Pap smears should be followed up vigilantly with colposcopy and biopsy to confirm the diagnosis and determine the extent of atypia. These lesions can eventually progress to invasive and metastatic disease. They may also regress. Treatment depends on the stage and extent of dysplasia; partners should also be examined for clinical and subclinical HPV disease.

Pelvic Inflammatory Disease (PID). This infection of the uterus, ovaries, fallopian tubes, and pelvic peritoneum is usually sexually transmitted. As PID can result in ectopic pregnancy or involuntary infertility due to scarring in the fallopian tubes, as well as chronic pain, it is a major cause of morbidity in female adolescents. Acute complications include tubo-ovarian abscesses and perihepatitis (Fitz-Hugh-Curtis syndrome).

Pelvic inflammatory disease is a polymicrobial infection. Pathogens such as *C trachomatis* or *N gonorrhoeae* ascend from the cervix along the endometrium to the fallopian tubes and peritoneum. This results in inflammation with an ensuing polymicrobial infection. Anaerobes are most frequently isolated. Nongonococcal, nonchlamydial anaerobes and aerobes can also initiate infection; the pathogenesis of these infections is poorly understood.

The typical signs and symptoms include lower abdominal pain, vaginal discharge, cervical motion tenderness, and uterine and adnexal tenderness. Guidelines for clinical diagnosis are presented in Table 2–13. Treatment should be considered whenever there is a high index of suspicion for PID, even when strict criteria are not met. The differential diagnosis is broad and includes most acute abdominal and pelvic processes (see Table 2–12).

Treatment requires broad-spectrum antibiotics because of the polymicrobial nature of infection; it should be instituted immediately, and the clinical course followed closely.

Proctitis. Proctitis, or inflammation of the rectal mucosa, may occur as an STD in male adolescents or female adolescents participating in anal intercourse or oral-anal activities, or by self-inoculation in women with cervical infections. The condition usually is painless unless the anus is also involved. Symptoms may include mucus or blood in the stools, loose stools, cramping, itching, or tenesmus and pain with defecation, which may lead to constipation. Physical examination may reveal a tender, inflamed anus with mucopurulent or bloody discharge. There is a wide variety of potential pathogens, including *C trachomatis, N gonorrhoeae, T pallidum,* and HSV, as well as food-borne enteric pathogens when anal intercourse is involved.

Table 2–13. Guidelines for the diagnosis of acute pelvic inflammatory disease.[1]

All three should be present:
Lower abdominal tenderness
Cervical motion tenderness
Adnexal tenderness (may be unilateral)
One of the following should be present:
Temperature ≥ 38 °C
White blood cell count ≥ 10,500/μL
Purulent material obtained by culdocentesis
Inflammatory mass present on bimanual pelvic exam ± sonogram
Erythrocyte sedimentation rate > 15 mm/h
Evidence of *Neisseria gonorrhoeae* or *Chlamydia trachomatis* in the endocervix
Gram stain with gram-negative diplococci
Monoclonal antibody for *C trachomatis*
> 5 white blood cells per oil-immersion field on Gram stain of endocervical discharge

[1]Reproduced, with permission, from Sweet RL: Pelvic inflammatory disease and infertility in women. Infect Dis Clin North Am 1987;1:199.

Numerous systemic illnesses may be contracted through sexual intercourse. These include, among others, syphilis, cytomegalovirus, hepatitis B, and HIV. HIV infection acquired in adolescence will most often be asymptomatic, unless the patient presents with acute retroviral syndrome during the initial phase of viremia. The course of illness in adolescents who acquire the infection more closely resembles that seen in adults than that of pediatric HIV infection. (For further discussion of HIV infections, see Chapter 9.) The clinician is wise to consider the possibility of an STD when evaluating an adolescent with systemic complaints.

APPROACH TO THE ADOLESCENT ENCOUNTER

INTRODUCTION

If it is to be successful, the nature of the physician-patient relationship changes to accommodate the developmental needs of the adolescent. As early adolescence involves individuation from the family, it is an appropriate time to begin seeing the patient alone for most of the visit. Often a transitional interview with the patient and parents is helpful at around 10 years of age, when these changes can be explained within a developmental context. Normal psychologic and physiologic development can be discussed, including the adolescent's need to take more responsibility and make decisions with adult guidance and support. Confidentiality is a critical component in the ensuing relationship; however, the limits should be made clear to the patient (see this chapter, Legal Issues). The interview should detail normal office procedures, which may include, depending on the age and interests of the patient and parental concerns, the adolescent initiating visits, taking an interval history from the parent and patient together and then each alone, examining the adolescent with the parent absent, and presenting findings and recommendations to the adolescent first. Successful health supervision necessitates respect for the adolescent's individuality, developing autonomy, and strengths.

The most pertinent elements of adolescent health care maintenance and screening are presented in Table 2–14. Salient features are discussed below. Yearly visits are indicated to monitor psychosocial development, support health-promoting behaviors, and screen for increasing participation in high-risk behaviors. Annual screening is also recommended for growth problems, iron deficiency, refractive errors, dental problems, scoliosis, hypertension, and thyroid disease. During any visit, whether for health assessment or care of a problem, it is crucial first to address the concerns of the adolescent.

Table 2–14. Most pertinent components of health supervision during adolescence.[1]

History
    Past medical history
        Immunizations: diphtheria-tetanus; poliovirus; measles, mumps, rubella; hepatitis B; Bacillus of
            Calmette-Guérin (tuberculosis vaccine)
        Chronic illness
    Family history
        Cardiovascular disease in parent or sibling who is younger than 55 years
    Review of systems (by history)
        Dietary habits and weight patterns
        Physical activity
        Dental history
        Menstrual history
    Psychosocial and medicosocial history
        HEADSS assessment[2] (see text)

Physical examination
    Height and weight with percentiles[2]; body mass index
    Blood pressure[2] and pulse
    Oral examination[2]
    Heart, lungs, and abdomen
    Spine (for scoliosis)[2]
    Breasts
    External genitalia
    Pelvic examination in girls (as indicated; see text)
    Skin, thyroid,[2] lymph nodes

Laboratory tests
    Hearing screening[3]
    Vision testing[2]
    Screen for iron deficiency[2,4]: complete blood count, transferrin saturation ratio, or free erythrocyte pro-
        toporphyrin[5]
    Tuberculosis skin test[6]
    Hyperlipidemia screening[7]

Sexually active adolescents
    Male adolescents
        Gonorrhea and chlamydia cultures[8,9]
        Syphilis serology (RPR or VDRL)[10]
        Hepatitis B surface antigen and antibody[10]
        HIV antibody[10]
    Female adolescents: Same as male adolescents, plus
        Papanicolaou smear[8]
        Wet mount for trichomonas[8]

Substance abuse
    Alcohol: liver enzymes (AST, ALT, GGT)
    Cigarettes: high-density lipoprotein cholesterol[10]
    Parenteral drugs: hepatitis B surface antigen and antibody, HIV antibody

[1]Adapted and reproduced, with permission, from Cromer BA et al: A review of comprehensive health screening in adolescents. J Adolescent Health 1992;13(Suppl 2):15S; Marks A, Fisher M: Health assessment and screening during adolescence. Pediatrics 1987;80(Suppl):135; Irwin CE Jr et al: The adolescent patient. Page 37 in: Rudolph AM et al (editors): *Rudolph's Pediatrics,* 20th ed. Appleton & Lange, 1996.
[2]Consider annual screening for all adolescents.
[3]If exposed to loud noises regularly or has recurrent otitis media.
[4]Minimally, females with moderate or heavy menses, chronic weight loss, malnutrition, or athletic activity should have annual hemoglobin or hematocrit.
[5]Consider serum levels of ferritin in competitive athletes.
[6]Perform annually in communities with prevalence greater than 1%, low socioeconomic status, exposure to tuberculosis, homelessness, Hispanic, black, Asian, Alaskan, and American Indian populations; among immigrant populations; among health care workers or history of incarceration; in all adolescents aged 14–16 years.
[7]Fasting serum lipid panel if positive family history for vascular disease before 55 years. Nonfasting total blood cholesterol minimally for adolescents older than 19 years or parental cholesterol of 240 mg/dL or greater.
[8]Annual screening.
[9]Leukocyte esterase by urine dipstick testing may be used as primary screening in males (with culture recommended if results are positive). Direct detection in clinical specimens also may be used, instead of culture, in areas with high rates of infection or without laboratory capability for culture.
[10]Consider in high-risk individuals; see text.
ALT = alanine aminotransferase; AST = aspartate aminotransferase; GGT = γ-glutamyltranspeptidase; RPR = rapid plasma reagin card test; VDRL = Venereal Disease Research Laboratories.

HISTORY

The psychosocial interview is foremost in the adolescent encounter. It is the means to assess the adolescent's progress with the tasks of this stage: separation and individuation from the family, development of a positive self-image and sexual identity, peer relationships, and a capacity for intimacy and planning one's future role in society. This interview is also used to screen for high-risk behaviors; one of the best predictors of these behaviors is the adolescent's intent to participate in them.

The psychosocial interview should be done in a direct, frank, and nonjudgmental manner, respecting the adolescent's need for privacy as much as possible. It is important to ask open-ended questions and to follow the flow of the conversation rather than cover an exact list of questions. For the younger adolescent, more sensitive areas, such as drugs and sexual practices, are best introduced within the context of the peer group (eg, "Some teenagers experiment with drugs or alcohol. Have any of your friends done this?"). Affirmative answers can be followed with direct questions about the individual.

A well-known, successful approach, known as the HEADSS method, structures the interview to move from more comfortable, less stressful topics to those that are most sensitive. The acronym stands for the following:

Home: Family structure, dynamics and relationships, general tone of the home environment, running away.

Education and employment: School performance and recent change thereof, relationships at school, employment part-time or as a substitute for school.

Eating: Weight changes and eating behaviors, both nutritional and social aspects; contribution of weight to self-esteem.

Activities: Peer-group fun, family, hobbies, sports, clubs, church, weekday and weekend, history of arrests.

Ambitions: Motivations, realistic educational and employment goals.

Affect: Frequent or marked mood swings; observe affect during interview.

Drugs: Alcohol, tobacco, and illicit drug use by peers, family, and patient, including amount and frequency, driving under the influence.

Sexuality: Orientation, practices, number of partners, history of pregnancy, STDs or abuse, contraception use, comfort and pleasure with sexual activities, associated drug use.

Suicide and depression: Suicidal ideation (specifics), history of attempts or depression, current signs or symptoms of depression, including depressive equivalents, such as somatoform symptoms.

Within a topic, questioning should move from more socially accepted behaviors (eg, alcohol) to the less accepted (eg, illicit drugs). Adolescents often deny sexual activity as well as drug use despite their participation in these behaviors. It may be helpful to reiterate a statement of confidentiality before the most sensitive questions pertaining to drugs and sexual behavior.

PHYSICAL EXAMINATION

The physical examination should be directed toward the nature of the complaint, if present. Examinations should be done with the parent absent, unless otherwise specified by the adolescent. It is appropriate to offer to have a same-sex assistant or chaperone present for more sensitive parts of the examination, (eg, genitalia or pelvic examinations, particularly for early adolescents). The examination may be used to offer reassurance about the normalcy of the adolescent's body, as many will have, but may not verbalize, such concerns. This time may be similarly used for demonstration of self-examination of breasts or testes, although the clinical utility of breast self-screening in this age group has been called into question. It may be educational to have adolescents stage their own sexual maturity with diagrams before the physical examination.

Other components of the examination that may be different from that of a younger child include skin examination for acne, oral examination for periodontal disease, Tanner staging, breast and pelvic examinations in girls, genitalia examinations in boys, thyroid palpation, scoliosis screening, muscle strength and joint flexibility, mental status examination for signs of depression or substance abuse, and detection of any other signs associated with high-risk behaviors, including trauma or sexual activity. Body mass index (BMI) should be determined, and the adolescent referred for dietary assessment and counseling for BMI either 95% or greater or 5% or lower for age and sex. A BMI of 85–95% indicates counseling for obesity.

Whereas external female genitalia are always examined, a pelvic examination is indicated for the sexually active adolescent, for evaluation of menstrual disorders, pelvic or lower abdominal pain, abnormal vaginal discharge or secondary dysmenorrhea, on request by the patient, or for routine health assessments in the older adolescent. Pelvic examination includes (1) external inspection, (2) speculum examination of the vagina and cervix, (3) bimanual vaginal-abdominal examination, and, if necessary, (4) rectovaginal-abdominal palpation of uterus and adnexae. Rectal examination is otherwise indicated in either sex for lower gastrointestinal complaints or a history of anal intercourse. Examination of male genitalia includes a thorough visual inspection of the penis and scrotum, retraction of the foreskin if present, compression of the glans to inspect the urethral meatus, palpation of scrotal contents, illumination of any intrascrotal masses, and assessment for the presence of a hernia at the inguinal ring.

LABORATORY EVALUATION

Screening tests and procedures for the well adolescent are summarized in Table 2–14. In addition, all sexually active teenagers should be screened for the presence of STDs. Specifically, as a minimum, male adolescents should be screened for urethritis and female adolescents for cervicitis and trichomonal infection. Testing for HIV antibody should be offered to all adolescents at risk, with appropriate pre- and post-test counseling; this includes those with multiple partners (including sequential monogamy), those with a history of STD, homosexual or bisexual males and their female partners, parenteral drug users and their sexual partners, those who engage in sex in exchange for drugs or money, those who are homeless, those who have received blood transfusions between 1977 and 1985, and anyone asking to be tested. Syphilis screening should occur in high-risk individuals as well, although the exact population that merits screening is controversial. Minimally, it includes male homosexuals, prostitutes, and sexually active adolescents in endemic areas; it also may include sexually active teens with a history of substance use or risk factors for HIV, except for blood transfusions. Screening for hepatitis B should be done in this same population. Sexually active females should be screened annually for cervical abnormalities with a Pap smear.

Screening for substance use is indicated for intoxications or other acute behavior changes, psychiatric symptoms, or accidental trauma. Screening is otherwise controversial, even to substantiate suspected use, as there is little to gain if the adolescent is not engaged in treatment and more to lose in terms of the physician-patient relationship. If there is known substance use, however, it may be useful to screen for sequelae such as liver damage with habitual alcohol use.

IMMUNIZATIONS

Most teenagers have received primary immunizations before starting school. Every effort should be made to obtain these records, as parental recall has been shown to correlate poorly with immune status. For those adequately immunized before school entrance, boosters may be required for tetanus and diphtheria (Td) and measles, mumps, rubella (MMR); primary hepatitis B virus vaccine should be administered if not done so previously. Td toxoid is recommended at 10-year intervals and so typically is due to be given at the 14- or 16-year visit, unless additional doses were given earlier for wound management. Current recommendations for MMR vaccines include a two-dose regimen, with the second dose to be given either before school entrance or during early adolescence, no later than 12 years of age. As this recommendation is relatively recent, many older adolescents may currently lack this MMR booster.

Pneumococcal, influenza, and either oral or inactivated poliomyelitis vaccines may all be indicated in special circumstances. Further information on immunizations is presented in Chapter 1.

PREVENTION

Risk-taking behaviors, as the major cause of injury and death in teenagers and young adults, are the primary target of health counseling in this age group. Modifiable risk factors for cardiovascular disease, a major killer of adults, are also important targets. Accordingly, national public health initiatives have established six priority behaviors for adolescents as the most effective, achievable lifetime behaviors to reduce potential life lost:

1. Use seat belts.
2. Do not drink (or use drugs) and drive.
3. If you have sex, use condoms.
4. Do not smoke.
5. Eat a low-fat diet.
6. Get regular aerobic exercise.

Other areas of anticipatory guidance to consider at appropriate ages are pubertal changes, nutrition, dental hygiene, contraception, avoidance of alcohol and drugs, safe use of recreational vehicles, and sports safety. Because behavior does not necessarily correlate with knowledge, the healthcare provider is wise to address resources and motivation as well. Resources might include condom supplies or refusal skills; motivation might include family rules requiring seat belts or behavioral contracts negotiated between the health care provider and the teenager, in which desired behaviors and rewards are documented. Encouraging and reinforcing healthy choices helps adolescents develop the self-responsibility necessary for personal health, school achievement, and job performance.

LEGAL ISSUES

Three primary areas of legal concern often arise in caring for adolescents: consent for treatment, confidentiality, and responsibility for payment of services. Refer to Chapter 24 for a full discussion of consent and confidentiality and ethical and legal issues involving the adolescent patient. Specific circumstances usually are governed by state laws, and clinicians should be informed of applicable laws in their state.

Responsibility for payment of services is usually that of the parent, unless the adolescent has sought care independently. In this case, the adolescent usually depends on public or private insurance or a variety of publicly funded programs; generally these sources are inadequate to ensure full access to care.

REFERENCES

Braverman PK, Strasburger VC: Why adolescent gynecology? Pediatricians and pelvic examinations. Pediatr Clin North Am 1989;36:471.

Cromer BA et al: A critical review of comprehensive health screening in adolescents. J Adolesc Health 1992;13(2 Suppl):1S.

Elster AM, Kuznets NJ: *AMA Guidelines for Adolescent Preventive Services (GAPS): Recommendations and Rationale.* Williams & Wilkins, 1993.

Farrow J: Adolescent medicine. Med Clin North Am 1990;74: 1085.

Green M (editor): *Bright Futures: Guidelines for Health Supervision of Infants, Children, and Adolescents.* National Center for Education in Maternal and Child Health, 1994.

Hatcher RA et al: *Contraceptive Technology, 1994–1996,* 16th ed. Irvington Publishers, 1994.

Irwin CE Jr et al: The adolescent patient. Page 37 in: Rudolph et al (editors): *Rudolph's Pediatrics,* 20th ed. Appleton & Lange, 1996.

Litt IF: *Evaluation of the Adolescent Patient.* Hanley & Belfus, 1990.

Rogers PD, Werner MJ: Substance abuse. Pediatr Clin North Am 1995;42:241.

Speroff L et al: *Clinical Gynecologic Endocrinology and Infertility,* 4th ed. Williams & Wilkins, 1989

3

Developmental & Behavioral Pediatrics

Tina Gabby, MD, MPH

Surveys reveal that parents are often more concerned about their children's behavior than about their physical well-being. To respond to the frequent challenges posed by behavioral problems in pediatrics, clinicians must remain attentive to a child's physiologic and psychological needs and to their interactions. Appreciating a child's developmental age and abilities will enhance understanding of problem behaviors. Because behavioral problems in children are influenced by their psychosocial environment, and family members are directly affected by a child's behavior, the evaluation and treatment plan should include the entire family.

The first section of this chapter focuses on understanding normal childhood behaviors. Common functional concerns relating to behavioral regulation will also be discussed. The next section is devoted to developmental and behavioral dysfunction seen in the classroom setting, followed by an overview of major psychopathologic disorders that affect children and adolescents. The final section reviews psychosocial issues that affect children and families in our society today.

COMMON FUNCTIONAL CONCERNS

CRYING & COLIC

Excessive crying or colic is one of the most common complaints during the first 3 months after birth and creates significant anxiety in parents. No comprehensive theory exists to explain colic, and reliable clinical treatment is not available to cure it. In 1962, T.B. Brazelton observed that median duration of crying in normal infants was 2.75 hours each day. Colic occurs in 15–30% of infants and is characterized by unexplained intermittent crying that lasts 3 hours a day for at least 3 days a week. Colic typically presents by 3 weeks of age and lasts until 3–4 months regardless of the management strategy used. Crying often occurs during the evening hours, but there may be no predictable pattern.

Colic is most likely of multifactorial etiology. Brazelton proposed that colic may serve as a normal physiologic function or a precursor to sociability. Others suggest that colic is a sign of neurologic lability or immaturity. The associated symptoms of abdominal distention, increased flatus, and flexing of the legs suggest to some that the infant is in pain. Accordingly, colic may indicate a painful disturbance of the gastrointestinal tract. (The term itself is derived from the Greek word meaning colon.) Gastrointestinal causes that have been suggested include abnormal peristalsis, increased flatus, gastrospasm, gastroesophageal reflux, visceral pain, and carbohydrate malabsorption. Only a few children with colic actually have lactose intolerance or a milk-protein allergy. Other explanations attribute colic to an intrinsically difficult temperament in the child or to a caretaker maladapted to parenting. Parents' perceptions of their baby's crying may be affected by prior expectations about what is normal. Colic affects parents with feelings of hopelessness, frustration, diminished confidence in parenting skills, and occasionally anger.

Evaluation of colic includes a thorough medical history; a description of the onset, duration, and character of crying; attempted approaches to manage crying; parental coping abilities; available family supports; and environmental stressors. A crying diary may be helpful in elucidating the patterns of crying. A thorough physical examination to exclude organic causes of infant irritability is a prerequisite to the diagnosis of colic (Table 3–1). This examination may provide credible reassurance to parents if no pathologic explanation is found.

An approach to the clinical management of an infant with colic is outlined in Figure 3–1. Just as one etiology cannot be determined, no single intervention will be effective for all infants with colic. Management begins by assuring parents that nothing is physically wrong with their child. Parents should be counseled on normal crying pat-

Table 3–1. Differential diagnosis of the irritable infant.

Gastrointestinal disorders
  Gastroesophageal reflux
  Volvulus
  Intermittent intussusception
  Constipation
  Anal fissure
  Milk allergy
  Carbohydrate intolerance
  Underfeeding/malnutrition
  Incarcerated hernia

Infections
  Urinary tract infection
  Sepsis
  Meningitis
  Osteomyelitis
  Otitis media

Neurologic disorders
  Subdural hematoma
  Skull fracture
  Central nervous system infections/meningitis
  Degenerative diseases

Cardiovascular disorders
  Congestive heart failure
  Cardiomyopathies
  Supraventricular tachycardias
  Cyanotic congenital heart disease
  Anomalous origin of coronary artery

Metabolic disorders
  Hyperthyroidism
  Hypoglycemia
  Hypocalcemia
  Inborn errors of metabolism

Psychosocial factors
  Child abuse/neglect
  Psychosocial deprivation
  Maternal depression

Miscellaneous
  Colic
  Testicular torsion
  Hair strangulation of digit
  Corneal abrasion
  Narcotic withdrawal syndrome
  Glaucoma
  Deafness

terns, the natural history of colic, and normal temperamental variation in infancy. Families should be reassured that infants cannot be spoiled. Because the number of infants with an actual milk allergy is small, switching formulas should be reserved for those infants with significant evidence of gastrointestinal distress. In most cases, parents should be discouraged from switching formulas, because of both the misconception that their child is allergic to cow's-milk formulas and the expense of alternative formulas. Medications, including antiflatulents and sedatives, are too frequently prescribed for the colicky infant and should be reserved for the most extreme cases.

Behavioral interventions should be encouraged with all colicky infants. Carrying the baby in a front-pack and the use of rockers, infant swings, strollers, and car rides often provide some relief. Monotonous noise, music, or singing also may be helpful. In attempting to calm the infant, caretakers may actually overstimulate the child; therefore, gentle handling should be encouraged. Parents should be encouraged to give each other "breaks" by taking turns during crying episodes as well as to plan for quality time together away from the infant. Parental support and respite are essential for parents who are emotionally and physically exhausted by the demands of an infant with colic. The time-limited nature of this problem is a relief to both parents and physicians.

SLEEP PROBLEMS

Sleep problems, which are among the more common behavioral concerns in early infancy and childhood, create exhaustion and frustration for parents. An understanding of normal sleep patterns and cycles is essential in helping parents deal with a child who has a disordered sleep pattern. Sleep regulation is dictated by neurophysiology, and sleep patterns are determined by parental, socioeconomic, and cultural factors as well.

Although the newborn infant sleeps 2–4 hours at a time throughout the day, nighttime sleep becomes consolidated and usually lasts 6–8 hours by 4 months of age. By 6 months, infants sleep 10–12 hours each day. Normal sleep is composed of two different states: rapid eye movement (REM) and non-REM sleep. Non-REM sleep is deep sleep from which it is difficult to arouse, whereas REM sleep is characterized by irregular pulse and respirations, rapid eye movements, and dreaming. The cycling between REM sleep, non-REM sleep, and waking shows major developmental progression in infancy and childhood. Premature infants spend 80% of sleep time in REM sleep, as opposed to 50% in term newborns and 25% in adults. Compared with adults, young children cycle rapidly through the different stages of sleep, and infants frequently arouse from REM sleep to awakening.

Because infants cycle quickly through their sleep, parents often misinterpret their child's groaning and movements during REM sleep with arousal and awakening. After 4–6 months of age, parents actually may reinforce a child's wakening if they intervene, pick up the child, and offer food. Breast-fed babies often wake more frequently during the night to feed, but whether differences in night wakening are caused by breast-milk composition, the body contact involved, or the mother-infant relationship is unclear.

Cultural differences in child rearing strongly influence sleep patterns. Few cultures, with the exception of the industrialized West, expect children to fall asleep independent of the caretakers. Many sleep problems that clinicians encounter involve children who have difficulty falling asleep at bedtime or awake in the middle of the night for parental attention. Co-sleeping, or least occasional sleeping in the parental bed, is often reported. Most studies reveal that children awaken more frequently when

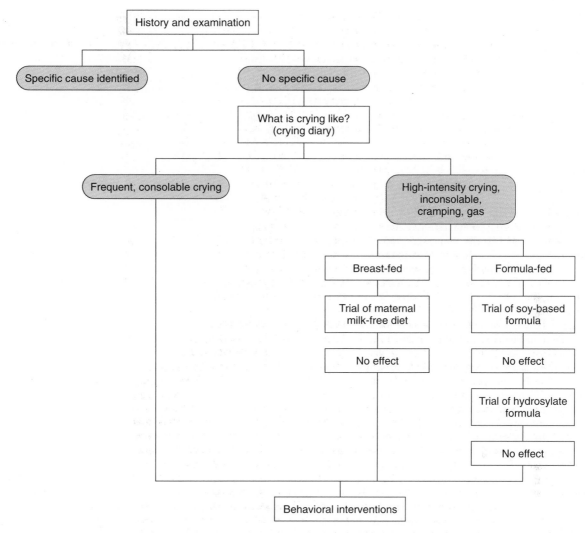

Figure 3–1. A clinical approach to colic. (Adapted and reproduced, with permission, from Geertsma MA, Hyams JS: Colic—a pain syndrome of infancy? Pediatr Clin North Am 1989;36:905.)

co-sleeping. Discussions with parents regarding nighttime awakening should include economic pressures (eg, only one bed in a family) and cultural expectations; caution should be exercised before labeling a child as having difficult sleep behavior.

Trouble going to sleep and night wakening may continue in the older toddler as well. Developmentally, parents and toddlers seem at odds; the toddler does whatever he or she can to stay awake, experience the world, and maintain contact with parents, whereas the exhausted caretaker wants only to sleep. As a child's imagination flourishes, the threat of monsters and other evils becomes very real at bedtime. Elaborate routines are often needed to reassure children that their room has been eradicated of potential threats.

Parasomnias

Parasomnias are events that occur during sleep or are induced or exacerbated by sleep. They often begin around the third year. When **nightmares** occur, a child wakes and expresses distress about the dream. Twenty-five to 50% of children aged 3–5 years will experience nightmares. Recurrent nightmares in later life often indicate stress or distress during a child's daytime life. **Night terrors** occur when a child appears to awaken in a frightened state, often yelling and flailing, but does not respond to caregivers. The child is amnestic of the event if asked about it the next morning. Night terrors represent a rapid transition from non-REM sleep to near arousal. They occur in up to 6% of children and are more common in boys. A family history is often elicited. Parents should be reassured that night terrors do not represent nightmares and will resolve of their own accord with time.

Somnambulism (sleep walking) and **somniloquy (sleep talking)** also occur. Sleep walking occurs between 4 and 8 years of age; 15% of children are affected before puberty. Sleep talking occurs during any stage of sleep, is likely underreported and very common, and is present throughout the life span. Parents can be reassured that a child's vocalizations do not imply awakening nor require intervention.

ENURESIS

Enuresis, the involuntary passage of urine, although usually benign in early childhood, may create significant distress in a child and family. Enuresis is more common in boys than in girls and is categorized as **primary** if a child has never been continent of urine, or **secondary** if incontinence develops after a period of at least 6 months of bladder control. Because 3-year-old children typically have the capacity to retain urine in their bladders, and 4-year-olds can voluntarily start and stop their urinary stream, lack of daytime bladder control after these ages indicates diurnal enuresis. About 90% of children are dry during the day by 4 years of age. **Nocturnal enuresis,** which is more common than diurnal enuresis, is defined as the involuntary passage of urine during the night in girls older than age 5 and boys older than age 6 years. Approximately 75% of children are dry during the night by age 4, increasing to 90% by age 8 years. The spontaneous cure rate of nocturnal enuresis is 15% per year; enuresis in adolescents is rare.

Etiology

Most causes of enuresis appear to be neuromaturational, but in about 5% of children there may be an organic, potentially treatable, etiology. Disorders involving increased bladder irritability, abnormal sphincter control, structural problems, or increased urinary output may lead to enuresis (Table 3–2). Enuresis appears to have a genetic component, because 75% of patients have a positive family history. Factors associated with enuresis include small bladder capacity, a tendency for bladder spasms, and central nervous system factors, as evidenced by the increased incidence of urinary incontinence in children with neurodevelopmental problems. Clinical data suggest that acute stressors, such as moving, marital discord, or the birth of a sibling, may exacerbate enuresis.

Evaluation

A careful history should include inquiry into family history, developmental milestones, significant life events, prior treatments, and symptoms of dysuria, urinary frequency, or hematuria. A thorough physical examination should be performed. Abdominal examination may reveal bladder distention or fecal impaction. The lower back may reveal lumbar anomalies. The external genitalia of girls

Table 3–2. Differential diagnosis of enuresis.

Increased bladder irritability
Urinary tract infection
Bladder spasms
Abnormal sphincter control
Bladder innervation problems
Neurogenic bladder
Spinal cord anomalies
Sphincter weakness
Structural problems
Urinary tract structural anomaly
Ectopic ureter
Epispadias
Vaginal reflux
Small bladder volume
Constipation
Vulvitis or vaginal trauma
Increased urinary output
Diabetes mellitus
Diabetes insipidus
Sickle cell anemia or trait
Emotional problems
Psychosocial stress
Psychosocial or social abuse
Regressive behavior
Other
Immature sleep patterns

[handwritten margin notes: • SZ's @ night; Drugs; • Li²⁺]

and the urethral meatus of boys should be closely inspected. A child's urinary stream should be observed if the history indicates. A rectal examination may reveal intrapelvic masses. Perianal sensation, anal tone, and gait are important elements of the neurologic examination.

Laboratory workup includes a screening urinalysis, including urine specific gravity, and urine culture. A sonogram, voiding cystourethrogram, or other urodynamic studies are indicated only in the few patients with a suspected organic etiology. Sickle cell disease should be excluded, because it may affect the ability to concentrate urine; thus, these children void frequently.

Treatment

Treatment of enuresis should focus on the underlying cause. Several behavioral techniques may assist in treatment of a child with neuromaturational enuresis. Because children are often embarrassed by their enuresis, they are often highly motivated to resolve their problem. The pediatrician should encourage them to participate actively in curing the problem. Parents should be advised to discourage fluid intake by the child after dinner. If feasible, parents should wake the young child several hours after sleep to void. Children should be expected to take responsibility for changing their linens, although never as a form of punishment. Incentive techniques are often helpful, such as star charts or positive reinforcements. Bladder stretching exercises of delayed micturition and the practice of starting and stopping streams have been helpful in children with small bladder capacities. If the above behavioral techniques fail despite adequate trials, an enuresis alarm may be used. These alarms are relatively inexpensive and rely on the principle of behavioral conditioning. Seventy-five percent of children with enuresis are dry within 4 months after beginning use of the alarm, although up to 20% may relapse. If enuresis persists, imipramine, a tricyclic antidepressant that has anticholinergic action on bladder muscle, may be effective, but relapse is common after discontinuation of the drug. Intranasal desmopressin, although expensive and controversial, may be used for short-term purposes, such as sleeping away from home.

ENCOPRESIS

Encopresis is defined as fecal soiling with formed or semi-formed stool after 4 years of age. This devastating problem is reported to occur in 1.5% of second-grade children and occurs much more commonly in boys than in girls (male-female ratio, 6:1). Encopresis is primary when a child has never achieved bowel control, or secondary when a child has had a period of successful bowel competency, although this distinction is often unclear. Afflicted children experience poor self-esteem and are prone to social withdrawal. Because encopresis creates stress within the family and exposes a child to peer ridicule, its management entails a comprehensive approach to the child and family.

Etiology

Encopresis may be attributed to somatic predispositions, genetic factors, inappropriate toilet-training techniques, and psychosocial influences. Early colonic inertia, a tendency toward immature or inefficient intestinal motility, often distinguishes the child who has had constipation since early infancy. A positive family history is found in 15% of patients with encopresis. Bowel dysfunction may also present at the time of toilet training, a time characterized by a child's autonomy and independence. Parents with coercive or extremely permissive toilet-training styles may potentiate a child's problem with bowel control. This is a time at which the withholding of stool and negative associations or avoidance of the toilet may develop.

By preschool age (3–4 years), some children may have an idiosyncratic avoidance of toilets, especially at school or in other public places. Out of fear, children may avoid using a toilet at school and consciously "hold" their stool. After a time, such a child loses the urge to defecate and develops constipation. Fecal impaction causes stretching of the colon and a loss of normal muscular control over the bowels. When defecation later occurs, it may be incomplete, resulting in constipation and incontinence.

Defecation may also be incomplete in children with attention deficits or hyperactivity, because they have a pervasive difficulty in finishing many tasks of daily living.

Encopresis may also be a manifestation of family problems, inconsistent parenting, abuse, or neglect. Some children with neuromotor problems, cerebral palsy, or spinal cord problems are especially prone to encopresis. Other medical problems such as Hirschsprung disease (aganglionic colon) or hypothyroidism need to be considered in any child with early constipation, although incontinence is relatively rare.

Assessment

Important historical information includes age of onset, habits of toilet use and training, and frequency of incontinence. Questions regarding current diet, psychosocial environment (marital strife, sibling issues, abuse, or neglect), social and attentional capacities, and peer and parental responses to the child's problem may reveal factors contributing to encopresis. A thorough physical examination should be performed with special attention to the child's abdominal and rectal examination. In uncomplicated encopresis, one typically finds a tubular mass of stool in the left lower abdomen along the course of the descending colon, a normal anal sphincter tone, and a dilated rectal vault with large fecal impaction on digital examination. Careful neurologic examination may reveal spinal cord lesions. A plain x-ray view of the abdomen may be helpful to assess the degree of stool retention before implementing vigorous catharsis. Rectal manometry is rarely indicated to rule out Hirschsprung disease.

Management

Treatment of encopresis should be initiated with a sensitive explanation of the pathophysiology of the problem to the child and family. Demystification of the problem is essential, and reviews of the etiology may be needed throughout therapy. Parents and children need reassurance that many other children experience similar problems, and feelings of guilt or blame should be assuaged. Commonly, parents of a child with encopresis exert inappropriate control over their child and become very involved in the problem. In these cases, further psychological counseling may be indicated to assist parents in allowing children to regain control of their own bodily functions.

Various approaches to the management of encopresis include relief of stool retention, encouragement of regular bowel habits, and restoration of normal neuromuscular bowel function (Table 3–3). Therapy is initiated with vigorous initial catharsis. Depending on the extent of fecal impaction, large doses of mineral oil may be used. Enemas and bisacodyl suppositories may be needed alternately for several cycles to ensure adequate clean-out. After initial catharsis is complete, a training routine should be established. Maintenance therapy with daily mineral oil should be instituted, and regular visits to the toilet—10 minutes after each meal—should be required. Positive reinforcement enhances increased bowel autonomy. Close follow-up for up to 6 months is essential because compliance problems and relapses are common.

Table 3–3. Management of the encopretic child.[1]

Initial counseling
Education and demystification of the problem
Removing blame
Explaining treatment plan
Initial catharsis
For severe retention: enemas × 3
Bisacodyl suppositories as supplement
For moderate retention: mineral oil (1–2 oz 2 × day)
Maintenance therapy
Mineral oil (tapered over 4–6 mo)
Child sits on toilet 2 × day for 10 min
Multiple vitamins between mineral oil doses
Adding roughage to diet (bran, cereal, vegetables)
Increasing fluid intake
Ongoing counseling
Repeated explanations
Positive reinforcement
Monthly visits to assess compliance
Attending to associated psychological issues

[1]Adapted and reproduced, with permission, from Levine M: Encopresis. Page 394 in: *Developmental-Behavioral Pediatrics,* 2nd ed. Saunders, 1992.

PAIN IN CHILDHOOD

Only recently has the clinical importance of pediatric pain been emphasized. Pain in neonates and children has been underreported, misunderstood, and undertreated. Because young children are often nonverbal and cannot complain about the extent of their pain, it has been assumed that children do not experience pain to the same degree as adults.

Fear of using powerful narcotics or the risk of addiction has also led clinicians to steer away from using appropriate pain management in children. A general discussion about the assessment and treatment of pain and the chronic pain syndromes of childhood follows.

Certain myths persist that contribute to the undertreatment of pain in childhood. Children's immature nervous systems and their lack of memory for pain have been rationales for not treating children in pain. Cutaneous sensory perception develops between the 7th and 20th weeks of gestation. Recent convincing anatomic and physiologic research exists to show that even premature infants undergoing procedures in the intensive care nursery experience pain. Neonates undergoing heel lancing and circumcision have distinct cries, changes in heart rates, and body movements. Even young children develop anticipatory fear of pain, often seen in the pediatric office as children return frequently for immunizations in the first few years of life. As children mature cognitively and verbally, they are better able to express their pain.

In interpreting children's pain, it is important to consider a child's developmental understanding of pain. In early infancy, children have no apparent understanding of pain, but memory for pain likely exists. As the infant ages, pain response includes sadness and anger. Between 1 and 2 years of age, children develop both fear of painful situations and the ability to localize and verbalize pain (eg, "owie" and "boo-boo"). Between 2 and 3 years of age, children develop increasing abilities to cope with pain and describe external causes of their pain. After 3 years, children are better able to discuss the intensity of pain and to use cognitive coping strategies or distractions to deal with pain. Not until age 7–10 years can children explain why a pain hurts. The importance of understanding a child's development in the expression and interpretation of painful events cannot be overestimated. Equally important are familial and cultural influences on a child's response to pain. Children vary in their response to pain just as adults do. The stoic child may be responding in an expected manner just as the "hysterical" child may have learned the behavior from other family members.

Psychological and socioeconomic factors are also important determinants of a child's response to pain. Despite our knowledge about developmental and cultural influences on pain, children continue to be poorly informed about pain, its significance, and ways to deal with it.

Physiologic measurements, including heart rate, blood pressure, palmar sweating, and serum levels of cortisol, have been used to assess the pain response in children. More often, clinicians rely on behavioral assessments (eg, cry, facial expression, and body movements) and physical signs of sympathetic activity to assess pain. Subjective self-report methods for pain assessment are often used in children older than 6 years. In less verbal children, pain assessment scales, which include drawings of cartoon faces with varying facial expressions from smiling to crying, are projective measures.

Treatment

Although specific pharmacotherapeutics are not discussed here, certain principles of drug management are important to review. Clinicians need to think of pain as a priority.

Dosing of pain medication should be fixed and not written "as needed" or "prn" in a postoperative patient, as children may not be capable of, or comfortable, asking for pain medication. Patient-controlled anesthesia may be useful in more mature children with chronic pain. The clinician should not be consumed with worry about addiction in children. Help should be sought from experienced professionals in the selection of appropriate drugs and dosages for children.

Nonpharmacologic techniques of pain management may be especially useful in clinical settings with anxious children. Clinicians should keep the child and parents informed about what to expect in preparation of a painful procedure. Distractions, relaxation therapies, deep-breathing exercises, and guided imagery may be useful tools at the bedside. Hypnotherapy can be useful in children with chronic pain as hypnotic susceptibility increases with age. With training, a school-aged child or adolescent can practice self-hypnosis to induce relaxation, focus attention, and create distraction from pain. Acupuncture is not well studied in children but has been found to be of benefit in adults with neuropathic pain, chronic headaches, and chest pain.

Recurrent Pain Syndromes in Childhood

Complaints of recurrent pain present a frustrating dilemma to clinicians, children, and parents. Costly laboratory, radiographic, and other diagnostic testing must be undertaken prudently to exclude organic causes. Because exhaustive studies may provide no answers, children and parents may become frustrated. Important days at school and work may be missed, and a child's normal activity level is usually diminished. Chronic pain is often accompanied by symptoms of depression, which further contribute to the diminished functioning of the child and family. When no organic etiology is detected, it is essential that the clinician understand that the pain is real to the child. The pain may represent other stresses in the child's life and may serve as a way for the child to receive attention for these problems. The most common of all the pain syndromes is chronic abdominal pain; however, the spectrum of pain syndromes in childhood is extensive (headaches, chest pain, limb pain). (See Chapter 13 for a discussion on chronic abdominal pain.)

DEVELOPMENTAL VARIATION IN THE SCHOOL-AGED CHILD

ATTENTION-DEFICIT HYPERACTIVITY DISORDER

Definition & History

This popular German children's rhyme by Hoffman, *Struwel Peter,* quoted by M. Stewart, reveals the characteristic nature of the child with attention-deficit hyperactivity disorder (ADHD):

> Fidgety Phil
> He won't sit still
> He wiggles
> He giggles. . . .

Although ADHD presents a characteristic clinical profile (Table 3–4), understanding of the etiology is elusive, and successful treatment is often difficult. Many terms have been used to describe the syndrome, including **minimal brain dysfunction, hyperkinetic child syndrome,** and the **hyperactive child,** yet none adequately describes the constellation of findings. Children with ADHD typi-

Table 3–4. Diagnostic criteria for attention-deficit hyperactivity disorder (ADHD).[1]

A. Either (1) or (2), of at least 6 months' duration:
  1. Six or more of the following symptoms of inattention:
     a. Fails to give close attention to work
     b. Difficulty sustaining attention in tasks or play activities
     c. Often does not seem to listen when spoken to directly
     d. Trouble following through on directions or fails to finish schoolwork
     e. Difficulty organizing tasks and activities
     f. Reluctant to engage in tasks that require sustained mental effort
     g. Often loses things necessary for school activities
     h. Easily distracted by extraneous stimuli
     i. Often forgetful in daily activities
  2. Six or more of the following symptoms of hyperactivity-impulsivity:
     Hyperactivity
     a. Often fidgets with hands or feet and squirms in seat
     b. Often leaves seat in classroom when remaining seated is expected
     c. Often runs or climbs excessively
     d. Often has difficulty playing or engaging in leisure activities quietly
     e. Often "on the go" or "driven by a motor"
     f. Often talks excessively
     Impulsivity
     g. Often blurts out answers before questions completed
     h. Often has difficulty awaiting turn
     i. Often interrupts or intrudes on others (in conversation or games)
B. Symptoms present before age 7 years
C. Impairment from symptoms in two or more settings (school and home)
D. Symptoms not accounted for by other diagnoses (eg, pervasive developmental disorder, schizophrenia, or anxiety disorder)

[1]Modified and reproduced, with permission, from *Diagnostic and Statistical Manual of Mental Disorders,* 4th ed. American Psychiatric Association, 1994.

cally are of normal intelligence but have abnormal behavior characterized primarily by inattention, distractibility, impulsivity, and hyperactivity. They often perform poorly at school and have learning disabilities, poor peer relationships, aggressive behavior, and emotional lability.

An estimated 3–5% of children in the United States have ADHD, making this the most common behavioral disorder of childhood. Boys are more frequently affected than girls (male-female ratio, 6:1). Hyperactivity often presents in early childhood. Parents describe their infants as excessively active, restless, and irritable. Older children typically have difficulty sitting still, although their activity level may fluctuate. A child's hyperkinesis usually resolves by age 12, with residual symptoms of short attention span and social immaturity. Learning disabilities including dyslexia, aphasia, or dyspraxia are present in 25–50% of these children, imposing serious burdens on the school system.

Diagnosis & Testing

A careful history is essential to formulate the diagnosis of ADHD. Interviews with all caretakers, teachers, or day-care workers are important, because a child with ADHD symptoms at home, but not at school, suggests some family dysfunction. A thorough evaluation of home and school environment, as well as study of a child's developmental history, may reveal complicating behavioral factors. Various assessment procedures may be indicated, including parent and teacher questionnaires, formal neuropsychological testing, or educational testing. A physical and neurologic examination is essential. Currently, no laboratory studies confirm the clinical diagnosis of ADHD, although screening tests for lead or iron-deficiency anemia should be considered in the young child. A hearing screen or formal audiometry evaluation may be indicated; electroencephalography, magnetic resonance imaging, and computed tomography have not proved helpful.

Treatment

Because ADHD is influenced by physical, psychological, and social factors, successful treatment depends on a comprehensive approach to the child, including family counseling. Explanations regarding the neurodevelopmental basis of this disorder may help relieve parental guilt. These children thrive on order and structure in their environment, so that developing routines and consistency in discipline is of utmost importance. A dynamic, individualized school program with small teacher-pupil ratio is optimal. Pediatricians should be available to discuss strategies for optimal performance with school professionals, and frequent reassessments of the child are necessary.

Central nervous system stimulant medication has a striking beneficial effect on the behavior of approximately 75% of children with ADHD. Because deficient dopaminergic transmission has been proposed as an explanation for the etiology of ADHD, methylphenidate hydrochloride (Ritalin) and dextroamphetamine sulfate (Dexedrine) are commonly used to treat ADHD. These drugs facilitate the synthesis and release of norepinephrine and dopamine and inhibit monoamine oxidase. Stimulants may improve attention span and fine motor and social skills and diminish impulsive behavior. Handwriting often improves. The effects of stimulant medication on academic performance are less clear. Many of the medications used to treat ADHD have adverse side effects. Parents should be counseled that increased hyperactivity, lethargy, emotional lability, anorexia, insomnia, and growth retardation may be seen. If therapy with methylphenidate exacerbates a previously unknown movement disorder, especially tics or Tourette syndrome, medication should be discontinued immediately. Because studies have not substantiated diet as a factor in the etiology of ADHD, parents should be counseled that most dietary manipulations (eg, restricting sugar) will neither hurt their child nor contribute to the disorder.

SCHOOL PROBLEMS & LEARNING DISABILITIES

Learning problems can be attributed to numerous causes operating independently or in combination. Learning disabilities, mental retardation, attentional or behavioral problems, neurologic and sensory impairment, and physical disabilities or chronic illness may affect school performance. Family dysfunction, psychological problems, and social stressors also may contribute to school problems.

An estimated 5–10% of children in the United States have some type of learning disability (LD). Specific disabilities or specific developmental disorders in the *Diagnostic and Statistic Manual of Mental Disorders (DSM IV)* are divided into learning disorders, communication disorders, and motor skills disorders. Learning disorders involve difficulties with reading, arithmetic, and expressive writing. Communication disorders primarily involve expressive and receptive language difficulties. Motor skill disorders involve problems with fine and gross motor functioning. Children may have subtle or obvious deficits in functioning, and children often may have more than one area of disability noted in their LD profile.

Learning differences may be organized according to difficulties with input, integration or processing, and output of information (Table 3–5). Difficulties with auditory discrimination or listening comprehension, if severe, are often easily identifiable. These children may understand only very concrete language and may have limited verbal expression. Students with such receptive language disorders may have behavioral problems outside the classroom as they may not understand conversations with peers and may have difficulty with verbal instructions and socializ-

Table 3–5. Description of specific learning disabilities.

A. Input disabilities
    1. Visual perceptual disabilities
       a. Perception with letters rotated or reversed
       b. Errors in judging depth or distance
    2. Auditory perceptual disabilities
       a. Difficulty distinguishing subtle differences in sounds
B. Integration disabilities
    1. Stimuli needs to be processed, organized, and comprehended
       a. Sequencing (disorganized recall of story events)
       b. Abstraction (unable to derive meaning from a particular word or symbol)
       c. Organization (impaired facility with acquired concepts)
C. Memory disability
    1. Short-term memory (more common)
    2. Long-term memory
D. Output disabilities
    1. Language disability
       a. Spontaneous language
       b. Language "on-demand"
    2. Motor disabilities
       a. Fine motor (paper-pencil tasks)
       b. Gross motor (coordination, balance)

ing in general. Children with oral expressive language disabilities may have difficulty retrieving words to use in sentences, much like the adult **aphasic** patient who has impaired speech secondary to a stroke in the dominant language centers of the brain. They may have difficulty using multisyllabic words and organizing their ideas in response to questions. Other language problems include difficulty with pragmatics, or the use of language in context. Children may also have poor nonverbal communication; they may lack appropriate eye contact or gestures that accompany speech or may use inappropriate rhymes, inflections, or loudness when speaking.

Articulation problems, if severe, may result in learning difficulties. **Dysarthria** is a disturbance in articulation because of problems in the neurologic control of the oromotor muscles used for speech production.

One of the most common problems associated with learning disabilities is **dyslexia.** Developmental dyslexia implies failure to acquire reading skills along the usual developmental time course. Reading is crucial to success in school; therefore, acquisition of knowledge is seriously impaired if a child has reading difficulties.

The primary defect appears to be in verbal coding; reliable recall and linking of specific speech sound units (phonemes) with their representative written letters, or vice versa, is often impaired. Dyslexia is thought to be a familial disorder of varying degrees of severity and affects boys and girls equally. Many children with dyslexia have excellent oral language; others, however, have language problems like those described above. In addition to reading problems, many individuals with dyslexia have problems with spatial relationships, directionality, and left-right discrimination.

Some professionals also use the term dyslexia to refer to difficulties in written language. Handwriting problems usually are readily identifiable as early as kindergarten. It is essential to determine whether writing difficulties are maturational or caused by developmental factors, rather than secondary to learning difficulties. Often, poor handwriters have other visual-spatial difficulties, including some aspects of math, drawing, and self-help skills such as tying shoes. Spelling problems are common developmentally, but some children write as words sound or have limited visual memory.

Mathematical skills, like other forms of symbolic behavior, also may be impaired. Memory deficits, faulty instruction, anxiety, lack of motivation, or lower intelligence may affect math skills. If oral language, visual-spatial, or memory deficits are present, math will be affected. Some students may have global symbolic deficits, and reading and math may be affected simultaneously.

Recently, the term "nonverbal" learning disorders has emerged. These "right-brain" disorders have in common deficits in spatial cognition and analysis. Social problems abound as these children have difficulty interpreting or using nonverbal communication, including body language, gestures, and facial expressions. These children seem to lack "common sense" in assessing social situations and responding appropriately.

Diagnosis

One must rely on the medical and developmental history and on physical and neurologic examinations to rule out neurologic insults as a basis for the suspected LD. Evaluation of the child's social history is essential to identify stresses at home. After reviewing a child's school performance with teachers, inconsistencies in performance should be noted (Table 3–6). Physical examination should include assessment of "soft" neurologic signs, (eg, poor fine-motor coordination, finger agnosia, and right-to-left disorientation). Although these signs may represent normal variation, they may represent neurologic dysfunction when seen in school-aged children with learning difficulties. Further diagnostic testing is essential. Psychoeducational testing reveals a child's cognitive style, strengths and weaknesses, and ability to develop and implement strategies to learn. Psychological assessment may consist of neuropsychological, clinical, or educational psychological evaluation.

Management

Clinicians should be aware of Public Law 94-142, the Education for Handicapped Children Act. This national legislation mandates that children with neurologically based LDs or significant school failure be provided with educational services appropriate to their needs. Parents are entitled to request and receive an evaluation of the child's learning needs free of charge; if found to qualify, the child will obtain special education services. Pediatricians play an essential role in educating families about their rights and serving as advocates throughout this sometimes cumbersome, bureaucratic process. Children with significant LDs who qualify for special education services may receive resource specialist help, specialized tutoring, or special day classes. Educational interventions should be

Table 3–6. Recognizing a child with learning problems.

Classroom Behavior	Academic Problems	Motor Skills
Moves constantly	*Reading*	Poor coordination
Quiet or withdrawn	Dysfluencies	Problems with
Disorganized	Poor compre-	balance
Poor peer relation-	hension	Confuses right
ships	Letter reversals	and left
Misunderstands	Story problems	Poor muscle
often	*Arithmetic*	strength
Distractible	Confuses sym-	Lacks rhythm
Daydreams	bols	Poor handwriting
Reluctant participa-	Poor math con-	Poor drawing
tion	cepts	Poor copying
Poor planning skills	*Writing*	
Incomplete projects	Difficulty copying	
Disturbs classmates	Slow in completion	
Unpredictable	Cannot stay on line	

individualized to take advantage of a child's cognitive strengths. Information garnered from educational testing will be helpful to teachers in highlighting strategies that may be taught to bypass the LD. Positive reinforcement is important to all children and especially to those with LD who may have poor self-esteem. Psychological counseling may be necessary in the child whose psychosocial situation contributes significantly to learning problems. Parents should be encouraged to avoid the many unsubstantiated treatments that have been touted as cures for LDs (eg, diets, vision training, hypnosis, and antihistamines).

SCHOOL PHOBIA

Most children, at some point in time, express reluctance to attend school. In comparison, the child with school phobia, school refusal, or the school avoidance syndrome often misses weeks or months of school because of complex psychosocial factors. Although actual prevalence figures are unknown, this condition is estimated to occur in 0.4% of all school children. Boys and girls are affected equally, and the condition is most often seen in the early teenage years. The onset of school avoidance may occur after a period of illness or a holiday or during periods of family stress or upheaval. The child may express anxiety in the morning, which will dissipate as the day progresses. Somatic complaints are common, ranging from nonspecific feelings of illness to specific chronic complaints of headache or abdominal pain. Unlike school phobia, truancy refers to the antisocial child who attempts to stay away from home or school and conceal the absence from parents. The differences between school phobia and school truancy are highlighted in Table 3–7.

Children with school refusal are often perceived by overprotective caretakers as being exceedingly vulnerable and dependent. They may be extremely manipulative, perfectionistic, depressed, or deprived. Severely disturbed children with dysfunctional families also may avoid school for long periods of time. Many children with school avoidance have associated psychiatric problems, including anxiety disorders, depression, and separation anxiety disorder.

Because most cases of school refusal represent some

Table 3–7. Features of school phobia and truancy.

School Phobia	School Truancy
Most common in early teen years	Common throughout adolescence
Child remains home with parents' knowledge	School absence concealed from parents
Parents attempt to have child return to school	Parents ineffective in ensuring attendance
No antisocial behavior	Often severe antisocial behavior
Child fearful at thought of going to school	No fears of school
	Child appears apathetic, bored

family problem, it is essential to include the family in the treatment plan. A sensitive clinician, or a therapist trained in more complicated cases, should inquire about legitimate threats at school and review for signs of child abuse and neglect. If there is a specific threat at school, the health professional may recommend that the school experience be adapted or structured to diminish the threat (eg, change seating or physical education classes). Somatic complaints should be taken seriously, and a medical workup should be pursued as indicated by the history. The child should be given positive reinforcements to return to school, and the clinician should work cooperatively to facilitate reentry. When anxiety appears generalized, ongoing counseling or psychotherapy may be needed. Medications may be needed in extreme cases to relieve anxiety.

PSYCHOPATHOLOGY

AUTISM

Definition & Etiology

Autism, the most severe form of pervasive developmental disorder (PDD), is a behaviorally defined disorder that presents before 30 months of age and is characterized by three primary features: impaired social interactions, impaired communication and language, and marked restriction in activity and interests. The three defining characteristics of autism vary considerably in severity depending on the child's intelligence, language abilities, and personality. Diagnostic criteria for autism are shown in Table 3–8.

Autism is relatively uncommon, affecting approximately 2–5 per 10,000 children. It is more common in males (male-female ratio, 3:1), and manifests in all races and social classes. Thirty-three percent of autistic children are severely retarded (IQ < 40), 38% have mild to moderate retardation (IQ 40–70), and 29% have borderline to normal intelligence (IQ > 70). The child with autism and severe mental retardation typically has dramatic behavioral manifestations, including stereotypic motor behaviors such as spinning, flapping hands, and rocking.

Early theorists popularized the notion that autism resulted from parental unresponsiveness or rejection. It is now apparent that deviant child-rearing practices do not account for autism, although parents of autistic children may experience appreciable stress, anxiety, or depression. Autism is familial, as reflected in the increased risk in siblings of autistic children. (Monozygotic twins have a concordance rate of 64% versus 9% in dizygotic twins.) Potential genetic mechanisms include autosomal recessive inheritance, X-linked inheritance, and sporadic chromosomal anomalies. Children with the specific chromosomal

Table 3–8. Criteria for autistic disorder.[1]

A. A total of six or more items from (1), (2), and (3) below, with at least 2 from (1) and one each from (2) and (3):
  1. Qualitative impairment in social interaction:
     a. Marked impairment in nonverbal behaviors, such as eye-to-eye gaze, facial expression, body postures to regulate social interaction
     b. Failure to develop peer relations appropriate to developmental level
     c. Lack of spontaneous seeking to share enjoyment, interests, or achievements with other people
     d. Lack of social or emotional reciprocity
  2. Qualitative impairments in communication:
     a. Delay in, or total lack of, development of spoken language
     b. When speech is present, marked impairment in ability to initiate or sustain a conversation with others
     c. Stereotyped and repetitive use of language or idiosyncratic language
     d. Lack of varied, spontaneous make-believe play or social imitative play appropriate to developmental level
  3. Restricted, repetitive, stereotyped patterns of behavior, interest, and activities:
     a. Preoccupation with one of more stereotyped and restricted patterns of interest that is abnormal either in intensity or focus
     b. Inflexible adherence to specific, nonfunctional routines or rituals
     c. Stereotyped and repetitive motor mannerisms (eg, hand flapping)
     d. Persistent preoccupation with parts of objects
B. Delays or abnormal functioning in at least one of the following areas, with onset before 3 years of age: (1) social interaction, (2) language as used in social communication, or (3) symbolic or imaginative play.
C. Does not meet the criteria for Rett disorder or childhood disintegrative disorder.

[1]Adapted and reproduced, with permission, from *Diagnostic and Statistical Manual of Mental Disorders,* 4th ed. American Psychiatric Association, 1994.

abnormality fragile X have an increased incidence of autism. Accordingly, a careful physical examination and chromosomal analysis should be performed. Recently, a neurodevelopmental abnormality in the biochemistry or anatomy of the brain has been thought to contribute to autistic features. An increased incidence of seizures, especially in autistic adolescents, support a neurologic etiology.

Clinical Description

Reports of parents reveal that autistic infants often have unusual patterns of development. Infants may fail to respond to social gestures or to make eye contact and may not appear to be attached to the primary caretaker. Peer relationships may be lacking, and autistic children often prefer solitary play. Within the first 2 years after birth, these children typically show delayed speech and language development; language may be unusual in rate, rhythm, and intonations. Echolalia, poor semantic development, and inappropriate nonverbal communication (absence of pointing, eye movements, gestures) are commonly seen.

Autistic children have impaired imitation, a feature of normal child development that is critical for language acquisition. They may have repetitive body movements, such as spinning, flapping, and rocking, and ritualistic behaviors, such as lining up toys, repetitive routines, and turning lights on and off. Higher-functioning autistic children may have "idiot savant" abilities and may have one specific area of developmental genius (eg, musical or numerical abilities). Self-injurious behaviors, such as head banging, make the low-functioning, older autistic child difficult to manage.

Prognosis & Management

The prognosis of autism depends on a child's intelligence, language abilities, personality, and family factors. Children with the lowest IQs have the worst outcomes. One third of autistic children become capable of some degree of self-sufficiency as adults, although residual difficulties in social relationships and communication may persist. Special education efforts may improve long-term adaptability.

Unfortunately, autism has no cure. Moreover, uniform approaches to managing the autistic child have not been established. Advocacy for patients and their families is a critical part of the management of any child with autism or PDD. Behavioral techniques in educational remediation may be needed in the lower-functioning child with severe behavioral problems. Intensive therapies targeting communication and social skills have shown dramatic improvements in higher-functioning autistic children. National and local autism societies and parent support groups are available to provide support to families with autistic children. Pharmacologic therapies have a limited role in the management of autistic children. Neuroleptic medication (tranquilizers) may decrease the problem behaviors and activity level that interfere with learning. Trials of the antipsychotic medication haloperidol have also resulted in improved behavioral performance and learning in some autistic children.

DEPRESSION IN CHILDHOOD & ADOLESCENCE

According to the *DSM-IV,* depression is characterized by a pervasive sadness, diminished interest, or loss of pleasure in nearly all activities. In children, the mood may be irritable rather than sad. The depressed child experiences profound helplessness, frustration, and failure at home and school. Depression in childhood is most common in female adolescents. Estimates of the incidence of depression vary: 5–20% for adolescents, 1–5% for prepubertal children, and 0.5–1% for preschool children. Depression is more common in children with attentional deficits, learning disabilities, and chronic illness.

Evidence suggests that depression is genetically determined. Depressed children often have mothers with a history of depression or other family members with bipolar disease. Monozygotic twin studies reveal a concordance rate of 76%, compared with a 19% concordance rate for dizygotic twins. Psychobiologic parameters also may contribute to depression. A dexamethasone suppression test (DST) is positive in 50% of depressed adults and adolescents; the DST normalizes after treatment. Environmental factors influence the expression of depression, as evidenced by the 67% concordance rates in monozygotic twins reared apart. Associated findings of marital discord, family violence, and child physical or sexual abuse are often noted in children with depression.

Clinical Manifestations

The clinical spectrum of depression varies according to the child's age (Table 3–9). Typically, depressed infants have lost their primary caretaker or have had insufficient nurturing; they may eat and grow poorly, appear apathetic, and have a watchful gaze. Older children may be sad, moody, and irritable and may cry easily. Children may speak in negative terms: "I'm stupid" or "No one loves me." Frequent somatic complaints, school avoidance, or poor school performance are hallmarks of the depressed school-aged child. Symptoms in older children and adolescents are similar to those in adults. Along with suicidal ideation or attempts, change in sleep and appetite patterns may occur. Depressed teenagers may have escalated high-risk behaviors of promiscuity and of drug and alcohol abuse.

Management

A thorough medical history and physical examination are important. Thyroid studies should be performed if the clinical examination is consistent with hypothyroidism. Major goals of acute management involve determining suicidal potential, precipitating factors, and appropriate disposition. Individual or family therapy and educational assessment and planning are components of successful long-term management programs.

Some depressed individuals respond dramatically to tricyclic antidepressants, despite limited scientific evidence to support medications as superior to other modalities of treatment. Major side effects of medications should be reviewed. Drowsiness and anticholinergic effects (dry mouth, constipation, and blurred vision) are common, but rarely severe enough to discontinue the medication. Imipramine may cause cardiac conduction slowing and arrhythmias. Accordingly, a baseline electrocardiogram should be obtained and monitored with changes in dose.

Outcomes

Depressive disorders often run a chronic, recurrent course. Even after recovery from depression, children may show serious social impairment. Adult sequelae of childhood depression include drug use, antisocial behavior, and increased risk of suicide.

MUNCHAUSEN SYNDROME BY PROXY

Munchausen syndrome by proxy (MSBP) is a complex, difficult problem for clinicians to manage. This relatively uncommon disorder is a variant of the classic Munchausen syndrome of adults, in which the individual fabricates elaborate physical symptoms. These patients often undergo extensive medical evaluations and hospitalizations. MSBP is a form of child abuse in which the caretaker, typically the mother, persistently fabricates symptoms on behalf of the child. The severity of the syndrome and the extent of the fabrication are variable. Some mothers report false symptoms, and their children are only subjected to diagnostic testing. In most extreme cases, children may be physically harmed or even killed. Often difficult to diagnose, MSBP may go undetected for years. Warning signals that should alert the clinician include illness that is unexplained, prolonged, and often extraordinary; signs and symptoms that are incongruous or inappropriate; symptoms only in the presence of the parent (usually the mother is the perpetrator); ineffective or poorly tolerated treatments; a mother who appears less worried about the child's illness than is the clinician; a mother who forms unusually close, dependent relationships with the staff; a mother with nursing or medical experience who has extensive medical problems; and families in which prior episodes of abuse or sudden infant death have occurred.

Treatment of MSBP is extremely difficult. Once the diagnosis is definitive, the physician must confront the perpetrator. Protective service agencies need to be notified in most cases in which the child has been abused and requires continued protection. The perpetrator should then be required to undergo psychiatric evaluation and treatment.

Table 3–9. Signs of depression.

Infants	Childhood	Adolescents
Poor weight gain	Sadness	Change in sleep patterns
Listlessness	Somatic complaints	Change in appetite
Watchful gaze	Poor school performance	Suicidal ideation/attempts
Passive, quiet	Low self-esteem Cries frequently	Psychomotor agitation
		Psychomotor retardation

PSYCHOSOCIAL ISSUES

DIVORCE

As early as the 19th century, when divorce was uncommon, the consequences of marital dissolution for children were debated. None of the participants in these debates ever contemplated an era when divorce would be as prevalent as it is today. The social changes of the past 30 years in the United States are reflected in decreasing marriage rates, increasing rates of childbirth outside marriage, and increasing rates of divorce; consequently, increasing numbers of children are living in single-parent households.

Currently, more than 50% of first marriages are expected to end in divorce. Seventy-five percent of African-American children will experience their married parents' divorce before the age of 18 years. Each year since the 1970s, more than 1 million children were affected by divorce. The impact of divorce persists; in 50% of families that experience divorce, another major transition, remarriage, occurs within 5 years. Despite the frequency with which divorce occurs, many pediatric care providers fail to provide guidance during this critical process.

Only now is a consensus beginning to emerge among social scientists about the effects of divorce on children. Children from divorced families differ little from children from married families on objective psychological measures. Most children continue to function competently after divorce, although at some personal cost. On average, children from divorced families experience more problems, often before the divorce is final. They have a lower level of well-being, including lower academic achievement, more behavioral problems, more negative self-concepts, and more problematic social relationships. Divorce also creates economic uncertainties for families. The average income for a woman experiencing divorce declines significantly. Poor financial support from the nonresident parent contributes to the economic decline. One study revealed that 44% of minority women experienced poverty after divorce. Children living in poverty are at increased risk for a variety of medical, behavioral, and developmental consequences.

The parent-child relationship is often affected by parents' emotional state and level of parental conflict. Depression and "self-focus" are common as parents look to understand their failed marriages. This, in turn, may make parents less emotionally available or able to attend to their child's needs. Poorer outcomes are seen in children who experience high levels of parental conflict throughout the divorce process.

A child's cognitive or developmental level affects the psychologic reactions to parental separation. Infants and toddlers are often too young to understand the full implications of their parents' separation. They are more affected by the changes in daily routines, the consistency of care, and the emotional availability or attachment of their primary caregiver. Preschool children, with their rich fantasy lives, often feel responsible for the divorce and react strongly to their parents' arguments. School-aged children begin to understand the causes of the divorce concretely and often have conflicting loyalties to each parent. School problems and aggression, especially in boys, are common during this time. Pre-adolescents may react more emotion-

ally, with psychosomatic complaints and behavioral noncompliance. As adolescents are in the process of developing a sense of identity and autonomy, and experiencing intimacy for the first time, they seem particularly vulnerable to the effects of divorce. Teens may become depressed, engage in high-risk behaviors, or become overprotective of other family members. Adult "children" may experience difficulty with commitment and intimacy. As time passes, all children are better able to cope with divorce, and behavioral problems lessen. It is important to reiterate that most children who experience divorce are resilient and do not have long-term problems.

Pediatricians should inquire about any changes in caretaking of the child on an annual basis. Most parents appreciate the understanding and information their health care provider can offer. Discussions with families should include how to talk to children about the separation, the impact of conflict on the children, and the importance of consistency in visitation or custody arrangements. Reading resources for children should be explored. Parents may be reassured that most children adjust well to divorce and do not need special therapeutic interventions. Counseling or referrals for family therapy for the parents should be initiated early if conflict continues. When a particularly volatile or difficult separation is occurring, mediation with a focus on the child's needs should be offered.

DEATH & DYING IN CHILDHOOD

Children's Understanding of Death

Unfortunately, a clinician caring for children will occasionally encounter a child with a terminal illness, a family of a deceased child, or a child whose parent is terminally ill. The clinician should anticipate a child's reaction to his or her dying or to the death of others by understanding the developmental stage of the child. Children younger than 3 years of age are indifferent to death but react strongly to separation. Children aged 3–5 years are prone to magical thinking and have no sense of causality. Although children 5–10 years of age may be very concrete in their thinking (eg, they may believe that death is a punishment for their wrongdoing), some may have a precocious understanding of death depending on their prior experience. By 7 or 8 years, most children can understand the irreversibility and nonfunctionality of death. By early adolescence, death is perceived as a final, inevitable process.

Common Grief Reactions

The grief process for dying individuals and their survivors (parents, siblings, and friends) follows a common progression as described by Kübler-Ross. Denial and isolation, anger and guilt, bargaining, depression, and finally acceptance are feelings commonly seen. Parents of a dying child often experience various somatic disturbances, diminished day-to-day functioning, and a great deal of guilt. Marital discord is common, and communication between family members frequently becomes strained. Children who are dying or who have experienced the death of a loved one may display emotional and behavioral adjustment disorders. They may develop acute fears on separation and regress in developmental milestones. Changes in eating and sleeping habits, nightmares, signs of withdrawal, hyperactivity, and aggression may occur.

The Clinician's Role

The sensitive clinician should invite family discussion when a parent has a fatal illness. In the case of a parent's death, the clinician should ensure that the child has received prompt and accurate information regarding the death. The child should participate in family grieving and attend the funeral if the presence of a comforting adult can be ensured.

When a child dies, clinicians should allow parents to express as much grief as they are willing to share. Parents should be encouraged to view the child's body and to talk about the child. Parents may have many questions regarding the medical circumstances surrounding the death of their child but may not be able to understand the information fully until a period of grieving has passed. A sensitive clinician should arrange follow-up calls or visits to provide ongoing support and to answer questions.

When a sibling dies, it is important to acknowledge the relationship the sibling had with the deceased. The child may develop extreme guilt, anxiety, and feelings of hostility common to normal sibling rivalry. Parents may need help in recognizing the surviving child's needs, because they may be absorbed in their own grief. If a clinician was actively involved in the care of a child who dies, he or she should be available to attend the funeral (Table 3–10).

Table 3–10. Helping children cope with death.

General guidelines	
	Openly discuss events surrounding death.
	Allow children to ask questions and give developmentally appropriate answers.
	Explain child's developmental understanding of death to parents.
	Encourage child to attend funeral if supportive adult can accompany child.
	Encourage family to discuss feelings of guilt and anger.
	Recognize one's own feelings of loss and sadness.
	Encourage follow-up visits after funeral to assess family adjustment.
Specific guidelines	
Infancy:	Avoid frequent changes in caretakers.
	Ensure consistent care.
Toddlers:	Encourage play regarding loss/separation.
	Help identify feelings of sadness, loss, and loneliness.
	Avoid misleading terms (he "went to sleep," he "went on a trip").
	Continue secure, consistent discipline.
School age:	Encourage discussion regarding death and loss.
	Attend to changes in behavior or school performance.
Adolescence:	Encourage grieving.
	Help identify feelings of loss.
	Respect autonomy.

Prolonged mourning with poor social functioning for more than 6–8 months is an indication for a mental health referral. Extended guilt, continued denial of the reality of death, or continued apathy or hostility toward the deceased are warning signs for a maladaptive grief process.

REFERENCES

Barakat LP et al: Management of fatal illness and death in children or their parents. Pediatr Rev 1995;16:419.

Bauer S: Autism and the pervasive developmental disorders. Pediatr Rev 1995;16:130, 168.

Boyce WT, Shonkoff JP: Developmental-behavioral pediatrics. Page 87 in: Rudolph AM et al (editors): *Rudolph's Pediatrics,* 20th ed. Appleton & Lange, 1996.

Diagnostic and Statistical Manual of Mental Disorders, 4th ed. American Psychiatric Association, 1987.

Emery RE, Cairo MJ: Divorce: Consequences for children. Pediatr Rev 1995;16:306.

Fletcher JM et al (editors): Learning disabilities. J Child Neurol 1995;10:S1.

Geertsma MA, Hyams JS: Colic—a pain syndrome of infancy? Pediatr Clin North Am 1989;36:905.

Kain ZN Rimar S: Management of chronic pain in children. Pediatr Rev 1995;16:218.

Levine MD et al: *Developmental-Behavioral Pediatrics,* 2nd ed. Saunders, 1992.

4

The Perinatal Period

Augusto Sola, MD, Marta R. Rogido, MD, & John Colin Partridge, MD, MPH

PERINATAL HISTORY

The care of the newborn, particularly the sick newborn, has evolved significantly over the past 20 years. Eighty to 90% of infants admitted to hospitals in the United States are healthy. Nonetheless, the neonatal period is important because many conditions that originate during this period can have a major impact, not only on infant mortality but also on future development of the infant.

Infant mortality, the death of infants from birth to 12 months of age, is now fewer than 9:1000 live births in the United States. More than 60% of these deaths occur during the neonatal period; the more frequent causes of neonatal death are perinatal asphyxia, prematurity, respiratory distress syndrome (RDS), congenital malformations, and infections. Infant mortality is inversely proportionate to birth weight. Even though the specific rate of infant mortality for any birth weight category under 2500 g is lower for blacks than for whites, the overall mortality among black infants is twice that among white infants because of the higher percentage of black low-birth-weight (LBW) infants. The interplay between multiple factors—environmental, behavioral, psychosocial, biologic, and clinical—affects birth weight and prematurity.

Morbidity is also higher in the neonatal period than during the rest of the first 12 months of life. Many neurologic abnormalities that manifest themselves during infancy or childhood, such as hearing deficits, vision deficits, cerebral palsy, and mental retardation, are secondary to injuries to the nervous system that occurred during labor and delivery or during the neonatal period.

At the time of birth, many physiologic changes must occur for the fetus to adapt from intrauterine to extrauterine life. Among these changes, the most immediate is the transfer of the function of gas exchange (oxygen uptake and carbon dioxide removal) from the placenta to the lungs. This requires that rhythmic ventilation of the lungs and an adequate pulmonary blood flow be established.

To evaluate the newborn completely, a detailed prenatal history should be elicited (Table 4–1); this includes a paternal and maternal history and a history of the neonate during intrauterine life. Risks to a neonate can often be identified during pregnancy or labor. About 20% of all pregnancies are considered to be "high risk," and they account for approximately 55% of fetal-neonatal (perinatal) morbidity and mortality. An additional 10% of high-risk infants can be identified during labor and represent 20–25% of perinatal morbidity and mortality. Thus, 75–80% of perinatal morbidity and mortality could be identified before birth; the remainder occurs with apparently normal pregnancy and labor.

ADAPTATION TO BIRTH

EFFECTS OF LABOR

During labor, repetitive stresses are placed on the fetus because uterine contraction results in a temporary reduction in uterine blood flow, thus interfering with oxygen supply to the fetus. The more severe and prolonged the contraction, the greater is the effect on oxygen delivery. Although the normal fetus can tolerate considerable reductions in oxygen delivery for fairly prolonged periods, labor may have a deleterious effect on the fetus that is already compromised because the placenta is abnormal or because the mother has a condition further influencing uterine blood flow. Fetal hypoxemia and acidemia develop, resulting in changes in fetal heart rate, blood pressure, and distribution of blood flow to the fetal body and organs. Uterine contraction during labor may also produce

Table 4–1. Neonatal risks associated with various prenatal and perinatal factors.

Family history
  Genetic abnormalities, congenital malformations, multiple pregnancies.
 	
History before this pregnancy
  Lower socioeconomic class: Prematurity, fetal growth retardation, infection.
  Maternal history: Diabetes; infections; hypertension; renal, cardiovascular or pulmonary disease; smoking; alcohol intake; medications; street drugs; Rh disease.
  Maternal age: Adolescent, fetal growth retardation; older age (> 36 y), chromosomal anomalies.
  Previous pregnancies: Abortions, prematurity, neonatal deaths, malformations.
 	
History of labor and delivery
  Medications during labor: Prolonged anesthesia or analgesia may cause hypotension, hypothermia, CNS or respiratory depression.
  Prolonged labor: Fetal distress, trauma, or death.
  Rapid labor and delivery: Hemorrhage, trauma.
  Cord prolapse, tight nuchal cord, real knot of the cord: Fetal distress, anemia, death.
  Uterine tetany: Fetal distress, death.
  Abnormal signs of fetal well-being (ultrasound, fetal monitoring, scalp pH): Fetal distress, death.
  Meconium-stained amniotic fluid: Fetal distress, intrapartum death, meconium aspiration syndrome, persistent pulmonary hypertension syndrome.
  Premature birth: All problems associated with prematurity.
  Post-term birth: Fetal distress, meconium, hypoglycemia, polycythemia, hyperthermia, prenatal or postnatal death.
	History of this pregnancy
	  Prenatal visits: Optimum is 8–10.
	  Urinary tract infection: Prematurity, neonatal sepsis.
	  Hemorrhage: Prematurity, fetal distress, fetal death, neonatal anemia.
	  Isoimmunization (Rh and others): Fetal death, fetal hydrops, neonatal anemia, hyperbilirubinemia.
	  Prolonged rupture of membranes: Chorioamnionitis, prematurity, neonatal sepsis, oligohydramnios, pulmonary hypoplasia.
	  Multiple pregnancy: Prematurity, fetal growth retardation, fetal distress, anemia, hypovolemia, obstetric trauma.
	  Medications during pregnancy: Many congenital anomalies can be ascribed to various drugs (see Chapter 5).
	  Polyhydramnios: Anencephaly, gastrointestinal obstruction, omphalocele, gastroschisis, renal tumors, fetal hydrops, chromosomal abnormalities, diaphragmatic hernia, fetal anemia.
	  Oligohydramnios: Placental insufficiency, renal malformations, fetal growth retardation, pulmonary hypoplasia.
	  Abnormal fetal position: Cord prolapse, placenta previa, obstetric trauma, congenital malformations.
	  Decreased fetal growth: Small-for-gestational-age infants, congenital malformations.
	  Increased fetal growth: Obstetric trauma, neonatal hypoglycemia, polycythemia, infant of diabetic mother, congenital malformations.
	  Decreased fetal movements: Death before or during labor, CNS and neuromuscular diseases.

CNS = central nervous system.

adverse effects on the fetus by causing head compression in the pelvis and, possibly, by compressing the umbilical cord if it is in the pelvis.

Fetal bradycardia occurs during uterine contraction, probably because of chemoreceptor stimulation by the hypoxemia or because of head compression if the fetal head is in the pelvis. Although deaths before labor outnumber those occurring during labor by approximately 3:1, no other comparable period contributes as heavily to fetal mortality and morbidity. The occurrence of intrapartum fetal deaths is usually stated as 1.5–4:1000 fetuses, but a specific cause can be identified in only about 50% of cases. Fetal scalp blood sampling to measure acid-base status and continuous monitoring of fetal heart rate and uterine contractions have been useful in assessing fetal well-being during labor. Recently, Doppler ultrasound studies of umbilical blood flow velocity and cerebral arterial blood flow, percutaneous blood sampling from the umbilical cord, and fetal electrocardiographic (ECG) changes have contributed significantly to fetal assessment.

Drugs administered to the mother during labor may have significant effects on both the fetus and on the newborn infant. Ritodrine, a β_2-receptor antagonist, may decrease uterine blood flow and cause fetal tachycardia. Magnesium sulfate tocolysis, used to inhibit uterine contractions during premature labor, may induce vasodilatation, hypotonia, hyporeflexia, and apnea in the neonate.

Indomethacin therapy for premature labor has been shown to cause constriction of the ductus arteriosus in approximately 50% of fetuses. Local anesthetics used for epidural analgesia are rapidly transferred across the maternal circulation to the fetus and may cause fetal or neonatal seizures. In addition, most analgesic or hypnotic drugs administered to the mother cross the placenta and may result in central nervous system (CNS) depression in the newborn, with respiratory compromise.

TRANSITION TO NEONATAL LIFE

In most cases, the fetus changes from the intrauterine environment to the extrauterine one and becomes a normal neonate without any difficulty. However, this transition is a fairly complex physiologic process involving many changes in organ and system function. The most significant of these changes are summarized in Table 4–2. The most important fetal physiologic functions necessary for normal growth and development are to pump blood to the placenta and to collaborate in some endocrine functions. Most of the organic functions, such as respiration, nutrition, metabolism, excretion, and even defense against infection, are performed by the placenta and the mother. To survive after birth it is mandatory that the neonate, regardless of degree of maturity, adapts satisfactorily to the

Table 4–2. Changes during fetal-neonatal transition.

Cord clamping
  Placental circulation disappears
  Hormonal concentrations increase
  Peripheral vascular resistance increases

Breathing
  Increased alveolar P_{O_2}
  Release of vasoactive substances
  Decrease of pulmonary vascular resistance
  Increase of pulmonary blood flow

Decrease of pulmonary fluid
  During labor and after birth; mostly through capillary circulation

Circulatory changes
  Closure of ductus arteriosus: Bidirectional shunt initially followed by functional closure and complete closure (term neonate, 10–12 days for anatomic closure)
  Closure of foramen ovale: Immediate closure due to changes in right and left atrial pressures
  Closure of ductus venosus: Closes within 2–7 days after birth

Endocrine changes
  Increase in catecholamine concentration
  Increase in vasopressin and renin-angiotensin concentrations
  Decrease in prostaglandin concentration

new demands that are imposed by the extrauterine environment.

Intrauterine Status

Early in pregnancy, the lungs start to produce a fluid similar to plasma but with significantly less protein. Toward the end of gestation, the volume of this lung fluid is approximately the same as the functional residual capacity found soon after extrauterine spontaneous respirations (30–35 mL/kg). The secretion of pulmonary fluid decreases during the hours that precede birth. During labor, a significant portion of this fluid is resorbed into the circulation in preparation for birth; this resorption of fluid continues after birth. The lymphatic drainage of this fluid is minimal, as is the quantity of fetal pulmonary fluid that is eliminated through the compression of the thorax during the fetal passage across the birth canal. In birth by cesarean section without preceding labor, plasma colloid oncotic pressure is low. Infants born by cesarean section without labor do not reabsorb pulmonary fluid as rapidly as those born by vaginal delivery or those born by cesarean section after preceding labor. In some infants, this slow resorption of fetal lung fluid causes transient respiratory distress.

The fetus exhibits rapid, oscillatory thoracic respiratory movements in utero. These movements are important for adequate lung growth and development. Fetal breathing movements are a useful clinical tool to assess fetal well-being (respiratory activity increases after meals or administration of glucose to the mother): Smoking and alcohol intake decrease fetal breathing movements.

The fetal circulation and its changes after birth are discussed in Chapter 17.

Pulmonary Adaptation After Birth

Respiratory movements after birth appear in response to multiple stimuli. During normal labor, partial pressure of arterial carbon dioxide (Pa_{CO_2}) increases modestly, and partial pressure of arterial oxygen (Pa_{O_2}) and serum pH decrease. Through the peripheral and central chemoreceptors, there is stimulation of the respiratory center. Furthermore, there are sensory stimuli from light and noise, pressure at various sites of the body, and a rapid decrease in body temperature. The first inspiration originated by a rapid descent of the diaphragm generates a negative intrapleural pressure of approximately 35–40 cm water. These initial high transpulmonary pressures are needed to overcome the resistance generated by the elevated surface tension at the air-fluid interface and the high viscosity of the fluid that fills the airways. In addition, these negative pressures cause alveolar fluid to move into the interstitial space. For air to be distributed appropriately in the lung and for a normal functional residual capacity to develop, surface tension in the alveoli needs to be low, and the pulmonary fluid has to be eliminated. Pulmonary surfactant decreases surface tension during expiration, maintaining alveolar stability and avoiding collapse; subsequent inspirations therefore require significantly less transpulmonary pressures. The lack of surfactant causes RDS or hyaline membrane disease (HMD), in which alveolar stability is decreased and interstitial fluid passes into the alveoli.

Expansion of the lungs and removal of alveolar fluid significantly decrease pulmonary vascular resistance. Mechanical expansion of the lung causes a decrease of pulmonary vascular resistance by release of prostaglandin I_2 (PGI_2; prostacyclin). Oxygen or air causes pulmonary vasodilation through release of endothelial-relaxing factor (EDRF), or nitric oxide (NO). This induces a massive increase in pulmonary blood flow. Simultaneously, systemic pressure increases as a result of umbilical cord clamping, release of hormones, and possibly other mechanisms. During fetal life, pulmonary blood flow is low (approximately 20 mL/kg/min) and increases 5–10 times with adequate alveolar ventilation after birth. When pulmonary vascular resistance does not decrease and the normal increase in pulmonary blood flow does not occur after birth, the infant is said to have the syndrome of persistent pulmonary hypertension of the neonate (PPHN), or **persistent fetal circulation.**

Perinatal Endocrine Responses

Concentrations of several hormones increase during the transition from the intrauterine to extrauterine environment. This increase may be due to physiologic stress secondary to the mild to moderate fetal hypoxia, uterine contractions, and compression of the fetal head in the birth canal. These hormonal responses may help the fetus to tolerate the stress of labor and promote neonatal adaptation to the extrauterine environment.

Corticotrophic hormone and glucocorticoid concentrations increase 2–3 days before birth in some species, and this is probably responsible for maturation of many enzyme systems. During labor, antidiuretic hormone (vasopressin) and renin and angiotensin concentrations increase; these hormones assist in achieving the increase in vascular resistance that occurs after birth.

Catecholamine concentrations increase after birth. The fetus responds to stress with an increase in norepinephrine concentrations, with a minor increase in epinephrine concentrations. Catecholamines are important in increasing the energy supply for maintenance of body temperature after birth by stimulating release of fatty acids into the circulation from brown fat. Furthermore catecholamines stimulate the conversion of T_4 to T_3. Thyroid stimulating hormone (TSH) increases in concentration at the time of birth because of an increase in thyrotrophin releasing hormone (TRH). The increase in TRH is mediated through α-adrenergic stimulation. TSH concentrations return to low basal levels within 2–3 days after birth. In congenital hypothyroidism, when concentrations of thyroid hormones are low, TSH levels remain elevated. Growing preterm infants, with low metabolic rates, have lower than normal serum concentrations of T_4 and T_3 but their TSH concentration is not elevated. This is usually a transient, self-resolving condition; in some instances, however, treatment with thyroid hormones is indicated to avoid poor long-term outcome.

Temperature Regulation

In the intrauterine environment, the fetus does not need to produce heat to maintain body temperature. The fetus is surrounded by amniotic fluid with a temperature only 0.2 °C less than fetal body temperature. Thus, there are no losses by radiation or evaporation, and losses of heat by conduction and convection from the fetal skin are minimal. Fetal temperature does not increase because heat produced is lost by convection through blood flow in the placenta. A decrease of placental blood flow can produce an increase in fetal temperature. This may occur in small-for-gestational-age (SGA) infants who have low placental blood flows and, as a result, are often born with rectal temperatures of 38.0–38.5 °C. Fetal temperature may also increase with maternal fever because heat loss to the mother is reduced. The fetus does not possess defense mechanisms against temperature increases, and severe prolonged maternal hyperthermia could be dangerous for fetal survival and development.

Thermal Instability of Newborn & Premature Infants. Environments with temperatures that are comfortable for adults may be inappropriate for newborn infants. At 22 °C (72 °F) there is a significant and rapid decrease in the neonate's body temperature because neonates lose heat easily and have limited ability to increase heat production in cold environments. Part of the rapid heat loss is associated with their large body surface-body volume ratio. A term infant with a birth weight of 3 kg has a body surface : body volume ratio 3 times greater than that of an adult, and a premature infant with birth weight of 1500 g has a ratio 4 times greater. The neonate also has a thinner skin and subcutaneous fat layer; this is even more marked in premature infants. Skin of the newborn and premature infant has greater thermal conductance than that of the adult; they consequently lose more heat per unit of surface area than does the adult.

In addition to producing heat by movement, as in the adult, the neonate has a well-developed mechanism to increase the production of heat in cool environments through energy metabolism in brown fat. Nevertheless, the thermal-regulating ability of the neonate is less efficient than in the adult and can be further impaired by hypoxia, sedatives, and anesthetic drugs. In suboptimal environments, newborn body temperature can decrease rapidly (up to 0.3 °C/min), reaching 33–35 °C. Therefore, newborn infants should be kept in a **neutral thermal environment,** which is defined as that environment in which heat losses are equivalent to the minimum metabolic needs of the infant. In this environment, oxygen consumption is minimal, as is the thermal regulatory water loss. This environment is usually achieved with a relative humidity of 50% and with an environmental temperature of 31–34 °C when the infant is naked. When the infant is dressed, the necessary environmental temperature is about 25 °C in term infants. The level of neutral thermal environmental temperature decreases with postnatal age and is always higher in infants of lower gestational age.

Infants exposed to temperatures below the neutral thermal environment may have cold stress, which induces increased oxygen consumption and elevated circulating catecholamine concentrations. Cold stress may cause a rapid decline in a neonate's health status (Table 4–3). To prevent cold stress, infants should be dried immediately after birth, with particular attention to the head and face, which represent a large proportion of total body surface area. Body temperature should be checked soon after birth, at least twice in the first hour and then every 1–2 hours in the first 8 hours. During physical examination, the neonate should not be placed on a cold surface or exposed to air conditioning or air currents. A radiant source of heat should be used if the environment is not warm enough. Normal neonatal body temperature should be 36–37.5 °C.

The neonate also should not be exposed to environments in which the temperature is much higher than neutral thermal environment. Newborn infants cannot lose heat efficiently; premature neonates cannot sweat, and full-term neonates have a limited capacity to perspire.

Table 4–3. Effects of cold stress.

Increased O_2 consumption	Increased circulating catecholamines
Increased fat metabolism	
Increased surfactant consumption	Increased fatty acids
	Metabolic acidosis
Hypoxia	Hypoglycemia
Pulmonary vasoconstriction	Peripheral vasoconstriction
Persistent pulmonary hypertension	Apnea
	Cyanosis
Respiratory distress	

Therefore, with temperatures above the neutral thermal environment, skin temperature increases. Environmental hyperthermia is a common cause of hyperthermia in the neonate; usually rectal temperature does not increase significantly. Thus, rectal temperature is a useful parameter in excluding nonenvironmental causes of hyperthermia. Neonates lose large amounts of water through their thin skin by evaporation and, if exposed to heat, may become dehydrated.

Table 4–4B. Causes of low Apgar scores.

Asphyxia
Maternal drugs: Anesthetics, sedatives, opiates, drugs of abuse
Central nervous system disease
Congenital muscular disease
Prematurity
Fetal sepsis

ASSESSMENT OF NEWBORNS

APGAR SCORES

In 1953, Virginia Apgar introduced a simple, systematic assessment of intrapartum stress and neurologic depression at birth. Five variables—heart rate, respiratory effort, muscle tone, reflex irritability, and color—are evaluated at 1 and 5 minutes after birth, and each one is scored from 0 to 2, as described in Table 4–4A. The final score is the sum of the five individual scores, with 10 representing the optimal score. Although the Apgar score is useful in evaluating the acute status of the infant at birth, it has limitations, because several factors other than asphyxia can affect the score; these are summarized in Table 4–4B. Regardless of the cause, a persistent very low score indicates the need for resuscitation. Scoring should continue every 5 minutes until a final score of 7 or more is reached.

The Apgar score should not be used to establish long-term prognosis. Only the clinical neurologic status at the time of hospital discharge has been clearly associated with poor prognosis related to asphyxial encephalopathy.

MATURITY–GESTATIONAL AGE

Several clinical methods have been described to assess gestational age in the neonate on the basis of external physical characteristics and neuromuscular evaluation. Although there may be an error of 1–2 weeks, trained and experienced physicians can closely estimate gestational age. External characteristics include the plantar creases, skin texture, skin opacity, lanugo, nipple formation and breast size, and evaluation of the ears and genitalia. Neurologic status is not always easy to evaluate and can change in relation to the state of the infant (quiet sleep, crying, etc), if there is CNS depression due to drugs or asphyxia, or if the infant is critically ill. Ballard has devised a simplified method that includes six parameters of neuromuscular maturation and six physical characteristics (Figure 4–1). Each receives an individual score; gestational age is determined from the sum of these scores. When the gestational age—determined from the first day of the last menstrual period—is 37–42 weeks (259–294 days), the newborn infant is considered to be at term. **Preterm** infants are those with less than 37 completed weeks (< 258 days), and **post-term** infants those with gestational age greater than 42 weeks (> 294 days).

Normal weight, length, and skull circumference at different gestational ages are shown in Figure 4–2. When fetuses grow normally, birth weight for a particular gestational age lies within 2 SD of the mean, and the infant is considered **appropriate for gestational age (AGA)**. Infants can be born preterm, at term, or post-term and be AGA. SGA is defined as birth weight less than 2 SD below the mean, and it suggests intrauterine growth retardation. **Large for gestational age (LGA)** is defined as birth weight greater than 2 SD above the mean. Infants born at term with appropriate weight for gestational age have the lowest neonatal risk. Morbidity and mortality rates are higher with both LGA and SGA infants (see this chapter).

Table 4–4A. Apgar scoring system.[1]

	Score		
Variable	**0**	**1**	**2**
Heart rate	Absent	Less than 100 beats/min	More than 100 beats/min
Respiratory effort	Absent	Slow, irregular	Good, crying
Muscle tone	Limp	Some flexion of extremities	Active motion
Reflex irritability (in response to catheter in nose)	Absent	Grimace	Grimace and cough or sneeze
Color	Blue, pale	Body pink, extremities blue (acrocyanosis)	Completely pink

[1]Reproduced, with permission, from Apgar V: A proposal for a new method of evaluation of the newborn infant. *Curr Res Anesthesiol* 1953;32:260.

Neuromuscular maturity

Score	−1	0	1	2	3	4	5
Posture 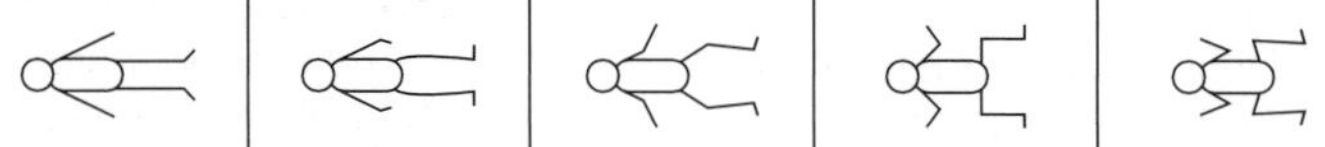							
Square window (wrist) 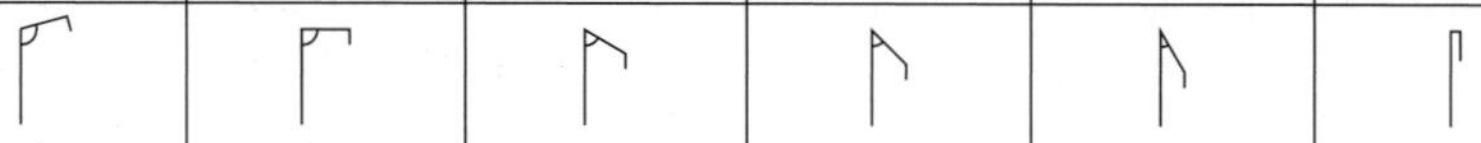	> 90 degrees	90 degrees	60 degrees	45 degrees	30 degrees	0 degrees	
Arm recoil 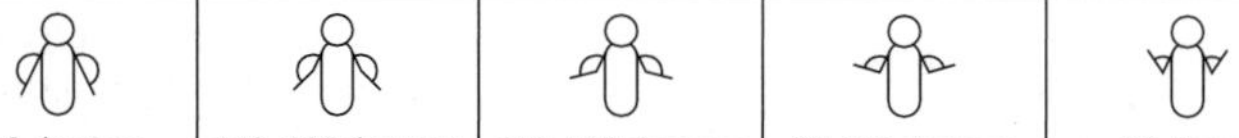		180 degrees	140–180 degrees	110–140 degrees	90–110 degrees	< 90 degrees	
Popliteal angle 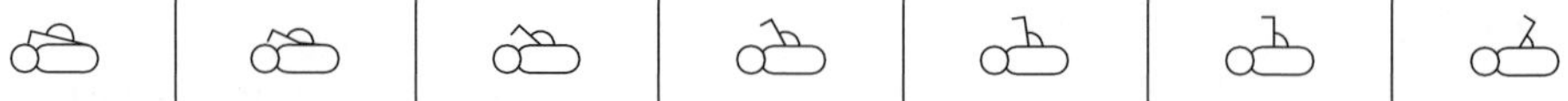	180 degrees	160 degrees	140 degrees	120 degrees	100 degrees	90 degrees	< 90 degrees
Scarf sign 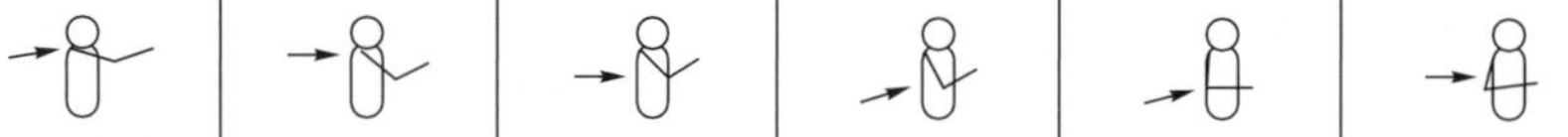							
Heel to ear 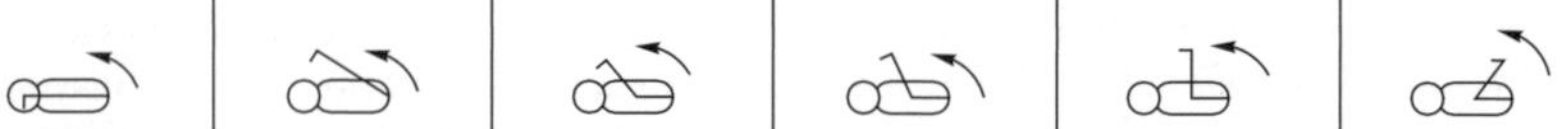							

Physical maturity

Score	−1	0	1	2	3	4	5
Skin	Sticky, friable, transparent	Gelatinous, red, translucent	Smooth pink, visible veins	Superficial peeling or rash, few veins	Cracking, pale areas, rare veins	Parchment, deep cracking, no vessels	Leathery, cracked, wrinkled
Lanugo	None	Sparse	Abundant	Thinning	Bald areas	Mostly bald	
Plantar surface	Heel–toe 40–50 mm: −1 < 40 mm: −2	> 50 mm no crease	Faint red marks	Anterior transverse crease only	Creases anterior two thirds	Creases over entire sole	
Breast	Imperceptible	Barely perceptible	Flat areola, no bud	Stippled areola, 1–2 mm bud	Raised areola, 3–4 mm bud	Full areola, 5–10 mm bud	
Eye/ear	Lids fused Loosely: −1 Tightly: −2	Lids open, pinna flat, stays folded	Slightly curved pinna; soft; slow recoil	Well-curved pinna; soft but ready recoil	Formed and firm; instant recoil	Thick cartilage, ear stiff	
Genitals (male)	Scrotum flat, smooth	Scrotum empty, faint rugae	Testes in upper canal, rare rugae	Testes descending, few rugae	Testes down, good rugae	Testes pendulous, deep rugae	
Genitals (female)	Clitoris prominent, labia flat	Clitoris prominent, small labia minora	Clitoris prominent, enlarging minora	Majora and minora equally prominent	Majora large, minora small	Majora covers clitoris and minora	

Maturity rating

Score	−10	−5	0	5	10	15	20	25	30	35	40	45	50
Weeks	20	22	24	26	28	30	32	34	36	38	40	42	44

Figure 4–1. Newborn maturity rating and classification. (Adapted and reproduced, with permission, from Ballard JL et al: New Ballard Score, expanded to include extremely premature infants. J Pediatr 1991;119:417.)

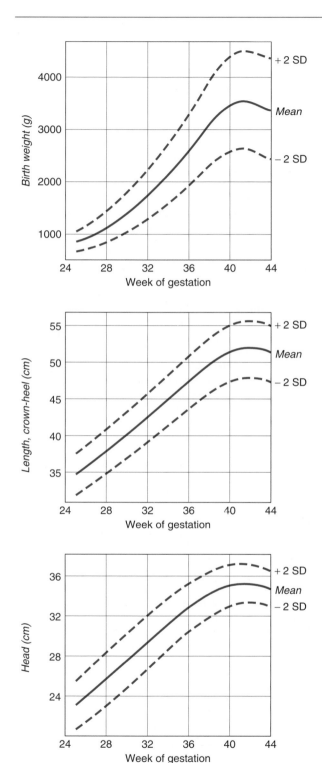

Figure 4–2. Intrauterine growth charts showing the normal values of body weight, length, and head circumference for infants born at different gestational ages at sea level (Montreal). (Data, with permission, from Usher R, McLean F: Intrauterine growth of live-born Caucasian infants at sea level: Standards obtained from measurements in 7 dimensions of infants born between 25 and 44 weeks of gestation. J Pediatr 1969;74:901.)

Regardless of gestational age, an infant with a birth weight less than 2500 g is considered a LBW infant. A LBW infant (eg, 2000 g) can be AGA, SGA, or LGA, according to the gestational age at birth. Infants born at less than 1500 g are considered **very-low-birth-weight (VLBW),** and infants born at less than 1000 g are considered **extremely low-birth-weight (ELBW).** By definition, regardless of gestational age, an infant with a birth weight greater than 4000 g is considered a high birth weight infant. As discussed later, infants with abnormalities of **maturity** (premature or postmature infants) are clinically very different from infants who have abnormalities of **growth** (SGA and LGA infants).

PHYSICAL EXAMINATION OF THE NEWBORN INFANT

Initial Evaluation

The changes in practice that have led to early hospital discharge of mothers and newborn infants after birth pose a new challenge to pediatricians, viz, how to make sure that the newborn is healthy. When this cannot be assured by observation and detailed physical examination at different postnatal ages in the hospital, arrangements must be made for providing the same outside the hospital setting. The transitional period from fetal to neonatal life is one of many changes. Some abnormal conditions can and must be recognized during this period to improve outcome, but others will not become apparent until later. Because of this, there is a need to observe and examine newborn infants, as summarized in Table 4–5 and described in the subsequent section. The neurologic examination completes the evaluation of the infant.

In the first few minutes after birth, a partial physical examination is performed when Apgar scores are assigned. Subsequently, within 24 hours after birth, a detailed physical examination must be performed to confirm the presence or absence of congenital malformations, traumatic injuries, or any other manifestation of neonatal disease. Before the first physical examination at birth, one should be familiar with the prenatal and perinatal history. The examination should be performed after the infant has been dried and stabilized; as previously mentioned, heat loss should be minimized during this examination.

Specific Findings

General Appearance. The general appearance of the neonate is observed to assess spontaneous activity, passive muscle tone, respirations, and abnormal signs, such as cyanosis, retractions, or meconium staining. Vital signs should be included in the examination, and accurate measurements of weight, length, and head circumference are plotted according to gestational age to determine whether the infant is appropriately grown (Table 4–5).

Skin. Skin texture differs with gestational age, being softer and thinner in premature infants. Post-term infants may have dry, scaly skin. The skin is covered with lanugo

Table 4–5. Observation and examination of newborns during first postnatal week.

Initial examination at birth
  Apgar scores
  Rule out major anomalies that are detectable at birth, eg, choanal atresia, major limb defects, omphalocele, congenital diaphragmatic hernia, meningomyelocele, anal atresia, ambiguous genitalia, hypospadias
  Detailed *observation:* skin, craniofacial, neck, chest, back, extremities; rule out cyanosis and respiratory distress
  Vital signs: length, weight, head circumference

Detailed examination: first 6–12 h after birth   Include all details of neonatal examination, from craniofacial to extremities; establish successful early transition; rule out early jaundice, gastrointestinal obstructions, abdominal masses, hip abnormalities, some cardiac diseases; verify pulses in lower extremities
Another detailed examination: 36–48 h   Same as before; rule out exaggerated jaundice and weight loss; complete neurologic examination if not done before
Observation at 72–96 h   Appropriate weight loss and intake; rule out exaggerated jaundice; check pulses in lower extremities, vital signs
Another detailed examination: 6–10 d   Include neurologic examination

hair in preterm infants; this is minimally present in term babies. The skin may be covered in some areas by **vernix caseosa,** a thick, white, creamy material in term babies. In preterm infants, vernix caseosa covers large areas of the skin; it is absent in post-term infants. The normal color of the skin a few hours after birth is pink, but **acrocyanosis** (cyanosis of the hands and feet) is frequent during the first 48 hours and can last in some babies throughout the first month of life, particularly when the infant is cold. Acrocyanosis and **cutis marmorata** (mottling of the skin with venous prominence) are frequent intermittent signs of the vasomotor instability characteristic of some infants. However, mottling could be a serious sign in some instances, such as with infection. Pallor can be a sign of neonatal asphyxia, shock, or chronic anemia. Jaundice is always abnormal if detected within the first 24 hours after birth. Subsequently, it is frequently seen during the first few days after birth, but usually is not associated with serious disease.

Mongolian spots, dark blue areas over the lumbosacral area and buttocks, are transient, hyperpigmented macules that have no pathologic significance and occur predominantly in Asians, blacks, and Latinos. **Erythema toxicum,** a rash resembling flea bites, is noted in up to 50% of full-term infants but is found much less frequently in preterm infants. It can be found on the trunk and also on the arms and legs but not on soles and palms. It occurs more frequently in the first 72 hours after birth but sometimes may last up to 10–15 days. No treatment is required. **Milia,** tiny, whitish papules that are seen over the nose, cheeks, forehead, and chin, are very small cysts formed around the pilosebaceous follicles or sudoriparous glands.

The condition is frequent and usually disappears in a few weeks without treatment.

"Birth marks," or **nevus simplex,** are pink macular hemangiomas found on the neck, upper lip, and eyelids and above the nose. They are usually transient. Capillary hemangiomas of more significance are the so-called port-wine stains, or **nevus flammeus.** These usually are located over the face and trunk, become darker with increasing postnatal age, and may be associated with intracranial or spinal vascular malformations, seizures, and intracranial calcifications. **Cavernous hemangiomas** occur in approximately 10% of infants and are often first noticed a few days after birth. They increase in size after birth and usually resolve within 18–24 months (see Chapter 12). **Pustular melanosis** consists of small, dry vesicles over a dark macular base. These are also benign lesions, which occur more frequently in black infants, but must be differentiated from viral infections, such as herpes simplex, or bacterial infections, such as impetigo.

Craniofacial. The skull may show molding; this is seen particularly after prolonged labor with vertex presentation, in which the vertical diameter of the head becomes elongated and the parieto-occipital area becomes prominent. **Caput succedaneum** is diffuse edema or the swelling of the soft tissue of the scalp that crosses the cranial sutures and usually the midline. With bruising, the area of caput will have a bluish discoloration. Caput succedaneum usually disappears in 2–3 days, and molding in 5–6 days. In general, head circumference immediately after birth is 1–2 cm different than it is 3–4 days later. **Cephalhematomas** are subperiosteal hemorrhages, usually involving the parietal or occipital bones. The head is typically elongated in its anterior posterior diameter in breech presentation and fairly round in those infants born by cesarean section without labor. The posterior portion of the skull is often depressed in infants born by persistent occipitoposterior delivery.

The **anterior fontanelle** is situated between the coronal and sagittal sutures, has a diamond shape, and measures approximately 1.5–2 × 1.5–2 cm. At birth, the anterior fontanelle may not be evident because of overriding of skull sutures or, less often, because of an abnormality such as premature fusion of the sutures or cranial synostosis. Causes of large fontanelles are listed in Table 4–6. Infants with intrauterine growth retardation (IUGR), in whom the skull may grow more slowly than the brain tissue, may show widely split sutures and large fontanelles.

Table 4–6. Causes of large fontanelle.

Hydrocephalus Rickets Hypothyroidism Achondroplasia Osteogenesis imperfecta Cleidocranial dysplasia Hypophosphatasia Intrauterine growth retardation

These findings may become more noticeable a few days or weeks after birth. This does not represent an abnormality and does not indicate hydrocephalus. The posterior fontanelle, located between the sagittal and lambdoid sutures, is usually barely palpable at birth. In some infants, the metopic suture can be felt over the frontal bone as an extension of the sagittal suture.

A head circumference below the 10th percentile can be due to a familial trait but can represent fetal-neonatal pathology (Table 4–7). **Craniotabes,** soft areas with a ping-pong ball feel, may occur in the parietal bones parasagittally; they are not related to rickets and disappear in weeks or months. In infants in whom a scalp electrode was applied for intrauterine monitoring during labor, this area should be inspected carefully and cleaned appropriately. Other signs of trauma or lacerations should also be detected at the time of birth.

The face should be examined in detail. The infant delivered by a face presentation may have edema of the eyelids and face, and, if bruising is severe, an ecchymotic mask may be present. This feature may also be present in infants who have had the umbilical cord tightly wrapped around the neck. The presence of dysmorphic features allows for diagnosis of genetic anomalies or classic chromosomal syndromes (see Chapter 5). An asymmetric facies may be due to seventh cranial nerve palsy or, if the asymmetry occurs only with crying, to congenital absence or hypotonia of the depressor muscle at the angle of the mouth.

Ears. The ears should be examined to assess maturity. By term, the ears are firm and have assumed their characteristic shape. Low-set ears can be normal but frequently are a feature of genetic syndromes. Normal infants hear at birth and may startle or have a complete Moro reflex with a sudden noise. The ears should also be inspected for preauricular tags or sinuses.

Eyes. The eyes open spontaneously soon after birth, particularly when the infant is awake and in the upright position. After several hours, the eyelids may develop edema, which may make spontaneous opening difficult. Subconjunctival hemorrhage due to rupture of scleral capillaries is common and results from compression of the head during labor and delivery; the lesion disappears in a few weeks. Epicanthal folds, slanted palpebral fissures, and hypertelorism may be normal variations; however, they should alert the examiner to the possibility of other anomalies. Nystagmus or fixed strabismus should be ex-

cluded; the pupils should be symmetric and respond to light.

The iris, in general, is hypopigmented at birth, often presenting a grayish or bluish color. By 6 months of age, most infants have a more definite color. The iris should be examined to rule out coloboma, which may be associated with intrauterine infections or malformations.

Aniridia is rare but may be associated with Wilms tumor. Nonfixed strabismus that persists more than 30–45 days requires careful ophthalmologic evaluation. Microphthalmia suggests other malformations or intrauterine infections, such as rubella or toxoplasmosis.

A mucous ocular drainage is common in the first 2 days after birth; it should not be confused with conjunctivitis. However, if the eyelids are swollen and red, ocular infection is likely. Constant tearing a few days after birth usually represents a blockage of the nasolacrimal duct. In general, this resolves spontaneously; however, sometimes recurrent conjunctival infections develop, and probing of the duct is necessary.

The red reflex of the retina is easily observed when examining with the ophthalmoscope 10–20 cm from the infant's eye. If there is obstruction to the passage of light, the red reflex will not be seen, and a white reflex will be present. This is abnormal and may be due to corneal opacification, crystalline opacification (cataracts), retinoblastoma, or severe chorioretinitis; if it appears a few weeks after birth it could be due to retinopathy of prematurity.

Cataracts, in which the iris is seen clearly and the pupil appears whitish, are frequent in congenital rubella and other intrauterine infections. When there is corneal opacity, the iris is partially occluded; this may occur in glaucoma of any etiology. Corneal diameter greater than 11–12 mm is suggestive of congenital glaucoma.

Nose. The nose should be examined immediately to rule out unilateral or bilateral choanal atresia. If this is suspected, it can be excluded by passing a nasogastric tube through each nostril. The tube should also be advanced to the stomach to exclude the presence of esophageal atresia. In the neonate, nasal obstruction of any origin may result in serious respiratory distress, not only because the diameter of the upper airway is normally small, but also because neonates have difficulty breathing through the mouth. The nose may be compressed or deformed by pressure before birth. Rarely, the nasal septum is dislocated. Correction should be performed to prevent permanent deformities. A flat and broad nasal bridge, a beaked nose, or anteversion of the nostrils and a long philtrum may be normal but could be part of a congenital syndrome.

Mouth. The mouth should be examined with the infant at rest and also during crying. The newborn infant may open the mouth when gentle digital pressure is applied on the lower lip or chin. Micrognathia should be noted. If there is cleft lip, the presence of a dimple in the lower lip indicates the presence of an autosomal-dominant condition. This increases the risk of cleft palate in future off-

Table 4–7. Causes of neonatal microcephaly.

Familial: Autosomal dominant trait (normal intelligence); autosomal recessive; X-linked (eg, Paine syndrome)
Structural brain malformations (ie, lissencephaly)
Chromosomal and malformation syndromes (eg, trisomy 13, deLange syndrome)
Maternal: Radiation exposure, alcoholism, phenylketonuria, infections (toxoplasmosis, cytomegalovirus)
Posthypoxic encephalopathy

spring from 4 to 50%. Clefts of the soft and hard palate are easily noted by inspection, but submucous clefts in the soft portion of the palate should be ruled out by digital palpation. These clefts may be isolated or associated with other dysmorphic features. A high-arched palate is, in general, an isolated finding. Retrognathia and/or micrognathia, together with cleft palate, glossoptosis, and obstruction of the upper airway, can be found in Pierre Robin anomaly or sequence. Macroglossia is characteristic of the Beckwith-Wiedemann syndrome, which presents with omphalocele, macrosomia, and hypoglycemia. Although not as significant, macroglossia can be present in Down syndrome, hypothyroidism, and gangliosidosis G_{M1}.

Rarely, neonatal teeth may be seen, usually in the area of the medial lower incisors. Sometimes they are not white, but covered with pink, membranous tissue. It is recommended that they be removed because of the risk of aspiration when they fall out spontaneously. White, small epidermoid-mucoid cysts on both sides of the hard palate (Epstein pearls) are found normally; they also may be present in the gum or in the floor of the oral cavity and disappear in a few weeks. Salivary secretion is scant in the neonate; therefore, saliva should not accumulate in the oral cavity unless there is an abnormality in swallowing or esophageal atresia. Some infants have a short lingual frenulum; this does not usually interfere with feedings or speech, and treatment usually is not necessary. A strong cry is a sign of well-being in neonates. A high-pitched cry can be present in CNS conditions and in some congenital syndromes; a catlike cry is seen in cri du chat syndrome; and a dysphonic cry with inspiratory stridor suggests upper airway problems.

Neck & Clavicles. The neck in an infant at term is short and symmetric. To examine the neck, the head should be extended and rotated to observe the lateral border of the sternocleidomastoid muscle. Cysts or sinuses may be due to branchial clefts. The sternocleidomastoid muscle may be shortened owing to a fixed position in utero or to a postnatal hematoma resulting from birth injury. This produces neonatal torticollis. Clefts or masses in the midline may be due to cysts of the thyroglossal duct or to goiter secondary to maternal antithyroid medication or transplacental passage of long-acting thyroid stimulating antibodies. Edema and webbing of the neck suggest Turner syndrome, but other syndromes, such as Noonan, Klippel-Feil, and pterygium-multiplex, are also associated with a short neck. Both clavicles should be examined routinely to rule out fractures. Cystic hygromas occur in the supraclavicular area.

Cardiothoracic. During examination of the chest, inspection of the breast tissue aids in determining gestational age. Accessory nipples, which could be present along the anterior axillary or midclavicular lines, should be noted because they may later grow owing to the presence of glandular tissue. In some term infants, breast engorgement develops, either unilaterally or bilaterally, at 3–5 days after birth as a result of stimulation by maternal estrogen. Sometimes there is milk secretion. Both male and female infants may be affected; no treatment is necessary. Milk expression should not be attempted because it enhances the risk of infection.

Congenital deformities of the thorax, such as pectus-carinatus and pectus-excavatus, and asymmetry due to absence of the formation of ribs or to the agenesis of the pectoralis muscle (Poland syndrome), should be ruled out. The thorax may be small in some skeletal dysplasias, causing respiratory distress.

Evaluation of the lung and upper airway requires detailed inspection of respiratory mechanics. Tachypnea, deep respirations, cyanosis, expiratory grunting, and intercostal or sternal retractions are all signs of respiratory distress. The respiratory rate is normally 40–60 breaths/min, but most neonates, particularly preterm infants, breathe irregularly with short, apneic bursts that last less than 5–10 seconds and have no clinical significance. Breath sounds should be equal in both sides of the chest, and, after the first 2–4 hours, rales should not be present. A scaphoid abdomen and decreased breath sounds on one side suggest the diagnosis of congenital diaphragmatic hernia. Soon after birth, bowel sounds may be heard over the involved side of the chest. Other causes of diminished or absent breath sounds on one side are pneumothorax, pleural effusion, or agenesis of the lung. In all these conditions, the chest may appear asymmetric on inspection.

The cardiac impulse is usually maximal at the fourth intercostal space between the sternum and the midclavicular line, but it shifts in cases of pneumothorax, pneumomediastinum, diaphragmatic hernia, and dextrocardia. The normal heart rate varies between 95 and 180 beats/min and changes when the infant is feeding, sleeping, or crying. If the heart rate exceeds 200 beats/min at rest, an ECG should be performed to exclude arrhythmias (see Chapter 17). If the heart rate is less than 70–80 beats/min, an ECG is useful to differentiate between pathologic sinus bradycardia (as seen in CNS lesions, severe perinatal hypoxia, etc) and specific bradycardias, such as atrioventricular block.

The second heart sound is normally loud and not split in the first 3 hours after birth because pulmonary arterial pressure is still high; it becomes split in 75% of neonates by 48 hours. A single second sound persists in PPHN, pulmonary atresia, and transposition of the great vessels. Frequently, systolic heart murmurs are heard immediately after birth and during the first 2 days, but they disappear within a few days. Many infants with severe congenital heart disease do not have heart murmurs soon after birth. Peripheral pulses should be palpated in all four extremities. In the neonate in whom symptoms develop, symptoms that could be associated with congenital heart disease or cardiac failure, as well as in neonates with a persistent heart murmur, blood pressures should be measured in all four extremities. The infant with coarctation of the aorta or arch interruption may have consistently high upper-extremity blood pressure.

Abdomen. The abdomen in the neonate is prominent

because of poor development of the abdominal wall muscles, the relatively larger liver, and diaphragmatic movements during respiration. The lack of this normal abdominal prominence is seen in diaphragmatic hernia or in esophageal atresia without tracheoesophageal fistula. Lack of abdominal prominence is also noted in SGA and post-term infants. The liver edge is usually felt about 2 cm below the right costal margin, and the kidneys may be palpable. Normally, peristaltic movements are observed on the abdominal wall. If the liver is felt in the midline or to the left, situs inversus, asplenia, or polysplenia syndrome is suggested. Abdominal masses may represent hydronephrosis, multicystic kidneys, ovarian cysts, or other lesions (see this chapter, Approach to Abdominal Masses, for a detailed discussion). Midline abdominal defects, such as diastasis-recti or an umbilical hernia, usually require no therapy. More significant lesions, such as **omphalocele** (a herniation of the abdominal contents through the umbilicus) or **gastroschisis** (herniation of the bowel through the abdominal wall 2–4 cm lateral to the umbilicus) are readily apparent. A flaccid abdominal wall, associated with complete or almost complete absence of abdominal muscle, is part of the prune-belly syndrome. These infants also have bladder dilation, hydroureter, hydronephrosis, and cryptorchidism.

The **umbilical cord** should be inspected to confirm the presence of two arteries and one vein and the absence of a urachus. The presence of only one umbilical artery may indicate other, particularly renal, congenital malformations. Infants of diabetic mothers tend to have a thick umbilical cord with increased Wharton jelly; a thin cord is frequently noted in infants with IUGR. Postmature infants and those that have had fetal distress may have a meconium-stained cord. Bleeding from the cord suggests a coagulation disorder. The umbilical cord usually dries and falls off about 7–14 days after birth. When this is delayed or if there is erythema around the umbilicus, omphalitis may develop. Sometimes when the cord falls off, granulation tissue may be noted in the umbilical base with minimal amounts of secretion. Usually no treatment is required. A chronic discharge suggests the presence of a granuloma of the umbilical stump or, on rare occasions, a draining omphalomesenteric cyst. A persistent omphalomesenteric duct usually drains a pink, mucoid or fecoid secretion over a shiny red polyp. In cutaneous umbilicus the skin of the abdominal wall extends 2–3 cm or more around the cord; when the cord falls off, a prominent cutaneous area is left, but this tends to disappear slowly. With persistent urachus, urine may drain from the umbilicus, particularly when pressure is applied over the bladder.

The **anus** should be examined for patency; on rare occasions, an imperforate anus may not be visible. Anal patency can be confirmed with careful introduction of either a soft rubber catheter into the anus or by using a rectal thermometer to determine the initial temperature. Intestinal obstruction should be suspected if there is a history of polyhydramnios; if, soon after birth, gastric content exceeds 15 mL or is bilious stained; or if there is abdominal distention associated with vomiting or decreased number of meconium stools. A nasogastric tube should be passed immediately, and further studies performed. Meconium peritonitis is the result of prenatal intestinal perforation due to intrinsic or extrinsic congenital mechanical obstructions. Calcification in the abdomen is a characteristic finding on the abdominal radiograph. Pneumoperitoneum may occur in infants with necrotizing enterocolitis (NEC) or in infants with pulmonary air leaks in which the air dissects into the abdomen.

Hirschsprung disease does not usually present immediately after birth but can cause abdominal distention in the neonate. Meconium plug and meconium ileus, which can be the first manifestations of cystic fibrosis, cause delay in the elimination of meconium, resulting in abdominal distention. Normally, meconium stool is passed within 24 hours after birth in 90% of term infants and within 48 hours in 99%.

Genitalia. The genitalia should be examined to assess gestational age and to exclude anomalies. At term, the labia majora covers the labia minora and the clitoris, but in preterm infants the labia minora and the clitoris are evident. A hymenal appendix may protrude externally from the vaginal floor. This and mucoid cysts, which may be present around the vaginal orifice, disappear within a few weeks after birth. Associated with maternal hormone withdrawal is the presence of a milky-white vaginal discharge, sometimes stained with blood, during the first week after birth; it usually disappears in 1–2 weeks. A hypertrophied clitoris can result from virilization due to androgen excess associated with virilizing adrenal hyperplasia; the presence of ambiguous genitalia is a real medical and social emergency. Hydrometrocolpos is due to an imperforate hymen with retention of vaginal secretions; it presents as a lower midline abdominal mass or as a small cyst between the labia.

In male infants at term, the testes should be descended into a well-formed and pigmented scrotum. In preterm infants, the testes may be in the abdomen or in the inguinal canal, and the scrotum will be small with less rugae and pigmentation. In most cases of undescended testes, the testes descend spontaneously before 12 months of age. Undescended testes or cryptorchidism must be differentiated from retractile testes, which are intermittently absent from the scrotum but which are always distal to the inguinal ring. Cryptorchidism may be associated with inguinal hernia, genitourinary malformations, hypospadias, and other syndromes. The prepuce in normal newborns is tight and should not be retracted. The penis may be small or more frequently appears small because of the presence of pubic fat. Micropenis is frequently associated with chloacal extrophy or may be due to primary or secondary hypogonadism; it is also associated with Prader-Willi syndrome. The urethral meatus should be at the end of the penis. In epispadias, the meatus is in the dorsal area of the penis and is usually associated with bladder extrophy. In hypospadias, the meatus is on the ventral part of the penis in different locations along the shaft; it is not associated with increased incidence of urinary malformations. Perineal hypospadias presents as ambiguous genitalia; if both testes are within the scrotum, there is no doubt about the genetic sex (see Chapter 20). Scrotal swelling may be present in hydrocele or in cases of testicular torsion. Hydroceles can be unilateral or bilateral and are more frequent in term infants. They are caused by persistence of the processus vaginalis; they may also be associated with inguinal hernia. The hydrocele may communicate with the abdominal cavity, and its size may change. Isolated hydroceles usually cause no clinical problems and often disappear spontaneously in a few weeks. Inguinal hernias are usually easily reducible, but because the internal inguinal ring is narrow, the risk of strangulation is high and surgery should be performed early.

Extremities & Back. The extremities should be examined to detect anatomic and functional abnormalities. The lack of spontaneous movements in the upper extremities may suggest fractures, infection, or brachial plexus injury. When the upper extremity is moved by the examiner, the infant will show signs of pain in cases of fracture or in congenital syphilis. Partial or complete absence of the clavicles, as in cleidocranial dysostosis, allows the shoulders to be flexed forward without limitation. Congenital abnormalities of the elbow, radioulnar synostosis, and absence or hypoplasia of the radius are usually unilateral and limit pronation and supination movements. Absence or hypoplasia of the radius may be associated with syndromes such as thrombocytopenia, Fanconi anemia, and Holt-Oram syndrome. The hands and fingers should be inspected carefully for indications of chromosomal malformations. Polydactyly can occur as an isolated anomaly or as part of a syndrome. Rudimentary fingers are often adjacent to the fifth finger. Syndactyly is frequently an isolated finding of the second or third fingers and may be inherited as an autosomal dominant trait. Normally, the tibias are curved laterally and internally rotated, and the toes may overlap, which does not require treatment. Edema of the feet with hypoplastic nails is characteristic of Turner and Noonan syndromes. Rocker-bottom feet are frequently seen in trisomy 18.

The hips should be examined for congenital dysplasia. In about 1–1.5% of infants, there will be either an unstable hip (much more frequent) or a completely dislocated hip (see Chapter 23).

The spine should be examined for the presence of hair tufts, nevus, or even lipomas in the lumbar-sacral area, which may suggest the presence of spina bifida. If there is a sacrococcygeal pilonidal dimple, a careful attempt to identify the base should be made to rule out a neurocutaneous sinus tract. Myelomeningoceles are usually obvious at the time of birth.

NEUROLOGIC & BEHAVIORAL EXAMINATION

Newborn infants demonstrate considerable cortical control. They show directed responses in social interaction with a nurturing adult or in response to an attractive auditory or visual stimulus. When positive rather than intrusive stimuli are used, neonates have amazing capacities for alertness and attention. They can respond and interact with the environment from birth with very predictable behavior and can suppress interfering reflex responses to attend to more "interesting stimuli," such as a human face or voice, a soft rattle, or a light caress. This complex interaction of visual, auditory, and motor behaviors to respond to a human stimulus is managed by normal neonates despite the enormous physiologic demands of labor and transition to neonatal life.

Behavioral States

Observation of the spontaneous state of consciousness or "state" of the infant is an important part of the neurologic and behavioral examination. Sleep is categorized as quiet or active sleep or a drowsy state. Wakefulness is classified as quiet alert, active alert, fussing, and crying. Full-term infants spend about 80% of the time in a sleep state and rise to light sleep in a cyclic fashion every 3–4 hours. Active, or rapid eye movement (REM), sleep is predominant in the healthy term newborn. Preterm infants spend more time sleeping, and a higher percentage of this is REM sleep. State also depends on physiologic variables, such as hunger, nutrition, degree of hydration, and illnesses, but it is also clearly related to the time within the wake-sleep cycle of the neonate.

Optimal sensory responses are best exhibited during the state of quiet alertness. Neonates respond to a bright light not only with a pupillary response but also with withdrawal. Repeated stimulation is likely to result in neurologic habituation; this explains the lack of response of infants housed in noisy, brightly lit nurseries to sound or light stimuli. Sharply contrasting colors, large squares, and bright objects appeal to neonates and keep them in a prolonged alert state of fixation.

The neonate's auditory responses are specific and well organized. The infant may respond to auditory stimuli with changes in respirations and eye blinks, as well as with more obvious behavioral startles. In addition, alerting and head turning are likely to occur in response to the source of sound. Habituation to repeated auditory stimuli also occurs normally and can be a good test of CNS function because behavioral inhibition is not likely to occur when the cortex is damaged.

Newborn infants can differentiate taste and smell; they respond differently to acetic acid or alcohol than to sweet odors, such as milk and sugary solutions. By 5 days, they can reliably distinguish their own mother's breasts from those of other lactating mothers.

Infants are very sensitive to touch. A quiet baby becomes alert with a rapid, intrusive tactile stimulus. When the infant is upset, a slow, modulated tactile stimulus can reduce activity. A lack of response to soothing tactile stimuli in the neonate should raise suspicion of irritability due to CNS disturbance.

Important information about the neonate's status can be

gleaned from simple observation of how the infant moves the extremities, the kind of movements made, and, in particular, whether the movements are random startles or seem to be purposeful. Careful assessment of resting muscle tone and responsive motor activity may be the best evidence of CNS disorder. Table 4–8 summarizes movement patterns that are significant in predicting risk in CNS development. They can all be assessed by careful observation.

Assessment of the neonate's behavioral responses should be part of every pediatric examination because it reflects the capacity for integration of the CNS and, therefore, is an accurate way of assessing the well-being of the newborn. The Brazelton Neonatal Behavioral Assessment Examination is a detailed behavioral examination that includes 26 behavioral items, which are assessed during specific states of sleep or wakefulness.

Neurologic Examination

Neurologic function changes considerably during the last 3 months of gestation. Increase in flexor tone begins in the lower extremities and progresses cephalad between 28 and 40 weeks of gestation. This progression correlates with increasing myelination of subcortical pathways originating in the brainstem. For example, the infant at 28 weeks lies with both upper and lower extremities fully extended, and there is little or no resistance to passive movement of the extremities. By 34 weeks the lower extremities are flexed at the knees and the hips. By 36 weeks, there is flexion of the upper extremities. After 40 weeks, a gradual loss of the resting flexion posture begins in the upper extremities. Deep tendon reflexes, such as the biceps and the patellar, can be elicited in normal term infants. Ankle clonus is normally present but not sustained in the neonate.

The neurologic examination should be performed in detail with newborn infants. A screening test designed by Prechtl (Table 4–9) is useful to identify obvious disturbances.

The baby should be examined in a warm environment, preferably 2–3 hours after feeding. The state of sleep or wakefulness and the resting posture should be observed. In the supine position, the posture is normally symmetric with the limbs semi-flexed and the lower limbs in slight abduction at the hips. Abnormal signs include opisthotonos, constant turning of the head toward one side with asymmetric body posture. Spontaneous motor activity,

Table 4–8. Movement patterns suggestive of central nervous system disturbance in the neonate.

Constant lateralized asymmetry of reflex motor responses
Athetoid movements
Obligatory tonic neck responses
Constant strabismus of eyes
Hypertonic/hypotonic muscular responses
Obligatory thumb in fist
Persistent abnormal reflexes (eg, sucking, Moro)

Table 4–9. Minimal neurologic examination of the newborn.

State at beginning of examination
Posture: Limbs, trunk, head
Overall assessment of tone
Eyes: Centered, constant deviation, constant strabismus
Spontaneous motor activity: Symmetry, intensity, speed, tremors, overshooting, jerks, convulsions
Resistance to passive movements: Neck, trunk, arms, legs
Flexion tests: Resistance in arms and legs; head control
Suck reflex
Moro response: Complete, symmetric, without tremors
A careful assessment of resting muscle tone and responsive motor activity may be the best way to detect evidence of central nervous system disorder.

presence of athetoid postures and movements, jitteriness, rhythmic twitching of the face or tongue, or frank convulsions should be noted. Skull examination should include head circumference and inspection of the fontanelles and sutures.

Reflexes. Reflex responses should be tested. The **lip reflex,** protrusion of the lips with tapping of the upper or lower lip, is elicited readily in normal sleepy babies. The **glabella reflex,** brisk closure of the eyes of short duration, is elicited by tapping sharply on the glabella. In facial paresis, an asymmetric response is noted. A strong response occurs in hyperexcitable infants, and the reflex is absent or barely discernible in babies with CNS injury. Constant strabismus is abnormal, as is sustained nystagmus after slight movement of the head. Pupils should be of equal shape and size and should be reactive to light. Asymmetry of the pupils or poor response to light suggests neurologic dysfunction. The **optical blink reflex,** quick closure of the eyelids, is elicited by suddenly shining a bright light into the eyes. An absent response suggests impaired light perception or CNS dysfunction. The **acoustic blink reflex,** elicited by clapping the hands about 30 cm away from the infants head, may be absent with impaired auditory system. The **corneal reflex,** closure of the eyes on touching the cornea, is absent in lesions of the fifth cranial nerve. The **dolls' eyes test** is performed by turning the head slowly to the right and left; normally, the eyes do not move with the head but lag behind. With CNS anomalies the eyes will move with the head, and in abducens nerve paresis there is asymmetry in the response. This reflex disappears as fixation develops.

Tonic neck reflex is best examined in the supine position by turning the face slowly to the right side and holding it in the extreme position with the jaw over the right shoulder. The arms and leg of the face side will extend, and the "occipital" arm will flex at the elbow. The reflex is then performed toward the left. The response may or may not be present in the newborn, but a constantly present, well-marked tonic neck reflex, even at rest, may be a sign of neurologic dysfunction. The resistance against passive movements, power of active movements, and range of movement should be examined in the supine position with the head in the midline to avoid the tonic neck reflex. This can be evaluated by moving both the upper and lower limbs rhythmically and simultaneously through their full range of movement. During this examination, no undue force should be used.

The palmar grasp is elicited by placing the index fingers into the infant's hands and pressing the palmar surface; the dorsal side of the hands should not be touched. The normal response is flexion of all fingers around the examiner's finger. Difference of intensity of grasp between the two sides suggests an anomaly. If the grasping reflex is absent or weak, sucking should be stimulated because this facilitates grasping. If sucking has no effect, the cause of the absent palmar grasp is probably peripheral and not central. In Erb palsy or in clavicular fracture, for example, asymmetry is present; in infants with CNS depression, the response is weak or absent bilaterally.

The rooting response is produced by stroking one corner of the mouth while the head is kept midline to avoid the asymmetric tonic neck reflex. The normal response is a directed head turn toward the stimulated side. With stimulation of the upper lip at the corner of the mouth there is opening of the mouth and retroflexion of the head. After stimulation of the lower lip, the mouth opens and the jaw drops. In all instances, the infant tries to suck the finger applying the stimulation. This reflex is absent with generalized CNS depression. The sucking reflex is elicited by introducing the index finger 2–3 cm into the infant's mouth; the normal response is a rhythmic sucking movement. All phases of sucking should be evaluated, including the stripping action of the tongue, forcing upward and back, the rate of suctioning, the negative pressure developed, and the grouping of the sucks. Premature infants and those with CNS depression, which may be induced by drugs such as barbiturates, will have poor or absent sucking.

The Moro response should be obtained with the infant in a symmetric position and the head in the midline. The back is supported by one of the examiner's hands, and the head is held by the other. The head is then lowered a few centimeters when the neck muscles are relaxed. A complete Moro response consists of abduction of the upper limbs at the shoulder, extension of the forearms at the elbow, and extension of the fingers followed by adduction of the arms at the shoulder. The threshold for the Moro response should be noted because the reflex may be elicited very easily but may have a medium or high threshold. An absent or constantly weak Moro response indicates serious CNS disturbances; asymmetries occur with Erb palsy and clavicular fractures.

The infant should also be turned onto the stomach to be examined in the prone position. The vertebral column should be palpated with the first and second fingers, and the skin should be inspected. Normally, the head may be lifted off the table for a few seconds and turned from side to side. Lifting of the head several centimeters for 10 seconds or longer suggests hypertonia or opisthotonos. Crawling can be observed spontaneously or with reinforcement by pressing the hands gently on the soles of the feet (Bauer response). If a stimulus is applied along the paravertebral line, about 3 cm from the midline from the shoulder down to the buttocks, the trunk normally curves with the concavity on the stimulated side; this is the normal incurvation of the trunk response. This response is absent below the level of a lesion of the spinal cord.

One should note whether the thumb is held in an adducted position, buried in the hand, in the so-called thumb-in-fist position. If this is persistent, it represents an unfavorable CNS sign. Babies with different types of neurologic abnormality cry differently than do normal infants. High-pitched or weak cries are almost certainly abnormal, as well as whining and a catlike cry.

Finally, the infant should be examined upright to test the placing response, which is elicited by holding the baby with both hands under the arms and around the chest and stimulating the dorsal part of the foot by making it touch a protruding edge such as a table top. The feet will be lifted by simultaneous flexion of the knees and hips. This response is absent in paresis of the lower limbs. Subsequently, by allowing the soles of the feet to touch the surface of the table, the infant will show alternating stepping movements. This response is also absent with paresis of the lower limbs, in infants born by breech presentation, and in infants with CNS depression.

The cremasteric reflex is absent in spinal cord lesions. The anal reflex, elicited by scratching the perianal skin with a pin, is characterized by a contraction of the external anal sphincter. An absent reflex may be associated with damage to the sacral cord.

A normal neurologic assessment within the first week of life of the term newborn is a strong predictor of later normalcy. Similarly, for the premature newborn who has reached 40 weeks' postconceptual age, a normal neurologic assessment is a better guarantee for a normal outcome than the absence of visible damage on brain imaging. Further details of neurologic disturbances in the neonate are presented in Chapter 21. Some of the reflexes present in the neonate and their changes during maturation are shown in Table 4–10.

Prechtl has proposed clustering abnormal neurologic signs into diagnostic syndromes. **Hyperexcitable** infants are characterized by the presence of tremor of low frequency and high amplitude, very active tendon reflexes, and low threshold to the Moro reflex. The **apathy syndrome** is characterized by reduced responsiveness, decreased resistance to passive movements, and long periods of quiet wakefulness. Hyperexcitability is associated with mild sequelae in a small percentage of infants who have had perinatal asphyxia, but apathy is followed by moderate sequelae in a larger percentage of infants. The **hemisyndrome** is characterized by at least three findings of asymmetry in motility, posturing, or response to stimulation; this correlates with unilateral neurologic findings in childhood. The syndrome of severe CNS **depression or coma** is associated with slow or abnormal respiration and depressed response to stimuli; seizures are frequently present. More than 50% of survivors with this syndrome have severe sequelae.

Table 4–10. Strength of eight reflexes in infants between 28 and 40 weeks' gestation.

	Weeks						
	28	30	32	34	36	38	40
Sucking	Weak, not really synchronized with swallowing		Stronger and better synchronized with swallowing		Perfect		
Palmar grasp	Present but weak			Stronger		Excellent	
Response to traction	Absent		Begins to appear	Strong enough to lift part of body weight		Strong enough to lift all of body weight	
Moro reflex	Weak, obtained just once, incomplete		Complete reflex				
Crossed extension	Flexion and extension in random pattern, purposeless reaction		Good extension but no tendency to adduction		Tendency to adduction, but imperfect	Complete response with extension, adduction, fanning of toes	
Automatic walking	—		Begins tiptoeing with good support on sole and righting reaction of legs			An infant born prematurely who reaches 40 wk walks in toe-heel progression on tiptoes	
				Quite good; very fast tiptoeing		A full-term newborn of 40 wk walks in heel-toe progression on whole sole of foot	
Root	Good with reinforcement		Good (no reinforcement)		Good	Good	Good
Pupillary response			Present	Present		Present	Present

ABNORMALITIES OF GROWTH

Adequate fetal growth is dependent on provision of substrates for fetal consumption, but tissue growth also depends on an appropriate fetal endocrine milieu. Insulin has been implicated as the growth hormone of the fetus; because it does not cross the placenta, it must be secreted by the fetus. In the absence of fetal insulin production, as in transient neonatal diabetes mellitus, congenital absence of the islets of Langerhans, or pancreatic aplasia, fetal growth is impaired. Hyperinsulinism in utero, as occurs in infants of mothers with diabetes, is associated with increased adipose and muscle tissue mass and excessive birth weight. C peptide, a cleavage protein of proinsulin, is also reduced with IUGR and increased with fetal macrosomia. Growth hormone and thyroid hormones do not affect fetal growth. Other hormones, such as insulin-like growth regulatory factor 2, have anabolic and growth functions.

SMALL-FOR-GESTATIONAL-AGE INFANTS

Infants that are born with a weight below the 5th percentile for corresponding gestational age are considered SGA. This is a sign that intrauterine growth has either stopped or slowed significantly some time during pregnancy. Growth failure can be symmetric; that is, the weight, length, and head circumference are approximately in the same percentile. IUGR can also be asymmetric; the head circumference can be either normal or less affected than length or weight. The length, in turn, may be affected similarly or less than the weight. Causes and types of SGA infants are shown in Table 4–11. When growth is af-

Table 4–11. Etiology of intrauterine growth retardation.

Type I: Early interference with fetal growth (from conception to 24 weeks' gestation)
Chromosomal anomalies (trisomy 21, 13–15, 18, etc)
Fetal infections (cytomegalovirus, toxoplasmosis, rubella, herpes)
Maternal drugs (chronic alcoholism, heroin)
Maternal chronic hypertension; severe diabetes

Type II: Chronic intrauterine malnutrition (24–32 weeks' gestation)
Inadequate intrauterine space (multiple pregnancies, uterine tumors, uterine anomalies)
Placental insufficiency: Maternal vascular disease (renal, chronic essential hypertension, collagen diseases, pregnancy-induced hypertension)
Small placenta with abnormal cellularity

Type III: Late intrauterine malnutrition (after 32 weeks' gestation)
Placental infarct or fibrosis
Pregnancy-induced hypertension
Maternal hypoxemia (lung disease, smoking)
Postmaturity
Maternal small stature or malnutrition

fected early in gestation, type I SGA, the growth retardation will be symmetric. In many of these infants, cell number is decreased in most organs. Head circumference is smaller than in other types of IUGR, and these infants typically have poor long-term outcomes. Infants that are SGA because they were subjected to chronic intrauterine hypoxia associated with uterine placental insufficiency (type II) have a normal number of cells that are reduced in size; they are at increased risk for perinatal problems (Table 4–12). Type III SGA (late intrauterine malnutrition) infants usually do well in long-term follow-up. In addition, if an infant is small because family members are small, outcome is good.

The ponderal index measures the relationship between weight (g) and length (cm): (weight/length) × 100. In normal infants, it is 2.32–2.85. In type I SGA infants, this index is normal; however, in type III it is less than 2.32. The lower the index, the more significant the asymmetry in intrauterine growth.

LARGE-FOR-GESTATIONAL-AGE INFANTS

Infants may be large for gestational age but not show high birth weight (> 4000 g). LGA infants, with or without high birth weight, frequently demonstrate hypoglycemia and polycythemia. Infants of diabetic mothers (IDMs) also have a higher incidence of RDS and sudden intrauterine death. Inappropriately increased weight for gestational age is often associated with congenital malformations. The more common causes of increased weight and LGA infants are listed in Table 4–13.

Infants of Diabetic Mothers

IDMs are large because of increased body fat and visceromegaly, primarily of the liver, adrenals, and heart. The skeletal length is increased in proportion to weight, but the head and face appear disproportionately small. The umbilical cord and placenta are also enlarged. Maternal hyperglycemia causes fetal hyperglycemia and fetal hyperinsulinemia. This causes increased hepatic glucose uptake and glycogen synthesis, accelerated lipogenesis, augmented protein synthesis, and macrosomia. In women with severe vascular complications, however, infants may be SGA secondary to placental insufficiency. IDMs appear plethoric with round facies. They are at considerable risk for the perinatal difficulties summarized in Table 4–14. Hypoglycemia occurs frequently after birth in these

infants, and prompt recognition and treatment is important (see Chapter 20).

Evaluation of fetal lung maturity is very important in mothers with diabetes because RDS develops in many with a normal lecithin-sphingomyelin (LS) ratio; evaluation of amniotic fluid phosphatidylglycerol concentration is a more reliable predictor of lung maturity (see later in this chapter, Respiratory Distress Syndrome). High fetal insulin concentrations delay the appearance of lamellar bodies in type 2 cells and increase glycogen content of the alveolar lining cells. If they do not lack pulmonary surfactant, many of these infants have respiratory distress because of transient tachypnea or PPHN. In some infants, hypertrophic cardiomyopathy develops; this is often manifested on echocardiography by asymmetric septal hypertrophy as well as thickening of the ventricular wall. This condition is usually benign and resolves spontaneously, but the findings could be interpreted as idiopathic hypertrophic subaortic stenosis.

A condition occurring exclusively in IDMs is the neonatal small left colon syndrome. This presents with failure to pass meconium, abdominal distention, and, in some infants, bile-stained vomitus. Barium enema shows a decreased caliber of the left colon. The syndrome is transient, but some infants improve slowly and require a transient colostomy. Congenital anomalies are two to four times more frequent in IDMs than in normal infants (Table 4–14). Maternal glycohemoglobin concentration (HbA$_{1C}$) has been shown to correlate with poor diabetic control and with an increased incidence of congenital malformations. When maternal HbA$_{1C}$ concentration is less than 8.5% in the first trimester of pregnancy, there is a low incidence of congenital malformations. Many of the problems in IDMs are related to less than adequate diabetic control during the preconceptual period and throughout pregnancy.

Table 4–13. Large-for-gestational-age infants: Causes.

Genetic/racial	Maternal drugs, such as tocolytic sympathomimetics
Infants of diabetic mothers	
Beckwith-Wiedemann syndrome	Rh immunization
	Prader-Willi syndrome
β-Cell nesidioblastosis spectrum	
Functional β-cell hyperplasia	

Table 4–12. Perinatal problems in small-for-gestational-age infants.

Perinatal asphyxia	Hypocalcemia
Hypothermia	Meconium aspiration syndrome
Hypoglycemia	Intrauterine fetal death
Polycythemia	Hypermagnesemia (maternal MgSO$_4$
Thrombocytopenia	therapy)

Table 4–14. Problems in infants of diabetic mothers.

Sudden intrauterine death	Hypertrophic cardiomyopathy
Large for gestational age	Persistent pulmonary hypertension of the newborn
Birth trauma	
Increased rate of cesarean section	Respiratory distress syndrome
	Congenital malformations: Cardiac, central nervous system, musculoskeletal
Asphyxia	
Hypoglycemia	
Polycythemia	
Hypocalcemia	

Treatment of IDMs includes careful monitoring of blood glucose concentrations, early feeding, and treatment of respiratory or cardiac insufficiency. Many infants require intravenous fluids with glucose for several hours after birth to prevent hypoglycemia. In infants of well-controlled diabetic mothers, not only is the neonatal morbidity rate significantly decreased, but also physical and mental development is essentially normal in long-term follow-up. The incidence of subsequent overt diabetes in women who have diabetes during pregnancy is 0.5–1% in most studies, but rates as high as 10% have been reported.

ABNORMALITIES OF MATURITY

PREMATURITY

A **preterm** delivery is defined as one occurring after less than 37 completed weeks of gestation from the first day of the last menstrual period. Approximately two thirds of neonates with birth weights less than 2500 g are preterm; few premature infants weigh more than 2500 g. The incidence of preterm delivery is higher in lower socioeconomic populations and in women who do not receive prenatal care. Approximately 7% of births are preterm, but this figure varies widely across the country and across the world. VLBW infants (those < 1500 g) constitute approximately 1.2% of all births in the United States but account for more than 40% of neonatal deaths. Perinatal care and improved survival rates of these VLBW infants have had a major impact on total neonatal and infant deaths. Furthermore, the decreasing mortality rate has not been associated with a significantly increased morbidity rate. The problems that the premature infant may face from the time of birth to the first several weeks of life are listed in Table 4–15.

Respiratory insufficiency is very common in preterm infants because they have less pulmonary compliance, qualitative and quantitative surfactant deficiency, increased compliance of the airway and rib cage, incomplete

Table 4–15. Frequent problems in preterm infants.

Increased incidence of neonatal death	Patent ductus arteriosus
Perinatal asphyxia	Intracranial hemorrhage
Hypothermia	Necrotizing enterocolitis
Hypoglycemia	Infection
Hypocalcemia	Retinopathy of prematurity
Respiratory distress syndrome	Bronchopulmonary dysplasia
Fluid and electrolyte abnormalities	Disrupted mother-father-infant interaction
Indirect hyperbilirubinemia	

development of respiratory muscles, and immaturity of mechanisms involved in respiratory control. Many of these infants require intubation and ventilation immediately after birth. The issues of temperature regulation and many other difficulties faced by preterm infants are discussed elsewhere in this chapter.

POSTMATURITY

The other extreme of maturation is the **post-term** pregnancy, lasting more than 42 weeks beyond the onset of the last menstrual period. The fetus of the post-term pregnancy may continue to grow in utero and therefore may become unusually large. If the uterine environment is unfavorable for fetal growth, the infant at birth may have significant loss of subcutaneous fat and muscle mass. In severe cases, meconium staining of the skin, nails, and umbilical cord; loss of vernix caseosa; and patchy or scaly skin are evident. The term **postmature** has been applied to these infants. **Dysmaturity** refers to infants who are born after sustaining placental insufficiency. The smaller, postmature infants are at great risk for fetal death and distress in labor; by 43 weeks' gestation, perinatal mortality rate doubles, and by 44 weeks it triples, compared with full-term infants at 39–41 weeks' gestation. Neonatal morbidity is also high because of fetal asphyxia, meconium aspiration syndrome (MAS), polycythemia, and hypoglycemia. Prolonged gestation may be secondary to anencephaly or to placental sulfatase deficiency. Because of the high perinatal morbidity of postmaturity, induction of labor is suggested after 42 weeks and definitely recommended after 43 weeks.

APPROACHES TO COMMON NEOTATAL CLINICAL PROBLEMS

CYANOSIS

Cyanosis is a bluish discoloration of the skin and mucous membranes. Some ancient cultures considered it a sign of divinity. In the neonate, it always constitutes an emergency, requiring immediate diagnosis and treatment. Clinical detection of cyanosis depends on the experience and ability of the observer, as well as on the environmental lighting. Cyanosis does not always indicate hypoxemia (low Pao_2). More important, infants may be severely hypoxic (low oxygen delivery to the tissues) without showing clinical cyanosis.

The interactions between hemoglobin (Hb) and oxygen are well described in physiology texts. Hb combines rapidly and reversibly with oxygen as long as its iron is in the ferrous state. Cyanosis is directly related to an absolute concentration of unoxygenated or reduced Hb. It is evident when more than 3 g/dL of Hb in arterial blood is reduced, or more than 5 g/dL in capillary blood. Fetal and adult Hb differ in their binding capacity for oxygen. The P_{50}, or Pao_2 at which Hb is 50% saturated with oxygen, in adult human blood is about 27 mm Hg. The P_{50} for fetal Hb is about 20 mm Hg. The Hb oxygen dissociation curve for HbF is thus shifted to the left, so that at the same Po_2, oxygen saturation is higher in fetal than in adult blood. In venous blood, in which Po_2 is about 30–35 mm Hg, Hb oxygen saturation in the neonate is about 80%; however, in the adult it is 70% or less. The Pao_2 necessary to produce oxygen desaturation of a degree to show cyanosis in the neonate is approximately 38–39 mm Hg, but in the adult it is 52–54 mm Hg.

Thus, cyanosis will develop in neonates at a lower Pao_2 than that necessary to produce cyanosis in older children or adults. The Hb dissociation curve can shift to the left or right for reasons other than Hb type (Table 4–16).

With low total Hb concentration, as in anemia, a higher percentage of desaturation is needed to cause cyanosis. In the normal neonate, the usual Hb concentration is 17 g/dL. When oxygen saturation is approximately 82%, more than 3 g/dL of Hb is reduced (18% of 17 g/dL), and cyanosis is evident. (The Pao_2 necessary to produce cyanosis in this case is approximately 38–39 mm Hg.) Many infants, particularly those who are premature, have Hb concentrations of 12 g/dL or less. In such cases, the desaturation needs to be 25% (saturation as low as 75%, Pao_2 30 mm Hg) to produce a reduced Hb concentration greater than 3 g/dL and, therefore, cyanosis.

When the total concentration of Hb is increased, as in polycythemia, the amount of reduced Hb in arterial blood will be higher even with only small reductions of oxygen saturation; cyanosis may be evident at saturations of 85–92%. In polycythemia, hyperviscosity may decrease the velocity of capillary blood, which may increase reduced Hb to more than 5 g/dL in the capillary bed even with normal arterial oxygen saturation, and cause peripheral cyanosis.

The major pathophysiologic mechanisms for cyanosis are shown in Table 4–17. In some conditions, several pathophysiologic mechanisms may be responsible for cyanosis. Oxygen saturation, Pao_2, and $Paco_2$ vary according to the cause of cyanosis. For example, if an infant's blood is dark with a very low saturation but with a normal Pao_2, the diagnosis is a decreased affinity of Hb for oxygen (eg, methemoglobinemia). When an infant is cyanotic and the $Paco_2$ is increased, cyanosis is likely to be respiratory in origin.

Immediate treatment of cyanosis may be necessary; this includes administration of oxygen and rapid correction of abnormalities of temperature, hematocrit, and glucose and calcium concentrations. In severely cyanotic infants, intubation and mechanical ventilation may be necessary.

Although the cause of cyanosis is usually apparent, sometimes it is difficult to differentiate between a pul-

Table 4–17. Pathophysiologic mechanisms of cyanosis and corresponding clinical entities.

Alveolar hypoventilation
Lung parenchyma: RDS, pulmonary edema, pulmonary hypoplasia, MAS.
Space-occupying lesions of the chest: Pneumothorax, interstitial emphysema, congenital lobar emphysema, congenital diaphragmatic hernia, pleural effusion, abdominal distention.
Obstructive lesions: Choanal atresia, vocal cord paralysis, vascular rings, stenotic lesions, membranes, and cysts, Pierre Robin syndrome.
Central nervous system: Infection, hemorrhage, asphyxia, seizures, apnea, malformations, tumors.
Neuromuscular: Phrenic nerve palsy, thoracic dystrophies.
Metabolic: Hypoglycemia, hypocalcemia.
Cardiovascular: Heart failure (PDA, supraventricular tachycardia, congenital AV block).

Right-to-left shunt
Intrapulmonary: MAS, respiratory distress syndrome; also may have alveolar hypoventilation.
Persistent pulmonary hypertension of the newborn (PPHN): may have alveolar hypoventilation.
Cardiac: Decreased pulmonary blood flow (tetralogy of Fallot, tricuspid atresia, pulmonary atresia), normal or increased pulmonary blood flow (transposition of the great vessels, truncus arteriosus, anomalous pulmonary venous return).

Abnormal ventilation-perfusion ratios
Lung parenchyma: Atelectasis, MAS, infections, pulmonary hemorrhage.

Abnormal diffusion
PIE, aspirations, pulmonary hemorrhage.

Decreased hemoglobin O_2 affinity
Methemoglobinemia (nitrites, sulfonamides, other drugs, congenital).

Decreased peripheral circulation (peripheral cyanosis)
Low cardiac output (hypocalcemia, pneumopericardium, cardiomyopathies, etc), shock of any etiology, polycythemia, hypothermia, hypoglycemia.

AV = atrioventricular; MAS = meconium aspiration syndrome; PDA = patent ductus arteriosus; PIE = pulmonary interstitial emphysema; RDS = respiratory distress syndrome.

Table 4–16. Causes of shift in hemoglobin dissociation curve.

To the Left (Lower P_{50}, more O_2 affinity)	To the Right (Higher P_{50}, less O_2 affinity)
HbF	HbA
Alkalosis	Acidosis
Hypocarbia	Hypercarbia
Decreased 2,3-DPG concentration	Increased 2,3-DPG concentration
Hypothermia	Hyperthermia
Carbon monoxide	Anemia
Hexokinase deficiency	Hypoxia
	Increased catecholamine concentration
	Pyruvate kinase deficiency

DPG = diphosphoglycerate; Hb = hemoglobin.

monary and a cardiac condition. A low Pao_2 with a low or normal $Paco_2$ suggests the presence of a right-to-left shunt that can be associated with congenital heart disease, pulmonary disease, or PPHN. In most infants with pulmonary disease, the $Paco_2$ will be elevated. An **oxygen** test may be useful in differentiation.

In infants who have cyanotic congenital heart disease with reduced pulmonary blood flow, administering 100% oxygen will increase the Pao_2 only slightly, usually less than 10–15 mm Hg. With lung disease, the Pao_2 usually increases considerably, often reaching levels greater than 150 mm Hg. In infants with cyanotic congenital heart lesions associated with normal or increased pulmonary blood flow, Pao_2 usually increases more than 15–20 mm Hg with 100% oxygen, but levels above 150 mm Hg are unusual. Some infants with severe lung disease or with PPHN may have large right-to-left shunts through the foramen ovale or ductus arteriosus, and Pao_2 therefore may not increase by more than 10–15 mm Hg with 100% oxygen.

Simultaneous measurement of oxygen saturation in the right arm and the leg may be useful. This can be done with skin surface oxygen saturation measurement or by direct sampling from a right radial artery and an umbilical arterial catheter in the descending aorta to measure Pao_2. Right-to-left shunting through the ductus arteriosus results in a lower oxygen saturation in the lower body. This may occur in congenital cardiac lesions such as interrupted aortic arch, in pulmonary diseases, and commonly in PPHN. In PPHN, the difference in Pao_2 may increase dramatically with 100% oxygen administration, reaching levels considerably higher than 100–150 mm Hg in the right radial artery, whereas descending aortic Pao_2 increases only slightly.

RESPIRATORY DISTRESS

Respiratory problems are among the most significant causes of morbidity and mortality during the neonatal period. MAS and PPHN in the full-term infant and RDS or HMD in the preterm infant are the more common pulmonary causes of respiratory distress. In general, infants with respiratory distress have tachypnea, decreased air entry or gas exchange, retractions (which may be intercostal, subcostal, or suprasternal), grunting, stridor, flaring of the alae nasae, and cyanosis. Many of these signs are nonspecific responses of the newborn to serious illnesses, and any of the conditions listed in Table 4–18 can cause respiratory distress. Thus, many conditions that produce neonatal respiratory distress are not primary diseases of the lungs. The differential diagnosis involves multiple organ systems.

The prenatal and perinatal history must be reviewed in detail, particularly in relation to diabetes, the presence of oligohydramnios or polyhydramnios, Rh or blood group incompatibility, maternal hemorrhage, premature rupture of the membranes (PROM), perinatal asphyxia or acido-

Table 4–18. Differential diagnosis of respiratory distress in neonates.

Respiratory	
Lung	Respiratory distress syndrome, meconium aspiration syndrome, persistent pulmonary hypertension of the newborn, pneumonia, transient tachypnea, pulmonary air leaks, pleural effusions, chylothorax, tumors, pulmonary hypoplasia, congenital lobar emphysema, congenital cystic adenomatoid malformation or the lung, lymphangiectasia, bronchopulmonary dysplasia
Airway	Nasal or choanal atresia, Pierre Robin syndrome, laryngotracheomalacia, membranes or stenosis of larynx or trachea; vocal cord paralysis, hemangiomas, lymphangiomas, massive aspirations, bronchopulmonary dysplasia
Cardiovascular	
Heart failure (congenital heart disease, cardiomyopathy)	
Myocarditis	
Tachyarrhythmias or bradyarrhythymias	
Patent ductus arteriosus	
Peripheral: Shock	
Nervous system	
Central	Meningoencephalitis, intracranial hemorrhage, congenital lesions, tumors
Peripheral	Phrenic nerve paralysis, vocal cord paralysis
Muscular-Skeletal	
Malformations	Thoracic dystrophies (dysplasias, osteogenesis, hypophosphatasia, Jeune syndrome, trisomy D and E)
Diaphragm	Eventration, hernia, paralysis
Hematologic	
Anemia	
Polycythemia	
Metabolic	
Hypoglycemia (infants of diabetic mothers)	
Hypocalcemia	
Hypothermia	
Inborn errors of metabolism	
Acidosis (organic, lactic, glycogenesis)	
Infections	
Sepsis, bacteremia	
Pneumonia	
Meningitis	
Drugs	
Any that depress central nervous system or induce acidemia or tissue hypoxia	
Abdominal	
Omphalocele	
Gastroschisis	
Ascites	
Significant distention	
Tumors	
Congenital anomalies	
Other	
Erythroblastosis fetalis	
Nonimmune hydrops	

sis, and the need for resuscitation. Oligohydramnios secondary to renal disorders or amniotic leakage could lead to pulmonary hypoplasia, Potter facies, malposition of the extremities, and growth retardation. Esophageal atresia or atresia of the upper gastrointestinal tract should be suspected with polyhydramnios. However, congenital diaphragmatic hernia, Rh incompatibility, mesoblastic nephroma, and nonimmune hydrops are also associated with polyhydramnios. The possibility of infection or pneumonia should be considered with prolonged rupture of membranes. Respiratory distress is more likely to occur in infants born by cesarean section. The risk of respiratory distress is 11 times greater in infants born by cesarean section than in those delivered vaginally. When a cesarean section is performed without preceding labor, more fluid remains in the lungs after birth; its absorption results in lower plasma colloid oncotic pressures compared with those of infants born by cesarean with previous labor. Furthermore, pulmonary vascular resistance is increased in these infants. Thoracic gas volume is diminished during the first 6 hours after birth, and less pulmonary surfactant is secreted.

The time of onset of respiratory distress is important. Absence of respiratory distress during the first few hours excludes RDS, MAS, transient tachypnea, severe diaphragmatic hernia, choanal atresia and other congenital anomalies, and most cases of PPHN. Table 4–19 classifies respiratory distress according to the time of onset of symptoms and clinical course.

In the infant with respiratory distress, an attempt should be made to differentiate between intrathoracic and extrathoracic causes. Intrathoracic causes include abnormalities of lungs, heart, diaphragm, rib cage, or airways. Extrathoracic causes include neurologic, abdominal, hematologic, and metabolic abnormalities; shock; infection; drugs; and those related to the upper airway obstruction. Usually, extrathoracic causes can be excluded readily from the history, physical examination, hematocrit, and blood pressure values. Abdominal causes usu-

ally can be diagnosed by inspection and palpation of the abdomen. Neurologic causes can be detected by history, examination, and imaging procedures. Extrathoracic obstruction of the airway usually causes inspiratory difficulty and stridor, because the normal reduction in extrathoracic airway diameter during inspiration is exaggerated. Suprasternal retraction may also be noted. Obstruction of the intrathoracic airways is unusual in the immediate neonatal period and is related to anatomic or spasmodic narrowing of the small airways during expiration; therefore, it is associated with a prolonged expiratory phase and wheezing. This usually occurs with bronchopulmonary dysplasia (BPD), bronchiolitis, and, occasionally, massive aspiration of meconium. If the obstruction is located in the intermediate segment of the airway, both inspiratory and expiratory stridor may occur.

Although a chest radiograph may not be diagnostic soon after birth, it may document such conditions as pneumothorax, pulmonary agenesis or hypoplasia, diaphragmatic hernia, and thoracic cysts. It is useful to classify intrathoracic causes of respiratory distress in the newborn by chest radiograph according to the intrathoracic volume (Table 4–20).

Evaluation

Assessment of the infant with respiratory distress includes a detailed history and examination; a chest radiograph; and measurement of arterial blood gases, Hb, hematocrit, and glucose and calcium concentrations. Depending on the clinical features, blood cultures and leukocyte and platelet counts should be included. An ECG, echocardiogram, and neurologic imaging procedures may also be indicated.

Management

As with all sick newborns, infants with respiratory distress should be placed in a neutral thermal environment with humidification; intravenous fluids and glucose should be administered. Oxygen should be given for hy-

Table 4–19. Causes of respiratory distress according to time of onset and clinical course.

Onset of Symptoms	Acute Course	Progressive Course
At birth	Pneumothorax, apnea, asphyxia, maternal drugs, choanal atresia and other congenital anomalies, diaphragmatic hernia, pulmonary hypoplasia	Respiratory distress syndrome, transient tachypnea, persistent pulmonary hypertension of the newborn, pneumonias, meconium aspiration; aspiration of clear or bloody amniotic fluid; rarely, congenital heart disease (CHD).
0–7 d	Pulmonary air leaks (pneumothorax, pneumomediastinum, pneumopericardium) apnea, sepsis, hypoglycemia, intracranial hemorrhage, pulmonary hemorrhage, aspiration	Pulmonary interstitial emphysema (PIE), pneumonias, congenital intrathoracic lesions; some CHD; abdominal distension, omphalocele, gastroschisis, neuromuscular disease, metabolic acidosis, patent ductus arteriosus (PDA).
After 7 d	Same as above	PIE, pneumonias, PDA, bronchopulmonary dysplasia, diaphragmatic eventration, phrenic palsy, congenital lobar emphysema, congenital cystic adenomatoid malformation of the lung, other intrathoracic abnormalities, some CHD.

Table 4–20. Chest radiograph classification according to intrathoracic volume.

Increased intrathoracic volume
Transient tachypnea of the newborn
Aspiration
Pneumothorax and other pulmonary air leaks
Cystic malformations
Congenital lobar emphysema
Diaphragmatic hernia
Some congenital heart diseases
Some cases of persistent pulmonary hypertension of the newborn (PPHN)
Bronchopulmonary dysplasia

Decreased intrathoracic volume
Respiratory distress syndrome
Atelectasis
Other: Pulmonary edema, hemorrhage, hypoplasia

Normal intrathoracic volume
Pneumonias
Some congenital heart diseases
Asymmetric intrathoracic volume
Pleural effusions
Chylothorax
Diaphragmatic eventration and paralysis
Congenital lobar emphysema
Pulmonary cysts
Diaphragmatic hernia
Pneumothorax

Variable intrathoracic volume
Pulmonary edema
Congenital heart disease
PPHN
Mediastinum tumors

poxemia. Heart rate and respirations, as well as oxygen saturation or Pao_2, should be monitored continuously by noninvasive methods. Serial blood gas determinations may be indicated; if repeated measurements are necessary, an indwelling radial arterial or umbilical arterial catheter should be placed. Infants whose condition continues to deteriorate, with increasing respiratory acidosis or significant hypoventilation or apnea, require endotracheal intubation and mechanical ventilation. Respiratory acidosis (decreased pH with elevated $Paco_2$ and no reduction in the bicarbonate concentration) is frequently noted in infants with pulmonary insufficiency associated with lung disease, upper airway abnormalities, malformations of the thoracic rib cage or diaphragm, neurologic abnormalities, and phrenic nerve palsy. Treatment requires assisted ventilation and *not* intravenous alkali such as sodium bicarbonate. Some infants with pulmonary insufficiency have increased $Paco_2$ and decreased pH but also have reduced bicarbonate concentration (mixed metabolic and respiratory acidosis). In addition to mechanical ventilation, tris(hydroxymethyl) aminomethane (THAM) may be used to correct the metabolic component in these infants. Hypoventilation due to central depression from transplacental passage of narcotics used during labor should be treated by assisted ventilation and narcotic antagonists, such as naloxone.

In the immediate neonatal period, the normal blood pH is greater than 7.30 and the normal base excess is about –4. Metabolic acidosis is considered to be present when pH is less than 7.30 and base excess is –5 or greater. The $Paco_2$ will decrease if the lungs and CNS are functioning appropriately to compensate for the decrease in pH. Usually, bicarbonate should not be given intravenously unless the infant is critically ill, the pH is less than 7.25, and the base deficit is greater than 10.

Continuing management of acidosis should be determined on the basis of the pathophysiologic mechanisms involved. If the infant has respiratory distress with a low Pao_2 and low $Paco_2$, the problem is likely to be cardiac. If the Pao_2 is normal and the infant is hypotonic or hyporeflexic, the cause may be infectious or, less commonly, an inborn error of metabolism. There are also nutritional, renal, hematologic, or iatrogenic causes of metabolic acidosis during the neonatal period.

Additional therapeutic procedures may be necessary. Blood volume expansion should be instituted for hypovolemic shock, and packed red blood cells should be provided for anemia. Inotropic cardiac support may also be indicated. If metabolic acidosis persists and the pH is less than 7.25, sodium bicarbonate in a solution that contains 0.5 meq/mL may be given by slow intravenous infusion. The dose of bicarbonate in milliequivalents in neonates is derived from the following formula:

$$0.7 \times \textbf{body weight (grams)} \times \textbf{base excess}$$

where 0.7 is an estimated constant for the distribution space of bicarbonate. Only half the calculated dose should be given initially; the acid-base status is then reviewed, and additional amounts of sodium bicarbonate may be given. Sodium bicarbonate may cause complications, particularly hypervolemia and hypernatremia. When sodium bicarbonate is used, the serum calcium and particularly ionized calcium concentrations should be monitored carefully, and calcium administered as needed.

NEONATAL ANEMIA

Hematopoiesis

Hematopoiesis begins in the embryo by approximately the 20th day of gestation in blood islands in the yolk sac. The site of erythropoiesis changes during gestation; in the second trimester it occurs primarily in the liver and spleen, and toward the end of the last trimester the bone marrow becomes the predominant site of erythropoiesis. The Hb concentration is usually 8–10 g/dL by 12 weeks' gestation and continues to increase until approximately 33 weeks in male fetuses, and 38–39 weeks in female fetuses. Newborn girls normally have lower values of Hb than do boys between 30 and 38 weeks. A full-term male infant with a Hb of 13 g/dL or less at birth should be considered to have anemia, but this is within normal limits for a female infant born at 30 weeks' gestation. The following formula is useful for estimating Hb concentration in relation to gestational age in female infants at birth: Hb concentration = lunar months of gestation + 7. For example, if the duration of gestation was 32 weeks (8 lunar months), the approximate value for a normal Hb concentration would be 15 g/dL. By this time, male fetuses have almost achieved values that are normally accepted for term infants (at 33 weeks the normal value for male infants is already 16.5–17.5 g/dL).

After birth, Hb levels increase transiently by 6–12 hours because of loss of water from the intravascular space. Subsequently, Hb concentration decreases, achieving a nadir by 3–6 months in full-term infants and by 6–10 weeks in preterm infants. Fetal and neonatal red blood cells are larger than adult cells, with a mean corpuscular volume of 110–120 fL, and they have a shorter half life of 70–90 days versus 120 days for adult cells. By 2 months after birth, normal full-term infants maintain a hematocrit of about 35%, with a red blood cell mass of only 80% of that at birth. However, a premature infant born at 1500 g would require a red blood cell mass of 130% of that at birth to achieve a hematocrit of 35% by 2 months. Premature infants are not able to increase the red blood cell mass so that their hematocrits are much lower at 2 months of postnatal age. Clinical signs of anemia are evident only when it is severe enough to affect oxygen delivery to the tissues. Hematocrit and Hb values vary with the site from which they are obtained. In general, values are higher in central venous than in arterial samples, and during the first few days after birth, capillary samples obtained by heel stick have higher values than central venous samples. In edematous infants, values are lower in the capillary samples.

Fetal HbF represents 65–90% of total Hb concentration at birth but normally decreases to less than 5% by 4 months of age. Fetal Hb values decline rapidly in infants that receive multiple transfusions or exchange transfusions. HbF is composed of two α chains and two γ chains; adult HbA is composed of two α-globin and two β-globin chains. HbF has a lower P_{50} compared with HbA. The release of oxygen to the tissues is less with HbF than with HbA. For this reason, at the same total Hb concentration and oxygen content of arterial blood, tissue oxygen uptake will be more greatly impaired with higher concentrations of HbF.

The blood volume of the term infant is approximately 85 mL/kg, and it is greater than 90 mL/kg in the preterm infant. The total fetal-placental blood volume is 25–35 mL/kg greater. At the time of birth, the relative blood volumes in the placenta and the infant can vary with position and time of cord clamping. Thus, if the baby is above the level of the placenta and the umbilical cord is clamped early, neonatal blood volume will be relatively lower. It is recommended that the infant be kept at the level of the placenta and the cord clamped about 30 seconds after delivery to avoid hypovolemia with subsequent anemia.

Etiology

Anemia is suspected by the presence of pallor, a heart murmur, poor peripheral perfusion, and tissue hypoxia with metabolic acidosis or, more frequently, is detected by a low hematocrit value or a low Hb concentration. The diagnosis of anemia from Hb and hematocrit values must take into account gestational age, sex, and postnatal age.

The common causes of neonatal anemia are blood loss and isoimmune hemolytic conditions. Table 4–21 lists the causes of neonatal anemia. Severe minor group incompatibilities, severe Rh disease, α-thalassemia, and congenital perinatal infections present soon after birth. ABO hemolytic disease (when the mother's blood type is O, and she carries high IgG titers of either anti-A or anti-B) usually presents more than 48–72 hours after birth with hyperbilirubinemia and decreasing Hb and hematocrit. β-Thalassemia major and sickle cell disease do not commonly manifest anemia during the neonatal period. The cause of blood loss differs in term and preterm infants, as does the time of manifestation of anemia. Early anemia in the term infant due to blood loss is usually related to obstetric conditions (eg, fetal-maternal bleeding, placenta previa, and cord conditions), whereas in the preterm infant

Table 4–21. Causes of neonatal anemia.

	Blood Loss	Hemolysis	Decreased Production	Other

Common	Fetal-maternal transfusion
	Placenta previa
	Abruption of placenta
	Twin-twin transfusion
	Organ hemorrhage
	  (cranial, hepatic, adrenal)
	Blood withdrawal
		ABO incompatibility
		Minor group incompatibility
			Intrauterine congenital
			  infection
				Anemia of prematurity
				  (multifactorial)

Uncommon	Vasa previa
	Cord accidents (knots,
	  nuchal rupture)
	Placental severage during
	  C-section
		Rh incompatibility
		Enzyme deficiency
		Abnormal hemoglobin
		Membrane abnormalities
		Lupus and other maternal
		  autoimmune conditions
		Disseminated intravascu-
		  lar coagulation
			Congenital aplasia
			Congenital leukemia
			Neuroblastoma
			Osteopetrosis	

the anemia is usually due to blood withdrawal for laboratory studies or to organ bleeding (eg, intracranial hemorrhage). The most common cause of anemia in a full-term 2–6-month-old infant is an undetected obstetric blood loss.

Early anemia of premature infants is usually associated with repeated blood sampling for laboratory tests; it usually presents with respiratory distress. Because the blood volume of a 1000-g infant is about 85–90 mL, the infant often loses almost half the blood volume in the first 3–7 days of hospitalization. Loss of 1 mL of blood in a 1000-g infant is equivalent to a loss of 55–70 mL in an adult. Other forms of blood loss, such as intracranial or gastrointestinal hemorrhage or disseminated intravascular coagulation, may cause anemia during the first month in premature infants. In preterm infants 2–4 months after birth, the most common cause of late anemia is the so-called anemia of prematurity.

Clinical Features

The signs of anemia vary with the cause and the rapidity with which it occurs. Acute blood loss due to a fetal-maternal hemorrhage, rupture of the umbilical cord, or any other obstetric accident presents immediately after birth with pallor and signs of shock (eg, decreased peripheral pulses, poor peripheral perfusion, and metabolic acidosis). In addition, red cell size, and Hb concentration and hematocrit, may be normal. Chronic blood loss is not associated with shock, but Hb and hematocrit values are reduced, and red cell morphology may be abnormal. Hepatic and splenic enlargement are also common, as is presence of a cardiac systolic murmur. Fetal-maternal hemorrhage occurs in more than 50% of pregnancies, but the fetal blood loss varies widely from 1–100 mL. Diagnosis of fetal-maternal bleeding is confirmed by an acid elution test on the mother's blood. Because HbF is resistant to acid elution, but HbA is not, the maternal cells are discolored and the fetal blood cells remain pink in the maternal peripheral blood smear. This test (Kleihaur-Betke) is currently available as a kit (Fetal Dex).

Reticulocyte counts are normally 4–12% during the first few days after birth, representing the active erythropoiesis present in utero. After birth, with the increase in arterial blood oxygen, erythropoietin concentrations decrease, as do erythropoiesis and reticulocyte counts. Hemolytic anemias are classically recognized by reticulocytosis and high bilirubin concentration. In all patients with hemolysis or anemia of indefinite cause, a complete blood count, peripheral blood smear, reticulocyte count, red blood cell indices, blood type, direct Coombs test, and bilirubin concentration should be performed in the initial evaluation. Reticulocytosis and anisocytosis are found with isoimmune Rh incompatibility in which hyperbilirubinemia and anemia develop within the first 24 hours after birth. Spherocytes are commonly observed with ABO incompatibility. Determination of the blood type and Coombs test and, in some cases, indirect Coombs or circulating antibody titer determination will help to establish an accurate diagnosis by identifying the antigen and antibody responsible for the hemolysis in isoimmune conditions. If the antibodies are not readily identified, rare cases of non-isoimmune hemolysis must be explored. This necessitates a more extensive workup, including red cell enzyme assays, Hb electrophoresis, red cell membrane tests, and autoimmune testing in mother and infant. Blood loss also may be associated with reticulocytosis, and, in cases of internal hemorrhage, jaundice may be present as the hemorrhage is reabsorbed. An algorithm for a diagnostic approach to neonatal anemia is shown in Chapter 14.

Management

Transfusion with cross-matched red blood cells is the treatment for severe acute blood loss. If isoimmune hemolysis is present and the infant needs a transfusion or an exchange transfusion, the cells must be cross-matched against both maternal and neonatal plasma. All blood used for transfusions should be screened for HIV, hepatitis B, and syphilis; for small neonates, cytomegalovirus (CMV)-negative blood is used. In infants with severe hydrops with hemolysis and anemia, it is advisable, as a first step, to do an exchange transfusion with packed red blood cells to increase the Hb concentration without increasing blood volume. Later, exchange transfusions may be necessary if severe hyperbilirubinemia develops. With ABO incompatibility, the blood for exchange should consist of type O red cells suspended in type AB plasma. Blood is irradiated to prevent graft-versus-host disease.

Premature infants who are very ill in the early neonatal period may be anemic and hypovolemic. In addition, the lower the birth weight, the lower the Hb concentration. It is common practice to provide transfusions with 10 mL/kg of packed red cells to maintain the hematocrit at about 45%. An accurate record should be kept of all blood extracted from the infant to replace the blood volume. As the infant improves and can tolerate feeding, rapid growth occurs and iron stores may be inadequate. It is important to provide all elements needed for erythropoiesis, such as folic acid, vitamin E, and iron. These should be provided no later than 30–45 days after birth. By 3–6 weeks after birth, hematocrit and Hb concentrations decrease in growing infants. Normally, this stimulates endogenous erythropoietin production; however, if transfusions are provided (with adult Hb), this will be suppressed, and reticulocytosis will not occur. The greater the number of transfusions, the more the Hb concentration will decrease, because with a higher percentage of HbA there is more oxygen available to the tissues, and symptoms of anemia are therefore less likely to occur. In preterm infants in the first few postnatal weeks, symptoms of anemia include apnea and bradycardic episodes, abnormal weight gain, poor feedings, and tachycardia. The appearance of a heart murmur also can be associated with early signs of anemia. A blood transfusion with packed red blood cells should be provided only when these signs are present in association with a low Hb concentration. Currently, trials with human recombinant erythropoietin (500 mg/kg/wk) are being conducted in premature infants, with the aim of decreasing the number of blood transfusions and preventing severe intermediate and late anemia of prematurity.

All premature infants should receive at least 50 mg of folic acid and 5 IU of vitamin E per day. Iron needs for full-term infants are 1 mg/kg/d continuing throughout the first year. Premature infants should receive at least 2 mg/kg/d, and premature infants with ELBW (less than 30 weeks' gestation) should receive at least 4 mg/kg/d of iron. In the trials with erythropoietin, it has been shown that for erythropoiesis to be maintained adequately, 6 mg/kg/d of iron is needed in VLBW infants.

BACTERIAL INFECTIONS

Compared with the adult, neonatal immune function is deficient in several aspects: types of specific antibodies, phagocytic and bactericidal function, opsonization, circulating complement, and ability to increase neutrophil production in response to infection. Therefore, the neonate should be considered a "compromised host." The incidence of infections during the newborn period is 1–2:1000 live births. Neonatal infections have three temporal patterns of presentation: early-, intermediate-, or late-onset. The causative organisms and the primary site of involvement vary somewhat in relation to the time of onset and whether the infant acquires the infection at home or in hospital (Table 4–22). **Early-onset** infections most frequently involve bacteremia with or without pneumonia and are caused by group B hemolytic streptococci (GBS) and *Escherichia coli*. Urinary tract infections and meningitis are unlikely in these early-onset infections. Infections that appear after 2 weeks in the hospital are often caused by *Staphylococcus epidermidis*, fungi, or some gram-negative organisms. In the infant at home, **late-onset** syndrome is usually caused by GBS or *Listeria monocytogenes;* 85% of these infants have meningitis. Most neonatal infections occur early or in hospitalized infants, particularly in LBW infants. Fatality rates are 15–40%, and there is substantial morbidity in surviving infants. Prompt diagnosis and appropriate medical management are essential.

Several perinatal conditions are associated with increased risk of early-onset sepsis (Table 4–23). These factors are used to select infants to be evaluated and treated until infection is ruled out. Maternal risk factors include vaginal streptococcal colonization, intrapartum fever, prolonged rupture of the membranes (> 18–24 hours), prolonged second stage of labor, and chorioamnionitis or a history of urinary tract infection. Early-onset sepsis is also more frequent with prematurity, twin gestation, congenital anomalies, perinatal asphyxia, and male sex. Perinatal risk factors are unusual in late-onset infections, but other factors, such as prolonged intravascular access and prolonged or repeated courses of antibiotics, are frequently noted in nosocomial infections.

Signs of Neonatal Sepsis

Early diagnosis is usually made when there is a high index of suspicion. The early signs of neonatal sepsis are subtle and nonspecific; a common early presentation is that the infant "does not look well" and has poor feeding or intolerance to feedings, irritability or lethargy, and temperature instability. By the time the infant manifests multiple and overt signs of sepsis, the morbidity and mortality have increased significantly. Various signs are shown in Table 4–24. Meningitis occurs in 10–30% of early-onset

Table 4–22. Organisms, risk factors, and choice of initial antibiotics in relation to time of onset and place of occurrence of neonatal sepsis.

Onset	Early 0–3 Days	Intermediate 4–14 Days	Late 14–28 (or more) Days	
Place of occurrence	Hospital (home unusual)	Hospital or home	Home	Hospital
Type	Early-onset syndrome	Systemic Urinary tract Skin/joints	Of late onset; 85% will have meningitis	Systemic Pneumonia
Organisms involved	GBS, *Escherichia coli* Other gram-negative organisms *Listeria monocytogenes*	Gram-negative *Staphylococcus* *aureus/epidermidis*	GBS *L monocytogenes* (Other)	*Staphylococcus epidermidis* Fungus (Gram-negative)
Risk factors	Perinatal	Unusual perinatal Other: GU anomaly Surgical procedures Very low birth weight	Unusual	Prolonged central IV access Repeated courses of antibiotics Very low birth weight
Initial treatment	Ampicillin and gentamicin	Ampicillin and gentamicin	Ampicillin and gentamicin	Ampicillin and gentamicin
Possible alternatives (positive blood culture, sensitivities, no response to treatment)	Individualized	First to third generation cephalosporins Vancomycin		Vancomycin Amphotericin B Second to third generation cephalosporins

GBS = group B streptococcus; GU = genitourinary; IV = intravenous.

Table 4–23. Risk assessment in neonatal sepsis.

Clinical Risk Factor	Incidence of Proven Sepsis (%)	Incidence of Proven and "Suspected" Sepsis (%)
Early-onset		
PROM > 18–24 h	1	1–2
Maternal GBS colonization	0.5–1	1–2
PROM + maternal GBS	4–6	7–11
Maternal GBS + fever	3–5	6–10
PROM and chorioamnionitis	3–8	6–10
PROM or GBS in preterm infant	4–6	7–11
PROM and Apgar < 6 at 5 min	3–4	6–10
Male gender	4-fold ↑	4-fold ↑
Nosocomial		
Low birth weight, intravascular access, multiple courses of antibiotics, etc	10–15	25

GBS = group B streptococcus; PROM = prolonged rupture of membranes.

infection. In late-onset sepsis, particularly with GBS or *L monocytogenes,* the incidence of meningitis is about 85%, in contrast with the low rate in early-onset infections. Newborn infants do not usually manifest the classic signs of meningitis described in older children and adults (see Chapter 9).

Many neonatal conditions may mimic the clinical presentation of neonatal sepsis. These include viral infections, congestive heart failure, congenital heart disease, NEC, and metabolic, endocrine, or chromosomal disorders.

When to Evaluate for Sepsis?

Because the initial clinical manifestations are often nonspecific, the early clinical diagnosis of neonatal sepsis is difficult. The decision to perform a partial or extended evaluation and to institute antimicrobial therapy remains a matter of clinical judgment. The presence of risk factors, inadequate treatment of maternal infection, and whether the infant is preterm should be noted when considering the diagnosis of early-onset sepsis. As shown in Figures 4–3

Table 4–24. Clinical signs in neonatal sepsis and meningitis.

Early Onset	Later Onset
"Infant Does Not Look Well"	
Grunting	Temperature instability
Tachypnea	Poor feeding
Cyanosis	Weak suck
Poor perfusion	Vomiting or gastric residual
Hypotonia	Abdominal distention
Lethargy/apnea	Lethargy/apnea
Jaundice (< 24 h)	Tense fontanelle/convulsions
Shock	Shock

and 4–4, some infants may require careful observation with or without a sepsis screen, whereas others require an immediate, complete sepsis workup, and still others are given antibiotics pending results of studies. Indications for performing a sepsis workup and for instituting empiric therapy vary, depending on the relative risk. Most clinicians recommend starting antibiotic treatment in infants with neonatal respiratory distress requiring oxygen or ventilatory support, particularly in infants older than 34 weeks' gestation, in whom RDS is unlikely. Symptomatic infants with signs consistent with sepsis, regardless of risk factors and gestational age, should be promptly evaluated and started on antibiotic therapy (see Figures 4–3 and 4–4).

The Sepsis Workup

The perinatal history, physical examination, and course should be carefully evaluated. Complete blood and differentials counts are often useful; although not specific for sepsis, the association of leukopenia (< 6000 mL), neutropenia (< 1700/mL, according to postnatal age), and left shifts defined by an immature-total neutrophil ratio of greater than 0.2, have a very good negative predictive value. If none of these is present, the likelihood of sepsis is small. Predictive accuracy is significantly improved by repeat analysis in 8–24 hours. Thrombocytopenia, toxic granulation, vacuolization, and Döhle bodies are other nonspecific alterations that help to exclude sepsis if they are absent. Leukocytosis and neutrophilia are *not* good indicators of neonatal sepsis.

Latex agglutination testing for the presence of GBS antigens is usually done on urine. However, false-positive results can occur in more than 10% of cases. Microsedimentation rate, C-reactive protein, fibronectin, and haptoglobin measurements have low positive predictive accuracy and specificity.

A more complete sepsis workup includes chest radiograph and blood culture. When an infant is at risk for infection but is younger than 72 hours of age and is **asymptomatic,** a urine culture and a spinal tap need *not* be performed. An infant in these circumstances is unlikely to have meningitis without having positive blood cultures. However, if the blood culture is positive, cerebrospinal fluid (CSF) should be analyzed. If CSF culture is positive or if there are clear signs of meningitis even with negative cultures, the antibiotic therapy must be prolonged. After the first 72 hours after birth or when there is a strong suspicion of sepsis, a suprapubic bladder tap and a spinal tap must be performed. Some critically ill infants, particularly those of LBW, may be given antibiotics before a spinal tap is performed. If antibiotics are started, the cultures should be incubated for 72 hours to provide enough time for the organism to grow before the culture is considered negative and the intravenous antibiotic therapy discontinued. Blood cultures are only 82–90% sensitive in neonates. Therefore, with strong clinical suspicion of sepsis and an abnormal white cell count, the infant may need

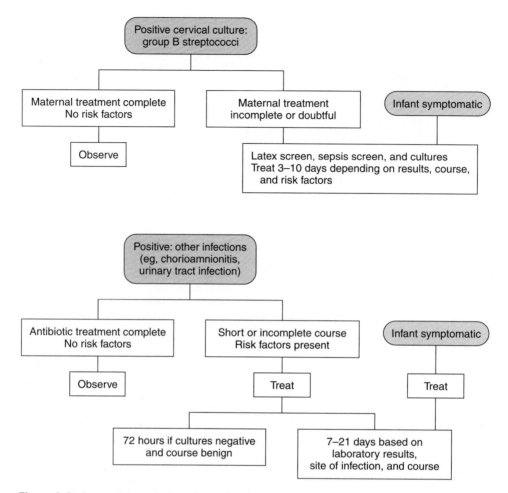

Figure 4–3. Approach to evaluation of neonate when mother has been infected and treated for sepsis.

to be fully treated with antibiotics even with negative blood cultures (see Figures 4–3 and 4–4).

CSF examination is often difficult to interpret in the newborn. A normal CSF may have up to 32 white cells per milliliter with up to 60% polymorphonuclear cells. The CSF glucose concentration is variable in neonates but, in general, is greater than 40% of serum glucose concentrations. Protein content may be as high as 180 mg/dL normally, or even higher in preterm infants. Organisms should be looked for on Gram stain.

Management

When sepsis is strongly suspected, some tests should be performed promptly and intravenous antibiotic therapy started immediately. Antibiotics are continued until the results of cultures are available and the clinical response to intervention is evaluated. Initially, the infection is treated empirically with a penicillin and an aminoglycoside to provide broad-spectrum coverage against both gram-positive and gram-negative organisms (see Table 4–22). When

an organism is identified, antibiotic coverage may need to be changed. The duration of therapy varies with the focus and etiologic agent, the infant's clinical status, and the response to therapy. Sepsis and bacteremia without a focus are usually treated for 7–10 days; pneumonia, 10 days; and meningitis, 14–21 days. Cultures should be repeated to document adequate response; persistent positive cultures warrant an investigation for occult foci, such as abscesses, ventriculitis, or a recurrent portal of entry such as a pilonidal sinus.

Because of the difficulty in diagnosis and the high risk of neonatal sepsis, many infants are overevaluated and empirically overtreated on the basis of "possible infection." Although approximately 10% of all newborns receive some antibiotics, only 1:11–25 treated infants eventually has infection documented by a positive culture. Therefore, if cultures prove to be negative at 72 hours and if the clinical assessment (examination, blood count, and risk factors) suggests low risk for infection, antibiotics may be discontinued (see Figures 4–3 and 4–4). Infants

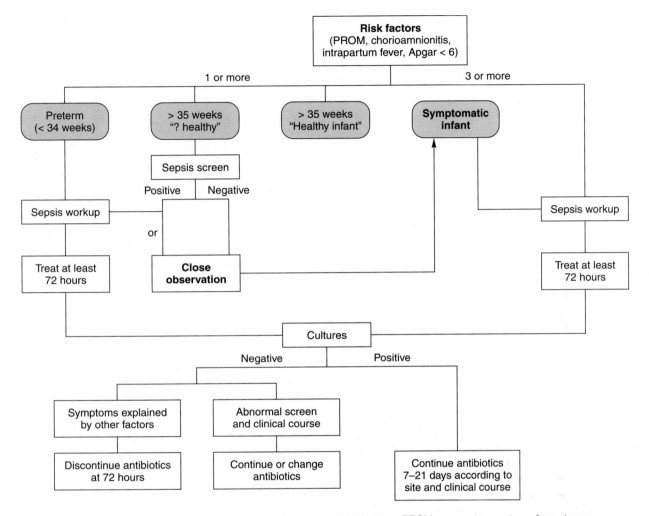

Figure 4–4. Steps in the evaluation of suspected early neonatal infections. PROM = premature rupture of membranes.

with high risk factors, abnormal sepsis screen, and a strong clinical suspicion of sepsis may be treated for 7–10 days even if cultures are negative (see Figures 4–3 and 4–4).

All infants with suspected sepsis should be hospitalized and monitored continuously. Some therapies have been proposed as adjuncts to antibiotic therapy; these include administration of blood products, such as fresh frozen plasma, white cell transfusions, whole blood transfusions, exchange transfusions, and, recently, intravenous γ-globulin. These therapies are still controversial and await evaluation in controlled studies.

Prolonged or repetitive antimicrobial administration increases the risk of altering normal flora and the development of superinfection with resistant bacterial organisms or with fungi, especially in LBW infants.

In infants receiving aminoglycosides or vancomycin, serum concentrations should be monitored and maintained

in both the safe and therapeutic range by modifying the dose and dosage interval as needed. All infants with prolonged aminoglycoside therapy or with meningitis should undergo hearing assessment.

ABDOMINAL MASS

Palpation of the abdomen during physical examination of the newborn is not difficult. Allowing the infant to suck or flexing the infant's hips decreases abdominal tone. If the abdomen is distended, nasogastric suction may be indicated to relieve possible functional or anatomic obstruction of the gastrointestinal tract. In the normal newborn, the liver may be palpated 1–3 cm below the right costal margin. The spleen tip is felt less frequently; it is enlarged if it extends 1 cm or more below the left costal margin. The lower poles of both kidneys are usually palpable; the right kidney is typically lower than the left. Uncommon renal anomalies that may be diagnosed by palpation include horseshoe kidney, pelvic kidney, and unilateral agenesis. Other structures that normally may be palpable in the newborn are the aorta, feces in the colon, and a full bladder.

Etiology

Abdominal enlargement may be due to abdominal distention from obstruction to the gastrointestinal tract. Associated signs are vomiting, distention, and absence of stool. Possible causes of intestinal obstruction include atresia (duodenal, jejunal, ileal, or colonic), meconium ileus, malrotation with midgut volvulus, Hirschsprung disease or imperforate anus, annular pancreas, and, at a later age, pyloric stenosis and intussusception. Compressive external abdominal masses or functional obstructions may also lead to abdominal distention.

Clinical Features

Evaluation of an abdominal mass not associated with obstruction includes definition of its mobility, location, characteristics, and associated symptoms. Mobility of the mass distinguishes intraperitoneal from retroperitoneal lesions. Masses in the flank tend to arise from the urinary tract, although adrenal hemorrhage or, rarely, neuroblastoma may displace the kidney. One half of all abdominal masses discovered in the newborn are of renal origin; hydronephrosis and multicystic kidney are the most frequent abdominal masses in the newborn. Obstruction early in renal development results in multicystic kidney, whereas obstruction, either unilaterally or bilaterally, after nephron development results in hydronephrosis. The hydronephrotic kidney is smooth and firm, whereas the multicystic kidney, which is usually nonfunctional, is irregular and cystic. Review of the prenatal history may help determine the cause of an abdominal mass, eg, when there is a history of inherited kidney disease (infantile polycystic disease). Renal vein thrombosis, rarely bilateral, usually occurs in the IDM or after polycythemia and severe dehydration; it is often associated with hematuria. Mesoblastic nephroma, a renal hamartoma, is the most common solid tumor in the infant kidney and may be associated with polyhydramnios. It must be distinguished from Wilms' tumor, which is rare in the newborn.

Masses in the right upper quadrant must be distinguished from liver enlargement. Masses involving the liver may be associated with a history of jaundice (choledochal cyst) or birth trauma (subcapsular hematoma). A smooth lower midline abdominal mass may be due to hydrometrocolpos in a female infant (from an intact hymen or lower vaginal atresia) or bladder distention. A distended bladder in a male infant is most commonly due to posterior urethral valves. Neuroblastoma, the most common congenital malignant tumor, arises from the adrenal cortex or along the sympathetic chain. The mass is stony hard and frequently crosses the midline.

Mobile midline cysts may be due to gastrointestinal du-plication or lymphatic abnormalities in the mesentery. In the female infant, stimulation by circulating hormones from the mother or chorion may result in ovarian, follicular, or theca lutein cysts. All these mobile cysts are smooth. Ovarian tumors are rare and are usually solid and fixed.

The investigation of choice after clinical evaluation is ultrasonography. Plain radiographs of the abdomen may be performed if there is concern for intestinal obstruction. In the past, owing to the high incidence of renal lesions, the study of choice for an abdominal mass was intravenous pyelography. Today, such studies with contrast materials can be avoided or delayed when ultrasound is used to identify a mass that arises outside the urinary tract. Nuclear scanning of kidney function, computed tomography (CT), or magnetic resonance imaging (MRI) may be indicated. Laboratory evaluation depends on the nature of the mass (eg, cystic versus solid). Many of the abdominal masses reviewed above require surgical intervention.

SEIZURES

The identification and classification of seizures is a difficult but important clinical problem in the newborn period. The typical unambiguous tonic-clonic seizure pattern seen in older children and adults is not evident, perhaps because of the immaturity of the newborn nervous system. Neonatal seizures frequently are subtle and difficult to distinguish from common, benign newborn activities, such as jitteriness or clonus. It is important to identify seizures correctly because they are frequently associated with underlying disorders requiring specific, prompt treatment. Recent evidence suggests that seizure activity that is allowed to persist without treatment may result in brain injury.

In the newborn, jitteriness may be confused with seizures. Many of the metabolic problems that underlie neonatal seizures, such as hypoglycemia, hypocalcemia, asphyxia, and drug withdrawal, are also associated with jitteriness. Premature infants and IDMs, even those without any of the previously mentioned metabolic problems, frequently have jitteriness. Several characteristics that can help distinguish jitteriness from seizures are presented in Table 4–25.

The prenatal, perinatal, and postnatal history and a detailed physical examination often provide the necessary information for establishing the etiology of neonatal seizures. Emphasis should be placed in identifying any family history of "unexplained" infant death, such as inherited metabolic disorders, in utero exposure to drugs of abuse (methadone, heroin, barbiturates, cocaine, and ethanol), inadvertent injection of local anesthetic agents into the fetus after paracervical or pudendal blocks for maternal analgesia, hypoxic events and perinatal asphyxia, maternal/perinatal infection, neonatal medications such a high doses of aminophylline, or rapid withdrawal after administering narcotics liberally. It is important to note the type and age

Table 4–25. Jitteriness and seizures compared.

Characteristic	Jitteriness	Seizure
Abnormal eye movements	No	Yes
Elicited with stimulation or passive stretch	Yes	No
Ceases with passive flexion	Yes	No
Dominant movement	Very rapid, rhythmic	Fast and slow components
Electroencephalogram	Normal	May be abnormal

of onset of the seizure (see below). Clinically, there are four major seizure types in the newborn period: subtle, tonic, clonic, and myoclonic. The additional adjectives focal, multifocal, and generalized describe the site(s) involved in the seizure activity. When several sites are involved, the activity may be either synchronous (generalized) or asynchronous (multifocal). Examination revealing a tense or bulging anterior fontanelle suggests intracranial hemorrhage or meningitis, and pupils may be fixed or asymmetric as a result of significant intracranial pathology. Posture, muscle tone, and reflexes should be evaluated carefully and frequently. A significant decrease in hematocrit may result from intracranial hemorrhage, and a high hematocrit (> 70%) may be associated with cerebral infarction. Hypoglycemia and hypocalcemia are the most frequent metabolic disorders that cause neonatal seizures. Extreme sodium imbalance can also cause seizures. Significant hypernatremia increases CNS irritability and thus may induce seizures. Hyponatremia decreases CNS excitability, but if sodium concentration decreases rapidly, cerebral edema and seizures may result. Hypernatremia must therefore be corrected slowly to avoid a rapid decrease in serum sodium concentration. A lumbar puncture is necessary to obtain CSF to diagnose meningitis usually caused by group B streptococcus or *E coli*. Examination of the CSF may also help to diagnose encephalitis resulting from viruses such as herpes simplex, enterovirus, or rubella or parasites such as toxoplasmosis. Evaluation of serum pH and base deficit may lead to the diagnosis of amino or organic acidopathies; in addition to seizures, these present with recurrent or persistent metabolic acidosis and signs of neurologic dysfunc-

tion. When early neonatal seizures are resistant to all usual therapeutic medications, pyridoxine dependency should be ruled out by a therapeutic trial with intravenous injection of 50–100 μg of pyridoxine while an electroencephalogram (EEG) is being performed. Normalization of the EEG immediately after the injection confirms the diagnosis. If it is apparent that seizures are not readily attributable to asphyxia, a metabolic problem, drugs, or infection, it is then necessary to perform imaging procedures. Head ultrasound examination can be used to diagnose intraventricular hemorrhages, but CT or MRI scans are usually necessary for diagnosing other lesions and cerebral cortical malformations, such as disorders of neuronal migration. In some infants with neonatal seizures an EEG can be very useful; it may determine the diagnosis in paralyzed or "jittery" newborns and can also provide information regarding the prognosis. (When the interictal EEG is abnormal, the risk of poor neurologic outcome is high with most seizure types). The EEG findings vary in relation to the different convulsive clinical types (Table 4–26), and several of the clinical phenomena classified as seizures in the newborn are not associated with synchronous EEG seizure activity. This may occur with many subtle seizures, particularly in the full-term infant, and with focal clonic and generalized tonic seizures when the electrical discharges do not accompany the clinical seizures (Table 4–26). Whether some of these seizures are associated with neural electrical discharges that are not recorded by the surface electrodes of current EEG equipment is unclear.

The clinical seizure type and the postnatal age at which the seizures are first detected bear a strong association with the possible etiology. The most important etiologies with the associated common seizure types and usual age of onset are shown in Table 4–27. Hypoxic-ischemic encephalopathy, usually after perinatal asphyxia, is a very common cause of early neonatal seizures. These seizures can be very difficult to control and often evolve into status epilepticus despite adequate doses of anticonvulsant medication.

Treatment

Urgent treatment of metabolic disorders such as hypoglycemia or hypocalcemia is crucial to prevent complications and sequelae. Hypoglycemia is treated with intravenous glucose solution, 10%, in a dose of 200 mg/kg followed by continuous glucose infusion. Hypocalcemia

Table 4–26. Classification of neonatal seizures.

Type	Manifestation	Common EEG Findings
Subtle	Paroxysms of ocular, oral, buccal, or lingual movements; apnea	Frequently abnormal
Focal clonic	Rhythmic twitching of one extremity	Focal sharp activity
Multifocal clonic	Sequential twitching of several limbs	Multiple foci of sharp activity
Focal tonic	Sustained asymmetric extensor posturing	Typically abnormal
Generalized tonic	Mimics decerebrate or decorticate posture	Discharges do not accompany clinical seizures
Focal myoclonic	Rapid, rhythmic jerks of flexion	Discharges do not accompany clinical seizures
Generalized myoclonic	Asynchronous jerking of several limbs	Burst suppression pattern

EEG = electroencephalogram.

Table 4–27. Relation of etiology to seizure type and onset.

Etiology	Seizure Type	Age of Onset
Hypoxic-ischemic	Subtle, tonic (premature), or clonic (full-term)	First 24 h
Intracranial hemorrhage	Subtle or focal clonic	First 3 days
Metabolic	Clonic or generalized tonic	First 3 days or > 5 days (late hypocalcemia or acidopathy)
Infection	Focal tonic or clonic	> 3 days
Cerebral malformation	Focal clonic or myoclonic	Any time from birth on
Drug withdrawal	Clonic or generalized tonic	> 2 days but depends on drug(s) of abuse
Systemic injection of local anesthetic agents	Generalized tonic	First 6 h

is treated with 200 mg/kg calcium gluconate in a 10% solution intravenously. If the diagnosis of pyridoxine deficiency is established (see above), treatment requires sufficiently high doses of vitamin B_6.

Inadvertent injection of local anesthetic agent into the fetus with resultant early seizures, usually at less than 6 hours after birth, has most commonly been described after paracervical or pudendal blocks for maternal analgesia. These seizures require vigorous treatment with anticonvulsants, and the infants usually recover completely and have a perfectly normal long-term follow-up.

For intracranial hemorrhage and meningitis, as well as in any case in which the cause of the seizure is not both readily apparent and amenable to specific treatment, anticonvulsant medication should also be initiated promptly. Phenobarbital is the most common first-line therapy, given intravenously as a loading dose of 20 mg/kg. When seizures are difficult to control, as is often the case in hypoxic-ischemic seizures, repeated doses up to 40–50 mg/kg total dose may be necessary in the first 4–24 hours of therapy. Maintenance doses are usually 3–4 mg/kg/d. When this single therapy is inadequate, phenytoin is usually considered next, with a loading dose of 20 mg/kg and a maintenance dose of 3–4 mg/kg/d intravenously. Diazepam and lorazepam, two benzodiazepines, are not used for maintenance therapy and are of limited usefulness in the management of neonatal seizures. For seizures that are refractory and difficult to manage, there has been some success with short-term use of intravenous lorazepam, 0.05 mg/kg.

DISORDERS OF THE NEWBORN

RESPIRATORY DISORDERS

APNEA IN THE PREMATURE INFANT

Apnea is defined as a respiratory pause without airflow lasting more than 20 seconds or as a pause of any duration accompanied by bradycardia and cyanosis or oxygen desaturation, as evidenced by pulse oximetry monitoring. Apnea in neonates can be **central,** with a complete cessation of chest wall movements and no airflow. Apnea also may be due to **airway obstruction;** in this circumstance, chest wall movements or respiratory efforts continue, but there is no airflow. The commonly available monitors do not record obstructive apnea because they continue to detect chest wall movements. A combination of central and obstructive apnea constitutes **mixed apnea,** the most frequent type encountered in premature infants.

When apnea is diagnosed, an immediate evaluation must be made to determine the etiology. Possible causes of apnea in preterm infants are presented in Table 4–28. The incidence of apnea increases with decreasing gestational age. **Idiopathic apnea of prematurity** occurs in the absence of any identifiable cause. It usually appears after 24 hours' postnatal age and during the first week after birth; it usually resolves by 38–44 weeks of postconceptual age (gestational age at birth plus weeks of postnatal age).

Management

An approach to management of apnea is shown in Table 4–29. Recurrent apnea can be treated with continuous positive airway pressure (CPAP) of 3–6 cm water. Methylxanthines stimulate central inspiratory drive and increase sensitivity of the respiratory center to carbon dioxide. Caffeine is the drug of choice because there is a wide separation between therapeutic (4–18 µg/mL) and toxic (≥ 50 µg/mL) serum concentrations. The usual oral dose is as follows: loading, 10 mg/kg caffeine base; maintenance, 2.5 mg/kg/d. The caffeine citrate loading dose is 20 mg/kg, and maintenance is 5 mg/kg/d, given once daily. Theophylline can be used, but the toxic and therapeutic concentrations are much closer. Toxic manifestations include tachycardia, irritability, tremors, seizures,

Table 4–28. Causes of apnea in preterm infants.

Infection	Hypoglycemia
Lung disease	Airway obstruction
Hypothermia/hyperthermia	Feedings
Patent ductus arteriosus	Bowel movement
Seizures	Intraventricular hemorrhage
Maternal drugs	Drug withdrawal
Gastroesophageal reflux	Anemia
Idiopathic apnea of prematurity	

Table 4–29. Management of apnea in premature infants.

Search for specific etiology	
Temperature	Avoid low temperature and rapid warming Maintain neutral thermal environment (lowest normal)
Oxygen	Do not use routinely Treat hypoxia (but avoid hyperoxia)
Airway	Put infant in prone position Place head and neck in neutral position Suction secretions as needed Remove orogastric or nasogastric tubes
Stimulation	Proprioceptive (eg, rocking or waterbeds) Cutaneous
Medications	Caffeine Theophylline Phenytoin Doxapram
Ventilation	Bag-and-mask (for a severe apneic episode) Continuous positive airway pressure Intermittent mechanical ventilation

and fever. Gastric residual may increase, with vomiting; in addition, hyperglycemia and polyuria may occur. If apnea is associated with seizures, methylxanthines are contraindicated because they may increase the risk of seizures.

RESPIRATORY DISTRESS SYNDROME

Lung Development During Fetal Life

Knowledge of lung development allows an understanding of the preterm infant's ability to maintain adequate respiratory function at different gestational ages. At 3–4 weeks of gestation, the trachea develops from the esophagus, and pulmonary arteries originate from the sixth aortic arch. By 14 weeks, the lung develops as an outpouching of the embryonic gut. By 16 weeks, bronchial segmentation is complete, and the canalicular stage begins with acinar formation and cuboidal cells in the epithelium. A vascular network develops in the mesoderm and proliferates around the potential airspaces. By 20–22 weeks, osmophilic lamellar inclusion bodies appear in the epithelial cells. The development of terminal air sacs begins at 24 weeks, and there is a closer approximation between the respiratory epithelium and the capillaries. The epithelial type II cells have an active endoplasmic reticulum in which phospholipids are synthesized, mainly dipalmitoylphosphatidylcholine (DPPC). Also by this time, the type II cells begin to differentiate into thinner type I epithelial cells. During this stage of lung development, gas exchange is possible, but the distance between the capillaries and the airspaces is still three times greater than in adults. By 26 weeks' gestation, there are larger airspaces in close

contact with capillaries but still no true alveoli; gas exchange, however, may be adequate during air breathing. By 28 weeks, alveolar ducts and respiratory bronchioles are easily distinguishable, with an increase in the area for diffusion. By 30 weeks, the subdivision of terminal bronchioles into respiratory bronchioles has almost ended, and alveoli are actively formed; this stage is completed by 34 weeks. Pulmonary surfactant, the surface-active material that decreases surface tension and prevents atelectasis, is first noted at approximately 23–24 weeks' gestation, with the appearance of the osmophilic inclusion bodies in the type II alveolar cells. However, a sufficient quantity of surfactant is produced only after 30–32 weeks' gestation; beyond this period, the incidence of RDS decreases significantly. Pulmonary surfactant is composed of phospholipids, mainly DPPC, and surfactant proteins A (SPA), B (SPB), and C (SPC). It is secreted into the alveolar lumen and into the tracheal fluid, which flows out of the nose and mouth into the amniotic cavity. Pulmonary maturity can be assessed before birth by determining presence of surfactant in amniotic fluid obtained by amniocentesis. In the "shake" test described by Clements, diluted amniotic fluid is shaken in a test tube; the stability of the bubbles is directly related to the presence of surface-active material. A ratio of lecithin (DPPC) to sphingomyelin (L:S ratio) greater than 2:1 or the presence of phosphatidylglycerol (a minor phospholipid in surfactant) is also an indicator of fetal lung maturity.

Clinical Manifestations

RDS occurs in approximately 0.5% of neonates and is the most frequent cause of respiratory distress and insufficiency in preterm infants. The incidence is as much as 50% before 30 weeks' gestation but less than 10% at 35–36 weeks. The risk factors for RDS are summarized in Table 4–30. The syndrome results from deficiency of pulmonary surfactant, resulting in atelectasis with decreased functional residual capacity, lung compliance, and lung volume. The alveolar collapse causes abnormalities in ventilation-perfusion relationships with intrapulmonary right-to-left shunt with hypoxemia. In severe cases, alveolar ventilation is greatly decreased with resultant hypercarbia and respiratory acidosis.

Clinical signs of RDS may develop at birth or a few hours after birth. The infants usually show increasing distress during the first 24–48 hours, with tachypnea, retraction of the chest wall, expiratory grunting, and cyanosis. The chest radiograph may show diffuse atelectasis with

Table 4–30. Risk factors for respiratory distress syndrome (RDS).

Asphyxia	Male sex
Cesarean section without labor	Prematurity Previous preterm infant with
Hypothermia	RDS
Immature L-S ratio	Second of twins
Infants of diabetic mothers	White race

L-S = lecithin-sphingomyelin.

an increased density in both lungs and a fine, granular, "ground-glass" appearance of the lungs. The small airways are filled with air and are clearly seen surrounded by the increased density of the pulmonary field, the so-called air bronchograms. Lung volume is usually decreased, and the diaphragms are somewhat elevated. These x-ray findings may be more noticeable by 24 hours after birth. Arterial blood gases show decreased Pa_{O_2} with elevated Pa_{CO_2} in more severe cases.

The clinical features are more severe and prolonged in preterm infants less than 31 weeks' gestation. Hyperkalemia and metabolic acidosis develop in many of these infants. Peripheral edema commonly develops. Hypoxia, hypercapnia, and acidosis combine to act on the function of the type II cells, further decreasing surfactant production. Respiratory insufficiency develops in infants with severe RDS, and mechanical ventilation becomes necessary. Pulmonary arterial hypertension may result from hypoxic and acidemic pulmonary vasoconstriction.

With active and adequate treatment in an intensive care nursery, most infants with RDS survive. Clinical improvement may be evident by 48–72 hours after birth when oxygen and respirator requirements stabilize, diuresis occurs, and edema diminishes. The clinical course of RDS has changed dramatically since the advent of exogenous surfactant. Clinical features and physiologic disturbances in RDS are summarized in Table 4–31.

Several complications may occur during the course of RDS (Table 4–32). Infants with RDS frequently have a left-to-right-shunt across a patent ductus arteriosus (PDA), usually when the lung disease begins to improve. Some infants are very ill for 2–3 weeks, and chronic complications, such as BPD, may develop.

Management

Since 1991, two products to replace deficient surfactant have been approved for use in the United States. One is synthetic (Exosurf); the other is a natural product obtained from bovine lungs (Survanta). The use of these products has significantly decreased mortality associated with RDS and also long-term morbidity such as BPD and intraventricular hemorrhage. These exogenous surfactants are administered into the trachea; even in the smallest infants, they can be administered prophylactically immediately after birth, before respirations are established. Currently,

Table 4–31. Clinical features and physiologic disturbances in respiratory distress syndrome.

Tachypnea	Atelectasis
Nasal flaring	Ground-glass appearance in chest
Retractions	radiographs
Expiratory grunting	Decreased compliance
Cyanosis	Increased physiologic dead-space
Hypotonia	Decreased lung volume
Decreased urine output	Hypoxemia/hypercarbia
Edema	Acidemia
Hyperkalemia	Hypotension

Table 4–32. Complications in respiratory distress syndrome.

Pneumothorax	Endotracheal tube–related:
Pulmonary interstitial emphysema	Extubation: misplacement
Intraventricular hemorrhage	Mucous plugs
Sepsis	Vocal cord damage
Patent ductus arteriosus	Subglottic stenosis
	Bronchopulmonary dysplasia
	Retinopathy of prematurity

however, surfactant is used more frequently after RDS has become established. The dose is approximately 3–5 mL/kg/dose given at 12-hour intervals; at least two doses must be administered. Even though this replacement therapy has greatly improved survival and morbidity, infants with RDS continue to require intensive care with general supportive measures and skillful ventilatory management.

Larger premature infants with mild to moderate disease may be stabilized by providing an increased concentration of oxygen, administered by hood using warm, humidified gas. Skin surface oxygen saturation or Pa_{O_2} should be monitored continuously, and arterial blood gases measured intermittently. In larger infants, the Pa_{O_2} should be maintained at 50–70 mm Hg, but in smaller infants a Pa_{O_2} of 45–60 mm Hg is acceptable. The pH should be maintained above 7.25 and the Pa_{CO_2} below 50 mm Hg. In some infants, metabolic acidosis with a base excess of –5 to –8 develops; this does not require treatment with alkaline solutions such as sodium bicarbonate or THAM. If hypercarbia with respiratory acidosis develops, mechanical ventilation should be instituted promptly. If the Pa_{CO_2} and pH are normal but the infant has hypoxemia with a fraction of inspired oxygen (Fi_{O_2}) greater than 0.7, CPAP should be added by nasal prongs, nasopharyngeal tubes, or endotracheal intubation using end-expiratory distending pressures of 6–10 cm water. If mechanical ventilation is needed, it is usual to start with an Fi_{O_2} of 0.5–1, peak inspiratory pressures of 20–28 cm water, a positive end-expiratory pressure (PEEP) of 4–6 cm water, and a respiratory rate of 40–60 breaths per minute. The inspiratory time should be about 0.35 seconds. Even though there has been extensive debate in the literature, it seems more prudent to use faster respiratory rates with smaller tidal volumes. Newer techniques of mechanical ventilation include high-frequency ventilation, which provides 150–600 breaths per minute, and oscillator ventilation, which provides up to 3000 breaths per minute. Even though these techniques may be useful for infants with severe hypercarbia resistant to conventional ventilation and for infants with pulmonary interstitial emphysema, they have not proved to be better than conventional ventilation for most infants.

Mechanical ventilation for long periods may cause lung damage. Furthermore, high concentrations of oxygen in inspired air can result in severe lung damage when used over prolonged periods. For this reason, it may be advisable to accept blood gas values that are considered borderline, rather than increasing ventilation or FiO_2, with risk of lung injury. PaO_2 and $PaCO_2$ can be manipulated by altering ventilator settings to satisfy the needs of each infant. Thus, PEEP, respiratory rate, tidal volume, and inspiratory duration, as well as FiO_2, all can be altered for optimal effect.

In infants with RDS, lung compliance changes with the clinical course, postnatal ages, and the use of exogenous surfactant. The ventilator settings—and particularly the mean airway pressure and respiratory rate—should be adjusted promptly to adjust for these changes. Failure to do so could result in pneumothorax, decreased venous return, hypoxemia, and hypercarbia.

Most clinicians obtain cultures and administer antibiotics in infants with RDS (usually ampicillin and gentamicin) because some pneumonias, particularly group B streptococcus infection, are difficult to differentiate from RDS. In general, antibiotics are administered for 3 days until the culture results are negative.

MECONIUM ASPIRATION SYNDROME

Meconium staining of amniotic fluid is noted at delivery in about 15% of pregnancies. The amniotic fluid may remain watery and be stained slightly green, or it may become thick and dark green. Meconium is often passed during intrauterine stress but not before 34–35 weeks' gestation, because meconium does not reach the rectal ampulla until that time. If the fetus becomes hypoxic and deep respiratory movements or gasps develop, meconium can reach the distal airway and alveoli in utero. Infants with MAS aspirate meconium at the time of birth when taking the first inspirations. The usual clinical symptoms are those of mild to moderate respiratory distress, but some infants have severe symptoms, requiring vigorous respiratory support or extracorporeal membrane oxygenation (ECMO). The clinical signs and physiologic changes in MAS are summarized in Table 4–33.

During birth, suctioning the upper airway before the shoulders are delivered and performing endotracheal suctioning immediately after birth decrease the incidence of MAS in infants born with meconium-stained amniotic fluid. This approach is recommended for all infants with thick, particulate, or "pea-soup" meconium, regardless of the Apgar score or need for resuscitation at birth. When the infants have a 1-minute Apgar greater than 8, with thin, watery meconium, endotracheal suctioning is not usually recommended. The overall reported incidence of MAS in infants born with meconium-stained amniotic fluid is 2–10%; however, the incidence is 2–4% in infants in whom endotracheal suctioning is performed immediately. The reported mortality for MAS varies from 0 to 30%. The wide variability is related to delivery room care. In our center, every infant with moderate or thick meconium-stained amniotic fluid is intubated and suctioned immediately. In the past 6 years (1989–1992), with more than 10,000 deliveries, no infant died nor required ECMO for treatment of MAS.

Infants with severe MAS often have PPHN, which usually presents with cyanosis and tachypnea. Pulmonary vascular resistance is increased, and pulmonary blood flow decreased. Untreated hypoxemia or acidosis accentuates these problems (see below).

PERSISTENT PULMONARY HYPERTENSION OF THE NEWBORN

Several structural anomalies of the heart cause pulmonary hypertension. Total anomalous pulmonary venous return sometimes poses a difficult differential diagnosis with PPHN; in certain cases, color flow Doppler studies, cardiac catheterization, or angiography are needed to localize the pulmonary veins. Perinatal asphyxia and meconium aspiration are common causes of PPHN, but there are many other causes (Table 4–34). There is often a large right-to-left shunt through the ductus arteriosus in these infants; therefore, there is a large difference in the PaO_2 between blood obtained from preductal aortic branches, such as the temporal or radial arteries, and postductal (descending aortic) blood as obtained from the umbilical arterial catheter or femoral artery. Right-to-left shunting through the foramen ovale is also common. The clinical and laboratory signs of PPHN are summarized in Table 4–35. Characteristic of these infants is respiratory lability,

Table 4–33. Clinical signs and physiologic changes in meconium aspiration syndrome.

Clinical	Lungs	Blood Gases	Other
Term/post-term	Mechanical obstruction	Hypoxemia	Extrapulmonary shunt
Pallor/cyanosis	Chemical inflammation	Hypocarbia/hypercarbia	Myocardial dysfunction
Barrel chest	Air tapping	Acidemia	Renal failure
Tachypnea/retractions	Atelectasis		Coagulopathy
Diffuse rales/ronchi	Uneven ventilation		Seizures
Air leaks	Intrapulmonary shunting		
Persistent pulmonary hypertension of the newborn	↑ Expiratory resistance		
	↓ Surfactant function		
	Mismatched V̇/Q̇		

$\dot{V}/\dot{Q}$ = ventilation/perfusion.

Table 4–34. Causes of persistent pulmonary hypertension syndrome in the newborn.

Increased development in smooth muscle of pulmonary vessels
  Chronic fetal hypoxia
  Fetal systemic hypertension with associated pulmonary hypertension
  Intrauterine constriction of the ductus arteriosus
 	
Decreased cross-sectional area of pulmonary vascular bed
  Pulmonary hypoplasia
  Diaphragmatic hernia
  Pulmonary cysts
  Drugs and congenital infections
 	
Abnormal levels of vasoactive agents
  Increased availability of pulmonary vasoconstrictors before or after birth
  Decreased availability of vasodilators before or after birth
	Decreased pulmonary blood flow with normal pulmonary vascular bed (with or without vasoconstriction)
	  Perinatal and postnatal asphyxia
	  Meconium aspiration syndrome
	  Upper airway obstruction
	  Lung disease
	  Pneumonia (group B streptococcus)
	  Central nervous system depression (hypoventilation)
	  Polycythemia
	  Hypothermia
	  Infant of diabetic mother
	  Postmature infants
	  Cardiomyopathies (ischemic, viral)
	  Shock
	  Pulmonary microthromboembolism
	  Hypovolemia-anemia

with large shifts in Pa_{O_2}. This is related to acute changes in pulmonary blood flow with changes in the degree of pulmonary vasoconstriction. This lability may persist even after the condition of these patients begins to improve, requiring prompt increase in respiratory settings and Fi_{O_2}. The chest radiograph is variable because of the many causes of this syndrome. Usually, pulmonary vasculature markings are decreased initially in infants with idiopathic PPHN without MAS or perinatal asphyxia.

Treatment is summarized in Table 4–36. The cornerstone of therapy is to prevent hypoxemia, maintain a high-normal Pa_{O_2} and a normal or above-normal pH, while avoiding extreme hypocarbia. Pulmonary vasodilator drugs (eg, tolazoline and prostaglandin E_1) have been tried, but no drug has yet been effective. Recently, promising results have been achieved with inhalation of NO in some infants with PPHN. NO is released from endothelial cells and has a vasodilator action on pulmonary vessels. A controlled multicenter trial is currently under way. In those infants who do not respond to these approaches, ECMO has been instituted. Criteria for starting ECMO are still not definitive and vary in different institutions. ECMO requires insertion of large catheters into a carotid artery and jugular vein; the frequency of complications attributable to this procedure varies from one institu-

tion to another. ECMO has proved effective in managing selected patients.

PERINATAL ASPHYXIA

Asphyxia is defined as hypoxemia with subsequent metabolic acidosis. Hypercarbia may occur in the fetus when the placental blood flow is affected. After birth, asphyxia usually involves inadequate pulmonary gas exchange that leads to hypercarbia and hypoxemia. The risk factors for asphyxia are summarized in Table 4–1. During labor, placental gas exchange may be disturbed by reduction of uterine or umbilical blood flow and cause fetal asphyxia. The healthy fetus uses several mechanisms to respond to hypoxia and asphyxia. However, maternal, placental, or fetal problems can compromise these responses, so that the fetus is incapable of responding adequately.

During the initial stage of asphyxia, the cardiac output remains stable but is redistributed. Vasoconstriction of the skin and the renal and mesenteric vascular beds results in a marked decrease in blood flow to these organs. In con-

Table 4–35. Features of persistent pulmonary hypertension of the newborn.

Perinatal history of fetal distress	S_2 loud and not split
Term or post-term pregnancy	Preductal and postductal difference in Pa_{O_2}
Cyanosis	Chest radiograph: variable lung parenchyma; ± cardiomegaly
Tachypnea (± tachycardia)	ECG: RV overload
Spontaneous swings in Pa_{O_2}	Echocardiography: shunting, RV dilation, tricuspid and pulmonic valve regurgitation
Significant decreases in Pa_{O_2} in response to Fi_{O_2} changes or stimulation	
Systolic murmur (50%)	

ECG = electrocardiogram; RV = right ventricle.

Table 4–36. Treatment of persistent pulmonary hypertension.

General Measures	Specific Measures
Avoid hypothermia	Maintain oxygenation
Correct promptly any abnormalities in glucose, calcium, potassium, hematocrit	Avoid hypoxia
	Maintain preductal Pa_{O_2} 100–150 mm Hg
Correct acidosis (sodium bicarbonate or THAM)	Initiate mechanical ventilation early
Maintain systemic arterial blood pressure (volume or vasoactive drugs)	Sedation—muscle paralysis
	Maintain normal or alkalotic pH
Avoid unnecessary stimulation, agitation, or crying	Administer pulmonary vasodilators
	Begin ECMO

ECMO = extracorporeal membrane oxygenation; THAM = tris(hydroxymethyl) aminomethane.

trast, blood flow to the myocardium, brain, and adrenal glands is increased. This redistribution of blood flow, as well as the increase in systemic arterial pressure and bradycardia, results from chemoreflex response, adrenal catecholamine release, and angiotensin and vasopressin response.

Redistribution of cardiac output is an attempt to maintain oxygen supply to vital organs. As oxygen delivery decreases to less than critical levels, metabolism becomes increasingly anaerobic; anaerobic glycolysis results in increased lactic acid production with development of metabolic acidemia. Hypoxemia also results in marked pulmonary vasoconstriction. Metabolic acidemia greatly exaggerates the increase in pulmonary vascular resistance associated with hypoxemia.

The redistribution of cardiac output and the increase in systemic vascular resistance are responsible for many of the clinical signs observed in asphyxiated patients (pallor, decreased urine production, intestinal necrosis). With severe asphyxia, myocardial function may be depressed; this may compromise umbilical-placental flow and thus further interfere with gas exchange. The decreased myocardial performance may persist into the newborn period.

Asphyxial events are better tolerated during the fetal and neonatal periods than during any other period of life. A possible explanation for this increased tolerance is that a large proportion of fetal and neonatal oxygen demand is facultative or nonessential for survival functions, such as growth and thermoregulation. In organs with high metabolic activity, such as the heart and brain, the amount of oxygen expended for growth is a very small percentage of the total oxygen requirement. Because the heart has little reserve in terms of increasing oxygen extraction, it depends on increased blood supply during asphyxia to sustain normal function. Table 4–37 summarizes the effects of asphyxia on various organ systems. The CNS effect of asphyxia or ischemia can be of varying degrees and usually begins during the final stages of a severe episode or after repetitive episodes.

During the early stages of asphyxia, the fetus and newborn may make vigorous breathing efforts; however, if hypoxia continues, the ventilatory center becomes depressed. During terminal stages of asphyxia, gasping efforts can be seen, but they are not useful to establish adequate inflation of the lungs. Absence of breathing (apnea) is a frequent finding in asphyxiated newborns.

CARDIOPULMONARY RESUSCITATION OF THE NEWBORN

The goal of cardiopulmonary resuscitation (CPR) is to protect the CNS during asphyxia. This is possible by reversing the pathophysiologic events that occurred during asphyxia. The first step in CPR is anticipation: This includes knowledge of the maternal personal and obstetric history; history of the pregnancy, including labor; preparation of the delivery room (eg, materials, equipment, and, drugs); and, most important, the presence of a trained team in the delivery room at the moment it is needed.

Immediately after birth, the infant's skin should be dried vigorously with prewarmed towels, and the baby placed in a radiant warmer to avoid loss of body temperature. This also provides external tactile and sensorial stimulation that can help to initiate ventilation after birth. The immediate use of suction catheters to clear the airways is not recommended unless there is obstruction by meco-

Table 4–37. Effects of asphyxia on organ systems.

Cardiovascular
  Regional blood flow redistribution (selective ischemia)
  Hypertension (by increased peripheral vascular resistance)
  Diminished glycogen reserves in myocardium
  Myocardial ischemia—cardiogenic shock (hypotension)
  Myocardial necrosis (subendocardial, papillary muscle)
  Massive tricuspid valve regurgitation
  Conduction abnormalities (bradycardia, first- and second-
    degree heart block)
  Persistent pulmonary hypertension
  Hypervolemia (less frequently hypovolemia)

Gastrointestinal system
  Necrotizing enterocolitis
  Perforation—mucosal ulceration

Kidney
  Medullar and tubular necrosis
  Stimulation of renin-angiotensin system
  Oliguria
    Renal failure
    Bladder paralysis

Central nervous system
  Loss of autoregulation of blood flow
  Cytotoxic and vasogenic edema
  Ischemia—necrosis
  Hypoxic—ischemic encephalopathy (irritability, hypotonia,
    seizures, coma)
  Intracranial hemorrhage

Respiratory system
  Increased pulmonary vascular resistance
  Decreased pulmonary surfactant
  Edema (alveolar edema, interstitial/perivascular)
  Hypoventilation (secondary to central nervous system depres-
    sion)
  Apnea
  Meconium aspiration (prenatal or postnatal)
  Persistent pulmonary hypertension

nium, blood, or amniotic fluid. Evaluation of the baby should begin immediately after birth rather than waiting for the 1-minute Apgar score. Figure 4–5 summarizes the steps of evaluation-action-reevaluation recommended by the American Heart Association and the American Academy of Pediatrics.

Most infants are blue at birth and become pink after effective ventilation is established. If central cyanosis persists when the baby is breathing adequately and the heart rate is normal, 100% free-flowing oxygen over the nose and mouth should be administered. If the newborn is apneic or fails to sustain effective ventilation (heart rate < 100 even when ventilatory movements are present), initiating artificial ventilation with mask-and-bag is mandatory. Special attention should be paid to the position of the head and neck to ensure adequate lung expansion. An increase in heart rate and reperfusion of the skin signal the adequacy of ventilation, unless severe metabolic acidosis and myocardial failure are present. An oro-

gastric tube must be inserted after 2 minutes of mask-and-bag ventilation to eliminate accumulated gastric air. Mask-and-bag ventilation is contraindicated when congenital diaphragmatic hernia (CDH) is suspected. Endotracheal intubation should be performed in the presence of CDH and in all infants in whom mask-and-bag ventilation is not effective, or when it is required for more than 2–3 minutes.

If the heart rate remains low after 30–60 seconds of effective ventilation, the infant requires external cardiac massage at a rate of 100–120 times per minute. The effectiveness of cardiac massage must be evaluated by palpation of femoral or carotid pulses or by measuring arterial blood pressure. In the unusual case that bradycardia persists after all these resuscitation efforts, further measures are instituted. Ventilation, cardiac massage, and drugs should all be initiated at once when the newborn has asystole. Table 4–38 summarizes the drugs most frequently used during CPR.

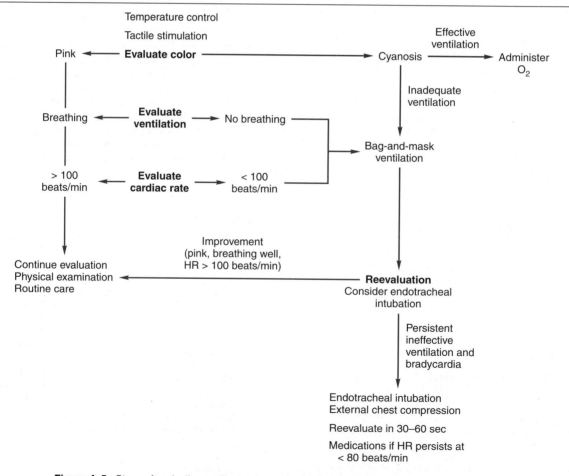

Figure 4–5. Steps of evaluation, action, and reevaluation in perinatal asphyxia. HR = heart rate.

Table 4–38. Medications used during neonatal resuscitation.

Drug	Indications	Dosage	Route	Effect
Epinephrine	Asystole	0.01 mg/kg (0.1 mL/kg) 1:10,000 dilution	ET, IV	↑ Heart rate ↑ Myocardial contractility ↑ Arterial pressure
Sodium bicarbonate	Metabolic acidosis (documented)	1–2 meq/kg diluted 1:2 (very slowly)	IV	Corrects metabolic acidosis Improves cardiac output and peripheral perfusion
Naloxone	Maternal administration of opiates + apneic infant	0.1 mg/kg	IV, SC, IM	↑ Ventilatory rate
Fluids (packed red cells, albumin 5%, normal saline)	Hypovolemia	10–20 mL/kg	IV slowly	↑ Blood pressure Improves tissue perfusion

ET = endotracheal; IM = intramuscular; IV = intravenous; SC = subcutaneous.

OTHER DISORDERS

POLYCYTHEMIA

Polycythemia, defined as a central venous hematocrit greater than 65%, is present in 2–4% of infants born at sea level. It may result from increased placental transfusion (delayed cord clamping) or from increased red blood cell production by the fetus in response to hypoxemia and increased erythropoietin secretion caused by placental insufficiency. Polycythemia is associated with several complications of pregnancy (Table 4–39) and also with SGA and LGA infants.

The pathophysiologic effects of polycythemia are related to blood hyperviscosity or hypervolemia. Blood viscosity depends on hematocrit values, blood flow velocity, and protein content of plasma (especially fibrinogen). The relationship of viscosity to hematocrit is exponential. Below a venous hematocrit of 65%, viscosity changes only modestly with red blood cell mass. Above 65%, increases of hematocrit result in dramatic increases in viscosity. This increased viscosity leads to a slower blood flow in tissues. At any given hematocrit, viscosity is higher with lower flow rates or higher protein content of plasma. Premature infants who have lower concentrations of plasma proteins have higher flow rates than do term infants, even at the same hematocrit values. After birth, fluid is redistributed between plasma and tissues, so that plasma water content decreases. Hematocrit values are highest at 2–6 hours after birth and decrease thereafter.

Diagnosis

Clinical features of hyperviscosity are shown in Table 4–40. Capillary hematocrits should be obtained routinely approximately 4 hours after birth for screening purposes, but infants with known perinatal risk factors for neonatal polycythemia (see Table 4–39) should be screened within 2 hours. If hematocrits exceed 65%, a venous blood sample should be obtained with minimal or no tourniquet or compression and free-flowing blood. If the values are borderline, measurement should be repeated after 2–4 hours. Coulter counter hematocrits are usually lower (5–6 points) than spun values. Infants with hematocrits of 60–65% and symptoms attributable to polycythemia should be considered polycythemic and managed accordingly.

Treatment

Standard accepted treatment for neonatal polycythemia is partial exchange transfusion. Blood is removed and re-

Table 4–39. Infants at risk for neonatal polycythemia.

Small-for-gestational-age infants
Large-for-gestational-age infants
Infants with birth weight > 4000 g
Infants of diabetic mothers
Infants born at high altitude
Infants born to hypertensive mothers (even if average for gestational age)
Infants with Down syndrome
Rarely, infants with congenital heart disease; adrenogenital syndrome

Table 4–40. Signs and symptoms of polycythemia.

Skin	**Renal**
Plethora	Hematuria
Cyanosis	
	Hematologic
Gastrointestinal	Thrombocytopenia
Poor feeding	
Feeding intolerance	**Cardiovascular**
	Poor perfusion
Respiratory	Ventricular failure
Tachypnea	Acidosis
Respiratory distress	
Persistent pulmonary hypertension	
Central nervous system	
Lethargy	
Hypotonia	
Jitteriness	

placed by the same volume of plasma or plasma substitutes in a stepwise manner. Hematocrit is thus reduced without further compromising blood flow. Simple phlebotomy or volume infusions alone are not recommended for polycythemic infants, because they will decrease or increase total blood volume.

To establish the volume of blood to exchange, the following formula is used:

$$\text{Volume (mL)} = \left(\frac{\text{Initial Hct} - \text{Desired Hct}}{\text{Initial Hct}} \right) \times \text{Wt (kg)} \times 90 \text{ (mL/kg)}$$

(Hct = hematocrit; Wt = body weight)

Desired hematocrits are 50–55%, and 90 represents the average blood volume (in mL/kg) for most newborn infants. Partial exchange transfusion can be safely performed with crystalloid solutions (eg, normal saline).

Infants with polycythemia should be carefully observed for 24–48 hours after partial exchange transfusion. Repeat hematocrits should be obtained 2–4 and 12 hours after the partial exchange transfusion. In infants with perinatal risk factors and in babies with Down syndrome, hematocrits should also be obtained 24 and 48 hours after treatment because they may continue to have increased red blood cell production. Occasionally, more than one partial exchange transfusion may be required to maintain appropriate hematocrits.

Hypoglycemia, hypocalcemia, and hyperbilirubinemia may be associated with polycythemia and require management (Table 4–41).

Outcome

Short-term outcome of polycythemic infants is usually good; the most troubling complication is NEC—although its exact relationship to polycythemia is not known.

Long-term outcome is still controversial. In reported studies, no attempt has been made to separate "normal" infants from those with IUGR, nor to separate infants who receive treatment from those who do not. In some recent studies, no difference in long-term outcome has been found between treated and untreated polycythemia, suggesting that there may be no advantage to treating this condition. However, until more reliable studies are conducted, exchange transfusion remains the standard treatment.

Table 4–41. Potential complications of polycythemia.

Hyperbilirubinemia	Transient feeding intolerance
Hypocalcemia	Necrotizing enterocolitis
Hypoglycemia	Irritability
Thrombocytopenia	Intracranial hemorrhage/infarct
Transient hematuria	Abnormal development
Renal failure (thrombosis)	

CONGENITAL INFECTIONS

Perinatal viral, bacterial, or protozoal infections of the mother can be transmitted to the fetus or to the newborn infant. The acronym TORCH was coined in 1974 to cover toxoplasmosis, rubella, CMV, herpes simplex virus (HSV), and other agents. However, an increasing list of maternal pathogens has been recognized that can infect the fetus and newborn infant transplacentally, hematogenously, or via contact with the colonized birth canal (Table 4–42). Transmissibility and the severity of the disease in infected infants vary according to the pathogen and the timing of the maternal infection during gestation. Many of the pathologic agents cause abortion or stillbirth; some lead to congenital anomalies (see Chapter 5).

Clinical Features

Maternal infections with TORCH agents are often asymptomatic, despite the frequency with which these organisms attack pregnant women. Similarly, most congenital infections are asymptomatic in the newborn infant. The clinical manifestations that suggest congenital infection are similar for many infecting agents. Some congenital infections may have recognizable patterns in the neonate (Table 4–43).

Clinical suspicion should be based on specific data from the maternal history and a combination of physical signs in the mother and the infant. Laboratory studies, including specific cultures and serologic testing, are required to confirm the diagnosis and identify a specific pathogen.

Diagnostic Evaluation

Diagnostic workup (Table 4–44) includes viral culture (oropharynx, urine, and rectum), serologic testing for antigens or antibodies to specific congenital pathogens, and microscopic examinations for herpes or syphilis (dark

Table 4–42. Organisms causing congenital infections.

Transplacental fetal infections	
Cytomegalovirus	*Plasmodium*
Enteroviruses	Rubella
Herpes simplex virus, types 1 and 2	*Staphylococcus aureus*
	Toxoplasma gondii
HIV	*Treponema pallidum*
Listeria monocytogenes	Varicella zoster
Measles	
Mumps	
Ascending infections	
Bacteroides	Enterobacteriaceae
β-Hemolytic streptococci	*Escherichia coli*
Candida	
Natal acquisition from maternal birth canal	
Candida	Herpes simplex virus
Chlamydia trachomatis	*L monocytogenes*
Cytomegalovirus	*Neisseria gonorrhoea*
Hepatitis B virus	

Table 4–43. Patterns of fetal and infant morbidity in some congenital infections.

Pathogen	Fetus	Congenital Defects	Neonatal Disease	Late Sequelae
Treponema pallidum	Stillbirth, hydrops fetalis	—	Skin lesions, rhinitis, hepatosplenomegaly, jaundice, hemolytic anemia, bone lesions	Interstitial keratitis, frontal bossing, saber shins, tooth changes
Toxoplasma gondii	Abortion	Hydrocephalus, microcephaly	Low birth weight, hepatosplenomegaly, jaundice, anemia, intracranial calcifications	Chorioretinitis, mental retardation
Rubella	Abortion	Heart defects, microcephaly, cataracts, microphthalmia	Low birth weight, hepatosplenomegaly, petechiae, osteitis	Deafness, mental retardation, diabetes, degenerative brain lesions
Cytomegalovirus	—	Microcephaly, microphthalmia, retinopathy	Anemia, thrombocytopenia, hepatosplenomegaly, jaundice, encephalitis, cerebral calcification	Deafness, psychomotor retardation
Varicella zoster virus	—	Limb hypoplasia, cortical atrophy, cicatricial skin lesions	Low birth weight, chorioretinitis, congenital chickenpox or disseminated neonatal varicella	Potential for fatal outcome due to secondary infection
Herpes simplex virus	Abortion	Possible microcephaly, retinopathy, intracranial calcifications	Disseminated disease, multiple organ involvement (lung, liver, CNS), vesicular skin lesions, retinopathy	Neurologic deficits
Hepatitis B virus	—	—	Asymptomatic HBsAg-positive infection, low birth weight, rarely acute hepatitis	Chronic hepatitis, persistent positive HBsAg, cirrhosis, hepatocellular carcinoma
HIV	—	—	Pediatric AIDS	Pediatric AIDS
Enteroviruses	Abortion	Myocarditis, possible congenital heart disease	Mild febrile disease, exanthems, aseptic meningitis, gastroenteritis or multiple organ involvement (CNS, liver, heart)	Neurologic deficits

CNS = central nervous system; HBsAg = hepatitis B surface antigen.

field, fluorescent antibody stain, or Tzanck preparation) from skin lesions. CMV and HSV infections are diagnosed predominantly by culture; syphilis, toxoplasmosis, and hepatitis B virus (HBV) predominantly by serologic tests; and rubella by both serologic and culture techniques.

Table 4–44. Diagnostic tests in congenital infection.

Nonspecific Tests	Specific Tests
Complete blood count and platelets	Viral culture:
	Oropharynx, urine, rectum
Lumbar puncture	Blood for HIV
Large bone radiographs	Cerebrospinal fluid or conjunctiva are optional
Cerebral imaging	Smears of skin lesions (herpes,
Computed tomography	syphilis):
Magnetic resonance imaging	Fluorescent antibody stain
	Darkfield examination
Ultrasound	Tzanck smear
Ophthalmologic evaluation	Serologic tests for:
Audiologic evaluation	Rubella
	Toxoplasma
	Syphilis
	Hepatitis B and HIV

The presence of thrombocytopenia or hemolytic anemia may suggest the diagnosis of a congenital infection. Radiographic indications of congenital infections include cerebral calcifications and abnormal ossification of long bones (celery-stalking, periostitis, and metaphyseal lucencies). Cerebral CT or MRI may also demonstrate white matter alterations, hydrocephalus, cortical atrophy, and cystic lesions of the cortex. Ophthalmologic evaluation is important in detecting chorioretinitis, as well as cataracts and glaucoma caused by congenital infections. Brainstem auditory-evoked responses may detect early hearing deficits that progress after congenital infection by rubella or CMV. Lumbar puncture should be performed on all infants being evaluated for congenital infection. Elevated protein concentration and pleocytosis in the spinal fluid are important confirmatory findings of meningoencephalitis in congenital syphilis and rubella or in natally acquired herpes simplex encephalitis.

Antibody titer determination in perinatal infections is complicated by transplacental passage of maternal IgG and the technical difficulties of specific IgM tests. Total serum IgM concentration has been used in the past as a screening test for congenital infection but is neither sensitive nor specific. Specific IgM titers for toxoplasmosis, rubella, syphilis, and CMV exhibit excellent specificity but are not highly sensitive.

General Management

Universal body substance precautions obviate the need for isolation or separation of the neonate from the mother in most cases. However, untreated tuberculosis, infectious syphilis, and intrapartum varicella may be indications for temporary separation from the mother. Neonates with congenital rubella and possibly HSV should be admitted to isolation rooms to prevent nosocomial spread; other infections are not likely to be spread if universal body substance precautions are followed. In all cases, special care must be taken by pregnant health care providers when handling infants with congenital infections.

Breast-feeding is not recommended in HIV-infected mothers or in untreated mothers with tuberculosis. Also, CMV and HBV can be transmitted by breast-feeding during the acute infection. No consensus exists regarding the risks of chronic HBV carriers. Otherwise, maternal infection does not preclude breast-feeding.

Recognition of congenital infections, such as varicella, HIV, syphilis, gonorrhea, tuberculosis, and HBV, should initiate the investigation of other family members at risk.

Treatment

Perinatal bacterial infection may be treated with appropriate antibiotics (see Chapter 9). Congenital syphilis or neurosyphilis is treated with penicillin for a 10-day course. Toxoplasmosis can be treated with pyrimethamine and sulfadiazine. HSV infection should be promptly treated with acyclovir. Ganciclovir treatment for CMV infections is still under investigation. The infant born to an HIV-infected mother should receive specific diagnostic testing and, once proved infected, be treated with zidovudine, immunoglobulin, and prophylactic trimethoprim-sulfamethoxazole.

Prevention

Cesarean delivery is indicated for women experiencing primary herpetic infection at the time of delivery, except when the fetus has been exposed to the birth canal after rupture of membranes for more than 4–6 hours. Recurrent herpes is not an absolute contraindication to vaginal delivery and carries a low risk of HSV infection in the neonate. Maternal chickenpox infection in the last 5 days of pregnancy or first 2 days after delivery is an indication for treatment with varicella zoster immunoglobulin. Neonatal chlamydia exposure after vaginal delivery may be an indication for prophylaxis with erythromycin. Natal acquisition of hepatitis B can be prevented to a significant degree by passive immunization with hepatitis B immunoglobulin and active vaccination with recombinant hepatitis vaccine. Neonatal acquisition of tuberculosis can be prevented by isoniazid or by passive immunization with bacillus Calmette-Guérin (BCG) vaccine.

Other methods to prevent congenital infections include maternal education about infectious exposures during pregnancy, rubella vaccination of all nonimmune women in their childbearing years, screening of blood products (for CMV, HIV, HBV, and syphilis), and universal neonatal eye prophylaxis (with silver nitrate or erythromycin ointment).

BIRTH TRAUMA

Mechanical forces applied to the fetus during labor and delivery can produce traumatic lesions, such as hemorrhage, edema, tissue laceration, fractures, or organ damage, at different sites. Risk for obstetric trauma is increased in primigravidas, abnormal presentations, fetal-maternal disproportion, multiple pregnancies, forceps and vacuum extraction, oligohydramnios, and internal version maneuvers. VLBW infants (< 1500 g) with breech presentation are subject to high risk because the cranium is easily deformable and is large in proportion to the body.

Subdural Hemorrhage

Subdural hemorrhage should not occur with obstetric improvements of the past decade; subarachnoid hemorrhage is much less severe and is more frequent in preterm infants. Spinal cord lesions may occur in frontal and face presentation or when shoulder dystocia is present with cephalic presentation. The incidence of spinal cord damage is very high in cases of breech presentation with neck hyperextension. High spinal cord or brainstem lesions may be associated with severe respiratory depression and shock from the time of birth. The lesion may be epidural or intraspinal edema or hemorrhage, or even complete cord transection. Usually the cervical vertebrae are normal in routine radiographs; the brachial plexus is affected in about 20% of cases. The differential diagnoses include intraspinal or extraspinal tumors, such as neuroblastoma, spina bifida with tethering cord, and severe hypoxic-ischemic encephalopathy.

Facial Palsy

Facial palsy is usually due to excessive pressure over the nerve, which can be induced by the maternal sacrum, a forceps blade, or the fetal shoulder. In complete peripheral palsy, the affected side shows no movement, the palpebral fissure remains open, and the facial folds are less noticeable. With crying, there is muscular contraction only on the healthy side, and the angle of the mouth deviates toward that side. Rarely, facial palsy may be of central origin. In these cases, frontal and ocular muscles are not affected, and there are usually other associated manifestations of intracranial lesions. Peripheral lesions recover partially or completely within weeks. To protect the eye from damage, artificial tears should be used.

Brachial Plexus Palsy

Brachial plexus palsy is secondary to difficult delivery

in either cephalic or breech presentations of mature infants. Clinical presentations are related to sites of injury. **Superior brachial palsy** (C-5 and C-6: Duchenne-Erb syndrome) is the most frequent and affects the shoulder and arm muscles. The affected upper extremity remains in abduction, extension, and internal rotation; the forearm is in pronation, and the wrist flexed, with very few spontaneous movements. The fingers move normally, and the palmar grasp reflex is normal. Moro reflex is abnormal, and movements of the shoulder are absent or diminished; phrenic nerve palsy can be associated with this lesion. **Inferior brachial palsy** (C-8, T-1: Klumpke syndrome) is rare. In this condition, wrist drop is present, and the fingers are separated. Frequently, Horner syndrome occurs on the same side (myosis, ptosis, and enophthalmos) because of lesions of the cervical sympathetic fibers of the first thoracic root. A **complete brachial palsy** is usually serious. The extremity is flaccid with no movement, all reflexes are absent, and there is also a sensory deficit. Superior brachial palsy shows good recovery in approximately 80% of cases, and inferior palsy shows recovery in around 40% of cases; however, in complete palsy, total recovery is rare. Other lesions, such as cerebral lesions, cervical column lesions, clavicle fracture or dislocation, and fracture of the head of the humerus, need to be excluded. Treatment for brachial plexus palsy is symptomatic, keeping the extremity in physiologic position over the chest during the first 2–3 weeks. Subsequently, physical therapy to maintain mobility of joint and avoid contractures and deformities is instituted.

Phrenic nerve palsy is associated with lesions of the nerve roots of C-3, C-4, and C-5 usually after lateral hyperextension of the neck in complicated labors (usually breech presentation). The lesion is unilateral, is associated with superior brachial palsy, and presents with apnea, cyanosis, chest retractions, and asymmetric respiration. Atelectasis is common, and pneumonia may develop. Chest radiograph shows a raised hemidiaphragm, with deviation of the mediastinum and heart. Ultrasound or fluoroscopy reveals paradoxical movement of the paralyzed diaphragm, which ascends in inspiration and descends in expiration. Treatment includes oxygen if necessary, and some infants require CPAP; in severe cases, mechanical ventilation may be indicated. A surgical procedure to stabilize the diaphragm is required in some infants.

Trauma to Other Sites

Intra-abdominal structures, particularly the liver or spleen, may rupture during traumatic deliveries, particularly in infants with breech presentation, in large fetuses, or in those with enlarged viscera due to hydrops fetalis or congenital infections. The clinical features are abdominal distention with progressive hypovolemic shock.

Lesions in the skull include caput succedaneum, which is of no clinical consequence and disappears in the first few days after birth, and **cephalhematoma,** which is a hemorrhagic collection caused by subperiosteal vascular rupture. This lesion appears after 24–48 hours, is unilateral, and is found over the parietal area. Cephalhematomas are limited to the area of the affected bone, do not cross the cranial sutures, and, in 15% of cases, are associated with an underlying skull fracture. Complications such as anemia and hypovolemic shock are rare, but large cephalhematomas can induce disseminated intravascular coagulation, hyperbilirubinemia, infection with osteomyelitis, sepsis, or meningitis. Most cases of cephalhematoma resolve spontaneously over the first few months of life, some with some degree of calcification. If there are signs of local infection or abscess formation, the cephalhematoma should be drained for appropriate treatment and to obtain cultures.

Trauma to the sternocleidomastoid muscle may cause an intramuscular hematoma, which subsequently leads to fibrosis and muscle contractures. Necrosis and edema can also develop in this muscle because of venous obstruction during labor. Clinically, the infants have torticollis with a small mass felt medial to the border of the muscle, becoming evident by 10–20 days after birth. Neck movement becomes increasingly limited. The typical position for these infants is with the chin rotated toward the contralateral shoulder and the head tilted over the contractured muscle. If physical therapy is not provided, the face may become asymmetric because of flattening on the facial side of the lesion.

Fractures are infrequent except for clavicular fracture. This type of fracture occurs in either vertex or breech presentation but is more common in large fetuses. In general, the movement of the shoulder and arm are not affected, and the Moro reflex could be entirely normal. Often it is noted in a chest radiograph obtained for other reasons. Treatment consists of decreasing pain by immobilizing the arm in a physiologic position. The prognosis is good.

INTRACRANIAL HEMORRHAGE

Intracranial hemorrhage, a significant cause of neurologic morbidity in the newborn, can be classified according to the anatomic space involved (Table 4–45). Subdural, subarachnoid, and intracerebellar hemorrhages are rare in full-term infants and result from birth trauma.

Periventricular-Intraventricular Hemorrhage

Periventricular-intraventricular hemorrhage (PV-IVH) is a frequent cause of neonatal morbidity and mortality in preterm infants. PV-IVH occurs in approximately 40% of infants with birth weights less than 1500 g but is uncommon in infants born after 34 weeks' gestation. Its incidence appears to have declined over the past decade. The risk of PV-IVH is highest in the most immature infants.

The typical site of bleeding in PV-IVH is the subependymal germinal matrix, a highly cellular region immediately ventrolateral to the lateral ventricle in the developing brain. This tissue is gelatinous with an elaborate, but immature, capillary bed. From 10 to 20 weeks'

Table 4–45. Classification of neonatal intracranial hemorrhage.

Type of Hemorrhage	Clinical Setting	Clinical Presentation	Complications
Subarachnoid	Asphyxia, coagulopathy	Asymptomatic with bloody CSF, seizures	Rarely problems but possible hydrocephalus
Subdural	Birth trauma, difficult delivery	Early—shock, stupor Late—macrocephaly	Subdural effusion requiring surgical evacuation
Intracerebellar	Breech delivery, forceps extraction, asphyxia, prematurity	Blood loss, apnea, or incidental finding on ultrasound or CT scan	Motor deficits, possible hydrocephalus
Periventricular-intraventricular	Trauma, asphyxia, prematurity	Neurologic dysfunction	Posthemorrhagic hydrocephalus

CSF = cerebrospinal fluid; CT = computed tomography.

gestation, the germinal matrix is the source of neuroblasts that migrate to the cerebral cortex. After 20 weeks, this tissue begins to involute over the next 12–15 weeks but remains a source of cerebral glial precursors until near term. During this involution, the capillary bed of the germinal matrix apparently is prone to disruption and hemorrhage, which frequently extends locally from the matrix through the ependyma into the lateral ventricles. The quantity of blood determines whether there is acute ventricular dilation. Blood can spread throughout the ventricular system and potentially obstruct ventricular CSF outflow or impair its absorption by arachnoid villi. Hydrocephalus, either acute or chronic, may then result. In approximately 15% of cases of PV-IVH, blood is found in the parenchyma of the cerebral cortex. Experimental and clinical evidence suggest that intraparenchymal hemorrhage is not merely an extension from the initial germinal matrix bleeding but results from a venous infarction believed to follow the same event causing PV-IVH.

Pathogenesis

The pathogenesis of PV-IVH is related to sudden disturbances in cerebral blood flow and increases in central venous pressure. The premature infant less than 34 weeks' gestation appears to be particularly vulnerable to alterations in systemic blood pressure, which may be associated with a number of conditions, including breech delivery and prolonged labor. Mechanical ventilation, asphyxia, RDS, pneumothorax, overzealous volume expansion, PDA, and agitation are considered to be risk factors.

Clinical Features

The initial bleeding of PV-IVH usually occurs 12–72 hours after birth. The clinical manifestations are related to blood loss and neurologic dysfunction. These include hypotension, bradycardia, apnea, lethargy, fixed pupils, seizures, and coma. In addition, coagulopathy, thrombocytopenia, and hyperbilirubinemia may occur. Many infants with small hemorrhages are totally asymptomatic, whereas others show intermittent hypotonia, apnea, or changes in heart rate and blood pressure; this has been called the "saltatory" presentation.

Diagnosis

Real-time cranial ultrasound scanning through the anterior fontanelle is the diagnostic tool of choice for evaluation of LBW infants and others at risk for PV-IVH. Several different schemes to grade the severity of PV-IVH have been proposed, but a **severe hemorrhage** is one with intraventricular hemorrhage, ventricular dilation, or intraparenchymal hemorrhage. Because 90% of cases of PV-IVH are evident within the first 4 days, one or two ultrasound scans are typically performed in the first week. Repeat ultrasound scans are used to follow progress and to assess subsequent neuropathology. This is important in prognosis and further management. For example, if posthemorrhagic hydrocephalus is progressive, agents to decrease CSF production, such as furosemide and acetazolamide, or serial lumbar punctures, may be indicated.

Outcome

The outcome associated with PV-IVH is not universally poor. The incidence for major neurodevelopmental handicaps at 2 years of age for premature infants with grade 1 or grade 2 hemorrhage is about 10%, which is similar to that for comparable infants with no hemorrhage. With increasing severity of hemorrhage, the risk of poor neurologic outcome increases; this appears to depend largely on the extent of associated parenchymal lesions. Posthemorrhagic hydrocephalus, however, does not appear to increase the risk of poor outcome independent of the severity of hemorrhage.

Prevention

Recently, major efforts have been directed toward preventing PV-IVH. Several approaches are currently being evaluated. Fresh frozen plasma has been used to correct coagulopathy; muscle relaxants or phenobarbital have been given in an attempt to reduce fluctuation in cerebral blood flow and blood pressure; vitamin E has been used for its potential antioxidant properties; and ethamsylate has been used in an attempt to stabilize capillaries in the immature vascular bed. The most promising approach has been the use of indomethacin, which induces cerebral vasoconstriction. The possibility that the decrease in cerebral blood flow could have late adverse effects requires further evaluation before indomethacin can be widely recommended.

INFANTS OF DRUG-ABUSING MOTHERS

Drug exposure of a developing fetus is thought to occur in approximately 15% of pregnancies in the United States, but the true number of pregnancies with substance abuse is perhaps higher. Although cocaine use by women has decreased in the past 7 years since the introduction of crack cocaine, opiate use by women appears to have increased. Most women who use illicit drugs use multiple drugs; thus, a causal relationship between a specific drug exposure and outcome is difficult to establish.

Drugs (particularly illicit drugs) may have serious consequences for the pregnant woman and her fetus. Risks include maternal drug and obstetric complications, impaired fetal somatic and brain growth, congenital malformations, clinical intoxication, and withdrawal symptoms. Use of alcohol, cocaine, amphetamines, phencyclidine (PCP), and narcotics may compound the fetal risk of tobacco, caffeine, and other illicit or prescribed drugs. Perinatal morbidity and mortality rates are higher for drug-exposed infants, as are long-term neurodevelopmental sequelae, later growth abnormalities, and increased risk for sudden infant death. Clinical manifestations in the neonate include irritability, tremulousness, feeding intolerance, and wakefulness. Because they are difficult to take care of, infants of drug-abusing mothers are at risk for child neglect or abuse when discharged home. Because of these increased risks for perinatal complications, pregnancies in which drugs are used should be identified prenatally and attempts made to control the exposure of the fetus. Infants born to women using drugs should be identified early in the neonatal period and observed for complications and withdrawal effects. A summary of the complications associated with substance abuse in both mother and infant is presented in Table 4–46.

Neonatal Identification of Drug Exposure

Because mothers frequently deny their drug use and be-

cause the onset of effects in the neonate can be delayed (depending on the specific drug, time of exposure, and half-life of the drug), identification of the exposed infant can be difficult. All women should be assessed for substance use during pregnancy by standardized interview techniques; the yield in identification improves with the depth of the risk assessment of a drug history. The substance-using woman and her exposed infant may also be identified from physical signs and reported symptoms in the mother.

Screening for drugs may identify drug exposure in the neonate and mother. This is usually performed on urine; the method provides quantitative information about recent substance use but has high rates of false-negative results and misses cases in women who abstain in the days before delivery. Use of newly devised techniques to test for drugs in meconium or in neonatal or maternal hair may improve the likelihood for an accurate diagnosis because they can detect earlier exposure during gestation. Thus, negative toxic screening results and denial of substance abuse during pregnancy do not exclude exposure of the infant. Screening is recommended in conditions in which there is suspicion of toxic abuse, in both the mother and the neonate. Mothers should be informed whether screening is to be done on their urine because they have the right of refusal. Because many mothers deny substance abuse, we do not advocate obtaining consent for testing the infant, although informing the mother is necessary. Testing is best performed on both the mother's and the infant's urine to obtain as many positive results as possible. A summary of the factors that should alert the clinician to perform toxic screening is presented in Table 4–47.

Neonatal Signs

The signs of drug effects vary with the specific drug, some of which cause both intoxication and a withdrawal syndrome. The most common signs are jitteriness and hyperreflexia; their presence in neonates should alert the clinician to the possibility of drug exposure.

Mortality rates range from 3 to 10%, and fetal demise

Table 4–46. Perinatal complications associated with substance abuse.

Neonatal Effects	Pregnancy/Mother
Intrauterine growth retardation	Inadequate prenatal care
Prematurity	Anemia
Birth defects	Endocarditis/hepatitis
Microcephaly	Urinary tract infection/ pneumonia
Antenatal cerebral infarctions	Tuberculosis/HIV
Small central nervous system bleeds	Venereal diseases
Respiratory depression at birth	Low self-esteem/depression
Infections/necrotizing enterocolitis	Low maternal weight gain
Poor feeding	Abruptio placentae
Abstinence/withdrawal syndrome	Possible precipitous delivery
Neurobehavioral abnormalities	Preterm labor and delivery

Table 4–47. Representative criteria for considering toxic screening.

Maternal and family history

Abruptio placentae	History of incarceration
Limited or no prenatal care	Maternal history of sexually transmitted disease
Intrauterine growth retardation	
History of substance use or alcohol use	Maternal history of prostitution
Maternal psychiatric history	

Neonatal history—three or more of the following:

Tremulousness/jitteriness	Sneezing, sweating, yawning
Hypertonia, hyperreflexia	Temperature instability
Irritability, incessant crying	Apnea
Unexplained depression, lethargy	Seizures or other neurologic signs
Increased sucking	Fetal alcohol syndrome
Vomiting, diarrhea	

can occur in utero from withdrawal. Causes of morbidity include perinatal asphyxia and congenital anomalies. Neurodevelopmental delay, specific neurologic deficits, and sudden infant death syndrome (SIDS) occur with increased frequency in opiate-exposed infants.

Cocaine is currently the illicit drug most commonly used during pregnancy. Symptoms are usually less severe than those with opiate exposure. Infants may be SGA with CNS, skull, eye, gastrointestinal, and genitourinary abnormalities; they may also be at increased risk for SIDS.

Fetal alcohol syndrome is characterized by IUGR, microcephaly, and dysmorphic features, including short palpebral fissures, microphthalmia, and flat nasal bridge. Congenital heart disease occurs in up to 40% of these infants. Chronic alcohol exposure causes neonatal depression and hypoglycemia in addition to a mild withdrawal syndrome in chronically exposed infants. Neurodevelopmental delay and growth failure usually are also noted.

PCP is associated with abnormal limb and eye movements and disordered regulation of sleep-wake states. Recently, fine motor control and subsequent behavioral disturbances have been reported in PCP-exposed infants. Microcephaly also has been noted.

Perinatal Management

Attempts should not be made to detoxify women who use opiates during pregnancy because of the risk of fetal withdrawal syndrome. These women should be maintained on methadone at the lowest dose tolerated. Neonatal care should be provided for the potential intrapartum complications, such as meconium aspiration, perinatal asphyxia, prematurity, IUGR, neonatal depression from maternal opiate use, or shock or asphyxia associated with abruptio placentae. Naloxone is not recommended, as it may abruptly induce acute withdrawal in opiate-habituated infants, producing seizures. When neonatal respiratory depression is associated with unknown substance exposure or known opiate exposure, ventilation should be supported to allow for gradual withdrawal from drug after birth.

Neonatal Management

Supportive care of the drug-exposed infant includes swaddling, limited sensory stimulation, and other comforting measures such as rocking, cuddling, pacifiers, warm baths, or gentle massage. The increased metabolic demands and oxygen consumption of the infant during withdrawal may require a caloric intake greater than 120 calories/kg/d to establish appropriate weight gain. Careful evaluation of symptoms (every 2–4 hours) is necessary to make decisions about pharmacologic therapy. The drugs most frequently used to treat withdrawal symptoms are presented in Table 4–48.

Several other issues need to be considered in caring for infants of drug-abusing mothers. Because breast milk contains drug, breast-feeding may prolong the withdrawal phase. In addition, there is an increased risk for HIV or hepatitis B infection in these infants because drug-abusing mothers may also have these infections. It is often necessary to provide careful home follow-up because of the adverse social circumstances associated with drug abuse.

NECROTIZING ENTEROCOLITIS

NEC is the most common acquired gastrointestinal disorder encountered in the neonatal intensive care unit. NEC predominantly affects premature infants and usually occurs as a complication of such conditions as RDS and PDA, but it occasionally occurs in full-term infants stressed by cyanotic congenital cardiac defect, asphyxia, anemia, or polycythemia.

Epidemiology

The incidence of NEC varies widely. In a collaborative study including several neonatal centers, the prevalence of proven NEC was 10.1%, and an additional 17.2% of infants had suspected NEC. The risk was greater in black boys and in infants with birth weights less than 1500 g. Significantly increased risk was associated with prolonged rupture of membranes, birth weight less than 1000 g, asphyxia, and maternal hemorrhage, whereas good prenatal care was associated with reduced risk. Ninety percent of cases occur in infants born at less than 36 weeks' gestation. The disease usually develops during the first 2 weeks after birth; it is uncommon before 5 days or after 1 month. The more immature the infant, the later is the onset of NEC.

Pathogenesis

The cause of NEC is not known. The most likely fac-

Table 4–48. Pharmacologic treatment of drug withdrawal symptoms.

	Phenobarbital	Diluted Tincture of Opium[1]	Diazepam
Comments	Useful but does not control diarrhea. Predictable decrease in serum levels when discontinued (10–20%/d)	Pharmacologic "replacement." Controls diarrhea. Requires very slow tapering	Works poorly alone. Does not control diarrhea
Dosage	Loading: 10–20 mg/kg Maintenance: 4–12 mg/kg/d orally (q 8 h)	0.8–2.0 mL/kg/d orally (q 4–6 h)	1.5–3.0 mg/kg/d orally or intramuscularly (q 6 h)

[1]Tincture of opium diluted in a concentration of 1:25 with H_2O.

tors contributing to NEC are bowel/blood flow, feeding disturbances, and infection.

Hypoxic-Ischemic Injury. Interference with gastrointestinal blood flow has been considered an important potential initiating factor in NEC. This may result from vasoconstriction caused by severe fetal or neonatal hypoxemia or from hypotension, shock, sepsis, PDA, congestive heart failure, and congenital heart disease with aortic arch obstruction. Vasospasm or thrombosis of the mesenteric circulation can also occur with umbilical arterial catheterization. Mucosal injury with necrosis and ulceration may ensue. Recently, it has been suggested that tissue damage may be aggravated by free oxygen radicals released during reperfusion after ischemia.

Bacterial Colonization. The gastrointestinal tract is usually sterile at birth. Within the first postnatal week, the gut normally becomes colonized with aerobic and anaerobic bacteria. However, colonization may be delayed by early antibiotic therapy, cesarean birth, or delayed enteric feeding; alternatively, the gut may become colonized with pathogenic bacteria in these conditions.

The role of bacterial infection in NEC is not resolved. It is possible that damaged bowel is secondarily infected. However, epidemic occurrences of NEC have suggested that infection may be the primary etiology. Epidemics have been associated with *E coli, Klebsiella pneumoniae, Staphylococcus epidermidis, Clostridium butyricum,* and some viruses (eg, enterovirus, coronavirus, and rotavirus).

Luminal Substrate. More than 90% of infants in whom NEC develops had received enteral feedings. Excessive and rapid increases of volume have been suggested as a risk factor for NEC, but this could merely contribute to an already damaged bowel.

Inflammatory Mediators. The physiologic events of NEC can be explained by the effects of inflammatory mediators, such as tumor necrosis factor produced by endo-toxin-stimulated macrophages, platelet-activating factor, and leukotrienes. The role of these mediators in endo-toxin-induced ischemic bowel necrosis has been confirmed in an animal model.

Clinical Manifestations

The earliest clinical manifestation of NEC is evidence of increased gastric residual volume during gavage feeding. NEC should also be suspected if an infant has abdominal distention or tenderness, bilious vomiting, and occult or frank blood in the stool. Other signs are nonspecific: apnea, bradycardia, cyanosis, lethargy, thermal instability, poor peripheral perfusion, hypoglycemia, jaundice, and shock.

The most common laboratory findings are metabolic acidosis, leukopenia, thrombocytopenia, anemia, electrolyte disturbances, reducing substances in stool, and, in severe cases, evidence of disseminated intravascular coagulation. The diagnosis of NEC is confirmed by evaluation of erect and recumbent abdominal radiographs. Bowel distention may be the earliest radiologic sign of NEC; other nonspecific findings include air-fluid levels within the intestine, thickening of the bowel wall, and a fixed dilated loop of intestine that persists in the same location in serial radiographs. **Pneumatosis intestinalis,** bubbles of subserosal air in the bowel wall that result from bacterial gas production, is considered pathognomonic of NEC. Pneumoperitoneum is a sign of intestinal perforation and indicates the need for immediate surgical intervention. The clinical staging criteria for NEC developed by Bell and coworkers are a useful guide to establish severity, treatment, and prognosis (Table 4–49).

Treatment

The goals of medical treatment are to stabilize the infant and to prevent progression of the disease. When NEC

Table 4–49. Modified Bell staging criteria for necrotizing enterocolitis (NEC).

Stage	Classification	Systemic Signs	Intestinal Signs	Radiologic Signs
I	Suspected NEC	Temperature instability, apnea, bradycardia, lethargy	Increased gastric residuals, mild abdominal distention, emesis, guaiac-positive stool	Normal; dilation; mild ileus
IIA	Proven NEC—mild	Same as above	Same as above, plus absent bowel sounds, with or without abdominal tenderness	Pneumatosis intestinalis, intestinal dilation, ileus, edema of bowel wall
IIB	Proven NEC—moderate	Same as above, plus mild metabolic acidosis and mild thrombocytopenia	Same as above, abdominal tenderness, with or without abdominal cellulitis or right lower quadrant mass	Same as above with or without portal venous gas and ascites
IIIA	Advanced NEC—severe; bowel intact	Same as above, plus hypotension, bradycardia, apnea, metabolic acidosis, thrombocytopenia, neutropenia, with or without DIC	Same as above; generalized peritonitis with marked distention of abdomen	Same plus ascites
IIIB	Advanced NEC—severe; bowel perforation or gangrene	Same plus DIC	Same as above	Same plus pneumoperitoneum or fixed bowel loop

DIC = disseminated intravascular coagulation.

is suspected, enteral feedings should be discontinued immediately and the intestinal tract decompressed by nasogastric or orogastric suction. Fluid and electrolytes should be administered to maintain urine output, blood pressure, and tissue perfusion. In addition, intravenous broad-spectrum antibiotics should be provided promptly. Frequent clinical and radiographic assessments are needed to recognize clinical deterioration early. Serial abdominal radiographs, including left lateral decubitus films to detect free air from intestinal perforation, should be repeated every 4–8 hours until the infant is stable. Parenteral nutrition should be initiated because oral intake is usually withheld for at least 10–14 days.

The timing and extent of surgical intervention in NEC is controversial. Definite indications are pneumoperitoneum, fixed loop on serial radiographs, or brown discoloration or presence of bacteria in peritoneal fluid withdrawn by paracentesis. Less definitive indications include abdominal erythema, abdominal mass, severe gastrointestinal bleeding, marked abdominal tenderness, thrombocytopenia, and clinical deterioration.

The most common late complication of NEC is colonic stricture, which occurs in 15–35% of recovered patients. Adhesions, abscesses, or fistulas may occur. Malabsorption or cholestasis also may occur. Short gut syndrome is a serious problem if a long segment of small bowel had to be removed surgically. It may require long-term parenteral nutrition. Mortality in NEC is high, approximating 10% in stages I and II and 55% in stage III.

THORACIC & GASTROINTESTINAL NEONATAL SURGICAL CONDITIONS

Approximately 1 of every 200 newborns requires a surgical procedure because of anomalies in the thorax, gastrointestinal tract, genitourinary system, or nervous system. Immediate neonatal care has been improved considerably by prenatal diagnosis of many of these anomalies. The more common thoracic and gastrointestinal conditions that require surgical repair during the neonatal period are reviewed.

Esophageal Atresia & Tracheoesophageal Fistula

Esophageal atresia and tracheoesophageal fistula is characterized by separation between the proximal and distal ends of the esophagus. The anomaly presents as five different types (Figure 4–6). The most common (type III) is associated with a tracheal fistula of the distal esophagus; it occurs in 1:3000 infants and is often associated with polyhydramnios. Owing to the esophageal obstruction, oropharyngeal secretions are copious because saliva cannot be swallowed. Choking and aspiration pneumonia may occur, particularly if feeding is attempted. In addition, air from the lungs crosses through the fistula to the distal esophageal segment inducing gastric distention, which in turn can stimulate regurgitation of gastric con-

tents through the fistula into the lungs. Aspiration from the upper airway or gastric contents entering the lungs through the fistula will cause respiratory distress.

To establish the radiographic diagnosis with certainty, no radiopaque substances are needed. An oral gastric tube is inserted until a stop is felt. A chest and abdominal radiograph will show the tube in the upper part of the thorax; air is seen in the stomach crossing through the distal fistula to the trachea.

Approximately 50% of infants with esophageal atresia have associated malformations, including congenital heart disease, anorectal, skeletal, and renal malformations, and the VACTERL association; the latter, present in 5–10% of infants, includes vertebral, anorectal, cardiac, tracheoesophageal, renal, and limb malformations.

General Management. Before surgery, the infant should be placed in an infant seat or the head and trunk elevated to avoid gastric reflux into the airway. Attempts to feed the infant should be stopped immediately, and continuous, gentle suction of the proximal esophageal pouch instituted. If the infant has respiratory distress due to aspiration, antibiotics should be started promptly. Cardiac and abdominal ultrasound studies should be performed to rule out associated anomalies. Surgical repair consists of closure of the fistula and anastomosis of the two esophageal segments. In the immediate postoperative period, infants are kept on mechanical ventilation for at least 24–48 hours, and parenteral nutrition is provided until appropriate calories can be administered enterally.

Complications include stenosis at the anastomotic site and prolonged difficulty in instituting oral feeding because of disturbed esophageal motility. Many of these infants also have respiratory distress and stridor because of associated tracheomalacia. The prognosis is most favorable in mature infants who have no associated congenital anomalies, who do not have respiratory distress, and who have no other severe congenital anomalies.

Congenital Diaphragmatic Hernia

The diaphragm develops between the fourth and eighth weeks of gestation. Abnormalities in its development may allow herniation of the abdominal contents into the thorax, which in turn impairs appropriate growth and maturation of the lungs. Most cases are in the left diaphragm in the posterior and lateral area. This condition occurs in 1:4000–5000 live births. The diagnosis can now be made in utero by ultrasound; if the lesion is found before 25 weeks' gestation, the prognosis is poor. Fetal surgery may become a solution for these cases.

The newborn with abdominal contents in the thorax and with pulmonary hypoplasia has severe respiratory insufficiency from birth, with severe hypoxemia and acidosis. The diagnosis can be made clinically by the presence of a scaphoid abdomen, because of abdominal organ displacement into the chest. Chest radiograph reveals little or no gas in the abdomen, absence of the diaphragmatic dome, significant mediastinal shift to the contralateral side (usu-

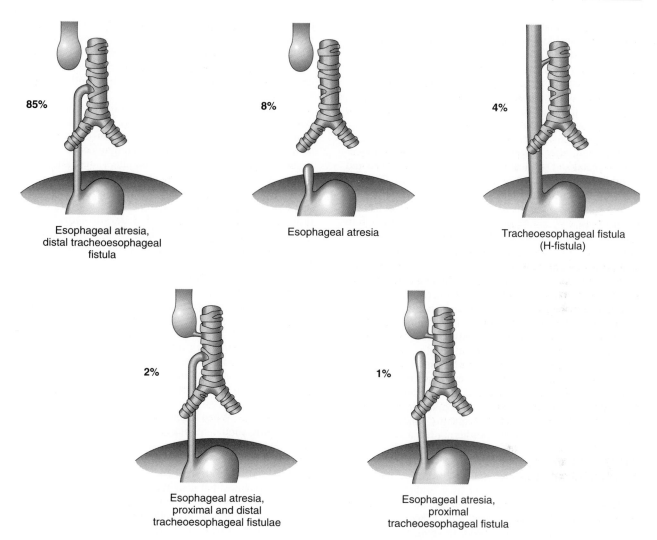

Figure 4–6. The major types and approximate incidence of tracheoesophageal malformations in newborn infants. (Reproduced, with permission, from Rudolph AM [editor]: Vanderhoof JA: Page 996 in: *Rudolph's Pediatrics,* 19th ed. Appleton & Lange, 1991.)

ally to the right), and bowel loops in the thorax, usually on the left side. PPHN also occurs frequently.

Management. If the diagnosis has been made before birth, the infant should be intubated immediately, preferably before spontaneous respiratory efforts or crying occur, to avoid gastrointestinal distention. A nasogastric tube should be inserted for continuous suction. *Bag-and-mask ventilation should not be used* because this may distend bowel and increase compression of the lung. Some infants do not improve with aggressive ventilatory treatment but may be helped by high-frequency or oscillatory ventilation; some require ECMO before surgery. If lung immaturity has been documented, artificial surfactant may be useful. Because the lung is hypoplastic, ventilatory pressures should be as low as possible to achieve adequate

blood gases. Slow lung reexpansion is important to avoid sudden mediastinal shifts and pneumothorax. Once the infant is stabilized, the condition is managed surgically by reduction of the hernia and closure of the diaphragmatic defect. This is usually performed by an abdominal or combined thoracoabdominal approach. When the defect is large, it may be necessary to place a plastic membrane over the abdomen to contain the reduced abdominal organs temporarily. The most serious complications, before or after surgery, are PPHN, pneumothorax, and gastrointestinal or hematologic complications.

Differential Diagnosis. Differential diagnoses of diaphragmatic hernia include congenital lobal emphysema and congenital cystic adenomatoid malformation of the lungs. The prognosis of infants with congenital diaphragmatic hernia is related to the size of the defect, the volume of the hernia inside the thorax, and the duration of the hernia in utero; these factors are associated with the degree of pulmonary hypoplasia. Clinical signs that have been associated with poor prognosis include early fetal diagnosis at less than 25 weeks' gestation, presence of liver and stomach in the thoracic cavity, significant polyhydramnios, early and severe neonatal symptoms, severe hypoxemia and acidosis, development of pneumothorax, and lack of improvement after surgery. With appropriate and aggressive neonatal and surgical care, survival has improved and is now greater than 80%. However, fetal and neonatal mortality is much higher for infants in whom the condition is diagnosed before 25 weeks' gestation, and many infants born with severe diaphragmatic hernias die before they are transported to a tertiary care facility.

Abdominal Wall Defects

By the 10th week of gestation, the midgut enters the abdomen. If this process is disturbed, an abdominal wall defect associated with a decrease in intra-abdominal volume results. The more common defects are **omphalocele, umbilical cord hernia,** and **gastroschisis.**

Omphalocele occurs in approximately 1:6000–8000 live births. The defect is localized centrally in the abdomen, the umbilical ring is missing, and the umbilical cord is inserted at the vertex of the sac. Abdominal organs other than bowel, such as liver, spleen, and pancreas, can be found in the hernia. It is frequently associated with other anomalies. Umbilical cord hernia has a diameter of less than 4 cm, and the sac contains only bowel.

Gastroschisis is a congenital fissure of the anterior abdominal wall; the umbilical cord is to the left of the defect and is separated from the defect by a bridge of skin. In gastroschisis there is no true hernia sac; the small bowel herniates and becomes thickened with adhesions because of contact with the amniotic fluid. In some cases, the intestine is infarcted and may be atretic. The abdominal cavity is often developed better than with large omphaloceles. Table 4–50 lists the principal differences between omphalocele and gastroschisis. Extraintestinal anomalies associated with omphalocele include imperforate anus with colon agenesis; pentalogy of Cantrell with sternal, pericardial, and cardiac defects; and Beckwith-Wiedemann syndrome. Congenital heart anomalies may occur in association with omphalocele; tetralogy of Fallot and atrial septal defects are the most common defects. Some cases are associated with trisomy 13 or, less frequently, with trisomy 18.

Treatment is surgical. Sometimes primary closure is not possible because forcing abdominal contents into the small cavity displaces the diaphragm, causing respiratory distress. In addition, bowel ischemia may occur when introducing the bowels under tension into a small abdominal cavity, sometimes resulting in compromised venous return and bowel ischemia. In such cases, a Silastic pouch is sutured to the skin around the defect. The size of this sac is progressively decreased every 1–3 days to introduce the bowel slowly into the abdominal cavity; this may take 10–15 days. Infection is a frequent complication.

Intestinal Obstruction

Intestinal obstruction may be acquired or congenital, and mechanical or functional (Table 4–51). The prenatal history may reveal polyhydramnios. In the immediate neonatal period, there may be abdominal distention, bilious vomiting, and lack of meconium passage. However, passage of meconium does not rule out the presence of obstruction. In more proximal obstructions, vomiting is the earliest sign; in distal obstruction, abdominal distention is marked.

Diagnosis. When intestinal obstruction is suspected, a gastric tube should be placed for immediate decompression, and abdominal radiographs obtained. Anteroposterior views should be taken with the infant supine and in right or left lateral decubitus; a cross-table lateral view is also useful. Intestinal distention with air-fluid levels, and sometimes the level of the obstruction, may be seen. Air reaches the rectum by 12 hours in term neonates and before 48 hours in preterm infants. Therefore, lack of distal

Table 4–50. Differences between omphalocele and gastroschisis.

	Omphalocele	Gastroschisis
Position	Central abdominal	Right paraumbilical
Hernia sac	Present	Absent
Umbilical ring	Absent	Present
Umbilical cord insertion	At the vertex of the sac	Normal
Herniation of other viscera	Common	Rare
Extraintestinal anomalies	Frequent	Rare
Intestinal infarction, atresia	Less frequent	More frequent

Table 4–51. Intestinal obstruction in neonates.

I. Mechanical
  A. Congenital
    Intestinal atresia or stenosis
    Meconium ileus
    Meconium plug
    Malrotation (with or without volvulus)
    Duplication
    Incarcerated hernia
    Annular pancreas
    Preduodenal portal vein
    Intestinal cysts
  B. Acquired
    Intussusception
    Adhesions
    Stenosis from necrotizing enterocolitis
    Lactobezoar
II. Functional
  Hirschsprung disease
  Hypoplastic left colon
  Other neuronal dysplasias or muscular diseases

air suggests intestinal obstruction. A barium enema is sometimes indicated; this will define the position of the cecum and thus detect malrotation. It can also be useful in cases of Hirschsprung disease or in congenital left microcolon syndrome.

Causes. Intestinal atresia is the most common cause of obstruction in the neonatal period. It can occur in the small or large bowel. Duodenal atresia may be intrinsic or extrinsic and is caused by malrotation, annular pancreas, or abnormal preduodenal portal vein. More than 50% of infants with duodenal atresia are SGA and have an increased incidence of cardiac, renal, and anal-rectal anomalies. Down syndrome is associated in 30–40% of cases. The diagnosis can be made prenatally by ultrasound or by abdominal radiograph, in which the typical "double-bubble" sign is noted. Treatment consists of resection of the area with duodenal-duodenal or duodenal-jejunal anastomosis.

Infants with jejunum-ileal atresias usually have no associated malformations. The cause is probably linked to a mesenteric vascular ischemic accident in utero. Bilious vomiting and abdominal distention vary with the level of obstruction. The abdominal radiograph shows multiple fluid-air levels with absence of distal air. A barium enema may show a very small colon. There are four different anatomic types of atresia. Type 1 is a simple atresia of the mucosa. In type 2, the most frequent, there is interruption of the mesentery and of the bowel wall, but the intestinal length is usually normal. Type 3 refers to multiple intestinal atresias, and in type 4, the so-called apple peel form, there is significant shortening of the bowel with a large mesenteric defect and ischemia of the small bowel.

Management. Treatment of jejunum-ileal atresias is surgical. The prognosis is related to the remaining length of intestine and to the presence or absence of the ileocecal valve after surgery. Morbidity and mortality are greatest in types 3 and 4, because short bowel syndrome and malabsorption are likely to develop in these infants. Parenteral nutrition has been a great aid in the management of these infants.

Meconium Ileus. Meconium ileus is a manifestation of cystic fibrosis during the neonatal period. Abnormal accumulation of intestinal secretions and deficiency of pancreatic enzymes presumably cause increased viscosity of meconium, which leads to occlusion of the distal ileum. Clinical features include abdominal distention, lack of meconium passage, and vomiting. Abdominal radiograph reveals distention with minimal or narrow air-fluid levels. Air remains trapped in the meconium; thus, there is no definite air-fluid interface. Fine gas bubbles may be seen mixed with meconium, producing a characteristic "soap-bubble" appearance. A barium enema may show a small colon secondary to the ileal obstruction. Early diagnosis and treatment are important to avoid perforation, meconium peritonitis, and volvulus. In some cases, however, these complications are present at the time of birth. Many newborns may respond to hyperosmolar enemas with iodine radiopaque substances, which are used in both diagnosis and treatment. These substances introduce water into the gastrointestinal tract, soften the meconium, and facilitate its elimination. If this procedure is performed, intravenous fluids should be provided appropriately to avoid dehydration and serum hyperosmolarity. If this approach is not successful, surgery is indicated to perform an ileostomy and, sometimes, ileal resection. N-acetylcysteine irrigations into the ileum may be useful for meconium dilution and bowel cleansing.

Intestinal Malrotation. Intestinal malrotation causes symptoms because of the presence of volvulus or because of intestinal obstruction secondary to bands. Circulation to the rotated segment is restricted, leading to intestinal gangrene. Volvulus presents with sudden onset of bilious vomiting with abdominal distention, profuse rectal hemorrhage, peritonitis, and shock. The cecum is displaced from its normal location in the right lower quadrant. When a diagnosis of intestinal volvulus is suspected, immediate surgical treatment is required: the volvulus is reduced by rotating the bowel loops counter-clockwise, and the gangrenous bowel is resected. Anastomosis may be performed and the intestine fixed in position surgically.

Anorectal Malformations. Anorectal malformations occur in approximately 1:5000 live births; the incidence is higher in male infants. Half these infants have associated anomalies, esophageal atresia, and genitourinary, skeletal, or cardiovascular malformations. If the defect is **low** it can produce anal stenosis, anal cutaneous fistula, anterior perineal anus, and, in girls, a vulvar anus. When the lesion is **intermediate,** the intestine ends above the elevator of the anus. These lesions include anal agenesis with or without rectal vaginal fistula and anal-rectal stenosis. When the defect is **high,** it produces anal-rectal agenesis and rectal atresia. Fistulas may be rectourethral, rectovaginal, or rectocloacal. The best diagnostic study is perineal examination; x-ray studies are useful to determine the level of the lesion. When there are fistulas, a fistulogram is useful before surgery. The initial treatment in the high and intermediate types is colostomy. By 1–2 years of age a final repair is performed, preserving the function of the sphincter. In the low lesion, perineal anoplasty is performed.

Hirschsprung Disease. Hirschsprung disease, or congenital aganglionic bowel disease, is rare, occurring in approximately 1:5000 live births. It is five times more frequent in male infants, and in 80% of cases there is a family history. The condition is due to lack of caudal migration of the ganglion cells from the neural crest; this produces contraction of a segment, causing obstruction with proximal dilatation. Vomiting, abdominal distention, and constipation are the classic clinical signs.

FREQUENT ELECTROLYTE & METABOLIC ABNORMALITIES

Hypoglycemia

Hypoglycemia is common in newborn infants. The actual serum glucose concentration defining hypoglycemia

is debatable but is generally agreed to be below 40 mg/dL. It is common practice to measure whole blood glucose concentration with test strips using a glucose oxidase method. Plasma glucose levels are approximately 14% higher than those of whole blood; therefore, a low glucose concentration by test strip should be confirmed by measuring the serum concentration. Hypoglycemia is suggested by an abnormal cry, diaphoresis, jitteriness, and seizures; other features include tachypnea, tachycardia, hypothermia, feeding problems, and, rarely, myocardial failure.

Hypoglycemia may be caused by conditions resulting in insulin excess, defective mechanisms of glucose homeostasis, defective carbohydrate or amino acid metabolism, or diminished substrate for gluconeogenesis (see Chapter 20).

Insulin Excess

Insulin excess occurs most commonly as a transient finding in the IDM. Maternal hyperglycemia results in fetal hyperglycemia and β-cell hyperplasia with elevated fetal insulin concentration. When the maternal-placental source of glucose is removed at the time of birth, hypoglycemia occurs in about 50% of IDMs in the first 24 hours after birth. β-cell hyperplasia is also implicated in the hypoglycemia observed with erythroblastosis fetalis and Beckwith-Wiedemann syndrome. β-Sympathomimetic drugs used for tocolysis cross the placenta and stimulate insulin release, causing transient hypoglycemia. Persistent hypoglycemia may result from insulin-producing tumors and usually requires subtotal or total pancreatectomy.

Diminished Glucose Production or Substrate Supply

Growth-retarded and preterm infants frequently have hypoglycemia because hepatic glycogen stores are limited and gluconeogenesis is poorly developed. Hypoglycemia may also occur after stress of asphyxia, polycythemia (hyperviscosity), congestive heart failure, infection, and cold. Inborn errors of metabolism causing hypoglycemia include galactosemia, hereditary fructose intolerance, glycogen storage disease Type I (von Gierke disease), and aminoacidopathies. Endocrine causes of hypoglycemia include growth hormone deficiency, panhypopituitarism, adrenal insufficiency, hypothyroidism, and glucagon deficiency.

The most important aspect of the medical management of neonatal hypoglycemia is appropriate anticipation and prevention in the infant at risk. Treatment is directed at increasing oral feeding, if possible. In the acute situation, glucose should be administered intravenously as a bolus (200 mg/kg as 2 mL/kg of 10% dextrose) followed by 5–8 mg/kg/min as a continuous infusion. If hypoglycemia persists, an endocrine evaluation should be instituted (see Chapter 20).

Hyperglycemia

Hyperglycemia, defined as a blood glucose concentration greater than 150 mg/dL, often results from excessive parenteral glucose administration but may occur with infection, during acute asphyxia or cold stress, and after surgery. Some drugs, such as theophylline and corticosteroids, may cause hyperglycemia. Transient diabetes mellitus occurs during the first 2 postnatal weeks in some SGA babies. Insulin therapy is usually required, although recovery in the first year is expected.

The major problems associated with hyperglycemia are hyperosmolarity and osmotic diuresis. Increased risk of PV-IVH and dehydration may result. If plasma glucose concentration is greater than 300 mg/dL or there is glycosuria, parenteral glucose infusion should be decreased 10–20% every 4–6 hours while plasma glucose concentration and urine are checked frequently. Insulin therapy is rarely required except in diabetic states. Insulin infusion, in very low doses (0.04–0.07 U/kg/h), has been used with reported success to increase early caloric intake without resulting hyperglycemia in VLBW infants.

Hypocalcemia

Hypocalcemia in the newborn is defined as a total calcium serum concentration less than 7.0 mg/dL (1.75 mmol/L) or an ionized calcium concentration less than 4.4 mg/dL (1.1 mmol/L). The clinical features of hypocalcemia are nonspecific and include irritability, jitteriness, tetany, and seizures. Infants may have a high-pitched cry, and apnea may occur. The ECG characteristically shows a prolonged QT interval and flat T waves. Neonatal hypocalcemia is usually evident in the first few postnatal days. It is common in preterm infants, in IDMs, and after asphyxia. It may also result from infection or maternal hyperparathyroidism. Later onset may be related to use of furosemide for diuresis.

Treatment of hypocalcemia depends on the clinical setting. Calcium gluconate, 10%, can be added to the intravenous solution. Each milliliter of 10% calcium gluconate (100 mg) provides 9 mg of elemental calcium. The dose ranges from 3 mL/kg/24 h to 12–15 mL/kg/24 h. With severe symptoms such as seizures, 10% calcium chloride is given by slow intravenous infusion in a dose of 25 mg/kg, or 10% calcium gluconate in a dose of 200 mg/kg, while the ECG and heart rate are monitored closely. Bradycardia or other cardiac arrhythmias can occur with rapid calcium infusion. A potentially serious complication of parenteral calcium chloride administration is extravasation into subcutaneous tissue, with skin sloughing. For chronic conditions, once the infant is feeding, oral calcium gluconate can be used.

Abnormalities in Serum Sodium Concentration

In full-term infants, hypernatremia occurs occasionally in breast-fed infants who have had very little intake over 5–7 days. However, hypernatremia and hyponatremia are more common in sick premature infants. In these infants,

serum sodium concentration is the best indicator of water balance during the first 7–14 days. It increases with water deficit and decreases with water excess; for this reason, serum sodium concentration may not accurately reflect total body sodium. **Hyponatremia** by definition is a serum sodium level below 130 meq/L. If hyponatremia develops acutely, cerebral edema and seizures may result. However, hyponatremia usually develops progressively, with clinical manifestations of hypotonia, hyporeflexia, and apneic episodes. The mechanisms responsible for hyponatremia and an approach to diagnosis are outlined in Figure 4–7. The treatment of hyponatremia is outlined in Table 4–52.

Hypernatremia, by definition, is a serum sodium concentration above 150 meq/L associated with excessive sodium intake or negative water balance. Usually in the neonate, excessive sodium intake is associated with an excess in total body water; thus, serum sodium concentration is normal. When hypernatremia is due to excessive sodium intake, sodium intake should be restricted and diuretics administered. When it is due to water deficit, it is associated with weight loss and negative water balance. The clinical manifestations of hypernatremia include hyperexcitability and hyperreflexia. One of the most serious risks in hypernatremia is the rapid correction of the serum sodium concentration. The brain cells contain osmols that prevent intracellular dehydration. If the serum sodium is decreased rapidly, these intracellular osmols draw water into the cells and generate edema, resulting in seizures. This complication is avoided if the serum sodium concentration does not decrease more than 10 meq/L in 6–8

Table 4–52. Treatment of sodium imbalance.[1]

Symptomatic hyponatremia
Fast correction (when serum [Na+] below 120 meq/L):
$(125 - \text{serum [Na}^+]) \times 0.8 \times \text{weight} = \text{total Na}^+$ (meq) to be given over 2–3 h.

Asymptomatic hyponatremia
Na+ deficit:
$(140 - \text{serum sodium}) \times 0.8 \times \text{weight} = \text{total meqs of Na}^+$ to be given over 12–36 h (added to Na+ maintenance).
Water excess
Calculate by weight curve or: $0.8 \times \text{weight} \times (1 - \text{serum [Na}^+]/140) = \text{H}_2\text{O}$ liters in excess.
Provide: Negative water balance, with sodium maintenance.

Hypernatremia
Calculate water deficit by weight curve or

$$0.8 \times \text{weight (kg)} \times \left(\frac{\text{serum Na}^+}{140} - 1 \right) = \text{H}_2\text{O deficit (liters)}$$

Provide free water plus maintenance fluids to decrease serum sodium not faster than 10 meq/L/6 h.

[1]The constant 0.8 in the formulas estimates the space of distribution of sodium.

hours. When there is water deficit, the treatment consists of adequate administration of free water to correct the negative water balance slowly (see Table 4–52).

Abnormalities in Serum Potassium Concentration

Hypokalemia may be due to excessive loss, as occurs with diuretics, or with inadequate K+ intake or metabolic

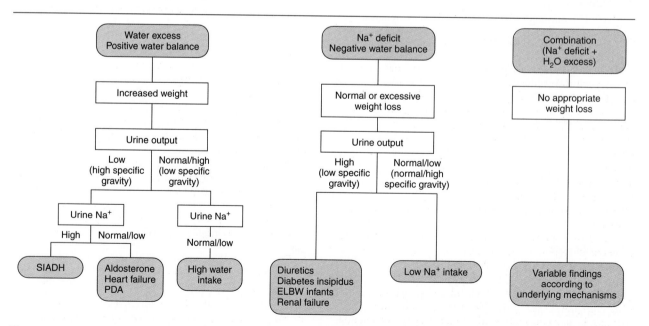

Figure 4–7. Mechanisms and diagnostic steps in hyponatremia. ELBW = extremely low birth weight; PDA = patent ductus arteriosus; SIADH = syndrome of inappropriate antidiuretic hormone secretion.

alkalosis. Treatment consists of increasing K^+ in the intravenous fluids and correcting alkalosis.

Hyperkalemia can occur in full-term infants with adrenogenital syndrome. It is very common in ELBW infants; as many as 50% of neonates less than 28 weeks' gestation show serum potassium concentrations greater than 6.5 meq/L. The cause has not been defined, but it could be due to low urinary output in the first 24–48 hours after birth, as well as to tissue damage at birth, acidosis, intracranial hemorrhage, and hemolysis. Neonates are more resistant to cardiac arrhythmias associated with hyperkalemia than are older children. Treatment is indicated when the serum potassium concentrations exceed 7 meq/L. Acidemia, if present, should be corrected, because this increases transfer of potassium from the extracellular

to the intracellular compartment. In addition, the serum calcium concentration should be maintained at normal levels to reduce the risk of arrhythmia. Potassium exchange resins, given by enema, may be indicated. Diuretics and dopamine infusion increase urinary output, and thus augment potassium excretion. Glucose and insulin are useful in decreasing serum potassium concentration, but can cause serious problems in VLBW infants. Peritoneal dialysis or continuous arterial venous hemofiltration are rarely required in neonates.

Electrolyte abnormalities usually can be prevented in VLBW infants by careful administration of fluids without sodium and potassium during the first 48–96 hours after birth, with frequent assessments of the glucose and fluid balance.

REFERENCES

PERINATAL HISTORY

Phibbs RH: The newborn infant. Neonatal mortality and morbidity. Page 197 in: Rudolph AM et al (eidtors): *Rudolph's Pediatrics,* 20th ed. Appleton & Lange, 1996.

Effects of Labor

Marsal K, Lindblad A: Fetal and placental circulation during labor. In: Polin R, Fox WW (editors): *Neonatal and Fetal Physiology.* Saunders, 1992.

Moise KJ et al: Indomethacin in the treatment of premature labor. Effects on the fetal ductus arteriosus. N Engl J Med 1988;319:327.

Transition to Neonatal Life

Bland R: Formation of fetal lung liquid and its removal near birth. In: Polin RA, Fox WW (editors): *Neonatal and Fetal Medicine, Physiology and Pathophysiology.* Saunders, 1992.

Rudolph AM: Circulation in the fetal-placental unit. In: Cowett RM (editor): *Principles of Perinatal-Neonatal Metabolism.* Springer-Verlag, 1991.

Temperature Regulation

Bruck K: Neonatal thermal regulation. In: Polin RA, Fox WW (editors): *Neonatal and Fetal Medicine: Physiology and Pathophysiology.* Saunders, 1992.

Saver PJJ: Neonatal thermoregulation. In Cowett RM: (editor): *Principles of Perinatal-Neonatal Metabolism.* Springer-Verlag, 1991.

ASSESSMENT OF NEWBORNS

Apgar Scores

Apgar V: A proposal for a new method of evaluation of the newborn infant. Curr Res Anesthesiol 1953;32:260.

Jacobs MM, Phibbs RH: Prevention, recognition, and treatment of perinatal asphyxia. Clin Perinatol 1989;16:785.

Nelson KB, Leviton A: How much of neonatal encephalopathy is due to birth asphyxia? Am J Dis Child 1991;145:1325.

Sykes GS et al: Do Apgar scores indicate asphyxia? Lancet 1982;1:494.

Maturity–Gestational Age

Ballard JL et al: A simplified score for assessment of fetal maturation of newborn infants. J Pediatr 1978;95:769.

Dubowitz LMS et al: Clinical assessment of gestational age in the newborn. J Pediatr 1970;77:1.

Physical Examination of the Newborn Infant

Charlton VE, Phibbs RH: Examination of the newborn. Page 208 in: Rudolph AM et al (editors): *Rudolph's Pediatrics,* 20th ed. Appleton & Lange, 1996.

Koop CE: *Visible and Palpable Lesions in Children.* Grune & Stratton, 1976.

Scanlon JW et al: *A System of Newborn Physical Examination.* University Park Press, 1979.

Neurologic Examination of the Newborn

Amiel-Tison C: Newborn neurologic examination. Page 218 in: Rudolph AM et al (editors): *Rudolph's Pediatrics,* 20th ed. Appleton & Lange, 1996.

Brann AW, Schwartz JF: Assessment of neonatal neurology function. In: Fanaroff AA, Martin RJ (editors): *Neonatal-Perinatal Medicine.* Mosby-Year Book, 1992.

Prechtl H, Beintena D: The neurological examination of the full-term newborn infant. *Clinics in Developmental Medicine,* #12. Heinemann, 1975.

ABNORMALITIES OF GROWTH

Cowett RM: Hypo and hyperglycemia in the newborn. In: Polin RA, Fox WW (editors): *Neonatal and Fetal Medicine: Physiology and Pathophysiology.* Saunders, 1992.

Kliegman R: Intrauterine growth retardation: Determinants of apparent fetal growth. In: Fanaroff AA, Martin RJ (editors): *Neonatal Perinatal Medicine.* Mosby-Year Book, 1992.

Ogata ES: Carbohydrate metabolism in the fetus and neonate

and altered neonatal glucoregulation. Pediatr Clin North Am 1986;13:2351.

ABNORMALITIES OF MATURITY

Clifford SH: Post-maturity with placental dysfunction. J Pediatr 1954;44:1.

Stubblefield G, Berek JS: Perinatal mortality in term and post-term births. Obstet Gynecol 1980;56:676.

Westgren M et al: Intrauterine asphyxia and long-term outcome in preterm infants. Obstet Gynecol 1986;67:512.

APPROACHES TO COMMON NEONATAL CLINICAL PROBLEMS

Cyanosis

Hoffman JIE: Right-to-left shunts. Page 1493 in: Rudolph AM et al (editors): *Rudolph's Pediatrics,* 20th ed. Appleton & Lange, 1996.

Kitterman JA: Cyanosis in the newborn infant. Pediatr Rev 1982;4:13.

Tooley W, Stanger P: The blue baby. Circulation or ventilation or both. N Engl J Med 1972;2878:983.

Respiratory Distress

Hazinski TA: The respiratory system. Page 1569 in: Rudolph AM et al (editors): *Rudolph's Pediatrics,* 20th ed. Appleton & Lange, 1996.

Swischuk L: Radiology of pulmonary insufficiency. In: Thibeault DW, Gregory GA (editors): *Neonatal Pulmonary Care,* 2nd ed. Appleton & Lange, 1986.

Swyer PR: Respiratory disorders in the neonate. In: Shoemaker W (editor): *Textbook of Critical Care.* Saunders, 1989.

Neonatal Anemia

Keyes WG et al: Assessing the need for transfusion of premature infants and role of hematocrit, clinical signs, and erythropoietin level. Pediatrics 1989;84:412.

Shannon KM et al: Enhancement of erythropoiesis by recombinant human erythropoietin in low birth weight infants: A pilot study. J Pediatr 1992;120:586.

Stockman JA: Anemia of prematurity: Current concepts in the issue of when to transfuse. Pediatr Clin North Am 1986; 33:111.

Bacterial Infections

Gerdes JS: Clinicopathologic approach to the diagnosis of neonatal sepsis. Clin Perinatol 1991;18:361.

Klein JO: Current antibacterial therapy for neonatal sepsis and meningitis. Pediatr Infect Dis 1990;9:783.

McCracken GH Jr, Frei BJ: Perinatal bacterial diseases. In: Feigin RD, Cherry JD (editors): *Textbook of Pediatric Infectious Diseases.* Saunders, 1987.

Abdominal Mass

Hartman GE, Shochat SJ: Abdominal mass lesions in the newborn: Diagnosis and treatment. Clin Perinatol 1989;16:123.

Koop CE: Abdominal mass in the newborn infant. N Engl J Med 1973;289:569.

Wilson DA: Ultrasound screening for abdominal masses in the neonatal period. Am J Dis Child 1982;136:147.

Seizures

Maytal J et al: Lorazepam in the treatment of refractory neonatal seizures. J Child Neurol 1991;6:319.

Painter MJ, Gaus LM: Neonatal seizures: Diagnosis and treatment. J Child Neurol 1991;6:101.

Volpe JJ: Neonatal seizures: Current concepts and revised classification. Pediatrics 1989;84:422.

DISORDERS OF THE NEWBORN

Apnea

Gerhardt T et al: Effects of aminophylline on respiratory center and reflex activity in premature infants with apnea. Pediatr Res 1983;17:188.

Miller MJ, Martin RJ: Pathophysiology of apnea of prematurity. In: RA Polin, WW Fox (editors): *Neonatal and Fetal Physiology.* Saunders, 1992.

Respiratory Distress Syndrome

Avery ME, Merritt TA: Surfactant replacement therapy. N Engl J Med 1991;324:910.

Hazinski TA: Acute respiratory distress syndromes in the newborn. Page 1597 in: Rudolph AM et al (editors): *Rudolph's Pediatrics,* 20th ed. Appleton & Lange, 1996.

Phibbs RH et al: Initial clinical trial of EXOSURF, a protein-free synthetic surfactant, for the prophylaxis and early treatment of hyaline membrane disease. Pediatrics 1991; 88:1.

Meconium Aspiration Syndrome & Persistent Pulmonary Hypertension of the Newborn

Bartlett RH et al: Extracorporeal circulation in neonatal respiratory failure: A prospective randomized study. Pediatrics 1985;76:479.

Fox WW, Duara S: Persistent pulmonary hypertension in the neonate: Diagnosis and management. J Pediatr 1983; 103:505.

Gregory GA et al: Meconium aspiration in neonates: A prospective study. J Pediatr 1974;85:848.

Wiswell TE, Henley MA: Intratracheal suctioning, systemic infection, and the meconium aspiration syndrome. Pediatrics 1992;89:203.

Perinatal Asphyxia & Resuscitation

Gregory GA: Resuscitation of the newborn. Page 237 in: Rudolph AM et al (editors): *Rudolph's Pediatrics,* 20th ed. Appleton & Lange, 1996.

Jacobs MM, Phibbs RH: Prevention, recognition and treatment of perinatal asphyxia in critical issues in intrapartum and delivery room management. Clin Perinatol 1989;16: 785.

Neonatal Cardiopulmonary Resuscitation Manual. American Heart Association, American Academy of Pediatrics, 1989.

Polycythemia

Black V et al: Developmental and neurologic sequelae of neonatal hyperviscosity syndrome. Pediatrics 1982;69:426.

Hathaway WE: Neonatal hyperviscosity. Pediatrics 1983;72: 567.

Kurlat I, Sola A: Risk of neonatal polycythemia in infants of hypertensive mothers. Acta Paediatr 1992;81:662.

Wiswell TE et al: Neonatal polycythemia: Frequency of clinical manifestations and other associated findings. Pediatrics 1986;78:26.

Congenital Infections

Alford CA et al: Congenital and perinatal cytomegalovirus infections. Rev Infect Dis 1990;12:S745.

Alpert G, Plotkin SA: A practical guide to the diagnosis of congenital infections in the newborn infant. Pediatr Clin N Am 1986;33:465.

Freij BJ et al: Maternal rubella and the congenital rubella syndrome. Clin Perinatol 1988;15:247.

Perlman JM, Argyle C: Lethal cytomegalovirus infection in preterm infants: Clinical, radiological, and neuropathological findings. Ann Neurol 1992;31:64.

Sever JL et al: Toxoplasmosis: Maternal and pediatric findings in 23,000 pregnancies. Pediatrics 1988;82:181.

Toltzis P: Current issues in neonatal herpes simplex virus infection. Clin Perinatol 1991;18:193.

Birth Trauma

Boome RS, Kaye JC: Obstetric traction injuries of the bracheal plexus. Natural history, indications for surgical repair and results. J Bone Joint Surg [Br] 1988;70:571.

Mangurten HH: Birth injuries. In: Fanaroff AA, Martin RJ (editors): *Neonatal Perinatal Medicine: Diseases of the Fetus and Infant,* 5th ed. Mosby-Year Book, 1992.

Intracranial Hemorrhage

Guzzetta F et al: Periventricular intraparenchymal echodensities in the premature newborn: Critical determinant of neurological outcome. Pediatrics 1986;78:995.

Papile L et al: Relationship of cerebral intraventricular hemorrhage and early childhood neurologic handicaps. J Pediatr 1983;103:273.

Volpe JJ: Intraventricular hemorrhage in the premature infant—current concepts. Part I. Ann Neurol 1989;25:3.

Volpe JJ: Intraventricular hemorrhage in the premature infant—current concepts. Part II. Ann Neurol 1989;25:109.

Infants of Drug-Abusing Mothers

Committee on Drugs, American Academy of Pediatrics: Neonatal drug withdrawal. Pediatrics 1983;82:895.

Hoegerman G et al: Drug-exposed neonates. Addiction Medicine (special issue). West J Med 1990;152:559.

Khalsa JH, Gfroerer J: Epidemiology and health care consequences of drug abuse among pregnant women. Semin Perinatol 1991;15:265.

Ostrea EM Jr, Welch RA: Detection of prenatal drug exposure in the pregnant woman and her newborn infant. Clin Perinatol 1991;18:629.

Necrotizing Enterocolitis

Bell MJ, Temberg JL et al: Neonatal necrotizing enterocolitis. Therapeutic decisions based upon clinical staging. Ann Surg 1978;187:10.

Kleinhaus S et al: Necrotizing enterocolitis in infancy. Surg Clin North Am 1991;72:261.

Uauy RD et al: Necrotizing enterocolitis in very low birth weight infants: Biodemographic and clinical correlates. National Institute of Child Health and Human Development Neonatal Research Network. J Pediatr 1991;119:630.

Thoracic & Gastrointestinal Neonatal Surgical Conditions

Hazebroek F et al: Congenital diaphragmatic hernia, impact of preoperative stabilization. J Pediatr Surg 1988;12:1138.

Meller JL et al: Gastroschisis and omphalocele. Clin Perinatol 1989;16:113.

Reyes H et al: Management of esophageal atresia and tracheoesophageal fistula. Clin Perinatol 1989;16:79.

Frequent Electrolyte & Metabolic Abnormalities

Costarino A, Baumgart S: Modern fluid and electrolyte management of the critically ill premature infant. Pediatr Clin North Am 1986;33:153.

Loughead J et al: Serum ionized calcium concentrations in normal neonates. Am J Dis Child 1988;142:516.

Ogata ES: Carbohydrate metabolism in the fetus and neonate and altered neonatal glucoregulation. Pediatr Clin North Am 1986;33:25.

Schaffer SG, Weismann DN: Fluid requirements in the preterm infant. Clin Perinatol 1992;19:233.

5

An Approach to Clinical Genetics

Cynthia R. Curry, MD

Clinical genetics is a rapidly expanding field that is broad in its scope and diversity and has wide applicability to both health and disease in pediatrics. From the principles of human heredity set forth by Gregor Mendel in 1865, which went unrecognized for several decades, to the current intense scientific efforts to map the entire human genome by the beginning of the 21st century, we have witnessed the growing impact of genetics on all fields of medicine. Nowhere is this more important than in pediatrics, as fully one third of hospitalized children are admitted as the consequence of genetic disease. With attention focused on the prenatal status of the fetus, and on causes of its death before birth, the fetus also has become a patient. As our technologic capabilities increase, we are aware of the many ethical and practical issues surrounding screening for prenatal, newborn, and childhood inherited disorders. We recognize the importance of accurate determination of risks and recurrence risks for children and their parents. In the following section, a categoric approach to genetic disease is presented with an emphasis on disorders likely to be encountered in pediatrics.

ELEMENTS OF THE GENETIC EVALUATION

A genetic evaluation consists of three principal elements:

1. Determination of the correct diagnosis
2. Estimation of risk
3. Supportive counseling that allows the family to use the information provided.

THE PEDIGREE

The first step in the collection of appropriate information is the construction of a family tree or pedigree. Underused by most medical personnel, the pedigree is a valuable record of genetic and medical information, which is much more useful in visual form than in list form. The use of uniform symbols is helpful, and common ones are denoted in Figure 5–1. An example of a family pedigree is shown in Figure 5–2.

Tips for pedigree preparation include the following:

- Start in the middle of the page to allow enough room for expansion. Start with a proband—his or her siblings and parents. The proband is the individual(s) through which the family genetic history was ascertained and should always be indicated by an arrow. Concentrate on one side of the family at a time to avoid confusing yourself and the person providing the history.

- Inquire about miscarriages, stillbirths, and neonatal deaths. This is frequently overlooked and may provide crucial information.

- Always ask about consanguinity. Sometimes the question "Are you (the parents) related by blood?" will result in laughter but yields often potentially useful clues suggesting autosomal-recessive inheritance. Families with multiple marriages or consanguinity can complicate pedigree preparation, but understanding these pedigrees is still simpler and visually clearer than trying to explain the situation in words.

- Even if the disease in question appears to be coming from one side of the family, always get the basic facts about the other side of the family as well. Sometimes unrelated data may be very important in interpreting the family's overall situation. In addition, obtaining data from both sides may avoid an inference of blame being placed on one family member.

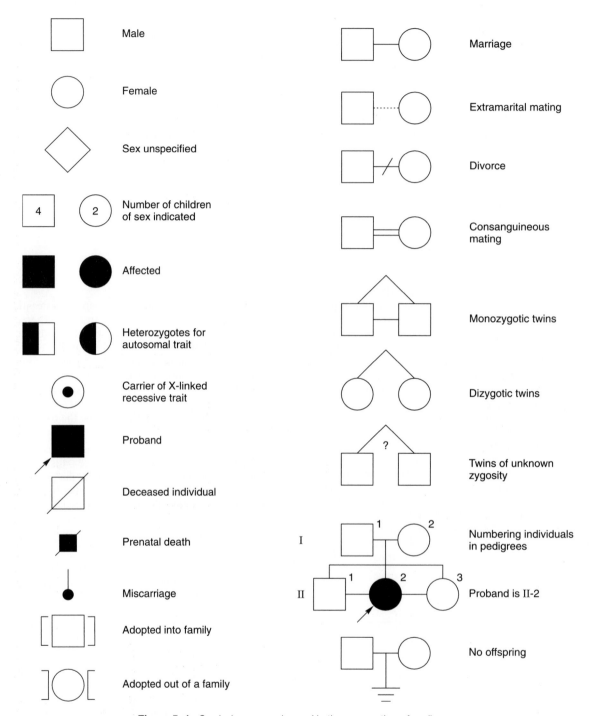

Figure 5–1. Symbols commonly used in the preparation of pedigrees.

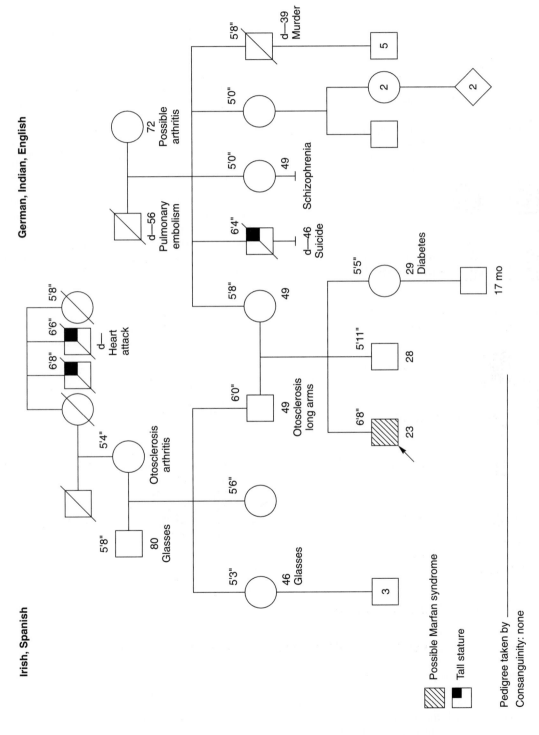

Figure 5–2. Pedigree chart of a family in which the proband (indicated with **arrow**) is being evaluated for possible Marfan syndrome. d = deceased.

- Obtain the maiden names of women in the family, particularly when investigating an X-linked pedigree.

- Ascertain the ages of living persons and dates of death for deceased family members.

- Place the name of the person obtaining the pedigree and the date recorded at the bottom of the sheet.

THE DIAGNOSTIC PROCESS

The diagnostic process may be complex and is somewhat different from that used with general pediatric problems. When an infant or child is the proband, obtaining a complete prenatal and perinatal history, as well as information regarding developmental milestones, is an important part of the medical history. Special attention needs to be placed on elements of the prenatal history, such as maternal illnesses, onset and quality of fetal movements, presence of oligohydramnios or polyhydramnios, fetal presentation (vertex versus breech), and ultrasound abnormalities in the pregnancy. Licit or illicit drug use, as well as alcohol and tobacco use, should be queried. In dealing with the family with a disorder such as Duchenne muscular dystrophy or adult-type polycystic kidney disease, it may be difficult to verify the exact diagnosis. The individuals of interest may be long since deceased or may have died without appropriate investigation. In this case, medical records should be requested whenever possible. Even in living affected individuals, a diagnosis can be difficult. For biochemical and DNA studies, pictures, radiographs, and samples of urine and blood, for example, can sometimes be obtained and shipped for evaluation or analysis to appropriate reference laboratories even when relevant family members live far from the evaluation site.

A complete genetic evaluation emphasizes components beyond the routine pediatric physical examination. Key elements include the following:

1. Growth parameters (height, weight, and head circumference) need to be plotted on the appropriate growth curves and, if possible, compared with earlier parameters.
2. Features that can be measured should be measured! There are established standards for inner canthal distance, interpupillary distance, ear length, hand length, middle finger length, foot length, penis length, etc.
3. The child's features should be compared with those of parents and siblings (use photographs if available).
4. The child's features should be analyzed over time by examining earlier chronologic photographs.
5. Clues should be sought that help date the onset of the problem, eg, altered palmar and phalangeal creases (see below).

APPROACH TO THE CHILD WITH STRUCTURAL DEFECTS

When confronted by a child with either single or multiple birth defects, the physician may be perplexed and unsure how to proceed. The diagnostic process, however, is not mysterious, and a correct diagnosis can usually be made by observing the patient's findings carefully and knowing where to look for additional information.

The first step in the diagnostic process is to determine the type of problem in morphogenesis. Is it an error in embryogenesis (ie, a malformation)? Is it a **deformation,** in which extrinsic forces have altered previously normally formed body parts? Is it a **disruption,** in which a normal fetus has been altered by a destructive process that may be mechanical, infectious, or vascular in etiology? Is the problem prenatal or postnatal in origin? Is there a single localized defect in morphogenesis or are there secondary anomalies? When a single error causes a cascade of subsequent defects, the pattern is known as a **sequence** (see Figure 5–3). Patients with multiple structural defects that cannot be explained on the basis of a cascade of events (sequence) are said to have a **malformation syndrome.** Usually such patterns are secondary to single causes, such as chromosomal abnormalities, single congenital defects, or teratogens. Many syndromes, however, have no known cause. Examples of malformations, deformations, disruptions, and syndromes are given in Table 5–1. By using these descriptors, pediatricians can categorize most structural defects.

Minor malformations are found in less than 4% of the normal population and are usually of no cosmetic or functional importance to the individual. Examples of minor congenital anomalies are presented in Table 5–2. Despite their lack of significance by themselves, the pattern of such abnormalities may be crucial in the recognition of specific syndromes. Many important syndromes with major functional significance for the individual involved are recognized primarily by their distinctive pattern of minor anomalies. For example, most of the features seen on physical examination in Down syndrome, Williams syndrome, and Smith-Lemli-Opitz syndrome are minor anomalies. In general, minor anomalies in an otherwise normal child are probably not significant and do not warrant further investigations, but when the anomaly is one of several or when there are growth or developmental problems, further studies are usually indicated.

It is important to be familiar with several principles and concepts that are useful in evaluating the child with birth defects. A discussion of these follows.

Concept of Variability

Structural defects and their associated patterns are highly variable among individuals who have the same condition. Within a given syndrome, it is rare to find a specific feature in 100% of affected patients. In Down syndrome, for example, mental retardation is seen in all patients, and hypotonia is very frequent; however, other

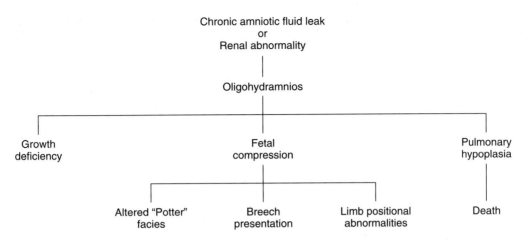

Figure 5–3. A sequence is a cascade of events with a single initiating problem, as exemplified by the condition of oligohydramnios.

specific features, such as Brushfield spots and redundant neck skin, are seen in fewer than 80% of these patients. The diagnosis is based on the overall pattern of abnormality. In addition, some patients with the same condition are severely affected, whereas others are very mildly affected, and the condition is therefore sometimes difficult to recognize. This is particularly true with teratogenically induced syndromes, such as fetal alcohol syndrome, in which the effects may range from neonatal death to mild neurologic dysfunction without physical stigmata.

Concept of Changing Phenotype

The presentation of specific conditions and syndromes may change with time, and the diagnosis may be relatively easy or more difficult to determine as the child ages. For example, in mucopolysaccharidosis, facial coarsening and organomegaly are progressive with time. In Noonan syndrome, the face changes rather dramatically in infancy through middle childhood and into adulthood. In Beckwith-Wiedemann syndrome, the condition of an infant who has been severely affected may appear normal by the time he or she reaches middle childhood.

Concept of Heterogeneity

Similar clinical phenotypes may result from different etiologies. This is obviously very important in terms of diagnosis, prognosis, and recurrence risk counseling. For example, the phenotype of Noonan syndrome can be caused by an autosomal-dominant gene or by exposure to alcohol or phenytoin. A Marfan-like phenotype can be seen not only with true Marfan syndrome, which is autosomal dominant, but also with homocystinuria, which is autosomal recessive. A similar Marfanoid phenotype may also be seen in some X-linked syndromes. The history and overall pattern of abnormalities need to be carefully considered before rendering a specific diagnosis.

Concept of Most Obvious Versus the Most Frequent Abnormalities

Certain syndromes are distinguishable by their striking features, but if one relies only on these features, most patients with the syndrome will be missed. For example, the white forelock and heterochromia of Waardenburg syndrome are distinctive but not nearly as common as lateral displacement of the inner canthi and hypoplastic alae nasi. Similarly, although cleft lip and palate and scalp defects are easily recognizable features of trisomy 13, they are much less common than the characteristic nose that is nearly always present.

Concept of Dating the Onset

Frequently, a specific diagnosis may not be possible. It is not rare for the child's problems to be ascribed to some perinatal event. Attempts should be made to date the onset

Table 5–1. Examples of structural defects caused by different mechanisms.

Malformations	Deformations	Disruptions	Syndromes
Cleft lip and cleft palate	Plagiocephaly	Amniotic bands	Down
Transposition of great vessels	Torticollis	Jejunal atresia	Cornelia de Lange
Polydactyly	Limb bowing	Congenital rubella	Williams
Anencephaly	Prune belly	Unilateral limb reduction defects (some)	Noonan
Omphalocele	Scoliosis (some)	Gastroschisis	Fetal alcohol
Renal agenesis			

Table 5–2. Minor malformations.

Darwinian tubercle	Preauricular pits
Double occipital hair whorls	Single umbilical artery
Flat nasal bridge	Supernumerary nipples
Micrognathia	Syndactyly: two to three toes
Nevus flammeus	Transverse palmar crease

as prenatal, perinatal, or postnatal. For example, abnormalities in hair patterning date from approximately the 10th to 15th week of fetal life. Similarly, palmar crease and dermal ridges form between the 13th and 19th fetal week and, if significantly altered and not present in other family members, offer valuable clues as to the timing of the insult affecting the child. Problems occurring after 20 weeks' gestation, no matter how severe, will not affect the dermal crease patterns because they are already formed. The presence of a thumb held in the palm (ie, "cortical thumb") may be seen in cases of birth asphyxia, but when thumb positioning is prenatal in origin, a web of skin will have formed and the thumb may be hypoplastic. This type of observation may be particularly important in the current legal climate, in which families may seek compensation for their damaged child by blaming events around the time of the delivery. Metabolic errors may occasionally present with structural defects, but children with inborn errors usually appear normal at birth with only gradual development of a specific phenotype. Examination of serial photographs may be particularly useful in documenting that facial changes are postnatal.

Concept of Using Rarest Feature for Quick Identification

Common functional abnormalities, such as short stature and mental retardation, are seen in a vast array of conditions and syndromes and thus are almost diagnostically useless. Features that are uncommon or rare are much more likely to lead to the correct diagnosis. The appendices in *Smith's Recognizable Patterns of Human Malformation* (1988) are useful. The rarer the finding, the more likely this resource is to be helpful. For example, the findings of scalp defects, lens dislocation, or choanal atresia yield relatively short lists of possible diagnoses. The same principle holds true when using any of the diagnostic computer programs in common use today. Research on computer-aided diagnoses in the field of malformation syndromes began in the 1980s and was at first restricted to relatively few users. More recent versions have brought these facilities to a broad audience. The programs most widely in use include OMIM (McKusick's Catalogue of Mendelian Inheritance in Man, on-line: http://www3.ncbi.nlm.nih.gov/omim/), the London Dysmorphology Database (LDD), pictures of standard syndromes and undiagnosed malformations (POSSUM), and SYNDROC. Because of the proliferation of syndromes, computer-as-

sisted diagnosis has been welcomed by clinical geneticists as an extremely valuable reference. Attempts are being made to evaluate the utility of these computer programs in clinical practice. Even with the computer programs, the concept that the rarer the abnormality the more likely one is to make a diagnosis remains unchanged. Unfortunately, this means that for the patient with mental retardation, short stature, and a flat nasal bridge as the only identifiable features, a specific diagnosis may be unlikely unless laboratory testing provides additional clues.

THE COUNSELING PROCESS

After the initial pedigree preparation and review of the history and physical examination, it is often necessary to obtain additional records or to order specific tests. Indicated testing may frequently include cytogenetic studies (ie, chromosomes), skeletal radiographs, and urine or serum biochemical studies (ie, organic acids, lysosomal enzymes, etc). During the initial visit, it is important to indicate to the family how long it may take to obtain a diagnosis, how many visits may be needed, and how likely it is that a diagnosis will actually be established. It is also important to relieve guilt at this initial meeting, even though no diagnosis may yet be apparent. Parental anxiety is usually great, and almost all parents fear that something they have done, either real or imagined, has caused the child's problems. Only rarely is this true. In clear-cut situations, counseling and recurrence risk information can be given at the initial visit; even in these situations, however, parents may be overwhelmed and require a second visit. Usually during a second visit, issues of recurrence risk need to be dealt with as objectively as possible. In addition, information on modalities that may be available to help them monitor for, or modify, these risks should be discussed. In the initial and subsequent visits, it is important to determine how the family perceives their child (ie, do they love and accept him or her, or is the child an intolerable burden?). It is important to understand how the family will view the concept of risk. For some families, risks are best presented as either high or low. For others, detailed explanations, including derivation of empiric risks, is appropriate. Usually, risks are given as odds or percentages. Some counselors quote odds, such as 1:10, 1:50, 1:100, whereas others use figures, such as 10%, 2%, or 1%. Sometimes these methods are used interchangeably and adapted to the requirements of the individual family.

In conveying the risk information, certain points need to be kept in mind:

- It is important to emphasize that "chance has no memory." Odds refer to future occurrence, not to past occurrence. For example, when there is a 1:4 chance of recurrence, the fact that the first child was normal does not guarantee that the next three will be normal, nor does the fact that one family has had two affected children in a row make it more or less likely that the next will be affected.

- Parents may reverse the risks in their head when told that they have a 2% chance of recurrence risk and may interpret this as a 2% chance of having a normal child.

- Each family has its own idea of what constitutes a high or low risk, and the interpretation of risk often has more to do with the disease in question than the actual risk. For example, parents may readily accept a 3% chance for recurrence for cleft lip and cleft palate, whereas the same risk for having a child with mental handicap and some associated physical abnormalities may be viewed as intolerable.

- The baseline risk for congenital anomalies facing any couple needs to be stressed and spelled out for the parents.

- It is important that genetic counseling information be given in a nondirective manner.

Although physicians may think that they know what is best for the patient, this is usually not the case. The physician's role is to ensure that families have the facts that will permit them to make their own decisions. These include a knowledge of the disorder, the genetic risks involved, and the possible steps that can be taken to ameliorate the condition or detect it in utero. Although some patients may beg for advice, and in these instances it may often be tempting to comply, it is almost always inadvisable. Certainly, there are genetic counselors whose orientation toward genetic risks is either more positive or more negative. For example, some may tend to stress the 25% chance of recurrence, whereas others may stress the 75% chance that the child will be normal. Usually, the approach is tempered by the counselor's knowledge of the disease in question. In the end, however, it is important that parents and individuals make their own decisions and understand that there is no right or wrong answer. Moreover, support should continue to be offered to families regardless of their decisions regarding future childbearing.

Part of the process of a genetic evaluation involves referral of the child and family to appropriate agencies for follow-up treatment or support. Consequently, geneticists often find themselves in the role of care coordinators. Follow-up contact with families is almost always necessary because the stress of receiving prognostic and genetic information often renders recall difficult or impossible. When new information becomes available, such as a specific molecular diagnostic test, it is important to call the family back to discuss these findings. Options such as adoption, sterilization, and artificial insemination by a donor need to be discussed when appropriate. Families should be asked to contact the genetic counselor should they again become pregnant because new information may drastically alter pregnancy monitoring.

MENDELIAN INHERITANCE PATTERNS & COMMON PEDIATRIC DISORDERS

As of January 1996, Victor McKusick's catalog, *Mendelian Inheritance in Man* listed more than 6500 entries in which the mode of inheritance is presumed to be autosomal dominant, autosomal recessive, X-linked dominant, or X-linked recessive. These disorders are caused by single genes, determined by a single allele at a single locus on one chromosome or a pair of chromosomes. When both alleles in a pair are identical, the individual is **homozygous.** When the alleles differ at the same locus, the individual is **heterozygous.** The inheritance pattern is usually diagnosed by (1) recognition of the condition and knowledge of its mode of inheritance and (2) analysis of the pedigree and the pattern of transmission in the family. When the case is "isolated" and no diagnosis is apparent, several possibilities need to be considered (Figure 5–4). When more than one family member is affected, the pedigree can be analyzed and decisions made regarding the likely mode of inheritance. This process is outlined in Figure 5–5.

AUTOSOMAL-DOMINANT INHERITANCE

Disorders showing autosomal-dominant inheritance generally are expressed when only one gene in the pair is altered (ie, the individual is heterozygous). Homozygous states of autosomal-dominant disorders are rare and usually severe or lethal (ie, homozygous achondroplasia). Rarely, homozygosity may be indistinguishable from heterozygosity (eg, Huntington disease). In typical autosomal-dominant disorders, counseling is straightforward (Figure 5–6). The risk for affected individuals' offspring is one half or 50/50, regardless of sex. However, risks alone do not tell the whole story in autosomal-dominant disorders. Several factors may modify the clinical presentation; these include the following:

Age of Onset. Certain important genetic diseases, such as adult-type polycystic kidney disease and Huntington disease, do not usually manifest until later in life. Thus, individuals have often passed their reproductive years before they become aware that they have the disease. Molecular diagnostic methods may be able to give information early in life, or even prenatally, but the ethical issues raised by presymptomatic testing are serious and must be approached with caution.

Lack of Penetrance. Some dominantly inherited disorders may show absolutely no evidence of the disorder by conventional clinical tools, yet clearly the patient must have the gene if he or she has an affected parent and transmitted the disorder to an offspring. Occasionally, a disor-

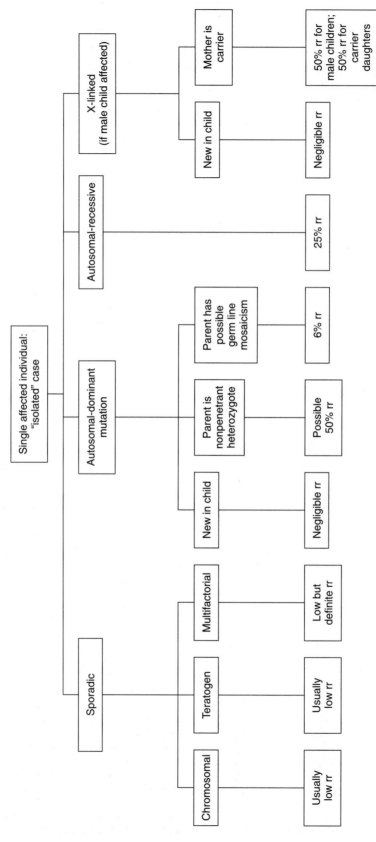

Figure 5–4. Recurrence risks (rr) for parents of a child who is the only affected family member.

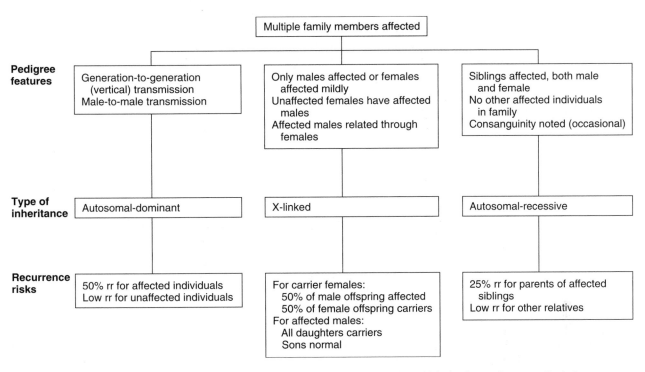

Figure 5–5. Possible modes of inheritance and recurrence risks (rr) when multiple family members are affected.

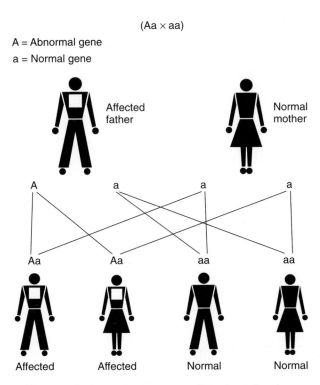

Figure 5–6. Counseling in autosomal-dominant disorders.

der can be found to be penetrant if one looks carefully with biochemical or radiologic studies. For example, adult-type polycystic kidney disease may appear to be nonpenetrant on the basis of clinical examination, but a renal ultrasound study may reveal renal cysts indicating the presence of the gene. In some situations, specific molecular testing may allow determination of the presence or absence of the gene, thus defining penetrance at a different level.

Variability. Dominant disorders are characterized by marked variability, and this factor has to be taken into account both when the physician assesses an individual for the presence or absence of the condition and when the physician wants to provide accurate genetic counseling. For example, an individual with tuberous sclerosis who has seizures, ash leaf spots, and mental retardation is unlikely to be missed. An intellectually normal parent may be erroneously assumed to be unaffected yet careful ophthalmologic, dermatologic, and radiologic studies may reveal subtle evidences of the gene's presence (eg, renal hematomas or subtle skin changes such as ash leaf spots, adenoma sebaceum, or a shagreen patch). Individuals who are mildly affected are much more likely to reproduce. Their chances of having a moderately or severely affected child need to be explored in the counseling setting, and the entire spectrum of the disorder explained. Because more than half the listings in McKusick's catalog are autosomal dominant in etiology, it is not possible to discuss these disorders in detail. Table 5–3 presents information on some of the more common autosomal-dominant disorders. Table 5–4 lists some malformation syndromes displaying autosomal-dominant inheritance.

AUTOSOMAL-RECESSIVE INHERITANCE

Autosomal-recessive phenotypes account for about one third of mendelian disorders. They occur when both parents are heterozygous carriers. Each parent passes either a normal or an altered gene to the child who is affected in 25% of conceptions. Consanguinity increases the risk for autosomal recessive disorders, as does reproduction among genetically isolated populations, particularly for rare recessive disorders such as Tay-Sachs disease. In an individual family, it may be difficult to determine whether a condition is autosomal recessive because often the affected children are the only ones in their families with the disorder. When the diagnosis is definite, counseling is relatively clear-cut (Figure 5–7). The recurrence risk for each sibling of the proband is 25%, or one in four. Both male and female siblings are equally affected. Recurrence risks for other relatives are very low. When one's sibling is affected with an autosomal-recessive disorder, the risk of being a carrier is two thirds. In contrast to autosomal-

Table 5–4. Clinical features in several common malformation syndromes with autosomal-dominant inheritance.

Syndrome	Primary Features
Stickler	Marfanoid habitus, myopia, cleft palate, arthritis
Noonan (some cases)	Short stature, ptosis, pulmonary valve stenosis, learning disabilities
Nail-patella	Absent patellas, nail dysplasia, renal disease
Treacher Collins	Downslanting palpebral fissures, ear malformations, malar hypoplasia, lid colobomas
Holt-Oram	Cardiac defects, radial defects
Waardenburg	Increased inner canthal distance, heterochromia, white forelock, congenital hearing loss
Van der Woude	Cleft lip ± cleft palate; lip pits

dominant disorders, many recessive disorders involve aberrant enzyme activities that block pathways crucial to normal metabolic function. Important autosomal-recessive disorders in pediatrics are listed in Table 5–5. Syndromes that are inherited in an autosomal-recessive fashion are probably also caused by alterations in basic regulatory or metabolic pathways even though the exact cause in many of these syndromes is not known (Table 5–6). Autosomal-

Table 5–3. Clinical features in several common diseases with autosomal-dominant inheritance.

Disease	Gene Localization	Disease Incidence	Clinical Features	Prenatal Diagnosis
Neurofibromatosis type I	17q11.2	1:3000–5000 (many cases are new mutations)	Café-au-lait spots, neurofibromas; malignancy (5%); mental retardation (5%); learning disabilities (15%)	Possible in some families using linked DNA markers
Myotonic dystrophy	19q13	New mutations rare	Muscular weakness: myotonia onset childhood → adult. Endocrine abnormalities; cardiac conduction defects; cataracts. Congenital presentation: hypotonia, clubfeet, respiratory problems	Possible with DNA technologies
Familial hypercholesterolemia	19q13	Heterozygotes 1:500 Homozygotes 1:1,000,000	Elevated LDL, xanthomas, early coronary artery disease, homozygotes; death due to coronary disease in childhood	? DNA technologies
Tuberous sclerosis	9q 16p	High mutation rate	Hypopigmented skin macules; seizures; mental retardation; renal, cardiac, and CNS hamartomas	DNA techniques in appropriate families
Huntington disease	4p16	4–8:100,000 (new mutations rare)	Dementia; chorea; usually onset in 5th decade	Possible using linked DNA markers
Marfan syndrome	15q	1–2:100,000 (new mutations 15–30%)	Tall stature, arachnodactyly; lens dislocation; aortic root dilatation, mitral valve prolapse	Possible in future using DNA markers

CNS = central nervous system; LDL = low-density lipoprotein.

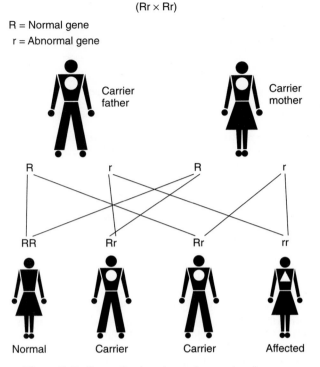

(Rr × Rr)

R = Normal gene
r = Abnormal gene

Carrier father

Carrier mother

R   r   R   r

RR   Rr   Rr   rr

Normal   Carrier   Carrier   Affected

Figure 5–7. Counseling in autosomal-recessive diseases.

recessive metabolic disorders with known abnormalities in mucopolysaccharide, amino acid, or organic acid metabolism are discussed in Chapter 6.

X-LINKED INHERITANCE

More than 300 genes have been mapped to the X chromosome. X-linked mutations are fully expressed in male carriers. Female carriers are functionally mosaic, with two cell populations—one carrying the normal X chromosome and the other carrying the altered X chromosome. This characteristic is due to X inactivation that occurs randomly early in embryonic development. As a result of X inactivation, both male and female carriers have only one X chromosome active in each cell. X inactivation is random and, therefore, by chance female carriers may have more of their normal X chromosomes inactivated and display some symptoms of an X-linked disorder, either clinically or biochemically.

In general, X-linked–recessive disorders affect men more than women. An affected man will transmit the gene to all of his daughters and none of his sons. Affected men in a family are related through women in the family. Male-to-male transmission never occurs. Female carriers are usually asymptomatic, but, as discussed, some may have mild symptoms of the disorder. The approach to counseling is diagrammed in Figure 5–8.

X-linked–dominant disorders are regularly expressed in females, although the distinction between X-linked–dominant and X-linked–recessive disorders blurs as our ability to detect manifestations in female carriers improve. Pedigrees of X-linked–dominant disorders demonstrate that affected men have daughters who are affected and sons who are never affected. This feature distinguishes

Table 5–5. Clinical features in several diseases with autosomal-recessive inheritance.

Disease	Gene Localization	Incidence	Clinical Features	Prenatal Diagnosis
Cystic fibrosis	7q31; single mutation in 70% (Δ F508)	1:2000 in whites	Pulmonary disease; pancreatic insufficiency	Yes: DNA
Tay-Sachs disease	15q23–q24	1:3600 in Ashkenazi Jewish populations; rare in other populations	Severe mental retardation and CNS deterioration; death by age 2–3 y	Yes: enzyme analysis (hexosaminidase A) or DNA
Sickle cell anemia	11p	1:400–600 African-Americans	Severe hemolytic anemia; splenomegaly; infections	Yes: DNA
α-Thalassemia	16p13.3	1:1600 Southeast Asians; frequent in descendents of Mediterranean countries, the Philippines	Deletion of all four alpha chains; hydrops fetalis (death) Three gene deletions: hemoglobin H disease Two gene deletions: silent carrier	Yes: DNA
Werdnig-Hoffmann disease	5q12–q13	1:10,000	Severe hypotonia; anterior horn cell disease; death by age 1–2 y Some forms have later onset and slower progression	Yes: DNA

CNS = central nervous system.

Table 5–6. Clinical features in selected malformation syndromes with autosomal-recessive inheritance.

Syndrome	Clinical Findings	Clinical Outcome	Prenatal Diagnosis
Zellweger	Deficiency of peroxisomes, hypotonia, hepatomegaly, stippled epiphyses, hydrocephalus	Lethal by 1–4 mo	Yes: analysis of amniotic fluid; very long chain fatty acids in amniotic fluid; ultrasound
Meckel-Gruber	Encephalocele, polydactyly, polycystic kidneys, congenital heart disease	Lethal soon after birth	Yes: ultrasound and α-fetoprotein in amniotic fluid
Ellis–van Creveld	Short limbs, natal teeth, congenital heart disease, polydactyly	About 50% die in infancy	Yes: ultrasound second trimester
Smith-Lemli-Opitz	Mental retardation, two- to three-toe syndactyly, genital abnormalities, polydactyly, cleft palate	Some neonatal deaths; some long-term survivors	Yes: dehydrocholesterol levels in amniotic fluid
Seckel	"Bird-headed" dwarfism; primordial short stature, severe microcephaly	Survival	Yes: No good data. Ultrasound third trimester
Ataxia-telangiectasia	Ataxia, immune deficiency, elevated risk for lymphoreticular malignancy, chromosome breakage	Death in 20s–30s, usually secondary to malignancy	Yes: chromosome breakage analysis in amniotic fluid or fetal blood

X-linked–dominant inheritance from autosomal-dominant inheritance. Women with X-linked–dominant disorders will transmit the trait to half their offspring regardless of sex. X-linked–dominant disorders are rare. One example is X-linked hypophosphatemic rickets. Although classified as a dominant disorder, the rickets is much less severe

in female than male offspring. There are several examples of probable X-linked–dominants that are lethal in male offspring. An example is ornithine transcarbamylase (OTC) deficiency, which leads to lethal hyperammonemia in affected male offspring. Female carriers may show protein intolerance and episodes of lethargy and may occasionally present with a Reye syndrome–like picture. Rett syndrome, characterized by severe mental retardation and seizures, is seen only in female children and is thought to be the result of a new mutation occurring only in the affected child. Another syndrome affecting only female children is Aicardi syndrome, in which there is absence of the corpus callosum, severe seizures, hemivertebrae, and unusual lacunar-like defects in the retina. Several important X-linked disorders are presented in Table 5–7.

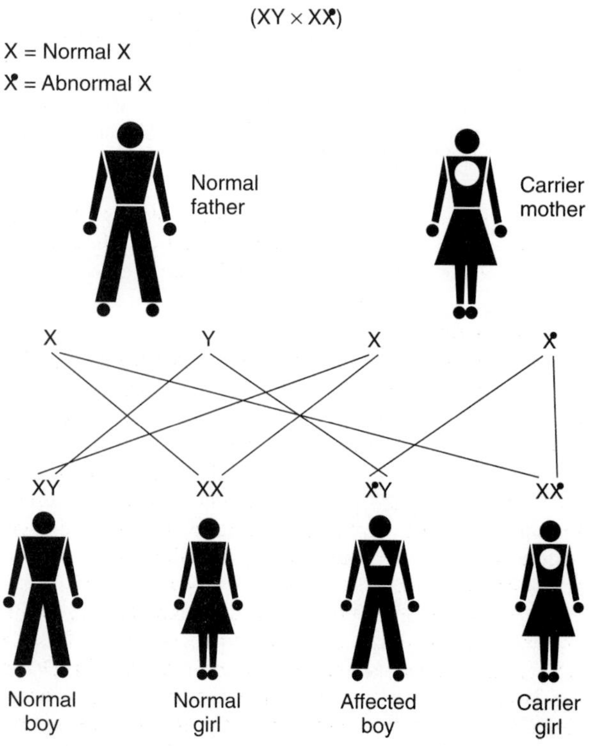

$(XY \times X\textbf{X})$

X = Normal X
X = Abnormal X

Figure 5–8. Counseling in X-linked recessive disorders.

CHROMOSOMAL ABNORMALITIES

Chromosomal disorders form a very important category of genetic disease and are responsible for a high percentage of pregnancy loss and congenital malformations and mental retardation in surviving children. Whereas approximately 60% of first trimester pregnancy losses are secondary to chromosomal imbalance, only about 0.6% of liveborn children have chromosomal abnormalities.

Advances in cytogenetic technology have blurred to some extent the distinctions between mendelian and chromosomal disorders, and this trend is likely to continue. In fact, some malformation syndromes previously thought to be due to an inherited single gene have now been found to be secondary to loss of cytogenetically detectable chromosomal material. Conversely, molecular geneticists have

Table 5–7. Clinical features in several important X-linked disorders.

Disease	Gene Localization	Incidence	Clinical Findings	Prenatal Diagnosis
Hemophilia A	Xq28 (large gene; many mutations)	1:10,000 male carriers (rare in female carriers)	Prolonged bleeding; bruising; joint and muscle hemorrhages; deficiency of factor VIII	Yes: DNA
Duchenne muscular dystrophy	Xp21 (large gene; many mutations)	1:3000–3500 (one third are new mutations; two thirds have carrier mothers)	Progressive muscle weakness; calf pseudohypertrophy; elevated CPK; death in teens to 20s; absent protein; dystrophin in muscle	Yes: in most cases using DNA
Becker muscular dystrophy	Xp21 (gene allelic to Duchenne dystrophy)	Rare	Milder course, but similar to Duchenne dystrophy; survival to middle age; elevated CPK	Yes: DNA
Ocular albinism	Xp21	Rare	Decreased visual acuity, nystagmus, strabismus, iris transillumination defects; female carriers show tigroid mosaic pattern in retina	Yes: DNA, but most families would not use
Lesch-Nyhan syndrome	Xq26–27	Rare	Mental retardation; choreoathetosis; self-destructive biting of fingers and lips; uric acid stones	Yes: enzyme (HPRT) in chorionic villus biopsy, amniocentesis, or preimplantation embryos

CPK = creatine phosphokinase; HPRT = hypoxanthine phosphoribosyl transferase.

now been able to show that some cytogenetically detectable disorders (ie, fragile X syndrome) are secondary to specific patterns of altered DNA.

Chromosomal abnormalities may be numeric or structural and may involve autosomes, sex chromosomes, or both. When there are too many or too few chromosomes, an individual is said to have **aneuploidy.** The most common form of aneuploidy is trisomy, in which there are three instead of the normal two of any one particular chromosome. Monosomy for specific chromosomes is rare, except monosomy X (ie, Turner syndrome). Structural rearrangements account for about 40% of all chromosomal abnormalities, and most of these are balanced (ie, there is no detectable loss or gain of chromosomal material). These rearrangements, however, when transmitted at conception in an unbalanced form, may cause miscarriage, stillbirth, or offspring with abnormal phenotypes and mental retardation. The nomenclature used to describe various chromosomal abnormalities can be confusing.

In general, the following rules are applied when describing a karyotype:

- The total chromosome number is given first, ie, 46.

- The sex chromosome constitution is written next (either XX, female, or XY, male).

- The arms of the chromosomes are indicated by the letters "p" for short arm and "q" for long arm.

- Additional or missing chromosomal material is indicated by a plus or a minus sign (ie, 46,XY,5p– equals

deletion of the short arm of chromosome 5, which is indicative of cri du chat syndrome).

- A translocation is indicated by the letter "t" with a description of the involved chromosomes in brackets (ie, t[13q;14q]).

AUTOSOMAL TRISOMIES

The autosomal chromosome abnormalities of trisomy 21, 18, and 13 are described below, and details are presented in Table 5–8 and depicted in Figure 5–9.

Down Syndrome

As the most common of the autosomal trisomies, this disorder should be familiar to the clinician. This syndrome usually is recognized at birth, although, rarely, diagnosis can be delayed. Hypotonia is universally present, and there are characteristic craniofacial features, including brachycephaly, small ears, upslanting palpebral fissures, Brushfield spots in light-eyed children, flat nasal bridge, underdeveloped midface, and protruding tongue. The hands and feet are usually distinctively broad with transverse palmar creases, fifth finger clinodactyly, and an increased space between the first and second toes. Despite significant intellectual limitations, individuals with Down syndrome are usually happy and productive and, occasionally, can live semi-independently. In addition, antibiotics and cardiac surgery have increased the life span of these individuals. Findings of premature senility charac-

Table 5–8. Clinical features in trisomies 21, 18, and 13.

	Incidence (in live births)	Mean Birth Weight (g)	Prenatal Survival	Life Expectancy	Clinical Features	Chromosome Findings	Recurrence Risk
Trisomy 21	1:800	2900	Spontaneous abortion in 75%	25% with congenital heart disease die before age 1 y (without surgery); 50% live to > 50 y	Hypotonia, typical face, congenital heart disease (40%, AV canal, VSD), IQ 25–50; Alzheimer disease in older patients	Trisomy 21 (95%) Translocation (4%) Mosaicism (1%)	Trisomy: ~ 1% overall Age-specific risk: > 35 years old Translocation: (4;21): maternal 5%, paternal 2%
Trisomy 18	1:8000	2240	Spontaneous abortion in 95%	90% die first month	Hypertonia, typical face, clenched hands with second and fifth overlapping third and fourth fingers, short sternum, nail hypoplasia	Trisomy 18 (> 90%) Translocation (< 5%) Rarely mosaicism	< 1%
Trisomy 13	1:25,000	2600	Spontaneous abortion in most	100% lethal by 6 mo	Severe CNS abnormality; microphthalmia, cleft lip and palate, polydactyly	Trisomy (75%) Unbalanced translocation (20%) Mosaicism (5%)	< 1%

AV = atrioventricular; CNS = central nervous system; VSD = ventricular septal defect.

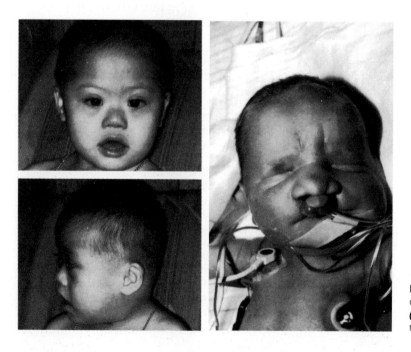

Figure 5–9. Facial appearance in Down syndrome in a Southeast Asian boy, aged 19 months *(upper and lower left)* and trisomy 13 *(right)* in newborns.

teristic of Alzheimer disease affect individuals with Down syndrome much earlier than the typical age of onset of Alzheimer disease in the general population.

Molecular studies of Down syndrome have localized a Down syndrome "critical region" to 21q22.2 to 22.3. Most of the characteristic phenotypic findings are produced by an extra dose of chromosomal material in this region, as exemplified in some patients with partial trisomy 21.

Prenatal diagnostic efforts (chiefly amniocentesis) have been targeted at women older than 35 years who are at an increased risk to have a Down syndrome fetus. Currently, more accurate identification of fetuses at risk through serum marker studies, including α-fetoprotein (AFP), human chorionic gonadotropin (hCG), and unconjugated estriol ("triple screen"), should help identify women of all ages who may be at increased risk to have a child with Down syndrome.

Trisomy 18

Trisomy 18 is much rarer than trisomy 21. It is more frequently identified prenatally on the basis of abnormal ultrasound findings of intrauterine growth retardation and an increased frequency of congenital anomalies, such as omphalocele and esophageal atresia. The characteristic triangular face, small mouth, short sternum, abnormal hand positioning, absent distal flexion creases, and nail hypoplasia aid in the diagnosis of this disorder in the newborn. Infants with this problem are almost always transferred to tertiary care centers because of problems in neonatal adaptation or because of congenital abnormalities. The mortality rate in the first 48 hours is more than 50%. Serum screening of pregnant mothers with triple screening will also detect many fetuses with trisomy 18.

Trisomy 13

Infants with trisomy 13 almost always die in the immediate neonatal period, and the phenotype of such infants tends to be dominated by severe congenital anomalies, including bilateral cleft lip and cleft palate, congenital heart disease, microphthalmia, and central nervous system defects, especially holoprosencephaly. The face of infants with trisomy 13 is notably different from that of infants with trisomy 18. The bulbous nasal tip is particularly distinctive. Other helpful diagnostic findings, when present, may include polydactyly and punched-out scalp defects at the vertex.

AUTOSOMAL DELETIONS

Most autosomal deletions are quite rare or their phenotypes are poorly delineated. An exception is **5p– (cri du chat syndrome).** This condition was given its name because affected infants have a peculiar high-pitched cry similar to that of a mewing cat. The craniofacies is characterized by microcephaly and hypertelorism. Most infants are small at birth, and all exhibit slow postnatal growth and mental deficiency. The distinctive cry becomes less

pronounced with age; thus, this diagnosis is less likely to be made in the older child. The critical deleted region missing in all patients with cri du chat syndrome includes the chromosome band 5p1.5.

SEX CHROMOSOME ABNORMALITIES

Sex chromosomal aneuploidy is relatively common, with an overall frequency of about 1:500 births. These disorders are, in general, less severe than autosomal aneuploidy. The reasons for this are probably related to X chromosome inactivation and to the relatively low number of genes thought to be contained on the Y chromosome. Only XO Turner syndrome is associated with an increased frequency of spontaneous abortion. In this situation, more than 99% of all XO conceptions end in pregnancy loss related to severe fetal hydrops. This is of great interest because the clinical phenotype in surviving XO female infants is relatively mild (Figure 5–10). Nearly all sex chromosome abnormalities tend to occur as isolated events without predisposing factors, although some are related to maternal age and errors in maternal meiosis I.

Turner Syndrome (45,X & Others)

About 50% of girls with Turner syndrome have a 45,X karyotype. The rest have other karyotypes or mosaicism. Approximately 10% of these girls have 46,X,iso(Xq). Mosaic Turner syndrome may have a somewhat milder phenotype, whereas ring X patients have a higher incidence of mental retardation. The characteristic phenotype of Turner syndrome includes short stature, infertility with gonadal dysgenesis or streak gonads, and an increased frequency of renal and cardiac anomalies, especially coarctation of the aorta (20%). There are mildly unusual facial features, with laterally protruding ears, uplifted lobules, and lower canthal folds; neck webbing; and a low posterior hairline. Edema of the hands and feet is often present at birth and may persist into early childhood. Approximately 18% of all chromosomally abnormal spontaneous abortions are found to have a 45,X karyotype.

Short stature and infertility are the constant sequelae of an XO karyotype. Hormonal treatment at puberty will produce adequate feminization and menstruation. However, stature remains a difficult clinical problem, as does infertility. Multiple studies of growth in patients with Turner syndrome have used growth hormone injections and androgens singly and in combination. Results have been inconclusive, although all methods seem to have short-term positive effects on growth velocity. Intellectual function is nearly always normal in Turner syndrome, although spatial relations and perceptual motor organization skills are frequently impaired, lowering the nonverbal IQ.

Klinefelter Syndrome (47,XXY)

Usually this disorder is not diagnosed until puberty, when hypogonadism becomes apparent. Long legs, a thin

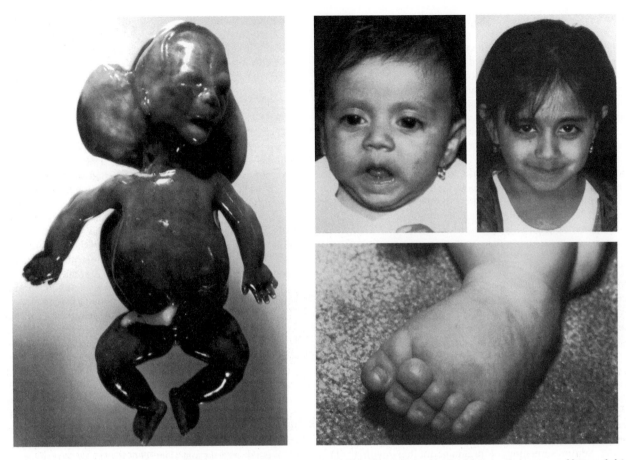

Figure 5–10. XO Turner syndrome. ***Left:*** Fetus that spontaneously aborted at 16 weeks and had a large cystic hygroma. ***Upper right:*** Child with XO Turner syndrome as an infant and at age 6 years. She has a relatively mild phenotype but has had coarctation of the aorta and a horseshoe kidney. Note very mild ptosis and laterally protruding ears. ***Lower right:*** Note the edema of the toes and nail hypoplasia.

habitus, and small testes may cause suspicion of this diagnosis in the prepubertal male. The IQ in Klinefelter syndrome is consistently reduced only mildly, with about two thirds of patients exhibiting learning problems such as dyslexia. Psychosocial adjustment problems are frequent, and infertility is to be expected.

47,XYY

Accurate assessment of the phenotype of XYY has been complicated by the early observation of an increased frequency of XYY individuals in maximum security prisons. Analysis of prospective data suggests that XYY boys are tall and have an increased risk of psychosocial adjustment problems despite intelligence in the low normal range (usually about 15 points below that of normal siblings). Although aggressive behavior and temper tantrums are definitely increased in XYY boys, the exact risk of deviant behavior in the individual identified with XYY either prenatally or in postnatal life is difficult to predict.

XXX (47,XXX)

The phenotype of XXX remains incompletely understood, although there seems to be a significant risk of developmental and learning problems in these individuals. The exact prevalence of mental retardation is not precisely known, but prospective studies have shown that the mean IQ of XXX girls is 10–25 points below that of their normal siblings. Both receptive and expressive language development are delayed. The phenotype of XXX is usually normal, although stature is increased as compared with that of normal siblings. In some instances, the head circumference is reduced. The majority of XXX women are probably fertile, but menstrual abnormalities, sterility, and early-onset menopause have been commonly reported.

MICRODELETION SYNDROMES

High-resolution chromosome banding techniques have greatly increased the ability to reveal abnormalities too small to be seen in ordinary chromosome preparations. These improved techniques have led to delineation of several clinical dysmorphic syndromes. Molecular techniques using fluorescence in situ hybridization (FISH) have further extended our understanding of these syndromes by precise identification of the genes responsible for certain aspects of the clinical phenotype. Evolving molecular information has brought closer to reality correlations between genotype and phenotype. Several examples of microdeletion syndromes are shown in Table 5–9.

Prader-Willi Syndrome & Angelman Syndrome

These two prototype microdeletion syndromes involve chromosomal deletions of bands 15q11 through 15q13. These deletions appear indistinguishable in cytogenetic and FISH studies. At the molecular level, it is likely that Prader-Willi and Angelman syndromes are caused by two closely linked, but distinct, genes or gene clusters. These very different clinical syndromes were the first two human diseases that demonstrated the principle of genomic imprinting. Genomic imprinting refers to the process whereby specific genes are differentially marked during parental gametogenesis, resulting in the differential expression of these genes in the embryo and adult. This concept is difficult because we are accustomed to the rules of mendelian inheritance. Imprinting implies that there is differential modification of genetic material depending on whether the genetic material is passed from the mother or the father. This concept is exemplified in Prader-Willi and Angelman syndromes.

Prader-Willi syndrome, first described clinically more than 30 years ago, is characterized by significant hypotonia in infancy followed by an evolving pattern of overeating and obesity that appears between 6 months and 2 years of age, variable mental retardation, characteristic facies, small hands and feet, and hypogonadism. Twenty-five years ago, Angelman described children with severe mental retardation, seizures, ataxia, and a "puppet-like" gait who had happy dispositions and were prone to episodes of unprovoked laughter. Recently, the P gene, which is involved in the biosynthesis of melanin, has been found to be responsible for the hypopigmentation that is seen in some Prader-Willi and Angelman syndrome patients, as well as for oculocutaneous (tyrosinase-positive) albinism. This is the only component of the Prader-Willi syndrome and Angelman syndrome phenotype for which the responsible gene is known at this time. However, this gene is not imprinted, probably explaining its presence in both syndromes.

Both syndromes are associated with abnormalities in the inheritance of chromosome 15q11 through 15q13. In Prader-Willi syndrome, a cytogenetically or molecularly demonstrable paternal deletion is responsible for 75% of cases. Twenty-five percent of patients with this syndrome have two normal copies of chromosome 15, but there is absence of the paternal chromosome 15 through either nondysjunction or an error in early embryonic development. This is termed "maternal uniparental disomy." In Angelman syndrome, a deletion accounts for 75% of cases, and paternal uniparental disomy accounts for only 2%. The end result is the loss of a functional paternal gene(s) for Prader-Willi syndrome or a functional maternal gene(s) for Angelman syndrome. In Angelman syndrome, a mutation of the maternally active gene may cause this syndrome to occur sporadically. This group of patients includes a significant number of familial cases. Rarely, a mutation may occur in Prader-Willi syndrome as well.

The concept of genomic imprinting may help explain unusual pedigrees in which parents with apparently balanced chromosome rearrangements have abnormal children with the same rearrangements. In addition, genomic imprinting eventually may explain some family histories in which a disease skips generations or is assumed to be multifactorial. Preliminary work indicates an important role of imprinting in tumorigenesis, particularly of childhood tumors, such as Wilms tumor and retinoblastoma. The concept of imprinting challenges our understanding of traditional mendelian inheritance and suggests the need to ask how many other diseases or syndromes might also be caused by this mechanism.

22q11 Deletion Syndromes (Velocardiofacial Syndrome, DiGeorge Syndrome, & Conotruncal Face Syndrome)

The velocardiofacial syndrome (VCFS) was first described in 1978 by Robert Shprintzen. This is the most

Table 5–9. Well-recognized chromosomal microdeletion syndromes.

Deletion	Chromosomal Segment Deleted	Clinical Features
Prader-Willi syndrome	15q11–q13	Hypotonia, obesity, hypogonadism, developmental retardation
Angelman syndrome	15q11–q13	Seizures, ataxia, inappropriate laughter, developmental retardation
Smith-Magenis syndrome	17p11.2	Abnormal behaviors, developmental retardation
Miller-Dieker syndrome	17p13.3	Lissencephaly, seizures, dysmorphic, developmental retardation
Chondrodysplasia punctata (XL)	Xp21	Bone dysplasia, short stature, cataracts, ichthyosis, developmental retardation
Retinoblastoma	13q14	Retinoblastoma, thumb hypoplasia, developmental retardation
DiGeorge, velo-cardiofacial syndromes	22q11	Congenital heart disease, immune deficiency, hypocalcemia, developmental retardation

common syndrome associated with cleft palate and is estimated to have an incidence of 1 in 5000. Patients with VCFS exhibit a large spectrum of anomalies, of which the most frequent are cleft palate and velopharyngeal insufficiency, seen in about 90% of patients. Conotruncal heart defects (truncus arteriosus, interrupted aortic arch, tetralogy of Fallot, and ventricular septal defect) are seen in about 30% of these patients. A characteristic facial appearance (Figure 5–11), learning disabilities, and mild retardation are common. Some patients have more complex phenotypes, with delayed growth, immunologic deficiencies, hypocalcemia, microcephaly, and psychiatric disorders. Newly recognized features of VCFS occurring in greater than expected frequencies include growth hormone deficiency and juvenile rheumatoid arthritis.

Several years ago, the spectrum of abnormalities in VCFS, particularly the conotruncal heart defects, suggested to investigators a possible link between the DiGeorge sequence, in which this type of heart defect predominates, and VCFS. Indeed, there are several instances of VCFS and DiGeorge sequence occurring in the same family in an autosomal-dominant pattern of transmission. It is now established that both VCFS and DiGeorge sequence are associated with submicroscopic deletions of 22q11, diagnosed with the use of a specific FISH probe. Patients with VCFS likely represent the mild end of the phenotypic spectrum, and those with DiGeorge sequence the more severe end, with more serious heart defects and a higher incidence of thymic and parathyroid hypoplasia. To date, there is no clear molecular distinction between the various clinical phenotypes described in 22q11 deletions. The clinical spectrum of 22q11 deletions and their molecular correlates will continue to demand much attention from both clinical and molecular geneticists for some time in the future. Pediatricians should be aware of the wide clinical variability in patients with 22q11 deletions. In patients with conotruncal heart lesions or cleft palate, a high degree of suspicion is warranted to rule out this important microdeletion syndrome.

FRAGILE X SYNDROME

For years, investigators have noted an excess of male children among the mentally retarded population. This is due primarily to an excess of X-linked genes causing mental retardation. Overall, about 25% of mental retardation is thought to be X-linked. Fragile X syndrome, the most common of the X-linked disorders, was so named because of the appearance of a specific cytogenetically detectable heritable fragile site at the end of the long arm of chromosome Xq27.3 in affected individuals. A fragile site is a specific region on a chromosome that fails to condense normally during mitosis and is characterized by a nonstaining gap or constriction. Fragile X is the most common cause of mental retardation and the second most common chromosomal cause of mental retardation after Down syndrome. Its incidence is slightly greater than 1:2500, with a frequency in female carriers of 1:1500.

The fragile X phenotype is subtle and usually unremarkable to those who are not familiar with the syndrome. Lack of phenotypic clarity has contributed to the failure to appreciate this syndrome fully as a major cause of inherited mental retardation. The features are difficult to recognize in infancy and usually evolve with time. Most male children are bigger than their normal siblings and have prominent jaws and foreheads and large ears. Macroorchidism is usually detected only after puberty. Hyperextensibility, high-arched palate, flat feet, and mitral valve prolapse are relatively common features, suggesting that this syndrome has components of a connective tissue dysplasia. IQ is usually reduced to the 30–65 range, and behavior may be dominated by hyperactivity, attention deficit disorder, or, occasionally, autism. Approximately 20% of fragile X male carriers are clinically and intellectually normal and have no obvious cytogenetic abnormality but can transmit the disorder to their daughters.

Female carriers may be either normal (one third), learning impaired (one third), or mildly retarded (one third). Approximately 30% of female carriers also show some features similar to those in male carriers, such as a long narrow face and large ears.

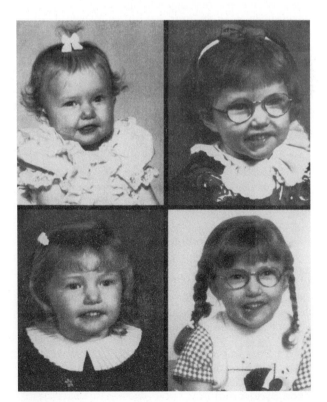

Figure 5–11. Characteristic facial appearance in velocardiofacial syndrome.

Before 1991, the usual diagnostic test for fragile X was a cytogenetic study using specific cell-culture conditions to enhance identification of the fragile site. Almost all affected fragile X males exhibit the fragile site, as do affected females and a small proportion of female carriers. In the past, unfortunately, accurate genetic counseling of families with this disorder frequently was complicated by inconclusive cytogenetic results.

In 1991, the mutation response for the fragile X syndrome was identified as an expansion of the trinucleotide sequence CGG within a gene designated as fragile X mental retardation-1 (FMR1). This CGG repeat in normal human beings ranges in size from 6 to 52 repeats. In affected patients with fragile X, this repeat has undergone expansion to hundreds and sometimes thousands of CGG repeats. If the trinucleotide repeat of the FMR1 gene exceeds approximately 230 repeats, the DNA of the entire 5' region of the gene becomes abnormally methylated, resulting in lack of transcription of FMR1 messenger RNA and the absence of its encoded protein. The length of the amplified CGG segment predicts relatively accurately the severity of the clinical phenotype (eg, affected male, affected female, female carrier, male carrier). Understanding the molecular basis of fragile X has allowed us to understand the unusual patterns of inheritance seen in this condition. When a mother carries a premutation (a CGG repeat length ranging from 50 to 230 repeats), this expansion can change in meiosis to a different and usually larger expansion, expanding to the full mutation and causing the full expression of the syndrome in an affected male child. In contrast, a male who carries the premutation (50–230 repeats) will transmit a repeat size only in the premutation range, which will not expand to cause the disorder in offspring. This explains why the condition may appear to skip generations. Knowledge of the size of the mutation in the individual at risk can allow for more accurate predictive counseling. The larger the mutation, the more likely it is to expand in the mother's children. Prenatal diagnosis is available for the fragile X syndrome; many laboratories now perform appropriate DNA testing (Southern blot and polymerase chain reaction) and can determine an individual's status with regard to fragile X with great accuracy. Cytogenetic testing for fragile X may still be appropriate in X-linked pedigrees when molecular studies for FMR1 are normal. At least two other recently identified fragile sites on the X chromosome near the site associated with fragile X are associated with syndromes that are phenotypically similar to those in classic fragile X.

The fragile X syndrome should be considered in any child with developmental delay or mental retardation in which the diagnosis is unknown. The clinical phenotype may be so mild that exclusion of fragile X on clinical grounds alone is not warranted. Once an individual is identified with fragile X, relevant family members should be evaluated with the use of molecular studies. An approach to a child with possible fragile X or another X-linked cause of mental retardation is presented in Figure 5–12.

MULTIFACTORIAL INHERITANCE

Although advances in the molecular genetics of single-gene disorders have been "headline grabbers" and progress has been dramatic in understanding cytogenetic disorders, most birth defects and common diseases that run in families are not caused by single-gene errors or chromosome imbalance and are poorly understood genetically. These are termed **multifactorial disorders,** indicating that they are caused by multiple factors, both genetic and environmental. These disorders recur in families but do not show particular patterns in the pedigree. Because they are common, epidemiologic studies have allowed estimation of empiric recurrence risks for individual defects. Some multifactorial traits, such as tall and short stature, are merely extreme variations of normal, and others, such as neural tube defects and congenital heart disease, are not thought to manifest until a certain threshold is exceeded. This threshold may vary by the sex of the affected individual, the severity of the defect, the number of family members affected, and several other factors. Another group of multifactorial disorders includes those diseases common to adult life, such as diabetes mellitus, hypertension, common psychiatric disorders, and many forms of cancer and coronary artery disease. Major genetic factors are undeniable in several of these diseases, but environmental risk factors are also important.

Common multifactorial birth defects are listed in Table 5–10 along with the approximate recurrence risks for first-degree relatives (siblings, sons, or daughters). Many of these traits have a strong predilection for one sex, ie, fewer genetic factors are needed to cause the defect in the sex that is affected more often. Therefore, when a child with a particular disorder is of the sex that is usually less often affected, more genetic factors are presumed to be present. Recurrence risks for first-degree relatives of this child are higher. For example, boys are five times as likely as girls to have pyloric stenosis. When a girl is affected, her parents' risk of having another affected child is much higher than if a boy had been affected. The severity of the defect also affects recurrence risks. For example, the recurrence risk is less when a child has unilateral rather than bilateral cleft lip. Pertinent information on important multifactorial defects is discussed below.

Neural Tube Defects

Neural tube defects, eg, anencephaly and spina bifida, are considered to have a common pathogenesis—failure of neural tube closure between 23 and 28 days' gestation. Failure of the neural tube to close in the cranial region results in anencephaly with absence of the forebrain, meninges, and vault of the skull and skin. Spina bifida results from failure of the fusion of the arches of the vertebrae, typically in the lumbar region. The severity differs

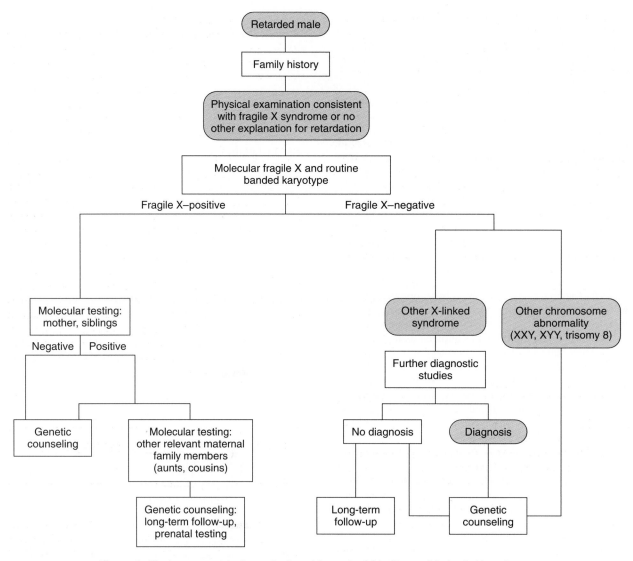

Figure 5–12. An approach to the evaluation of the male child with possible fragile X syndrome.

depending on whether the defect is open or closed, the involvement of neural elements, and the location of the defect. Spina bifida is a major cause of developmental retardation and motor handicap in surviving infants. The incidence varies significantly between populations, occurring in nearly 1% of live births in Ireland and in less than 0.2% in the United States. Certain ethnic populations, such as the Sikhs in British Columbia and Hispanics in rural counties in the United States, have an increased risk.

Several studies have suggested the important role of nutritional factors, and much attention has focused on the possible preventative action of folate. Folate supplementation (4 mg/d) has been recommended beginning before conception and continuing for the first 3 months of pregnancy in women who have already had a child with a neural tube defect. The Centers for Disease Control and Prevention has recently recommended that all women of reproductive age take supplemental vitamins containing small amounts of folate (0.4 mg) on a daily basis. As a public health measure, this seems to be a much more reasonable approach to the prevention of neural tube defects, because most children with neural tube defects are born into families with an entirely negative history.

Neural tube defects rarely are associated with chromosome disorders. Women receiving the anticonvulsants valproic acid (Depakene) and carbamazepine (Tegretol) have an increased risk for having a child with a neural tube defect. In general, however, they are isolated defects with presumed multifactorial inheritance.

Neural tube defects are prenatally detectable in several

Table 5–10. Recurrence risks in first-degree relatives in common multifactorial birth defects.

Defect	Sex Ratio (M:F)	Recurrence Risks (%)
Pyloric stenosis	5:1	Male affected: 2–5 Female affected: 7–20
Cleft lip ± cleft palate	1.6:1	Unilateral: 4 Unilateral + P: 4.9 Bilateral: 6.7 Bilateral + P: 8
Cleft palate	1:1.14	3.5
Anencephaly/spina bifida	1:1.5	2–3
Congenital heart disease	1:1	
Ventricular septal defect		3
Patent ductus arteriosus		3
Hypoplastic left heart syndrome		2

ways: by maternal serum AFP screening, by ultrasound, and by measurement of AFP in the amniotic fluid.

Cleft Lip & Cleft Palate

Cleft lip, with or without cleft palate, is genetically distinct from cleft palate alone. In families in which a child has been born with cleft lip and cleft palate, there is a recurrence risk for cleft lip, either alone or with cleft palate, but not for cleft palate alone. Parents of children with isolated cleft palate have a recurrence risk for cleft palate, but not cleft lip. Cleft lip with or without cleft palate is a heterogeneous defect. Numerous single-gene syndromes and chromosome disorders are associated with oral clefting. Teratogens, such as phenylhydantoin, can cause this defect. In contrast to the multifactorial model, some researchers have proposed that there are major genes for this disorder. Most data, however, fit best within the multifactorial threshold trait model, and empiric recurrence risks are appropriately used when more complex patterns of malformation have been ruled out.

Cleft palate also occurs frequently as a component of syndromes. The Pierre Robin sequence is not a specific syndrome but is a feature of more than 60 conditions. The Pierre Robin sequence consists of a small mandible, which is thought to be primary, and a U-shaped cleft palate, which is caused by the tongue falling back and preventing palatal closure. The Pierre Robin sequence is a frequent feature of the autosomal-dominant Stickler syndrome. Because the Stickler syndrome is common, many geneticists recommend that all infants with isolated cleft palate be screened ophthalmologically because severe myopia, which can result in retinal detachment, is an important feature. Cleft palate is also a common feature of the velocardiofacial syndrome (see Microdeletion Syndromes).

Congenital Heart Defects

Congenital heart abnormalities are very common, seen in 4–8:1000 livebirths. Heart defects are also common components of multiple syndromes and are increased in frequency in nearly all chromosome disorders. It is therefore important to determine whether the child has an isolated heart defect before using empiric recurrence risks. Certain heart defects, such as patent ductus arteriosus and patent foramen ovale, are essentially normal in premature infants and do not represent real birth defects. Congenital infections, such as rubella and maternal diabetes, and anticonvulsant drugs significantly increase the risk for congenital heart disease. Most defects, however, are isolated. Recurrence risks have been subdivided by type of defect and are generally low. Hypoplastic left heart syndrome, coarctation of the aorta, atrial septal defect, and pulmonary valve stenosis may have a stronger predisposition to family recurrence. Mothers who have had a previous child with congenital heart disease, who have a positive family history of congenital heart defects, or who are in a high-risk group (eg, those with insulin-dependent diabetes and those who are receiving anticonvulsant drugs) should be offered fetal echocardiography during pregnancy to monitor for occurrence or recurrence. Major structural defects of the heart can be detected prenatally, although subtle lesions may be missed.

APPROACH TO DISPROPORTIONATE SHORT STATURE

Pediatricians are usually rightfully confused when confronted with the differential diagnosis of the disproportionately short infant or child. This confusion stems from the nomenclature, which is a mixture of eponyms, Greek terminology, and a classification based on the part of the skeleton that is affected radiographically. There are also clinical classifications based on the location of shortening (ie, limb or spine), the age of onset, the presence of associated anomalies, and the mode of inheritance. The confusion has been compounded by the growing recognition of the genetic, molecular, and clinical heterogeneity of many bone dysplasias. There are more than 100 distinct bone dysplasias recognized today. Obviously no pediatrician can be an expert on all these! The purpose of this section is to introduce the classification and suggest an approach to these children.

Most experts rely on radiographic abnormalities as the basis of classification. This method notes which parts of the long bones are abnormal and whether the spine is involved. Thus a disorder may be classified as primarily involving the epiphyses, the metaphyses, the diaphyses, or the spine (**spondylo-**). Various combinations are possible, such as spondyloepiphyseal and spondylometaphyseal. Clinically, there are discrepancies between the lengths of the limbs and trunk in disproportionate short stature. Limb shortening can be further defined by noting which segment of the limb is primarily involved. If the shortening is chiefly proximal (ie, humerus and femur), it is termed **rhizomelic;** if it involves the middle segment (ie, radius, ulna, tibia, and fibula), it is termed **mesomelic;** and if the distal segments (ie, hands and feet) are involved, it is termed **acromelic.** Some bone dysplasias combine elements of altered bone growth with true malformation syndromes. For example, in camptomelic dysplasia, there are abnormalities of the brain and heart in association with sex reversal in genetically male infants. An International Nomenclature of Constitutional Diseases of Bone was proposed in 1970 and most recently updated in 1992. On the basis of this system, skeletal disorders have been divided into five major groups as follows:

1. **Osteochondrodysplasias,** in which there is abnormal growth and development of cartilage and/or bone. The osteochondrodysplasias include disorders evident at birth, such as achondroplasia; those that may both manifest before birth or be delayed in onset, such as osteogenesis imperfecta; and those that appear in early childhood such as hypochondroplasia.
2. **Dysostoses,** in which there are malformations of individual bones, either alone or in combination.
3. **Osteolytic disorders,** in which there is multiple or focal resorption of bone.
4. **Skeletal abnormalities,** which are associated with chromosome disorders.
5. **Primary metabolic disorders,** such as the Morquio and type I Gaucher syndromes.

With the increased routine use of ultrasonography, evaluation of the patient with disproportionate short stature often begins before birth with the recognition of short limbs in utero. The diagnostic process in the fetus and newborn are similar and complex.

To determine an accurate diagnosis, clinicians will require the assistance of a radiologist and a geneticist, who, because of the individual rarity of these conditions, may often need to consult with experts in the skeletal dysplasias. Gathering appropriate data so that the diagnosis can be made is crucial. Appropriate radiographs must be obtained (eg, long bones, the spine, the skull, and the hands and feet). As in other genetic evaluations, the family history, developmental history, and age when the problem of short stature was first noticed are important. This physical examination should include measurements of arm span and upper-lower segment ratio (measured from the level of the symphysis pubis). Short-limbed dwarfs will have increased upper-lower segment ratios (normal is approximately 1.7 at birth and decreases to 1.0 by age 8 years), and their arm span will be less than the height. Short-trunk dwarfs will have decreased upper-lower segment ratios and increased arm span. Assessment of the

primary location of shortening (ie, rhizomelic, mesomelic, acromelic) can be important. Nonskeletal clinical abnormalities may also be helpful to note, such as cleft palate and myopia in Kniest dysplasia, natal teeth and preaxial polydactyly in Ellis-van Creveld syndrome, and "hitchhiker's" thumbs and swollen ear pinnae in diastrophic dysplasia.

Several dwarfing conditions are fatal either before or shortly after birth. Additional diagnostic studies can be of crucial assistance in making an appropriate diagnosis and in providing for family counseling when an infant with dwarfism has died. These studies require obtaining bone specimens for biochemical and ultrastructural analysis. Usually a piece of costochondral junction should be flash frozen, a piece fixed for electron microscopy, and sections prepared for routine histologic studies. Bone or skin should be grown in tissue culture for later molecular analysis.

A virtual explosion of knowledge in the general field of the chondrodysplasias has been based in large part on advances related to the human genome project. Although a full discussion of the molecular basis of these defects is beyond the purview of this chapter, pediatricians should be aware of the tremendous and rapid advances in this field, which allow children and adults with disproportionate short stature to be classified much more precisely and their specific molecular error identified. Eventually, knowledge of the specific gene defect in each individual should allow for much more precise counseling regarding etiology and natural history. The original classifications of bone dysplasia based on such factors as radiologic features and time of onset, have been redefined substantially on the basis of our current knowledge of the mutated genes involved.

The first of these disorders delineated on a molecular basis was osteogenesis imperfecta (OI). Previously, OI had been divided clinically into four types, all characterized by increased fracturability. In type I there was normal stature with little deformity, blue sclera, and a high frequency of hearing loss. Type II, lethal in the perinatal period, revealed thickened bones, beaded ribs, and marked long-bone deformity. Type III was characterized by progressively deforming long bones, variably blue sclera, dentinogenesis imperfecta, and extreme short stature. Type IV was characterized by normal sclera, mild to moderate bone deformity, and variable short stature. Work in many different laboratories has identified more than 150 specific gene mutations that cause OI. All the mutations are either in the gene for the pro-α-1(I) chain of type I procollagen or the pro-α-2(I) chain for the same protein. Ninety percent of patients with OI have mutations in either of these two genes. In more than one third of the mutations that cause the mildest form of OI (type I), there is decreased expression of the gene for the pro-α-1(I) chains. Most mutations in the more severe forms of the disease cause synthesis of structurally abnormal but partially functional pro-α-chains. In general, these abnormal chains exert their effects by changing the configuration of procollagen or by forming abnormally thin and irregular fibers. Any mutation that drastically reduces the amount of collagen or distorts the normal geometry of collagen fibers weakens the entire collagen structure, which is responsible for the structural strength of bone. For all four clinical forms of OI, the most likely inheritance is autosomal dominant. Rarely, types II and III may be caused by autosomal-recessive genes. In counseling families, therefore, it is extremely important to obtain a complete family history and examine relatives. Molecular analysis can clarify this process and allow for refinement of recurrence risks. For parents who are clinically normal but have an affected child, the recurrence risk for OI in a subsequent pregnancy is approximately 6%, on the basis of the possibility that one of the parents is carrying a germ-line mutation for the defect.

It has recently been recognized that three quite dissimilar disorders—thanatophoric dysplasia, achondroplasia, and hypochondroplasia—all are caused by defects in fibroblast growth factor receptor 3 (FGFR III). It is of great interest that more than 98% of cases of achondroplasia analyzed to date reveal the same amino acid substitution. This situation is remarkably different from the mutational heterogeneity seen in other disorders. Several different mutations in FGFR III have been described in thanatophoric dysplasia and hypochondroplasia.

Several years ago, it was predicted that defects in type II collagen would be found primarily in disorders affecting cartilage, the nucleus pulposus, and the vitreous humor of the eye. Indeed, these molecular defects of type II collagen, termed the "type II collagenopathies," have been found in a large group of patients with phenotypes ranging from severe achondrogenesis type II to hypochondrogenesis, to the spondyloepiphyseal dysplasias and the spondylometaphyseal dysplasias through Kniest dysplasia, and Stickler syndrome. Other identified gene defects in the bone dysplasias include abnormalities in the sulfate transporter gene on the long arm of chromosome 5, causing diastrophic dysplasia, atelosteogenesis II, and achondrogenesis IB. The X-linked form of chondrodysplasia punctata, which is mapped to the short arm of the X chromosome (Xp22.3), has been found to contain mutations in previously unrecognized enzymes of sulfate metabolism termed aryl sulfatase E (ARSE), D, and F. Several patients with X-linked recessive chondrodysplasia punctata have been found to have mutations in ARSE. Campomelic dysplasia, a disorder associated with sex reversal, was localized to an area on chromosome 17q24.1-225.1. in 1993. In 1995, the gene SOX 9 was characterized and mutations identified in a number of patients with classic campomelic dysplasia who were chromosomally normal. These patients were therefore found to be heterozygous for their mutations, invalidating the previously proposed autosomal-recessive inheritance pattern for this disorder. This, therefore, appears to be a dominant disorder with a very low recurrence for normal parents with an affected child. The pathogenetic mechanism of the SOX 9 mutation dysplasia in campomelic dysplasia is still unknown.

We can expect that progress in identifying the genes responsible for many other skeletal dysplasias will continue rapidly. It will be increasingly important for pediatricians caring for children with disproportionate short stature to be in close communication with a tertiary-level genetic center to provide families with the most current information regarding their child's defect and its likely recurrence risk.

In the surviving child with a bone dysplasia, all efforts are usually warranted to allow the child to lead as normal a life as possible. This requires considerable knowledge of the natural history of the disorder so that appropriate anticipatory guidance can be provided. For example, avoidance of early sitting and weight bearing in children with achondroplasia can reduce the chance of significant gibbus formation and spinal cord compression later in life. Vision and hearing screening are extremely important in children with the spondyloepiphyseal dysplasias because severe myopia and hearing loss are frequent. Surgical bone-lengthening procedures may greatly increase the self-esteem, employability, and even general health of individuals with bone dysplasias. To date, these procedures have been used mostly in achondroplasia but are likely to be extended to other bone dysplasias as well. Referral of individuals with bone dysplasias to support groups is of inestimable help. The largest of these, Little People of America, provides an educational, social, and employment network for parents and affected individuals. Provision of accurate genetic counseling is a crucial element to the complete evaluation of a dwarfed individual and is sometimes overlooked because of the complexities of daily management.

Clinical details on several important lethal and nonlethal skeletal dysplasias are presented in Tables 5–11 and 5–12.

APPROACH TO THE STILLBORN INFANT

The birth of a stillborn infant is often an unexpected event for the pediatrician who may be unprepared with strategies to help the family cope and unsure of the appropriate diagnostic approach. Pregnancy loss is no longer an easily accepted consequence of childbearing. Families now expect answers to such questions as "Will it happen again?" and "Did I do something to cause this to happen?" Too often the answers to these questions are not available, and families then make reproductive decisions with little knowledge of real recurrence risks or understanding of possible prenatal monitoring in subsequent pregnancies. Given a uniform rational approach to the stillborn infant, a diagnosis can be anticipated in a high percentage of cases.

Table 5–11. Clinical and radiographic features in selected lethal skeletal dysplasias.

Diagnosis	Mode of Inheritance	Clinical Features	Radiographic Features
Achondrogenesis I (A&B)	AR	Extremely short limbs, frequent hydrops	Incomplete spine ossification
Achondrogenesis II (hypochondrogenesis)	AD (probable)	Short limbs, fetal hydrops	Poor spine ossification, metaphyseal abnormalities
Thanatophoric dysplasia	AD	Relatively large cranium, short limbs, spatulate fingers	"Telephone-receiver" femurs
Campomelic dysplasia	AD	Bowing of tibias with skin dimples, sex reversal in XY males, cleft palate, CNS and cardiac malformations	Bowing of the long bones
Rhizomelic chondrodysplasia punctata	AR	Cleft palate, cataracts, occasional ichthyosis, short limbs	Punctate epiphyseal calcifications; vertebral, coronal clefts
Atelosteogenesis syndromes	?	Very short proximal limbs, depressed nasal bridge, cleft palate, deviation of fingers	Short ribs, flat vertebrae, coronal clefts
Short-limb polydactyly syndromes	AR	Short limbs, polydactyly, heart and renal defects	Short horizontal ribs; wide, flat vertebral bodies
Jarcho-Levin syndrome	AR	Very short trunk, camptodactyly	Multiple vertebral segmentation defects, "crab-like" appearance of ribs
Osteogenesis imperfecta type II	AD (usual)	Very short bowed limbs, blue sclera, flat facies, hydrops	Multiple fractures, thick bones, beading of ribs

AD = autosomal dominant; AR = autosomal recessive; CNS = central nervous system.

The diagnostic and counseling process requires advanced planning and should involve the obstetrician, pathologist, nurses, geneticist, radiologist, and laboratory personnel.

Ideally, complete studies should be performed on all stillborn infants; however, practical issues, such as the yield of the test, the cost, and the impact on the family, need to be considered when choosing diagnostic studies. Sometimes the cause of fetal death is apparent (eg, cord accident, placental abruption, or acute infection). Even in these obvious cases, however, an autopsy and other stud-ies can be reassuring to families regarding the absence of other anomalies and the anticipated pathologic findings. Such studies are increasingly important in medicolegal defense. Often the cause of fetal death is not clear. In these cases, appropriate focused studies should be routine.

Fetuses that appear to have died soon before delivery are much more likely to have died acutely from a nonrecurring event, such as an ascending infection, cord accident, or placental abruption. These fetuses should be examined carefully, and, if no external malformations are

Table 5–12. Clinical and radiographic features in selected nonlethal bone dysplasias.

Bone Dysplasia	Mode of Inheritance	Age at Recognition	Clinical Features	Radiographic Features
Achondroplasia	AD	Birth	Relatively large head, characteristic face, rhizomelic shortenings of limbs, spinal stenosis, trident hand	Small sacrosciatic notches, decreased interpedicular distance, short pedicles, short, broad long bones
Asphyxiating thoracic dystrophy (Jeune syndrome)	AR	Birth	Narrow chest, occasional polydactyly, variable limb shortening, respiratory insufficiency, renal disease	Short ribs, square, short ilia, acetabular spurs, broad proximal femurs
Spondyloepiphyseal dysplasia congenita	AD	Birth	Short barrel chest, normal hands, slightly short limbs, myopia, retinal detachment, hearing loss, subluxation C1-2	Odontoid hypoplasia; flat, pear-shaped vertebrae; delayed ossification of epiphyses, hips, and knees
Hypochondroplasia	AD	About 2 y	Normal face; rhizomelic shortening of limbs; short, broad hands; mild short stature	Short, wide long bones; lumbosacral interpedicular narrowing; short pedicles
Pseudoachondroplasia	AD	About 2 y	Normal face; long trunk; very short limbs; severe joint problems; small, broad hands	Platyspondyly, epiphyseal, and metaphyseal dysplasia; marked hand involvement

AD = autosomal dominant; AR = autosomal recessive.

apparent and there is no history of recurrent loss, appropriate studies may consist of an autopsy, an examination of the placenta and cord, and photographs.

Macerated fetuses, which are precisely those least likely to be studied, are more likely to have such findings as malformations, syndromes, and chromosome abnormalities. A complete evaluation should always be performed on these infants. Complete studies should also be performed on infants with an external or suspected internal structural malformation (eg, cleft lip, with or without cleft palate, ear anomalies, extra or missing digits, or imperforate anus) or those with abnormal prenatal ultrasound examinations. Other infants who warrant complete investigation are those with intrauterine growth retardation, as these infants are significantly more likely to have chromosomal errors or severe placental abnormalities. When no cause of death is apparent or with a history of previously unexplained fetal or neonatal loss, a full investigation should be conducted.

THE STILLBORN PROTOCOL

An algorithm for the evaluation of a stillbirth or neonatal death is shown in Figure 5–13. A complete protocol for the investigation of a stillborn infant includes the following:

1. History of the unsuccessful pregnancy
2. Family history
3. External clinical examination of the infant
4. Photographs
5. Chromosome cultures (via cord or cardiac blood, skin biopsy, or placenta and fetal membranes)
6. Skeletal radiographs (mandatory when short limbs or a dwarfing condition is suspected)
7. Fetal autopsy
8. Examination of the placenta and cord
9. Special studies such as cord blood TORCH titers and cord IgM levels in suspected in utero infections, hemoglobin electrophoresis in cases of suspected hemoglobinopathy or thalassemia, and skin biopsy for enzymatic and DNA studies in suspected storage or metabolic disorders
10. Counseling, which may be provided by the pediatrician in straightforward situations or by a geneticist or genetic counselor.

All the data should be reviewed with the family and appropriate options for prenatal monitoring in subsequent pregnancies discussed. The family should have a clear idea of the recurrence risks involved. Supportive grief counseling and referral to pregnancy loss support groups are appropriate in all cases.

COMMON DIAGNOSES IN STILLBORNS

Although it is beyond the scope of this chapter to discuss the myriad conditions presenting as stillbirth, certain conditions are so common to the pediatric experience that they deserve additional discussion.

Chromosome disorders frequently result in stillbirth and neonatal death. About 6% of stillborns and 5.5% of neonatal deaths are chromosomally abnormal. Presentation of the fetus with a chromosome disorder may differ greatly from that seen in newborns or older infants. Relatively small fetal size may make appreciation of dysmorphic features difficult. This is particularly true for Down syndrome. The overturned ear helices, upslanted palpebral fissures, and midface hypoplasia are often not obvious. Fetal maceration can also obscure subtle dysmorphic features as can fetal hydrops or swelling, which is relatively common in Down syndrome and trisomy 18. Fetal swelling is the hallmark of XO Turner syndrome, in which it is associated with nuchal cystic hygroma. Chromosomally abnormal stillborns tend to have more severe and obvious malformations than those seen in liveborn infants. For example, neural tube defects are not uncommon in stillborn fetuses with trisomy 18, whereas they are rare in liveborn infants with trisomy 18.

Amniotic Bands

Amniotic bands in the liveborn child usually consist of characteristic asymmetric involvement of limbs and digits with occasional facial clefting. Frequently, vestigial fibrous bands remain on the digits at the time of birth and are helpful diagnostically. These children usually are entirely normal apart from their disruptive and deformational defects. This is in marked contrast to the phenotypic picture in the stillborn, which tends to be much more severe and in which body wall clefts (the so-called limb-body wall complex), exencephaly, acrania, scoliosis, short cord, and internal malformations may occur (Figure 5–14). Often in these situations, there is no direct evidence of amniotic bands, but examination of the placenta can help establish the diagnosis because the chorial plate is mostly devoid of amnion. These bizarre body wall defects are frequently diagnosed prenatally and probably result from very early disruption of the amnion, although the exact pathogenesis remains somewhat obscure.

Potter Phenotype

Severe oligohydramnios, from whatever cause, produces the Potter phenotype, which is characterized by an aged facial appearance, lower canthal folds, depressed nasal tip, micrognathia, loose skin, and limb abnormalities secondary to chronic in utero constraint. Death occurs postnatally because of pulmonary hypoplasia. Infants are severely depressed at birth and cannot be successfully ventilated. The overall pattern of the anomalies may not become evident for several hours, when the lack of response to mechanical ventilation becomes progressively

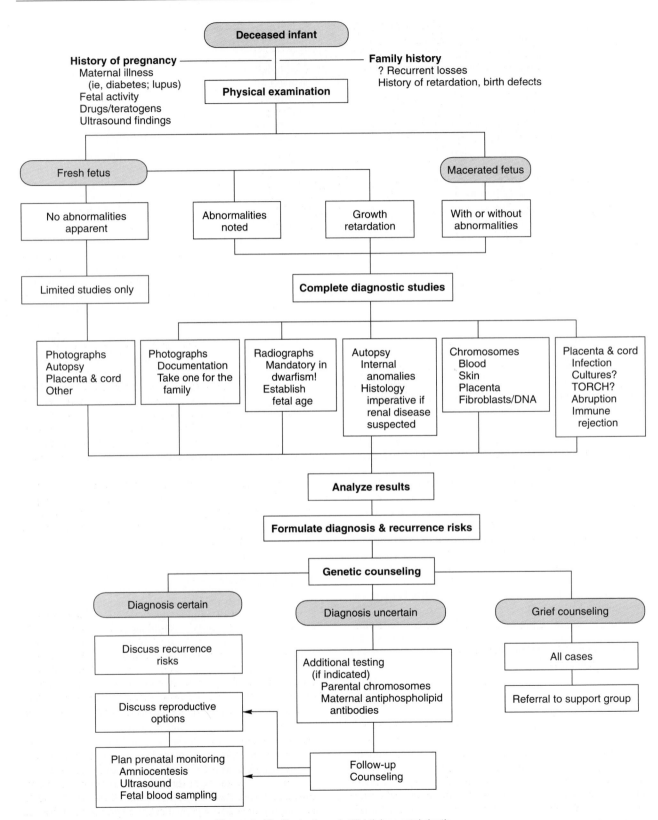

Figure 5–13. Evaluation of stillbirth/neonatal death.

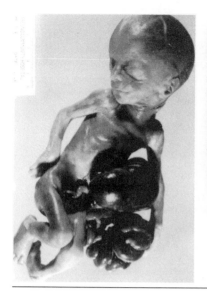 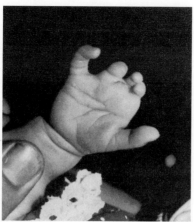

Figure 5–14. Early amnion rupture sequence may result in severe limb and wall defects **(left)**, or be limited to distal limb amputations **(right).**

apparent. Although the Potter phenotype can occur secondary to a chronic amniotic fluid leak or severe intrauterine growth retardation, renal causes are frequent and mandate evaluation of renal histology. Possible renal findings include bilateral renal agenesis or cystic dysplastic kidneys, obstructive uropathy, and type 2 autosomal-recessive infantile polycystic kidney disease. Rarely, type 1 autosomal-dominant adult-type polycystic kidney disease may present with the Potter phenotype. These disorders carry different genetic recurrence risks, which may vary from 3.5% for bilateral renal agenesis in parents with normal renal ultrasounds, to 25% for type 2 infantile polycystic kidney disease.

After complete evaluation, an accurate diagnosis can be anticipated in most stillborn infants and children dying neonatally. Advances in prenatal diagnosis, especially use of DNA techniques, make accurate investigation of fetal or neonatal death increasingly relevant.

IMPORTANT TERATOGENS IN PEDIATRICS

A **teratogen** is an agent that can cause abnormalities in form and function (ie, birth defects) in an exposed fetus. Teratogens act in a relatively limited number of ways by producing cell death, altering tissue growth, or interfering with differentiation. As these are basic functions of growing cells and developing organisms, there is commonly more than one effect observed in the developing fetus. Certain characteristics are common to teratogenic agents: infertility

or fetal wastage, prenatal onset growth deficiency, alterations in morphogenesis, and alterations of organ system function, including central nervous system performance.

There is a wide variability in the effect of the teratogenic agent on the fetus; this has undoubtedly delayed recognition of many human teratogens. Factors accounting for variability include the dose of the agent, the timing of the exposure, the host's susceptibility (ie, maternal and fetal genetic factors), and interactions with other environmental agents.

Teratogens include infectious agents; drugs and chemicals; physical agents, such as radiation; and maternal metabolic disorders, such as insulin-dependent diabetes mellitus and phenylketonuria. Major teratogens, together with their effects, are presented in Table 5–13.

INFECTIOUS AGENTS

Recognized effects of viruses, bacteria, and parasites include fetal death, growth retardation, birth defects, and mental retardation. In most instances, the fetus is directly invaded with secondary inflammation of fetal tissues and cell death. Symptoms characterizing prenatal infections include microcephaly, mental retardation, cerebral palsy, seizures, and visual and hearing defects (see Chapter 4). In general, structural defects such as polydactyly are not seen.

Rubella Virus
Rubella virus is the best studied infectious agent. The severity of fetal effects varies significantly according to the month of gestation at the time of infection. Of infants infected during the first trimester, 15–25% are found to have symptoms of congenital rubella syndrome. After the first trimester, the incidence of severely affected children

L

Table 5–13. Important human teratogens and their major clinical effects.

Teratogen	Susceptible Period (Trimester)	Fetal Effects
Infections		
Rubella	First	Cararacts, congenital heart disease, hearing loss, mental retardation
Cytomegalovirus	First and second	Microcephaly, mental retardation, chorioretinitis, seizures, hearing loss
Toxoplasmosis	First to third	Hydrocephalus, mental retardation, microcephaly, chorioretinitis
Drugs		
Warfarin	First	CNS defects, nasal hypoplasia
Isotretinoin	First	Cardiac, ear, and CNS
Lithium	First	Cardiac (Ebstein anomaly), overgrowth
Anticonvulsant drugs		
Diphenylhydantoin	First to third	Characteristic face, nail hypoplasia, ↑ risk cleft lip ± palate, developmental problems
Valproic acid	First to third	Neural tube defects, characteristic face, learning problems
Carbamazepine	First to third	Neural tube defects, learning problems
Chemical/physical agents		
Hyperthermia	First	Neural tube defects, microcephaly
Radiation	First month	Therapeutic radiation only; microcephaly Diagnostic: low risk
Alcohol	First to third	Wide spectrum of effects; CNS functional impairment most important

CNS = central nervous system.

decreases; however, hearing loss and mental retardation can occur in children exposed in the fourth and fifth months of pregnancy. Congenital rubella syndrome is characterized by growth retardation; failure to thrive; congenital anomalies, including cataracts, pigmentary retinopathy, microphthalmia, and glaucoma; cardiovascular malformations, especially patent ductus arteriosus, pulmonary valvar and arterial stenoses, atrial septal defect, and ventricular septal defect; neonatal myocarditis; and central nervous system abnormalities. Sensorineural hearing loss is frequent. Hepatosplenomegaly, thrombocytopenia, chronic rash, chronic diarrhea, and immune defects are also seen. Prevention of congenital rubella is possible through the routine use of effective rubella vaccines. Attenuated live rubella vaccines are known to cross the placenta, and the virus has been recovered from abortus material. However, inadvertent vaccination of a pregnant woman appears to pose a very low risk to the fetus.

Cytomegalovirus

Possibly 5–6% of all pregnant women become infected with cytomegalovirus. Risks to the fetus appears to be confined mainly to those women with primary infection. The overall risk for a woman with primary infection to have an infected fetus is approximately 30–40%. Approximately 10–15% of these infants show some symptoms, although most infants are clinically asymptomatic. Severe congenital cytomegalovirus infection causes diffuse central nervous system damage, including microcephaly, associated with paraventricular calcifications; rarely hydrocephalus; hearing loss; mental retardation; and seizures. Ocular involvement with chorioretinitis, optic atrophy, and microphthalmia can produce severe visual impairment. Infants may present with the so-called blueberry muffin syndrome with hepatosplenomegaly, jaundice, thrombocytopenia, petechiae, or hemolytic anemia.

Herpes Simplex Virus

Most of the risk associated with the herpes simplex virus has been attributable to infants acquiring infection at or around the time of birth. Nevertheless, herpes simplex infection in early pregnancy may result in fetal loss and, rarely, in microcephaly and microphthalmia. Intracranial calcifications, retinal dysplasia, patent ductus arteriosus, vesicular cutaneous lesions, and hypoplastic distal phalanges have also been reported. Perinatal transmission can often be avoided by appropriate obstetric precautions.

Congenital Varicella

Congenital varicella (chickenpox) syndrome resulting from infection of the pregnant mother appears to occur infrequently (± 2%). The crucial period for fetal infection appears to be the third and fourth month. Affected children may show growth deficiency, microcephaly, peripheral nerve palsy, ocular involvement, and limb anomalies, including distal phalangeal hypoplasia or hypoplasia of an entire limb. Cutaneous abnormalities include scars, vesicles, and underdevelopment of the skin, possibly secondary to in utero ulceration.

Human Immunodeficiency Virus (HIV)

HIV has been suggested as a cause of altered growth and development and as a cause of dysmorphic facial features. The bulk of evidence suggests, however, that the virus is not teratogenic, although it may be transmitted transplacentally, causing AIDS in fetuses and infants.

Parvovirus B19

Since its discovery in 1975, human parvovirus (B19) has been shown to cause a diverse spectrum of clinical manifestations, including the childhood illness fifth disease (erythema infectiosum), aplastic crises in patients with chronic hemolytic anemia, chronic anemia in immunodeficient patients, and arthritis. In 1984, reports appeared of intrauterine death associated with B19 infections. Approximately 50% of adult women are immune to parvovirus. The transplacental infection rate has been estimated to be about 33%, although precise information on fetal risk has been difficult to obtain because B19 infection rarely persists throughout the pregnancy. Therefore, measuring B19 IgM in cord blood of surviving infants is not a reliable method for detecting intrauterine infections. Maternal B19 infection, usually asymptomatic, is most often followed by the delivery of a normal infant. However, fetal loss can occur at all stages of pregnancy; the highest risk occurs during the first 20 weeks, especially between weeks 10 and 20, with hydrops and ascites developing rapidly. Various studies have reported overall fetal risk to be approximately 4–16%.

In the fetus, B19 infection causes a maturational arrest in the development of red blood cells. Because the fetus is rapidly expanding its red blood cell volume and has a short red blood cell lifespan, it is particularly vulnerable to this type of insult. Anemia results, which is thought to cause cardiac failure, ascites, pleural effusions, and edema of the skin. Myocarditis and liver disease also have been reported, as have meconium peritonitis and, rarely, congenital malformations, although this association has not been proved.

When a mother is known or thought to have been exposed to parvovirus, the first step is to determine her immune status. If her parvovirus IgG findings are positive and her IgM negative, she can be assumed to be immune. If her IgG and IgM findings both are negative, testing should be repeated serially to rule out newly occurring infection. In a woman whose IgG and IgM results are positive, the mother should be assumed to be infected and the fetus monitored appropriately. Serum AFP has been suggested as a means of detecting early fetal involvement. However, weekly ultrasound examinations are currently recommended between 6 and 14 weeks' gestation, which represents the maximum interval between maternal illness and fetal death. Early detection of fetal ascites should lead to prompt referral to a center specializing in intrauterine blood transfusions, which have been a lifesaving approach in this form of anemia. In some situations, the ascites and hydrops caused by B19-induced anemia resolve spontaneously. Many issues have yet to be defined, including the role of intrauterine transfusion and the best method for monitoring women at risk.

Bacterial Agents

Among bacterial agents, only syphilis and possibly mycoplasmas are thought to have significant teratogenicity. Syphilis is the oldest of the known prenatal infectious teratogens, and, although rare, its frequency may be increasing. It is generally thought that infection of the fetus with syphilis does not occur until about the fourth month of pregnancy. If untreated, about 50% of infants will be affected with congenital syphilis, and the remainder will be stillborn or die in the perinatal period. Late infection with

syphilis results in only about a 10% risk of fetal infection. Infants with early congenital syphilis may present with fetal hydrops and evidence of generalized infection, as well as with hepatosplenomegaly, lymphadenitis, anemia, thrombocytopenia, rhinitis, and rashes. Inflammation of bone may be manifested by Parrot pseudoparalysis, which may mimic an Erb palsy or present as an irritable infant. Meningitis, nerve palsies, and progressive hydrocephalus may occur. Eye problems are frequent with chorioretinitis, uveitis, optic atrophy, glaucoma, and occasional chancres of the eyelid. Late manifestations of congenital syphilis, which occur after age 2 include Hutchinson teeth, interstitial keratitis, deafness, mulberry molars, and Clutton joints. Saddle nose deformity and linear facial scars around body orifices (*rhagades*) are late manifestations.

Toxoplasmosis

Toxoplasmosis is the major parasitic teratogen of concern to pediatricians. The major risk to the fetus occurs from acute toxoplasmosis infection during pregnancy. First-trimester infection is associated with a 15–20% risk of fetal transmission, whereas second- or third-trimester infections are associated with a 75% risk. Later infections most often result in clinically asymptomatic disease. Manifestations in the infant include microcephaly or hydrocephalus, as well as a range of systemic symptoms associated with generalized sepsis. Long-term follow-up of involved children reveals a high percentage of mental retardation, cerebral palsy, and visual and hearing deficits.

PHYSICAL TERATOGENS

The nuclear disaster in Chernobyl and episodes such as the Three Mile Island accident have raised concern regarding the role of radiation in human malformations. Experimental animal and epidemiologic studies suggest that high doses of radiation (> 200 rads) can produce prenatal onset growth deficiency, central nervous system damage, microcephaly, and ocular defects. The sensitive period for such abnormalities appears to be from about 2 to 5 fetal weeks. Therapeutic doses of radiation carry a significant risk of anomalies for the fetus only when delivered to the region of the developing embryo during the first month of pregnancy. Lower doses of radiation appear to have a low risk for malformations or functional abnormalities in humans at any time in pregnancy. There is also the theoretic risk of mutagenesis and carcinogenesis, but the magnitude of risk is quite low. Exposures to radiation should be avoided, but women undergoing diagnostic x-ray studies can generally be given significant reassurance regarding the risks to their fetuses.

Hyperthermia

There appear to be real risks to the fetus from sustained increases in body temperature from whatever cause. The most obvious cause of hyperthermia is maternal fever, but other sources include saunas, hot tubs, bathing, and prolonged exertion. Human data are limited, although laboratory animal data strongly support the role of heat as a teratogenic agent at critical stages in neural tube development. There are several anecdotal reports regarding the association of anencephaly and spina bifida with hyperthermia. In addition, microcephaly, mental retardation, and cerebral palsy have been reported in women who have had sustained, uncontrolled febrile episodes.

DRUGS & CHEMICAL AGENTS

Much attention was focused on drugs as a cause of malformations after the thalidomide disaster in the early 1960s. Good data on most drugs to which pregnant women may be exposed are not available. Unfortunately, because exposures may be rare and outcomes not reported, recognition of potential human teratogens may take years. Only a few of those drugs recognized as teratogens are discussed here.

The recognition of the adverse affects of **alcohol** on fetal growth and development was delayed for many years, in part because the effects on the fetus are diverse and the major effects are functional (ie, on the central nervous system). Infants with full-blown fetal alcohol syndrome are typically born to chronically alcoholic women who have a 40–50% risk of having infants with severe problems in growth and development. The full-blown syndrome is characterized by a distinctive facial appearance, with short palpebral fissures and long philtrum; prenatal onset growth deficiency; and an increased frequency of congenital abnormalities of the heart, skeleton, joints, and palate. The face, which may be characteristic in the young child, tends to normalize with time, making recognition in the adult difficult. Mental deficiency and learning disabilities, however, do not disappear with time. Consumption of alcohol by pregnant women is a significant public health concern and has led to warning labels on alcoholic beverages and in restaurants and bars. These warnings are perhaps effective for some portions of society, but for those women in which a pattern of heavy drinking has long been established, such measures may have little effect.

Pregnant women usually receive **anticoagulants** because of the presence of prosthetic heart valves or thrombophlebitis. Coumadin derivatives, particularly warfarin, are associated with an approximately 33% risk of death or malformations in infants exposed in the first trimester. The crucial period appears to be 6–9 weeks after conception. The facial and skeletal features resemble those seen in chondrodysplasia punctata, with stippling (like paint spatters) seen radiographically. Children may have severe nasal hypoplasia, occasional choanal atresia, microcephaly, absence of the corpus callosum, and ocular defects. Some survivors with major craniofacial involvement are mentally normal. The use of heparin is not thought to be teratogenic, but there is an increased risk of fetal loss with an approximate 15% rate of stillbirth and a 20% rate of prematurity. Overall, carefully monitored heparin administration is probably safer for the woman who must have continuous anticoagulation.

Women treated with **anticonvulsants** during pregnancy are clearly at increased risk for serious adverse fetal effects. How much of this risk is attributable directly to anticonvulsants is not clear, as the underlying seizure disorder or the mother's reason for seizures may contribute to the risk. Nonetheless, the pattern of anomalies associated with individual anticonvulsants supports the concept that these drugs are directly related to the adverse outcome. All of the anticonvulsant drugs, with the possible exceptions of phenobarbital and Mysoline, have been associated with significant teratogenic risks. The best studied of these, diphenylhydantoin (Dilantin), produces a recognizable pattern of defects in approximately 10% of exposed infants. Findings include underdevelopment of the midface, flat nasal bridge, occasional growth deficiency, increased risk of cleft lip or cleft palate, and hypoplasia of the distal phalanges with notably small nails. Overt mental deficiency is rare, but learning disabilities are frequent.

Valproic acid (Depakene) and carbamazepine (Tegretol) are both associated with an approximately 1% risk of neural tube defects. A specific pattern of minor facial anomalies, genital abnormalities, cardiac defects, and learning problems has also been recognized. Trimethadione (Zarontin) and related anticonvulsant drugs are significantly teratogenic. Exposed children have characteristic faces with V-shaped eyebrows, overturned ear helices, and a short upturned nose. Although no anticonvulsant drugs are "safe," this particular class of drug should be rigorously avoided during pregnancy.

Excessive doses of **vitamin A** and other **retinoids** have long been known to cause birth defects, but the recently released drug isotretinoin (Accutane) has been clearly established as a new human teratogen. Isotretinoin is used for cystic acne. The group most likely to use this drug are teenagers who are also at an increased risk for unplanned pregnancy. The highest fetal risk is associated with exposure at 2–5 fetal weeks, and the pattern of anomalies is characteristic, including microcephaly with serious central nervous system abnormalities, conotruncal cardiac abnormalities, and malformations of the ear. Death in infancy is common, and survivors have a high incidence of mental retardation. Isotretinoin has a relatively short half-life, but another related drug, etretinate, has a half-life of weeks to months. Children born long after this drug has been discontinued show characteristic birth defects. Use of reliable birth control is imperative in women being treated with these agents, and etretinate should be avoided entirely in women of reproductive age.

Cocaine is the most widely used illicit drug in the reproductive age group. Numerous adverse effects have been demonstrated in human pregnancy, including increased rates of spontaneous abortion, abruptio placenta, and premature delivery. The effects on the newborn include an increased incidence of intraventricular hemorrhage, gastrointestinal and genitourinary abnormalities, and limb reduction defects. Long-term neurologic and behavioral sequelae of maternal cocaine abuse have also been reported. There may possibly be a fetal cocaine dysmorphic phenotype consisting of periorbital and eyelid edema, flat nasal bridge with transverse crease, short nose, and large fontanelles. It is thought that most prenatal problems associated with cocaine relate to vasospasm from the sympathomimetic effects of cocaine and subsequent vascular disruption.

MATERNAL CONDITIONS

Maternal Diabetes

Maternal diabetes is a known human teratogen. It has been assumed that only women with insulin-dependent diabetes have an increased risk for fetal anomalies, but recent evidence suggests that women with gestational diabetes may also have some increased risk. When women have diabetes at the time of their first prenatal visit, it is difficult to know the status of their glucose control during the critical first few weeks of embryonic development. The specific defects of caudal regression and sirenomelia are definitely increased in infants of mothers with diabetes. The risk of neural tube defects, holoprosencephaly, congenital heart disease, and cleft lip and cleft palate is also significantly increased in these infants. Although available data are inconclusive, careful glucose control during the early weeks of pregnancy is thought to lower the risk of fetal malformations.

Maternal Phenylketonuria

Maternal phenylketonuria poses a definite risk to the fetus. Women who were treated for phenylketonuria with diet restriction as children are now of reproductive age, and, in many, dietary restriction was discontinued after age 10. Thus, in the pregnant mother with phenylketonuria, the fetus is exposed to very high serum levels of phenylalanine, phenylpyruvic acid, and other metabolites. Twenty-five percent of exposed fetuses have congenital abnormalities, and 90% are mentally retarded and microcephalic. Women with phenylketonuria should be treated with dietary restriction before and throughout pregnancy. Early follow-up studies have suggested greatly improved pregnancy outcomes with appropriate dietary management.

PRENATAL DIAGNOSIS

Prenatal diagnosis offers parents and physicians an assessment of the status and well-being of the fetus before birth. Advances in cytogenetic and DNA technology, the development of high-resolution ultrasonography, and new obstetric technologies are allowing parents an ever-in-creasing range of informed choices regarding the unborn child. In the past, families either could accept the risk of a handicapped child or could avoid childbearing altogether. Prenatal diagnosis offers reassurance to parents in high-risk groups and provides couples who might otherwise not attempt a pregnancy with information about the presence or absence of the genetic disorder in question. When the fetus is found to have a serious defect, the parents may elect to terminate or continue the pregnancy. Even when termination is not an option, parents may use the information to be fully prepared for their child's birth and postnatal care. They may wish to meet with other families who have similarly affected children and are often referred to surgeons or other neonatal specialists who will be involved in their newborn's care. In more than 98% of cases, however, prenatal diagnostic studies provide reassuring information that the baby is not affected by the condition under study.

Indications

The prenatal diagnosis of many disorders, including cystic fibrosis, the hemoglobinopathies, and inborn errors of metabolism, is now possible with the use of molecular techniques. However, the primary reason for a woman to seek prenatal diagnosis remains the detection of Down syndrome. With advancing maternal age, the risk of a chromosomally abnormal fetus increases. For example, the chance for a 35-year-old woman to have a child with Down syndrome is about 1:250 at the time of amniocentesis. At age 40, this risk increases to 1:75. Because chromosomally abnormal fetuses have an increased risk of loss during pregnancy, the birth incidence of Down syndrome is somewhat less than the risk cited above.

Other indications for prenatal diagnosis include the following:

A Previous Child With a Chromosome Abnormality. When a mother has had a child with Down syndrome and is younger than 35 years, her recurrence risk is somewhat increased as compared with other women her age. A general recurrence risk of 1% is usually quoted. Parents who have had children with other chromosome abnormalities, such as trisomy 18, trisomy 13, and deletions, may also seek the reassurance that prenatal testing can provide, even though recurrence risks are usually low.

One Parent Carries a Structural Chromosomal Abnormality. In these situations, the risk of having a child with birth defects and mental retardation significantly increases. For example, if a mother carries a 14/21 translocation, her chance of having a child with Down syndrome is about 5%. The risk is less (about 2%) when the father carries this translocation. Many other translocations carried in balanced form pose a risk to produce children with phenotypic abnormalities and retardation. The exact risk for each specific translocation is different, but in all cases, parents carrying these rearrangements are at a significantly increased risk and are eligible for prenatal testing.

Family at Risk for a Genetic Disorder That Can Be Diagnosed by Biochemical or DNA Testing. This category includes multiple disorders, many of which are inborn errors of metabolism. Most are single gene defects, with risks ranging from 25–50%. The list of defects for which enzymatic or DNA testing is possible is presented in Table 5–14.

Family History of an X-linked Disorder for Which There Is No Precise Prenatal Testing. Fetal sex determination may help families make decisions or plan delivery strategies. Fortunately, the list of X-linked disorders for which DNA diagnosis is now possible is increasing so that families do not need to make decisions solely on the basis of knowledge of the fetal sex. However, it still may save time and expense if fetal sex is determined before proceeding with DNA diagnostic studies in disorders such as Duchenne muscular dystrophy and hemophilia A and B.

Family Has a Risk for a Neural Tube Defect. In general, only first- and second-degree relatives of infants with spina bifida or anencephaly are considered candidates for amniocentesis and determination of amniotic fluid AFP. Most infants with neural tube defects are born to parents with no positive family history. Testing modalities for neural tube defects are discussed below.

Techniques

Chorionic Villus Sampling (CVS). In CVS, fetal trophoblastic tissue is aspirated from the villus area of the chorion either transcervically or transabdominally. It is usually performed at 10–12 weeks' gestation. This earlier test offers a family more time to make decisions regarding possible abnormal results. Concerns regarding limb reduction defects as a complication of CVS have been raised in several centers. This risk, although very low, may be related to operative inexperience and hemorrhagic lesions in the developing fetus. Most of these complications have occurred in procedures done before 9 fetal weeks. A disadvantage of CVS is that the amniotic fluid

AFP value cannot be provided and mothers will need to undergo later maternal serum AFP screening.

Fetal Blood Sampling (Periumbilical Fetal Blood Sampling [PUBS] or Cordocentesis). This procedure is used to obtain samples of fetal blood directly from the umbilical cord. Indications for fetal blood sampling include rapid karyotyping, obtaining a fetal hematocrit or white count in selected disorders, and obtaining antibody titers in suspected fetal infection. This procedure usually is not done until after 18 weeks' gestation and carries an increased risk of miscarriage (approximately 4%).

Ultrasonography. This procedure has become increasingly important in prenatal diagnosis for assessment of morphologic abnormalities that cannot be detected by amniocentesis, CVS, or AFP testing. Fetal age, multiple pregnancy, fetal viability, and fetal sex can be identified with a high degree of accuracy. It is the procedure of choice for the diagnosis of most skeletal dysplasias, several renal diseases, congenital heart defects, and cleft lip and cleft palate. A list of selected defects detectable by ultrasound is provided in Table 5–15.

Serum Screening for Neural Tube Defects & Chromosome Abnormalities

Maternal serum screening is a noninvasive method of obtaining information about the fetus. As in all medical screening, the object is to identify in a healthy population those who are at a sufficiently increased risk of having a particular disorder to be offered specific diagnostic testing. In prenatal screening, the biochemical screening markers are used to select women who may be offered ultrasound examinations, amniocentesis, and other studies to clarify their positive screen test results. Prenatal screening was initially confined to detect neural tube defects on the basis of elevated levels of AFP. AFP is produced in the fetal liver and is found in small amounts in the maternal serum and amniotic fluid. With the use of additional analytes, maternal serum screening has been expanded to include risk screening for fetal chromosome abnormalities and third-trimester obstetric complications. The combina-

Table 5–14. Examples of prenatal diagnosis of metabolic disorders with enzyme and DNA analysis.

Diagnosis by Enzyme Analysis	Diagnosis by DNA Analysis
Galactosemia	Cystic fibrosis
Glycogen storage disease (II, III, and IV)	Duchenne muscular dystrophy
Citrullinemia	Hemophilia A & B
Maple syrup urine disease	Sickle cell disease
Methylmalonic aciduria	Ornithine transcarbamylase deficiency
Propionic aciduria	α_1-Antitripsin deficiency
Tay-Sachs disease	Lesch-Nyhan syndrome
Hurler syndrome	Charcot-Marie-Tooth disease
Hunter syndrome	Huntington disease
Adenine deaminase deficiency	Myotonic dystrophy
Hypophosphatasia	

Table 5–15. Indications for ultrasound prenatal diagnosis.

Previous child with abnormality
Skeletal dysplasia
Congenital heart disease
Renal disease (absence/polycystic)
Central nervous system abnormalities
Neural tube defects
Cleft lip ± palate
Syndromes without chromosomal or biochemical marker

Abnormal pregnancy
Polyhydramnios
Oligohydramnios
Twins
Decreased fetal activity
Abnormal fetal growth
Maternal illness (eg, diabetes)

tions of three different markers are measured in maternal serum: AFP, hCG, and unconjugated estriol.

Maternal serum AFP has been used to screen for fetal abnormalities since around 1972. The basis for this screening test is that the level of AFP, which is strictly a fetal protein, is elevated when there is an open or non–skin-covered defect, such as meningomyelocele, omphalocele, or gastroschisis. In these situations fetal AFP leaks across the exposed capillaries into the amniotic fluid and across the placenta into the maternal circulation. Normal ranges for AFP have been well established for the gestational ages between 15 and 22 weeks, the time during which most women undergo prenatal testing. Considerable efforts have been undertaken to define cutoff points at which a relatively low number of open neural tube defects or abdominal wall defects are missed so that large numbers of women do not undergo unnecessary testing for false-positive results. In general, a woman who has a high AFP level is referred for high-resolution ultrasonography, which can determine the presence or absence of a neural tube defect with great reliability, as well as detect other defects, such as omphalocele and gastroschisis. When a high maternal serum AFP level is unexplained, there remains an increased risk for prematurity and late fetal death. Maternal serum AFP screening detects about 85% of cases of open fetal neural tube defects, including about 80% of fetuses with open spina bifida and 90% of those with anencephaly. A combination of AFP screening and ultrasound will detect more than 99% of the cases of anencephaly.

Some years after the association between neural tube defects and elevated AFP was reported, investigators noted the association between low maternal serum AFP and fetal chromosome abnormalities. Using the maternal serum AFP alone, about 20% of all fetuses with Down syndrome could be detected prenatally. During the past several years, other serum analytes have been reported to improve detection of chromosome abnormalities, particularly Down syndrome. The most useful is hCG, which is elevated in pregnancies of fetuses with Down syndrome. The addition of the serum analyte unconjugated estriol has helped reduce the false-positive rate and has helped detect trisomy 18. With the use of all three markers, the overall detection rate for Down syndrome is 60%; this rate increases with maternal age to approximately 75–90%. This screening method, if applied on a population basis, could reduce the incidence of amniocentesis in women older than 35 years; at present, however, serum screening would miss a number of affected pregnancies. Amniocentesis should therefore remain an option for all women of advanced maternal age.

Much effort currently is focused on the isolation of fetal cells in the maternal circulation. In pregnancy, small numbers of nucleated fetal red blood cells enter the maternal circulation and can be separated by sorting techniques. Once perfected, this procedure would allow determination of fetal chromosome abnormalities at very early stages of pregnancy without the use of invasive testing.

In Utero Fetal Treatment

Technologies for detection of fetal abnormalities have greatly exceeded our abilities to treat the fetus successfully. However, there have been numerous successful attempts at treating various conditions, and these are likely to increase in the coming years. Most of the conditions for which treatment can be considered are rare. Fetal treatment modalities are of several types, and the availability of these treatments underscore the need for early and accurate prenatal diagnosis.

Drugs. Occasionally, medications given to the mother can effectively treat a fetal condition. For example, when there is a fetal supraventricular tachycardia, digitalization of the mother may convert the arrhythmia. Other antiarrhythmic agents have also been tried with some success. Treatment of the mother with massive doses of vitamin B_{12} has been effective in prenatally detectable vitamin B_{12}-responsive methylmalonic aciduria. There are several other rare examples of treatment of this general type.

Transfusion. Fetal anemia is not an uncommon cause of hydrops fetalis and fetal death. Fetal anemia can result from several causes, the most common of which is fetal-maternal hemorrhage. Another relatively recently identified cause is hemolytic anemia secondary to maternal infection with human parvovirus B19. These fetuses are usually identified by ultrasound as having fetal ascites or hydrops. Direct transfusion of packed maternal cells via fetal vessels may be lifesaving. Such techniques are used only in settings with specialists highly experienced in reproductive genetics and fetal-maternal medicine.

Removal of Amniotic Fluid. Severe polyhydramnios may occur in a variety of clinical settings, and usually removal of fluid is indicated only for reasons of maternal comfort. Polyhydramnios is frequent in monozygotic twin pregnancies affected with twin-to-twin transfusion syndrome. This condition is often lethal. Several centers have reported improved survival rates with repeated removal of amniotic fluid from around the polyhydramniotic twin. Reasons for the success of this treatment are not entirely clear.

In Utero Transplantation. Bone marrow transplantation has been tried to treat several genetic disorders in children. Unfortunately, transplantation in the older child is often unsuccessful because of rejection phenomena. In addition, the transplantation may not have the desired effect because damage, especially to the central nervous system, may be irreversible. Before 22 weeks' gestation, the fetus does not have immunocompetence and therefore might be an ideal target for selected efforts in transplantation. Intraperitoneal transfusion of stem cells could genetically reconstitute fetuses affected with α-thalassemia, various mucopolysaccharidoses, and several other rare genetic disorders. To date, US federal laws have prevented full exploration of this exciting area of treatment.

Fetal Surgery. During the past several years, several centers have attempted direct surgical intervention for selected conditions—specifically, hydrocephalus, obstructive uropathy, and diaphragmatic hernia. Treatment for fetal hydrocephalus has been abandoned with the recognition that many infants with prenatally detected hydrocephalus have severe abnormalities in general brain development. Thus, even when their hydrocephalus is treated, mental deficiency remains. Surgical approaches for fetuses with urinary tract obstruction have included the placement of catheters in the fetal bladder to relieve distal obstruction and open surgery with the direct placement of small catheters in the ureters. Although these techniques are associated with significant morbidity and fetal mortality, there are several long-term survivors with good renal function.

REFERENCES

Cassidy SB: Uniparental disomy and genomic imprinting as causes of human genetic disease. Environ Mol Mutagenesis 1995;25(Suppl 26):13.

Curry CJR: Pregnancy loss, stillbirth, and neonatal death. A guide for the pediatrician. Pediatr Clin North Am 1992;39: 157.

De Grouchy J, Turleau C: *Clinical Atlas of Human Chromosomes,* 2nd ed. Wiley, 1984.

Evans CD: Computer systems and dysmorphology. Clin Dysmorphol 1995;4:185.

Graham JM Jr (editor): *Smith's Recognizable Patterns of Human Deformation,* 2nd ed. Saunders, 1988.

Hall CJ: Parvovirus B19 infection in pregnancy. Arch Dis Child 1994;71:F4.

Hall JG et al: *Handbook of Normal Physical Measurements.* Oxford, 1989.

Hanson JW: Teratogenic agents. In: Emery AE, Rimion DL (editors): *Principles and Practices of Medical Genetics,* 2nd ed. Churchill Livingstone, 1990.

Harper PS: *Practical Genetic Counselling.* Wright, 1988.

Harrison MR et al: *The Unborn Patient: Prenatal Diagnoses and Treatment.* Saunders, 1990.

Jones KL (editor): *Smith's Recognizable Patterns of Human Malformation,* 5th ed. Saunders, in press.

Kelly D et al: Confirmation that the velocardiofacial syndrome is associated with haplo-insufficiency of genes at chromosome 22q11. Am J Med Genet 1993;45:308.

Larson JW: Cytomegalovirus infection during pregnancy. Contemp Obstet Gynecol 1991;36:89.

McKusick VA: *Mendelian Inheritance in Man: Catalogs of Autosomal-dominant, Autosomal-recessive, and X-Linked Phenotypes,* 11th ed. Johns Hopkins, 1995.

Morrow B et al: Molecular definition of the 22q11 deletions in velocardiofacial syndrome. Am J Hum Genet 1995;56:1391.

Nichols RD: Invited editorial: New insights reveal complex mechanisms involved in genomic imprinting. Am J Hum Genet 1994;54:733.

Nora JJ, Nora AH: Update on counseling the family with a first degree relative with a congenital heart defect. Am J Med Genet 1988;29:137.

Prockop DJ et al: Molecular basis of osteogenesis imperfecta and related disorders of bone. Clin Plas Surg 1994;21:407.

Rimoin DL: Molecular defects in the chondrodysplasias. Am J Med Genet 1996;63:106.

Rose NC, Mennuti MT: Maternal serum screening for neural tube defects and fetal chromosome abnormalities. West J Med 1993;159:312.

Seaver LH, Hoyme HE: Teratology in pediatric practice. Pediatr Clin North Am 1992;39:111.

Shepard TH: *Catalog of Teratogenic Agents,* 6th ed. Johns Hopkins, 1989.

Spranger J: International classification of osteochondrodysplasias. The International Working Group on Constitutional Diseases of Bone. Eur J Pediatr 1992;15:407.

Tarleton JC, Saul RA: Molecular genetic advances in Fragile X syndrome. J Pediatr 1993;122:169.

Thompson MW et al: *Thompson & Thompson Genetics in Medicine,* 5th ed. Saunders, 1991.

Warren FT, Nelson DL: Advances in molecular analysis of Fragile X syndrome. JAMA 1994;271:536.

Wigglesworth JS: *Perinatal Pathology.* Saunders, 1984.

Winter RM et al: *The Malformed Fetus and Stillbirth: A Diagnostic Approach.* Wiley, 1988.

6

A Clinical Approach to Inborn Errors of Metabolism

John Christodoulou, MD, BS, PhD, FRACP, CGHGSA, & Roderick R. McInnes, MD, PhD

Inborn errors of metabolism are genetic diseases that disrupt normal metabolic function. Although the primary biochemical defect associated with a disease may not be known, there must be some knowledge of its associated metabolic abnormalities for it to be included in this group of conditions. This chapter describes the common clinical situations in which inborn errors should be considered and demonstrates that the clinical recognition of these conditions is not dependent on sophisticated biochemical analysis. Once laboratory corroboration of a suspected inborn error is obtained, however, optimal treatment often requires an uncommon degree of diagnostic precision, usually at the biochemical level.

More than 400 biochemically diverse inborn errors have been identified, but, despite their diversity, these diseases share a number of features. First, most patients with an inborn error present clinically with one of five general phenotypes (Table 6–1). Although these phenotypes provide a useful clinical guide, other clinical presentations occur, and some are specific to a single disease or group of disorders. Some of the most important of these distinctive phenotypes are listed in Table 6–1. Second, almost all inborn errors are recessive in inheritance, and most of these conditions map to one of the 22 autosomes; unless otherwise stated, the diseases reviewed here are autosomal recessive. Third, specific and effective treatment of inborn errors is often made possible by our understanding of their biochemical basis. Because inborn errors are genetic diseases, families with affected children can be informed of the risk of recurrence through genetic counseling. In many instances, presymptomatic treatment of affected relatives, carrier testing, and prenatal diagnosis can be offered.

WHICH PATIENTS MIGHT HAVE AN INBORN ERROR?

The crucial step in diagnosing any disease is considering the possibility that the patient may have the disorder. For inborn errors of metabolism, this step is particularly difficult for most physicians because few will have previously encountered a patient with one of these uncommon conditions. On the other hand, neither the patient with the uncommon disease nor the parents care about the rarity of the condition: They are interested only in correct diagnosis and treatment. These two difficulties can be largely reconciled if the physician recognizes that there may be a genetic basis to the patient's illness and that the clinical presentation is one commonly associated with an inherited metabolic disease (Table 6–1).

GENETIC EVIDENCE SUGGESTING AN INBORN ERROR

Two genetic clues should make one aware of the need to exclude a genetic disorder. First, a history of a similarly affected sibling or other affected relative strongly suggests a genetic disease. However, because most genetic metabolic diseases are autosomal recessive in their inheritance, there usually will not be any history of other affected members, apart from siblings. Second, if the parents are consanguineous (or if they come from the same small town or village or have the same surname), an autosomal-recessive disease must be carefully excluded. Although some cultures attach a stigma to consanguineous relationships, marriages between cousins are

Table 6–1. The common clinical presentations of inborn errors of metabolism.

Clinical Presentation	Diseases
Encephalopathy	
Acute encephalopathy	
Diseases of small diffusible molecules	Amino acid disorders (eg, maple syrup urine disease)
	Organic acid disorders (eg, methylmalonic aciduria)
	Fatty acid oxidation defects (eg, medium-chain acyl-CoA dehydrogenase [MCAD] deficiency)
	Hyperammonemias (eg, ornithine transcarbamylase deficiency)
	Lactate and mitochondrial disorders (eg, cytochrome oxidase deficiency)
	Encephalopathy with seizures (eg, nonketotic hyperglycinemia)
Chronic encephalopathy	
Diseases of small diffusible molecules	
Diseases of organelles	
Mitochondrial disorders: defects in pyruvate and electron transport bioenergetics	Electron transport chain defects (eg, cytochrome c oxidase deficiency)
	Defects of pyruvate metabolism (eg, pyruvate dehydrogenase deficiency)
Lysosomal storage disorders	Mucopolysaccharidoses (eg, Hurler disease)
	Glycoproteinoses (eg, α-mannosidosis)
	Gangliosidoses (eg, G_{M2} gangliosidosis)
	Other sphingolipidoses (eg, Gaucher disease)
	Leukodystrophies (eg, metachromatic leukodystrophy)
Peroxisomal disorders	Defects of peroxisomal biogenesis (eg, Zellweger syndrome)
	Defects of several peroxisomal proteins (eg, rhizomelic chondrodysplasia punctata)
	Defects of single peroxisomal proteins (eg, X-linked adrenoleukodystrophy)
Diffuse hepatocellular disease	
Acute or chronic liver disease	Defects of carbohydrate metabolism (eg, galactosemia)
	Defects of amino acid metabolism (eg, tyrosinemia)
	Defects of metal transport (eg, Wilson disease)
	Defects of protease inhibitors (eg, α1-antitrypsin deficiency)
Myopathy	
Skeletal myopathy	Acute rhabdomyolysis (eg, muscle phosphorylase deficiency)
	Chronic myopathy (eg, mitochondrial electron transport chain defects, fatty acid metabolism defects)
Cardiomyopathy	Lysosomal storage disorders (eg, Pompe disease, α-glucosidase deficiency)
	Disorders of fatty acid metabolism (eg, long-chain 3-hydroxyacyl-CoA dehydrogenase [LCHAD] deficiency)
Renal tubular disease	
Glomerular and tubular disease	Lysosomal storage disorder (eg, cystinosis)
	Enzyme defect (eg, oxalosis)
Transport defects	Defective transport of individual or groups of similar molecules (eg, cystinuria)
Disorders with distinctive phenotypes	
Hepatomegaly without dementia	Defects of gluconeogenesis (eg, glucose-6-phosphatase deficiency)
	Lysosomal storage disorders (eg, Gaucher disease [non-neuronopathic variant])
"Cerebral palsy" without a history of perinatal distress	Five different enzymopathies (eg, Lesch-Nyhan syndrome [HPRT] deficiency)
Stroke or thrombosis	Increased risk of thrombosis (eg, homocystinuria)
	Other diverse conditions (eg, MELAS syndrome)
Disorders causing facial dysmorphism or congenital malformations	Teratogenic metabolites (eg, maternal phenylketonuria)
	Impairment of cellular bioenergetics (eg, pyruvate dehydrogenase deficiency)
Premature atherosclerosis	Defects of lipoprotein metabolism (eg, familial hypercholesterolemia)
Menkes disease	A disorder of copper metabolism with a unique phenotype

CoA = coenzyme A; HPRT = hypoxanthine phosphoribosyltransferase deficiency; MELAS = *m*itochondrial myopathy, *e*ncephalopathy, *l*actic *a*cidosis, and *s*troke-like episodes.

commonplace in many ethnic groups. Marriage between first cousins almost doubles the risk of having a child affected with a genetic disease, from approximately 2% to approximately 4%; this increase always occurs with autosomal-recessive diseases.

Less often, metabolic genetic diseases are inherited in an X-linked or autosomal-dominant manner or manifest maternal inheritance. Disorders of the latter type are likely to be associated with a mutation in the mitochondrial genome, because only the mitochondria from the ovum—not the sperm—contribute to the mitochondrial DNA (mtDNA) of the zygote. Mutations in the mtDNA therefore are passed from one generation to the next strictly through the maternal line.

COMMON PRESENTATIONS
OF INBORN ERRORS

Five common clinical presentations (Table 6–1) should always suggest the possibility of an inborn error of metabolism. An important sixth category consists of disorders with distinctive phenotypes that invariably ought to suggest the possibility of an inborn error (Table 6–1).

ACUTE ENCEPHALOPATHY:
DISEASES OF SMALL MOLECULES

Encephalopathy is by far the most common clinical manifestation of inborn errors of metabolism. The encephalopathy can be acute, intermittent, chronic, or even nonprogressive (Figure 6–1), but only the inborn errors of small (ie, diffusible) molecules cause acute encephalopathy (Figure 6–2). Patients with acute encephalopathy are most often newborns or infants who have a severe enzyme defect that results in the accumulation of toxic metabolites early in life, although the small-molecule diseases may cause acute encephalopathy at any age (Figures 6–1 and 6–2). Consequently, the small-molecule defects must be excluded in any patient—even adults—with unexplained acute encephalopathy.

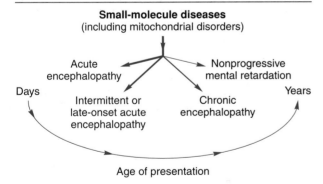

Small-molecule diseases
(including mitochondrial disorders)

Acute encephalopathy

Nonprogressive mental retardation

Days

Intermittent or late-onset acute encephalopathy

Chronic encephalopathy

Years

Age of presentation

Figure 6–1. Clinical presentations of inborn errors of small diffusible molecules. Acute encephalopathy is the most common presentation of the small-molecule diseases, as indicated by the thickness of the arrow, and is most common in the newborn or infant. The less severe presentations of the small-molecule diseases tend to occur later in life, even in adulthood. Less severely affected patients tend to have higher residual enzyme activity. The clinical features seen in the small-molecule disorders are due to an accumulation of toxic metabolites, a deficiency of a crucial product, or both.

CLASSIC CLINICAL PRESENTATION
OF ACUTE ENCEPHALOPATHY
IN THE NEWBORN & INFANT

Acute encephalopathy due to genetic metabolic disease usually results from a crucial accumulation of a small diffusible metabolite or substrate in the brain or from the deficiency of an essential product or transport process (Figure 6–3). Typically, the affected neonate will be well for several days to a week after birth, because the offending metabolite takes this time, or longer, to accumulate to toxic levels. Such infants are frequently discharged from the newborn nursery, apparently healthy, only to return— sometimes within 24 hours—with poor feeding, vomiting, lethargy, irritability, seizures, and, if metabolic acidosis is also present, tachypnea and hyperpnea. Cerebral edema is a frequent consequence of these conditions. Not surprisingly, given the disruption of metabolism, failure to thrive is invariably present in newborns and infants with small-molecule metabolic diseases that are severe enough to cause encephalopathy early in life. Hepatomegaly is also often present. The most common alternative diagnoses are infection and perinatal hypoxia, as well as trauma, intoxications, malformations, and malignant diseases. Failure to diagnose and treat the small-molecule inborn error, and reverse the acute encephalopathy, will result in severe neurologic damage or death.

Pathogenesis

Accumulation of Toxic Metabolites. The intoxicating molecules that accumulate in inborn errors include amino acids, organic acids, fatty acids, and ammonium (see Figure 6–2). Most small-molecule diseases affect "housekeeping" enzymes in catabolic pathways. Consequently, catabolic events, such as infections, will increase the amount of substrate delivered to the mutant enzyme. Other small-molecule diseases are caused by defects in the transport of small molecules across cell membranes. Although the enzymes implicated in these diseases are usually found in most or all tissues, they generally are most active in the liver. Hepatomegaly and signs of generalized hepatic dysfunction, particularly increased levels of serum glutamic pyruvic transaminase (SGOT; AST [aspartate aminotransferase]), and abnormalities of clotting function, are often seen. The involvement of the brain in the disease process reflects its vulnerability to metabolic disturbance, not necessarily the fact that the enzymatic activity is greater in the brain. As indicated in Figure 6–3, the substrate accumulation may inhibit other metabolic pathways to produce unexpected pathophysiologic and clinical effects.

Product Deficiency. The most serious disorders that result from product deficiency are those that impair energy production, ie, diseases due to defects in pyruvate metabolism or the function of the mitochondrial electron transport system. In contrast to most inborn errors that lead to acute encephalopathy, the pathophysiology of these conditions is probably associated with intracellular

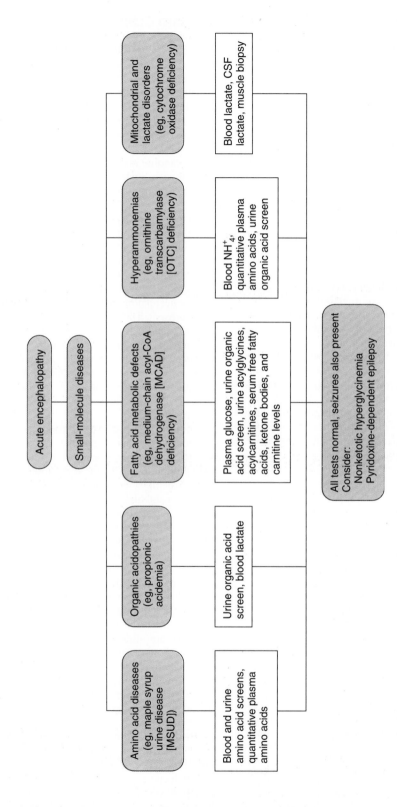

Figure 6–2. Biochemical evaluation of inborn errors causing acute encephalopathy. The four types of small molecules associated with metabolic defects that cause inborn errors are shown, together with the laboratory studies that are required to identify the diseases of each type. As the clinical presentation of these disorders is often similar, a series of screening investigations (square boxes) should be performed in all such children. CSF = cerebral spinal fluid.

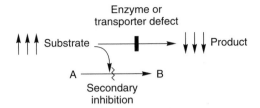

Figure 6–3. The pathophysiology of enzyme defects. The pathogenesis of all enzyme defects results from the accumulation of the unmetabolized substrate, the deficiency of the enzyme product, or some combination of these two events. The substrate accumulation may secondarily inhibit other metabolic pathways to produce unexpected pathophysiologic consequences. The inhibition of urea cycle enzymes in propionic acidemia and methylmalonic aciduria exemplifies this phenomenon.

depletion of the product of energy pathways (adenosine triphosphate [ATP]), rather than with accumulation of metabolites.

Catabolic Stress Initiates Small-Molecule Metabolic Crises

Inborn errors frequently present in the newborn period because this is a time of substantial catabolism—the normal newborn usually loses weight for several days before anabolism dominates. The catabolic breakdown of protein and fat results in increased delivery of the metabolite to the pathway blocked by the mutation and consequent elevations of the metabolite levels. Infants who escape a newborn presentation (often because they have slightly more residual enzyme activity with a less severe metabolic block) may present after the postnatal period when they are exposed to catabolic stresses, such as increased protein intake (eg, by a switch from breast milk to formula) or breakdown of body protein due to infection, starvation, or trauma (including surgery). Moreover, most of the encephalopathic metabolic crises that periodically affect even well-treated patients with inborn errors are precipitated by catabolic stress. The parents of older patients often recognize subtle signs (such as changes in behavior) of impending metabolic decompensation early enough to prevent progression of the episode to acute encephalopathy.

ACUTE ENCEPHALOPATHY IN CHILDREN OR ADULTS DUE TO SMALL-MOLECULE INBORN ERRORS

A child or adult with a small-molecule disease may have good health for years or decades and then unexpectedly manifest the metabolic defect, presenting with an acute encephalopathy. These patients have sufficient residual enzyme activity to catabolize the substrate when they are in good health. In the face of a catabolic stress, however, the residual enzyme activity is insufficient to prevent substrate accumulation. How these patients escape the metabolic crisis in the catabolic newborn period or on other occasions in childhood is unknown, particularly as the later episodes invariably are precipitated by catabolic events, such as viral infections, which the patient tolerated previously without having a metabolic crisis. One example is the **intermittent variant of maple syrup urine disease,** in which the child is biochemically normal except when challenged by the catabolism of intercurrent illness, at which time ataxia and decreased consciousness develops because of an accumulation of the branch-chain α-ketoacids.

Occasionally a patient with a disease of this type may not present until adult life. For example, the initial presentation of the X-linked urea cycle disorder **ornithine transcarbamylase (OTC) deficiency** in a female carrier of the disease may occur after she has given birth—a time of great catabolism. Older patients with small-molecule diseases may present with ataxia, disorientation, or frank psychosis, as well as loss of consciousness.

The intermittent or late-onset forms of the small-molecule inborn errors are commonly misdiagnosed as **Reye syndrome** because of the presence of encephalopathy, cerebral edema, and mild liver dysfunction (increases in SGOT [AST], with fatty degeneration of the liver, and hypoglycemia and hyperammonemia). Thus, the diagnosis of Reye syndrome should be made only after the exclusion of small-molecule inborn errors.

LABORATORY STUDIES TO EXCLUDE SMALL-MOLECULE DISEASES

Any newborn or infant with acute encephalopathy must quickly undergo investigations to exclude genetic metabolic conditions, because aggressive treatment is required to minimize permanent brain damage. The difficulty in remembering to consider genetic metabolic diseases is well illustrated here: Unresponsiveness and seizures are common in newborns, and the cause usually is not a genetic metabolic defect. Nevertheless, inborn errors must be excluded quickly by initiating the investigations outlined in Figure 6–2. Despite the variety of metabolic defects that may produce acute encephalopathy in the newborn and infant, the clinical presentation is often so similar that it is not possible to make a specific diagnosis without the aid of laboratory studies (Figure 6–2).

THE SMALL-MOLECULE INBORN ERRORS THAT CAUSE ACUTE ENCEPHALOPATHY

Aminoacidopathies

One group of inborn errors results from abnormalities in the metabolism or transport of amino acids. Amino acids are essential for protein synthesis. Once the anabolic needs are met, the surplus is degraded and used for energy. Intake of the amino acid at a rate that exceeds the capacity of the pathway affected by the mutation will lead to accumulation of the toxic metabolite. A classic disease of amino acid catabolism that causes acute encephalopathy is **maple syrup urine disease (MSUD).** The unusual urinary odor is derived from the accumulation of urinary α-ketoacids due to the deficiency of the α-ketoacid dehydrogenase (Figure 6–4). The increased levels of the α-ketoacids, rather than the amino acids, are the cause of the encephalopathy; for this reason, this disease can be regarded as either an aminoacidopathy or an organic acidopathy. Patients present with the classic acute encephalopathy phenotype described above. Ketoacidosis (the three accumulating branch-chain ketoacids are shown in Figure 6–4) is the predominant biochemical abnormality, and occasionally patients have hypoglycemia. A widely used but nonspecific test that detects the presence of ketoacids, including those accumulating in MSUD (Figure 6–4), is the 2,4-dinitrophenylhydrazine (2,4-DNPH) test. This test also detects ketonuria of any cause. Although screening tests of this type are of historical sig-

nificance, the diagnosis of inborn errors causing encephalopathy requires the specific tests indicated in Figure 6–2.

Organic Acidoses

A defect in an enzyme that degrades an organic acid will result in accumulation of the acid, often producing acidosis. The major clinical difference between aminoacidopathies and organic acidopathies is the metabolic acidosis that often results from the accumulation of organic acids in the latter conditions. An organic acidopathy should be considered in any patient with a metabolic acidosis. The acidosis causes hyperpnea, a compensatory physiologic response. Most organic acidopathies are caused by enzyme defects in the catabolic pathways of amino acids, as shown, for example, in the later steps of the breakdown of the carbon chain of the branched-chain amino acids (Figure 6–4). The different catabolic pathways of the various amino acids result in the formation of many different organic acid intermediates. Two classic inborn errors of organic acid metabolism are caused by defects in enzymes active in the metabolism of propionic acid (Figure 6–4), namely propionyl-coenzyme A (CoA)

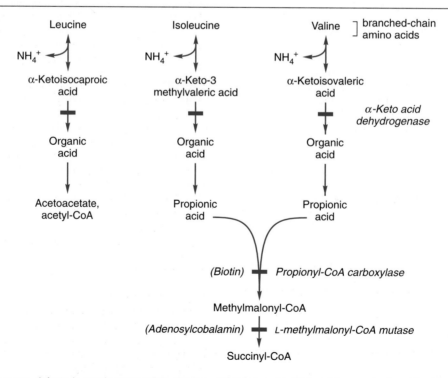

Figure 6–4. The enzyme defects in maple syrup urine disease and the organic acidopathies propionic acidemia and methylmalonic aciduria. Defects of many of the enzymes in these pathways cause organic acidopathies, all of which are autosomal recessive in their inheritance. The branch-chain amino acids are leucine, isoleucine, and valine. The relevant α-keto acids in this context are simply the amino acids from which the amino group has been removed. Biotin is a cofactor of propionyl-coenzyme A (CoA) carboxylase, and adenosylcobalamin, a vitamin B_{12} derivative, is a cofactor of methylmalonyl-CoA mutase.

carboxylase (a defect of which causes **propionic acidemia**) and L-methylmalonyl-CoA mutase (deficiency of which leads to **methylmalonic acidemia**). Propionic acid is a catabolic product of the amino acids isoleucine, valine, threonine, and methionine, as well as odd-chain fatty acids and cholesterol. In addition to having the classic encephalopathic phenotype described above and a metabolic acidosis, patients with either of these two enzymopathies often have moderate to severe hyperammonemia, the result of a secondary inhibition of the urea cycle by the accumulating organic acids. Less commonly seen are hypoglycemia, leukopenia, and thrombocytopenia.

The Anion Gap. A clue to the presence of an organic acid accumulation is an increase in the anion gap (Figure 6–5). A modest increase in the anion gap (up to 20 meq/L) usually is not significant in a patient who is seriously ill from any cause, but an increase greater than 20 meq/L requires that organic acid defects be excluded. Of course, most patients with an increased anion gap do not have an inborn error of metabolism; rather, they have an acquired acidosis, either from lactic acid accumulation secondary to hypoxia or from ketone body accumulation (ketoacidosis), as occurs in diabetes mellitus. On the other hand, a normal anion gap does not exclude significant lactic acidemia, as the gap remains normal until the blood lactate level exceeds approximately 6 mmol/L.

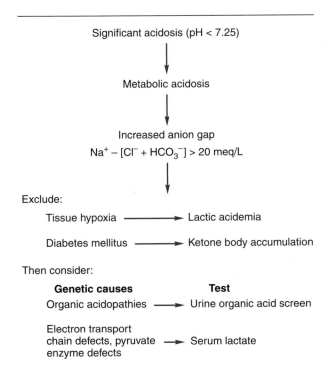

Significant acidosis (pH < 7.25)

↓

Metabolic acidosis

↓

Increased anion gap

$Na^+ - [Cl^- + HCO_3^-] > 20$ meq/L

↓

Exclude:

Tissue hypoxia ⟶ Lactic acidemia

Diabetes mellitus ⟶ Ketone body accumulation

Then consider:

Genetic causes	Test
Organic acidopathies ⟶	Urine organic acid screen
Electron transport chain defects, pyruvate enzyme defects ⟶	Serum lactate

Figure 6–5. Identification and investigation of an increased anion gap in metabolic acidosis.

Fatty Acid Oxidation Defects

A genetic defect of fatty acid β-oxidation (Figure 6–6) should be suspected in any child with fasting coma or lethargy and vomiting associated with fasting hypoglycemia; acute hepatomegaly is often noted. Alternatively, skeletal myopathy or cardiomyopathy may be the predominant clinical feature (see section on Myopathy). **Sudden infant death syndrome (SIDS)** also can result from defects in fatty acid oxidation; this group of metabolic disorders must be excluded in families with a history of SIDS or in patients in whom near-SIDS has occurred. As a consequence of prolonged fasting, hepatic glycogen stores become depleted, resulting in a shift by brain and muscle to increased use of the fatty acids liberated by lipolysis. Ketone bodies, which can be used directly by brain and muscle, are the product of fatty acid β-oxidation (Figure 6–6), but the decrease in their production in this group of diseases leads to hypoketotic hypoglycemia. Therefore, defects of fatty acid oxidation are usually exposed by fasting, a time when brain and muscle normally rely on ketone bodies as an alternative energy substrates.

Impaired fatty acid oxidation may result from a deficiency of the very–long-chain, long-chain, medium-chain, or short-chain acyl CoA dehydrogenases, or from any one of several other mitochondrial enzymes or transport functions essential for the transport of carnitine or long-chain fatty acid across the plasma membrane or one of the mitochondrial membranes (Figure 6–6). The most common defect in fatty acid oxidation, with an incidence of approximately 1/10,000–15,000 births, is **medium-chain acyl-CoA dehydrogenase (MCAD) deficiency.** The key diagnostic features of this disease, in addition to recurrent episodes of fasting hypoglycemia that usually first occur before age 2 years, are inadequate ketosis relative to the level of total serum free fatty acid levels (although some patients may produce moderate amounts of ketones in the fasting state), reduced levels of carnitine in body fluids, and abnormal fatty acid metabolites (organic acids, acylcarnitines, and acylglycines) in urine, detected by organic acid screening and acylcarnitine and acylglycine analysis (see Figure 6–2). Treatment consists of the avoidance of prolonged starvation. The value of a low-fat diet is uncertain. Carnitine administration may be beneficial, because the increased formation of acylcarnitines (Figure 6–6)—enhancement of a normal reaction—may augment the urinary excretion of toxic fatty acyl-CoA intermediates.

Hyperammonemia

An elevated blood ammonium level mandates that an inborn error of metabolism should be excluded as a matter of urgency, because ammonium is a potent neurotoxin. Moderate to severe hyperammonemia is often seen in the organic acidoses and fatty acid oxidation defects, reflecting a secondary inhibition of the urea cycle by the accumulating metabolites of those disorders. Genetic defects of ureagenesis (Figure 6–7A) most often present in the first week after birth. The most common such defect is OTC deficiency, an X-linked disorder that often manifests

Cytosol

Mitochondrial matrix

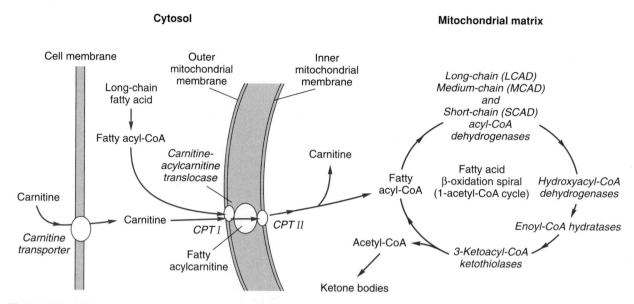

Figure 6–6. Transport and metabolism of fatty acids. To cross the mitochondrial membrane, long-chain fatty acids must be ligated to carnitine by carnitine palmitoyltransferase I (CPT I) and transferred by a translocase. Carnitine palmitoyltransferase II (CPT II) releases the acyl group from carnitine into the mitochondrial matrix. Medium- and short-chain fatty acids can enter the mitochondria freely and do not require the carnitine system. Fatty acids are oxidized in a cycle that removes one acetyl-coenzyme A (CoA) moiety per turn. Dehydrogenases specific to very-long-, long-, medium-, and short-chain fatty acids catalyze the first reaction. As described in the text, defects have been found in many of the transporters and enzymes shown. Ketone bodies are formed in the liver from acetyl-CoA moieties. All defects of fatty acid oxidation are inherited as autosomal-recessive diseases.

in carrier females and is usually very severe in affected males. Affected infants are well for the first day after birth; however, acute encephalopathy then develops, often within 24–48 hours but sometimes not until a week.

Two clinical clues of hyperammonemia in neonates are **respiratory alkalosis,** caused by stimulation of the respiratory center by ammonium, and **pulmonary hemorrhage,** caused by an unknown mechanism. Survivors in whom the disorder is diagnosed late are invariably neurologically impaired and are at risk for further encephalopathic episodes after excessive protein intake or during catabolic periods. Long-term treatment is directed toward reducing protein intake, giving urea cycle intermediates to replenish the cycle (eg, arginine administration in patients with argininosuccinate synthase and lyase deficiencies (Figure 6–7A)), and providing alternative pathways of ammonium excretion (Figure 6–7B).

Transient hyperammonemia of the newborn (THAN) is an acquired form of newborn hyperammonemia of unknown cause. It is observed in premature or low-birth-weight newborns, often in the presence of pulmonary disease. The other major clue to the diagnosis is the early postnatal onset of the hyperammonemia and encephalopathy, usually within 24 hours of birth, in contrast to the urea cycle defects. The elevation of ammonium can be as high as that seen in the most severe urea cycle defects (up to 2500 µM). There are no specific biochemical markers. The condition must be treated in the short term, as with a urea cycle defect (see below).

Lactic Acidosis: Defects in Three Classes of Enzymes

Inherited defects of pyruvate metabolism or of the mitochondrial electron transport chain should be suspected in any infant with the combination of acute encephalopathy and lactic acidosis, if poor tissue perfusion due to cardiac or pulmonary disease or some other cause of shock can be excluded as the acquired cause of increased lactate (Figure 6–8). Three classes of inherited diseases may be associated with encephalopathy (acute or chronic) and elevated levels of lactate. In addition, any metabolic defect severe enough to cause acute encephalopathy usually will be severe enough to elevate the lactate to levels that will cause metabolic acidosis and an increased anion gap. Occasionally, however, the acidosis may be mild and the anion gap normal.

Class I: Disorders of Pyruvate & Citric Acid Cycle Enzymes. Defects in enzymes that link glycolysis with the citric acid cycle, such as pyruvate dehydrogenase (PDH) or pyruvate carboxylase (PC), or enzymopathies of the citric acid cycle itself, are usually associated with severe impairment of neurologic function. PDH or PC deficiency always must be considered in the presence of elevated blood (or cerebrospinal fluid [CSF]) lactate lev-

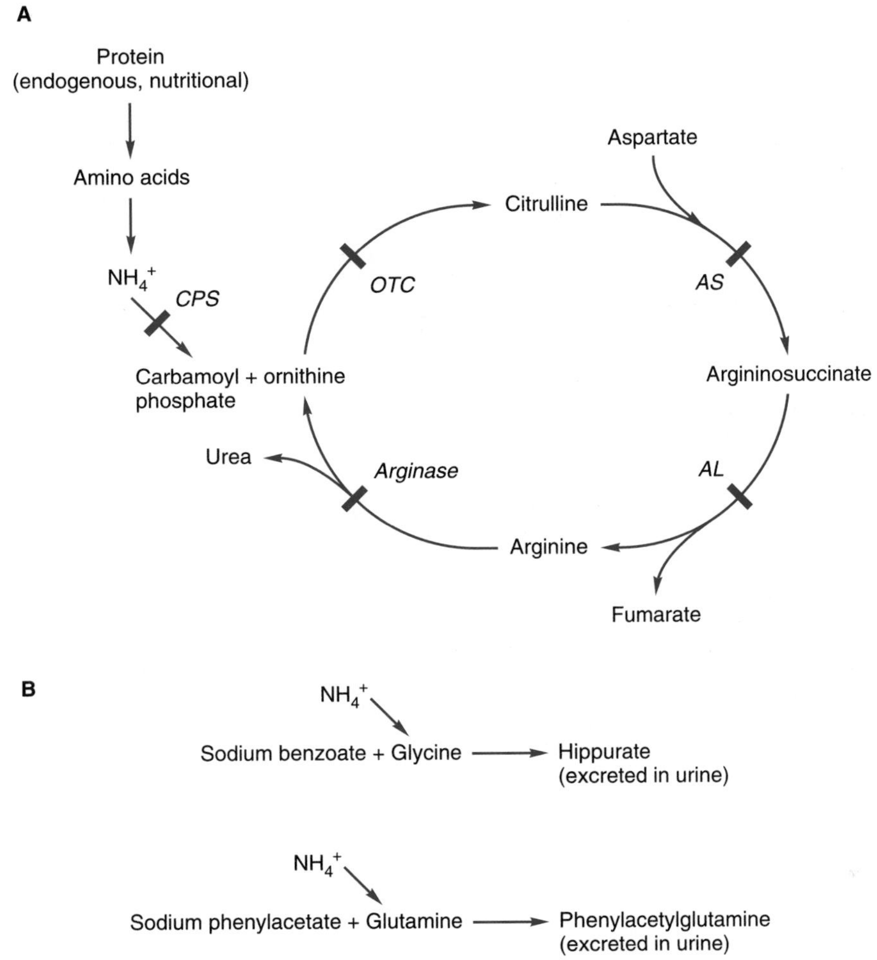

Figure 6–7. *A:* The urea cycle. The urea cycle converts ammonium, which is neurotoxic, to urea, which is nontoxic and excretable. In carbamoyl phosphate synthase (CPS) deficiency and ornithine transcarbamylase (OTC) deficiency, none of the amino acid intermediates of the cycle is increased. Citrullinemia is characteristic of argininosuccinate synthase (AS) deficiency, argininosuccinic aciduria of argininosuccinate lyase (AL) deficiency, and hyperargininemia of arginase deficiency. All defects of the urea cycle are autosomal-recessive, except for OTC deficiency, which is X-linked recessive. OTC carrier females may be affected. ***B:*** Treatment of hyperammonemia by using alternate pathways for the elimination of ammonium. Ammonium excretion can be enhanced very effectively by the administration of sodium benzoate and sodium phenylacetate. These compounds are conjugated to amino acids (glycine and glutamine, respectively), which therefore must be synthesized de novo to maintain normal body levels, consuming ammonium in the process. The products of the above reactions, hippurate and phenylacetylglutamine, are harmless excretable metabolites. For each mole of hippurate excreted, one mole of ammonium is consumed, and for each mole of phenylacetate used, 2 moles of ammonium are removed. These treatments are used both acutely and in long-term management.

els. Defects in the enzymes of the citric acid cycle are suggested by metabolic acidosis, and urine organic acid screen will reveal the identity of the accumulating organic acid (eg, fumarate in fumarase deficiency [Figure 6–8]). Enzymatic assay is required to confirm the specific diagnosis.

Class II: Defects of Gluconeogenesis. The second group comprises abnormalities in the enzymes of gluconeogenesis (Figure 6–8). Many of the reactions of glycol-

ysis can be reversed for gluconeogenesis, but four enzymes are unique to gluconeogenesis: PC, phosphoenolpyruvate carboxykinase (PEPCK), fructose 1,6 diphosphatase (F-1,6-diPase), and glucose-6-phosphatase (G-6-Pase) (Figure 6–8). Because gluconeogenesis (the formation of glucose from noncarbohydrate sources) is particularly important during fasting, the hypoglycemia that occurs with the defects of gluconeogenesis occurs only during fasting (although hypoglycemia is rare in PC

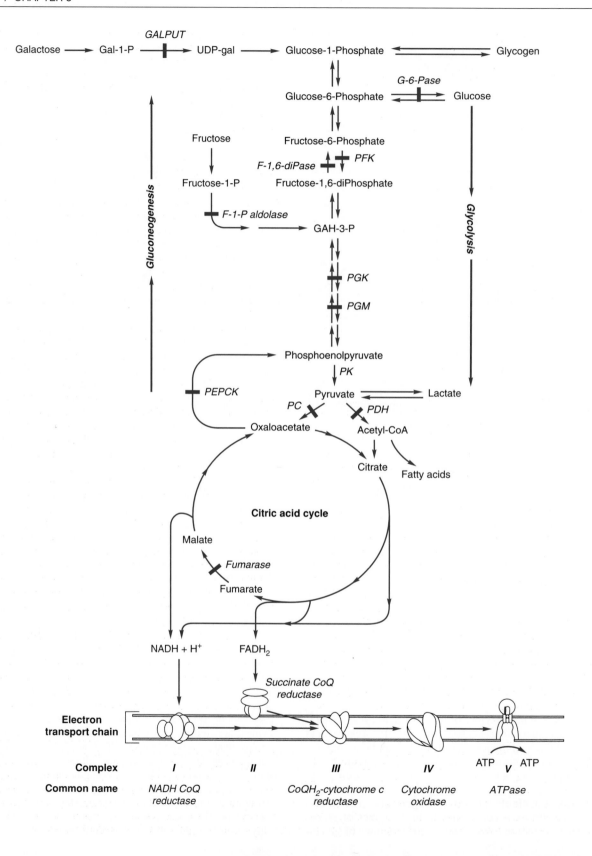

deficiency). Impaired gluconeogenesis leads to the accumulation of pyruvate (the initial compound in the gluconeogenic pathway) and therefore of lactate (Figure 6–8). Acute hepatomegaly is present, partly because of lipid accumulation from the increased fatty acid synthesis that is secondary to increased formation of acetyl-CoA from pyruvate (Figure 6–8). Ketoacidosis is often present, perhaps reflecting increased formation of acetyl-CoA and ketone body synthesis.

The most common of these disorders is G-6-Pase deficiency (von Gierke disease or Type 1 glycogen storage disease). These patients may present in the neonatal period with symptomatic hypoglycemia and pronounced hepatomegaly but only mild ketosis (a newborn with significant ketosis invariably has another serious genetic metabolic disease, such as an organic acid defect). Some patients present later in the first year with an enlarged liver, failure to thrive, and doll-like facies. Despite the presence of hypoglycemia, these patients may be asymptomatic because the brain has adapted to the use of ketone bodies rather than glucose as the primary source of energy. The diagnosis should be suspected on the basis of the hepatomegaly, increased lactate levels (usually with acidosis), hyperlipidemia, hypercholesterolemia, and hyperuricemia and can be confirmed directly by enzyme assay of liver tissue. Indirect confirmation can be obtained by the parenteral administration of glucagon. As shown in Figure 6–8, glycogen breakdown will increase the formation of G-6-Pase and ultimately of lactate, but free glucose cannot be released in the face of this enzyme defect. Thus, the designation of von Gierke disease as a glycogen storage defect actually is misleading, because it is really the prototypic gluconeogenic defect. Deficiencies of the other gluconeogenic enzymes share many of the features of G-6-Pase deficiency, although they may not be as dramatic in their presentation. The diagnosis of those deficiencies ultimately rests on specific enzyme assays.

Treatment of the gluconeogenic disorders during acute episodes centers on correction of hypoglycemia and acidosis. Long-term management aims to prevent hypoglycemia (and its attendant metabolic abnormalities) by frequent feeding, particularly of a slow-release glucose preparation such as uncooked cornstarch. With good metabolic control, the biochemical abnormalities return to normal, and growth is improved. The long-term prognosis is reasonably good, but hepatomas and glomerular insufficiency may develop in patients with von Gierke disease.

Class III: Disorders of Mitochondrial Respiratory Chain Proteins. The proteins of the respiratory chain (Figure 6–8) mediate energy production by mitochondria. Genetic abnormalities of these polypeptides may be associated with severe lactic acidosis and encephalopathy early in life, whereas less severe defects in electron transport can lead to chronic encephalopathy and other neurologic disturbances. This whole group of diseases is described below (see section on Chronic Encephalopathy due to Organelle Diseases).

Encephalopathy With Predominating Seizures

Four disorders—nonketotic hyperglycinemia, pyridoxine-dependent epilepsy, sulfite oxidase deficiency, and the molybdenum cofactor deficiency—are characterized by early seizures as the predominant feature and can be reminiscent of perinatal asphyxia, but without a supportive history. These disorders differ from the preceding ones, in which seizures often occur as a later and less predominant part of an acute encephalopathy. The screening tests for the other encephalopathic metabolic disorders are normal (see Figure 6–2).

Nonketotic hyperglycinemia (NKH) typically presents in the newborn period as a rapidly progressive disorder with profound hypotonia, progressive obtundation, seizures, and apnea, which is fatal without resuscitative treatment. Hiccups are a clue to the diagnosis. Survivors usually have profound intellectual handicap and poorly controlled seizures. This autosomal-recessive disorder results from defects in one of the four proteins of the glycine cleavage system (GCS) (Figure 6–9). Variant forms of the disease have been recognized, including a rapidly progressive disorder that first presents after the newborn period; an early-onset but slowly progressive disorder with moderate to severe intellectual handicap, with or without seizures; and a spinocerebellar degeneration phenotype with onset in the second or third decade. The diagnosis is strongly suggested by an elevation in the CSF–plasma glycine ratio and can be confirmed by measuring the activity of the GCS in liver or transformed lymphoblasts. Plasma glycine levels may be normal. There is no effective treatment, although the N-methyl-D-aspartate (NMDA) receptor channel antagonist dextromethorphan improves seizure control.

The classic form of **pyridoxine (vitamin B6)-dependent epilepsy** is a relentless seizure disorder that begins in the first week after birth (or even in utero). The seizures are poorly or not controlled by traditional anticonvulsants. B6-dependent epilepsy should be excluded in any infant or child with an unexplained seizure disorder. The diagno-

Figure 6–8. Inborn errors of energy metabolism. All the defects shown are of autosomal-recessive inheritance, except for deficiency of the E$_{1a}$ subunit of pyruvate dehydrogenase (PDH) deficiency and phosphoglycerate kinase (PGK), which are X-linked, and defects in the mitochondrial DNA, which are maternally inherited. Pyruvate carboxylase (PC), phosphoenolpyruvate carboxykinase (PEPCK), fructose-1,6 diphosphatase (F-1,6-diPase), and glucose-6-phosphatase (G-6-Pase) are enzymes unique to gluconeogenesis. ATP = adenosine triphosphatase; F-1-P = fructose-1-phosphate; FADH = flavin adenine dinucleotide reduced; GAH-3-P = glyceraldehyde-3-phosphate; Gal-1-P = galactose-1-phosphate; GALPUT = galactose-1-P uridyl transferase; NADH = nicotinamide adenine dinucleotide reduced; PFK = phosphofructokinase; PGM = phosphoglyceromutase; PK = pyruvate kinase; UDP-gal = uridine diphosphate-galactose.

$$\text{Glycine} \xrightarrow{\text{GCS}} CO_2 + NH_4^+ + C_1$$

Figure 6–9. The glycine cleavage reaction. Deficient function of this multiprotein complex causes nonketotic hyperglycinemia. Glycine is an inhibitory neurotransmitter. GCS = glycine cleavage system.

sis is based on the clinical and electroencephalogram (EEG) response to pyridoxine, which may be rapid (minutes). Even if there is no immediate improvement clinically or in the EEG, however, the patient should receive maintenance of B6 (75 mg twice a day for newborns) for a trial of at least 3 weeks. The site of the primary biochemical defect(s) is unknown.

A second group of children with B6-dependent epilepsy has other phenotypes. These children may have a later onset (as late as 18 months of age), they may be initially or partially responsive to other anticonvulsants, or they may have seizure-free periods without medications.

The outcome is variable. Some patients have had good seizure control and normal development, but many others have been intellectually impaired, although this may reflect late diagnosis.

A defect in an enzyme of cysteine catabolism, sulfite oxidase, or in the biosynthesis of its molybdenum cofactor, produces a remarkably similar phenotype, which most often has its onset in the neonatal period. Typical clinical features in the first 2 weeks after birth include refractory tonic-clonic seizures, axial hypotonia with peripheral hypertonia, and feeding difficulties. Infants who survive beyond the neonatal period have progressive destructive brain changes, choreoathetoid movements, and dislocation of the lens. Milder variants have also been described, with later onset of symptoms and less severe neurologic and somatic abnormalities.

Routine biochemical screening may miss these disorders, but dipstick screening of fresh urine for sulfite is highly suggestive. Specific testing of urine for increased S-sulfocysteine and thiosulfate levels is diagnostic. In addition, patients with the molybdenum cofactor defect also have low urinary and blood levels of uric acid because of the functional abnormality of another molybdenum cofactor–requiring enzyme, xanthine oxidase. The diagnosis of these autosomal-recessive disorders can be confirmed by enzyme assay in liver samples or cultured cells. There is no effective treatment for these disorders.

TREATMENT OF ACUTE ENCEPHALOPATHIES DUE TO INBORN ERRORS OF SMALL MOLECULES

Acute Resuscitative Therapy

The initial resuscitative phase of management must be initiated immediately, while the diagnostic workup is in progress. Initial treatment should include the following:

1. Good hydration and provision of fluid, electrolytes, and glucose (administration of the latter will help reduce catabolism). A useful initial fluid protocol is 10% dextrose in 0.2% saline, run at 150% of maintenance, supplemented with the daily requirement of potassium. This regimen provides approximately 9–10 mg/kg/min of glucose to neonates and infants. Fluid restriction may be necessary if cerebral edema is present.

2. Correction of the metabolic acidosis by sodium bicarbonate administration if the serum bicarbonate level is less than 15 meq/L. Beware of overcorrection: Stop once the bicarbonate level has reached 15 meq/L. Also beware of producing hypernatremia, although this may be unavoidable, and dialysis may be required.

3. Once these measures have been instituted, and even before a precise biochemical diagnosis has been made, begin hemodialysis or hemofiltration to remove the offending small molecule as quickly as possible if the patient is semi-comatose or comatose.

4. Provide specific therapy according to the disease, for example:

   • Nutritional modification, such as appropriate caloric supplements (eg, intralipid), and intravenous amino acid supplements free of the offending precursor amino acids (eg, leucine, isoleucine, and valine in MSUD [Figure 6–4])

   • Cofactor administration, which will sometimes improve the function of a genetically defective enzyme (eg, vitamin B12 in some cases of methylmalonic aciduria, because adenosylcobalamin is a cofactor for methylmalonyl-CoA mutase [Figure 6–4])

   • Metabolic manipulation, such as the administration of sodium benzoate in hyperammonemias (Figure 6–7B), to divert a toxic substrate to a benign excretable form

Dietary Therapy for Small-Molecule Diseases

Once the acutely elevated levels of the toxic small molecule have been reduced, dietary modification is instituted to maintain low levels of the toxic metabolite(s). For example, in patients with MSUD, leucine, isoleucine, and valine (all essential amino acids) are provided in amounts sufficient to allow normal growth. Levels in excess of this amount will be catabolized to form the toxic ketoacids. The objective of therapy, therefore, is to balance anabolic needs and catabolic capacity. Such diets are composed of an artificial formula of the other essential amino acids mixed together with other crucial nutrients (vitamins, minerals). The required leucine, isoleucine, and valine are provided by giving very small amounts of normal protein-containing foods, such as milk. Blood samples must be taken regularly to monitor the levels of the relevant amino acids. For many well-managed and compliant patients, the neurologic outcome may be normal or near-normal, depending on the degree and duration of the perinatal encephalopathy, the severity of subsequent encephalopathic episodes, and the quality of the chronic metabolic control.

CHRONIC ENCEPHALOPATHY: SMALL-MOLECULE DISEASES & DISEASES OF ORGANELLES

The dramatic clinical presentation of the acute encephalopathies makes it relatively easy to keep genetic metabolic diseases in mind when confronted with such patients. The diagnosis is difficult, however, in a child with the more common problems of slowly progressive or nonprogressive developmental delay or mental retardation or another chronic neurologic disorder. Although the etiology is often not determined in such patients, genetic causes must be excluded.

The inborn errors that can produce chronic encephalopathy can be divided into two broad groups: small-molecule diseases and diseases of organelles. The small-molecule diseases that cause chronic encephalopathy are of two types: the less severe variants of enzymopathies that are also associated with acute en-

cephalopathy (discussed above) and a quite distinct group of conditions, exemplified by phenylketonuria (PKU), that leads to chronic encephalopathy. The organelle diseases include the lysosomal storage diseases, diseases of mitochondrial energy metabolism, and peroxisomal disorders (Figure 6–10).

CHRONIC ENCEPHALOPATHY DUE TO SMALL-MOLECULE DISEASES

Small-Molecule Diseases That May Cause Either Acute or Chronic Encephalopathy

Patients with mild forms of many small-molecule diseases (Figures 6–1 and 6–2) may present with static or relatively nonprogressive developmental delay or mental retardation. Unlike patients who are more severely affected, these patients have avoided the extreme accumulations of metabolites, generally because they tend to have more residual enzyme activity. The evaluation outlined in Figure 6–2 for disorders of amino acid, organic acid, and ammonium metabolism should be completed on such patients. For example, with the intermediate variant of

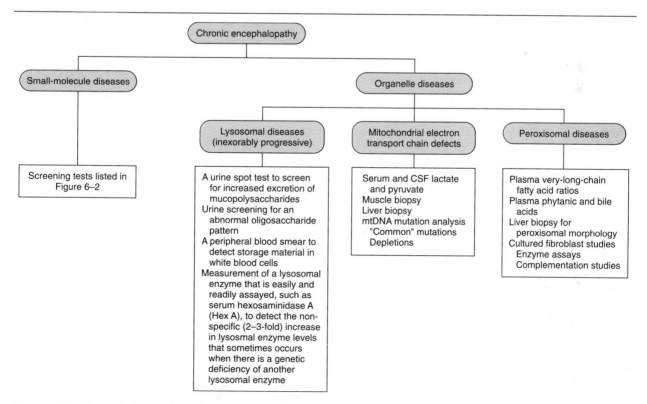

Figure 6–10. Biochemical evaluation of inborn errors of metabolism causing chronic progressive encephalopathy. CSF = cerebrospinal fluid.

MSUD, the amino and keto acids are chronically increased to a level that damages the brain but does not alter consciousness (except with a catabolic stress). Patients with less severe forms of organic acidopathies may never accumulate enough of the abnormal organic acid to become overtly acidotic; in those with mild urea cycle defects (eg, some carrier females with OTC deficiency), blood ammonia levels may be increased only postprandially (2–3 hours after finishing a protein-containing meal). A mitochondrial defect and disorders of pyruvate metabolism also must be excluded, particularly if there is any evidence of muscle weakness, by measuring serum levels of pyruvate and lactate. This latter group of conditions is discussed further below. Depending on the disease, patients with this group of chronic encephalopathies may have intellectual handicap, dementia, or motor deficits.

Small-Molecule Diseases That Cause Only Chronic Encephalopathy

Phenylketonuria. Some small-molecule inborn errors never cause acute encephalopathy but produce developmental delay and mental retardation. The classic example is PKU, which is caused by mutations in the gene encoding phenylalanine hydroxylase (Figure 6–11). Affected infants are normal at birth, but within the first 48 hours the plasma phenylalanine increases to high levels. This increase has no clinical effects in the short term, but the persistent elevation in levels of phenylalanine or its metabolites is neurotoxic, and the result is profound intellectual handicap, often with seizures and aggressive behavior. There are no other serious clinical manifestations. A diet restricting phenylalanine intake to the minimum necessary for normal growth prevents the intellectual handicap, provided treatment is instituted within the first weeks postnatally.

Newborn screening programs are widely used to detect PKU within the first weeks, with a dramatic reduction in the incidence of severe intellectual handicap. (Newborn screening has been initiated for other metabolic disorders, particularly congenital hypothyroidism, which is genetic

in origin in 10–15% of cases). Not all infants with increased postnatal phenylalanine will have classic PKU. About half have less severe disruption of phenylalanine hydroxylase function, and, provided that the blood phenylalanine level does not exceed a crucial threshold (probably approximately 400 μmol/L; normal, < 200), intellectual development will be normal. Such patients are said to have **benign hyperphenylalaninemia.**

Approximately 2% of patients with hyperphenylalaninemia have defects in the synthesis of the cofactor tetrahydrobiopterin (BH_4) or in its resynthesis from the oxidized form quininoid dihydrobiopterin (qBH2) by 4α-carbinolamine dehydratase and dihydropteridine reductase (DHPR) (Figure 6–11). Patients with hyperphenylalaninemia are routinely screened to identify those who have BH4 deficiency, because the treatment is very different from classic PKU.

Homocystinuria. A second important small-molecule disease that causes nonprogressive encephalopathy is the aminoacidopathy homocystinuria, caused by a defect in the enzyme cystathionine β-synthase (Figure 6–12). The clinical features of this disorder include eye abnormalities (high myopia, lens dislocation), skeletal anomalies (osteoporosis, Marfan syndrome–like habitus), and intellectual handicap; in addition, patients with homocystinuria are at increased risk of spontaneous venous or arterial thrombosis. In half the cases, the blood homocystine level can be normalized or greatly reduced by giving pharmacologic doses (up to 1 g/d in adults) of oral pyridoxine (Figure 6–12). Because the diagnosis (unlike that of PKU) usually is not made until the second year of life or later, attempts at dietary restriction of methionine usually are met with poor compliance because the older child finds the diet unpalatable. Supplementation with betaine, a methyl group donor that participates in the normal recycling of homo-

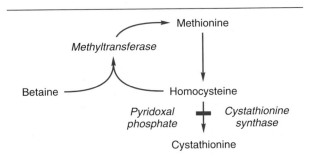

Figure 6–12. Cystathionine synthase deficiency and its treatment. Pyridoxal phosphate, derived from pyridoxine (vitamin B6), is the cofactor of cystathionine synthase. Administration of high doses of pyridoxine improves the function of the mutant enzyme in about 50% of patients with cystathionine synthase deficiency and is sufficient treatment for these B6-responsive patients. Patients who are not responsive to B6 patients are given a low methionine diet or high doses of betaine, which increases homocysteine methylation to form methionine, thereby reducing homocysteine levels.

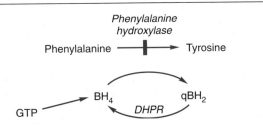

Figure 6–11. Phenylalanine hydroxylation. The conversion of phenylalanine to tyrosine requires both phenylalanine hydroxylase and its cofactor tetrahydrobiopterin (BH_4). Dihydropteridine reductase (DHPR) and 4α-carbinolamine dehydratase (4αCD) are required to recycle 4α-hydroxytetrahydrobiopterin ($4\alpha OHBH_4$) to quininoid dihydropbiopterin (qBH_2) and ultimately to BH_4.

cysteine to methionine (Figure 6–12), reduces the homocystine level, but its long-term efficacy remains to be established.

CHRONIC ENCEPHALOPATHY DUE TO ORGANELLE DISEASES

The diseases of organelles that must be considered in patients with slowly deteriorating or static neurologic dysfunction are those that impair the ability of mitochondria to produce energy, lysosomal storage diseases, and peroxisomal disorders (Table 6–1; Figure 6–10). As indicated in earlier sections, diseases of mitochondrial energy metabolism often present as acute encephalopathy, in addition to being responsible for much chronic neurologic disease. The lysosomal and peroxisomal diseases, in contrast, are usually associated only with chronic neurologic abnormalities.

Diseases of the Mitochondrial Respiratory Chain & Other Proteins of Pyruvate Metabolism

The major function of mitochondria is to produce energy in the form of ATP. Consequently, patients with defects in the respiratory chain and other key proteins of energy metabolism, particularly PDH and PC (Figure 6–8) often have abnormalities in organs that are heavily energy dependent, particularly brain and skeletal muscle; heart, kidney, retina, and other organs are less commonly affected. The mitochondrial respiratory chain consists of five major protein complexes (Figure 6–8), which together include approximately 70 different polypeptides. Abnormalities in the function of four of these complexes of the chain (Figure 6–8) have been demonstrated. Most respiratory chain proteins are encoded by the nuclear genome, and defects in these genes therefore are autosomal recessive or X-linked in inheritance. Defects in mtDNA, in contrast, are either maternally inherited or sporadic.

A wide range of clinical phenotypes have been observed in patients with diseases that impair bioenergetics (Table 6–2), but encephalopathy is by far the most common and obvious feature. **Leigh disease (subacute necrotizing encephalomyopathy)** is the most frequent of the severe bioenergetic disorders affecting the brain in infancy or later childhood. A progressive dementia begins within the first year after birth, in association with pyramidal signs, ataxia, movement disorders (dystonia, tremor), eye abnormalities (optic neuropathy, ophthalmoplegia, nystagmus, ptosis), and respiratory dysfunction (episodes of hypo- or hyperventilation). In addition, some affected individuals have a later age of onset and a more slowly progressive course. The neuropathology is characteristic, with symmetric regions of necrosis involving basal ganglia, pons, midbrain, thalamus, and optic nerves.

Many different biochemical defects of energy metabolism have been found to produce the Leigh syndrome phe-

Table 6–2. Clinical findings in patients with defects of mitochondrial bioenergetics.

General	Skeletal and muscle
Small stature	Hypotonia
Anorexia	Weakness
Central nervous system	Exercise intolerance
Neonatal acute	Rhabdomyolysis
encephalomyopathy,	Cardiac muscle
with severe lactic	Cardiomyopathy
acidosis	Cardiac conduction defects
Leigh disease (subacute	Kidney
necrotizing encephalo-	Renal Fanconi syndrome
myelopathy)	Liver
Developmental delay	Progressive hepatic failure
Dementia	Endocrine
Myoclonic seizures	Diabetes mellitus
Ataxia	Diabetes insipidus
Stroke-like episodes	Hematologic
(often reversible)	Sideroblastic anemia
Dysphagia	Neutropenia
Progressive external	Gastrointestinal
ophthalmoplegia	Malabsorption
Sensorineural hearing loss	Diarrhea
Retinal degeneration	
Optic atrophy	
Peripheral neuropathy	

notype, including abnormalities of the respiratory chain (eg, cytochrome c oxidase deficiency), mtDNA-encoded ATPase subunit 6, and PDH (Figure 6–8). The defect remains unidentified in approximately 60% of cases.

Mitochondrial DNA Mutations. Several more specific and memorable phenotypes have been found to result from mutations in mtDNA. The mitochondrial genome encodes 13 of the subunits found in four of the electron transport chain complexes, a complete complement of mitochondrial specific transfer RNAs (tRNA), and two mitochondrial-specific RNAs. In general, defects in the mitochondrial genome should be suspected in any infant or child with unexplained multisystem disease. The most notable phenotypes include *m*yoclonic *e*pilepsy and *r*agged-*r*ed *f*iber disease (MERRF); a syndrome with *mi*tochondrial *m*yopathy, *e*ncephalopathy, *l*actic *a*cidosis, and *s*troke-like episodes (MELAS); *L*eber *h*ereditary *o*ptic *n*europathy (LHON; late-onset optic nerve death, cardiac dysrhythmias); Pearson syndrome (sideroblastic or aplastic anemia, pancreatic exocrine insufficiency, and progressive liver failure); Alper disease (progressive infantile poliodystrophy; seizures in association with progressive brain and liver failure); and Kearns-Sayre syndrome (KSS; encephalopathy, ophthalmoplegia, ataxia, pigmentary retinopathy, and heart block). Some patients may have only chronic external ophthalmoplegia (CEO); in others, one phenotype can evolve into another (eg, CEO to KKS or Pearson syndrome to KSS). Single nucleotide substitutions of genes encoding respiratory chain subunits have been described in LHON and Leigh disease, and point mutations of one of the tRNAs have been described in the MERRF and MELAS syndromes. Deletions of mtDNA are the cause of Pearson syndrome, KSS, and CEO. Diseases due to substitutions of mtDNA are inherited maternally, whereas almost all cases of deletions in mtDNA are sporadic.

Blood & CSF Lactate. Many neonates with defects in the electron transport chain present with overwhelming lactic acidosis; in others, particularly those presenting later with chronic disease, the increase in blood lactate is often too low to produce acidosis or a noticeably increased anion gap. Thus, any persistent increase in blood lactate level (normal < 2.2 mmol/L) may be significant, and an increase in CSF lactate level almost always signifies a metabolic defect (except in the presence of meningitis); in some cases, only the CSF lactate level may be increased. Thus, a normal blood and CSF lactate level effectively excludes almost all bioenergetic defects.

Detection of an increased blood or CSF lactate level requires that attempts be made to identify the precise biochemical and genetic defects. This information may allow appropriate treatment and offers the possibility of precise genetic counseling and prenatal diagnosis. Muscle (usually of skeletal muscle, but of the myocardium if only cardiac involvement is suspected) and liver biopsy specimens provide tissue for biochemical and ultrastructural analysis. Structural abnormalities of the mitochondria are commonly found in these conditions. For example, ragged-red fibers have been found in the skeletal muscle of some patients. These fibers contain peripherally situated clumps of mitochondria that stain red with the modified Gomori trichrome stain used for light microscopy.

Lysosomal Storage Diseases

The lysosomal storage diseases are caused either by enzyme defects that impair the degradation of macromolecules in lysosomes or by disruptions in the efflux of molecules from the lysosome to the cytoplasm. Cell death results from the consequent intralysosomal "storage" of the undigested macromolecule or from the accumulation of a nontransportable substrate. Macromolecules are integral structural components of cells. The major function of the lysosome is to degrade such molecules, including gly-

cosaminoglycans, glycoproteins, gangliosides, and glycolipids (the latter two collectively known as sphingolipids) into their small-molecule components, which then can be recycled in metabolism and biosynthesis. In contrast to diseases that disturb the metabolism of small diffusible molecules, the pathology of the lysosomal diseases is restricted to tissues in which the macromolecule is normally degraded. Examples of lysosomal storage diseases include the mucopolysaccharidoses (MPS), the oligosaccharidoses, and the gangliosidoses (Figures 6–13 and 6–14). These conditions are all recessive and are either autosomal or X-linked in their inheritance.

Clinical Features. Most of these diseases are associated with clinically detectable storage in many organs and tissues. Clinical features often found (Figures 6–13 and 6–14) include neurologic deterioration culminating in dementia, coarse facial features, hepatosplenomegaly, retinal and peripheral nerve degeneration, and bony abnormalities collectively termed **dysostosis multiplex.** The nervous system is affected in most of these conditions and is the only affected system in many. Virtually any neurologic activity may be disrupted; the presentations commonly include seizures, dementia, blindness, deafness, ataxia, and hypotonia. Macrocephaly occurs in some of the conditions that affect the brain but is not a predominant or early feature in most of them.

The single invariant characteristic of the lysosomal storage diseases is their progressive nature. In many of these diseases, the deterioration is obvious from early in the course of the disease; in other instances, the deterioration may be much less evident, progressing with almost imperceptible slowness over years but eventually being undeniable. In obtaining the history, it is important to document the loss of developmental milestones or of intellectual or other neurologic functions to be sure that the condition is not static. A common diagnosis that can masquerade as progressive neurologic deterioration is uncontrolled seizures (pseudodementia). A complicating factor in considering this possibility is that many of the storage diseases are themselves associated with seizures.

Abnormalities diagnostic of storage diseases are often

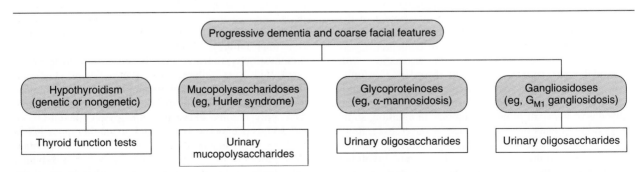

Figure 6–13. Biochemical evaluation of inborn errors causing chronic progressive dementia associated with coarse facial features. All these defects are autosomal recessive in their inheritance except Hunter syndrome, which is X-linked.

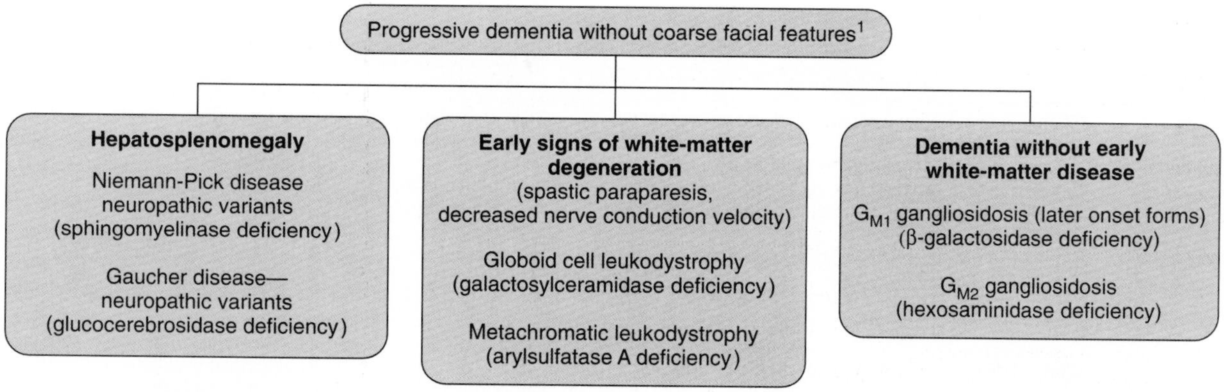

Figure 6–14. Biochemical evaluation of inborn errors causing chronic progressive dementia without coarse facial features. All these defects are autosomal recessive in their inheritance. [1]Patients with Sanfilippo syndrome have coarsening of facial features later in the course of their disease.

seen in the retina. Because it is the only clinically visible part of the central nervous system, it should always be examined carefully, preferably by an experienced ophthalmologist. Typical retinal abnormalities include the "cherry-red spot" (seen in Tay-Sachs disease and a few others), optic nerve atrophy, and macular degeneration.

White-matter degeneration is suggested by loss of peripheral nerve function (eg, hyporeflexia or areflexia), delayed nerve conduction velocity (NCV), abnormal auditory brainstem response (ABR) and visual evoked potential (VEP), and elevated CSF protein level. Gray-matter degeneration is more often associated with seizures and earlier loss of intellectual function, but both white- and gray-matter diseases eventually lead to intellectual deterioration. The EEG does not show a specific abnormality in these diseases.

Radiographs of the bones show changes of dysostosis multiplex in some conditions, most commonly in the MPS disorders such as Hurler syndrome. Features include thickened bones with coarse trabeculations and characteristic bone dysplasia, including the "beaked" vertebra, which results from hypoplasia of the anterior part of the vertebra.

If the clinical presentation, together with any of the screening tests (Table 6–3), suggests a storage disease, then specific enzymatic assays are performed, guided by the specific clinical findings.

Table 6–3. Screening tests for lysosomal storage disorders.

- Radiologic examination of skull, hands, vertebral column, and long bones
- Careful inspection of the retina and cornea, preferably by slit-lamp examination
- Nerve conduction velocity, ABRs, and CT or MRI scan for white-matter diseases
- Biochemical screening tests (see Figure 6–10)

ABRs = auditory brainstem responses; CT = computed tomography; MRI = magnetic resonance imaging.

Specific Lysosomal Storage Diseases.

Mucopolysaccharidoses. The MPS disorders should be considered in a child with coarse facies, mental retardation, or dysostosis multiplex (Figure 6–13; Table 6–4). Other common features include hepatosplenomegaly, thickening of skin and subcutaneous tissues, and reduced joint mobility. The six disorders are caused by abnormalities in enzymes that degrade glycosaminoglycans, which are macromolecular components of connective tissue. Phenotypic heterogeneity in the MPS diseases is broad (Table 6–4), ranging from a severe, relentless neurodegenerative and physically debilitating disease with progressive coarsening of facial features, as seen in Hurler syndrome; to disorders in which intellectual deterioration predominates, with initially little in the way of overt physical signs, as in Sanfilippo disease; to disorders in which intellectual function is unaffected, but severe physical effects occur, as in Maroteaux-Lamy disease and Morquio disease. Analysis of the urinary MPS pattern, followed by specific enzyme assay of leukocytes or fibroblasts, will establish the diagnosis. No effective therapy is currently available, although limited success has been achieved with bone-marrow transplantation in Hurler, Hunter, and Maroteaux-Lamy diseases. All the MPS disorders are autosomal-recessive in inheritance, except for Hunter disease, which is X-linked recessive.

Glycoproteinoses. In general, the glycoproteinoses resemble the MPS disorders, with coarsening of facial features, dysostosis multiplex, mental retardation of variable severity, and hepatosplenomegaly (Figure 6–13). In addition, some of these conditions have characteristic clinical features, eg, cherry-red spot and myoclonic seizures in **sialidosis** (sialidase deficiency), deafness in **α-mannosidosis** (α-mannosidase deficiency), and a telangiectatic skin rash, angiokeratoma corporis, in fucosidosis (α-fucosidase deficiency). Glycoproteins, which are widely distributed in the body, have a protein backbone, with

Table 6–4. Clinical and biochemical features of the mucopolysaccharidoses.

Syndrome	Clinical Features	Accumulated Substances	Enzyme Defect
Hurler	Coarse facies, corneas cloudy, dysostosis, dementia, hepatosplenomegaly	Dermatan sulfate Heparan sulfate	α-L-iduronidase
Scheie	As above but no dementia; normal intelligence	As above	As above
Hunter	Coarse facies, corneas clear, dysostosis, dementia (mild form has no dementia), hepatosplenomegaly, sensorineural deafness	Dermatan sulfate Heparan sulfate	Iduronate sulfatase
Sanfilippo (4 types)	Signs of "storage" only mild, difficult behavior (hyperactivity), dementia	Heparan sulfate	A; heparan-N-sulfatase B; α-N-acetylglucosaminidase C; acetyl-CoA:α-glucosaminide acetyltransferase D; N-acetylglucosamine 6-sulfatase
Morquio (2 types)	Skeletal dysplasia (including odontoid hypoplasia), normal intellect	Keratan sulfate Chondroitin 6-sulfate	A; galactose 6-sulfatase B; β-galactosidase
Maroteaux-Lamy	Skeletal dysplasia, normal intellect, corneal clouding	Dermatan sulfate	N-acetylgalactosamine 4-sulfatase
Sly	Coarse facies, corneas cloudy, dysostosis, mental retardation, hepatosplenomegaly; rarely, presents as neonatal hydrops; milder form has normal intellect	Dermatan sulfate Heparan sulfate Chondroitin 4-sulfate Chondroitin 6-sulfate	β-glucuronidase

oligosaccharide side-chains covalently attached; a series of enzymes systematically removes the oligosaccharides one by one. The urine of a patient with suspected glycoproteinosis should be screened for an abnormal oligosaccharide pattern, followed by specific enzyme assay in leukocytes or cultured fibroblasts. No specific treatment is available.

Gangliosidoses. The gangliosidoses highlight the important clinical principle that defects in a single biochemical function can be associated with extremely variable clinical phenotypes, although their common feature is progressive neurodegeneration (Figures 6–13 and 6–14). Neonates with G_{M1} gangliosidosis (β-galactosidase deficiency) have coarse facies, hepatosplenomegaly, dysostosis, cherry-red spot, and dementia; death occurs by 2 years of age (Figure 6–13). Patients presenting in later infancy or adolescence do not have facial coarseness or hepatosplenomegaly (Figure 6–14) and have only mild dysostosis; however, the neurodegenerative component remains prominent. Similarly, in G_{M2} gangliosidosis, the clinical phenotype is broad, ranging from infantile forms (Tay-Sachs disease [hexosaminidase A deficiency] and Sandhoff disease [hexosaminidase A and B deficiency]), to adult-onset variants. Specific clues suggesting infantile Tay-Sachs disease include an exaggerated response to sudden sounds (hyperacusis) and a cherry-red spot in the retina. In contrast to the storage diseases discussed above, coarse facies and hepatosplenomegaly are not usually features of the G_{M2} gangliosidoses (Figure 6–14). In the later-presenting forms, the course is milder, and the cherry-red spot is an inconsistent finding. The adult-onset form may have a psychiatric presentation or clinical features of a spinocerebellar disorder. Urinary oligosaccharides are not consistently abnormal; therefore, the diagnosis must be excluded by specific enzyme assays of serum, leukocytes, or cultured fibroblasts.

Other Classic Sphingolipidoses: Gaucher & Niemann-Pick Diseases. These two diseases are biochemically related to gangliosidoses (they are all sphingolipidoses) and have variants that also can cause progressive dementia. However, unlike many of the other sphingolipidoses, these conditions are not associated with coarse facial features (Figure 6–14). **Gaucher disease** (glucocerebrosidase deficiency), the most common of the lysosomal storage disorders, has both non-neuronopathic (most patients) and neuronopathic forms. The clinical features of the non-neuronopathic form result from accumulation of glucocerebrosides in the reticuloendothelial system. Consequently, the clinical signs, which can be extremely variable, include hepatosplenomegaly (massive splenomegaly may occur), pancytopenia, and degenerative bony changes. More severely affected patients have life-threatening anemia, thrombocytopenia, or liver disease, as well as bony "crises" similar to those seen in patients with sickle-cell anemia. In infants, the neuronopathic form of Gaucher disease is suggested by the triad of strabismus, trismus, and opisthotonus, occurring in association with a progressive spastic and seizure disorder. In both forms of Gaucher disease, the lipid-laden cells of the reticuloendothelial system have a characteristic "wrinkled tissue" appearance. The diagnosis can be confirmed by enzyme assay of leukocytes or cultured fibroblasts.

Bone-marrow transplantation has been used to treat the non-neuronopathic and the subacute neuronopathic forms of Gaucher disease, and trials are under way in the infantile neuronopathic form. An alternative treatment involves regular infusions of a chemically modified form of glucocerebrosidase, purified from human placenta. Initial trials suggest that this therapy has ameliorated the abnormalities in some patients, but further study is needed to determine whether this form of treatment will be of prophylactic value. In addition, gene therapy trials for Gaucher disease have recently begun.

Niemann-Pick disease is a second sphingolipidosis that has both neuronopathic and non-neuronopathic forms, but hepatosplenomegaly and lipid-containing "foam" cells in bone marrow are characteristic of both types. In the neuronopathic form, the neurologic deterioration is progressive but of variable severity and age of onset (Figure 6–14). Affected infants often have a neonatal "hepatitis," which is sometimes fatal. Some patients have a defect in the enzyme sphingomyelinase, which can be assayed in leukocytes or cultured fibroblasts; the defect in other patients is uncertain, although it may involve cholesterol esterification. There is no specific treatment for either form.

Leukodystrophies. The white-matter degeneration of the leukodystrophies is reflected initially by both upper motor neuron signs and peripheral neuropathy, first evident from reduced deep tendon reflexes (Figure 6–14). In the most common form of **metachromatic leukodystrophy** (arylsulfatase A deficiency), which has a late infantile onset between 1 and 2 years, early features include gait abnormalities, ataxia, clumsiness, weakness, and behavioral changes and developmental delay. Within a few years of onset, patients subsequently have spastic quadriplegia, optic atrophy and blindness, and dementia with seizures. Later-onset forms of the disease have a similar constellation of features, but the rate of progression varies. A second leukodystrophy, **globoid cell leukodystrophy,** or **Krabbe disease** (galactosylceramidase deficiency), has a similar array of clinical features. However, the onset of symptoms is usually within the first 6 months after birth, with rapidly progressive mental and motor deterioration and severe spasticity, culminating in a severe vegetative state with seizures, optic atrophy and blindness, and microcephaly in later stages. An unforgettable sign is that these infants are inconsolably irritable or "crabby."

In both leukodystrophies, NCV is delayed and the CSF protein level is elevated, although it may be normal in the early stages of the disease or in later-onset cases. Computed tomography and magnetic resonance imaging show atrophy of white matter. There are no screening tests, and confirmation of the diagnosis rests with enzyme assay of leukocytes or cultured fibroblasts. Treatment is largely symptomatic. Bone-marrow transplantation may ameliorate the natural course of the disease if performed early but is not curative. The γ-aminobutyric acid (GABA) transaminase inhibitor vigabatrin has been found to be effective in reducing the severe spasticity experienced in the terminal stages.

Peroxisomal Diseases

Peroxisomes participate in a number of unique anabolic processes, including bile acid and plasmalogen (ether phospholipids found in almost all membranes, most notably myelin) biosynthesis, and catabolic processes, including the oxidation of very-long-chain fatty acids (VLCFA) and pipecolic acid. More than a dozen peroxisomal disorders have been identified; on a biochemical basis, they can be divided into three groups, as outlined in Figure 6–15. Unfortunately, these diseases are almost uniformly untreatable. They are all autosomal recessive in their inheritance, except for X-linked adrenoleukodystrophy.

Clinical Presentation. The cardinal feature of most peroxisomal diseases is severe, progressive central nervous system dysfunction, usually evident in infancy. Other features that should raise suspicion of these diseases in early life are facial dysmorphism, hepatomegaly and liver dysfunction, hypotonia, renal cysts, and various ocular abnormalities. In older patients, the phenotype is more variable; in addition to the above findings, diverse manifestations of neurodegeneration, including ataxia and other signs of white-matter disease, may occur.

Group I: Defects of Peroxisomal Biogenesis. The defects of peroxisome biogenesis largely or completely impair the synthesis of structurally normal peroxisomes. Consequently, the activities of multiple peroxisomal enzymes are severely reduced. The classic member of this group is the **cerebrohepatorenal (Zellweger) syndrome.** Affected newborns have profound neurologic impairment, severe hypotonia and weakness, seizures, a typical facial appearance (including dolichocephaly, high narrow forehead, large fontanelle, epicanthic folds, external ear deformities), and eye abnormalities (including cataracts and corneal opacities), as well as hepatic dysfunction (particularly cholestatic jaundice) and renal cysts. More than half the affected infants have stippled calcification of the patella. Most die within the first 6 months. Other defects of peroxisomal biogenesis, however, may have limited facial dysmorphism or congenital malformations but still have a severe neurologic outcome, as seen in neonatal adrenoleukodystrophy. Mutations in at least 10 genes interfere with peroxisomal biogenesis, and 2 have been identified.

Group II: Peroxisomes Present, Many Enzymes Deficient. In some cases peroxisomes are present, but their distribution and structure are abnormal, and many, although not all, peroxisomal enzymes are deficient. One member of this group, **rhizomelic chondrodysplasia punctata (RCP),** presents in neonates with proximal limb shortening, cataracts, and severe dysplastic changes of endochondral cartilage; ichthyosis may also appear. Seizures may be prominent, and the condition is often fatal in early infancy. The primary biochemical abnormality is unknown, but unlike most peroxisomal diseases, VLCFA oxidation is normal. The incomplete pattern of enzymatic abnormalities differentiates this condition biochemically from the comprehensive defects of peroxisome biogenesis described above.

Group III: Defects of a Single Peroxisomal Enzyme. Some patients have a deficiency of only a single peroxisomal enzyme; the peroxisome number and structure are normal. The clinical phenotypes of this group vary greatly. Some of these infants are clinically indistinguishable from those with Zellweger syndrome, with a severe neonatal phenotype. One example is an abnormality

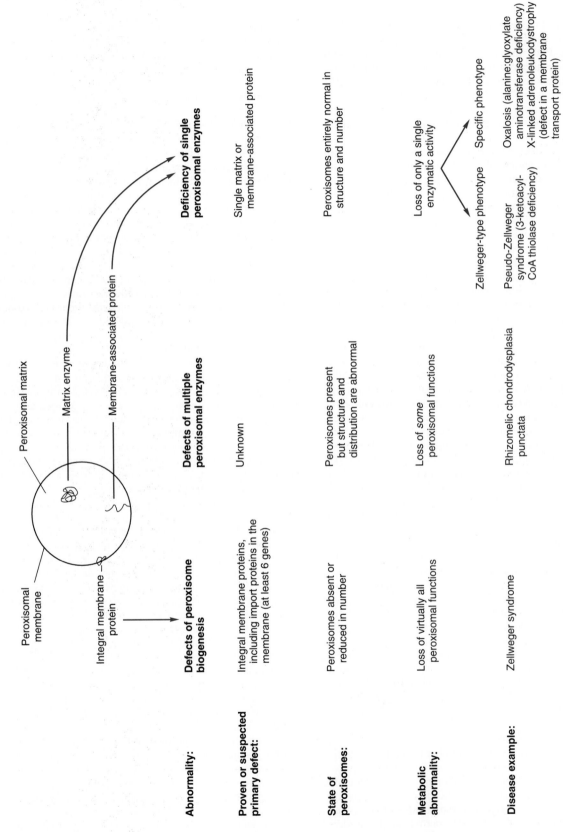

Figure 6-15. Pathogenesis of peroxisomal disorders. All defects are autosomal recessive in their inheritance, except for adrenoleukodystrophy, which is X-linked. CoA = coenzyme A.

of peroxisomal VLCFA oxidation, **3-ketoacyl-CoA thiolase deficiency** (pseudo-Zellweger syndrome). In contrast, patients with X-linked adrenoleukodystrophy may have a course similar to that seen in patients with metachromatic leukodystrophy. However, this disease also may present as behavioral changes and dementia in childhood or as spastic paraparesis in adolescents or adults; the degree of adrenal insufficiency is variable. Female heterozygotes of X-linked adrenoleukodystrophy may have neurologic disturbances. A peroxisomal enzyme defect that does not present in the newborn period, alanine-glyoxylate aminotransferase deficiency, causes hyperoxaluria and renal stones.

Biochemical Diagnosis. Patients with a suspected peroxisomal disease initially should undergo assay of plasma VLCFAs, which will show increases in most conditions (Figure 6–15). Plasma phytanic acid accumulates with time in many patients; plasma bile acid levels also may be elevated. Liver biopsy specimens are also useful in group I and II diseases, with electron microscopy showing absent or abnormal peroxisomes. The specific biochemical abnormality can be identified by enzymatic and immunologic studies of tissues or cultured skin fibroblasts. For other disorders, eg, hyperoxaluria, the diagnosis must be specifically considered, because the results of the usual peroxisomal screening tests are normal.

DIFFUSE HEPATOCELLULAR DISEASE

DIFFUSE LIVER DISEASE IN THE NEWBORN

A small group of inborn errors present with diffuse hepatocellular disease (Table 6–5). Three of these diseases—galactosemia, hereditary fructose intolerance, and tyrosinemia type I—usually manifest in the newborn period or infancy, but their presentation also may be later. Patients have hepatomegaly, jaundice (direct and indirect hyperbilirubinemia), a marked reduction of clotting factors (reflecting severe impairment of hepatic synthetic functions), increased liver enzymes (reflecting hepatocellular

Table 6–5. Important inborn errors presenting with diffuse hepatocellular disease.[1]

Disease	Primary Biochemical Defect	Hepatocellular Disease	Renal Fanconi Syndrome	Other	Laboratory Diagnosis
Galactosemia	Galactose-1-P uridyl transferase (GALPUT) deficiency (see Figure 6–8)	Invariable	Frequent	Retardation, cataracts,[2] hemolysis, *Escherichia coli* sepsis in neonates; hypoglycemia	RBC screening test and enzyme assay; urine reducing substances often negative[3]
Fructose intolerance	Fructose 1,6-diP aldolase deficiency (see Figure 6–8)	Invariable after fructose ingestion	Frequent	Vomiting; hypoglycemia; diagnosis often missed because history of fructose intake unrecognized	Enzyme assay of liver biopsy specimen; loading tests are dangerous; mutation analysis
Tyrosinemia type I	Fumaryl acetoacetate hydrolase (FAH) deficiency	May or may not manifest in neonates; inevitable	Inevitable; may be presenting feature in later-onset form	Occasionally no symptoms until teens; rickets	Detection of succinylacetone in urine; often extreme elevation of serum α-fetoprotein
α1-Antitrypsin (α1AT) deficiency	Mutations in the α1AT gene impair its hepatic synthesis or secretion	Cholestasis in some affected newborns; no liver disease in many patients	None	Adult-onset emphysema	PI typing of serum α1–AT
Wilson disease	Liver-specific copper transporter protein	Presents after ~ 6 y, not necessarily with liver disease	Variable occurrence and severity	Kayser-Fleisher corneal ring; hemolytic anemia; basal ganglia disease in teens and later	Low plasma ceruloplasmin; elevated urine and liver copper levels

[1]All five of these disorders are autosomal recessive in their inheritance.
[2]Only detectable by slit-lamp examination in early stages.
[3]These tests must be done before blood transfusion and at least 3 months after any previous transfusion. Urine screening for reducing substances is an unreliable method for excluding the diagnosis of galactosemia.
PI = protease inhibitor; RBC = red blood cell.

damage), and often hypoglycemia. The **renal Fanconi syndrome** is a feature of these three enzymopathies as well as Wilson disease (see below). This syndrome is characterized by the impaired proximal renal tubular transport of glucose, phosphate, amino acids, protein, bicarbonate, electrolytes, and other solutes; it can be detected by the increased urinary concentration of these substances, often simply by using a urine dipstick test. It is especially important not to miss the diagnosis of these four diseases, both because they are genetic and because they are treatable. In addition, defects of the mitochondrial respiratory chain, fatty acid β-oxidation, and Niemann-Pick disease may sometimes have neonatal hepatic dysfunction as a presenting feature.

Galactosemia. Many neonates with galactosemia present with gram-negative sepsis, well before the metabolic diagnosis is suspected; consequently, all newborns with sepsis should undergo biochemical screening for this disease (Table 6–5). Delayed treatment will result in mental retardation. The absence of galactose in urine (as a reducing substance) does not exclude the diagnosis, which can be done only by the red-cell metabolic or enzymatic assays. Galactosemia is effectively managed by dietary restriction of galactose- and lactose-containing products. However, despite early diagnosis and good dietary compliance, subtle defects in intellectual function frequently are present, and ovarian failure occurs in more than 80% of affected females.

Fructose Intolerance. Vomiting is the common presenting sign of fructose intolerance; in the infant or small child, vomiting is associated with hypoglycemia, gastrointestinal discomfort, failure to thrive, and rickets. The diagnosis of fructose intolerance is easily missed if a careful dietary history is not taken to establish that the symptoms began with the ingestion of fructose or sucrose. The most common sources are fruit, some proprietary formulas, and honey or sugar added to food. In older children with fructose intolerance, an aversion to sweet foods invariably develops. Fructose loading tests to demonstrate typical biochemical effects, such as hypoglycemia, are potentially dangerous and may not be diagnostic. Assay of the liver enzyme or mutation analysis of the fructose 1-phosphate aldolase gene is required (Figure 6–8); more than 95% of affected individuals have one of four mutations in the gene (Table 6–5).

Tyrosinemia. Patients with tyrosinemia type I who do not have acute liver disease in the first month present later, even after 1 year, with chronic liver disease or rickets caused by the renal phosphate loss. The deficient enzyme (Table 6–5) is in the tyrosine catabolic pathway. Dietary phenylalanine-tyrosine restriction improves the hepatic dysfunction in the short term, but liver transplantation offers the only cure at present. The drug 2-(2-nitro-4-trifluoromethylbenzoyl)-1,3-cyclohexanedione NTBC), which inhibits the enzyme three steps proximal to fumaroylacetoacetate hydrolase, namely 4-hydroxyphenylpyruvate dioxygenase, has been very effective in improving renal tubular and hepatic function. This drug should be used until liver transplantation is possible.

α1-Antitrypsin Deficiency. In contrast to the three conditions described above, α1-antitrypsin deficiency is usually associated with cholestatic jaundice. The liver disease improves without treatment in most patients, although about 5% progress to cirrhosis (Table 6–5). α1-Antitrypsin is a major protease inhibitor, and the most common disease-causing genetic variant, or protease inhibitor type, is the ZZ allele. The aggregation of this mutant polypeptide in the hepatocyte appears to cause the liver disease. The reduced secretion of the ZZ protein into plasma permits the unimpeded activity of neutrophil elastase in the lung. This process slowly destroys the alveoli, causing the most common presentation of α1-antitrypsin deficiency, premature emphysema in adults. Apart from hepatic transplantation, there is no treatment for the liver disease. Evaluation of the effect of regular injections of α1-antitrypsin on the progression of the pulmonary disease is under way.

Acid Lipase Deficiency (Wolman Disease). This disorder of lipid metabolism also presents with severe progressive liver failure within the first few weeks of life, in association with progressive neurologic deterioration. It is almost pathognomonic, with adrenal gland calcification detectable radiographically. The disease is usually fatal by 6 months of age. The enzyme defect leaves patients unable to hydrolyze cholesterol esters to free cholesterol:

$$\text{cholesterol esters} \longmapsto \text{cholesterol}$$

Diagnosis of this disorder hinges on having a high index of suspicion, as routine screening tests are not helpful. Liver histopathology shows characteristic abnormalities, and the diagnosis can be confirmed by specific enzyme assay in liver or cultured skin fibroblasts. Liver transplantation is effective in tyrosinemia but has been of no benefit in Wolman disease.

DIFFUSE LIVER DISEASE BEYOND THE NEWBORN PERIOD

Conditions Associated With Either Acute or Chronic Hepatocellular Disease. The five disorders discussed in the previous section (galactosemia, fructose intolerance, tyrosinemia, α1-antitrypsin deficiency, Wolman disease) can present as either acute or chronic hepatopathy. Wilson disease, a defect in copper metabolism, may also present with either acute or chronic liver disease. Unlike the above-mentioned conditions, however, the hepatic abnormalities in Wilson disease are rarely evident clinically before 6 years of age (see Table 6–5). The primary defect is now known to be in a liver-specific protein required for the biliary excretion of copper. The result is a damaging accumulation of copper in the liver and a secondary copper "spill over" to other tissues. Patients may have acute disease in childhood, with fulminant liver failure and hemolytic anemia, or may have more insidious disease in the second or later decades, with cirrhosis. After the age of 12 years, the presentation may be neurologic, with extrapyramidal or neuropsychiatric signs. The Kayser-Fleischer ring, a dull copper-colored granular deposit at the limbus of the cornea, is often seen. The diagnosis is made by finding low serum ceruloplasmin, high urinary copper excretion, and increased hepatic copper levels and can be confirmed by mutation analysis of the Wilson disease gene.

Conditions Associated Only With Chronic Hepatocellular Disease. Several inborn errors of glycogen and lipid metabolism are not associated with acute liver disease but cause a chronic process that ultimately produces cirrhosis. The classic example is **brancher enzyme deficiency** (glycogen storage disease type IV):

glucose-1,4-glucosidic ⟶ glucose-1, 6-glucosidic
linkages linkages

This disease presents in infancy with progressive liver failure and portal hypertension, failure to thrive, severe hypotonia, and absent deep tendon reflexes; most patients die before 3 years of age. Cardiomyopathy may occasionally be a prominent feature. The brancher enzyme is responsible for the transfer of glucosyl units from an α-1,4 to a 1,6 position in the glycogen molecule. Liver transplantation has been helpful in some cases.

MYOPATHY

Acute rhabdomyolysis, muscle cramps, muscle weakness and wasting, or cardiomyopathy, are the common presenting features of inherited metabolic diseases of muscle (Figure 6–16). Skeletal muscle relies on glucose as the major fuel for short-lived bursts of intense exercise; however, while resting muscle or during sustained exercise, free fatty acids are the main energy source. Consequently, defects that prevent the normal production or transport of these fuels (Figures 6–6 and 6–8) impair the function of skeletal muscle, the myocardium, or both. Myoglobinuria and elevated serum creatine kinase levels are the biochemical hallmarks of these events. As reviewed above, skeletal myopathy may be prominent in mitochondrial electron transport chain defects; infrequently, it may be the only clinical problem.

ACUTE SKELETAL MYOPATHY
(Rhabdomyolysis)

McArdle Disease & Defects of Muscle Glycolysis.
Recurrent rhabdomyolysis with myoglobinuria occurs with enzymopathies that reduce energy production from carbohydrate fuels. One major example is the glycogen

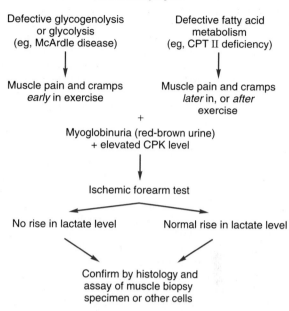

Figure 6–16. An overview of two inborn errors that cause acute skeletal myopathy. All the known defects are autosomal recessive. CPK = creatine phosphokinase; CPT II = carnitine palmitoyltransferase II.

storage disorder muscle phosphorylase deficiency (McArdle disease):

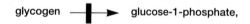

glycogen ⟶ glucose-1-phosphate,

Other examples include the defects of glycolysis, such as phosphofructokinase, phosphoglycerate mutase, and phosphoglycerate kinase deficiencies (Figure 6–8). The initial symptoms usually develop in childhood; pain, cramps, weakness, and myoglobinuria develop early in the course of intense exercise (Figure 6–16). Patients often learn to pace themselves until the "second wind" develops. The precise basis for the second wind phenomenon is not known but may be associated with the use of free fatty acids as fuel when exercise is sustained. Oliguric renal failure secondary to severe myoglobinuria must be prevented by good hydration and alkalinization of urine. Finally, mitochondrial respiratory chain defects may occasionally present with rhabdomyolysis.

Carnitine Palmitoyltransferase (CPT) II Deficiency. In contrast to defects of muscle carbohydrate metabolism, the initial symptoms of patients with CPT II deficiency (see Figure 6–6) usually occur both later in the course of exercise (when fat becomes the preferred fuel) (see Figure 6–16) and later in life. Patients with the milder form of CPT II deficiency (severe CPT II deficiency is discussed below) usually present after adolescence.

Weakness and myoglobinuria occur after prolonged exercise, particularly if there has been an inadequate caloric intake; other precipitating factors include exposure to cold, infection, and emotional stress. Muscle cramps are unusual, and the second wind phenomenon does not occur. For both groups of disorders, in most patients the physical examination findings between episodes are entirely normal, although some patients with CPT II deficiency have muscle weakness. Other disorders of fatty acid β-oxidation, such as deficiencies of long- and short-chain 3-hydroxyacyl-CoA dehydrogenase (LCHAD and SCHAD, respectively) or very-long-chain acyl-CoA dehydrogenase (VLCAD) (Figure 6–6) also may cause intermittent rhabdomyolysis, but these conditions usually have persistent muscle symptoms (see below).

Diagnosis of glycolytic defects (see Figure 6–8) and McArdle disease can be made by demonstrating that the serum lactate level does not increase normally during exercise, eg, during forearm exercise when the arterial blood supply is blocked by a blood pressure cuff (the ischemic forearm test). CPT II deficiency has no effect on lactate levels, but approximately half the patients have a delay or reduction in ketone body formation during a prolonged fast. Avoidance of extreme exercise is advocated for all patients with these myopathic defects. Treatment of CPT II deficiency includes avoidance of ketosis and other precipitating factors.

ISOLATED SKELETAL MUSCLE WEAKNESS

Patients who present with muscle weakness alone, or with a static or chronic progressive myopathy without myoglobinuria, may have one of the glycolytic defects, CPT II deficiency, a defect of one of the mitochondrial respiratory chain components discussed earlier, childhood or adult Pompe disease (see below), or one of a group of disorders that impair fatty acid oxidation and often cause cardiomyopathy (Table 6–6).

CARDIOMYOPATHY

Heart muscle is the principal tissue affected in Pompe disease, a classic disorder of glycogen metabolism. Dilated cardiomyopathy also may be a predominant feature of several inborn errors of fatty acid metabolism, although other features also may be seen initially in these conditions, as described above. The numerous diseases that may be associated with cardiomyopathy include glycogen storage disease types III (debrancher deficiency) and IV (brancher deficiency), defects of the mitochondrial respiratory chain, organic acidopathies (including propionic and methylmalonic acidemia), certain MPS disorders, and the carbohydrate-deficient glycoprotein deficiency syndrome (discussed below).

Pompe Disease (Glycogen Storage Disease Type II). This glycogen storage disease is associated with the accumulation of glycogen within the lysosomes of many organs, particularly the myocardium, skeletal muscle, and brain, because of lysosomal α-glucosidase deficiency (Figure 6–17). Glucose homeostasis is normal. The classic infantile form of this disease is characterized by development of congestive heart failure and extreme cardiomegaly, muscle hypotonia, weakness, and an enlarged tongue; the muscles often are hypertrophic and "rubbery" in consistency. The electrocardiogram (ECG) is character-

Table 6–6. Defects of fatty acid oxidation that cause cardiomyopathy.

Defect Impairing Fatty Acid Oxidation[1]	Presenting Abnormality					Biochemical Abnormalities	
	Cardiac Myopathy		Skeletal Myopathy		Fasting Coma	Abnormal Urine Organic Acids, Acylglycines, or Acylcarnitines	Plasma Carnitine
Carnitine cycle							
Plasma membrane carnitine transporter defect	+	and/or	+	and/or	+	no	↓↓↓
Carnitine-acylcarnitine translocase deficiency	+	and/or	+	and/or	+	no	↓↓
Carnitine palmitoyltransferase (CPT) II deficiency (severe form)	+	and/or	+	and/or	−	no	↓
β-Oxidation cycle							
Very-long-chain acyl-coenzymeA dehydrogenase (VLCAD) deficiency	+	and/or	+	and/or	+	yes	N or ↓[2]
Long-chain acyl-coenzymeA dehydrogenase (LCAD) deficiency	+	and/or	+	and/or	+	yes	↓
Long-chain 3-hydroxyacyl-coenzymeA dehydrogenase (LCHAD) deficiency	+	and/or	+	and/or	+	yes	↓

[1]Each of these biochemical functions is depicted in Figure 6–6.
[2]Fasting coma has been reported only in severe CPT II deficiency.
N = normal.

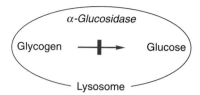

Figure 6–17. The enzyme defect in Pompe disease, α-glucosidase deficiency.

istic, showing a short PR interval, very large amplitude QRS complexes, and inverted T waves. There is no effective treatment, and death usually occurs in the first year. In contrast to the infantile form, the childhood and adult variants of α-glucosidase deficiency are slowly progressive disorders in which skeletal myopathy is the predominant feature.

Fatty Acid Oxidation Defects. Cardiomyopathy also may be a presenting feature of six disorders (Table 6–6) that either interfere with the cycling of carnitine back and forth across the inner mitochondrial membrane (Figure 6–6) or impair long-chain fatty acid oxidation. The existence of these disorders reflects the heavy dependence of the heart on fatty acids as a fuel. Affected infants usually present before 5 years of age, and the cardiomyopathy can be fatal. These conditions may also present with skeletal myopathy or fasting coma, as well as with the metabolic abnormalities characteristic of fatty acid oxidation defects in general, such as MCAD deficiency These abnormalities include hypoketotic hypoglycemia, hyperammonemia, and metabolic acidosis (Table 6–6). It is unclear why MCAD deficiency and other fatty acid defects do not generally affect heart muscle. Unlike MCAD deficiency, however, the urine organic acid profile of defects of carnitine cycling (Figure 6–6) is normal, whereas the urinary profile invariably is abnormal for long-chain β-oxidation defects. The enzymes or transport proteins involved in these diseases are required for the delivery of carnitine or long-chain fatty acyl-CoA into the mitochondrial matrix or for fatty acid oxidation (Figure 6–6). Treatment of these conditions has had limited success, apart from the reversal of the cardiomyopathy obtained with carnitine supplementation in the carnitine transporter defect. For the other diseases, the benefits of strategies such as the prevention of fasting or dietary supplementation with medium-chain fatty acids are unclear.

RENAL TUBULAR DISEASE

Loss of renal glomerular and tubular function may occur in many inborn errors in which other systems are the primary focus of clinically evident disease, including mitochondrial respiratory chain defects and peroxisomal diseases. Several inborn errors, however, are associated with more specific defects in renal function. For example, a decrease in most of the reabsorptive functions of the proximal tubule, ie, a renal Fanconi syndrome, occurs commonly in four of the disorders associated with diffuse liver disease (galactosemia, tyrosinemia, fructose intolerance, and Wilson disease) reviewed above. In other diseases, represented by cystinosis, the renal Fanconi syndrome is the major initial clinical problem. A final group of renal tubular disorders results from the defective transport of an individual solute, such as phosphate (in X-linked hypophosphatemic rickets) or bicarbonate (in one form of renal tubular acidosis), or from chemically similar solutes, such as cystine and the basic amino acids in cystinuria.

Cystinosis. This lysosomal storage disease is caused by an abnormality in the transport protein that mediates cystine efflux from the lysosome. Lysosomal cystine accumulation occurs in virtually all tissues but damages the renal tubule most quickly, producing the renal Fanconi syndrome. Renal parenchymal destruction gradually leads to renal failure by as early as 6 years of age. Most patients present in the first year with failure to thrive, dehydration, weakness due to electrolyte losses, acidosis, and rickets. Cystine crystal deposition in the cornea results in photophobia; in the retina, it results in a pigmentary retinopathy. The diagnosis can be established in the appropriate clinical setting by demonstration of cystine crystals in the cornea or bone marrow or in rectal biopsy specimens, but direct measurement of leukocyte cystine content is the definitive test. Symptomatic treatment includes the management of the electrolyte imbalances that occur. Renal transplantation corrects the renal defect, but the later development of hypothyroidism, diabetes mellitus, or central nervous system and liver disease is not prevented. Specific therapy to reduce the intracellular accumulation of cystine, using cysteamine, improves growth and delays the onset of renal failure if started early in the course of the disease; cysteamine eyedrops can totally clear cystine crystals from the cornea. Inside the lysosome, cysteamine and cysteine form a mixed disulfide that uses an efflux carrier distinct from that used by cystine.

Cystinuria. This relatively common disease, with a prevalence of approximately 1/7000, is caused by impaired renal transport of the structurally similar amino acids cystine, ornithine, arginine, and lysine (or COAL), which share a common carrier (a protein encoded by the *rBAT* gene) in both the proximal renal tubule and gastrointestinal epithelium. The only clinical consequence of this defect results from the low solubility of cystine, which causes renal stones. The stones may be multiple and can lead to infection and progressive renal damage; late complications are hypertension and renal failure. The diagnosis must be excluded in any patient with nephrolithiasis by quantification of urinary cystine. (Stone analysis is inadequate, because some stones in cystinurics contain only trace amounts of cystine.) Treatment, which is aimed at increasing the solubility of cystine, includes increased fluid intake and alkalinization of urine with regular doses of bicarbonate or citrate to keep the urine pH greater than 7.5. In those patients in whom stones have already formed, or in whom there is already significant renal damage, penicillamine or captopril are advocated. These drugs form soluble mixed disulfides with cysteine, and their use may lead to the dissolution of preexisting stones.

DISORDERS WITH DISTINCTIVE PHENOTYPES

A number of important inherited metabolic disorders have distinctive phenotypes that should immediately suggest the possible diagnosis (Table 6–1). The diagnosis may be missed, however, because many of the clinical features associated with these diseases are also found in other diseases. Examples include the apparent cerebral palsy that results from a number of enzymopathies and the dysmorphism and malformations that occur with a small number of inborn errors. Menkes disease, a classic defect of copper metabolism, requires astute clinical observation to be recognized.

HEPATOMEGALY WITHOUT DEMENTIA

As seen in many lysosomal storage diseases, metabolic disorders causing hepatomegaly are often associated with a neurodegenerative course. Two notable exceptions are the non-neuronopathic forms of Niemann-Pick and Gaucher diseases, the neuronopathic variants of which were reviewed above; in Gaucher disease, splenomegaly is predominant. Hepatomegaly is also a prominent feature of defects of gluconeogenesis, and in particular of G-6-Pase deficiency (glycogen storage disease type I or von Gierke disease) (Figure 6–8) and debrancher deficiency (glycogen storage disease type III), as discussed earlier.

"CEREBRAL PALSY" WITHOUT A HISTORY OF PERINATAL DISTRESS OR OTHER NEUROLOGIC INSULT

Cerebral palsy is the term used to describe a variety of nonprogressive neurologic syndromes with disordered movement or posture; mental retardation and seizures also may be present. The condition is the result of damage to the developing brain from such causes as hypoxia or infection; in many cases, however, no definitive cause can be ascertained. The four enzymopathies reviewed below should be considered in patients with this clinical presentation if no other clear cause has been established. In addition, infants with nonketotic hyperglycinemia (discussed above) who survive infancy have spastic cerebral palsy;

this disease also must always be excluded. Although the neurologic disability caused by these inborn errors often cannot be improved, recognition of the correct diagnosis will allow appropriate genetic counseling.

The **Lesch-Nyhan syndrome** is a rare X-linked disorder caused by a deficiency of hypoxanthine phosphoribosyltransferase (HPRT), an enzyme of purine metabolism. Affected boys have delayed motor development apparent in the first 6 months after birth and a movement disorder characterized by athetoid and choreiform movements, poor head control, and hypotonia within the first year. The degree of intellectual handicap, which may seem worse because of dysarthria, has probably been overestimated. Although some patients are definitely cognitively impaired, others are apparently normal. One unforgettable behavior, self-mutilation (eg, severe biting of lips, ear-banging), develops in most, but not all, affected patients. Hyperuricemia is not consistently present in all patients, but a normal urine uric acid–creatinine ratio will exclude the disease. The diagnosis can be confirmed by enzyme assay of erythrocytes or cultured skin fibroblasts. Gout and uric acid renal stones can be prevented by the administration of allopurinol, a drug that reduces the synthesis of urate. There is no therapy for the neurologic disorder.

Deficiency of the urea cycle enzyme **arginase** (Figure 6–7A) usually causes progressive spastic diplegia, intellectual handicap, and seizures. Acute hyperammonemic encephalopathy is a less common feature. The diagnosis is made by quantification of plasma arginine levels, and management is similar to that of the other urea cycle defects.

Fumarase deficiency is a rare defect of the citric acid cycle (Figure 6–8). It may present in early infancy as a severe progressive encephalopathic disorder with acidosis that leads to death in the first year, or as a static disorder with intellectual handicap and dysarthria that mimics cerebral palsy. A urine organic acid screen will detect increased fumarate levels. There is no specific treatment.

Glutaric aciduria type I is an organic acidopathy caused by a deficiency of glutaryl-CoA dehydrogenase, an enzyme of the lysine catabolic pathway. The main clinical features include dysarthria, dystonic "cerebral palsy," choreoathetosis, macrocephaly, and mental retardation. Episodes of ketoacidosis and vomiting may be seen (particularly during periods of catabolic stress). Urinary organic acid analysis usually, although not always, will show an elevation in levels of glutaric acid and related compounds. Attempts at therapy have been unsuccessful.

STROKE OR THROMBOSIS

Cerebrovascular accidents are sometimes seen as a complicating feature of homocystinuria caused by cystathionine β-synthase deficiency, organic acidopathies (eg, methylmalonic acidemia, propionic acidemia, isovaleric acidemia, and glutaric aciduria type I); defects of the mitochondrial electron transport chain (MELAS syndrome); the urea cycle disorders (particularly OTC deficiency); the carbohydrate-deficient glycoprotein deficiency syndrome (see below); the sphingolipidosis; Fabry disease (α-galactosidase deficiency); and inherited disorders of coagulation, such as antithrombin III deficiency and protein C or protein S deficiency.

PREMATURE ATHEROSCLEROSIS

The mendelian disorders of lipid metabolism are important and potentially treatable causes of premature atherosclerosis and myocardial infarction. They are characterized by elevations in levels of cholesterol, triglyceride, or certain plasma lipoproteins. Familial hypercholesterolemia (FH) is a particularly important example of this group: It was the first genetic disorder shown to predispose to myocardial infarction, and it is the prototypic genetic defect of receptor molecules. FH is characterized biochemically by elevated total plasma cholesterol and low-density lipoprotein (LDL) cholesterol (giving a type 2 lipoprotein pattern with electrophoretic studies). FH is inherited (autosomal dominant) and has a heterozygote frequency of 1/500, making it one of the most common mendelian defects. It is caused by mutations in the LDL receptor, which takes up LDL cholesterol from the extracellular fluid.

In the second decade, heterozygotes often have xanthomata caused by cholesterol deposition, particularly on the extensor tendons of the hands and on the Achilles tendon, as well as on the extensor surfaces of the elbows and knees. Cholesterol accumulation around the peripheral margins of the cornea (arcus corneae) and on the eyelids (xanthelasma) is seen later. Premature coronary artery disease and myocardial infarction may first become evident in patients aged 30–40 years or older. Homozygotes (prevalence, approximately 1/1 million) have a much more severe form of the disease, with cutaneous xanthomas often being present at birth and present in all patients by 4 years of age. The earliest recorded myocardial infarction in a homozygote is at 18 months, and few homozygotes survive beyond the age of 30 years.

The clinical diagnosis in homozygotes is confirmed by the finding of a plasma cholesterol level greater than 17 mmol/L in a child without jaundice. Both parents, of course, will be heterozygotes. The diagnosis in heterozygotes is more difficult, because only 5% of patients with an elevated plasma cholesterol level and a type 2 lipoprotein pattern have FH. The diagnosis should be strongly suspected in any individual with a type 2 lipoprotein pattern who also has tendon xanthomata. The diagnosis can be confirmed by assaying LDL receptor function in cultured skin fibroblasts.

Heterozygotes are treated with a combination of dietary cholesterol restriction, enhancement of intestinal bile acid excretion using resins such as cholestyramine, and inhibition of the rate-limiting step in cholesterol biosynthesis (3-hydroxy-3-methylglutaryl-CoA reductase) with inhibitors such as lovastatin. These maneuvers are much less effective in homozygotes, who may respond partially to portocaval shunting (for reasons that are unclear) and to regular plasma exchange. Liver transplantation has cured at least one child. Trials to assess the efficacy of LDL-receptor gene transfer into the liver are under way.

DISORDERS WITH FACIAL DYSMORPHISM OR CONGENITAL MALFORMATIONS

Inborn errors of lysosomes and peroxisomes are well-recognized causes of facial and other physical abnormalities in the newborn. In addition, defects in the metabolism of small molecules also may lead to facial dysmorphism and congenital malformations. Familiar examples include the endocrine disorders congenital hypothyroidism and congenital adrenal hyperplasia. More recently, it has been recognized that small-molecule diseases may cause facial dysmorphism or other malformations. These conditions impair fetal development either because they lead to the accumulation of teratogens, or because they impair cellular bioenergetics.

One such situation is illustrated by women with untreated PKU. When such women become pregnant (maternal PKU), the high maternal phenylalanine level acts as a teratogen on the fetus, causing mental retardation, microcephaly, poor growth, and congenital heart defects, particularly ventricular septal defect. Most such children are heterozygotes for phenylalanine hydroxylase deficiency. Compliance with a low-phenylalanine diet by women with PKU before conception prevents the fetal abnormalities. Examples of inborn errors that probably lead to malformations because they impair fetal energy production include PDH deficiency (see Figure 6–8) (facies like the fetal-alcohol syndrome, brain malformations) and severe CPT II deficiency (see Figure 6–6) (brain malformations, renal cysts).

More recently, two other dysmorphic/malformation syndromes have been identified for which the pathogenesis remains uncertain. Smith-Lemli-Opitz syndrome is an autosomal-recessive disorder notable for microcephaly, a dysmorphic facies, polydactyly, hypospadias, renal and heart malformations, cataracts, and intellectual disability. It is now known to be caused by a defect of cholesterol biosynthesis at the 7-dehydrocholesterol reductase step. The pathogenesis is uncertain but may be associated with cholesterol deficiency (which may lead to neuronal degeneration or abnormalities in myelination) or toxic effects of 7-dehydrocholesterol, the level of which is markedly elevated in plasma. There is no effective treatment, although a cholesterol-rich diet has been advocated by some.

The second new disorder is the carbohydrate-deficiency glycoprotein (CDG) syndrome. This autosomal-recessive multisystem disorder has several clinically recognizable phenotypes, with the most common variant characterized in infancy initially by failure to thrive, facial dysmorphism, lipodystrophic skin changes (including characteristic fat pads on the buttocks), hypotonia, multisystem failure (including pericardial effusions and liver dysfunction), and joint restriction. Later, patients may manifest severe intellectual disability, seizures, retinitis pigmentosa, peripheral neuropathy, and stroke-like episodes, whereas the lipodystrophic changes have a tendency to regress. The metabolic defect in the most common form (Type I CDG syndrome) involves an abnormality in the glycosylation of proteins by the enzyme phosphomannomutase, which is located within the Golgi apparatus. There is no effective treatment.

Small-molecule disorders, therefore, should be considered in infants with dysmorphism or malformations. The above conditions and others can be excluded in the infant by examining levels of blood amino acids, lactate, glucose, ammonium, CSF lactate, urine organic acids, and, if indicated, plasma phenylalanine in the mother. Screening for Smith-Lemli-Opitz syndrome should include measurement of plasma cholesterol and 7-dehydrocholesterol (the latter using gas chromatography-mass spectrometry). Plasma cholesterol and lipid levels also may be reduced in the CDG syndrome, as will be plasma levels of a number of glycoproteins including α1-antitrypsin, haptoglobin, thyroxine-binding globulin (giving abnormal thyroid function tests), coagulation factors, and apolipoproteins. Confirmation of CDG syndrome can be made by demonstrating an abnormal serum transferrin isoform pattern, which can be done on blood from dried newborn screening card blood spots.

MENKES DISEASE

The hallmarks of this X-linked defect of copper metabolism in infants are seizures, facial dysmorphism (abnormal eyebrows, pudgy cheeks, sagging jowls), hair fragility, connective tissue abnormalities (including ligamentous laxity, hernias, bladder diverticula, and arterial rupture), osteoporosis and fractures, a progressive neurodegenerative course, episodic hypothermia, and skin depigmentation. The basic defect is in a membrane copper-transporting ATPase present in most tissues except liver, which is similar in structure to the copper-transporting protein that is defective in Wilson disease. In Menkes disease, copper uptake into the cell is normal, but copper cannot be transported to sites of synthesis of copper-dependent proteins, such as lysyl oxidase (giving rise to the connective tissue abnormalities), dopamine β-hydroxylase (contributing to the autonomic dysfunction), and cytochrome c oxidase (possibly contributing to the neurologic disturbance). Copper accumulates in the gastrointestinal mucosa and kidney; paradoxically, however, copper levels are low in most other tissues, including liver. The diagnosis is established by demonstrating very low serum levels of copper and ceruloplasmin. Treatment with parenteral copper-histidinate makes little difference to the clinical course if brain damage has occurred, but may be of benefit if given to affected brothers in whom the disorder is diagnosed early, before the onset of symptoms.

REFERENCES

Fernandes J et al (editors): *Inborn Metabolic Disorders: Diagnosis and Management,* 2nd ed. Springer-Verlag, 1995.

Scriver CR et al (editors): *The Metabolic Basis of Inherited Disease,* 7th ed. McGraw-Hill, 1995.

Thompson MW et al (editors): *Thompson and Thompson Genetics in Medicine,* 5th ed. Saunders, 1991.

7

Immunologic Disorders

Anna Huttenlocher, MD, & Diane Wara, MD

Infections are commonly seen in children. These infections usually are self-limited and respond promptly to appropriate treatment. Some children present with recurrent infections that are difficult to treat and immediately recur when antibiotics are discontinued, suggesting the possibility of immunodeficiency. It may be difficult for the primary care physician to determine which of these children require evaluation for immunodeficiency and the extent of this evaluation. The primary immunodeficiencies are relatively rare disorders and occur in the population with a frequency of approximately 1/10,000; however, IgA deficiency may occur as frequently as 1/500. More than 50 disorders of the immune system have been described. These disorders reflect the heterogeneity of primary immunodeficiency disorders (Table 7–1). In recent years, the most common form of immunodeficiency in children is an acquired infection with HIV type I. Pediatric HIV is discussed later in this chapter.

Early detection of immunodeficiency, whether primary or secondary, is increasingly important. Therapy is available for many primary immunodeficiencies and usually is most effective when initiated before the onset of severe clinical disease. In the past few years, remarkable progress has been made in our understanding of the molecular mechanisms underlying primary immunodeficiencies. This progress has implications for new approaches to diagnosis and genetic counseling, as well as for potential development of new therapeutic interventions, such as gene therapy.

APPROACH TO THE PRIMARY IMMUNODEFICIENCY DISORDERS

The immune system has four main components: the B lymphocytes, or humoral immunity; the T lymphocytes, or cellular immunity; the phagocytic system; and the complement system. These components work together to produce an effective immune response (Figure 7–1). Dysfunction of the immune system may manifest itself either as a susceptibility to infections or, on the other extreme, as autoimmune disease. Although immunodeficiencies are best categorized according to the primary component of the immune system that is abnormal, dysfunction of one component of the immune system may disrupt normal functioning of other components; eg, normal B-cell function requires the participation of T cells.

CLINICAL FEATURES

The clinical manifestations of primary immunodeficiency are variable in terms of both the nature of the symptoms and the age of onset (Table 7–2). Patients with serious immunodeficiency usually present at an early age with recurrent infections. When to suspect an immunodeficiency in a child with frequent infections is often difficult to determine. Normal children may have one or more episodes of upper respiratory tract infection or otitis media per month, particularly during the winter months. Concerning features may include difficulty clearing infections with prescribed treatment or immediate recurrence of symptoms when antibiotic treatment is discontinued. In this era of aggressive antibiotic treatment, patients with immunodeficiency often present at older ages with different symptoms, such as arthritis, chronic diarrhea, or failure to thrive. In fact, immunodeficiency should be a diagnostic consideration in the child presenting with failure to thrive or chronic diarrhea. Particular immunodeficiencies may have unique symptoms suggestive of their diagnosis, including thrombocytopenia and eczema in Wiskott-Aldrich syndrome and ataxia and telangiectasia in ataxia-telangiectasia (Table 7–3).

The infections seen in patients with underlying immunodeficiency usually are common, eg, otitis media, sinusitis, and pneumonia. Organisms also are typically the commonly occurring encapsulated organisms, such as

Table 7–1. Primary immunodeficiency disorders.

B-Lymphocyte Abnormalities	T-Lymphocyte Abnormalities
Selective IgA deficiency	DiGeorge syndrome
X-linked agammaglobulin-emia	Chronic mucocutaneous candidiasis
Common variable immuno-deficiency	Purine nucleoside phosphor-ylase deficiency
Combined T- and B-lympho-cyte abnormalities	
Severe combined immuno-deficiency	
Ataxia-telangiectasia	
Wiskott-Aldrich syndrome	

Phagocytic Cell Abnormalities	Complement Deficiencies
Chronic granulomatous dis-ease	C1 deficiency
Neutropenia	C4 deficiency
Leukocyte adhesion defect	C2 deficiency
Chédiak-Higashi syndrome	

Streptococcus pneumoniae and *Haemophilus influenzae.* More severe infections, such as mastoiditis, bacteremia, osteomyelitis, and meningitis, also may occur. With major primary immunodeficiency, one of the infections usually is quite severe, involving unusual organisms or resulting in unexpected complications. The presence of opportunistic infections, such as *Pneumocystis carinii* pneumonia (PCP) or *Candida* esophagitis, is suggestive of a child with T-cell abnormality. An additional consideration is the onset of complications from immunization with live-virus vaccines, including paralytic polio after immunization with oral poliovirus vaccine (OPV), in patients with both B- and T-cell defects. On the other hand, patients with phagocytic disorders typically present with recurrent abscesses and distinctive organisms, such as *Staphylococcus aureus* and gram-negative organisms, such as *Serratia.* Finally, patients with complement deficiencies present with recurrent infections involving encapsulated organisms, such as pneumococcus and meningococcus. Several distinguishing features on history and physical examination should be emphasized when differentiating primary immunodeficiency from pediatric HIV (summarized in Table 7–4). Features on physical examination include the presence of lymphadenopathy and splenomegaly in HIV and their absence commonly in deficiencies of antibody or cell-mediated immunity.

LABORATORY EVALUATION

The complete evaluation of a patient with suspected immunodeficiency may be difficult to determine, but the initial screening tests are straightforward (Table 7–5). A lot of information can be obtained from a complete blood count (CBC) and erythrocyte sedimentation rate (ESR). For instance, an elevated ESR may be consistent with chronic infection. In the immunodeficient child, the CBC

may show anemia of chronic disease, thrombocytopenia suggestive of Wiskott-Aldrich syndrome, or a low absolute lymphocyte count (ALC) indicative of a possible T-cell–mediated defect. Normal values for ALC vary with age; an ALC less than 3000 may be abnormal in infancy, whereas an ALC less then 1200 is abnormal in older children. Neutropenia or neutrophilia may be suggestive of specific immunodeficiencies, including cyclic neutropenia and leukocyte adhesion deficiency, respectively. Additional laboratory tests to include in a screening evaluation are HIV antibody, CH50, delayed hypersensitivity skin tests, and isohemagglutinin and quantitative immunoglobulin levels. Low immunoglobulin levels suggest a specific immunodeficiency, whereas high levels may suggest HIV or chronic granulomatous disease. Determination of iso-hemagglutinin levels, which are IgM antibodies to A and B polysaccharide antigens, also is a useful screening test in children older than 2 years; this information assesses the ability to make specific IgM antibody. Finally, skin testing for specific antigens (mumps, *Candida,* and tetanus), which is useful only in children older than 2 years, is performed by intradermal injection and interpreted by determining the extent of induration. Induration greater than 10 mm at 48 hours makes a primary T-cell defect very unlikely. More extensive evaluation of immune function may be indicated when the screening tests yield abnormal results or if the clinical index of suspicion for immunodeficiency is high (Table 7–6).

DISORDERS OF ANTIBODY-MEDIATED IMMUNITY

DEVELOPMENT OF ANTIBODY-MEDIATED IMMUNITY

B-cell–mediated immunity develops in two stages. The first stage is antigen independent and involves rearrangement of activated immunoglobulin genes. This stage occurs in the fetus by 8 weeks' gestation. By 13 weeks, the fetus has B cells capable of undergoing the second stage of differentiation, which is antigen dependent and requires the binding of specific antigen to surface immunoglobulin. The second stage usually occurs after birth and requires multiple signals, including T-cell participation (see Figure 7–1). Ultimately, B cells differentiate into plasma cells that can secrete specific antibody, which acts with activated complement to coat or opsonize foreign antigen. Activated phagocytes engulf this complex through immunoglobulin and complement receptors on their surface, resulting in elimination of the foreign antigen.

Distinct classes of antibody play unique roles in the immune response and appear at different stages of develop-

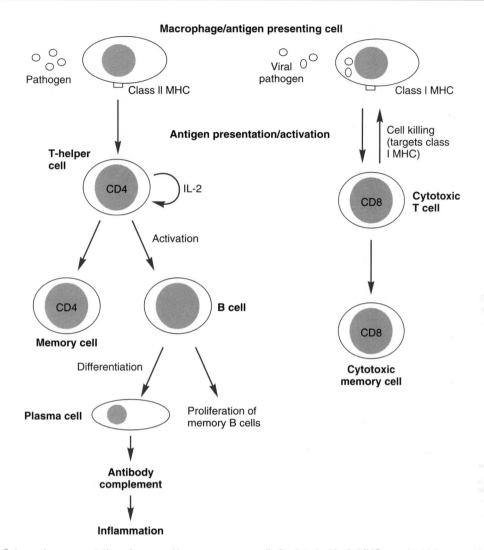

Figure 7–1. Schematic representation of a normal immune response. IL-2 = interleukin-2; MHC = major histocompatibility complex.

ment (Table 7–7). IgG, the only immunoglobulin class capable of transplacental passage, plays an important role in protecting the full-term newborn from infection during the first few months. This protective feature results in a delay in onset of clinical symptoms in patients with hypogam-

maglobulinemia until after they lose maternal immunoglobulin at 4–6 months after birth. Transplacental passage of IgG occurs at 30–32 weeks' gestation; therefore, premature infants may be deprived of the protective advantage of maternally acquired IgG. Because the half-life of IgG is approximately 25 days, normal infants may have a significant decrease in IgG concentrations (as low as 200 mg/dL) at approximately 3–4 months of age, be-

Table 7–2. Clinical features consistent with primary immunodeficiency.

Chronic or recurrent infection (more than expected for age)
Incomplete response to treatment
Unusual infections (opportunistic: eg, *Pneumocystis carinii*)
Chronic thrush
Chronic diarrhea
Failure to thrive
Recurrent abscesses

Table 7–3. Features of specific primary immunodeficiencies.

Ataxia or telangiectasia (ataxia-telangiectasia)
Eczema or thrombocytopenia (Wiskott-Aldrich syndrome)
Tetany (DiGeorge syndrome)
Endocrinopathy (chronic mucocutaneous candidiasis)

Table 7–4. Clinical signs and symptoms in primary immunodeficiency disorders.

Clinical Signs/Symptoms	Deficiency of Antibody-Mediated Immunity	Deficiency of Cell-Mediated Immunity	Pediatric HIV Infection
Increased sinopulmonary disease	Common	Common	Common
Increased infection with encapsulated organisms	Common	Common	Common
Increased infection with opportunistic organisms	Rare	Common	Common
Oral candidiasis	Rare	Common	Common
Systemic fungal infections	Rare	Unusual	Common
Pneumocystis carinii pneumonia	Rare	Common	Common
Tonsil/lymphoid tissue	Decreased or absent	Frequently absent	Frequently enlarged
Liver and spleen	Normal	Usually normal	Frequently enlarged

fore they synthesize their own IgG. Premature infants who lack maternally acquired IgG may have a significant decrease to concentrations as low as 60 mg/dL at age 4 months. Transient hypogammaglobulinemia of infancy (THI) must be considered in the differential diagnosis of a patient presenting with low immunoglobulin levels in infancy. Unlike infants with hypogammaglobulinemia, those with THI are capable of making specific antibodies to diphtheria and tetanus toxoids by age 6–10 months. There are four IgG subclasses, which may be selectively deficient and result in disordered immunity. IgG_1 and IgG_3 subclass concentrations follow the pattern of total IgG in the infant, with a decrease during the first 3–6 months and a subsequent gradual increase to adult concentrations. IgG_2 and IgG_4 subclasses increase more slowly and do not reach physiologic concentrations until 2–3 years of age. IgG_1 antibodies are produced in response to protein antigens, whereas IgG_2 antibodies are produced in response to polysaccharide antigens. IgG_3 antibody is responsible for the primary antibody response to many viruses.

IgM concentrations at birth usually are low because IgM does not cross the placenta; however, IgM synthesis can be increased in utero in response to intrauterine infection. In the initial immune response, the first antibody to be produced is IgM antibody, which is of relatively low affinity. Subsequently, after activation of B cells, there is isotype switching to higher affinity antibodies, such as IgG and IgA. Both IgG and IgM, but not IgA, can bind complement. IgM antibody remains confined to the intravascular space in contrast to IgG antibody, which is in both the intravascular and interstitial spaces. IgA antibody is primarily found in secretions such as saliva, nasal secretions, sweat, and breast milk. IgA antibody provides local immunity and prevents systemic access of foreign antigens. Secretory IgA, primarily IgA subtype 1, is found in very high concentrations in breast milk and provides an important protective function against infection for breast-feeding infants. Normal plasma levels of IgG, IgA, and IgM at different ages are shown in Table 7–8.

Table 7–5. Initial workup for suspected immunodeficiency.

Complete blood count with differential (absolute lymphocyte count)
HIV antibody (if positive in child < 15 mo; HIV polymerase chain reaction to confirm)
Quantitative immunoglobulin levels (IgG, IgA, IgM, and IgE)
Isohemagglutinin levels (> 2 y)
Skin testing for candida, mumps, and tetanus (> 2 y)
CH50 (quantitates complement component activity)

Table 7–6. Evaluation of immune system.

	Quantity	Function
B cell	IgG, IgM, IgA, IgE IgG subclasses ($IgG_{1, 2, 3, 4}$) B cell numbers (CD19)	Isohemagglutinins Specific antibody response to tetanus (protein) and Pneumovax In vitro proliferation to PWM
T cell	Absolute lymphocyte count Chest radiograph (thymus) T-cell numbers (CD3+) T-cell subsets (CD4, CD8)	Delayed hypersensitivity skin testing (candida, mumps, tetanus) T cell in vitro proliferation to mitogens (PHA, concanavalin A) T cell in vitro proliferation to antigens (candida, tetanus) ADA/PNP concentrations Cytokine production
Complement	C3, C4 Concentration of specific components (C7, 8, 9)	CH50 Hemolytic activity of other complement components
Phagocytic	Absolute neutrophil count	NBT reduction Enzyme assays (MPO, G-6PD) Bacterial killing Chemotaxis assays

ADA/PNP = adenosine deaminase/purine nucleoside phosporylase; NBT = nitroblue tetrazolium; PHA = phytohemagglutinin; PWM = pokeweed mitogen.

Table 7–7. Immunoglobulin classes (isotypes).

	IgG	IgM	IgA
Percentage of total immunoglobulin	70–80	5–10	10–15
Mean adult value	1200 mg/dL	150 mg/dL	300 mg/dL
Distribution	Intravascular/interstitial spaces	Intravascular	Secretions/intravascular
Transplacental passage	Yes: after 30–32 wk	No	No
Synthesized in utero	No	Yes	Yes (late)
Activates complement	Yes	Yes	No
Subclasses	4	0	2

CLINICAL DISORDERS

The more common forms of antibody-mediated immunodeficiency are discussed in this section. By far the most common form of B-cell–mediated immunodeficiency is **IgA deficiency,** occurring at a frequency of as high as 1/500, as compared with **agammaglobulinemia,** occurring at a frequency of approximately 1/50,000. Diagnosis of **hypogammaglobulinemia** is suggested by low concentrations of immunoglobulins (usually < 250 mg/dL) and an inability to make specific antibody. Not all patients presenting with low immunoglobulin concentrations in infancy have hypogammaglobulinemia. Those with THI are capable of making specific antibodies to diphtheria and tetanus toxoids by age 6–10 months. Treatment involves replacement therapy with intravenous γ-globulin. An approach to the evaluation of disorders of antibody-mediated immunity is shown in Figure 7–2.

X-Linked Agammaglobulinemia

X-linked agammaglobulinemia (XLA) is the most common form of hypogammaglobulinemia. Male infants typically present with recurrent infections within the first year. The primary defect is caused by a developmental arrest in B-lymphocyte differentiation as a result of a mutation in the gene for Bruton tyrosine kinase.

Affected male infants usually are well during the first few months, when they are protected by maternal IgG. When maternal IgG is catabolized and infants are unable to synthesize their own IgG, recurrent infections, frequently sinopulmonary infections, develop. If treatment is prompt or if exposure to infections is minimal, individual infections may be no more severe than in the general population. The infections usually are chronic or recurrent, with symptoms recurring shortly after antibiotic treatment is discontinued. The most frequent infectious agents are common pyogenic bacteria, including *S aureus, S pneumoniae,* and *H influenzae;* later in the course, mycoplasma may be an important pathogen in patients with chronic lung disease. Septicemia, bacterial meningitis, and osteomyelitis occur in as many as 10% of male infants who do not receive treatment. Affected infants usually are not susceptible to opportunistic infections, although they may have sensitivity to enteroviruses, including vaccine-related complications or severe echovirus meningoencephalitis, despite normal T-cell function. Findings on physical examination include absence of adenoids, tonsils, and lymph nodes.

Laboratory studies in patients with XLA show a total immunoglobulin concentration of less than 250 mg/dL, with absence of B cells in the peripheral blood. Patients are unable to make a specific antibody response, although they have normal T-cell function. Early diagnosis and initiation of replacement immunoglobulin (IVIG) are essential to prevent complications, including the development of chronic pulmonary disease. Despite the use of IVIG, some patients may still have chronic sinusitis and otitis media. Risks of IVIG are discussed in the section on Treatment. Prophylactic antibiotics are now generally discouraged because of the emergence of antibiotic-resistant bacteria. Patients with XLA frequently require more aggressive treatment to clear infections. For example, the treatment of pneumonia may require prolonged administration of intravenous antibiotics. With early diagnosis and appropriate treatment, children with XLA can survive into adulthood without significant morbidity.

Common Variable Immunodeficiency

Common variable immunodeficiency (CVI) is a primary immunodeficiency with hypogammaglobulinemia that is distinct from XLA. Distinguishing features include the presence of B cells in the peripheral blood, autoimmune disease, and later age of onset. CVI is a heterogeneous group of disorders without a unifying pathogenesis. The disease frequently is caused by an intrinsic B-cell defect, although abnormalities of cytokines or T-B cell interaction also have been implicated. In addition, there is no clear mode of inheritance, although CVI may cluster in families.

Table 7–8. Normal plasma values for immunoglobulins at various ages.

Age	IgG (mg/dL)	IgA (mg/dL)	IgM (mg/dL)
Newborn	600–1670	0–5	6–15
1–3 mo	218–610	20–53	11–51
4–6 mo	228–636	27–72	25–60
7–9 mo	292–816	27–73	12–124
10–18 mo	383–1070	27–169	28–113
2 y	423–1184	35–222	21–131
3 y	477–1334	40–251	28–113
4–5 y	540–1500	48–336	20–106
6–8 y	571–1700	52–535	28–112
14 y	570–1570	86–544	33–135
Adult	635–1775	106–668	37–154

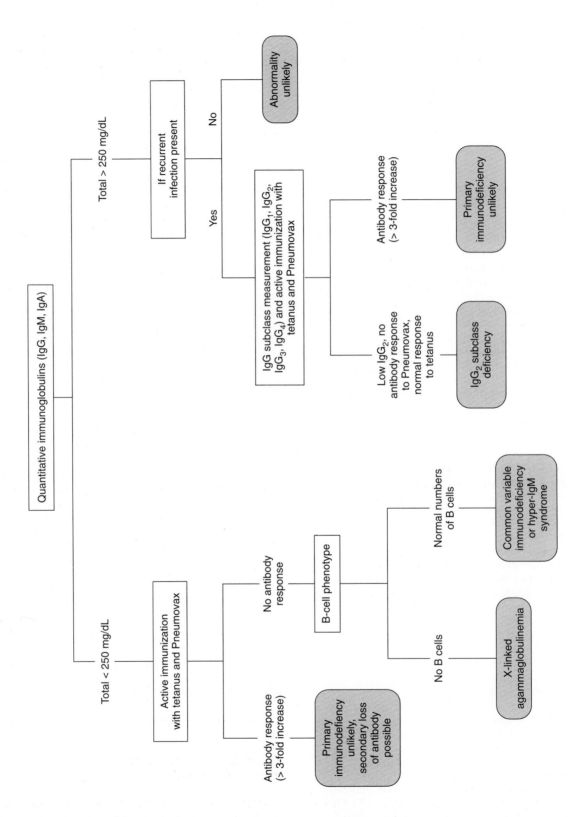

Figure 7–2. Algorithm showing an approach to the evaluation of clinical disorders of antibody-mediated immunity.

Most patients with CVI are well in early childhood, but recurrent infections develop during the second and third decades of life. The most common manifestations of CVI are chronic sinopulmonary infections from pyogenic bacteria and chronic diarrhea frequently due to *Giardia lamblia.* Malabsorption also is commonly seen; small bowel biopsy specimens show flattened villi. Additional features include autoimmune hemolytic anemia and thrombocytopenia, inflammatory bowel disease, gluten-sensitive enteropathy, and nodular lymphoid hyperplasia. Malignant neoplasms, including non-Hodgkin lymphoma, thymoma, and gastric adenocarcinoma, occur in approximately 10% of patients and increase in frequency with age. Physical examination of patients with CVI shows presence of lymph nodes and tonsils; splenomegaly is present in approximately 25% of patients. Laboratory evaluation shows hypogammaglobulinemia with typically normal T-cell function. The mainstay of treatment is intravenous γ-globulin and aggressive management of infections.

Hyper-IgM Syndrome

Hyper-IgM syndrome is characterized by low levels of IgG but normal to increased levels of IgM. It is typically X-linked, and the underlying molecular defect has recently been defined. Most patients with hyper-IgM syndrome have mutations in the gene for the CD40 ligand that is present on T cells. Absence of T-cell CD40 ligand results in abnormal T-B cell interaction and an inability of B cells to undergo isotype switching from IgM- to IgG- or IgA-producing cells. In addition, deficiency of CD40 ligand on T cells results in a partial T-cell defect and susceptibility of patients with hyper-IgM to opportunistic infections. Like patients with XLA, these patients usually become symptomatic within the first 6–12 months postnatally; sinopulmonary disease develops from common encapsulated bacteria. Distinctive clinical features include the presence of opportunistic infections such as *P carinii.* In addition, patients with hyper-IgM frequently have lymphoid hyperplasia and autoimmune diseases, such as hemolytic anemia, thrombocytopenia, and neutropenia. The results of laboratory studies reveal a deficiency in IgG and IgA but normal to increased levels of IgM. B cells are present in the peripheral blood, and patients usually have normal T-cell numbers and function. Treatment requires replacement therapy with IVIG and PCP prophylaxis with trimethoprim-sulfamethoxazole.

Selective IgA Deficiency

Selective IgA deficiency, the most prevalent primary immunodeficiency, occurs in approximately 1/500 individuals. Most cases occur sporadically, although risk is increased among family members. Most patients with IgA deficiency are healthy. Symptomatic patients present with recurrent sinopulmonary infections, allergy, gastrointestinal diseases, and autoimmune disorders. The age of onset of symptoms is variable. Laboratory study results include normal IgG and IgM with decreased IgA (< 10 mg/dL). Patients with IgA deficiency may have a coexisting IgG$_2$-subclass deficiency. Treatment with intravenous γ-globulin is not indicated; in fact, commercial γ-globulin preparations contain small amounts of IgA capable of sensitizing patients with IgA deficiency. On rare occasions, this sensitization results in an anaphylactic response to IVIG or blood transfusions.

IgG Subclass Deficiencies

Deficiencies in IgG subclasses may occur despite normal total IgG levels. The most common subclass deficiency is **IgG$_2$ deficiency.** Patients typically present with recurrent infections, including sinopulmonary infections and otitis media caused by pyogenic organisms. Laboratory evaluation usually reveals decreased IgG$_2$ levels and absence of a specific antibody response to immunization with polysaccharide vaccines, such as Pneumovax. Pre- and post-immunization titers are obtained at the time of and 3 weeks after immunization with Pneumovax. Normal response to immunization is a greater than threefold increase in antibody titer to three or more serotypes of *S pneumoniae* contained within the Pneumovax vaccine. Use of intravenous γ-globulin to treat IgG$_2$ subclass deficiency is controversial and is recommended only in patients with severe recurrent infections.

TREATMENT

Replacement therapy with intravenous γ-globulin remains the mainstay of therapy for disorders of antibody-mediated immunity. Risks of γ-globulin include those associated with the infusion of blood and blood products. Although there have been several reported cases of the transmission of hepatitis C, γ-globulin preparations currently are acid treated, making the transmission of hepatitis C less likely. There have been no reported cases of HIV transmission with IVIG. Additional treatment approaches for patients with hypogammaglobulinemia include aggressive treatment of infections with antibiotics. Patients with hypogammaglobulinemia should not receive live-virus vaccines, such as OPV or mumps, measles, and rubella vaccine (MMR).

DISORDERS OF CELL-MEDIATED IMMUNITY

DEVELOPMENT OF CELL-MEDIATED IMMUNITY

Differentiation of stem cells into a mature population of T lymphocytes occurs in the thymus. Prothymocytes colonize the fetal thymus at 8–9 weeks' gestation, initially entering the subcapsular region of the thymus. As the T cells move through the cortex to the medulla, they differentiate into mature T cells. Cell surface markers vary as the T cell matures, with early T-cell precursors coexpressing CD4 and CD8. As T cells differentiate, they acquire a mature T-cell receptor, as well as the cell-surface antigens CD3 and CD11. The presence of CD4 on mature T cells correlates with T-helper activity, whereas the presence of CD8 correlates with T-suppressor and T-cytotoxic activity. By 12 weeks' gestation, functioning T cells are present in the human fetus, and by 40 weeks the T-cell population generally is mature. This process of generating a mature T-cell population requires positive and negative selection in the thymus, with most T-cell precursors dying before maturity. At birth, the full-term newborn frequently has an elevated total lymphocyte count (mean, 4500/μL) with normal total T-cell numbers in the peripheral blood. In addition, CD4 cells make up 60% of peripheral T cells, and the CD4-CD8 ratio exceeds 3:1. The numbers of CD4 cells slowly decrease with age; by 6 years, 40% of the peripheral blood cells are CD4 cells, and the CD4-CD8 ratio reaches the adult value of 2:1. The changes in lymphocytes, T cells, and T-cell subpopulations are shown in Table 7–9.

The two main populations of T cells, CD4 and CD8 cells, have distinct functions. T-helper cells, or CD4 cells, play an important role in helping B cells produce antibody by generating stimulating cytokines, such as interleukin-2 (IL-2) (see Figure 7–1). The CD4-positive cells are stimulated by interacting with antigen in the context of major histocompatibility complex (MHC) class II molecules on antigen-presenting cells, such as dendritic cells and macrophages. Cytotoxic T cells, on the other hand, play an essential role in fighting infection that involves targeting and killing cells infected with viruses. This recognition process involves the direct interaction of CD8-positive T cells with viral antigen presented on cells in the context of MHC class I molecules.

CLINICAL DISORDERS

Although the clinical spectrum may vary depending on the severity of disease, patients with disorders of cell-mediated immunity tend to present earlier during infancy and usually require more aggressive treatment and interven-

tion for survival than those with isolated B-cell disorders. T cells play an important role in the organization and activation of other components of the immune response, such as B cell and macrophage response (see Figure 7–1). Abnormal antibody-mediated immunity is an important component of T-cell disorders.

Severe Combined Immunodeficiency Syndrome

Severe combined immunodeficiency syndrome (SCID) is a heterogeneous disorder characterized by the absence of functional T cells and abnormal antibody-mediated immunity. Progress has been made recently in defining the molecular defects underlying several forms of SCID. The defect in X-linked SCID, the most common form, has been identified as a mutation in the gene for the IL-2 receptor γ-chain. Other recently defined forms of SCID include a T-cell–receptor (TCR) signaling defect with mutations in the *ZAP70* gene, defective expression of CD3-TCR with mutations in the CD3 γ-chain, and defective IL-2 production. Approximately half the patients with the autosomal-recessive form of SCID have a deficiency in the enzyme adenosine deaminase (ADA), which results in the accumulation of metabolites toxic to the lymphocyte.

Infants with SCID usually present with serious or recurrent infections by 3–6 months of age. Other manifestations include failure to thrive and chronic respiratory, gastrointestinal, or cutaneous infections. However, the first indication of SCID frequently is pneumonia with an opportunistic organism, such as *P carinii* or cytomegalovirus. In addition, oral ulcers, oral esophageal candidiasis, severe varicella, and secretory diarrhea are commonly seen in infants with SCID. Laboratory evaluation reveals lymphopenia (< 1200/μL) in most patients, although a normal lymphocyte count does not exclude the diagnosis of SCID. Further evaluation for SCID should include quantitation of T-cell subpopulations and determination of T-cell function. Studies of T-cell function include T-cell proliferative responses to mitogens (phytohemagglutinin and concanavalin A), antigens (tetanus, candida), and alloantigens (mixed lymphocyte culture). Patients with SCID also have reduced serum immunoglobulin levels and an inability to form specific antibody.

Treatment of SCID varies depending on the pathogenesis of the disorder. The best treatment for most patients

Table 7–9. Peripheral blood lymphocytes, T cells, T-cell subpopulation by age.

	Lymphocyte Count (μL)	CD3 (% Lymphs)	CD4 (% CD3)	CD8 (% CD3)	CD4:CD8 Ratio
Third trimester early	—	—	80	15	5:1
Third trimester term/newborn	> 3000	55	60	20	3:1
Newborn to 2 y	> 2000	65	50	20	2:1
2–4 y	> 1500	65	40	20	2:1
4–6 y	> 1200	65	40	20	2:1
Adult	> 1200	65	40	20	2:1

with SCID is a histocompatible bone-marrow transplantation from a sibling. Success with bone-marrow transplantation, if performed early and before the onset of severe infections, may be seen in as many as 90% of patients. However, most patients do not have a matched donor for bone-marrow transplantation. Alternative therapeutic options include haploidentical bone-marrow transplantation, eg, from a parent, after depleting the bone marrow of mature T cells. Infants with enzyme deficiencies, such as ADA, may receive enzyme replacement therapy as an alternative. In some recent clinical trials, some patients with ADA deficiency have received stem-cell gene therapy, and the early results have been promising; these studies are still in progress. Gene therapy may become a more common therapeutic approach as the technology improves and additional molecular mechanisms are defined.

Infants with SCID should not receive live-virus vaccines because dissemination may occur resulting in vaccine-induced poliomyelitis after OPV. Close contacts of the patient also should receive killed poliovirus vaccine. All blood products should be irradiated to avoid graft-versus-host reaction and should be screened for cytomegalovirus. Intravenous γ-globulin and prophylaxis against PCP should be administered until bone marrow engraftment is complete.

DiGeorge Syndrome

DiGeorge syndrome is characterized by thymic hypoplasia, congenital tetany, abnormal facies, an increased susceptibility to infection, and congenital heart disease. Chromosomal deletions in 22q11 have been found, although the molecular defect has not been determined. Most cases are sporadic, with both male and female infants affected. DiGeorge syndrome results from a developmental defect that affects third and fourth pharyngeal pouch evagination at 6–8 weeks' gestation. This syndrome is therefore a multisystem developmental disorder affecting the thymus and parathyroid glands as well as certain aortic-arch structures, resulting in congenital heart defects.

The spectrum of immunodeficiency may vary, with some patients having "partial DiGeorge syndrome" and essentially normal immune function. On the other extreme, some patients have severe immunodeficiency with clinical presentation similar to SCID. Infants with DiGeorge syndrome usually are identified because of their congenital heart disease and hypocalcemia. In general, the thymic hypoplasia results in decreased but not absent T cells (30–40% CD3 cells). Serum immunoglobulin levels usually are near normal for age, and T-cell proliferative studies vary depending on the severity of the immunodeficiency. Patients with severe immunodeficiency have benefited from thymic transplants and human leukocyte antigen (HLA)–identical bone-marrow transplantation. The bone-marrow transplant cannot be depleted of T cells, as its success requires the presence of mature T cells from the donor because of the thymic hypoplasia seen in DiGeorge syndrome.

Wiskott-Aldrich Syndrome

Wiskott-Aldrich syndrome (WAS) is an X-linked disorder characterized by thrombocytopenia, eczema, and recurrent infections. Both cellular and antibody-mediated immunity are abnormal. The defective gene in WAS has been cloned recently and is known as *WASP; WASP* is important for normal immune cell development, but its precise function is unknown.

Patients typically present with eczema and bleeding in early infancy. Recurrent infections frequently develop later, often during the first 1–2 years. The infections usually are secondary to encapsulated organisms, such as *S pneumoniae,* although patients also are susceptible to opportunistic infections, including PCP. Patients with WAS also have an increased incidence of lymphoreticular malignant disease, autoimmune hemolytic anemia, and arthritis. Laboratory studies usually reveal absent production of antibody to polysaccharide antigens, elevated IgA and IgE, normal IgG, and low IgM concentrations. Isohemagglutinins are absent, and T-cell responses to mitogens are variable. The diagnosis is suggested by presence of thrombocytopenia and small platelets.

Survival into adulthood is rare, and the cause of death is commonly related to bleeding, infection, or malignant disease. Treatment is, at minimum, supportive with intravenous γ-globulin and aggressive management of acute infections. Patients may benefit from an HLA-mixed lymphocyte culture (MLC)–identical bone-marrow transplant. Successful bone-marrow transplant results in normalization of platelet count, reconstitution of the immune system, and improvement in eczema.

Ataxia-telangiectasia

Ataxia-telangiectasia (AT) is an autosomal-recessive disorder characterized by cerebellar ataxia, oculocutaneous telangiectasia, recurrent sinopulmonary tract infections, and variable immunodeficiency. The immunodeficiency may involve both antibody- and cell-mediated immunity. Patients with AT have defective mechanisms of DNA repair and increased susceptibility to chromosomal breaks and translocation after irradiation. The defect in AT has recently been discovered in a gene on chromosome 11q22-23, which encodes a phosphatidylinositol-3-kinase–like protein that is believed to be important in DNA repair.

Patients typically present at 3–6 years of age with progressive cerebellar ataxia and telangiectasia. The immune dysfunction usually develops later and is accompanied by recurrent sinopulmonary infections. Older patients with AT may have insulin-resistant diabetes mellitus and an increased incidence of malignant disorders, such as lymphosarcoma, leukemia, adenocarcinoma, dysgerminoma, and medulloblastoma. Diagnosis of AT is confirmed by an elevated serum α-fetoprotein level. The immunologic abnormalities are variable and may be progressive. Patients commonly have IgA deficiency and low IgG$_2$ subclass levels, with variable defects in ability to make antibody to specific antigens. Most patients have abnormal cell-mediated immunity characterized by cutaneous anergy and depressed, but not absent, T-cell function.

There is no specific treatment to limit progression of AT. Intravenous immunoglobulin may be indicated if there is IgG subclass deficiency and significant infections. Progression of the disease is variable, and many patients survive into adulthood.

Chronic Mucocutaneous Candidiasis

Chronic mucocutaneous candidiasis (CMC) is a rare disorder in which patients have persistent candida infection of the skin, mucous membranes, and nails. The pathogenesis of CMC is unknown, although family history may be present in as many as 20% of patients.

Approximately half the patients have an associated endocrinopathy, such as Addison disease, hypoparathyroidism, hypothyroidism, or diabetes mellitus. Patients with CMC are anergic on delayed hypersensitivity skin testing to *Candida* despite normal responses to mumps and tetanus. These results are supported by absent T-cell proliferative responses to *Candida* despite normal responses to mitogens and other specific antigens, such as tetanus. Patients with CMC have normal antibody-mediated immunity. Patients usually require systemic treatment with antifungal agents, such as fluconazole. They typically survive into adulthood with the primary complication being endocrinopathy, such as unsuspected adrenal insufficiency.

Hyper-IgE Syndrome

Hyper-IgE syndrome is a rare disorder characterized by recurrent staphylococcal skin infections, dermatitis, and a markedly elevated serum IgE level. The underlying cause of hyper-IgE syndrome is unknown. Patients typically present in childhood with recurrent staphylococcal infections of the skin and lung; complications include abscess formation and the development of pneumatoceles. Patients frequently have a chronic inflammatory skin condition similar to eczema. Laboratory studies reveal eosinophilia and elevated IgE levels with normal IgG, IgA, and IgM levels. T-cell function is variable with generally normal T-cell proliferative responses to mitogens but decreased responses to specific antigens. Some patients have abnormal phagocytic chemotactic responses, although this finding is not universal. Treatment is supportive with prophylactic antibiotics against staphylococcal infections and aggressive treatment of acute infections. Some patients have benefited from treatment with IVIG and γ-interferon.

TREATMENT

The ideal treatment for severe T-cell–mediated immunodeficiency is bone-marrow transplantation using an HLA-identical donor. Alternative treatments include bone-marrow transplantation from a haploidentical donor,

usually the child's parents, after depletion of mature T cells to prevent graft-versus-host disease. Less severe forms of T-cell–mediated immunodeficiency may be managed with the use of intravenous antibiotics, PCP prophylaxis, and supportive care as indicated. The patients should not receive live-virus vaccines, and blood transfusions should be negative for cytomegalovirus and irradiated. ADA deficiency is a unique form of SCID in which patients can receive enzyme replacement therapy. Early clinical trials using stem-cell gene therapy to treat ADA deficiency currently are in progress, with some evidence of potential therapeutic benefit.

DISORDERS OF THE COMPLEMENT SYSTEM

The complement system has more than 20 components, and deficiencies in many of these components have been reported. Most of these are inherited as autosomal-recessive traits, although C1 esterase inhibitor deficiency is autosomal-dominant. The most common defect in the complement system is C2 deficiency, occurring in 1/10,000 individuals.

The complement system plays an important role in host defense by (1) causing lysis of cells and bacteria, (2) mediating opsonization by coating foreign antigens with complement and thereby promoting phagocytosis, and (3) producing peptide fragments that generate an inflammatory response, including chemotactic and vasodilatory factors. The two major pathways of the complement system are the classic and alternative pathways. The classic pathway is activated by antibody and involves complement components C1, C4, and C2, which activate C3 and the terminal components of the complement cascade. The alternative pathway may function independently of antibody and includes factors B, D, and properdin, which subsequently activate C3 and the terminal components of the cascade.

Deficiency of Complement Components

Patients with complement deficiency have variable clinical presentations depending on the component that is deficient. Patients deficient in C1, C2, C3, or C4 have an increased susceptibility to encapsulated bacteria as well as to autoimmune disorders, such as systemic lupus erythematosus. On the other hand, patients with deficiencies of the terminal complement components C5–C9 have a selected susceptibility to meningococcal and gonococcal infections. Screening laboratory evaluation is best done by quantitation of hemolytic complement. This is a functional assay and requires the presence of functional complement components C1–C9. If hemolytic complement is decreased or absent, the quantity and function of each complement component should be determined.

There is no specific therapy for complement deficiencies. Treatment includes immunization against *H influenzae, S pneumoniae,* and *Neisseria meningitidis.* Prophylactic antibiotics using trimethoprim-sulfamethoxazole may benefit some patients. Children with deficiencies in early complement components should be observed carefully for the development of autoimmune diseases.

Deficiency of Mannose Binding Protein

Mannose binding protein (MBP) plays an important role in the immune response by acting as an opsonin and activating the classic complement pathway. Recent studies have suggested that low serum levels of MBP may be associated with recurrent infections in childhood. As many as 25% of children with unexplained recurrent infections may have deficiencies in MBP. Children typically present at 6–18 months of age with recurrent otitis media, sinopulmonary infections, skin infections, and diarrhea. Reports have indicated that the spectrum of clinical involvement may be variable, with some patients having more severe infections, including chronic cryptosporidial diarrhea and meningococcal meningitis. Treatment usually is supportive and similar to the approach used with patients deficient in components of the complement cascade.

DISORDERS OF THE PHAGOCYTIC SYSTEM

Infants with defects in phagocyte function typically present with recurrent infections in the first year of life. The clinical disorders of phagocytes can be divided into those with decreased neutrophil counts and those with normal or increased neutrophil counts but abnormal neutrophil function.

The phagocytic system is made up of a number of different cell types, including neutrophils and macrophages, which play an important role in host defense. Phagocytes play a role in the immune response by accumulating in areas of inflammation and participating in the local inflammatory response. They also play an important role in host defense through phagocytosis and, subsequently, by killing certain types of pathogens.

Leukocyte Adhesion Deficiency

Leukocyte adhesion deficiency (LAD) is a rare disorder characterized by abnormal phagocyte adhesion and migration. The more common form of the disease, LAD type I, is caused by a deficiency in the cell-surface β_2 integrin CD11/CD18. As a result of this autosomal-recessive disorder, immune cells are unable to attach to, and subsequently migrate through, the endothelial surface and accumulate in sites of inflammation. Patients present with delayed separation of the umbilical cord (> 3 weeks), poor wound healing, and recurrent infections. The more common infections include skin abscesses, otitis media, perirectal abscesses, bacteremia, and pneumonia. The organisms typically seen are *S aureus, E coli,* and *Pseudomonas aeruginosa.* Severity of disease may vary depending on the levels of integrin present on the cell surface. Patients with complete absence of CD11/CD18 usually present with severe recurrent infections and die within the first few years of life. Bone-marrow transplantation has been successful in some of these patients.

Chédiak-Higashi Syndrome

Chédiak-Higashi syndrome is a rare autosomal-recessive disorder characterized by recurrent pyogenic infections, partial albinism, platelet storage pool defect, and the presence of giant cytoplasmic granules in granulocytes. The pathogenesis of this disorder is not well understood. Patients have a lysosomal storage defect as well as abnormal phagocyte chemotaxis. Children present with recurrent pyogenic sinopulmonary infections, skin infections, and subcutaneous abscesses. They have increased susceptibility to *S aureus* and streptococci as well as to gram-negative organisms and fungi. The diagnosis is made by identifying the giant granules in myeloid cells on the peripheral smear. Treatment is supportive, with aggressive treatment of acute infections. Some patients have had a successful response to bone-marrow transplantation.

Chronic Granulomatous Disease

Chronic granulomatous disease (CGD) is an inherited disorder caused by an abnormal respiratory burst in phagocytes. The phagocytes are unable to generate oxygen radicals such as superoxide anion and, as a result, have defective intracellular killing. There is an X-linked form of CGD, which is the more common, as well as an autosomal-recessive form. The X-linked form is caused by a defect in one of the membrane-associated NADPH subunits. The autosomal-recessive form is caused by a defect in one of the cytosolic components, which is also required for a normal oxidative burst.

Patients commonly present with recurrent infections caused by catalase-positive microorganisms. The most common organisms are *S aureus, Serratia marcescens,* and *Aspergillus* species. Patients frequently present with cutaneous abscesses, lymphadenitis, pneumonia complicated by empyema or lung abscess, and perirectal abscess. Patients also may have a chronic inflammatory disease, which may manifest itself as chronic lymphadenopathy and intermittent fevers with no identifiable microorganisms. Treatment usually is supportive, with aggressive treatment of infections as well as prophylaxis with trimethoprim-sulfamethoxazole. Many patients have benefited from γ-interferon; a significant reduction in recurrent infections has been noted in placebo-controlled clinical trials. The mechanism of action of γ-interferon in this disease is unknown, although it has been postulated to increase respiratory burst activity.

PEDIATRIC ACQUIRED IMMUNODEFICIENCY SYNDROME: APPROACHES TO DIAGNOSIS & TREATMENT

Pediatric AIDS is a leading cause of death in children throughout the world. The clinical signs and symptoms seen in children infected with HIV-1 are indistinguishable from those seen in children with inherited primary immunodeficiency disease (see Table 7–4). Because pediatric AIDS is a far more common disorder than any other inherited primary immunodeficiency disorder, it is important to examine all children with too many infections or unusual infections for HIV-1.

TRANSMISSION

Most children infected with HIV acquire the virus by transmission from an infected mother. The risk of transmission without intervention varies throughout the world from as low as 14.4% in Europe to more than 30% in coastal cities in the United States. Rates of transmission are dramatically decreased by the administration of zidovudine during pregnancy. Results of a randomized, placebo-controlled trial indicate that giving zidovudine to the mother orally during pregnancy (after 14 weeks' gestation), intravenously during labor, and to the infant for 6 weeks after delivery reduced transmission from 25% (placebo group) to 8% (zidovudine group). This treatment plan is now recommended for all pregnant women with HIV-1 infection in the United States and the developed world.

The transmission of HIV from mother to infant is multifactorial. Factors contributing to such transmission include advanced maternal disease, primary infection during pregnancy, high viral load during pregnancy, and low maternal CD4 count. Obstetric factors contributing to transmission include rupture of membranes longer than 4 hours, prematurity (< 32 weeks' gestation), and chorioamniocentesis, as well as "skin breaks" and bloody gastric aspirates in newborns. In twin births, the risk of transmission for the second-born child is 40% versus 24% in the first-born. It is likely that most (two thirds) infants with HIV-1 infection acquire their infection peripartum, as the infant passes through the mother's birth canal and is exposed to HIV-1 in the mother's blood and cervical vaginal secretions. Transmission also may occur in utero or postpartum in breast-fed infants.

A primary goal in HIV treatment is to develop strategies to prevent transmission from mother to child. Promising approaches include the treatment of HIV-1 infected mothers with zidovudine. Other areas of active investigation include HIV-specific vaccines in combination with specific monoclonal antibodies to be administered shortly after birth. The second strategy to prevent transmission includes a universal approach to offering HIV counseling and testing to pregnant women, regardless of the prevalence of HIV infection in their community or their perceived risk for infection. This uniform policy should reach HIV infected pregnant women in all populations and geographic areas of the United States. Although this universal approach will necessitate increased resources, the effect of implementation of HIV-1 counseling and testing services for pregnant women will result in medical interventions that will reduce HIV-related morbidity in women and their infants and should ultimately reduce medical costs.

DIAGNOSIS OF HIV INFECTION IN CHILDREN

The diagnosis of HIV-1 infection in infants and children is based on (1) epidemiologic risk factors, (2) clinical presentation, and (3) confirmation by serologic test or documentation of the presence of virus and/or genome in the peripheral blood. The "gold standard" for the documentation of genome in the peripheral blood remains DNA polymerase chain reaction (PCR), which detects the integration of viral genetic material into the human chromosome. The standard test for the diagnosis of HIV infection in adults is enzyme-linked immunosorbent assay (ELISA) IgG anti-HIV with confirmation using Western blot analysis. IgG antibody in infants born after 32 weeks' gestation and until age 18 months may reflect maternal antibody because of the active transport of IgG across the placenta at 32 weeks' gestation. Therefore, the documentation of HIV-1 infection in infants younger than 18 months is based on the identification of HIV-1 in peripheral blood mononuclear cells by culture or the identification of genome by DNA-PCR. The finding must be confirmed by repeating the HIV-1 culture or DNA-PCR within 1 month. With the use of DNA-PCR, it is now possible to distinguish those infants who have HIV-1 infection from those who are exposed but not infected in 96% of infants by age 28 days. The recommended schedule for testing infants at risk is as close to birth as possible (within 72 hours); if there is no evidence of virus by culture or DNA-PCR, these tests should be repeated at age 1 month and again at age 2–4 months. If there still is no evidence of virus, IgG anti-HIV (ELISA) should be obtained at age 12 and 18 months. However, if an infant has no evidence of virus or genome by culture or DNA-PCR on two occasions after age 1 month, there is greater than 96% certainty that the infant is not infected with HIV-1.

After HIV-1 infection is documented, baseline immunologic studies should be obtained. These include total T-cell count, percentage and total numbers of CD4 and CD8 cells, and quantitative immunoglobulin levels. In addition, the HIV-1 viral load should be quantitated by plasma RNA-PCR, which measures the circulating plasma virus not yet incorporated into the human genome.

CLINICAL MANIFESTATIONS

There are two risk populations for clinical progression in infants who acquire HIV from their mothers. The first group includes approximately 20% of infected infants. These infants have early onset and rapidly progressive disease, and most die by age 2 years. These infants likely acquire HIV in utero. The second and larger group has a longer incubation period, with the first signs of clinical disease at a median age of 6.1 years. These infants likely acquire HIV-1 infection perinatally.

The clinical features of AIDS in children, as well as the differences between children and adults, are shown in Table 7–10. Common clinical features include failure to thrive, developmental delay, oral candidiasis, diarrhea, chronic eczema, and intermittent fevers of unknown origin. Abnormal antibody-mediated immunity in HIV-infected children predisposes them to overwhelming infections with encapsulated organisms. Chronic sinopulmonary disease, as well as skin and soft tissue infections, is common. Physical examination findings may include splenomegaly and lymphadenopathy.

Children with HIV are susceptible to opportunistic infections, including *P carinii, Mycobacterium avium-intracellulare, Candida, Cryptosporidiosis,* and *Mycobacterium tuberculosis.* Chronic herpes simplex infection is common in HIV-1 infected children, and chronic vari-

cella frequently follows a primary infection. Pulmonary disease is common in children with AIDS. In a child with HIV-1 and pulmonary infiltrates, the differential diagnosis is broad and ranges from lymphocytic interstitial pneumonitis to acute bacterial pneumonia, viral pneumonia, fungal pneumonitis, and PCP.

HIV-1 infection of the central nervous system and developmental delay are among the most devastating complications of pediatric AIDS. Encephalopathy may be the first manifestation of HIV-1 infection; the rate of progression varies, and children may remain stable for several years or progress rapidly over a few weeks. Developmental delay and intellectual deterioration usually are accompanied by neurologic abnormalities, such as increased muscle tone, paresis, or Bell palsy. Acquired microcephaly may be the first sign of neurologic disease. Computed tomographic scans show atrophy of the brain with ventricular enlargement; calcifications and contrast enhancement in the basal ganglia and frontal lobes plus attenuation of white matter may be present.

Autoimmune disorders are common in children with HIV and probably reflect the early polyclonal activation of B cells and hypergammaglobulinemia. Immune-mediated thrombocytopenia occurs in up to 10% of infected children. Patients also may have a positive Coombs test result for hemolytic anemia. The role of autoantibody in the cardiovascular manifestations of HIV disease remains poorly defined. A relatively rare and usually mild autoimmune renal disease may also occur.

Most children currently infected with HIV-1 likely will live for extended periods of time. Before the institution of antiretroviral therapy, the median life expectancy after diagnosis of HIV-1 infection was approximately 35 months; the current median life expectancy with the use of three antiretroviral agents is unknown but is greatly improved.

MANAGEMENT

HIV-1 infection in children is a multisystem disorder and a chronic illness with acute exacerbations. Management includes providing specific treatment of HIV-1 and supportive care within a multidisciplinary setting. Prompt diagnosis and specific treatment of all infections is essential. Nutrition should be carefully followed, and nighttime enteral feedings or hyperalimentation should be used when failure to thrive is a major problem. Although there is no specific management for the central nervous system disease, treatment is directed at its neurologic manifestations. For example, as lower extremity neurologic signs develop, providing leg braces may allow for longer periods of normal ambulation.

The time for the initiation of antiretroviral agents, as well as the specific agents to use in infants, is controversial. Viral load, quantitated by RNA-PCR copy per milliliter, is substantially greater in children than in adults at the time of diagnosis; remains elevated for up to 2–3 years in children, compared with 2 months in adults; and sub-

Table 7–10. Clinical features of AIDS in children and adults.

Common in children and adults
Opportunistic infections (not CNS)
Chronic mucocutaneous *Candida*
Neurologic abnormalities
Chronic diarrhea
Chronic fevers
Diffuse adenopathy
Hepatosplenomegaly
Chronic eczema
Renal disease
Cardiomyopathy
More common in children
Recurrent bacterial infections
Chronic interstitial pneumonitis
Parotitis
Failure to thrive
Early onset developmental delay
More common in adults
Neoplasms
Opportunistic infections of CNS

CNS = central nervous system.

sequently declines to 100,000 copies rather than 10,000 copies as in adults. Therefore, the early initiation of antiretroviral therapy to control the high viral load is particularly important in children. Many now recommend initiation of combination antiretroviral therapy at the time of diagnosis and as early as age 28 days.

Zidovudine, a thymidine analogue and reverse transcriptase inhibitor, is safe in children. As a single agent, however, it reduces viral load modestly and only temporarily. When accompanied by a second nonthymidine analogue–reverse transcriptase inhibitor, such as dideoxyinosine or Epivir, the impact on viral load is greater and is sustained for longer periods of time. It also is likely that the addition of a protease inhibitor to the regimen will further improve the treatment of HIV-1 in children. Regardless of the therapy selected, it is important to monitor decreases of viral load by RNA-PCR in order to assess the effect of therapy and to adjust treatment appropriately.

Because PCP is the most common opportunistic infection in HIV-1 infected children, prophylaxis with trimethoprim-sulfamethoxazole is recommended for all HIV-exposed infants between age 6 weeks and 4 months. Prophylaxis should be continued between 4 and 12 months if HIV infection is indeterminate. However, if HIV infection has been reasonably excluded, prophylaxis should be discontinued. For those children in whom HIV-1 infection is documented between 1 and 5 years of age, prophylaxis should be initiated or continued if the absolute CD4 count is less than 500 cells/mL or the CD4 percentage is less than 15%. Between 6 and 12 years, prophylaxis should be continued if the CD4 count is less than 200 cells/mL or the CD4 percentage is less than 15%.

Childhood immunizations, including hepatitis B, should be provided. Inactivated poliovirus vaccine must be substituted for OPV in the patient as well as in all household contacts. HIV-1 infected children should receive both polyvalent pneumococcal vaccine (Pneumovax) and, if exposed to measles, immunoglobulin. Likewise, zoster immunoglobulin should be administered after exposure to varicella.

There has been significant progress recently in the prevention and treatment of pediatric AIDS, which has greatly improved prognosis. It is likely that many children with HIV-1 infection will live through adolescence and that new manifestations of this increasingly chronic illness will be identified during the next few years.

MOLECULAR MECHANISMS IN PRIMARY IMMUNODEFICIENCY DISORDERS

Remarkable progress has been made in our understanding of the molecular defects causing primary immunodefi-

Table 7–11. Molecular defects found in some of the primary immunodeficiencies.

Disorder	Classification	Molecular Defect
Ataxia-telangiectasia	Combined T/B cell	*ATM* gene (PI-3 kinase-like gene)
Agammaglobulinemia	B cell	Bruton tyrosine kinase
Hyper-IgM	B/T cell	CD40 ligand (on T cells)
SCID X-linked	Combined T/B cell	IL-2 γ-chain
SCID-AR	Combined T/B cell	ADA/PNP
SCID-AR	CD8 lymphopenia	ZAP-70
Wiskott-Aldrich	T/B cell	WASP protein, proline-rich

ADA/PNP = adenosine deaminase/purine nucleoside phosphorylase; AR = autosomal recessive; IL-2 = interleukin-2; SCID = severe combined immunodeficiency.

ciency disorders (Table 7–11). This information has improved our understanding of how the normal immune system functions and has guided our approach to treatment of primary immunodeficiency disorders.

Understanding molecular mechanisms has lead to new diagnostic approaches and has aided the development of new therapeutic interventions. Characterization of these defects at a molecular level has opened the door to sophisticated techniques to identify the precise genetic mutation and to identify family members at risk for passing the disorder onto their offspring. Involvement of genetic counselors may be very important for these families.

The recent progress in understanding molecular mechanisms also has led to the development of new therapeutic approaches. Newer treatments include the use of recombinant enzyme replacement therapies, such as polyethylene glycol-modified bovine adenosine deaminase (PEG-ADA) for ADA deficiency, and the use of recombinant cytokines, such as γ-interferon for CGD and hyper-IgE syndrome. Identification of the precise genetic defect is allowing the definition of genotype-phenotype associations for specific diseases. For example, definition of the precise abnormality in the *WASP* gene in a child with WAS allows prediction of the relative risk of severe thrombocytopenia versus the development of malignant disease. This knowledge can be used to guide therapy.

The ultimate treatment for many of these diseases would be to cure the illness with gene therapy. Because many of the primary immunodeficiencies currently are treatable by bone-marrow transplantation, a potential therapeutic approach is placement of the functional gene in bone-marrow stem cells. Gene therapy in autologous peripheral blood lymphocytes has been used successfully to treat ADA deficiency in patients whose condition was unresponsive to enzyme replacement. Some of these children have had good clinical responses to peripheral lymphocyte gene therapy, although frequent treatments are required because peripheral lymphocytes have a limited life span. Clinical studies using stem-cell gene therapy currently are under way, with the hope of providing a cure for patients with ADA deficiency. Preliminary results show that retroviral gene therapy may successfully transfer a gene into stem cells and that this gene remains expressed several years after initial treatment. It is not yet known, however, whether the patients have substantial therapeutic benefit from these treatments. Further studies are needed to develop efficient gene delivery systems, including viral vectors and liposomes, that are safe and allow for long-term expression of the desired gene in vivo.

REFERENCES

Auger I et al: Incubation periods for paediatric AIDS patients. Nature 1988;336:575.

Boyer P et al: Factors predictive of maternal-fetal transmission of HIV-1. JAMA 1994;271:1925.

Bryson Y et al: Establishment of a definition of the timing of vertical HIV-1 infection. N Engl J Med 1992;327:1246.

Buckley RH: Breakthroughs in the understanding and therapy of primary immunodeficiency. Pediatr Clin North Am 1994; 41:665.

Buckley RH: Immunodeficiency diseases. JAMA 1987;258: 2841.

Connor E et al: Reduction of maternal-infant transmission of human immunodeficiency virus type 1 with zidovudine treatment. N Engl J Med 1994;331:1173.

el Habbal MH, Strobel S: Leukocyte adhesion deficiency. Arch Dis Child 1993;69:463.

Mayaux M et al: Maternal factors associated with perinatal HIV-1 transmission: The French cohort study & years of follow-up observation. JAIDS 1995;8:188.

Nelson D, Kurman CC: Molecular genetic analysis of the primary immunodeficiency disorders. Pediatr Clin North Am 1994;41:657.

Pacheco SE, Shearer WT: Laboratory aspects of immunology. Pediatr Clin North Am 1994;41:623.

Savitsky K et al: A single ataxia-telangiectasia gene with a product similar to PI-3 kinase. Science 1995;268:1749.

Shearer W et al: Viral load and disease progression in infants infected with human immunodeficiency virus type 1. N Engl J Med 1997;336:1337.

Shyur SD, Hill HR: Immunodeficiency in the 1990s. Pediatr Infect Dis J 1991;10:595.

Summerfield J et al: Mannose binding protein gene mutations associated with unusual and severe infections in adults. Lancet 1995;345:886.

Wahn U: Evaluation of the child with suspected primary immunodeficiency. Pediatr Allergy Immunol 1995;6:71.

Wood RA, Sampson HA: The child with frequent infections. Curr Probl Pediatr 1989;19:229.

8

Rheumatic Diseases

Andrew Eichenfield, MD

Rheumatic, or connective tissue, diseases are conditions of unknown etiology that are characterized by inappropriate immune responses, resulting in inflammation and fibrosis. Although these diseases have a low incidence, they have serious clinical impact, given their potential for chronicity and engendering disability in childhood. Inasmuch as rheumatic diseases often present with musculoskeletal pain, it is useful to develop an organized approach to the evaluation of the child with limb pain.

THE CHILD WITH LIMB PAIN

Musculoskeletal aches and pains are among the most common of childhood complaints. Evaluation of children with limb pain involves careful history-taking, a thorough physical examination, and a few simple laboratory investigations. A list of some of the more prevalent causes of limb pain is presented in Table 8–1.

HISTORY

Nature of the Pain

Timing. The sudden onset of limb pain accompanies trauma but is also associated with septic arthritis, osteomyelitis, and, occasionally, occult malignant disease. Arthritis may have a more insidious onset, in which case a history of joint stiffness, most pronounced after periods of inactivity, serves to separate true arthritis from arthralgia (joint pain).

It is important to determine whether the child complains at any particular time of day. Pain that occurs after physical activity is suggestive of overuse and hypermobility syndromes. Diurnal variation in symptomatology (morning stiffness and evening pain after prolonged use)

is common in children with chronic arthritis. In such cases, a child may not complain of overt pain but may limp transiently on awakening. Pain severe enough to awaken a child from sleep is seen in both primary bone tumors and those that infiltrate bone (leukemia and neuroblastoma) and in osteomyelitis; however, it is also characteristic of growing pains, a completely benign condition.

Frequency & Duration. Relatively transient complaints that occur frequently, as in growing pains and hypermobility, are disconcerting to the family but are less likely to signify significant pathology than are symptoms that interfere with activities of daily living. Pain that is persistent or increases in intensity, frequency, or duration warrants investigation.

Trauma. A history of injury may be elicited but is often misleading (eg, toddlers fall on a regular basis). Young children are unlikely to sustain strains or sprains, owing to the greater flexibility of their tissues. A suspicion of child abuse is raised if the degree of injury is out of proportion to the history or is recurrent.

Location. The examination should determine whether the child can localize the pain to joint or muscle. Poorly localized pain involving the knees, shins, and ankles is characteristic of growing pains. Unilateral pain suggests a local cause, such as trauma or tumor. Consider the possibility of referred pain; recall that hip pathology (eg, slipped capital femoral epiphysis and avascular necrosis) may present with knee pain. Tenderness over the tibial tubercle or heel pain suggests osteochondrosis (Osgood-Schlatter and Sever diseases, respectively) but also may be an early sign of spondyloarthritis, secondary to inflammation of the infrapatellar or Achilles tendon insertions (enthesis).

Aggravating & Alleviating Factors. Rest alleviates the discomfort of chronic arthritis and overuse syndromes. Pain that occurs at rest is characteristic of bacterial infection or tumor. Nonsteroidal anti-inflammatory drugs (NSAIDs) are analgesics; do not presume that improvement after their use implies the presence of inflammation.

Associated Symptoms. The presence of precipitat-

Table 8–1. Common causes of limb pain in childhood.

Trauma
  Contusions
  Sprains, strains
  Fractures, subluxations
  Overuse syndromes (tennis elbow, Little League shoulder)
  Child abuse
Structural
  Slipped capital femoral epiphysis
  Avascular necrosis of bone
  Patellofemoral syndrome
  Hypermobility
Infection
  Osteomyelitis
  Septic arthritis
  Postinfectious (reactive) arthritis (enteric arthritis, rheumatic fever)
  Viral arthritis
  Lyme disease
  Disseminated gonococcal infection
  Cellulitis
  Diskitis
Hematologic/Oncologic
  Sickle-cell disease
  Leukemia
  Neuroblastoma
  Primary bone tumors
  Osteoid osteoma
  Hemophilia
Rheumatic diseases
  Juvenile rheumatoid arthritis
  Systemic lupus erythematosus
  Seronegative spondyloarthropathies
  Dermatomyositis
  Vasculitis (Henoch-Schönlein purpura, Kawasaki disease, polyarteritis nodosa, serum sickness)
Other
  Growing pains
  Psychogenic pain
  Reflex neurovascular dystrophy

ing factors (eg, illness, drug exposure, immunization, travel, and tick exposure) should be ascertained, as should a family history of arthritis or rheumatic disease. The presence of fever raises the question of infection, but fever often occurs in systemic lupus erythematosus (SLE), systemic-onset juvenile rheumatoid arthritis (JRA), and leukemia. An underlying systemic disease is suggested by a history of photosensitive or malar rash (SLE, dermatomyositis, parvovirus), Raynaud phenomenon (SLE, scleroderma), oral ulcers (SLE, inflammatory bowel disease [IBD]), weight loss (malignant disease, IBD), abdominal pain (SLE, Henoch-Schönlein purpura [HSP]), dysphagia (SLE, dermatomyositis, scleroderma), or eye inflammation (JRA, Reiter syndrome, IBD, spondyloarthritis).

PHYSICAL EXAMINATION

A complete physical examination is mandatory in the child with limb pain to corroborate findings suggested by history and to establish whether the pain is a localized or systemic process. Physical findings that suggest multisystem disease include hepatosplenomegaly, diffuse lymphadenopathy, and rash. Specifically, the extremities should be inspected for swelling and deformity. Any asymmetry should be noted; muscle wasting can occur after as little as 1 week of disuse. All the extremities should be palpated to confirm the presence of swelling that may not be obvious and to assess for tenderness (fracture, osteomyelitis). Range of motion, both active and passive, should be tested, as should muscle strength and deep tendon reflexes.

LABORATORY INVESTIGATIONS

Laboratory investigations in the child with limb pain are aimed at documenting the presence of inflammation and/or autoimmunity. The erythrocyte sedimentation rate (ESR), a simple test that indirectly reflects levels of fibrinogen and other acute phase reactants, can often distinguish children with arthritis from those with arthralgia. Joint swelling in the absence of an elevated ESR occurs in post-traumatic arthritis, occasionally in pauciarticular JRA, and in sickle-cell disease (sickling interferes with the test). The complete blood count will often provide useful clues to the presence of occult malignant disease (anemia, thrombocytopenia, lymphocytosis), acute osteoarticular infection (leukocytosis with a predominance of neutrophils and bands), and inflammatory joint disease (varying degrees of elevation in the white blood cell and platelet counts with or without associated anemia). If multisystem disease is suspected, urinalysis and screening blood chemistry panel will serve to establish the presence of renal or hepatic dysfunction. Although a positive fluorescent antinuclear antibody (ANA) is a sensitive indicator of humoral immune dysregulation, it is not specific for rheumatic disease. Specific associations between various ANAs and rheumatic conditions are discussed below. Rheumatoid factor (RF), which is IgM antibody against the Fc fragment of immunoglobulins, is positive in up to 80% of adults with rheumatoid arthritis; however, it is neither sensitive nor specific in the evaluation of children with arthritis.

Radiographs are indicated in patients with suspected orthopedic conditions (eg, trauma, tumor, avascular necrosis, and slipped capital femoral epiphysis). Comparison views of the contralateral extremity should always be obtained in growing children. Bone scintigraphy is useful in distinguishing between arthritis and occult malignant disease; the results are positive in osteomyelitis before radiographic changes occur.

IMPORTANT NONARTHRITIC CAUSES OF LIMB PAIN

Growing Pains

Growing pains have nothing to do with growth. They are troublesome nonarticular limb pains that affect up to

15% of school-aged children. Growing pains often are associated with physical activity and therefore tend to occur late in the day and early evening, after the child is no longer distracted by play. They often awaken the child from sleep and respond to analgesics and massage. The patient typically has difficulty localizing the pain, which may involve the thighs, knees, calves, and pretibial surfaces. Physical examination and gait are invariably normal, as are the results of laboratory investigations. Growing pains are never unilateral and do not cause the child to limp. Pain that is limited to joints or increases in frequency, duration, or intensity should be evaluated carefully to rule out inflammatory joint disease or occult malignant disease.

Generalized Hypermobility

The benign hypermobile joint syndrome of childhood is an extreme variation of normal joint range that occurs in the absence of a defined heritable disorder of connective tissue. Up to 12% of school-aged children have been found to have hyperextensible joints; it is more common in younger children and girls. Joint laxity is more prevalent among dancers, gymnasts, and instrumental musicians. It predisposes affected individuals to recurrent nonspecific limb pains, as well as to arthralgias, sprains, transient joint effusions, dislocations, and fibromyalgia. Children with hypermobility may also have mitral valve prolapse. Criteria for hypermobility are presented in Table 8–2. Management is conservative and includes curtailment of offending physical activities, physical therapy, and NSAIDs as required.

APPROACH TO ARTHRITIS

The presence of arthritis is considered in any patient with limb pain but especially in those with a history of pain limited to the joints. As already noted, it is the presence of joint stiffness after periods of inactivity that distinguishes arthritis from arthralgia. Children with inflammatory joint disease awaken with morning stiffness and often are noted to limp at that time; the stiffness improves with movement. In the child in whom more than one joint is involved, it is important to determine the mode of onset. Migratory arthritis refers to pain that resolves in one joint before going on to involve the next; this is classically seen in acute rheumatic fever but also in a number of other conditions. JRA tends not to migrate but to take on an additive pattern.

The presence of arthritis is established by the appearance of joint swelling or, in its absence, tenderness to palpation, reduced range of motion or pain on movement, and increased warmth. This may be difficult to ascertain in an uncooperative younger child. Pain out of proportion to objective physical findings is seen in children with acute rheumatic fever, occult malignant disease, and psychogenic conditions.

The differential diagnosis of joint inflammation in children is extensive. The pattern of joint involvement may help in distinguishing among the many causes of arthritis.

ACUTE ARTHRITIS

CAUSES OF ACUTE ARTHRITIS

Acute Monarthritis

Determining the duration and pattern of joint involvement is crucial in establishing a potential diagnosis. Monarticular arthritis and fever represents pyogenic infection until proved otherwise and is the only absolute indication for diagnostic arthrocentesis in a child (see Chapter 9). All joint fluids should be examined by Gram stain and cultured for bacteria, although the yield of synovial fluid culture in otherwise diagnosed septic arthritis is only 70–80%.

Monarthritis without fever lasting less than a week is a typical pattern in hemarthrosis; prolonged or unusual bruising should suggest a bleeding diathesis or child abuse. As noted above, children with hyperextensibility may present with joint pain and fleeting effusions. **Transient synovitis of the hip** is the most common nontraumatic cause of childhood arthritis. It more commonly affects boys aged 3–6 years, usually after an upper respiratory infection. The child either limps or refuses to bear weight and complains of pain in the groin, anterior thigh, or knee. Radiographs of both hips and knees should be obtained in any child complaining of knee pain in the absence of corroborative physical findings. The results of laboratory investigations usually are within normal limits. The condition is self-limiting, rarely lasting more than 10 days; management involves rest and analgesics. Recurrence with subsequent upper respiratory infections is not uncommon, but care should be taken to rule out avascular

Table 8–2. Criteria for joint hypermobility.[1,2]

1. Passive dorsiflexion of the fifth finger beyond 90 degrees with the forearm flat on a table
2. Passive apposition of the thumb to the flexor aspect of the forearm
3. Hyperextension of the elbow beyond 10 degrees
4. Hyperextension of the knee beyond 10 degrees
5. Forward flexion of the trunk so that the palms of the hands rest easily on the floor

[1]Reproduced, with permission, from Beighton P: The Ehlers-Danlos syndromes. Page 200 in: Beighton P (editor): *Heritable Disorders of Connective Tissue.* Mosby-Year Book, 1993.
[2]Presence of any three criteria establishes joint hypermobility.

necrosis of the femoral head (Perthé disease) when the limp persists.

Acute Polyarthritis

Acute polyarthritis of relatively short duration is often the presenting manifestation of rheumatic fever and features prominently in a number of vasculitic syndromes (HSP, serum sickness–like reactions, and Kawasaki disease). Other infectious causes result in an acute polyarthritis as well.

INFECTIOUS POLYARTHRITIS

Unlike other bacterial etiologies of arthritis, *Neisseria gonorrhoeae* often affects more than one joint and is often associated with tenosynovitis. Embolic skin lesions that can be mistaken for vasculitis are a feature of disseminated gonococcal and meningococcal infection. Lyme disease can affect more than one joint at a time, as can parvovirus B19.

POSTINFECTIOUS POLYARTHRITIS: RHEUMATIC FEVER

Rheumatic fever was once a common cause of polyarthritis. However, although its incidence has declined in the United States, the disease still occurs in epidemics, with peak ages of onset from 5 to 15 years. It is an example of molecular mimicry in which antibodies to group A streptococci cross-react with antigens in various tissues, resulting in inflammation.

Clinical Manifestations

The onset of rheumatic fever typically follows streptococcal pharyngitis after 1–3 weeks and is characterized by nonspecific malaise and fever. **Polyarthritis** is the most common major manifestation, occurring in up to 75% of patients. Articular pain often is severe and out of proportion to objective findings. The arthritis is frequently migratory, resolving in one joint after 3–10 days before going on to involve another. Large joints of the lower extremities tend to be affected more frequently. The arthritis is exquisitely sensitive to even low doses of aspirin; failure to respond to salicylates should suggest another diagnosis.

Carditis, present in 40% of patients, is suspected in children with resting tachycardia but is diagnosed with certainty in those with new heart murmurs. A systolic murmur suggesting mitral insufficiency is the most common of these; the next most common murmurs are a middiastolic rumble at the apex (Carey-Coombs murmur) and an early diastolic murmur of aortic regurgitation. Right-sided lesions are uncommon. Myocarditis (eg, resting tachycardia, cardiomegaly, and congestive heart failure) and pericarditis may accompany valvular involvement but rarely occur in isolation.

Less common manifestations of rheumatic fever include Sydenham chorea, which may occur in isolation weeks after the inciting infection or other signs of the disease. In fewer than 15% of patients, emotional lability and involuntary movements of the face and upper extremities develop. These disappear during sleep and are exacerbated by emotional factors, which may wrongly suggest a conversion reaction. **Erythema marginatum** is an evanescent, macular eruption with serpiginous borders and central clearing. It is virtually always associated with carditis but is uncommon, occurring in fewer than 10% of patients. **Subcutaneous nodules,** which are even rarer, are painless swellings less than 1 cm in diameter. They are found over bony prominences and extensor tendons.

Laboratory Findings

Establishing evidence of an antecedent streptococcal pharyngitis is a sine qua non for the diagnosis of rheumatic fever. Streptococci may be detected by rapid antigen tests or pharyngeal culture or by elevated serum levels of antistreptococcal antibodies. Antistreptolysin O (ASO) titers are elevated in 80% of patients when first measured. In those with normal ASO titers, antibodies to the streptococcal proteins hyaluronidase and deoxyribonuclease B will increase the yield to 90%. With the exception of isolated chorea, rheumatic fever is always associated with an acute phase response, so that the ESR or C-reactive protein level will be elevated.

Diagnosis

A diagnosis of rheumatic fever is established clinically through the application of the Jones criteria (Table 8–3). A few caveats are in order. Arthralgia cannot be considered a minor criterion if arthritis is the major one. The arthritis of rheumatic fever is not always migratory; monarthritis can occur after streptococcal pharyngitis, as can fixed polyarthritis lasting for months. Such children have been said to have "post-streptococcal reactive arthritis," an entity originally believed to be distinct from rheumatic fever. With reports of subsequent carditis in

Table 8–3. Criteria for the diagnosis of rheumatic fever.[1,2]

Major Manifestations	Minor Manifestations
Carditis	Clinical findings
Polyarthritis	Arthralgia
Chorea	Fever
Erythema marginatum	Laboratory findings
Subcutaneous nodules	Elevated acute phase reactants
	Erythrocyte sedimentation rate
	C-reactive protein
	Prolonged P-R interval

[1]Reproduced, with permission, from Dajani AS et al: Guideline for the diagnosis of rheumatic fever: Jones criteria, updated 1992. Circulation 1993; 87:302.
[2]Supporting evidence of antecedent group A streptococcal infection: positive throat culture or rapid streptococcal antigen test; elevated or increasing streptococcal antibody titer.

some patients, this is now believed to represent a variant of rheumatic fever.

According to the current version of the Jones criteria, echocardiographically documented but clinically inaudible valvular insufficiency is not sufficient evidence of carditis. Similarly, P-R prolongation on electrocardiogram is not diagnostic of cardiac involvement.

Treatment

Once a diagnosis is established, all patients should receive a full treatment course of penicillin, even in the absence of a positive throat culture. This is followed by continuous antistreptococcal prophylaxis administered as 1.2 million U of benzathine penicillin every 3–4 weeks. Oral prophylaxis with twice-daily penicillin is effective, but compliance is almost never completely attained. Relief of joint symptoms and fever typically is achieved rapidly with salicylates administered as aspirin, 60–100 mg/kg/d in four divided doses. Corticosteroids (prednisone, 2 mg/kg/d) are indicated for congestive heart failure.

Prognosis

Children without carditis fare well, although they are at risk for heart involvement with subsequent attacks; therefore, continuous antibiotic prophylaxis is crucial. Although up to 70% of those with heart involvement have no major sequelae, those with severe carditis are likely to have permanent valvular lesions.

VASCULITIS & ACUTE ARTHRITIS

Henoch-Schönlein Purpura

Polyarthritis is an important feature of HSP, an IgA-mediated vasculitis involving small blood vessels. Also known as anaphylactoid purpura, it is recognized by the association of typical rash, arthritis, abdominal colic, and renal involvement. The illness affects school-aged children and most often follows an upper respiratory infection or streptococcal pharyngitis. A typical presentation begins with the appearance of skin lesions that resemble urticaria but are fixed in location, predominating over the lower extremities and buttocks. Within a day or so, as the inflammatory response continues, damage to vessel walls results in hemorrhage into the skin and the appearance of palpable petechiae and purpura. The skin lesions occur in successive crops and tend to correlate with other manifestations of the disease. Angioedema of the hands and feet (occasionally periorbital and forehead) accompanies the rash in approximately half the affected children.

The arthritis of HSP affects up to 84% of patients and more often involves the large joints of the lower extremities. It may migrate and precedes the rash in a significant minority of cases. It may interfere with ambulation but leaves no permanent sequelae.

Gastrointestinal (GI) involvement occurs in 60–85% of patients and can also precede the rash. Crampy abdominal pain is related to vasculitis and bowel wall edema and hemorrhage. This results in clinical or occult GI bleeding. Intussusception, usually ileo-ileal, is a feared complication of HSP, as it can lead to bowel infarction and perforation.

Renal disease develops in 10–50% of patients and is associated with varying degrees of hematuria and proteinuria. Hypertension or marked proteinuria, sometimes at levels noted in nephrosis, are poor prognostic features. Other less frequent manifestations include scrotal edema and hemorrhage, pulmonary vasculitis and hemorrhage, and central nervous system involvement.

The entire illness typically lasts less than 6 weeks, although HSP can recur with subsequent infections. Management is symptomatic. NSAIDs are effective in controlling the arthritis of HSP but may confuse the picture, as they may engender abdominal pain. Although corticosteroids have never been subjected to rigorous study, they appear to be useful in managing GI involvement but are ineffective in preventing or controlling nephritis.

Serum Sickness–like Reaction

Serum sickness occurs when a foreign protein (classically horse serum) is administered, resulting in circulating antigen-antibody complexes that fix to the walls of blood vessels and initiate a vasculitis. Serum sickness–like reactions occur after exposure to a drug or virus and result in a leukocytoclastic vasculitis involving small blood vessels. Clinically, this is manifested as urticarial skin lesions and polyarthritis, often in association with fever. Commonly implicated drugs include antibiotics (eg, cefaclor, sulfonamides, and penicillins) and anticonvulsants (eg, phenytoin).

ARTHRITIS OF GREATER THAN 1 WEEK'S DURATION

JUVENILE RHEUMATOID ARTHRITIS

JRA is an umbrella term describing a group of disorders that have in common chronic joint inflammation. If a child's arthritis lasts longer than 7–10 days, JRA becomes a diagnostic possibility and is considered strongly with duration greater than 6 weeks. Because JRA is a diagnosis of exclusion, care must be taken to rule out any underlying infectious, inflammatory, or oncologic condition. It has been possible to identify a number of different patterns of joint involvement on the basis of numbers of joints involved, age of onset, and presence of fever.

Clinical Features of JRA by Subgroup

Pauciarticular JRA. This affects four or fewer joints and accounts for nearly 50% of cases of chronic arthritis in children. It can be subdivided into two subgroups, affecting young girls and older boys.

Type 1 typically involves girls, aged 2–3 years, who tend to have fair skin and hair. The arthritis involves large joints, commonly the knee, ankle, and wrist, and may be associated with few symptoms. A child may be noted to limp in the morning, or swelling may be noted by a parent at the time of a bath or diaper change. These children are at great risk for asymptomatic chronic iridocyclitis, a disease manifestation that is associated with the presence of ANAs. Children with pauciarticular JRA and positive ANAs should be screened by slit-lamp examination every 3–4 months to ensure early diagnosis and therapy.

Type 2 pauciarticular JRA affects boys more than girls and is characterized by an asymmetric arthritis of the lower extremities, often involving the hips and knees. These children are often HLA B27–positive and are more properly considered to have a form of spondyloarthropathy than rheumatoid arthritis. They need not, however, go on to have involvement of the axial spine. There usually are no associated autoantibodies. Uveitis, when it does occur, results in a symptomatic reddened eye.

Polyarticular JRA. This affects five or more joints and is also subdivided into two subgroups, depending on the presence or absence of RF. RF-negative children tend to be younger, and the course of their arthritis more variable. This subgroup accounts for approximately 20% of children with JRA. Some resemble girls with pauciarticular onset, varying only in the number and size of involved joints. These children, however, less often are ANA positive, but asymptomatic uveitis can also develop. RF-positive polyarthritis affects 5–10% of children with JRA and represents early-onset adult rheumatoid arthritis. As such, it also has a female predominance and is associated with those features common in adults with rheumatoid arthritis, including rheumatoid nodules and early progression to erosive disease. Eye inflammation is uncommon in these children.

Systemic-onset JRA. This is characterized by fever as high as 41 °C, typically as once or twice daily spikes, at which time the child is extremely irritable and may complain of arthralgia and myalgia. In more than 75% of patients, a salmon-colored macular eruption occurs at the time of the temperature spike, but this does not establish the diagnosis. Affected children present with fevers of unknown origin, because they may not have obvious arthritis. Inflammation of serosal surfaces can also occur, most commonly as pericarditis (15–30% of patients) and less commonly as pleuritis or peritonitis. Other systemic features include hepatosplenomegaly and generalized lymphadenopathy, which may prompt consideration of occult malignant disease or chronic viral infection (ie, HIV). Arthritis eventually becomes evident, often as the fevers are beginning to wane. Joint involvement may be pauciarticular or polyarticular, and permanent deformity develops in approximately 25% of patients. Hematologic features of systemic JRA include microcytic anemia, polymorphonuclear leukocytosis with left shift, and thrombocytosis. Other laboratory findings include markedly elevated acute phase reactants (ESR, C-reactive protein), hyperglobulinemia,

and, notably, absent autoantibodies (negative ANA and RF).

Treatment

Management of JRA is individualized according to the severity of the disease. In general, all children initially receive an NSAID. The NSAIDs approved by the Food and Drug Administration are listed in Table 8–4. Parents can be told to expect some amelioration of joint pain in the first 7–10 days, improvement in stiffness in the second week, and diminished swelling by the third week of therapy. Swelling continues to improve over a 6-week interval and then typically plateaus. Not all children will respond to the first NSAID used, but care should be taken to use a given NSAID to its maximum tolerated dose for at least 3–6 weeks before abandoning it in favor of another. Up to 50% of children with JRA will respond adequately to NSAIDs alone. Adverse effects common to all NSAIDs include GI intolerance (eg, gastritis and ulceration) and easy bruising.

If arthritis continues after several NSAIDs are tried, consideration should be given to the addition of disease-modifying drugs. These are also known as slow-acting antirheumatic drugs, as they take weeks to months to exert their effects. Injectable gold salts have fallen out of favor in many centers, owing to frequent side effects (eg, reversible bone marrow suppression, proteinuria, and dermatitis). They should not be administered to children with systemic JRA. Children with milder, persistent polyarthritis may respond to hydroxychloroquine or oral gold. Sulfasalazine appears to be most effective in children with

Table 8–4. Drug therapy of juvenile rheumatoid arthritis.

Nonsteroidal anti-inflammatory drugs approved by the Food and Drug Administration for use in children.	
Drug	**Dose**
Aspirin (or choline magnesium trisalicylate)	80–100 mg/kg/d ÷ 4 (max 4000 mg/d)
Ibuprofen	40 mg/kg/d ÷ 3 (max 3600 mg/d)
Naproxen	10–20 mg/kg/d ÷ 2 (max 1000 mg/d)
Tolmetin sodium	20–30 mg/kg/d ÷ 3 (max 2000 mg/d)
Indomethacin	2–3 mg/kg/d ÷ 3 (max 150 mg/d)
Disease-modifying antirheumatic drugs.	
Drug	**Dose**
Hydroxycholoroquine	6.5 mg/kg/d (max 400 mg/d)
Sulfasalazine	40–50 mg/kg/d ÷ 2 (max 3000 mg/d)
Intramuscular gold salts	1 mg/kg/wk (max 50 mg)
Auranofin (oral gold)	0.15 mg/kg/d initially, 0.2 mg/kg day if not effective after 6 months (max 9 mg/d)
Methotrexate	10–15 mg/m^2/wk (max 20 mg/wk)

HLA-B27–related disease. Low-dose methotrexate is the only disease-modifying agent that has been shown to be effective in JRA in a placebo-controlled study. It usually is reserved for children with aggressive polyarthritis and those with ongoing systemic features.

Corticosteroids are more potent anti-inflammatory agents than NSAIDs. However, these drugs are not believed to affect disease progression and are associated with many potential adverse effects, including growth retardation and osteoporosis. Indications for corticosteroid therapy in systemic JRA include fever unresponsive to NSAIDs, pericarditis, and disseminated intravascular coagulation. Consultation with a hematologist should be undertaken for any child with putative systemic JRA before steroid therapy is instituted to rule out occult leukemia or neuroblastoma. Other indications for steroid therapy include intractable uveitis unresponsive to topical steroids and inability to ambulate. Whenever possible, glucocorticoids should be given on alternative days, and the child should be weaned of the drug at the first opportunity. Corticosteroids can be directly injected into a persistently inflamed joint in children in whom NSAIDs are not well tolerated or are ineffective.

The importance of balancing rest (splinting of inflamed joints) and exercise (physical and occupational therapy) cannot be overemphasized. Swimming and cycling can be recommended as low-impact aerobic exercises that encourage full range of motion. In general, management of children with chronic arthritis is best carried out in specialized centers with interdisciplinary teams consisting of rheumatologists, nurse practitioners, occupational and physical therapists, and social workers, as well as orthopedic and ophthalmologic consultants. In this era of managed care, however, such arrangements may not be viewed as cost-effective.

Prognosis

Children with JRA, like those with any chronic condition, should be encouraged to lead as normal lives as possible. Support groups, such as the American Juvenile Arthritis Organization, provide families with an opportunity to network and share effective coping strategies. Whereas the prognosis for children with pauciarticular disease is excellent, 25–50% of those with systemic-onset disease and positive RFs may have aggressive erosive disease.

REACTIVE ARTHRITIS

Reactive, or postinfectious, arthritis refers to joint inflammation in association with infection in another part of the body. By definition, no organism can be recovered from the joint. Reactive arthritis can affect one or multiple joints and can occur after enteric infection with *Salmonella, Shigella, Yersinia,* or Campylobacter. Reactive arthritis after an episode of urethritis suggests Reiter syndrome, especially if there is associated conjunctivitis. In patients with post-dysenteric arthritis or Reiter syndrome,

the histocompatibility antigen HLA-B27 often is manifested. Monarthritis after group A streptococcal pharyngitis is considered by many to represent a variant of rheumatic fever (see above). Reactive arthritis typically lasts less than 6 weeks, effectively distinguishing it from JRA, and is often invoked as the etiology of short-lived arthritis of undetermined etiology.

SPONDYLOARTHRITIS

The seronegative spondyloarthropathies also should be considered when evaluating arthritis of one or a few joints of longer duration. Diseases in this grouping include ankylosing spondylitis, the arthritis of IBD, and psoriatic arthritis and are often associated with HLA-B27. It may be difficult to distinguish children with these disorders from those with JRA, but episodes of arthritis tend to be of shorter duration (weeks to months rather than months to years). Children with prodromal spondyloarthritis also can present with arthralgia and inflammation of ligamentous and tendinous insertion sites (enthesitis) without objective arthritis. Back pain and involvement of the sacroiliac joints are common but can take years to become apparent in children with ankylosing spondylitis. The arthritis of Crohn disease or ulcerative colitis is suggested by the presence of abdominal pain or history of bloody stools but can precede bowel symptoms. In such cases, a diagnosis of IBD should be considered in children with a positive family history, growth failure, or acute phase reaction out of proportion to physical findings. Psoriatic arthritis also can precede skin involvement and is suspected from the family history or the presence of nail pits.

OTHER CHRONIC MONARTHRITIS

In addition to pauciarticular JRA and the spondyloarthropathies, unusual causes of persistent monarticular arthritis include retained radiolucent foreign bodies (eg, plant thorns and sea urchin spines), synovial or cartilaginous tumors, and indolent infection. Relapsing monarthritis is typical in untreated Lyme disease. Radiographs, radionuclide studies, magnetic resonance imaging, and arthroscopic biopsy may prove helpful in establishing diagnoses in prolonged monarticular joint swelling of obscure etiology.

VASCULITIS

Inflammation of blood vessels of various sizes often is a major feature of immune-mediated diseases. Vasculitis may be triggered by infection (eg, group A *Streptococcus* and hepatitis B) and can accompany defined connective tissue disease; however, it can also occur in isolation. As already noted, HSP and serum sickness are leukocytoclastic vasculitides affecting small vessels and are commonly associated with joint inflammation. Involvement of small- to medium-sized vessels characterizes polyarteritis nodosa and Wegener granulomatosis, both of which affect adults more often than children. Takayasu disease is rare in childhood and typically involves medium and large vessels, including the aorta. Kawasaki disease is arguably the most common vasculitic syndrome of childhood and is notable for its predilection for the coronary arteries.

Diagnosis of vasculitis is based on clinical presentation and confirmed by biopsy for patients with small vessel disease and by angiography for those with larger vessel involvement. Antibodies to the cytoplasm of neutrophils are regularly detected in sera of patients with Wegener granulomatosis and appear to be directed at a serine proteinase. Other antineutrophil cytoplasmic antibodies (ANCA) have been documented to occur in virtually all vasculitides, as well as in IBD and autoimmune hepatitis.

KAWASAKI DISEASE

Kawasaki disease, or mucocutaneous lymph node syndrome, was first described in Japan in 1967. Kawasaki disease more commonly affects children younger than 5 years and boys more than girls and is most common in those of Asian ancestry. Although case clustering has been associated with residence near bodies of water and exposure to rug shampoo, the paucity of secondary cases within families suggests common exposure and not secondary transmission. Clinical resemblance of the illness to scarlet fever and toxic shock syndrome (fever, rash, desquamation) and laboratory evidence of elevation of multiple cytokines (interleukin-1, interleukin-6, tumor necrosis factor-α, interferon-γ) has suggested the possibility of a superantigen as the trigger for Kawasaki disease. A staphylococcal toxic shock syndrome exotoxin has been implicated but not established in this role.

Kawasaki disease is diagnosed according to well-established criteria (Table 8–5) and can be divided into three phases. The first, or acute, phase lasts about 10 days if untreated and is marked by a temperature as high as 40 °C, accompanied by a polymorphous exanthem. The rash can at times resemble scarlatina, measles, erythema multiforme, and Rocky Mountain spotted fever, illnesses for which Kawasaki disease may be mistaken. Other findings in the acute phase include conjunctival suffusion without discharge (sparing the limbus), marked erythema of the lips and oral mucous membranes, strawberry tongue, and indurative edema of the hands and feet. Cervical lymphadenitis, affecting fewer than 40% of children, may be mistaken for bacterial adenitis. Cardiac manifestations during this phase include tachycardia disproportionate to

Table 8–5. Criteria for the diagnosis of Kawasaki disease.

Fever of at least 5 days' duration, unresponsive to antibiotics (generally ≥ 40 °C)
and
Four of the following:
  Extremity changes: palmar and plantar erythema, indurative edema, desquamation of hands and feet, Beau lines (transverse ridges across nails months after resolution of illness)
  Polymorphous exanthem: earliest changes often seen in perineum, urticaria, morbilliform papules, scarletiniform erythroderma
  Lymphadenopathy: unilateral cervical, greater than 1.5 cm; firm, nonfluctuant
  Mucosal changes: erythema; dry, cracked, fissured lips; strawberry tongue; marked erythema of oropharyngeal mucosa
  Conjunctival injection: bilateral bulbar, limbal sparing; nonexudative; painless

fever, gallop rhythm, congestive heart failure, pericardial effusion, and arrhythmias.

Arthritis and arthralgia occur during the subacute phase, which is signaled by gradual subsiding of fever, marked thrombocytosis, and desquamation of the palms and soles beginning at the fingertips. Other organ systems may be involved in the first days to weeks. Nonspecific GI symptoms include abdominal pain, diarrhea, vomiting, and evidence of hepatic dysfunction. An enlarged, tender liver in a child with Kawasaki disease should raise the possibility of hydrops of the gallbladder (acalculias cholecystis), which can be confirmed sonographically. Children with Kawasaki disease are commonly very irritable; lumbar puncture often reveals a lymphocytic pleocytosis (aseptic meningitis). Urethritis, manifested as sterile pyuria, is the most frequent genitourinary finding. (This will be missed if the sample is obtained by catheterization or bladder puncture.)

Up to 40% of untreated patients have echocardiographically documented coronary artery dilatation and aneurysms in the convalescent phase, typically 3–6 weeks after the onset of symptoms. Coronary aneurysms have been reported in infants with prolonged febrile illnesses without rashes or conjunctivitis, so-called atypical Kawasaki disease.

Administration of intravenous immunoglobulin, 2 gm/ kg, in combination with high-dose salicylates (aspirin, 80–100 mg/kg/d) is effective in preventing coronary aneurysms in most patients and modifies the clinical picture of Kawasaki disease. When administered within 7–10 days of onset, defervescence occurs promptly, and clinical manifestations associated with the later stages of illness may not occur. High-dose aspirin is continued until signs of acute inflammation subside (usually 7–10 days) but should be reduced to 5–10 mg/kg/d when the platelet count begins to increase. Salicylates are discontinued once the platelet count normalizes but are continued indefinitely in those with coronary involvement.

CONNECTIVE TISSUE DISEASE

SYSTEMIC LUPUS ERYTHEMATOSUS

Clinical Features

SLE is the prototypical autoimmune disease, characterized by inappropriate production of antibodies to nuclear constituents and immune complex mediated vasculitis of virtually any organ. SLE is more common among those of African and Asian heritage. SLE develops in girls more frequently than in boys; the female-male ratio is 3:1 in the first decade of life and 6–8:1 thereafter. Experimental and circumstantial evidence indicates that estrogen is largely responsible for this sexual difference in incidence. It is not uncommon for SLE to present within the first few years after menarche, after institution of estrogen-containing oral contraceptives, or around pregnancy and delivery. Up to 12% of first-degree relatives of patients with SLE have the disease and up to 40% will have positive ANAs or other laboratory abnormalities without associated symptoms.

The American College of Rheumatology 1982 criteria for the classification of SLE are presented in Table 8–6. The presence of four criteria is 96% sensitive and specific. Among the most common symptoms of SLE are arthralgia and arthritis, fatigue, fever, headache, and weight loss. Cutaneous manifestations are frequent and include the classic butterfly malar eruption, generalized photosensitivity, alopecia, Raynaud phenomenon, and cutaneous vasculitis (palpable purpura, livedo reticularis). Renal involvement occurs in 50–70% of patients, ranging from minimal mesangial proliferation to diffuse proliferative glomerulonephritis on biopsy specimens. Inflammatory lesions can occur throughout the central nervous system, resulting in seizures, psychosis, stroke, and coma.

Laboratory Features

ANAs are found in 97% of patients with SLE. As such, the ANA is a good screening test for SLE but lacks specificity. It is possible to confirm a clinical diagnosis of SLE in the laboratory in most cases by demonstrating the presence of antibodies to native DNA or the extractable nuclear antigen Sm (Smith). Active SLE most often is accompanied by low levels of the complement components C3 and C4. The combination of a depressed complement level and elevated antibody to native DNA is 100% specific for SLE. Deficiencies of early complement components leading to lupus-like disease are suspected if the total hemolytic complement is persistently depressed. Hematologic features of SLE include leukopenia, lymphopenia, thrombocytopenia, and Coombs-positive hemolytic anemia. Patients with SLE and antiphospholipid antibodies or the lupus anticoagulant are prone to recurrent arterial and venous thromboses (stroke, thrombophlebitis) and miscarriage.

Table 8–6. American College of Rheumatology 1982 classification criteria for systemic lupus erythematosus.[1]

Criterion	Definition
Malar rash	Fixed erythema, flat or raised over malar eminences, sparing nasolabial folds
Discoid rash	Erythematous raised lesions with hyperkeratosis and follicular plugging; atrophic scarring
Photosensitivity	Cutaneous reaction to sunlight
Oral ulcers	Usually painless
Arthritis	Nonerosive involvement of ≥ 2 joints
Serositis	Pleuritis or pericarditis
Renal disorder	Proteinuria > 0.5 g/d or persistently greater than 3+ on dipstick *or* Cellular casts
Neurologic disorder	Seizures or psychosis
Hematologic disorder	Hemolytic anemia with reticulocytosis *or* Leukopenia < 4000/mm³ on ≥ 2 occasions *or* Lymphopenia < 1500/mm³ on ≥ 2 occasions *or* Thrombocytopenia < 100,000/mm³
Immunologic disorder	Positive lupus erythematosus (LE) preparation *or* Antibody to native DNA in abnormal titer *or* Antibody to Sm nuclear antigen *or* Chronic false-positive serologic test result for syphilis for at least 6 months with negative treponemal testing
Antinuclear antibody	Abnormal titer of antinuclear antibody by immunofluorescence in the absence of drugs known to be associated with "drug-induced LE"

[1]Reproduced, with permission, from Tan EM et al: The 1982 revised criteria for the classification of systemic lupus erythematosus. Arthritis Rheum 1982;25:1271.

Treatment

Treatment for SLE is based on the organ systems involved. Arthritis and mucocutaneous disease are manageable with nonsteroidal drugs and hydroxychloroquine. All children with SLE must wear sunscreens to avoid cutaneous and systemic flares. Estrogen-containing oral contraceptives should be avoided. Corticosteroids are indicated for any visceral involvement or severe hematologic derangement and typically are begun at a dose of 2 mg/kg/d of prednisone (maximum 60–80 mg/d). The dosage of medication is titrated on the basis of the patient's symptoms and objective measures of disease activity (physical examination, urinary sediment, and levels of C3, C4, and DNA antibodies). Whenever possible, steroids should be converted to alternate-day dosing in an effort to minimize side effects. Severe symptomatic flares (eg, onset of renal insufficiency, seizures, and coma) are managed with pulse methylprednisolone (30 mg/kg, up to 1000 mg). Immunosuppressive therapy is added in children with severe disease, such as with diffuse proliferative glomerulonephritis, in whom the steroid dose cannot be reduced. This is commonly administered as monthly intravenous cyclophosphamide. Azathioprine continues to be used as a steroid-sparing agent.

Prognosis

Ten-year survival rates for children with SLE typically are greater than 90%. Deaths occur primarily related to infections in immune-suppressed hosts but also as a result of pulmonary hemorrhage, severe central nervous system disease, and early myocardial infarction.

OTHER LUPUS SYNDROMES

Drug-induced Lupus

Symptoms of lupus (commonly arthritis, rash, oral ulcers) accompany drug-induced ANAs in patients with hypersensitivity reactions to various drugs, including anticonvulsants (phenytoin, phenobarbital), procainamide, and hydralazine. The finding of a positive ANA and symptoms of SLE in a patient with epilepsy raises the possibility that the seizures may have been the first manifestation of SLE. However, drug-induced disease is characterized by the presence of antihistone antibodies in the absence of any other lupus-specific antibodies (ie, negative anti-DNA and anti-Sm antibodies), so laboratory studies will usually distinguish between the two conditions.

Neonatal Lupus

Transplacental passage of maternal autoantibodies may result in neonatal lupus. Complete congenital heart block occurs when maternal anti-Ro antibody binds to the fetal conduction system and is permanent. Other infants may present with photosensitive skin eruptions after birth, as well as with thrombocytopenia and, occasionally, hepatitis. These manifestations wane as the titer of maternal IgG decreases during the first 6 months of life.

MIXED CONNECTIVE TISSUE DISEASE

Mixed connective tissue disease (MCTD) is one of the "overlap" syndromes with features of SLE, systemic sclerosis, myositis, and arthritis. It is defined by the presence of antibody to the extractable nuclear antigen ribonucleoprotein (RNP). Classically, children with MCTD present with Raynaud phenomenon, puffy hands, and arthritis. They are less likely to have significant renal involvement than children with classic SLE. Over time, they tend to have more features of scleroderma.

DERMATOMYOSITIS

Clinical Features

Dermatomyositis is a condition characterized by inflammation of skin and muscle. Arthritis occurs in up to 40% of patients. Temporal case clustering has suggested an infectious agent as a potential trigger, but no specific etiology has been determined. Although occult malignant disease is common in adults with dermatomyositis, it does not occur in childhood. Muscle biopsy specimens reveal inflammation and an obliterative endarteropathy in which capillary lumina are occluded by thrombi and fibrin. Other signs of vasculitis include nail-fold telangiectasias and ulcerative lesions of the skin and GI tract.

The cutaneous manifestations of the disease include Gottron papules, a psoriasiform eruption over the extensor surfaces of the knuckles, elbows, and knees, and the heliotrope rash, a purplish discoloration of the eyelids secondary to vasculitis at the lid margins. Photosensitive eruptions also occur on the face and extend down the upper trunk in a V- or shawl-distribution.

Muscle weakness usually begins insidiously. Common signs are the inability to perform a sit-up in physical education class and difficulty in stair-climbing, commonly manifested as difficulty in getting onto the first step of the school bus. Physical examination discloses a positive Gowers maneuver and diminished proximal muscle strength on manual testing. Deep tendon reflexes usually are preserved but may be diminished in intensity. Inflammation is limited to striated muscle, but palatal weakness and involvement of the diaphragm and accessory muscles can lead to respiratory embarrassment in severe cases. Esophageal dysmotility is not uncommon, and cardiac arrhythmias can occur.

A diagnosis of dermatomyositis is established by applying the criteria of Bohan and Peter (Table 8–7). If weakness is documented, the rash is classic, and serum muscle enzyme concentrations are elevated, a diagnosis may be confirmed through magnetic resonance imaging. This may obviate the need for muscle biopsy or electrophysiologic testing.

Treatment

High-dose corticosteroid therapy is the mainstay of therapy for dermatomyositis. Traditionally this is administered as prednisone, 2 mg/kg/d, in divided doses. In children with life-threatening illness, pulse methylprednisolone is administered. Corticosteroids are continued in high doses until muscle strength improves and serum muscle enzyme levels normalize and then are gradually tapered. It usually is not possible to convert to alternate-day dosing during periods of disease activity. Failure to respond to corticosteroids or the development of untenable side effects calls for the addition of immunosuppressive therapy, usually as methotrexate or cyclophosphamide. Cyclosporine and intravenous immunoglobulin have been reported to be effective anecdotally. Children in

Table 8–7. Criteria for the diagnosis of dermatomyositis.[1]

Diagnosis requires classic skin eruption and three of four other findings
Rash
Purplish, edematous discoloration of eyelids
Scaly eruption over metacarpal and proximal interphalangeal joints, knees, elbows, malleoli (Gottron papules)
Scaly erythema of face, neck, anterior chest, shawl area
Muscular weakness
Progressive symmetric involvement of proximal limb-girdle, anterior neck flexors, and abdominal musculature
Gowers sign, difficulty climbing stairs, arising from chair, combing hair
Muscle enzyme elevations
Creatine kinase
Aldolase
Aspartate aminotransferase
Lactate dehydrogenase
Electromyographic abnormalities
Insertional irritability
Spontaneous activity at rest
Short, small polyphasic motor units
Positive sharp waves
Muscle biopsy
Vascular compromise and capillary dropout
Perifascicular atrophy of type I and II fibers

[1]Reproduced, with permission, from Bohan A, Peter J: Polymyositis and dermatomyositis. N Engl J Med 1975;292:344, 403.

whom cutaneous involvement outstrips muscle disease can benefit from hydroxychloroquine.

Prognosis

Before corticosteroids came into routine use, the mortality rate for childhood dermatomyositis approached 33%. Death is now uncommon, occurring in children with fulminant disease on initial presentation or occasionally from infectious complications. More than 75% of children can be expected to have a monocyclic course lasting 2 years or less. Delay in diagnosis and effective therapy is correlated with the late development of dystrophic calcification of muscle and soft tissues.

SCLERODERMA

Scleroderma is a rare disease in children and is of unknown etiology. It is characterized by the increased deposition of collagen in skin and, on occasion, other organ systems. The most severe form, **progressive systemic sclerosis (PSS),** involves multiple organs. It occurs more frequently in females. Skin changes begin with edema and then are followed by induration, sclerosis, and eventually atrophy. The skin of the digits, hands, face, or arm usually is affected first; the disease then progresses proximally. Dysphagia results from thickening of the lower third of the esophagus. Hypertension, renal failure, pulmonary fibrosis, and cardiac involvement may also occur. This disease is commonly associated with the Raynaud phenomenon and tends to be relentlessly progressive. The diagnosis is based on clinical suspicion and may be confirmed by a biopsy specimen of affected tissue. No single laboratory test is useful for the diagnosis. The ANA and RF may be positive but usually have lower titers than those found in patients with SLE. Treatment is aimed at decreasing deposition of collagen (eg, using D-penicillamine) and controlling associated phenomena, such as hypertension and digital necrosis. The long-term prognosis for children with PSS is not well established and depends greatly on the extent of renal, cardiac, and pulmonary involvement.

Bands of localized thickened tissues are seen with **linear scleroderma.** This form usually is not associated with systemic involvement but may cause flexion contractures and growth abnormalities. The natural history varies from total spontaneous remission to progression of lesions over several years. Treatment emphasizes good physical therapy to soften the skin and maintain range and function. Drugs are occasionally indicated for more severe or rapidly progressive disease.

REFERENCES

Abu Arafeh I, Russell G: Recurrent limb pain in schoolchildren. Arch Dis Child 1996;74:336.

Cassidy JT, Petty RE: *Textbook of Pediatric Rheumatology,* 3rd ed. Saunders, 1994.

Dajani AS et al: Diagnosis and therapy of Kawasaki disease in children. Circulation 1993;87:1776.

Dajani AS et al: Guideline for the diagnosis of rheumatic fever: Jones criteria, updated 1992. Circulation 1993;87:302.

Gedalia A et al: Hypermobility of the joints in juvenile episodic arthritis/arthralgia. J Pediatr 1985;107:873.

Lang B, Silverman E: A clinical overview of systemic lupus erythematosus. Pediatr Rev 1993;14:194.

Lanzkowsky S et al: Henoch-Schoenlein purpura. Pediatr Rev 1992;13:130.

Lindsley CB: Uses of nonsteroidal anti-inflammatory drugs in pediatrics. Am J Dis Child 1993;147:229.

Pachman LM: Inflammatory myopathy in children. Rheum Dis Clin North Am 1994;20:919.

9

Infectious Diseases

Allan S. Lau, MD, FRCP(C), Alan Uba, MD, Deborah Lehman, MD, Francesca Geertsma, MD,
& Surachai Supattapone, MD, PhD, DPhil

This chapter provides a general approach to pediatric infections, from history-taking and physical examination to proper use of laboratory services and basic principles of antimicrobial therapy. Discussions of individual infections begin with the associated complaints or symptoms. Then, the pathogenesis and management of individual diseases with respect to the organ systems are presented. Individual pathogens are discussed according to the system in which the organism is most commonly found as the causative agent. Also included are sections on special topics, including tropical diseases relevant to immigrant children and infections of the immunocompromised host. Certain important childhood infections, such as bacterial endocarditis and congenital infections, are discussed in the respective chapters dealing with the particular organ system or age group. Throughout the text, tables and figures outline important points relevant to clinical practice. In general, dosing information regarding antimicrobial drug therapy and technical descriptions of laboratory tests are not provided in detail.

APPROACH TO THE CHILD WITH A POSSIBLE INFECTION

In approaching the child with a possible infection, a detailed history and thorough physical examination are essential to enable the development of a differential diagnosis. On the basis of the differential diagnosis, the clinician can formulate a plan of action to determine the causative agent and treat the disease appropriately.

MEDICAL HISTORY & PHYSICAL EXAMINATION

In the initial assessment of an ill child with a possible infectious disease, a detailed history must be obtained, followed by a careful and thorough physical examination. Although this process is true for all of pediatric medicine, nowhere is it more important than in the evaluation of a patient with a complex disease of infectious etiology. Knowledge of exposures, whether they involve household contacts, food, domestic pets or other animals, personal travels, or visitors from overseas, frequently holds the clues the clinician needs to make an accurate and timely diagnosis.

The medical history should begin with the nature of the illness, including the duration and severity. Historical points unique to infectious diseases include questions regarding immunization history, previous antibiotic use, and recent contacts and exposures to infectious diseases. Specific symptoms should direct the examiner through a series of historical questions.

The child with diarrhea should be questioned about food exposures, including raw meats and eggs. For example, hemolytic uremic syndrome has been associated with patients who consumed meat contaminated with specific strains of *Escherichia coli. Salmonella* is commonly found in poultry and dairy products. Travel history may reveal exposure to intestinal parasites, such as *Entamoeba histolytica* in Mexico or *Cryptosporidium,* reported in municipal water supplies in several US cities during 1995. History of animal contacts may reveal exposure to reptiles likely to carry *Salmonella.* The family should be questioned about day-care attendance, as *Giardia* and *Cryptosporidium* may be transmitted in day-care settings. Recent antibiotic use should prompt the clinician to consider *Clostridium difficile* colitis.

Pneumonia is caused most frequently by common viral and bacterial pathogens. However, if the symptoms are persistent and unresponsive to conventional therapy, a more extensive history may give clues to the infectious etiology of the pulmonary infiltrates. Tuberculosis is probably the most common and most frequently overlooked cause of persistent pneumonia. Every child with pneumonia should have a purified protein derivative (PPD) placed and should be questioned extensively about possible exposures to tuberculosis, including contacts with high-risk groups, such as those from endemic areas, as well as incarcerated and homeless individuals. Questions should extend beyond immediate family members to include unrelated child-care providers, such as nannies and caretakers in home day-care centers. *Legionella* is associated with known outbreaks in hospitals, hotels, and cruise ships via exposure to contaminated water and air-conditioning systems. *Chlamydia psittaci* causes pulmonary infiltrates and high fever after exposure to infected domestic birds. *Coccidiomycosis* is a common cause of lymphadenopathy and pneumonia and is contracted by inhalation of spores in the San Joaquin Valley, California. Similarly, *Histoplasmosis* and *Blastomycosis* may cause pneumonia in individuals exposed to the fungal spores in parts of the Midwest and Mississippi valley, respectively.

Patients with fever of unknown origin (FUO) should be questioned extensively regarding potential exposures (see below). Brucellosis may be acquired by drinking nonpasteurized milk. Malaria and other parasitic infections may be acquired during travel to endemic areas. Cat-scratch disease, now known to be caused by *Bartonella henselae,* is transmitted to humans by exposure to cats, most frequently kittens. This usually causes painless lymphadenopathy, but several reports have found serologic evidence of acute *B henselae* infection in children with FUO and liver or spleen lesions.

No medical history is complete without a thorough investigation of animal exposure. The examiner should ask specifically about pets, including dogs, cats, reptiles, rats, and birds. Other animals, such as bats, squirrels, and raccoons, can transmit serious infectious diseases; possible exposures should always be investigated when confronted with a seriously ill child.

Finally, every child with a persistent illness or an infection with an unusual organism should be evaluated for an underlying immunodeficiency. The most common immunodeficiency is infection with HIV. Transmission of HIV to children is now almost exclusively perinatal. Therefore, the pediatric medical history depends on the parents' medical and social histories as well.

A detailed medical history should be followed by a comprehensive and well-directed physical examination. The examiner should be especially attentive to lymphadenopathy, swollen joints, and skin lesions.

If the clinician obtains a complete history and performs a thorough examination, the differential diagnosis can be narrowed and the diagnostic investigations focused. If a clinician spends time with the child and family members to gather clues about the illness before ordering medical tests, the patient can be spared unnecessary procedures and the cost of investigations and hospitalizations can be minimized.

LABORATORY MEDICINE IN INFECTIOUS DISEASES

The laboratory can provide both supportive and definitive evidence for diagnosis of an infectious pathogen. Clinical judgment is always the most important and first approach in reaching a diagnosis of an infectious disease. However, a strong understanding of the general principles involved in modern laboratory medicine will aid the clinician greatly.

Basic Principles in Using Laboratory Services

Practitioners should understand the techniques involved and the time required for culturing pathogens and performing specialized tests. Many cultures are now actually completed much more quickly than in the past decade. With modern techniques, blood cultures are reportable within 48 hours, urine and throat within 1–2 days, and herpes simplex virus (HSV) and cytomegalovirus (CMV) cultures within 3 days. However, cultures for anaerobes, mycobacteria, and fungi continue to require longer incubation time.

When seeing patients with fever or suspected infections, physicians should identify the subset of patients whose diagnosis or management may be affected by results of microbiologic tests. If there is no clinical relevance for performing cultures and other diagnostic tests, testing is seldom indicated.

Excessive and unnecessary investigations are a common problem. For example, if an infection (such as upper respiratory tract [URT] infection of nonspecific etiology) is trivial or self-limiting, little effort should be made to prove a specific etiology. Other examples include the performance of six or eight blood cultures when one or two would have been sufficient, or ordering three stool examinations for parasites without waiting for the results of the first test. In addition to wasting resources, the indiscriminate use of the laboratory can lead to misuse of antimicrobial agents that are not indicated clinically.

Once a decision is made to perform a test, the physician is responsible for careful specimen collection under optimal conditions. Cultures from normally sterile sites, such as cerebrospinal fluid (CSF), blood, and joint fluid, must be collected using aseptic techniques. When samples are collected from skin or mucosal surfaces (eg, expectorated sputum or urine specimens), efforts should be made to minimize contamination. Urine specimens for bacterial culture are most reliable if collected by midstream void, catheter, or suprapubic puncture rather than by a plastic bag attached to the perineal skin. In general, body fluids and tissue are preferred over swab specimens; stool specimens are preferred over rectal swabs. Whenever possible, bacterial cultures should be obtained before beginning antimicrobial therapy.

After collection, specimens should be promptly transported to the laboratory or held at the proper temperature to avoid bacterial overgrowth or death of fastidious organisms. When in doubt, specimens should be held at refrigerator temperature. In some situations, especially for viral cultures, inoculation of specimens at the bedside or special transport media may enhance isolation.

To enhance the recovery of pathogens and save cost, clinicians should fully complete test request forms. The laboratory requisition should include the type of specimen, site, time of collection, patient's age, symptoms, clinical diagnosis, prior antibiotic treatment, and suspected agents. This information will guide the choice of laboratory media and procedures. If an unusual infection is suspected, the laboratory should be alerted and the clinical microbiologist or an infectious disease specialist consulted.

When results are reported to the clinician, they should be interpreted carefully on the basis of the nature of the specimen and the clinical history. All skin and exposed mucosal surfaces have their own normal bacterial and fungal flora, creating potential difficulties in interpreting the results of cultures. Without knowing the patient's clinical information and the method of specimen collection, it would be difficult to distinguish contamination from infection. Correct interpretation is easy when a single pathogen is recovered from a usually sterile site. Likewise, contamination should be suspected when multiple organisms of low virulence are found in urine or respiratory tract specimens. When a common contaminant is isolated in pure culture from a normally sterile site (eg, *Staphylococcus epidermidis* in CSF and blood cultures), proper interpretation of the results requires knowledge of the clinical setting and the medical history of the host. For example, the presence of a ventriculoperitoneal shunt (in the case of CSF culture) or cardiac disease with foreign graft materials (in the case of blood culture) increases the likelihood of a true *S epidermidis* infection. Likewise, if the patient is an immunocompromised host, isolation of a bacterial species of usual low virulence must be interpreted with care. In summary, judicious use of laboratory tests to aid diagnosis and management must be coupled with proper interpretation of the significance of the microbe identified.

Direct Demonstration of a Pathogen

Direct detection of infectious pathogens is of great value to the clinician because this method usually is quick and relatively inexpensive. Staining of clinical specimens is the most direct method to demonstrate a pathogen. Other methods involve culturing specimens and subsequent staining to identify the pathogen. In addition, detection of bacterial antigens or specific sequences of bacterial DNA provides direct evidence of the presence of a pathogen.

Gram stain is an old, time-tested method of staining bacteria that aids in the initial general identification of the organism. The result of the Gram stain often guides the initial choice of antibiotic; with anaerobic or extremely fastidious bacterial infections, it may provide the only clue that a pathogen is present.

Other stains used commonly in the clinical laboratory include Wright or Giemsa to identify malaria parasites from thick blood smears, silver stains to identify fungal elements, and Ziehl-Neelsen to identify acid-fast organisms, such as mycobacterium. Recently, aramine orange, a fluorescent dye that stains acid-fast bacilli, has been used in addition to the Ziehl-Neelsen stain. The bright fluorescence of this dye enhances identification of the bacteria.

Fluorescent antibody staining is a widely used technique used to identify pathogens from both specimens and cultures. A smear of the infected material is made on a glass slide, which is then coated with an antibody (typically a mouse monoclonal antibody) directed against a specific antigenic determinant of the pathogen. Unbound antibody is washed from the slide. If the monoclonal antibody is fluorescein tagged, the slide can be examined directly for antigen-expressing cells; this technique is called direct immunofluorescence. If the monoclonal antibody is not tagged, the slide can be stained with a fluorescein-tagged antibody directed against the species of the monoclonal antibody. The preparation can then be examined for fluorescence in a technique called indirect immunofluorescence. This approach offers the advantage of versatility without the need for different individual specific antibodies tagged with fluorescein, which is cost-saving. The major limitation of this technique is the subjectivity of slide interpretation; positive and negative control slides should be included for each determination. Laboratory personnel must be skilled in the interpretation of these slides. Antibody kits for immunofluorescent staining currently are available for the diagnosis of infection by respiratory syncytial virus (RSV), *Bordetella pertussis,* HSV, varicella-zoster virus (VZV), and *Chlamydia trachomatis.* Special tests for Rocky Mountain spotted fever (*Rickettsia rickettsii*) and typhus (*Rickettsia typhi*) are available from regional reference laboratories.

Direct identification of pathogens also can be made without the use of staining techniques. Samples are examined under a standard light microscope as a "wet preparation." For example, these preparations, with samples dissolved in potassium hydroxide (KOH), can be used to look for yeast or mycelial forms of fungus in skin scrapings or vaginal secretions. Unspun urine samples can be used to identify bacteria and white blood cells in the setting of urinary tract infections (UTIs) as well as to identify Trichomonas. Darkfield examination of suspected syphilitic lesions can be used to diagnose *Treponema pallidum* infections.

Major obstacles complicate the identification of viruses as etiologic agents. Viruses are not easily cultured, and some are impossible to grow in vitro. Polymerase chain reaction (PCR) assays and copy DNA (cDNA) probes are not routinely available for most viruses because of prohibitive costs and technical problems. However, examination of potentially infected materials (eg, stool) by electron microscopy remains a convenient tool to identify viruses as pathogens. In addition, gold-labeled antibodies specific for viral antigens permit visualization of antibody-viral binding and the establishment of a specific diagnosis. This technique is known as immunoelectron microscopy.

Identification of Pathogens by Culture. Identification by culture is traditionally considered the "gold standard" by which one establishes a diagnosis of a known pathogen from a usually sterile body site. Unfortunately, many varied factors come into play that may influence whether a pathogen will grow in culture. These include whether the correct medium has been used, whether the patient is receiving antimicrobial therapy, and which collection techniques are used.

Numerous protocols and algorithms are used by each laboratory in identifying a bacterial pathogen, including selective media, biochemical tests, morphology, and different environmental conditions. For instance, CSF cultures are usually plated onto 5% sheep blood agar and chocolate agar and grown in a carbon dioxide–enriched environment. Genitourinary cultures for *Neisseria gonorrhoeae* are plated on to antibiotic-containing agar (Thayer-Martin medium) for selective isolation. *Yersinia* species require incubation at colder temperature (4 °C) for growth and also favor iron supplement. Culture of unusual or fastidious organisms including *Mycobacterium tuberculosis, Legionella,* or *B pertussis* requires special media; laboratory personnel should be alerted and specific requests made. To identify the specific species of bacterial pathogen, various biochemical tests are performed on the isolated colonies, often on the basis of colony morphology or Gram stain result. At this time, antibiotic sensitivity tests can be performed to help the clinician in therapy options.

Many yeasts, especially *Candida* species, can be cultured on standard bacteria media. However, most mycelial organisms require the use of fungal medium, such as Sabouraud medium. The diagnostic laboratory should be informed when a fungal infection is suspected, and the sample should be handled appropriately with the proper culture media.

Viral cultures often are more labor-intensive and take longer to grow, because viruses must be grown in active cell cultures. Specific cell lines are needed for specific viruses; therefore, the laboratory must be aware of which viruses are suspected in a particular patient. Usually, the diagnosis of a viral infection is made by identification of specific change in the morphology of the host cells in culture. This **cytopathic effect (CPE)** provides evidence that the virus was present in the inoculated sample. Demonstration of CPE can take days to weeks for most viruses. However, recent use of monoclonal antibody tagged with fluorescein has enhanced the identification of the virus (eg, HSV and CMV) in the cultured cells, without the need to wait for the onset of a CPE. The fluorescein-labeled virus-containing cells are identified with the use of a simple light microscope.

Detection of Microbial Antigens & Antibodies. Detection of pathogen-specific antigens is a useful and usually fairly rapid method to support a suspected diagnosis. These techniques identify specific epitopes of a pathogen with the use of antibodies to the epitope.

Latex agglutination tests are used fairly commonly in pediatrics to help identify infections caused by *Hemophilus influenzae* type b (HIB), group B *Streptococcus, Streptococcus pneumoniae, Neisseria meningitides,* and *E coli.* These tests work by coating a tiny latex particle with the antibody to the pathogen-specific epitope. When these particles are mixed with the body fluid in question, they agglutinate by antigen-antibody bridging between the latex particles. This agglutination reaction is visible to the eye or by light microscope. A drawback to this technique is that false-positive results are common; other, more definitive tests probably should be used before a final diagnosis is determined.

The enzyme-linked immunosorbent assay (ELISA) is another antigen-antibody–based test that is performed easily and rapidly on clinical specimens. ELISA is inexpensive, sensitive, readily available, and easily quantifiable for measuring either a pathogen-specific antigen or antibody. Antigen detection is accomplished by immobilizing a specific antibody into the wells of a tissue culture plastic plate. The clinical sample to be tested is added, and the antigen contained therein is immobilized and subsequently recognized by a second pathogen-specific antibody. Finally, after washings, a third antibody (which is covalently linked to a chromophore or enzyme) is added to develop the color. The intensity of the color development in the reaction is directly proportional to the amount of antigen present in the clinical sample. Similarly, ELISA can be used to detect antibodies specific for the pathogen in question. In this scenario, antigens are used for immobilization on the plastic plate instead.

As an alternative to the plastic well technique, the primary antibody is immobilized onto a membrane and the sample, second, and third antibodies are added sequentially. This membrane ELISA forms the basis for most commercially available rapid group A streptococcal tests.

Detection of Pathogen-Specific Nucleotide Sequences by Molecular Biology Techniques. PCR is a new and increasingly available method of direct detection of pathogens. It involves identification of sequences of DNA that are specific to a certain pathogen in a specimen. PCR can be used with viral, fungal, bacterial, and parasitic pathogens. Briefly, two specific oligodeoxynucleotides that define the 5′ and 3′ ends of the DNA sequence of interest are added to total DNA extracted from the clinical sample. A special polymerase, Taq (from thermus aquaticus), is added; Taq has polymerase activity only at high temperatures. The mixture is repeatedly heated and cooled. This allows for a logarithmic amplification of the sequence of interest, if it is present in the sample. This amplified DNA sequence then can be identified by gel electrophoresis followed by nucleic acid hybridization assays as described below. In theory, this technique can detect a single copy of the sequence of interest. Because of the enormous sensitivity of the technique, inadvertent contamination with very minute amounts of DNA can give false-positive results; thus, strict quality assurance measures must be undertaken by any laboratory performing these assays. Currently, PCR techniques are available for detection of HSV, parvovirus, HIV, and other pathogens by many reference laboratories.

An alternative to this approach is nucleic acid hybridization (Northern analysis for RNA and Southern analysis for DNA), which is more cumbersome and far less sensitive than PCR. This technique may give false-negative results because relatively high concentrations of nucleic acids from the pathogen in question must be present.

Indirect Demonstration of an Infectious Agent

These techniques use identification of an immune response as indirect evidence that a specific pathogen was present in a patient. A caveat when using these techniques is that the patient must be able to mount an immune response to a pathogen. Thus, timing of the test, immune status, and nutritional status must be considered when using these methods.

Tzanck Smear. This technique involves identification of multinucleated giant cells from skin lesions. The presence of these cells is suggestive of a HSV or VZV infection. To perform this test correctly, one must scrape the base of a cutaneous vesicle and place the epithelial cells onto a glass slide. The dried slide is then stained with Wright, Giemsa, Papanicolaou, or other stains and examined under a light microscope.

Skin Test. Intradermal injection of an antigen preparation to look for delayed hypersensitivity response (erythema, induration) was once a widely used immunodiagnostic test in clinical medicine. Infectious concerns, problems with standardization of preparations, and improvement in other types of testing all have led to a general decrease in the use of these tests, with several exceptions.

The Mantoux tuberculin skin test still is widely used as a screening test for mycobacterial infections. Routine testing of children often begins at 1 year of age. Definitions of a positive responder are based on population/risk groups and are thoroughly outlined in the *Red Book* of the American Academy of Pediatrics. In the Mantoux test, 5 U of PPD is injected intradermally, and the site is checked for induration in 48–72 hours. Both children with tuberculous and those with nontuberculous mycobacterial infections may have positive reactions, although nontuberculous (atypical) mycobacterial infections classically demonstrate a smaller area of induration. The clinician should be aware that early in the disease, a child's test result may be negative and later, if repeated, may be positive. In addition, with active disease, generalized anergy to skin testing may exist, and a positive control to rule this out should also be performed.

Skin testing for coccidiomycosis occasionally can be helpful in a child whose clinical picture and history fit this diagnosis. Unfortunately, a positive skin test result may merely reflect past exposure or self-limited previous disease, instead of current active disease.

Antibody Testing. Quantification of serum antibody titers to a pathogen-specific antigen provides indirect evidence of a specific infection. As a general rule, paired serum samples are assayed with an "acute" serum sample obtained at the time of clinical presentation and a "convalescent" serum sample obtained 4–6 weeks later. If a fourfold or greater increase in antibody titer is exhibited, the test is considered positive for that pathogen. Another test for the presence of antibody against pathogen-specific antigens is performed by the ELISA method, mentioned above. Some of these assays can specifically measure IgM production against the antigens, thus making the test more specific for acute disease. Examples of pathogens detected by this method include Epstein-Barr virus (EBV), CMV, HIV, and *Mycoplasma.*

Western blots, or immunoblots, are qualitative tests used to detect antibody against pathogen-specific protein antigens. A mixture of these antigens is separated electrophoretically by molecular weight. The antigens are immobilized on a membrane, and the membrane is blocked to prevent nonspecific binding. The serum sample is then applied to the membrane, incubated, and washed. The blot is processed in a manner similar to ELISA. Positive blots yield darkly colored bands that correspond to the molecular weight of the desired antigen. This technique currently is used to confirm positive ELISA results for the diagnosis of HIV.

ANTIMICROBIAL THERAPY

In the second half of the 19th century, Louis Pasteur formulated the germ theory and postulated that severe infections are caused by microbial agents. This theory led to the introduction of the pasteurization process for dairy and other food products. In addition, these early works resulted in the introduction of vaccination against bacterial and viral pathogens. These advances in microbiology and disease pathogenesis laid the foundation for modern medicine. The control and management of infectious diseases are among the greatest achievements of medical science.

Using the historical work on germ theory as a basis, therapy directed against microbes was developed in this century. The first antibiotic to be discovered was penicillin, a natural product of *Penicillium* mold. Since then, innumerable microbial products have been investigated and chemically modified, leading to the generation of a great variety of antibiotics. These modified products, termed semisynthetic antibiotics, represent most antibiotics in use in current clinical practice. Beneficial effects of these semisynthetic products include increased antimicrobial activity, increased stability and solubility, and improved pharmacokinetics and bioavailability (ie, wider distribution and tissue penetration and longer half-life). Another important aspect of developing semisynthetic antibiotics is to custom-design new generations of antibiotics with high therapeutic efficacy and minimal undesirable effects. With the vast array of antibiotics, however, there are enormous concerns for their overuse and misuse, which would add unnecessary high cost to the health system, cause iatrogenic diseases due to toxicity, and induce microbial resistance.

Antibiotics are one of the most frequently prescribed classes of drugs, accounting for approximately 11% of all drug costs, or more than $80 billion in the United States. It has been estimated that two thirds of antibiotic prescriptions in hospitals are of questionable value. For example, clinical research data have determined that 50% of physicians prescribe antibiotics for the common cold. It is a common belief among the public that antibiotics are useful in preventing complications and treating viral diseases. Thus, pediatricians frequently face enormous parental pressure to relieve symptoms by prescribing antibiotics. Indiscriminate use of antibiotics can lead to iatrogenic diseases arising from adverse side effects and drug toxicity, emergence of resistant bacteria, and masking of more serious infections.

PRINCIPLES OF ANTIBIOTIC THERAPY

The decision to prescribe an antibiotic is based on proof or strong suspicion that the patient has a bacterial infection. If the patient has a noninfectious process or an infection of probable viral etiology, withholding an antibacterial agent is rational. However, if the patient appears to be septic and critically ill, empiric use of antibiotics is essential. The specific antibiotic chosen is based on knowledge of the pathogens likely to cause infection at a specific site in a specific host. Table 9–1 provides a list of clinical infections with the most likely etiologic organisms and recommended antibiotics for the respective bacteria.

To prescribe antibiotics appropriately, the clinician must know the likely antibiotic sensitivities of these pathogens. In addition, the tissue concentrations of the antibiotics at the site of the infection must be considered in selecting an appropriate agent. If more than one antibiotic is active against the likely pathogens at the site of infection, the specific agent should be chosen on the basis of relative toxicity, convenience of administration, and cost. Furthermore, preference will be given to the drug with the narrowest spectrum against that specific organism. If the site of presumed infection is readily accessible for sampling (eg, blood, urine, CSF), bacterial cultures should be performed to guide therapy. Once the infectious agent is identified, therapy should be directed specifically against the organism, and the spectrum of the antibiotics used should be narrow to avoid toxicity and emergence of resistance.

Route of Administration

Systemic antibiotics are given either orally or parenterally, by either the intravenous (IV) or the intramuscular route. Several factors should be considered when choosing the specific route of administration. To ensure direct delivery and enhance bioavailability of the drug, the IV route is commonly used with hospitalized patients. Antibiotics can be administered intramuscularly in patients who do not have an IV device in place, unless they have a bleeding disorder or are in shock. For outpatients, antibiotics are usually given orally. An exception would be a single intramuscular administration of an antibiotic in a child when family compliance is questionable or pending outcome of culture results. Another exception would be long-term IV antibiotics administered as part of a home therapy program.

In recent years it is becoming increasingly popular to give antibiotics initially by the parenteral route when the patient is relatively unstable during the initial phase of hospitalization. This is followed by the oral route when the patient is stable enough to complete the course of therapy. This practice is most common in treating osteomyelitis and septic arthritis. Although this innovative treatment protocol saves hospital cost and serves the patient well for early discharge, the patient must be monitored carefully with frequent clinical follow-up and physical examinations to ensure compliance and to avoid potential complications.

Duration of Therapy

The duration of antibiotic administration recommended for specific infections usually is arbitrary and empiric on the basis of historical experience in the past few decades. Recommendations are usually based on uncontrolled experience, not on controlled trials. Guidelines concerning the duration of therapy for most infections are discussed for individual syndromes. Therapy should be guided by clinical response rather than by an arbitrary number of days with a rigid duration of therapy.

Response to Therapy

The response of the patient to antibiotic therapy is monitored by clinical assessment and laboratory tests. Clinical monitoring involves sequential physical examinations with special attention to the site originally infected and vital signs, including body temperature. Signs of inflammation and fever should resolve within several days after appropriate antibiotics are initiated. Laboratory monitoring involves obtaining repeat bacterial cultures, when appropriate, during therapy to ensure sterilization. In addition, for severe infections, the peripheral white blood cell

Table 9–1. Antibiotics of choice: A prescribing guide for infectious diseases.[1]

Diagnosis	Probable Pathogen(s)	Recommended Antibiotic(s) Either	Or
Ears and sinuses			
Acute otitis media	*Streptococcus pneumoniae* *Haemophilus influenzae* (most strains not typable) *Moraxella catarrhalis*	Amoxicillin	Trimethoprim-sulfamethoxazole
Acute sinusitis	As above	Amoxicillin	Trimethoprim-sulfamethoxazole
Upper airway			
Pharyngitis			
Exudative	*S pyogenes* (group A *Streptococcus*)	Penicillin	Cephalexin
Membranous	*Corynebacterium diphtheriae*	Erythromycin	Penicillin
Epiglottitis	HIB	Cefotaxime	Ampicillin + chloramphenicol
Eyes			
Cellulitis			
Preseptal			
Spontaneous	HIB	Cefotaxime	Ampicillin + chloramphenicol
After trauma (especially penetrating trauma near the eye, eg, insect bites, scratches)	HIB *S aureus*	Cefotaxime ± nafcillin	Cefuroxime
Orbital	HIB *Staphylococcus aureus* *S pneumoniae*	Cefotaxime ± nafcillin	Cefuroxime
Conjunctivitis			
Neonate < 5 d	*Neisseria gonorrhoeae*	Penicillin	Ceftriaxone
Neonate > 5 d	*Chlamydia trachomatis*	Erythromycin	Sulfonamide
Central nervous system			
Meningitis			
Neonate	Group B *Streptococcus* *Escherichia coli* *Listeria monocytogenes*	Ampicillin + gentamicin	Ampicillin + cefotaxime
Infant or child	HIB *S pneumoniae* *Neisseria meningitidis*	Cefotaxime	Ampicillin + chloramphenicol
Abscess			
Without trauma	Microaerophilic streptococci Anaerobes	Penicillin + chloramphenicol	Metronidazole
With trauma (refers to penetrating trauma, including postneurosurgery)	Microaerophilic streptococci Anaerobes *S aureus*	Nafcillin + chloramphenicol	Nafcillin + metronidazole
Abdomen			
Peritonitis			
Primary	*S pneumoniae* *E coli*	Ampicillin + gentamicin	Cefotaxime
After perforation	Enterobacteriaceae Anaerobes	Clindamycin + gentamicin	Cefoxitin
CAPD (secondary to continuous ambulatory peritoneal dialysis)	Coagulase negative staphylococci Enterobacteriaceae Anaerobes	Vancomycin + cefotaxime	Cefazolin + gentamicin
NEC (necrotizing enterocolitis in neonates)	Coagulase negative staphylococci	Vancomycin + cefotaxime	Clindamycin + gentamicin
Kidneys			
Pyelonephritis	Enterobacteriaceae (most frequenty *E coli*)	Ampicillin + gentamicin	Cefotaxime
Cystitis and asymptomatic bacteriuria	Enterobacteriaceae (most frequently *E coli*) *S aureus*	Sulfisoxazole	Amoxicillin
Perinephric abscess	Enterobacteriaceae	Nafcillin + cefotaxime	Nafcillin + gentamicin

(continued)

Table 9–1 (cont'd). Antibiotics of choice: A prescribing guide for infectious diseases.[1]

Diagnosis	Probable Pathogen(s)	Recommended Antibiotic(s)	
		Either	**Or**
Skin and soft tissues			
Cellulitis			
Extremity	S aureus S pyogenes	Nafcillin + penicillin (to prevent treatment failure when S pyogenes is infective agent)	Clindamycin
Face (buccal cellulitis)	HIB	Cefotaxime	Ampicillin + chloramphenicol
Impetigo	S pyogenes S aureus	Cephalexin	Erythromycin
Fasciitis	S pyogenes	Penicillin	Clindamycin
Myositis	S aureus	Nafcillin	Vancomycin
Bones (osteomyelitis)			
In neonates	Group B Streptococcus S aureus Enterobacteriaceae	Nafcillin + gentamicin	Nafcillin + cefotaxime
Acute hematogenous	S aureus	Nafcillin + consider appropriate coverage for HIB in children < 24 mo	Clindamycin
In children with sickle cell anemia	S aureus Salmonella sp.	Nafcillin + ampicillin	Cefotaxime
After puncture wound to the foot	Pseudomonas aeruginosa	Ticarcillin + tobramycin	Ceftazidime
Joints			
Infections in neonates	Group B Streptococcus S aureus Enterobacteriaceae	Nafcillin + gentamicin	Nafcillin + cefotaxime
Infections in infants and children	HIB S aureus S pneumoniae	Cefotaxime ± nafcillin	Cefuroxime
Infections in adolescents	S aureus N gonorrhoeae S pneumoniae	Nafcillin + penicillin	Ceftriaxone + nafcillin
Postoperative infections	S aureus Coagulase negative staphylococci Enterobacteriaceae	Nafcillin + cefotaxime	Nafcillin + gentamicin
Blood (septicemia/bacteremia)			
In neonates < 7 d	Group B Streptococcus E coli L monocytogenes	Ampicillin + gentamicin	Ampicillin + cefotaxime
Nosocomial	Coagulase negative staphylococci S aureus Enterobacteriaceae	Vancomycin + cefotaxime	Vancomycin + tobramycin
In children	HIB S pneumoniae N meningitidis	Cefotaxime	Ampicillin + chloramphenicol
In adolescents	N meningitidis N gonorrhoeae S aureus	Penicillin + nafcillin	Cefotaxime
Pericarditis	S aureus	Cefotaxime ± nafcillin	Nafcillin + chloramphenicol

[1]Modified, with permission, from Prober CG: *Contemporary Pediatrics*, Medical Economics 1989;6:16.
HIB = *H influenzae* type b.

count and acute phase reactants (eg, erythrocyte sedimentation rate [ESR] or C-reactive protein) should be monitored until they normalize. Sometimes it may be necessary to determine that adequate concentrations of the antibiotic are achieved in vivo. This can be done by measuring the antibiotic concentration in the serum or, alternatively, assaying for serum bactericidal level, which is reflective of antibiotic killing effects on the organism. In general, a lack of clinical or laboratory response to therapy may mandate a change of antibiotics.

Mechanisms of Action

Antibiotics attack targets present in bacteria but absent or less vulnerable in human cells. This directed attack is referred to as selective toxicity. Four categories of sites of antibiotic action have been developed (Table 9–2).

Bacteriostatic Versus Bactericidal Antimicrobials

In addition to classifying antibiotics by mechanism of action, they may be classified as bacteriostatic or bacteri-

Table 9–2. Classification of antibiotics by mechanism of action.[1]

Inhibition of cell wall synthesis	Inhibition of protein synthesis
Penicillins	Aminoglycosides
Cephalosporins	Chloramphenicol
Vancomycin	Clindamycin
Aztreonam	Erythromycin
Imipenem	Spectinomycin
	Tetracyclines
Inhibition of nucleic acid synthesis	
Metronidazole	Inhibition of folate synthesis
Quinolones	Sulfonamides
Rifampin	Trimethoprim

[1]Adapted, with permission, from Prober CG: Antibacterial therapy. Page 499 in: Rudolph AM et al (editors): *Rudolph's Pediatrics,* 20th ed. Appleton & Lange, 1996.

cidal. Bacteriostatic agents inhibit bacterial cell replication but do not kill the organisms. In this case, they halt bacterial growth and allow the host's immune mechanisms to clear the infection. Theoretically, if host immunity is suppressed or the infection is in an area of poor immunologic surveillance (eg, CSF or vitreous humor), bacteriostatic agents may not be effective. Chloramphenicol and erythromycin are bacteriostatic against most bacteria, although chloramphenicol is bactericidal against the common and important pediatric pathogens including HIB, *S pneumoniae,* and *N meningitidis.* Examples of bactericidal antibiotics include penicillins, cephalosporins, vancomycin, and aminoglycosides. They cause microbial death by cell lysis. In addition, some antibiotics have dual properties and may be either bacteriostatic or bactericidal depending on the specific bacteria, concentration of the drug, and nature of the tissue environment. These antibiotics include the sulfonamides and tetracyclines.

Emergence of Antibiotic Resistance

The development of microbial drug resistance results from the widespread overuse and indiscriminate use of antimicrobial agents, coupled with the ability of bacteria to acquire and spread resistance and the capacity of humans to spread bacteria. Antimicrobial drug resistance is a major driving force behind the incessant search for newer drugs. Few antibiotics can escape bacterial ability to develop resistance. Development of resistance has resulted in major changes in the therapy of important pathogens for children, including *Staphylococcus aureus,* HIB, and *S pneumoniae.* For instance, infections caused by *S aureus* no longer can be treated with penicillin, and some strains are not even sensitive to methicillin. Another example is the emergence of penicillin-resistant pneumococci in many parts of the world.

Emergence of resistant organisms in the community, as well as in the hospital, results in longer hospital stays, frequent use of newer generations of expensive drugs, increased morbidity from these infections, and about a twofold increase in mortality rate. Resistance can result from a mutation or the insertion of foreign DNA by recombination. More often, however, resistance results from the transfer of genes carried on extrachromosomal resistance plasmids. Transfer of the plasmids is mediated most commonly by conjugation and followed by transformation, transduction, or transposon transfer. During the emergence of antibiotic resistance, it is quite common for clinical bacterial isolates to develop resistance to a number of antimicrobial agents, ie, multiresistance.

Mechanisms for the development of resistance include production of enzymes that inactivate or modify the antibiotic, decreased antibiotic uptake or an active efflux transport system, and alteration in antibiotic target. First, β-lactamase is probably the best known inactivating enzyme produced by resistant bacteria to inactivate penicillins and cephalosporins. Second, alterations in specific outer membrane proteins can result in decreased uptake or penetration of antibiotics into the bacteria. For example, certain bacteria change their uptake of imipenem. Third, an example of altered antibiotic target is the development of penicillin-binding proteins with markedly reduced affinity for penicillin, resulting in strains of *S pneumoniae* poorly killed by penicillin. Bacteria may develop resistance via more than one mechanism.

Combination Therapy With Antibiotics

In general, a single antibiotic should be used to treat an uncomplicated infection attributable to a single pathogen. The drug used should have the narrowest spectrum of activity specific for the targeted organism to avoid misuse and emergence of resistance. For certain clinical conditions, however, combination therapy is indicated. The most common reason for combining two or more antibiotics is to provide broad empiric therapy until the infecting pathogen has been identified. Combination therapy is also used when the infection is presumed or proved to be caused by more than one bacterium that cannot be adequately treated with a single agent. Examples of this include intrapelvic and intra-abdominal infections, which are usually caused by a mixture of organisms including aerobes and anaerobes. Combining two agents may at times prevent or delay the emergence of resistance. For instance, multiple drugs are used to treat mycobacterial infections. Management of most *Pseudomonas aeruginosa* infections requires the use of two drugs, such as tobramycin and piperacillin, for synergistic effects. In addition, antibiotics are prescribed in combination to provide greater inhibition or killing of the pathogenic bacteria than would occur with single-drug therapy. This is particularly important for the management of immunocompromised hosts with sepsis or episodes of fever and neutropenia (see below).

Although extensive in vitro data demonstrate synergism between various antibiotics, definitive proof of the clinical relevance of these interactions is generally lacking. Nevertheless, combination therapy is often advised for the following reasons:

1. clinical presentation suggestive of severe infection or septic shock

2. immunocompromised host with sepsis or febrile, neutropenic episodes
3. a relatively resistant organism.

The possible beneficial effects of combination antibiotic therapy should be weighed against possible harmful effects, including an increased incidence of superinfection and toxicity, increased cost, and potential antagonism.

Special Issues Relevant to Pediatrics

Antibiotics frequently are given intravenously to hospitalized children with serious infections. This route of administration appears to ensure drug delivery, but this is not always true. First, the stability of the specific antibiotic in the delivery solution must be considered. Second, drugs always should be given separately to avoid potential drug incompatibilities. If this is not possible, the compatibility of the mixed agents must be verified. An example is the inactivation of aminoglycosides by penicillins when they are allowed to mix before an infusion. It is therefore important to administer drugs in the appropriate solutions and only with compatible drugs. Third, the delivery system itself must also be considered because of the small amount in pediatric unit doses relative to the volume in the IV infusion system.

In pediatrics, food and beverages influence the successful use of oral antibiotics. In young children, unlike adults, how the antibiotics smell and taste are major factors in achieving compliance with therapy. Another important factor is concomitant food ingestion. Food may reduce the gastrointestinal discomfort generated by certain antibiotics and therefore indirectly enhance compliance. For certain antibiotics, however, the benefit of reduced gastrointestinal upset is outweighed by the decrease in bioavailability that results from the presence of food. Table 9–3 indicates which antibiotics should be taken on an empty stomach and which should be taken with food.

Other special issues in pediatrics include transplacental transfer of antibiotics, excretion in breast milk, and imma-

Table 9–4. Transplacental transfer of antibiotics.

Maternal Concentrations Attained in Fetus	Antibiotics
≥ 50%	Aminoglycosides Ampicillin Chloramphenicol Methicillin Nitrofurantoin Penicillin Sulfonamides Tetracyclines
< 20%	Cephalosporins Clindamycin Dicloxacillin Erythromycin Nafcillin Oxacillin

turity of the liver and kidney in neonates. It is well recognized that certain antibiotics cross the placenta and can be potentially toxic to the fetus (Table 9–4). In addition, an antibiotic can be excreted in breast milk (Table 9–5). These issues of transplacental transfer and breast milk excretion should be considered in the prescribing antibiotics to pregnant women and lactating mothers. For further discussion, see Chapter 11.

Neonates, especially those born prematurely, present special pharmacokinetic issues. Their hepatic and renal function is less mature than that of older children and adults. Therapy must be carefully guided, with special attention paid to antibiotics that have a narrow toxic-to-therapeutic ratio, such as aminoglycosides, vancomycin, and chloramphenicol. In patients with renal or hepatic impairment, the clinician must be aware of the pharmacologic properties of the drug and its route of excretion. For example, for the patient with significant renal failure, antibiotics that are excreted by the kidney must be administered carefully. The dosage of the drug should be adjusted appropriately to accommodate the residual function of the respective organ (Tables 9–6 and 9–7).

PHARMACOLOGY OF ANTIMICROBIAL AGENTS

The following discussion is an abbreviated review of antimicrobial agents, including antibacterial, antiviral, antifungal, and antiparasitic drugs. Readers are encouraged

Table 9–3. Antibiotic administration and food consumption.

Antibiotics that should be taken on an empty stomach
Clindamycin
Erythromycin base and stearate
Penicillins (except those listed below)
Rifampin
Tetracyclines (except those listed below)
Antibiotics that should be taken with food
Amoxicillin
Amoxicillin-clavulanic acid
Doxycycline
Erythromycin
Metronidazole
Minocycline
Penicillin V
Nalidixic acid
Nitrofurantoin
Sulfonamides

Table 9–5. Antibiotics excreted into breast milk.

Antibiotics excreted in substantial amounts	Aminoglycosides, chloramphenicol, erythromycin, metronidazole, sulfonamides, tetracycline, trimethoprim-sulfamethoxazole
Antibiotics excreted in only trace amounts	Acyclovir, cephalosporins, clindamycin, nitrofurantoin, penicillins

to consult major textbooks, such as *Rudolph's Pediatrics* (20th ed, 1996) for in-depth reading.

ANTIBACTERIAL AGENTS

On the basis of the mode of action, antibacterial agents can be divided into four categories:

1. cell wall synthesis inhibitors
2. protein synthesis inhibitors
3. nucleic acid synthesis inhibitors
4. antimetabolites (folate synthesis inhibitors).

Cell Wall Synthesis Inhibitors

β-Lactam Agents. Many different antibacterial agents contain a β-lactam, or monobactam, ring (Table 9–8) that contains an amide link. This is the site for β-lactamase action as well as for covalent binding to penicillin binding proteins (PBP). With the exception of the monobactams, all agents in this class have either a five-membered ring (penicillins) or a six-membered ring (cephalosporins) adjacent to the β-lactam structure.

Mechanism of Action. The cell wall of bacteria consists of peptidoglycans, protein receptors, enzymes, and lipopolysaccharides. The peptidoglycan, the major structural framework of the cell wall, is a network of alternating polysaccharide chains (glycans) that are cross-linked with short polypeptides unique for different species of bacteria. Peptidoglycans are synthesized by enzymes located on the inner membrane of the bacteria. In general, β-lactam antibiotics exert their action by binding to PBPs located on the inner membrane, causing inhibition of cross-linking of the polysaccharide chains. Different types of PBP exist in different bacteria.

Clinical Uses. Because of the relatively few toxicities

Table 9–6. Antibiotics in patients with renal failure.

Major decrease in dose
Aminoglycosides
Vancomycin
Trimethoprim-sulfamethoxazole
Minor decrease in dose
Penicillins
Cephalosporins
Tetracyclines
Erythromycins
No dose adjustments
Clindamycin
Chloramphenicol
Metronidazole
Rifampin
Avoid
Methenamine
Nalidixic acid
Nitrofurantoin
Polymyxin B
Spectinomycin

Table 9–7. Antibiotics in patients with hepatic failure.

Dose reduction required
Chloramphenicol
Clindamycin
Doxycycline
Erythromycin
Antibiotics to be used with caution
Rifampin
Tetracyclines

associated with these drugs, β-lactams are widely used in many clinical infections. The penicillins are active against a variety of aerobic and anaerobic gram-positive and gram-negative organisms. Penicillin G is active against gram-positive organisms, including the hemolytic streptococci, most isolates of *S pneumoniae,* non–β-lactamase-producing strains of *S aureus,* and most oral streptococci. Of the gram-negative aerobes, only *N meningitidis* and non–penicillinase-producing isolates of *N gonorrhoeae* are susceptible to this agent. Nafcillin and oxacillin have a spectrum of activity similar to penicillin G, with additional activity against β-lactamase–producing strains of *S aureus.*

The aminopenicillins, such as amoxicillin and ampicillin, are among the most commonly prescribed antibiotics in pediatrics. These agents have a spectrum of activity similar to penicillin G and also are active against non–β-lactamase-producing strains of *H influenzae, Listeria monocytogenes,* many strains of *E coli,* and *Moraxella catarrhalis.* Amoxicillin has been the initial drug of choice in the pediatric age group for outpatient management of otitis media, uncomplicated UTIs, and sinusitis. Because of its effects on *E coli,* group B streptococci, and *Listeria,* ampicillin is commonly used in neonatal anti-infective therapy. When used in combination, amoxicillin and the β-lactamase inhibitor clavulanic acid (Augmentin) provide an oral agent with all of the activity of ampicillin. This agent is also effective against the β-lactamase–producing strains of *H influenzae, M catarrhalis,* and *S aureus.*

Table 9–8. β-Lactam antibiotics.

Penicillin derivatives
Aminopenicillins: ampicillin, amoxicillin
Penicillinase-resistant penicillins: cloxacillin, methicillin, nafcillin
Antipseudomonal penicillin: carbenicillin, piperacillin, ticarcillin
Monobactam
Aztreonam
Carbapenem
Imipenem
Cephalosporins
First-generation: cefazolin, cephalexin, cepharoridine
Second-generation: cefoxitin, cefuroxime
Third-generation: cefotaxime, ceftriaxone, ceftizoxime, ceftazidime

The extended-spectrum penicillins include carbenicillin and piperacillin; they are hydrolyzed by β-lactamase. In general, these agents have expanded activity against gram-negative aerobes; they are active against many isolates of *P aeruginosa* and members of the Enterobacteriaceae family. These antibiotics are often used in combination with aminoglycosides for synergistic effects.

The cephalosporin derivatives are often divided into "generations." In general, the higher generation derivatives are more active against gram-negative bacteria with concomitant loss of activity against gram-positive organisms. For instance, the first-generation derivatives are active against most aerobic gram-positive cocci, β-lactamase–producing strains of *S aureus, E coli*, and *Klebsiella* species, with the important exception of the enterococci (group D streptococci). The second-generation agents have expanded anaerobic activity (cefoxitin) or expanded gram-negative activity against *H influenzae* and *M catarrhalis* (cefuroxime). Neither first- nor second-generation cephalosporins achieve adequate CSF concentrations for the treatment of meningitis or are active against organisms including *Listeria, Enterococci,* or *Pseudomonas.*

As compared with the earlier-generation agents, the properties of third-generation cephalosporins include improved penetration into the CSF, diminished gram-positive activity, and expanded gram-negative activity. Because of their increased activity against gram-negative pathogens such as HIB and *E coli,* cefotaxime and ceftriaxone are usually recommended for the treatment of meningitis and sepsis in children. In contrast to other cephalosporins, ceftazidime has expanded activity against *P aeruginosa* and *Pseudomonas cepacia.* Cephalosporins in general are not active against anaerobes, with the exception of cefoxitin, and have no activity against *Listeria.* Thus, ampicillin is needed in addition to cefotaxime-ceftizoxime or aminoglycoside for the management of neonatal meningitis.

Aztreonam has a narrow spectrum of activity covering only the Enterobacteriaceae and some members of the Pseudomonadaceae families. In contrast, imipenem has broad activity against many gram-positive and gram-negative organisms.

Side Effects. In general, β-lactam agents have few side effects. Type I hypersensitivity, manifested by urticaria and wheezing, is the most serious side effect of this class of agents. Extremely high doses or intraventricular administration of β-lactam agents can precipitate seizures. Prolonged high-dosage administration of any of these agents can result in a type-specific neutropenia, which is reversible after cessation of drug therapy. Many of these agents, particularly oxacillin and nafcillin, have been associated with dose-dependent elevations in serum hepatic transaminase activity as well as thrombophlebitis.

Vancomycin, a tricyclic glycopeptide antibiotic, is the only drug of this group approved for clinical use. It is active only against gram-positive aerobic and anaerobic organisms. Vancomycin inhibits cell wall synthesis by binding to the polypeptide side-chain of the peptidoglycan, thereby inhibiting polymerization necessary for elongation of the peptidoglycan. Clinical uses of vancomycin include gram-positive infections in penicillin-allergic patients and methicillin-resistant strains of *S aureus* and *S epidermidis* and penicillin-resistant strains of *S pneumoniae.* The major toxicity of vancomycin is cutaneous vasodilatation ("red man syndrome") and hypotension, which may result from rapid IV infusion. Nephrotoxicity is rare with modern formulations.

Protein Synthesis Inhibitors

Aminoglycosides. Commonly used antibiotics in this class include gentamicin, tobramycin, and amikacin. Others include neomycin, kanamycin, and streptomycin, which is used for unusual infections or resistant organisms, such as *M tuberculosis.* The toxicity of the latter three compared with that of newer agents precludes their generalized use.

Mechanism of Action. The cellular uptake of aminoglycosides in gram-negative bacteria involves several phases. The first phase is non–energy-dependent and involves binding of the cationic aminoglycoside to the anionic sites of lipopolysaccharide, phospholipids, and outer membrane proteins. This results in disruption of the outer membrane integrity. This phenomenon provides a molecular explanation for the synergy observed between certain β-lactam antibiotics and aminoglycosides. The other phases of drug uptake are energy dependent. Once entered into the bacterial cell, the aminoglycoside binds to the bacterial ribosomes (30S subunit). This leads to inhibition of protein synthesis, further destruction of the integrity of the outer membrane, and inhibition of DNA replication. All these events culminate in ultimate bacterial cell death.

Clinical Uses. The activity spectrum of aminoglycosides is limited to the treatment of gram-negative aerobic infections. These agents must be prescribed and monitored with caution because the therapeutic index of the aminoglycosides is narrow. Although not entirely related to high plasma concentrations of the drug, deafness may occur, usually at high drug concentrations (eg, 10–15 μg/mL of gentamicin), and is often irreversible. Nephrotoxicity is reversible but can create major problems in the management of seriously ill patients. As a rare complication, these agents can produce paralysis in patients with preexisting neuromuscular disease (notably myasthenia gravis). Thus, their use is usually reserved for empiric coverage of short durations or for UTIs. They may also be combined with a broad-spectrum β-lactam agent for the treatment of serious gram-negative infections.

Chloramphenicol. This lipophilic drug provides high concentrations in CSF even without meningeal inflammation. However, with the newer generation of cephalosporins available, this drug is not in common use in pediatrics for the treatment of sepsis and meningitis.

Mechanism of Action. Because it is highly hydrophobic, chloramphenicol appears to enter the bacterial cell by passive diffusion across the outer membrane. It inhibits protein synthesis by binding to the 50S subunit of the 70S ribosome. Many gram-negative aerobes "tolerate" this action by ceasing to grow without dying. Because of cross-reactivity and binding of the drug to 70S ribosomes in human mitochondria, prolonged administration of this agent results in bone marrow toxicity, including anemia, thrombocytopenia, and neutropenia. Significant poisoning of mitochondria in the myocardium produces generalized shock ("gray baby syndrome"). For certain individuals, irreversible aplastic anemia (bone marrow failure) develops after brief exposure to this drug. The incidence of this idiosyncratic complication is approximately 1 in 50,000; therefore, it is not as common as previously assumed.

Clinical Uses. Until recently, chloramphenicol was used extensively for the treatment of suspected *H influenzae* infections (sepsis, meningitis, pneumonia, and septic arthritis). The drug is also bactericidal against other typical childhood pathogens, including *S pneumoniae* and *N meningitidis,* and active against most anaerobic bacteria. The potentially serious toxicity of this drug has led to remarkably decreased use of chloramphenicol in recent years. Nevertheless, chloramphenicol remains a drug of choice for infections in children with type I β-lactam hypersensitivity and in the unusual circumstance in which oral therapy is needed for serious infections caused by susceptible pathogens. Because chloramphenicol achieves excellent concentrations in the vitreous of the eye and in brain tissue and because of its broad spectrum of activity against many aerobic and most anaerobic bacteria, this agent is still recommended for the treatment of bacterial endophthalmitis and for rickettsial diseases in children younger than 9 years.

Miscellaneous Protein Synthesis Inhibitors. Although chemically dissimilar, the tetracyclines, erythromycin, and clindamycin have similar sites of action but slightly different spectra of activity and clinical use.

Mechanism of Action. Tetracycline products prevent binding of transfer RNA (tRNA) to the 30S ribosome, whereas both erythromycin and clindamycin block protein synthesis by binding to the 50S ribosomal subunit.

Clinical Uses. Tetracycline is used for a variety of infections, including acnes, and it is the drug of choice for most rickettsial diseases in adults. Tetracycline is also active against the organisms that cause Lyme disease and nongonococcal arthritis. A common side effect for tetracycline is the yellow discoloration of teeth seen in some children after treatment. Thus, the drug should not be used in children younger than 8 years unless there are no other alternatives. Erythromycin is often used as an alternative to oral penicillins in allergic patients. This antibiotic is also the drug of choice for the treatment of Legionnaire disease, Campylobacter diarrhea, and pertussis. Clindamycin has excellent gram-positive and as well as anaerobic activity. However, clindamycin, unlike metronidazole and chloramphenicol, does not penetrate into CSF well.

Alterations of Nucleic Acid Synthesis
Rifampin (Rifamycin)
Mechanism of Action. Of all the rifamycin products, rifampin is the only member of this drug class used clini-

cally. Rifampin binds bacterial DNA-dependent RNA polymerase, effectively inhibiting transcription. Because it can induce hepatic microsomal P-450, patients receiving rifampin have altered liver metabolism of drugs, including anticonvulsants such as phenobarbital and antibiotics such as chloramphenicol.

Clinical Uses. Rifampin is an important antituberculous drug and is also active against some nontuberculous mycobacteria. Because it achieves high mucosal concentrations, rifampin is frequently used to eliminate carriage of *N meningitidis, H influenzae,* and *S aureus* in potential carriers. Except as a prophylactic treatment against *N meningitidis* or *H influenzae,* rifampin is not used as a single agent.

Quinolones. Nalidixic acid was the first member of this drug class to be used clinically. Because of the poor bioavailability and rapid development of bacterial drug resistance, this agent was limited to the treatment of UTIs. Recently, norfloxacin, ciprofloxacin, and other 6-fluorinated piperazinyl quinolones have been developed.

Mechanism of Action. The quinolones inhibit bacterial topoisomerase II (DNA gyrase). This enzyme introduces negative superhelical twists into double-stranded bacterial DNA, a requirement for DNA replication. These antibiotics inhibit the formation of a DNA-topoisomerase complex, resulting in inhibition of DNA synthesis.

Clinical Uses. The precise clinical role for the quinolones, particularly in pediatrics, is still controversial. The observation that drugs of this class inhibit cartilage formation in young animals currently precludes their use in children. The newer agents are active against a wide variety of aerobic gram-negative bacteria and are used occasionally against *S aureus.* The advantage of these drugs is that they are administered orally. However, resistance appears to develop rapidly, and these agents are not officially approved for general use in children. These agents have been used successfully in the treatment of non–life-threatening gram-negative infections (eg, osteomyelitis and UTIs) as an alternative to IV antibiotics with prolonged hospitalization.

Metronidazole
Mechanism of Action. Metronidazole is a hydroxy-aliphatic derivative of nitroimidazole, with unique spectrum of activity. It is active only against anaerobes and some protozoa. It requires bacterial nitroreductase, a unique enzyme produced exclusively by anaerobic bacteria and some protozoa, to convert the drug into its active form, an amine derivative. Its mechanism of action is probably via intracellular nitroreduction of metronidazole to generate unstable hydroxylamino and nitroso intermediates to interfere with synthesis of nucleic acids.

Clinical Uses. This agent has been used extensively to treat life-threatening anaerobic infections, including brain abscesses. It is also used for the treatment of vaginal *Trichomonas* and some protozoan infections. One major concern about this antibiotic is its potential mutagenic effects; therefore, it probably should not be used in pregnant women.

Antimetabolites

Folate Synthesis Inhibitors

Mechanism of Action. The sulfa agents are analogues of para-aminobenzoic acid, a necessary precursor for bacterial folate synthesis. Thus, they have specific antibacterial activity with relatively high therapeutic indices, because humans cannot synthesize folate. In addition, trimethoprim and pyrimethamine selectively inhibit dihydrofolate reductase, another enzyme necessary in the bacterial synthesis pathway of folates. The combination of trimethoprim with a sulfa drug (sulfamethoxazole) has synergistic effects. This combination is marketed commercially as Bactrim or Septra.

Clinical Uses. Sulfa drugs alone, or in combination with trimethoprim, are used for the outpatient treatment of a variety of non–life-threatening infections (eg, otitis media and UTIs). The combination of a dihydrofolate reductase inhibitor with sulfa has been used extensively for the treatment of a variety of parasitic infections, most notably malaria and *Pneumocystis carinii,* a common infection in AIDS.

ANTIVIRAL AGENTS

The development of antiviral therapy is still in its infancy despite recent advances. Most antiviral agents have spectra of activity limited to one or, at most, two viral genera. In general, antiviral agents may be divided into four types: (1) antimetabolites in nucleic acid synthesis, (2) specific antiviral antiserum, (3) natural immunomodulators such as interferons, and (4) miscellaneous compounds (Table 9–9).

Acyclovir

Acyclovir is a guanine derivative effective against HSV and VZV. Acyclovir is thought to be activated by viral thymidine kinase, thus ensuring its specificity against virus-infected cells only and sparing the normal host cells. After initial activation by viral thymidine kinase, the acyclovir monophosphate is converted by the host's cellular

Table 9–9. Antiviral agents.

Antimetabolites
Vidarabine
Acyclovir
Ganciclovir
Zidovudine (azidothymidine [AZT])
Dideoxyinosine
Ribavirin
Human antisera preparations
Hepatitis B immunoglobulin
Varicella zoster immunoglobulin
Human rabies immunoglobulin
Immunomodulators
Human interferon: α, β, γ
Other drugs
Amantadine, rimantadine

machinery into its triphosphate forms. These would compete with deoxyguanosine triphosphate for incorporation into viral genome via viral DNA polymerase. Viral DNA elongation is terminated because acyclovir triphosphate lacks a 3′-hydroxyl group. Consequently, the incomplete DNA polymer effectively inhibits viral DNA polymerase.

Acyclovir is the drug of choice for the treatment of all serious infections caused by HSV and VZV. In particular, acyclovir treatment reduces the morbidity and mortality of herpes encephalitis and neonatal herpes infection. It is also effective for primary and reactivated VZV infections in the immunocompromised host. Orally administered acyclovir is effective for the treatment of initial or recurrent episodes of genital herpes infections. The use of oral acyclovir for primary VZV infections in normal children is controversial because of the marginal benefits and high cost of the drug. Because of the specific nature of its activation process, as mentioned above, acyclovir is a relatively nontoxic agent. Although it has been implicated in a variety of symptoms of the central nervous system (CNS), including hallucinations cortical dysfunction, it is unclear whether acyclovir causes these side effects. One important issue is to maintain good hydration and urine output to prevent nephrotoxicity, which is a rare complication caused by crystallization of acyclovir in the renal cortex in the dehydrated patient.

Zidovudine

Zidovudine (AZT) was the first agent licensed and approved for the treatment of HIV infections. Unlike acyclovir, zidovudine is triphosphorylated by cellular kinases. The 5′-triphosphate derivative inhibits retroviral reverse transcriptase by prematurely terminating chain elongation of the viral DNA. At present, zidovudine is often used in the treatment of HIV-infected children and children with acquired immunodeficiency syndrome (see Chapter 11). Because of its mechanism of activation, unlike acyclovir, the drug has remarkable side effects with significant bone marrow suppression. This is manifested as neutropenia or megaloblastic anemia. Recent studies have demonstrated the gradual development of significant drug resistance among many clinical isolates of HIV. Recently, a new class of anti-HIV drug, protease inhibitor, has been introduced. This drug specifically interferes with the processing of viral proteins during replication resulting in inhibition of HIV replication.

Ribavirin

Ribavirin is a nucleoside analogue with relatively broad activity in vitro and in vivo against RNA viruses. Ribavirin has several potential modes of action, including inhibition of viral RNA polymerases and reduction of cellular pools of guanosine triphosphate, by competitively inhibiting cellular inosine monophosphate dehydrogenase activity. In the United States, ribavirin is used mainly for treating RSV infections in hospitalized, critically ill infants; it is administered by aerosol. Other potential uses of ribavirin are still under investigation.

Rimantadine & Amantadine

Rimantadine and amantadine are tricyclic aminohydrocarbons with antiviral activity directed uniquely against influenza A virus. These two compounds appear to have similar mechanisms of activity through the inhibition of early phases of viral replication by preventing uncoating of the viral genome and virus-mediated membrane fusion. Both agents have been used successfully to prevent and treat influenza A infections. Frequently, the use of empiric therapy with amantadine or rimantadine is determined on the basis of the local prevalence of influenza A and the clinical picture. Their therapeutic effect depends on the initiation of therapy within 48 hours of the onset of symptoms. The most common side effects of these agents involve the gastrointestinal tract and, mildly, the CNS.

ANTIFUNGAL AGENTS

Three classes of compounds are useful for the treatment of fungal diseases in children:

1. polyenes
2. antimetabolite flucytosine
3. imidazole derivatives.

Polyene Agents
Amphotericin B

Mechanism of Action. Amphotericin B binds to sterols, particularly ergosterol, on the fungal cell membrane. Probably because of the hydrophobic properties associated with the formation of ionic channels when amphotericin molecules are clustered, there is a consequent loss of membrane integrity resulting in leakage of intracellular constituents and osmotic lysis of the fungal cell. Recently, amphotericin B has also been shown to lyse cells by oxidant injury to the cell. Toxicity to human cell is caused by cross-over binding of the drug to cholesterol on human cells.

Clinical Uses. Amphotericin B is administered parenterally and is the drug of choice for most systemic fungal infections in children, including *Candida, Cryptococcus, Histoplasma, Blastomyces,* and *Coccidioides.* The relative toxicity of amphotericin B is significant; hypokalemia and oliguria are the most common complications. The syndrome of fever, chills, and rigors that accompanies drug infusion often can be modified or eliminated by pretreatment with meperidine and antihistamines. Phlebitis can be minimized by simultaneous infusion of hydrocortisone. Co-administration of blood leukocytes with amphotericin B is contraindicated because of the development of severe pulmonary injury.

Nystatin. Nystatin is a polyene antifungal agent with presumed mechanisms of action similar to amphotericin B. Nystatin is currently available only for nonsystemic use for the treatment of superficial mucosal *Candida* infections, eg, thrush.

Flucytosine

Flucytosine (5-fluorocytosine) is an antimetabolite with limited activity against human fungal infections. After entry into fungal cells, flucytosine is deaminated to form 5-fluorouracil, an inhibitor of DNA synthesis. Because of the rapid development of drug resistance to flucytosine, this agent is rarely used alone. Most studies have examined the use of flucytosine in combination with amphotericin B. This combination is recommended for the treatment of cryptococcal meningitis and candidal meningitis in the newborn. The major toxicity of flucytosine is myelosuppression. Because the drug is excreted by the kidney, changes in dosage are required in individuals with renal impairment.

Imidazoles

Ketoconazole, miconazole, and fluconazole are all systemically administered imidazoles with activity against pathogens, including *Candida* species, *Histoplasma capsulatum, Coccidioides immitis, Blastomyces dermatitidis,* and *Cryptococcus neoformans.* They affect membrane permeability by competitive inhibition of cytochrome P-450 enzymes. Ketoconazole has been used successfully for the treatment of many dermatomycoses and mucocutaneous candidiasis. Miconazole is available in over-the-counter preparations for the treatment of tinea pedis and tinea cruris. The use of fluconazole for the treatment of systemic and invasive candidal infections is currently being investigated; it has been approved for some indications. To varying degrees, these agents have gastrointestinal and hepatic toxicities. Nausea and vomiting are common with ketoconazole, whereas changes in liver function tests may occur with all these agents. Ketoconazole has been known to downregulate ergosterol synthesis; therefore, this class of compound should not be used in conjunction with amphotericin B.

ANTIPARASITIC AGENTS

Folic Acid Synthesis Inhibitors. A variety of sulfa drugs and dihydrofolate reductase inhibitors are useful for the treatment of selective parasitic infections. For example, pyrimethamine is a dihydrofolate reductase inhibitor that is often combined with sulfadoxine as a single medication (Fansidar) or used in combination with sulfadiazine. Either combination can be used to treat chloroquine-resistant falciparum malaria. Pyrimethamine is potentially hepatotoxic and may cause bone marrow suppression; the latter side effect may be prevented by co-administration of folinic acid.

Antimalarials. Chloroquine phosphate is the main antimalarial drug in use today. Chloroquine, a weak base, is actively taken up by the malarial parasites. Alkalinization of the food vacuoles presumably prevents subsequent hemoglobin hydrolysis by inhibiting the parasites' acid proteases and intracellular transport of macromolecules. Chloroquine is used for the prevention and treatment of most forms of malaria, except for infections caused by *Plasmodium falciparum.* Gastrointestinal and CNS side effects, although common, are dose dependent. Primaquine is used for eradication of extra-erythrocytic phase of malarial infections caused by *Plasmodium vivax* and *Plasmodium ovale.* Caution should be taken in using this agent, because it can precipitate hemolysis in patients with glucose-6-phosphate dehydrogenase deficiency. The combination of pyrimethamine and sulfadoxine is used for treatment of chloroquine-resistant falciparum malaria.

Antihelminthics. Mebendazole, pyrantel pamoate, and **niclosamide** are orally administered agents used for the treatment of most intestinal parasites encountered in the United States. However, they have different mechanisms of action. Mebendazole is the drug of choice for the treatment of pinworms (*Enterobius vermicularis*), ascariasis (*Ascaris lumbricoides*), *Ancylostoma duodenale,* and *Necator americanus* infections. Thiabendazole is recommended for the treatment of *Strongyloides stercoralis* infection and some infections caused by *Toxocara* species. Thiabendazole alone can be used in individuals coinfected with *Strongyloides* and some of the worms typically treated with mebendazole. Niclosamide and praziquantel are used for the treatment of *Taenia* infections, including neurocysticercosis.

Other Agents. Pentamidine is used as an alternative drug for the treatment of *P carinii* infections in individuals who are intolerant of or nonresponsive to trimethoprim-sulfamethoxazole therapy. **Furazolidone** is used for the treatment of *Giardia lamblia* infections in young children because this compound is available in liquid form and is well tolerated. **Praziquantel** is used for the treatment of a variety of fluke and schistosoma infections.

NATURAL IMMUNOMODULATORS

Cytokines are naturally occurring proteins that function as short-range signaling molecules to enhance cell-to-cell interactions. They are important in the regulation of immune responses, growth and development, and homeostasis. Recent advances in recombinant DNA technology have enabled the production of certain cytokines in mass quantities for their therapeutic applications. Some prototypes of this class of molecules are discussed below.

Hematopoietic Growth Factors

Both granulocyte-macrophage colony stimulating factors (GM-CSF) and granulocyte colony stimulating factors (G-CSF) are growth factors categorized on the basis of their biologic activity on the hematopoietic system. G-CSF is a late-acting hematopoietin; its effects are mainly restricted to the neutrophil lineage. In contrast, GM-CSF is a multilineage hematopoietin; it acts on multiple steps of myeloid differentiation from the early stem cell to mature macrophage cell functions. Human GM-CSF and G-CSF are used as adjunctive therapy; in many centers, they are used as standard therapy in recipients of

bone-marrow transplantation and cancer chemotherapy and in patients with dysfunctional hematopoiesis. Both GM-CSF and G-CSF have clearly reduced neutropenia and infection rate when given to patients after conventional cytotoxic chemotherapy and high-dose chemotherapy preceding autologous bone-marrow transplantation. Similar results have been described in other diseases, including aplastic anemia, myelodysplasia, drug-induced agranulocytosis, and chronic neutropenia. In general, the recipients showed increases in peripheral blood granulocyte counts, less opportunistic infection, and shorter period of hospitalization. Treatment appears to be well tolerated, despite the common occurrence of mild to moderate flulike symptoms and occasional fluid retention problems. The bedside use of these growth factors represents a major contribution of biotechnology to a difficult area of therapeutics in febrile, neutropenic patients.

Interferon

Interferons (IFNs) are naturally occurring proteins produced by mammals in response to detection of cancer cells and infectious pathogens, especially viruses. They possess antitumor and immunomodulatory activities in addition to their antiviral effects. IFNs can be divided into three major groups: α, β, and γ. By 1996, the US Food and Drug Administration had approved IFNs for a number of clinical indications in the United States, including hepatitis B and C virus and human papilloma virus (condyloma acuminata), and malignant neoplasms, including hairy cell leukemia, chronic myelogenous leukemia, and malignant melanoma, as well as Kaposi sarcoma in HIV-infected patients. IFN-γ is approved for prophylactic use in patients with chronic granulomatous disease to prevent recurrence of bacterial infections. IFN-β was approved for the treatment of patients with multiple sclerosis several years ago. In addition, IFNs have demonstrable efficacy in laryngeal papillomatosis, multiple myeloma, and basal cell and cutaneous squamous cell carcinoma. In some European countries, IFNs are approved for a number of these diseases. Although significant work has been done on the use of these drugs in children, most IFN clinical trials to date involve adults.

IFNs, GM-CSF, and G-CSF therefore serve as prototypes of naturally occurring immune proteins that can be produced in mass quantities by advanced biotechnology techniques. They can be used as therapeutic agents in the modulation of the immune system for the benefit of patient care.

Specific Immunoglobulins

Passive immunization using specific high-titer human IgG preparations is recommended for a variety of viral illnesses. For example, immunoglobulin preparations containing high titers of antibodies against respiratory syncytial virus have been approved recently for use in premature neonates at risk for the infection.

All these preparations are screened for the presence of high titers of specific antibody, and most are available through the Red Cross. The risk of infection, including HIV and hepatitis C, from any of these preparations is very low. Caution should be exercised in the administration of these preparations because anaphylaxis may occur. Care should also be used in administering any of these IgG preparations to patients with IgA deficiency because the minute quantities of IgA contained in each preparation may prompt the development of endogenous anti-IgA antibody, resulting in subsequent hypersensitivity reactions to transfusion of blood products.

APPROACH TO THE CHILD WITH FEVER

EVALUATION OF ACUTE FEVER

Fever is one of the most common complaints that prompt a telephone call or visit to a pediatrician. Although parents are often worried about the risks of the fever itself, physicians are more concerned about identifying the underlying cause of fever.

Fever may be a manifestation of many different disease processes, including most infectious illnesses. In the primary care setting, most children with fever have illnesses that are benign and self-limited. However, fever may be the initial sign of more serious or life-threatening illness. In addition, it is important to understand that neonates and young infants may not mount a fever in response to serious or even overwhelming infection, and may, in fact, become hypothermic. This is, in part, associated with immaturity of the immune system in this age group.

One general approach to the ill child with a history of fever is to ask a series of questions: Is fever present? Does the child appear "toxic"? Is there a source for the fever on physical examination? Are laboratory tests indicated? What is the risk of serious, life-threatening bacterial infection? Is treatment necessary?

Is Fever Present? The definition of fever is itself controversial. Normal body temperature demonstrates a diurnal variation with lowest values in the morning and highest values in the evening. Small differences in temperature exist depending on the patient's sex, ethnicity, and age. One recent study looked at temperatures in normal infants younger than 3 months and established values for 2 SD above the mean. In this study, such values increased with increasing age, from 38.0 °C in infants younger than 1 month to 38.2 °C in infants aged 2–3 months. In a study by Baraff, a survey of residency directors in pediatrics and emergency medicine produced a range of temperatures (37.4–38.6 °C) that were accepted as fever.

In addition, the measuring device and anatomic site used to determine temperature influence the interpretation of fever. In infants and young children, a rectal temperature with a glass-mercury or digital-electronic thermometer is considered the standard for taking temperatures. Axillary, oral, and tympanic temperatures may provide easier routes of measuring temperature in infants, but their accuracy in the outpatient setting is not without criticism. For example, axillary temperatures may be affected by skin perfusion or thickness. Oral temperatures may be affected by respiratory rate and the consumption of hot or cold liquids. A tympanic temperature is the newest route of thermometry, and reports have some conflicting results. For practical purposes, a rectal temperature of 38.0 °C probably qualifies as a fever in a young infant. Some clinicians use a temperature of 38.5 or 39.0 °C in older children or in the evening when body temperatures are at their peak.

Does the Child Appear "Toxic"? "Toxicity" refers to the severity of illness of a child on the basis of clinical observation and physical examination. It has been used to describe a child who appears to have sepsis or is at risk for it. McCarthy and colleagues at Yale designed the Infant Observation Scales to identify specific observational items that would aid the clinician in assessing risk of serious illness in a child (Table 9–10). This scale includes an evaluation of a child's cry, reaction to parents, state variation, and response to social overtures (eg, smile), in addition to skin color and hydration status. Children who are seriously impaired in these areas are believed to be much more likely to have serious illnesses when compared with children who are "well-appearing."

Is There a Source for the Fever on Physical Examination? After the fever is documented and the history reviewed, a thorough physical examination should be performed to identify a source of infection. Common sources include upper respiratory infections (URIs), such as colds and otitis media, and gastroenteritis. If no source is detected in this initial evaluation, further workup, including laboratory data and radiologic studies, must be considered. These children fall into the categories of fever without source, fever of unclear etiology, or fever without localizing signs. Fever of unknown origin is discussed below.

Are Laboratory Tests Indicated? In infants and children who lack an obvious source of infection on preliminary examination, the utility of other diagnostic tests must be considered. Serious bacterial infections may be present in the blood (eg, bacteremia or sepsis), CSF (eg, meningitis), lungs (eg, pneumonia), urinary tract (eg, lower or upper UTIs), or stool (eg, gastroenteritis). Therefore, further laboratory investigations are directed toward these specific areas. The clinician weighs the risk of complication, cost, and patient discomfort associated with performing tests versus the benefit of detecting a serious bacterial infection.

What Is the Risk? Further discussion of risk involves the likelihood of infection, seriousness of infection, and the risk of morbidity and mortality from serious infections

Table 9–10. The Yale observation scale.

Observation Item	Normal	Moderate Impairment	Severe Impairment
Quality of cry	Strong cry and normal tone OR content and not crying	Whimpering OR sobbing	Weak OR moaning OR high-pitched
Reaction to parent stimulation	Cries briefly then stops OR content and not crying	Cries off and on	Continual cry OR hardly responds
State variation	If awake → stays awake OR is asleep and stimulated → wakes up quickly	Eyes close briefly → awake OR awakes with prolonged stimulation	Falls to sleep OR will not rouse
Color	Pink	Pale extremities OR acrocyanosis	Pale OR cyanotic OR mottled OR ashen
Hydration	Skin normal, eyes normal, AND mucous membranes moist	Skin normal, eyes normal, AND mouth slightly dry	Skin doughy OR tented AND dry mucous membranes AND/OR sunken eyes
Response (talk, smile), anxiety to social overtures	Smiles OR alerts (≤ 2 mo)	Brief smile OR alerts briefly (≤ 2 mo)	No smile, face dull, expressionless OR no alerting (≤ 2 mo)

that may be undetected or untreated. For example, undetected or inadequately treated meningitis can result in permanent disability, including hearing loss and seizure disorder, or death. Undetected bacteremia can go on to cause septic shock and multisystem organ failure. Likewise, undetected UTIs can lead to renal scarring. Various protocols have been designed to assess risk. Of these, one of the most widely accepted is the Rochester Criteria, which combines the findings of history, physical examination, and laboratory evaluation (Table 9–11).

Table 9–11. The Rochester Criteria (modified).[1,2]

Goal	Defines febrile infant at low risk of serious bacterial infection if following criteria are met
History	
Previously healthy	Term infant, normal perinatal course, no antibiotics, no medical conditions, no hospitalizations
Physical examination	
Well appearing	
No focal bacterial infections	
Laboratory	
White blood cell count (WBC)	5000–15,000 cells/mm³
Band count (immature neutrophils)	< 1500 cells/mm³
Urinalysis	Normal (≤ 10 WBC/high-power field on spun urine sediment)
Stool WBC (if diarrhea is present)	< 5 WBC/high-power field

[1]Reproduced, with permission, from McCarthy PL et al: Observation scales to identify serious illness in febrile children. Pediatrics 1982;70:802.
[2]Examination of the stool was not a part of the initial Rochester Criteria.

Is Treatment Necessary? Once the initial evaluation has been completed, the next decision involves whether specific treatment is necessary. If antibiotics are to be administered empirically, the specific drug and route (oral, parenteral) must be determined, as well as whether the patient should be hospitalized or seen in the outpatient clinic.

Although the above outline may seem simple in theory, its application in the management of febrile infants and children continues to be controversial. Much of this is related to the difficulty in distinguishing children with benign, self-limited infections from those with occult, serious infections. In addition to the overlap in signs and symptoms of benign and serious illness, it is often difficult to judge the toxicity of infants and very young children. Younger infants have fewer social cues to assess (eg, smile), and the only signs of illness early in the course of a serious disease may be nonspecific (eg, fever and irritability). Finally, even the use of screening laboratory tests will not entirely eliminate risk of serious infection.

Recently, practice guidelines were published on the management of febrile illness in children. These guidelines were developed by an expert panel to outline a reasonable approach to this common clinical problem (Figure 9–1). Similar guidelines are currently being developed by the American Academy of Pediatrics.

SPECIAL CONSIDERATIONS

The Febrile Infant Younger Than 3 Months

The management of younger infants is complicated by the following limitations:

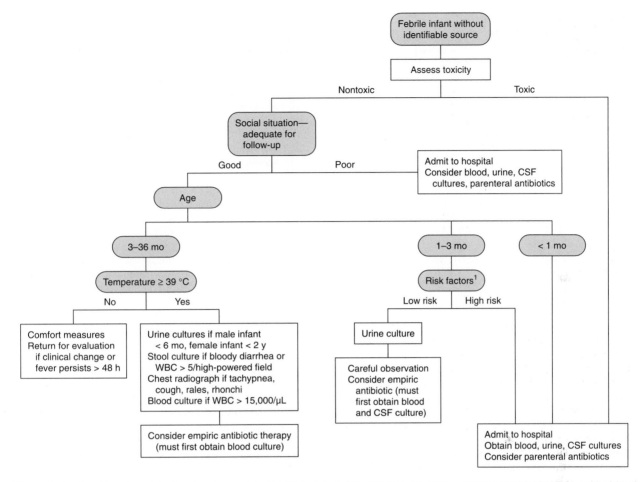

Figure 9–1. Algorithm demonstrating the approach to the febrile infant. [1]See Table 9–10. CSF = cerebrospinal fluid; WBC = white blood cell count. (Reproduced, with permission, from Baraff LJ et al: Practice guidelines for the management of infants and children 0 to 36 months of age with fever without source. Agency for Health Care Policy and Research. Ann Emerg Med 1993;22:1198.)

1. medical history provided by caretaker or parents without direct complaints from the patient
2. a more difficult examination because of limited cooperation and fewer signs for assessment
3. decreased or delayed host response because of the relative immaturity of the young infant's immune system
4. possibly higher risk of serious bacterial infections associated with febrile episodes.

On the basis of these limitations, it had been routinely recommended that all febrile infants younger than 3 months have the "rule-out sepsis" evaluation, including blood, urine, and CSF cultures and chest radiograph. These infants were admitted to the hospital and given empiric parenteral antibiotics until the results of the cultures were known. Because of costs, inconvenience, and nosocomial complications incurred during hospitalization, the management of the young, febrile infant has been readdressed (see below for treatment). With current manage-

ment guidelines, the opportunity for more choices in decision-making can be made on the basis of the clinician's assessment of the severity of illness.

Does the Young Infant Appear Toxic? At times, the only manifestation of serious illness in a young infant is increased irritability along with fever. Physicians use the accumulation of subtle and semi-objective signs as suggested by the Yale Observation Scale to assess toxicity and the need for further diagnostic evaluation. Unfortunately, the Yale Observation Scale may not be as sensitive in detecting ill infants in this age group as it is in older infants and children.

Is There a Source for the Fever on Physical Examination? A careful physical examination must be performed, with special attention to clues that may point to the source of fever. Tachypnea may signal a pneumonia that cannot be detected by auscultation. Decreased movement of an extremity may be an indication of an osteomyelitis or septic arthritis. A bulging fontanelle and nuchal rigidity are excellent indicators of CNS infection; however, the absence of these signs does not exclude the possibility of meningitis.

Are Laboratory Tests Indicated? The infant who has fever without localizing signs can have occult infection in the blood, urine, CSF, or lungs. A complete blood count (CBC) with white blood count (WBC) and differential, along with a blood culture, can be obtained simultaneously. Urine and CSF specimens can be examined for presence of white blood cells and bacteria, and samples of both can be sent for culture (Table 9–12). A chest radiograph can confirm the suspicion of pneumonia.

What Is the Risk? The incidence of serious bacterial infection in infants younger than 3 months has been estimated to be between 3 and 10%. In one study of "low-risk" infants aged 2–3 months with febrile episodes, 5.4% had a serious bacterial infection with roughly even distribution of bacteremia, UTIs, and bacterial gastroenteritis. This risk is significantly increased in toxic-appearing infants to more than 10%. The Rochester Criteria protocol has been used successfully to assign infants to high and low-risk categories.

Is Treatment Necessary? Any toxic-appearing infant or child should undergo a full evaluation for sepsis and meningitis and be hospitalized for treatment. Most clinicians suggest that infants younger than 1 month should be hospitalized and treated with parenteral antibiotics pending initial laboratory and culture results. Recently, there has been growing support for outpatient management of infants aged 1–3 months who meet low-risk criteria. Ceftriaxone, a third-generation cephalosporin, has been studied in the outpatient setting because of its activity against the common bacterial agents (including *S pneumoniae, N meningitides,* and *H influenzae*) seen in infancy, good penetration into the CSF, and longer half-life that enables once-daily dosing. If this management plan is selected, blood and CSF cultures should be obtained first to avoid possible future confusion in distinguishing a viral infection from a partially treated bacterial infection. In selecting outpatient management, close outpatient follow-up by the primary health care provider must be ensured. In addition to determining the patient's condition, it is important to assess factors that may impede compliance with follow-up (eg, access to health care, transportation, ability to be contacted by phone, and ability of the family to detect changes in the infant's medical condition).

Table 9–12. Initial laboratory investigations for possible sepsis.

Complete blood count, white blood cell count
Urinalysis
Blood culture
Urine culture
Cerebrospinal fluid (CSF) studies: cell count, glucose, total protein
CSF culture
Chest radiograph

Approach to the Older Febrile Infant (3–36 Months)

Febrile illnesses due to viral infections occur frequently in this age group, and temperatures as high as 39–40 °C may be encountered commonly. A series of questions should be asked after fever is documented.

Does the Child Appear Toxic? Any severely ill child with signs and symptoms of meningitis or cardiovascular instability suggestive of septic shock should be admitted to the hospital. Nontoxic-appearing children aged 3–36 months may be considered for outpatient management.

Is There a Source for the Fever on Physical Examination? The concept of occult bacteremia refers to infants and children who are well-appearing and have no source of fever detected by history or physical examination, but whose blood culture taken at the time of initial presentation subsequently grew bacteria. The most common reported pathogen is *S pneumoniae,* followed by HIB and *N meningitidis.* With the recent introduction of HIB vaccine, disease due to this organism is waning.

Are Laboratory Tests Indicated? If no source is identified after initial history and physical examination, the clinician must consider the role of further diagnostic testing. Blood, urine, and CSF are potential occult sites of infection along with pneumonia and osteomyelitis. Many experts have recommended further testing in children whose temperature is 39 °C or higher. In addition to blood cultures, urine cultures should be obtained in boys younger than 6 months and in girls younger than 2 years. Stool cultures and chest radiographs should be performed if there are any signs or symptoms suggesting a bacterial gastroenteritis or pneumonia.

What Is the Risk? The incidence of infections with bacteremia in this age group is similar to the incidence of serious bacterial infections in the younger infants, between 3 and 11%. Data suggest that this risk increases with increasing fever ($\geq$ 39 °C) and with elevated WBCs (> 15,000/mm^3). Unrecognized and untreated bacteremia is associated with a risk of developing otitis media, meningitis (7–9%), arthritis, pericarditis, and epiglottitis.

Is Treatment Necessary? The empiric antibiotic treatment of febrile children without an identifiable source remains controversial. Some discourage the use of antibiotics when there is no discernible focus of infection because of cost, potential for allergic reaction, and contribution to increasing bacterial antibiotic resistance. Others believe that empiric use of antibiotics can prevent serious infectious complications.

In patients who are subsequently found to have bacteremia, follow-up and clinical reassessment are essential. The child with *S pneumoniae* bacteremia, the most commonly isolated pathogen, who is well-appearing can be managed as an outpatient with antibiotic treatment and continued close follow-up. The child who is ill appearing or persistently febrile on reevaluation, or in whom *H influenzae* or *N meningitidis* is isolated from the blood, should be hospitalized for parenteral antibiotics.

As described in this section, the management of febrile infants and children provides a frequent and continuing challenge to clinicians. Of utmost importance is the individualized care of each patient. Guidelines can be extremely useful in outlining general principles and in providing expert opinion, which must then be tailored to a specific clinical situation. Finally, diagnostic investigations and therapy should not supplant the importance of follow-up (either in inpatient or outpatient setting) and support for family members, including education; all these elements are essential in the care of these patients.

FEVER OF UNKNOWN ORIGIN

In the broad sense, **fever of unknown** (unspecified, undetermined) **origin** could include fevers occurring for any duration of time. Traditionally, however, the clinical condition described by FUO applies to illnesses of a longer duration in which initial diagnostic evaluation has been unrevealing. It is the prolonged nature of the fever that differentiates FUO from the preceding discussion of fever without localizing signs.

In 1961, Petersdorf and Beeson published the classic paper detailing the results of evaluation of 100 adults with FUO. The authors defined a FUO as (1) an "illness of more than 3 weeks duration," (2) "fever higher than 100 °F on several occasions," and (3) "diagnosis uncertain after 1 week in hospital." In this study, infections, neoplasms, and collagen disorders made up, respectively, 36%, 19%, and 15% of diagnoses. Of additional significance was a reported mortality rate of 32%.

In the 35 years since this report, a number of studies have been published on FUO in the pediatric population. Data from seven of these pediatric case series, consisting of a total of 786 patients, are summarized in Table 9–13. The exact duration of fever, height of fever, and extent of diagnostic testing necessary to result in a diagnosis of FUO have varied from study to study.

In contrast to adult studies of FUO, most cases in children represent atypical presentations of common diseases. Infectious diseases account for more than half (52.3%) the cases, followed by collagen-vascular and inflammatory causes (11.5%). Malignancy represented only 5.0% of pediatric cases. Overall, 21.8% of cases remained undiagnosed. In one report, 67% of cases were undiagnosed. Of interest, HIV infection was reported in just one instance, but most of these studies predated clinical and serologic diagnosis of HIV.

Approach to the Child With Prolonged Fever

An approach similar to that for acute febrile illnesses can be used in the evaluation of children with prolonged fever.

Is Fever Present? The diagnostic evaluation of pro-

Table 9–13. Final diagnosis in children with fever of unknown origin.[1]

Diagnoses	No.	%
Total	786	100
Infection	411	52.3
Respiratory infections	114	14.5
Urinary tract infections	31	3.9
Bacterial meningitis	14	1.8
Tuberculosis[2]	15	1.9
Collagen-vascular/inflammatory	90	11.5
Juvenile rheumatoid arthritis	40	5.1
Systemic lupus erythematosus	11	1.4
Crohn disease	12	1.5
Malignancy	39	5.0
Leukemia	19	2.4
Lymphoma	8	1.0
Undiagnosed	171	21.8

[1]A composite summary based on published literature on fever of unknown origin, including Gartner 1992, Steele 1991, Feigin & Shearer 1976.
[2]Incudes pulmonary, meningitis, disseminated, and site unspecified.

longed fever begins with a documentation of fever and fever patterns. The degree of temperature that defines fever has been addressed above. The description of the fever should include the duration, timing (continuous or intermittent, day or night, daily or weekly), and height. Fevers can be continuous or sustained, intermittent or spiking, or relapsing. In some conditions, temperature may return to normal or even subnormal levels between fever spikes.

Although the determination and interpretation of fevers are important in the first step of the evaluation, limitations exist. The documentation of fever has become more difficult, as the evaluation of many of these patients has moved from inpatient to outpatient settings. Optimally, multiple daily temperature measurements should be recorded by an objective, trained individual. Parental reports may be complicated by intentional (eg, factitious fever, Münchausen syndrome by proxy) or unintentional (eg, misunderstanding of normal temperature) errors. In addition, it is not clear that the pattern of fever or response to antipyretics can be correlated with the severity of illness or ultimate diagnosis in a significant number of patients.

In addition to a description of the fever, a thorough history is the cornerstone of the evaluation of FUO. It should detail travel and exposure history. Examples of how historical factors may lead to specific diagnoses are listed in Table 9–14. Travel history should include all previous travel experiences (recent and distant past, domestic and foreign). Exposures include ill contacts, animals (domestic and wild), pica, water or food sources, medication, family history, and ethnicity.

Does the Child Appear Toxic? Does the patient appear acutely or chronically ill? A toxic-appearing patient requires immediate, thorough evaluation in the hospital setting. Patients who are otherwise well appearing are candidates for initial outpatient evaluation.

Table 9–14. Historical considerations in diagnosis of fever of unknown origin.

History	Diagnoses	Test
Medications	Drug fever	Stop medication
Animal exposure (wild and domestic)		
Rodent	Tularemia	Serology, culture
Rodent	Rat-bite fever	Serology, culture
Many species	Leptospirosis	Serology, culture
Dog	Visceral larva migrans	Stool for parasites: *Toxocara canis*
Travel history (endemic area)		
Foreign travel	Malaria	Thick blood smear examination
Southwestern United States	Coccidioidomycosis	Serology, culture
Central river valleys, United States	Histoplasmosis	Serology, culture, stains
Mississippi and Ohio river basins	Blastomycosis	Serology, culture, stains
Family history	Familial Mediterranean fever	Clinical diagnosis

Is There a Source for the Fever on Physical Examination? By definition, preliminary examination has failed to identify a source for fever. However, it is essential that careful physical examinations be repeated to observe for subtle or fleeting signs that can help lead to a specific diagnosis. Table 9–15 lists some of these physical examination findings.

Which Laboratory Tests Are Indicated? Usually, several screening laboratory tests already have been performed as part of the initial diagnostic evaluation. Typically, these have included a CBC and markers of inflammation (eg, ESR or C-reactive protein). The CBC can demonstrate abnormalities (increases or decreases) in white blood cell, red blood cell, or platelet count. A low hemoglobin concentration may reflect anemia of chronic disease or nutritional deficiencies. A decrease in multiple hematopoietic cell lines (anemia, leukopenia, and thrombocytopenia) may indicate primary marrow failure or a malignant neoplasm that is invading the bone marrow space. An elevation in ESR or C-reactive protein can suggest an ongoing inflammatory process, such as infection, collage vascular disease, or occult malignancy.

The clinical laboratory provides a large variety of tests that can be used to identify or exclude specific diseases. However, because of the wide range of conditions associated with fever, it is impractical to order tests to exclude

Table 9–15. Physical examination considerations in diagnosis of fever of unknown origin.

Physical Examination	Diseases	Diagnostic Studies
Ocular		
Conjunctivitis	Kawasaki disease	Clinical diagnosis
	Tularemia (oculoglandular type)	Serology, culture
	Leptospirosis	Serology, culture
	Histoplasmosis	Serology, culture
	Cat-scratch fever	Skin test, special stain, serology
	SLE	Clinical diagnosis, serology (ANA)
Fundoscopic	Toxoplasmosis, cytomegalovirus (congenital infections)	Chorioretinitis
Roth spots	Bacterial endocarditis	Blood culture, echocardiogram
Uveitis	Autoimmune disorders	Slit lamp
Hepatomegaly	Visceral larva migrans (toxocariasis)	Clinical diagnosis, histology, ELISA
	Hepatitis	Serology
Jaundice	Hepatitis	Serology
	Leptospirosis	Serology, culture
Lymphadenopathy	Cat-scratch	Skin test, serology
	Tularemia	Serology, culture
	Kawasaki	Clinical diagnosis
Arthritis	Autoimmune	Clinical diagnosis, serology (ANA)
	Septic arthritis	Culture
Bone pain or tenderness	Osteomyelitis	Culture
	Leukemia	Complete blood count, bone marrow aspiration
Skin		
Erythematous maculopapular rash	Kawasaki disease	Clinical diagnosis
Salmon-colored rash	Autoimmune (JRA, SLE)	Clinical diagnosis, serology (ANA)
Osler, Janeway lesions	Bacterial endocarditis	Blood culture, echocardiogram

ANA = antinuclear antibody; ELISA = enzyme-linked immunosorbent assay; JRA = juvenile rheumatoid arthritis; SLE = systemic lupus erythematosus.

all possibilities. Further diagnostic evaluations should be directed by clues obtained by history and physical examination and exclusion of the most common or most urgent causes of FUO (Table 9–16). Bacteremia, UTIs, and meningitis can be detected through appropriate analysis, culture, or both, as previously discussed. Skin testing with PPD can be performed for tuberculosis. A wide range of serologic tests are available. Elevations in antinuclear antibody (ANA) can support the diagnosis of systemic lupus erythematosus (SLE). Serologic titers can be obtained for EBV, tularemia, brucellosis, toxoplasmosis, salmonellosis, and Lyme disease, to name a few. Consultation with infectious disease, hematology-oncology, and/or rheumatology specialists can be useful in directing further workup.

Radiologic examinations are frequently part of the evaluation of patients with FUO. In particular, chest and sinus radiographs are important because of the frequency with which respiratory infections are a cause of pediatric FUO. Although more sophisticated imaging studies (eg, ultrasonography, computed tomography (CT) scans, magnetic resonance imaging (MRI), and nuclear medicine scans) are widely available, their usefulness as routine screening procedures for FUO is less certain. More invasive procedures, such as biopsies (eg, bone marrow, skin, lymph node, liver) and exploratory laparotomy, may be indicated in certain settings if patients remain febrile and sick.

What Is the Risk? Children with FUO are less likely than adults to have a life-threatening illness. Most children with FUO represent atypical presentations of common diseases. Infectious diseases and collagen-vascular and inflammatory diseases are the two most commonly identified classifications of disease. The risk of adverse outcomes varies from diagnosis to diagnosis. The mortality rate reported in two studies was 9–18%.

Is Treatment Necessary? Treatment must be disease directed. Because numerous infectious and noninfectious causes can produce prolonged fever, thorough investigation must precede attempts at empiric therapy. Empiric therapy with broad spectrum antibiotics can potentially

Table 9–16. Laboratory considerations in diagnosis of fever of unknown origin.

Screening laboratory
    Complete blood count
    Erythrocyte sedimentation rate or C-reactive protein
    Urinalysis and urine culture
    Blood culture
    Cerebrospinal fluid analysis and culture[1]
    Tuberculosis skin test
Serology
    Antinuclear antibodies
    Lyme titers
    Febrile agglutinins
Radiology
    Chest radiograph, sinus radiograph
    Others: ultrasonography, computed tomographic scan, magnetic resonance imaging, nuclear scan[1]

[1]When indicated.

mask infections and delay the diagnosis of meningitis, osteomyelitis, and endocarditis. When a diagnosis cannot be made, close follow-up and serial examinations and reevaluations are essential. In a significant number of cases, the etiology of FUO cannot be determined, and the fever resolves spontaneously without obvious sequelae.

Approach to the Child With Intermittent Fever

Children attending schools or day-care centers are exposed to a large number of community acquired infections. Most of these episodes are typically a series of unrelated, self-limited viral infections. A series of fever episodes may present as intermittent fever with irregular or regular patterns lasting several days to several weeks. Among the many causes of intermittent fever are the more common infections, including recurrent viral infections (eg, different serotypes of enterovirus causing aphthous stomatitis), viral and bacterial gastroenteritis, infections associated with lymphadenitis, recurrent URT infection caused by viruses, and recurrent otitis media. These benign infections must be differentiated from more ominous pathogens. Additional differential diagnoses of intermittent fever include malaria, relapsing fever, rat bite fevers, and cyclic neutropenia.

Brucellosis is caused by the non–spore-forming, gram-negative coccobacilli species, *Brucella.* In children, brucellosis frequently is a mild, self-limited disease, especially if caused by *Brucella abortus.* However, the infection can be severe with *Brucella melitensis,* commonly associated with nonpasteurized goat dairy products. The onset of disease may be insidious or acute, with fever, chills, weakness, malaise, weight loss, anorexia, arthralgia, and myalgia. In more severe cases, patients may present with abdominal pain, hepatomegaly, or splenomegaly. Rare complications include endocarditis, meningoencephalitis, pneumonia, and osteomyelitis. Diagnosis is determined by blood or bone-marrow culture, as well as by specific serologic tests. With appropriate treatment with tetracycline or trimethoprim-sulfa, patients usually recover without serious complications.

Malaria is one of the most common infectious diseases worldwide, although it is rare in the United States except in travelers returning from endemic areas. (See section on Tropical Diseases.) Infections with *Plasmodium* species are mosquito-borne, most commonly caused by *P falciparum, P vivax, P ovale,* and *Plasmodium malariae.* The infections are characterized by recurrent episodes of high fever, rigors, headache, and abdominal pain. The diagnosis of malaria should be suspected in patients with an appropriate history of travel and noncompliance with prophylaxis. The diagnosis is confirmed by visualizing parasites in a thick smear of blood. The drug of choice depends on the species and the pattern of drug resistance in different endemic areas. Medications used include chloroquine phosphate, quinidine gluconate, pyrimethamine-sulfadoxine, and primaquine.

Relapsing fever refers to an infection caused by *Borre-*

lia recurrentis. The microbe is transmitted to man by ticks (*Ornithodoros* species) or the body louse (*Pediculus humanus*). For tick-borne fever, rodents are the main reservoir in the western United States. Relapsing fever is characterized by sudden onset of high fever, photophobia, myalgia, arthralgias, headache, and gastrointestinal disorders, including hematemesis and pain. Maculopapular or petechial rash develops in 25% of patients. Diagnosis is confirmed by serologic tests. Management includes supportive therapy and the use of chloramphenicol, erythromycin, or tetracycline.

Other causes of rodent-transmitted diseases include streptobacillary (Haverhill fever) and spirillary (Sodoku) rat-bite fever. The former is caused by an aerobic gram-negative bacillus (*Streptobacillus moniliformis*), whereas the latter is caused by a spirochete (*Spirillum minor*). Both diseases are transmitted directly by the saliva of an infested animal and are usually inoculated to humans by a rat bite. The clinical presentation is associated with onset of fever, rigors, myalgia, arthralgia, and rash. Sodoku is typically associated with lymphadenitis and lymphangitis in contrast to Haverhill fever. Diagnosis can be confirmed by blood culture of the gram-negative bacterium or by dark field examination of spirochetes. Penicillin is the drug of choice for both organisms. In some cases of *Streptobacillus* infection, streptomycin may be needed to treat penicillin resistance.

Cyclic neutropenia, a rare disorder, is commonly associated with recurrent, regular fever episodes. The diagnosis is made by documentation of neutropenia during febrile episodes and normal neutrophil counts between febrile episodes. Granulocyte growth factors, including G-CSF and GM-CSF, may be used in the management of this syndrome.

EYE, MOUTH, & NECK INFECTIONS

EYE INFECTIONS

Eye swelling can be a manifestation of a variety of different clinical conditions in the pediatric age group. The loose connective tissue of the eyelid predisposes this area to swelling in response to a variety of disease states. When the swelling and redness is of acute onset, the principal diagnoses include allergic reactions, trauma, insect bites, and infection.

History and initial physical examination may support some of these diagnoses. A history of allergy (eg, allergic rhinitis) or injury can be important. Physical examination may reveal an insect bite mark in the center of swelling or signs of atopic disease (eg, allergic shiners, infraorbital folds or "Dennie lines," horizontal nasal crease). Even when other causes are suspected, it is always important to consider the possibility of periorbital and orbital infection. In some cases, an insect bite or trauma may be the precipitating event in periorbital cellulitis.

PERIORBITAL & ORBITAL CELLULITIS

Pathogenesis

The orbit is a bony cavity surrounded by the paranasal sinuses: medially by the ethmoid sinus, inferiorly by the maxillary sinus, and superiorly (in older children) by the frontal sinus. In some areas, only a very thin bony wall separates the adjoining spaces, eg, the lamina papyracea separating the ethmoid sinus and orbit. These close anatomic relationships are a factor in the development of many of these infections, especially orbital sinusitis. Thus, the area around the eye can be divided into two clinically important areas by a coronal fascial plane that runs from the bony orbital rim to the tarsal plate of the eyelid. The periorbital and orbital spaces are separated by the fibrous orbital septum, which serves as a barrier to edema and infection. Infections anterior to the orbital septum are classified as periorbital or preseptal cellulitis.

Several routes of entry have been hypothesized for periorbital and orbital infections:

1. direct inoculation (eg, trauma)
2. extension of infection from an adjacent site (eg, sinusitis, conjunctivitis, hordeolum)
3. deposition of organisms during bacteremia.

Etiology

The most frequently reported bacterial isolates in periorbital and orbital infections are HIB, *S aureus, S epidermidis,* and *Streptococcus* species (eg, *S pneumoniae*). In the past, *H influenzae* has represented half of all isolates in periorbital cellulitis. Many of these infections are presumed to have resulted from the hematogenous spread of *H influenzae.* In contrast, cases of periorbital cellulitis secondary to insect bites or trauma are more commonly caused by *S aureus* and *Streptococcus* species.

On the basis of the anatomic proximity to the sinuses, the bacteria responsible for orbital cellulitis are the same as those responsible for acute sinusitis. A relatively even distribution between *H influenzae, S aureus,* and *Streptococcus* species has been reported. Anaerobic and mixed infections may play a more frequent role in orbital, than in periorbital, infections.

Clinical Manifestations

Periorbital erythema and edema are the presenting signs in both periorbital (preseptal) and orbital cellulitis. Most patients with either periorbital or orbital infection present with fever. Table 9–17 compares some of the features of periorbital and orbital cellulitis.

Table 9–17. Comparison of periorbital and orbital cellulitis.

	Periorbital Cellulitis	Orbital Cellulitis
History		
Incidence	More common	Less common
Age	Toddler to preschool-age	School-age
Physical examination		
Fever	Usually present	Usually present
Periorbital swelling and redness	Present	Present
Chemosis	Present	Present
Conjunctival infection	Present	Present
Proptosis	Absent	Present[1]
Ophthalmoplegia	Absent	Present[1]
Visual acuity	Normal	Normal or impaired[1]
Pathogenetic mechanism		
Sinusitis	Common	Common
Trauma/skin infections	Common	Uncommon

[1]Features distinguishing orbital involvement.

Diagnosis

When evaluating the patient with the red and swollen eye, one of the primary efforts is to exclude the possibility of periorbital and orbital infection. A history of viral URI, trauma, insect bites, and allergies should be elicited. Evidence for sinusitis and dental infection should be identified on examination. Physical examination can be especially useful in distinguishing periorbital and orbital infection (see Table 9–17). Proptosis, ophthalmoplegia, and decreased visual acuity are hallmarks of orbital infection. These findings are absent in periorbital infection.

When the results of history and physical examination are equivocal, or whenever suspicion of orbital infection exists, radiologic imaging is indicated. Imaging of the orbits can be performed with CT scan or MRI. Both techniques can reveal the presence of an abscess and thickening of the extraocular muscles consisting with orbital involvement.

Other laboratory tests are of limited benefit. WBC and ESR, which are nonspecific, may be elevated. Positive blood cultures, primarily *H influenzae* and *S pneumoniae,* have been reported in roughly one fourth of patients. CSF analysis is more likely to be positive in disease caused by *H influenzae.*

Treatment & Complications

Treatment of both periorbital and orbital cellulitis consists of antibiotics aimed at the most common organisms. Traditionally, all patients who are toxic appearing or have evidence of orbital involvement are hospitalized. Outpatient therapy for periorbital cellulitis is possible for selected patients, eg, those with mild infections whose compliance with medications and close follow-up can be ensured. Antibiotic regimens may include an antistaphylococcal penicillin (eg, nafcillin) and an aminoglycoside or

third-generation cephalosporin. Surgery is indicated for abscess formation, sinus drainage, or lack of clinical response. Prevention of a significant number of these infections is now possible through the use of the HIB conjugate vaccines.

The most frequent complications of periorbital cellulitis are meningitis and lid abscess. Orbital cellulitis, although rare, can be complicated by periosteal abscess, meningitis, and cavernous sinus thrombosis.

SORE MOUTH OR THROAT

A large variety of infectious agents can produce inflammation in and around the oropharynx. In older children, this inflammation results in complaints of sore throat or dysphagia. In younger children, irritability, increased drooling, or decreased appetite may be the only symptoms of sore throat.

Sore throat due to the common respiratory viruses (eg, rhinovirus, coronavirus) can result in fever, rhinorrhea, and cough. Other infectious agents can produce relatively distinctive skin (exanthem) and mucous membrane (enanthem) eruptions. Examples include adenoviruses (pharyngoconjunctival fever), coxsackievirus (hand, foot, and mouth disease), and HSV (gingivostomatitis).

It has been reported that pharyngitis brings almost 1% of the population to a physician each year, making it one of the most common infectious diseases encountered in the office setting.

STOMATITIS & GINGIVOSTOMATITIS

In young infants, *Candida albicans* can produce whitish plaques on the tongue, palate, and buccal mucosa. Infection of the oral cavity with *C albicans* is referred to as **oral candidiasis** or **thrush.** Gentle brushing of the involved areas with a tongue blade can be used to distinguish between thrush and residual milk particles. Thrush will be more adherent to the underlying mucosa, and removal of the whitish plaques will reveal inflamed mucosal surfaces. Laboratory tests (wet mounts, Gram stains, and culture) are not usually necessary to make the diagnosis. Infection typically responds to the application of a topical antifungal agent (eg, nystatin).

In infants and young children, infection with coxsackievirus or HSV (primarily HSV-1) can produce vesicular oral lesions. These conditions may be classified as stomatitis, gingivitis, or gingivostomatitis depending on the site(s) of involvement.

HSV typically results in a cluster of vesicles around the lips, gingiva (ie, gingivostomatitis), and the anterior portion of the tongue. Primary infections with HSV may range from asymptomatic to severe. Symptomatic cases are associated with fever, irritability, dysphagia, and cervical lymphadenopathy. The vesicles eventually break and form ulcers. The diagnosis is usually a clinical one, although Tzanck smears (multinucleated giant cells and intranuclear inclusions) and viral cultures can be used to confirm the diagnosis. Treatment is aimed at pain relief (eg, acetaminophen or topical preparations using viscous lidocaine as analgesics) and prevention of dehydration. Antiviral agents, such as acyclovir, may be useful in specialized settings (eg, immunodeficiency states or severe disease). Recurrences have been attributed to a variety of physiologic stresses (eg, sun, febrile illness, emotional duress).

The vesicles of coxsackievirus have been characteristically described in the posterior aspect of the mouth, including tonsils and soft palate. These infections are transmitted by fecal-oral route. When lesions are limited to the mouth, infection with coxsackievirus is referred to as **herpangina.** Some serotypes of coxsackievirus (eg, coxsackievirus A16) are associated with other cutaneous manifestations. Oral lesions in combination with similar vesicular lesions on the dorsal aspect of the hands and feet describe the clinical condition known as **hand, foot, and mouth disease.** In these cases, maculopapular lesions on the hands, feet, and buttocks often become vesicular. The progression from vesicles to ulcers is similar to that seen in HSV infection. The diagnosis of coxsackievirus infection is made on clinical grounds and additional laboratory tests are usually not indicated. The disease is often self-limited and requires only symptomatic treatment.

PHARYNGITIS & TONSILLITIS

Etiology

In children, the etiology of pharyngitis (tonsillopharyngitis) can be divided into viruses, bacteria, and idiopathic causes. The actual frequency of the various causes is influenced by the age of the patient and the time of year. The viruses responsible for pharyngitis include adenovirus, parainfluenza virus, enterovirus, influenza virus, HSV, and EBV. Rhinovirus and coronavirus may produce sore throat in conjunction with other upper respiratory symptoms. Of the bacterial agents, group A Streptococcus (GAS) is the most frequent isolate. Other bacteria responsible for pharyngitis are non–group A streptococci (groups C, F, and G), *Arcanobacterium haemolyticum,* and *Neisseria* species (*gonorrhoeae* and *meningitidis*). *Mycoplasma pneumoniae* and *Chlamydia pneumoniae* are among the less common causes of pharyngitis.

The frequency with which viruses are responsible for pharyngitis decreases outside of the preschool age group. School-aged children represent the group most frequently infected with GAS. Outbreaks of groups C, G, and F streptococci have been reported in adolescents (eg, college students).

Diagnosis

Despite the variety of agents known to cause pharyngitis, the traditional approach to pharyngitis (tonsillopharyn-gitis) focuses on distinguishing GAS infections from all other causes. The importance given to GAS infection relates primarily to its association with rheumatic fever and the recent resurgence of this syndrome. In approaching the diagnosis of GAS pharyngitis, the clinician begins with the history and physical examination. However, because many clinical findings lack specificity or sensitivity, the laboratory plays a central role in the diagnosis of GAS pharyngitis.

The history and physical examination focus on factors that increase or decrease the likelihood of GAS infection (Table 9–18). Classic manifestations of GAS tonsillopharyngitis include the acute onset of sore throat, dysphagia, fever, headache, nausea, vomiting, and abdominal pain. On physical examination, the throat and tonsils are erythematous and covered with exudate. Palatal petechiae, although infrequently present, are very suggestive of GAS infection. The anterior cervical nodes are typically swollen and tender. Unfortunately, the classic manifestations may be present only in a minority of patients with GAS infection.

Signs and symptoms that diminish the likelihood of GAS include viral URI symptoms, conjunctivitis, viral exanthems or enanthems, myalgias, and diarrhea. The absence of fever, lymphadenitis, or tonsillar exudate may also decrease the likelihood of GAS.

The clinical laboratory provides several methods of establishing the diagnosis of GAS pharyngitis. Culture, rapid antigen assays, and serologic tests are all widely available (Table 9–19). In the clinic, a single throat cul-

Table 9–18. Comparison of group A streptococcal (GAS) and viral pharyngitis.

	GAS Infection	Viral Infection
History		
Sore throat	Yes	Yes
Rhinorrhea	No	Yes
Cough	No	Yes
Hoarseness	No	Yes
Headache	Yes	Yes or no
Stridor	No	Yes or no
Conjunctivitis	No	Yes or no
Stomachache	Yes	Yes or no
Exposures to GAS	Yes	No
Physical examination		
Fever	Yes[1]	Yes or no
Tonsillar exudates	Yes	Yes
Tender cervical adenopathy	Yes	Yes or no
Palatal petechiae[1]	Yes	No
Scarlatiniform rash[1]	Yes	No
Laboratory		
White blood cell count	Yes[2]	No

[1]Probably has the greatest specificity for GAS infection. However, the low frequency of this finding makes it insensitive for diagnosing GAS.
[2]Risk of GAS infection may be higher with higher elevations of white blood cell count (especially ≥ 20,500) and neutrophil predominance.

Table 9–19. Diagnostic tests for group A streptococcal pharyngitis.[1]

	Sensitivity	Specificity	Time for Result	Advantage	Disadvantage
Culture	Good	Good	24–48 h	Early diagnosis	Role of carrier
Rapid antigen assay	Fair	Good	Minutes	Earliest diagnosis	Less sensitive, ? more recurrence with early treatment
ASO titers[2]	Good	Good	Weeks	? Gold standard	Too late for therapy to prevent rheumatic fever

[1]Many diagnostic algorithms use a combination of rapid antigen and culture (see Figure 9–1).
[2]Acute and convalescent sera.

ture is the gold standard for GAS pharyngitis. Modifications of the culture technique (eg, use of multiple cultures, culture of surgical specimens) or documentation of an increase in antistreptolysin O (ASO) antibody titer can increase the detection rate of GAS. However, these techniques are neither useful, practical, nor available in the usual clinic setting. Isolation of GAS by throat culture for GAS usually occurs within 24–48 hours. A useful adjunct to the culture has been the development of antigen detection techniques based on detection of group A streptococcal carbohydrate by specific antisera. Rapid antigen tests for GAS have a lower sensitivity but good specificity when compared with culture. Antigen studies are popular because of their ease of use and the availability of immediate results. A positive antigen test can allow immediate initiation of antibiotic therapy. When a negative test result is obtained, however, a standard culture should be performed because of the lower sensitivity of the antigen tests (Figure 9–2).

Treatment

The goals of treatment of GAS pharyngitis are as follows:

1. bacteriologic cure
2. prevention of nonsuppurative complications (eg, acute rheumatic fever)
3. prevention of suppurative complications
4. hastening of clinical recovery
5. reduction of transmission.

Bacteriologic cure is, for the most part, readily achieved with the administration of any number of antibiotics. Prevention of acute rheumatic fever was demonstrated in the 1950s through treatment of GAS pharyngitis with benzathine penicillin. The incidence of suppurative complications, such as peritonsillar abscess or systemic infection (eg, sepsis), is likely to be reduced with antibiotic therapy.

The duration of symptoms of pharyngitis is shortened by 1–2 days in patients who receive treatment. Since the early studies, penicillin has remained the treatment of choice for GAS pharyngitis (Figure 9–2). Alternative antibiotics, including other penicillins (eg, amoxicillin, ampicillin, amoxicillin plus clavulanate), cephalosporins, clindamycin, and erythromycin, have been demonstrated to achieve bacteriologic cures. Erythromycin is a standard

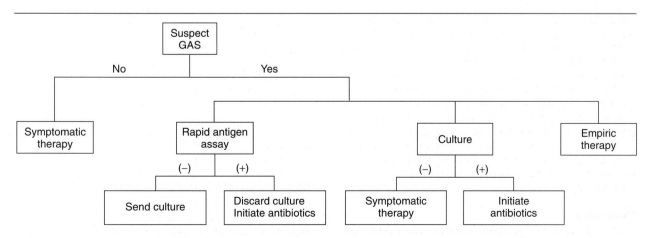

Figure 9–2. Management strategies in pharyngitis. GAS = group A *Streptococcus.*

recommendation for patients with penicillin allergy. The duration of antibiotic therapy is typically a 10-day course of oral antibiotics or a single dose of intramuscular benzathine penicillin G.

Symptomatic treatment involves the use of oral analgesic agents, such as acetaminophen, ibuprofen.

Treatment Failures & Carriers

Recurrent symptoms or repeated throat cultures positive for GAS can represent treatment failure, recurrent disease, or the GAS carrier state. **Antibiotic failure** is believed to occur in 10–30% of cases. Treatment failure can result from poor compliance (the most common cause), co-pathogens (other β-lactamase–producing bacteria in the oropharynx), antibiotic resistance or penicillin tolerance, and biologic properties of the bacteria. Penicillin tolerance exists when there is a large difference between the minimal inhibitory concentrations (MIC) and minimal bactericidal concentrations (MBC). Erythromycin-resistant GAS has been reported to represent 5% of cases in the United States and almost 50% in Finland and Japan in recent years.

Recurrent disease may represent up to half the "treatment failures." However, it is difficult to distinguish treatment failure from recurrent disease without knowledge of the serotypes of the organisms responsible for the initial and subsequent episodes. Recurrence may result from re-exposure and the high carrier rate. In addition, early treatment may suppress the development of protective antibodies, thus allowing reinfection.

The existence of the **GAS carrier state** has been known since 1947. GAS carriers are defined as individuals with positive throat culture results who demonstrate no increase in ASO titers. Carriers may be detected during episodes of pharyngitis from other causes (symptomatic) or during screening (asymptomatic). The symptomatic carrier cannot be differentiated from acute infection without the results of acute and convalescent titers. The carrier state is especially common in pediatric patients (an estimated 10–50% of school-aged children) and may last for weeks to months. The etiology of the carrier state is unknown, and neither host- nor organism-specific factors (eg, serotype) have been identified that predispose to this condition. After adequate treatment for the acute infection, no further antibiotic therapy is indicated for the chronic carrier state.

The management of treatment failures depends on the presumed cause. When compliance is a problem, a single intramuscular injection of benzathine penicillin is an effective choice. The therapy for compliant patients with recurrent or persistent disease, as well as for the GAS carrier state, is less easily defined. Usually, alternative antibiotics, such as erythromycin, amoxicillin-clavulanate, cephalosporins, or clindamycin, are used.

Complications

GAS pharyngitis can result in both suppurative and nonsuppurative complications. Suppurative complications include **peritonsillar abscess (or quinsy), retropharyngeal abscess, septicemia,** and **toxin-mediated shock.** Peritonsillar abscess is characterized by trismus, muffled voice, drooling, and asymmetric tonsillar enlargement with movement of the uvula away from the affected side. Retropharyngeal abscess usually extends anteriorly to form a bulge in the posterior pharynx that can be seen on physical examination or on lateral neck radiographs. It is usually associated with abrupt fever and severe dysphagia; in severe cases, the airway can become compromised, resulting in respiratory distress. Treatment involves antibiotic therapy and surgery. Sepsis and toxic-shock have been reported in association with the M serotype (types 1 and 3) of GAS.

Nonsuppurative complications include **acute rheumatic fever** and **acute post-streptococcal glomerulonephritis.** Acute rheumatic fever is the principal reason that so much time and effort is placed into identifying individuals with GAS pharyngitis. The incidence of rheumatic fever has been shown to be significantly diminished by antibiotic therapy for GAS pharyngitis. Acute rheumatic fever is associated with M types 3 and 18 serotypes. Unlike acute rheumatic fever, the incidence of glomerulonephritis does not appear to be reduced by treatment of GAS pharyngitis. Acute glomerulonephritis is associated with the M type 12 serotype. For additional discussion, Chapters 8 and 16.

PAROTITIS

Parotitis is an inflammation of the parotid salivary glands and must be distinguished from anterior cervical lymphadenopathy. On physical examination, parotid swelling is usually identifiable by location as a swelling centered above or at the angle of the jaw, often displacing the lobe of the ear. The two main causes are viral parotitis (eg, mumps) and acute suppurative parotitis.

Mumps is caused by a paramyxovirus. Viral parotitis can also be caused by coxsackievirus group A, EBV, influenza A, lymphocytic-choriomeningitis, parainfluenza virus, and, in the case of the immunocompromised patient, CMV. With mumps, the incubation is about 2–3 weeks after exposure. The child presents with pain and swelling of one or both parotid glands, which may develop within a few hours. The affected parotids usually are tender to palpation, and the child experiences pain on tasting sour substances. On examination, the Stensen duct is erythematous, and tonsils may be displaced medially from ipsilateral swelling of the affected salivary glands. The submandibular glands may also be involved, resulting in erythema of the Wharton duct. A mild to moderate fever may be present. The swelling resolves gradually over the next week. Complications of mumps include meningoencephalitis, pancreatitis, oophoritis, and orchitis and epididymitis (in up to one third of adolescent and adult males). Treatment is symptomatic. Analgesics may be helpful, and diet should be adjusted to accommodate the patient's ability to chew. The worldwide vaccination program, in which a live attenuated mumps virus is used, has markedly decreased the incidence of this disease.

Although considered in the differential diagnosis of parotid swelling, **acute suppurative parotitis** is a far less common condition in children. Predisposing factors are conditions that decrease salivary flow, such as dehydration, sialolithiasis, and certain medications. Bacterial seeding usually takes place from bacteremia or a local infection in the oral cavity. The most common organism is *S aureus.* Other common agents include *Streptococcus pyogenes* and α-hemolytic streptococci. Patients with the infection are often toxic and febrile. The swelling is unilateral and very tender. The opening of the Stensen duct is inflamed, and pus can be expressed from the duct on gentle palpation. Complications include rupture of the parotid with local spread of infection to the face, ear, or temporomandibular joint and development of osteomyelitis of the mandible. If pus can be expressed from the duct, Gram-stain results may be useful to direct initial therapy. In the absence of pus, needle aspiration of the gland may be necessary for cultures. Cultures should be sent for aerobes, anaerobes, fungi, and mycobacteria. Laboratory evaluation may show an increased ESR, WBC, and serum amylase level. Therapy consists of parenteral antimicrobial agents, and the initial empiric therapy should include coverage of *S aureus,* streptococcal species, and anaerobes. Surgical drainage is sometimes required.

ENLARGED LYMPH NODES

"Bumps in the neck," or enlarged cervical lymph nodes, are common complaints bringing children and adolescents to the pediatrician. Fortunately, most of these are self-limited or easily treatable. It is the task of the physician to determine which of these lymph nodes points to a more serious etiology and requires further, frequently invasive, evaluation.

To evaluate abnormal lymph nodes, consideration must be given first to normal lymph nodes in children. Compared with adults, children have larger, more easily palpable lymph nodes. Furthermore, children's lymph nodes typically mount a more exaggerated response to infection and other inflammatory stimuli. Normally palpated lymph nodes occur in cervical, inguinal, and occasionally axillary regions and usually are less than 1–2 cm in diameter. Lymph nodes found in the occipital, pre- or post-auricular, supraclavicular, epitrochlear, and popliteal areas usually are abnormal and indicate some intrinsic or adjacent inflammatory process. Furthermore, lymph nodes larger than 2 cm usually represent a pathologic process.

When evaluating a patient with lymphadenopathy, it is important to consider whether the lymph node is isolated or part of generalized lymphadenopathy. Generalized lymphadenopathy, enlarged lymph nodes in multiple loca-

tions, is usually a response to a systemic process involving the reticuloendothelial system and may be associated with liver and spleen enlargement. An enlargement of an isolated lymph node is frequently a local response to a nearby infection or an infiltrative process, such as *M tuberculosis* or lymphoma.

A detailed and complete medical and social history is essential in the initial workup of a child presenting with enlarged lymph nodes (Table 9–20). A review of systems should focus on overall health, fever, night sweats, weight loss, upper respiratory symptoms, cough, sore throat, rashes, and bone pain. Important historical facts can help direct the workup and diagnosis in cases of lymphadenopathy caused by *M tuberculosis, B melitensis, B henselae, Toxoplasma gondii, Francisella tularensis,* and HIV.

The history should focus on possible exposures, including ill contacts, pets, unpasteurized milk, and farm animals. A detailed travel history should be obtained, which may point the examiner toward coccidiomycosis, histoplasmosis, or tuberculosis. Recent dental work or history of dental pain may implicate an occult dental abscess with lymph drainage. Occasionally, *Actinomyces israelii* is isolated from a cervical lymph node draining an odontogenic infection.

A thorough physical examination may narrow the differential diagnosis (Table 9–21). When the adenopathy is associated with prolonged fever, conjunctivitis, mucous membrane erythema, and rash, Kawasaki disease should be considered. When exudative pharyngitis is present, reactive lymphadenopathy from such culprits as EBV, CMV, adenovirus, or *S pyogenes* is likely. Isolated conjunctival injection associated with cervical adenopathy is described in the oculoglandular form of tularemia, as well as in the Parinaud oculoglandular syndrome. The presence of a rash may suggest the diagnosis of a generalized viral process, such as measles, varicella, or rubella. When abdominal examination reveals hepatosplenomegaly, the lymphadenopathy may be due to a systemic process such as EBV, CMV, HIV, or malignant neoplasm; if the history is consistent, more unusual etiologies, such as brucellosis, should be considered.

Involvement of specific lymph nodes may help guide the diagnosis. Occipital and posterior auricular nodes are enlarged in rubella; occipital nodes may be enlarged in an infection with tinea capitis. Axillary and cervical lymphadenopathy are commonly involved in cat-scratch dis-

Table 9–20. Historical clues to diagnosis of infectious lymphadenopathy.

Exposure	Etiologic Organisms
Kitten	*Bartonella henselae*
	Toxoplasma gondii
Raw milk	*Brucella* species
Rabbits	*Francisella tularensis*
Rats/mice	Rat-bite fever
	Leptospirosis

Table 9–21. Most common causes of neck swelling.

Isolated lymphadenopathy bacteria	Viruses	Parasitic/fungal/other
Staphylococcus aureus	EBV	*Toxoplasma gondii*
Group A β-hemolytic *Streptococcus*	CMV	Kawasaki syndrome
Bartonella henselae (cat-scratch disease)	HSV	Coccidiomycosis
Mycobacterium tuberculosis	Adenovirus	
Mycobacterium avium-intracellulare		
Bacterial abscess		
Generalized lymphadenopathy	**Other causes**	
HIV	Tumor	
EBV	Congenital cysts	
CMV	Parotid swelling	
Rubeola		

CMV = cytomegalovirus; EBV = Epstein-Barr virus; HSV = herpes simplex virus.

ease. Knowledge of the body's lymphatic drainage can be helpful in identifying a source for lymph node enlargement. Epitrochlear nodes drain the ulnar side of the hand and forearm. Inguinal nodes drain the lower extremities as well as the genital regions.

The most common cause of enlarged lymph nodes is reactive lymphadenopathy responding to a systemic or local infection. Lymphadenopathy in the anterior cervical region most frequently is a reaction to pharyngitis, otitis media, or viral URI. These lymph nodes can be quite enlarged and tender, but usually have no overlying erythema and are not fluctuant. If cultured, these lymph nodes would be sterile, histologically showing an infiltration of benign lymphocytes. The lymph nodes are usually multiple and will decrease in size over the course of the illness. In general, the nodes themselves require no diagnostic intervention.

Occasionally one of these lymph nodes may become more tender and develop overlying erythema with or without being fluctuant. In these cases, the involved node has become superinfected and is termed cervical adenitis. The most common pathogens are *S pyogenes* and *S aureus*. These usually respond to warm soaks and oral antibiotics. The antibiotic chosen should cover the above pathogens, either a first-generation cephalosporin or an antistaphylo-coccal penicillin. Occasionally, and most frequently when an abscess has developed, oral antibiotics are unsuccessful and IV antibiotics are needed. The choice of IV antibiotics should mirror the oral antibiotics mentioned. If there is no response in 48 hours to the administration of parenteral therapy, a surgeon should be consulted for incision and drainage (Table 9–22).

Although gram-positive organisms are most commonly encountered in cervical adenitis, others should be considered in every diagnostic workup. Cervical adenitis caused by *M tuberculosis* is referred to as *scrofula.* It frequently presents as a nontender, mobile, unilateral cervical lymph node. Placement of a PPD is mandatory in any workup of cervical lymphadenitis. If scrofula is diagnosed, treatment

involves antituberculous chemotherapy and surgical excision. A diligent search for the source case should be undertaken.

Nontuberculous mycobacterial infection of cervical lymph nodes is by far the most common cause of lymphadenopathy. This usually occurs in younger children, most of whom are younger than 5 years. These nodes usually are unilateral but can be of significant size. The overlying skin frequently is erythematous with a bluish hue. As with the nodes in tuberculous adenitis, these nodes are nontender. A minimally reactive PPD may be present. Definitive diagnosis is made surgically, and treatment ideally involves complete surgical excision, not chemotherapy.

Cat-scratch disease is a very common cause of chronic lymphadenitis in children. The organism responsible is *B henselae,* a small pleomorphic gram-negative bacillus. Cat-scratch disease typically presents as an enlarging nontender lymph node, frequently located in the cervical, axillary, or inguinal regions. After the scratch of a kitten, a papule develops at the site of the scratch, and then the lymph node draining the involved area becomes enlarged within 2–3 weeks. The disease is self-limited and requires no intervention, although the node may remain enlarged for several months and eventually may suppurate. Needle biopsy has been reported to create sinus tracts that are dif-

Table 9–22. Indications for biopsy of a lymph node.

Persistent enlargement despite empiric therapy
Persistent enlargement or no improvement with negative workup results
Solid fixed mass
Mass located in supraclavicular area
Accompanying constitutional signs of persistent fever, weight loss

ficult to treat and thus should be avoided. If the node is removed surgically, a Warthin-Starry stain will reveal the bacillus. Diagnosis is best made by serology, which is now commercially available. Usually no treatment is needed, as the enlarged nodes usually resolve in a few months. Although antibiotics usually are not effective, some previous reports indicated that trimethoprim-sulfamethoxazole may be useful.

Certain congenital lesions may become secondarily infected and present as acutely enlarged neck mass resembling lymph nodes. These include branchial cleft cyst, cystic hygroma, thyroglossal duct, and dermoid cyst.

The workup of a child or adolescent presenting with an enlarged lymph node or a group of enlarged lymph nodes should proceed in a step-wise fashion. Empiric therapy with antibiotics is appropriate if the node appears to be superinfected. If after cessation of a superinfection the node persists or continues to enlarge, a more thorough workup should be undertaken to rule out less common causes of lymphadenopathy. Serologic evaluation for cat-scratch disease should be made if the history is compatible. Serologic tests for EBV, HIV, and toxoplasmosis may be appropriate as well. A chest radiograph is frequently indicated to evaluate for mediastinal adenopathy and pulmonary nodules. Regardless of exposure history, a PPD should be placed as a clue toward mycobacterial node infection. Other unusual etiologies include fungal pathogens such as *H capsulatum, Aspergillus* species, and *C neoformans.* Less commonly encountered bacteria include *Yersinia, Actinomyces,* and oral anaerobes, such as *Peptostreptococcus.* Finally, noninfectious etiologies should be considered, especially if the enlarged node is accompanied by systemic symptoms, such as fever and weight loss. These would include lymphoma, histiocytosis X, and metastatic tumors.

RESPIRATORY INFECTIONS

Respiratory infections can be classified according to the symptom complexes associated with upper, middle, and lower airway involvement. In early childhood, infections of the respiratory tract are most often due to viruses, followed by bacteria. These common complaints usually start after the first few months postnatally, when the protective immunoglobulins, transferred prenatally from the mother, start to wane. Thereafter, the child undergoes natural immunization with the various respiratory pathogens. It is not uncommon for a young child to have six to eight URI infections a year. The most common infections are associated with nasal congestions and rhinorrhea. These include simple URIs (eg, the common cold), sinusitis, and otitis media.

UPPER RESPIRATORY TRACT INFECTIONS

THE COMMON COLD

The common cold is a minor illness that poses a major nuisance to society. Colds are important not so much for the quality (ie, severity) of illness, but for the quantity (ie, prevalence). The Public Health Service has reported that half the population experiences a cold during a single winter season. Children, especially preschool children, are susceptible to recurrent colds. Reasons underlying this high frequency may include attendance in day care, resulting in increased exposure to colds.

The high prevalence of the common cold generates great costs to society. Colds are responsible for more missed school and work than any other illness in the United States, with estimates near 50 million days per year. In addition to absenteeism, colds generate health care costs related to physician visits and the use of prescription and nonprescription medications.

Pathogenesis & Etiology

Transmission of cold viruses is believed to occur primarily through direct (sneezing, hand-to-nose) or indirect (fomites) contact with nasal secretions. Children literally pick up cold viruses from school or day care and bring them home to other family members. Inoculation with a virus is followed by invasion of epithelium of nasopharynx, sinuses, and URT. The typical incubation period is 2–5 days. Viral replication results in cholinergic stimulation, direct cellular damage, and the release of inflammatory mediators and cytokines, which in turn affect vascular permeability, mucosal edema, and mucus production.

Numerous viruses are responsible for producing symptoms of the common cold. Rhinovirus and its many serotypes have been the most commonly identified agent, representing approximately one third of all cases. Other viral causes include parainfluenza, RSV, coronavirus, adenovirus, and influenza virus.

Clinical Manifestations

The principal manifestations are nasal congestion and rhinorrhea. Sore throat, sneezing, cough, and hoarseness may be associated. The symptoms usually last for around 1 week, although considerable variation may occur. In addition to costs to society in wages and cold remedies, colds also can produce medical complications. In children, the common cold is a frequent precipitant of otitis media, sinusitis, and asthma exacerbations.

The diagnosis of the common cold is made on history and physical examination. Because of the mild and self-limited nature of the disease, specific diagnostic evaluations usually are not warranted. A variety of viral culture and antigen techniques are available in specialized circumstances.

Treatment

Currently, the most effective management of the common cold is to educate parents regarding the natural course of the infection. This includes a discussion of the expected course of illness, signs and symptoms that would require physician evaluation, and methods to limit transmission (eg, hand-washing). Other than education, many therapies have been advocated to prevent or treat the common cold. Humidification, hydration, saline nose drops, and bulb suctioning of the nostrils may loosen nasal secretions and provide relief in some patients. In addition, families may use a range of traditional over-the-counter (OTC) preparations, as well as alternative and folk medicines. Alternative remedies include herbs and teas, chicken noodle soup, vitamin C, and homeopathic medicines.

In the United States, the market for OTC cold preparations represents $2 billion in annual sales. Patient requests for recommendations on the hundreds of OTC cold remedies necessitate that physicians familiarize themselves with their ingredients. Despite the large assortment of preparations, usually there are only four types of active ingredients: antihistamines, decongestants, expectorants, and cough suppressants. The mechanisms of action of these compounds are often theoretical, and their clinical effects are speculative and anecdotal. Many preparations contain combinations of these four ingredients, and some also contain antipyretics-analgesics (eg, acetaminophen, ibuprofen). Antihistamines (eg, diphenhydramine, brompheniramine, chlorpheniramine) block H-1 receptors and may produce some anticholinergic effects. Although histamine may play no role in the pathophysiology of the common cold, anticholinergic effects of the antihistamines may reduce mucous secretion. Decongestants (eg, phenylephrine, phenylpropanolamine, pseudoephedrine) are sympathomimetics that can produce vasoconstriction through α-adrenergic stimulation. Vasoconstriction could reduce mucous-membrane swelling and mucous secretion. Expectorants (eg, guaifenesin) have been suggested to act by thinning respiratory tract secretions. Cough suppressants (eg, codeine, dextromethorphan) may act on the medullary cough center to reduce cough.

With respect to current therapeutics for the common cold, it is unclear whether any of the cold or cough ingredients, individually or in combination, is effective in providing relief from common cold symptoms in children. Despite the widespread use of these preparations, few, if any, scientific data from the pediatric literature support their use. In addition, cough and cold preparations have the risk of adverse effects (eg, sedation, respiratory depression, sleeplessness, agitation, hypertension, tachycardia, mucus plugging). Prolonged use of topical nasal decongestants can produce rebound congestion secondary to local irritation or ischemia. The high prevalence of these compounds in homes contributes to their not uncommon role in intentional and unintentional drug poisonings.

Families should be educated on the use and misuse of these preparations. Attention should be paid to appropriate indications, dosing (age- and weight-dependent), and potential adverse effects. Currently, antibiotics and antiviral agents have no role in the therapy of the common cold. Despite a flurry of interest in vitamin C for prevention and therapy of the common cold, little scientific evidence supports its use. Researchers previously have reported some success with intranasal α-2 interferon in preventing colds due to rhinovirus; however, general use of the cytokine for the common cold is not indicated at present.

EAR PAIN

Ear aches are one of the most frequent presenting complaints to the primary care physician's office. Although infectious causes predominate, other conditions can produce direct or referred pain in this area. Among these are foreign bodies, local trauma, and temporomandibular joint pain. A host of infectious processes of the ear and nearby structures can present with ear ache: otitis media, otitis externa, myringitis, mastoiditis, cervical lymphadenitis, folliculitis, furunculosis, and cellulitis of the outer ear structures (Table 9–23). Because of the frequency of otitis externa and acute otitis media, the following discussion focuses on these conditions.

Otitis Externa

Otitis externa refers to an inflammatory process involving the external ear structures—external auditory canal and auricle. An intact epithelial lining and acid pH normally contribute to the local defense of the external auditory canal. The pathophysiology of otitis externa centers primarily on alterations in these local defenses, and in some cases on systemic host immunity. High humidity, frequent or prolonged water immersion ("swimmer's ear"), local trauma, or underlying dermatitis each can compromise local defenses and lead to infection and inflammation of the external ear. *P aeruginosa* and *S aureus* are common bacterial isolates from cases of otitis externa. Streptococci, mycoplasma, and fungi (eg, *Candida* species) also can cause otitis externa. The primary symptom of otitis externa is ear pain. Ear discharge (otorrhea) can

Table 9–23. Differential diagnosis of earache.

Otitis media
Otitis externa
Myringitis
Mastoiditis
Folliculitis and furunculosis
Cervical lymphadenitis
Cellulitis of the outer-ear structures

also be reported. Systemic signs such as fever are uncommon.

History and physical examination usually are sufficient to make the diagnosis of otitis externa. The hallmark of this condition is pain with manipulation of the external auricle or pressure on the tragus. This pain results from stretching of the inflamed auditory canal. Otoscopy reveals erythema, edema, and exudate in the auditory canal. Laboratory evaluation, such as cultures, may be indicated in unusually severe cases or treatment failures. Otitis media with perforation of the tympanic membrane can produce ear pain and otorrhea.

Treatment of otitis externa consists of topical drops containing a combination of antibiotic and steroid ingredients (eg, Cortisporin otic suspension, which contains neomycin, polymyxin B, and hydrocortisone). Prevention of recurrent episodes of otitis externa involves avoidance of precipitating factors (eg, swimming, local trauma from cotton swabs) and/or prophylaxis therapy. Prophylaxis with topical solutions containing alcohol or preparations of boric or acetic acid have been used. These compounds act by sterilizing the auditory canal and restoring the normally acid pH.

Acute Otitis Media

Otitis media refers to an inflammation of the middle ear. In fact, otitis media represents a spectrum of disease of both acute and chronic nature (Table 9–24). The frequency with which otitis media occurs creates a major challenge to pediatricians, patients, families, and society. The National Center for Health Statistics reported 24.5 million office visits for otitis media in the United States in 1990. It represented the most frequent diagnosis in children younger than 15 years. A study from Boston (Teele, 1989) reported more than 80% of children had an episode of otitis media by 3 years of age. Nearly half of this same group (46%) had three or more ear infections.

Otitis media produces short-term costs related to physician visits, antibiotic prescriptions, school absenteeism, and work loss by parents. In 1986, more than 40% of prescriptions for antibiotics in children younger than 10 years of age were used for otitis media. Long-term costs secondary to otitis media are placement of myringotomy tubes, the need for hearing evaluations, and speech and language therapy. In addition, the development of bacterial antibiotic resistance caused by the routine administration of antibiotics is of increasing concern throughout the world.

Certain factors are associated with increased risk of recurrent otitis media. These include young age at first ear infection, male gender, family history of recurrent ear infections, participation in day care, and exposure to cigarette smoke. Individuals of Native American or Eskimo ancestry, as well as individuals with cleft palate or Down syndrome, may be particularly susceptible to severe or persistent otitis media. In contrast, there are data to support the hypothesis that breast feeding may have protective effects against the development of ear infections.

Pathogenesis. The middle ear is an air-filled cavity lined by respiratory mucosa and connected to the nasopharynx via the eustachian tube. The pathogenesis of acute otitis media begins with dysfunction and obstruction of the eustachian tube. Obstruction of the eustachian tube allows negative pressure to develop within the middle ear. Negative pressure, along with the inability to drain, allows the collection of fluid within this space. Bacteria colonizing the nasopharynx can reflux into the fluid-filled middle-ear space. The proliferation of bacteria and host inflammatory response produce the signs and symptoms of acute otitis media. It is believed that the shorter, more horizontal orientation of the eustachian tube, along with more frequent viral URIs, contributes to the higher incidence of acute otitis media in childhood.

The most common organisms isolated in otitis media are *S pneumoniae, H influenzae,* and *M catarrhalis* (Table 9–25). Most of the *H influenzae* are nontypable strains. Although a respiratory virus (eg, RSV, rhinovirus, adenovirus, parainfluenza virus) may be a frequent inciting event in otitis media, isolation of virus without bacterial coinfection has been reported in fewer than 10% of cases.

Table 9–24. Spectrum of middle-ear infections.

	Description	Otoscopy	Tympanometry	
			Compliance	Pressure[1]
Otitis media without effusion	eg, myringitis	Erythematous, opaque TM; bullae may be present	Normal	+
Acute otitis media (suppurative otitis media, purulent otitis media)	Implies rapid onset of local and/or systemic illness	Erythematous, opaque, bulging TM	Decreased	+
Otitis media with effusion (secretory, serous, or nonsuppurative otitis media)	Implies presence of effusion in an asymptomatic patient	Translucent or opaque TM; bubbles or air fluid levels may be seen	Decreased	+ or −

[1]Implies positive or negative pressure within the middle-ear space relative to atmospheric pressure.
TM = tympanic membrane.

Table 9–25. Etiology of acute otitis media.

Organisms	Percent of Infections[1]	β-Lactamase-Producing (%)
Streptococcus pneumoniae	38	None[2]
Haemophilus influenzae (nontypable)	27	20–40[3]
Moraxella catarrhalis	10	> 90[3]

[1]Barnett 1995.
[2]Resistance of S pneumoniae mediated by alterations in penicillin-binding proteins.
[3]Bluestone and Klein 1995.

Clinical Manifestations. Classically, the child with acute otitis media presents with the history of a prodromal viral URI followed by the development of ear pain (otalgia) or pulling on the ear. Fever, increased irritability, and anorexia may be present. These later, less specific signs may be the only indicators of acute otitis media in younger infants. Otorrhea may be seen if the tympanic membrane has been perforated by the buildup of inflammatory material within the middle ear.

In acute otitis media, the diagnosis can be strongly suspected on the basis of history. With otoscopy, it is crucial for students of pediatrics to be familiar with the normal landmarks (eg, the cone of light, location of the malleus, and neutral position of the tympanic membrane) in order to recognize pathologic changes. In acute otitis media, the tympanic membrane may appear erythematous, opaque, and bulging or retracted. The light reflex may be diminished or absent, and air-fluid levels may be visualized. If perforation of the tympanic membrane has occurred, purulent exudate can be seen in the external canal.

Pneumatic otoscopy and tympanometry are additional techniques that can be used to detect changes in compliance of the tympanic membrane (see Table 9–24). Compliance of the tympanic membrane is reduced by the presence of fluid in the middle-ear space. In addition, the tympanogram can verify the presence of a perforated tympanic membrane or patent ventilating tube by demonstrating dramatic increases in canal volume (caused by the combined measurement of both canal and middle-ear spaces).

Treatment. At present, antibiotics are the treatment of choice for acute otitis media in the United States. The selection of antibiotics is based on the usual bacteria isolated during studies of otitis media. Therapy is empiric in most cases, because rarely is middle-ear fluid collected for culture and antibiotic sensitivities. Additional factors that influence antibiotic selection are cost, availability of an oral suspension for younger children, palatability (ie, taste), and dosing frequency. Traditionally, amoxicillin has been the initial drug of choice. Second-line antibiotics include a variety of penicillin, erythromycin, sulfa, and cephalosporin-type antibiotics. The choice of antibiotic in a given community depends on the common agents and antibiotic resistance patterns seen in the area. Acute otitis media usually responds to a 10-day course of oral antibi-

otics. Adjunctive therapies (eg, decongestants) generally are not believed to be effective.

It is of interest that some pediatricians do not immediately prescribe antibiotic therapy for this disorder. The widespread use of antibiotics for acute otitis media is no doubt contributing to the alarming increase in the frequency of bacterial antibiotic resistance. These concerns, as well as the costs and side-effects of antibiotic therapy, are generating interest in the fact that some countries (eg, the Netherlands) prescribe antibiotics much less frequently than does the United States.

Recurrent infections are treated with separate courses of antibiotics. **Persistent** infections are treated with changes in antibiotics. Differentiation between recurrent and persistent infections requires that the patient has documented clearing of infections. For chronic middle-ear effusions, tympanocentesis may be diagnostic (with fluid sent for culture) and therapeutic (allowing drainage of the middle-ear space). Prophylaxis against recurring infections has been demonstrated with the use of daily, low-dose antibiotics (commonly amoxicillin or sulfisoxazole). Selection of appropriate patients for prophylaxis is based on the number of infections experienced in a given time frame (eg, three infections within 6 months). Ventilating tubes (eg, "pressure-equalizing" [PE] tubes) to minimize fluid accumulation in the middle-ear cavity represent another alternative for prevention of recurrent infections or treatment of persistent middle-ear effusion. Ventilating tubes allow drainage of the middle-ear space by bypassing the obstructed eustachian tube. National guidelines do exist concerning the management of persistent middle-ear effusions. The use of oral corticosteroids (eg, prednisone) in persistent effusion is controversial; these drugs should not be prescribed routinely.

Follow-up & Complications. In otitis media, pain and fever should improve within 2–3 days of appropriate therapy. A treatment failure should be considered if symptoms persist despite good compliance with initial therapy. A change in antibiotic therapy should be considered in these patients. If symptoms resolve, options for follow-up range from no additional visits (except for routine health supervision) to follow-up at 2–6 weeks after diagnosis. Patients at risk for persistent or recurrent infections should be monitored more closely.

Complications of acute otitis media include perforation of the tympanic membrane, mastoiditis, lateral sinus thrombosis, meningitis, and abscess formation. The long-term effects of persistent middle-ear effusion include conductive hearing loss and speech delay.

ACUTE SINUSITIS

The paranasal sinuses (maxillary, ethmoid, sphenoid, and frontal) are air-filled cavities lined by ciliated columnar epithelium and mucus-producing goblet cells. The coordinated action of cilia allows drainage of these spaces into the nasopharynx through a series of ostia. Developmentally, the maxillary and ethmoid sinuses are present at birth, whereas the sphenoid and frontal sinuses appear later in childhood.

The actual incidence of sinusitis in the pediatric age group is unknown. Some estimates can be made on the basis of the frequency of viral URIs. Sinusitis is estimated to complicate URIs in 0.5–10.0% of cases, a 20-fold range. Because preschool-aged children have an average of five to eight colds per year, this could translate into almost one episode of sinusitis per child per year using the highest estimates of 10%.

Pathogenesis & Etiology

Sinusitis results from the impaired drainage of the sinus and subsequent accumulation of fluid in the sinus cavity. As in otitis media, bacteria can enter and multiply within the enclosed space of the sinuses, resulting in infection. Impaired drainage of the sinuses can occur through alterations in the character of mucus, decrease in ciliary activity, and obstruction of the sinus ostia. Sinus infection may occur as a complication of allergy (eg, allergic rhinitis) or viral URI (eg, the common cold).

The common respiratory pathogens are the typical cause of acute sinusitis: *S pneumoniae,* nontypable *H influenzae,* and *M catarrhalis.* Respiratory viruses (adenovirus, parainfluenza virus, influenza virus, and rhinovirus) are responsible for fewer than 10% of acute sinusitis.

Clinical Manifestations

Bacterial sinusitis must be distinguished from allergic conditions and recurrent viral URIs. The clinical differentiation of these conditions can be difficult. The most common manifestations of sinusitis—rhinorrhea, cough, and fever—are not particularly specific or sensitive. These signs and symptoms can be shared with a variety of URIs. In acute sinusitis, the rhinorrhea may be clear or purulent. In general, the patient presents with cough during both day and night. Fever that is high or occurs late in the course of respiratory symptoms is also suggestive of bacterial sinusitis. Painless, periorbital edema occurring in the morning and malodorous breath may be reported. The facial pain and frontal headache commonly described by adults are uncommon complaints in children with sinusitis.

Although the duration and severity of symptoms are nonspecific in sinusitis, they may assist in the diagnosis. The clinical diagnosis of sinusitis should be supported by persistent respiratory symptoms (ie, lack of improvement by 10 days) or severe symptoms (ie, temperature ≥ 39 °C and purulent nasal discharge). In comparison, the expected course of the common cold is one of significant improvement over a week. History of atopic disease (eg, eczema, asthma), nasal itching, and seasonal occurrence may suggest the diagnosis of allergic rhinitis.

On examination, the nasal mucosa in acute bacterial sinusitis typically are inflamed. Allergic rhinitis classically results in pale, boggy mucous membranes. The presence of allergic shiners, allergic nasal crease, and Dennie lines also can support the diagnosis of atopic disease. In chil-

dren, palpation over the sinuses, although helpful in making the diagnosis, rarely elicits facial tenderness.

Transillumination of the maxillary sinuses with a light source placed on the inferior orbital rim has been recommended in older children (> 10 years). If the light transmitted through the palate is markedly diminished on one side, this may support the diagnosis of sinusitis.

The radiologic evaluation of sinusitis includes either the traditional plain film sinus series (three views—anteroposterior, lateral, occipitomental) or CT scan. Both can be used to demonstrate opacification, mucosal thickening (≥ 4 mm), and the presence of air-fluid levels within the sinuses. The specificity and sensitivity of radiologic studies in diagnosing bacterial sinusitis have been questioned by some authors.

Aspiration of the maxillary sinuses is the gold standard for diagnosing acute bacterial sinusitis. Because it is an invasive procedure, it is usually reserved for severe or atypical cases or treatment failures.

Treatment

The treatment of sinusitis centers on antibiotic therapy. The choice of antibiotics is similar to the selection of antibiotics in other respiratory infections, including otitis media. The prevalence of resistant organisms should be considered. In addition, a cure rate of 40–50% without antibiotic therapy has been reported. As in otitis media, amoxicillin is often considered the initial agent. Second-line agents, including amoxicillin-clavulanate (Augmentin), erythromycin ethylsuccinate-sulfisoxazole (Pediazole), and cephalosporins may be indicated in areas with high rates of β-lactamase–producing organisms or in patients with complicated disease or treatment failures.

Symptoms should improve within 2–3 days of appropriate antibiotic therapy. The duration of therapy depends in part on the individual patient's rate of clinical response. Children who respond rapidly to antibiotics probably require shorter schedules, whereas slow responders may benefit from longer duration of therapy. Overall, typical regimens vary from 10 to 21 days. It has been recommended that antibiotics be continued for 7 days after the resolution of symptoms in patients who have had a slow response to antibiotics.

Additional medical therapies, such as decongestants and antihistamines, have not proved effective in children with sinusitis. The value of using nasal steroid preparations to prevent sinusitis also is not proved.

MIDDLE RESPIRATORY TRACT INFECTIONS

FEVER & STRIDOR

Because of the potentially life-threatening nature of stridor, patients presenting with this complaint warrant careful evaluation and follow-up. Noninfectious etiologies represent a range of anatomic, functional, and allergic causes. Congenital and acquired anatomic abnormalities can reduce the caliber of the airway from intrinsic or extrinsic compression. Examples of anatomic abnormalities include enlarged lymph nodes, neoplasms, hemangiomas, aberrant vascular structures, laryngeal polyps or papillomas, foreign bodies, and subglottic webs. Vocal cord paralysis, allergic conditions (eg, angioneurotic edema, anaphylaxis), trauma, and burns also can produce upper airway obstruction.

Infectious etiologies of stridor are croup (or laryngotracheitis), epiglottitis, bacterial tracheitis, diphtheria, peritonsillar abscess, and retropharyngeal cellulitis or abscess. In addition, these infections may present as a membranous swelling in the oropharynx (Table 9–26). The following discussion focuses on croup, bacterial tracheitis, and epiglottis. These three conditions produce inflammation of the upper or middle airway, resulting in signs and symptoms of upper airway obstruction, which potentially can cause life-threatening respiratory failure.

Croup
(Acute Laryngotracheitis)

Of the three conditions—croup laryngotracheitis, epiglottitis, and bacterial tracheitis—croup is the most common by far. The peak incidence occurs in children aged 1–2 years, and it has been reported in 14.9–47 cases per 1000 children. Boys have a higher frequency than girls by a ratio of 1.5:1. The seasonal occurrence of croup mirrors the appearance of respiratory viral infections during fall and winter.

The parainfluenza viruses types 1, 2, and 3 are the most common causes of croup, accounting for 50–75% of cases. RSV and influenza virus (types A and B) are the next most frequent causes of croup. Croup also has been reported as a frequent manifestation of measles infection.

Croup occurs as a result of inflammation of the subglottic area. The typical case of croup begins with symptoms of a viral URI—rhinorrhea and fever. Hours to days later, symptoms of upper airway obstruction develop. A "barking" or "croupy" cough, inspiratory stridor, and hoarseness are the hallmarks of croup. The amount of respiratory distress can range from mild to severe, depending on the degree of airway obstruction.

Of note, attempts are often made to distinguish between **viral croup** and **spasmodic croup**. Spasmodic croup

Table 9–26. Differential diagnosis of "oropharyngeal membrane" or swelling.

Diphtheria
Enlarged tonsils, tonsillitis, peritonsillar abscess
Retropharyngeal abscess
Laryngeal papillomatosis
Tracheitis, bacterial
Epiglottitis
Trauma, hematoma

probably lies along a spectrum of illness with viral croup. Allergy, viral infection, and muscle spasm all have been postulated in the pathogenesis of spasmodic croup. Patients exhibit the typical barking cough and stridor; however, the symptoms traditionally occur at night, and fever and URI symptoms are lacking. Recurrences of spasmodic croup are not uncommon and may represent an element of airway hypersensitivity.

Epiglottitis
(Supraglottitis)

In 1941, Sinclair was one of the first to describe a bacterial infection of the epiglottis. This account and others confirmed the association of epiglottitis with infection by HIB. Epiglottitis (or supraglottitis) is characterized by inflammation of the epiglottis and adjacent structures, including the aryepiglottic folds. The incidence of epiglottitis has decreased dramatically since the vaccine for HIB first became available in the United States in the past decade.

Epiglottitis presents with the acute onset of fever, toxicity, and respiratory distress. Although viral URI symptoms may precede some cases, the progression of illness and upper respiratory obstruction typically is more rapid than that seen in viral croup or bacterial tracheitis. Unlike croup, cough is usually absent, and drooling, dyspnea, respiratory distress, apprehension, and toxicity are the prominent signs.

Bacterial Tracheitis

Nondiphtheritic bacterial infections of the URT were common at least through the early 1900s. Reports on these bacterial infections gradually disappeared from the literature until 1979, when separate groups described children with upper airway obstruction caused by an exudative tracheitis. This condition has been called bacterial tracheitis, or membranous or pseudomembranous laryngotracheobronchitis.

The incidence of bacterial tracheitis is much lower than that of viral croup. Cases occur most frequently in preschool-aged children, and boys are more commonly affected than girls.

Most evidence suggests that an initial insult to the airway predisposes to bacterial infection. The most common inciting event is viral croup, although other airway injuries (eg, endotracheal intubation) have been associated with bacterial tracheitis. Patients with Down syndrome also may be at higher risk for development of this condition, possibly through alterations in immunity or airway anatomy.

S aureus is the major isolate from these patients. Other common respiratory pathogens (eg, streptococcal species, *Hemophilus* species, and *M catarrhalis*) have also been isolated. In a number of patients with bacterial tracheitis, viruses responsible for croup (eg, parainfluenza, influenza, RSV, and measles) have been identified.

Bacterial tracheitis shares features of both viral croup and epiglottitis. In many cases, symptoms of viral URI are followed by barking cough. In general, fever is higher and the patient is more ill appearing than in the typical case of croup. Upper airway obstruction may develop rapidly, although drooling may be less common than in epiglottitis.

Diagnosis. The history should explore allergic reactions, foreign body aspiration, and trauma. A comparison of croup, bacterial tracheitis, and epiglottitis is presented in Table 9–27. Initial diagnosis and management of the patient with stridor is directed at distinguishing patients in need of immediate airway management (eg, intubation) from all others. Any number of infectious and noninfectious causes of acute stridor can produce complete obstruction of the upper airway. Therefore, assessment of the general state of the patient and patency of the airway is essential. Does the child appear toxic (severely ill, obtunded)? What is the work of breathing? Is there evidence of respiratory fatigue? These questions can be addressed by observing and monitoring the patient's level of consciousness, degree of stridor, respiratory distress (eg, retractions), air movement, and color. Patients who appear toxic or at risk of complete airway obstruction should be treated without delay for unnecessary diagnostic procedures.

The need for serial reexaminations cannot be overestimated. Selection of initial therapy, response to therapy, requirement for additional therapy, and/or hospitalization all will be directed by changes in the patient status.

In general, the laboratory plays a limited role in the evaluation of patients with stridor. Marked elevations in WBC, C-reactive protein, or ESR will suggest bacterial infection. However, these tests are not diagnostic and usually add little to the diagnostic evaluation. Microbiologic studies for bacterial pathogens (eg, Gram stains, cultures, antigen detection) are useful in cases of severe disease but usually are obtained only after the airway has been secured. Viral studies (eg, cultures, antigen detection, serology) usually are not indicated.

Radiologic studies, although helpful, probably are indicated infrequently in the evaluation of upper airway obstruction. In viral croup, the diagnosis is primarily clinical. In bacterial tracheitis and epiglottitis, the importance of securing the airway outweighs any benefit of radiologic imaging. If radiographs are obtained, the pathognomonic findings of epiglottitis is the "thumb sign." This sign is the result of inflammatory swelling from infection, which gives the epiglottis the appearance of a thumb. The AP neck radiograph of patients with severe croup reveals a tapering subglottic narrowing from soft-tissue edema resembling a "steeple" (see Table 9–27). In addition to these findings, neck radiographs can demonstrate evidence of retropharyngeal cellulitis or abscess (thickening of the prevertebral space) and radiopaque foreign bodies.

The definitive diagnosis of bacterial tracheitis and epiglottitis is made by direct visualization by an otolaryngologist or anesthetist. Laryngoscopy can be both diagnostic and therapeutic by documenting the location and severity of airway injury and allowing removal of a foreign body or purulent secretions.

Of interest, the clinical response to treatment with racemic epinephrine also may help distinguish between viral croup and bacterial tracheitis in some patients. A number of authors have commented on the lack of improvement after administration of inhaled racemic epinephrine in patients with bacterial tracheitis. Another distinguishing feature is that patients with bacterial tracheitis appear to be more toxic, with high fever and leukocytosis.

Treatment. In patients with marked stridor, regardless of cause, the treatment is aimed at airway management. Most patients with bacterial tracheitis and epiglottitis, as well as a small percentage of those with croup, require placement of an artificial airway. Therefore, patients should be managed in a controlled setting by experienced personnel with a plan for emergency airway assistance.

Antibiotic therapy is crucial for both epiglottitis and bacterial tracheitis. The selection of antibiotics is aimed toward the likely organisms; for example, treatment of bacterial tracheitis includes antistaphylococcal antibiotics, such as nafcillin or vancomycin. Before antibiotics are administered, blood and tracheal aspirate cultures should be performed to guide definitive therapy. Antibiotics usually are not indicated in patients with viral or spasmodic croup.

Table 9–27. Comparison of infectious causes of stridor.

	Croup	Bacterial Tracheitis	Epiglottitis
Age	Infant to preschool	Infant to preschool	Older infant to preschool
Prodrome	Viral URI	Viral URI	Usually none
Toxicity	Variable mild to severe	Severe	Severe
Drooling	No	Yes or no	Yes
Microbiology	Viral, ? role of allergy in spasmodic croup	*Staphylococcus aureus*	*Haemophilus influenzae* type b
Radiographic findings	Subglottic narrowing ("steeple sign" on AP), dilated hypopharynx, air trapping	Subglottic narrowing, irregular tracheal margin, intratracheal membranes	"Thumb" sign, thickened aryepiglottic folds
Treatment	Variable depending on severity (see text)	Artificial airway, antibiotics	Artificial airway, antibiotics

AP = anteroposterior view; URI = upper respiratory infection.

Management of epiglottitis includes the possibility of intubation because of the aggressive nature of epiglottitis, which often progresses quickly to airway obstruction. When the diagnosis of epiglottitis is suspected, care must be taken not to irritate the patient and precipitate obstruction. Anesthesia and otolaryngology services should be consulted, and emergency procedures should be readily available for immediate intubation or tracheostomy if the need arises. Antimicrobial therapy must include coverage for *H influenzae,* usually a third-generation cephalosporin or ampicillin plus chloramphenicol. As mentioned above, invasive infections due to *H influenzae* have been decreasing since the introduction of the vaccine for this organism.

In patients in whom the diagnosis of viral croup has been made, therapy depends on the severity of clinical findings. Many of these therapies are controversial. Humidified air (eg, by baths, showers, croup kettles, and croup tents) has been the mainstay therapy. The exact mechanism of action (eg, loosening of secretions, reducing irritation, action of laryngeal receptors) is unknown. The use of humidified air has been supported primarily by anecdotal evidence, and the limited research studies in this area have not been able to document benefit. Mist therapy is often considered "reasonable" if it does not interfere with observation of the patient or result in increased agitation.

The use of corticosteroids in viral croup has been debated for more than 40 years. Like humidified air, the exact mechanism of action of corticosteroids in croup is unclear, although effects on local inflammation, capillary permeability, and allergic responses have been postulated. The onset of activity of corticosteroids is believed to be within hours of administration. A meta-analysis of nine randomized studies reported fewer intubations and greater clinical improvement at 12 and 24 hours after treatment with corticosteroids when compared with controls. The choice of corticosteroid and the dose, route, and duration of therapy have varied from study to study. Oral, parenteral, and nebulized corticosteroids have been used. Traditionally, corticosteroids have been used in patients ill enough to be hospitalized, although increasing evidence is being reported from the outpatient setting.

Inhaled racemic epinephrine (via nebulizer or intermittent positive pressure breathing) has been used in croup for 30 years. Although racemic epinephrine (equal quantities of levorotatory and dextrorotatory isomers) has been used primarily, there is evidence to suggest that L-epinephrine may be equally effective. The α-adrenergic action of epinephrine is believed to result in vasoconstriction and the reduction of edema in the subglottic area. The rapid onset of action (10–30 minutes) has made it a useful therapy in emergency departments. However, its short duration of activity (2 hours) and risk of rebound swelling have restricted the use of epinephrine primarily to hospitalized patients. Combination therapy (racemic epinephrine and corticosteroids) has been used successfully in a few outpatient studies of croup. In contrast, patients with bacterial tracheitis are usually unresponsive to treatment with racemic epinephrine.

DIPHTHERIA

Diphtheria was recognized as a clinical syndrome early in the 19th century. The bacillus responsible, *Corynebacterium diphtheriae,* was identified in the latter part of the century. Until the early part of this century, laryngeal diphtheria was the leading serious infection of the larynx and infraglottic airway. At that time, the term croup was synonymous with diphtheria. The advent of diphtheria antitoxin, antibiotics, and immunizations against diphtheria have dramatically reduced the number of cases of laryngeal diphtheria. Clinically, laryngeal diphtheria is similar to bacterial tracheitis and is notable for producing a fibrinous tracheal exudate.

Diphtheria occurs throughout the world and at any time of the year, although it is most common in winter. Humans are the only known reservoir of *C diphtheriae.* Sources of infection include discharges from the patient's nose, throat, eye, and skin lesions. Transmission results from direct contact with a patient, rarely through fomites and animals. As a result, attack rates are high in households and crowded living conditions. In temperate climates, the skin lesions are superficial, rather insignificant sores that resemble impetigo. Toxic manifestations usually do not develop in individuals with skin lesions, but these lesions can be epidemiologically important as sources of new respiratory tract disease.

The incidence of diphtheria is inversely related to the percentage of immune individuals in an area. It remains common in countries without effective immunization programs. In the United States, the incidence of diphtheria has declined dramatically since the 1950s, with only a few cases reported annually. However, the potential for outbreaks continues if segments of a community are not immunized, as demonstrated by the 1970 outbreak in San Antonio, Texas.

Pathogenesis

Diphtheria is caused by *C diphtheriae* and characterized by a localized pseudomembranous infection in the URT, which can cause obstruction, and by toxic damage to visceral organs and the nervous system. The organisms are gram-positive, slender, pleomorphic rods that lack spores or a capsule. There are three types of organism: *Corynebacterium gravis, Corynebacterium intermedius,* and *Corynebacterium mitis.* All are capable of elaborating an exotoxin. The diphtheria toxin is a cytotoxic protein that interferes with protein synthesis by the host cells. The ability of a strain of *C diphtheriae* to produce toxin is conferred by a bacteriophage that carries the gene for toxin production.

Pseudomembranous lesions, a hallmark of the infection, are commonly found on the mucous membranes of the pharynx, tonsils, and uvula and less frequently in the nose, larynx, and lower respiratory tract. Sometimes the infection extends to the middle ear or to the esophagus and stomach, as well as to the skin or the mucosa of the genital organs. The pseudomembrane consists of necrotic epithelium embedded in inflammatory exudate that has co-agulated on the surface. Although the bacilli remain in these surface lesions, the diphtheria toxin is absorbed from the local lesion, causing damage in distant organs and tissues. The changes are degenerative rather than inflammatory, with myocarditis being most common. Other organs susceptible to the toxin include liver, spleen, kidney, adrenal gland, and brain. Degenerative changes in the nervous system occur in nearly all fatal infections.

Clinical Presentations

The incubation period of diphtheria is usually 2–5 days, but sometimes longer. The clinical features depend on the primary site of infection in terms of local signs and symptoms, but the toxic manifestations are the same regardless of the primary site of proliferation of the organism. The patient presents with a low-grade fever and the gradual manifestation of a pharyngeal membrane over 1–2 days (Table 9–26). The tonsils are the most common site of infection, commonly with spread from the primary site. The infection usually presents as membranous nasopharyngeal and/or obstructive laryngotracheobronchitis.

For tonsillopharyngeal diphtheria, the onset of symptoms is usually insidious, in contrast to streptococcal sore throat. There is mild sore throat with slight redness and low-grade fever. Systemic signs of illness are absent in the early stages. Within 1–2 days, spots of pale yellowish–white exudate appear and coalesce to form a shiny, sharply outlined pseudomembrane. In those lacking immunity to diphtheria, the pseudomembrane may spread to the soft palate and to the posterior pharynx. The breath sometimes has a faint odor resembling garlic. The cervical lymph nodes are only mildly enlarged in many patients. With extensive membrane formation, dysphagia and drooling ensue. After approximately 5 days, the pseudomembrane changes to a grayish color and starts to slough. Ten percent of patients have an acute presentation with high fever, systemic toxicity, rapid proliferation of the pseudomembrane, marked edema of the face and neck, and cerebral obtundation. This is referred to as "bull neck" diphtheria and has a grave prognosis.

In fewer than 5% of patients, diphtheria of the laryngotracheal area occurs with tonsillopharyngeal involvement. Varying degrees of hoarseness, stridor, and respiratory distress occur, depending on the extent and thickness of the membrane in relation to the caliber of the airway. Young children are at particular risk of respiratory compromise because of their small airways. Rarely, the membrane extends into the bronchi, resulting in airway obstruction, which is almost invariably fatal.

Less commonly, the infection presents as cutaneous, vaginal, conjunctival, or otic infection. In tropical areas, cutaneous lesions appear to be more common. Life-threatening complications of diphtheria include thrombocytopenia, myocarditis, and neurologic manifestations of vocal cord paralysis and ascending paralysis similar to that of Guillain-Barré syndrome

Diagnosis can be accomplished by culturing the bacte-ria from lesions in the throat, nostrils, and skin. For better yield, materials should be obtained from beneath the membrane as well as directly from the membrane. Because special media are required, the laboratory should be notified. In remote areas, throat swabs can be placed in the silica gel packs and sent to regional reference centers for culture. Direct staining and immunofluorescence antibody staining are not reliable.

Treatment

Management of the patient is targeted at neutralizing the diphtheria toxin as well as rendering the patient noncontagious with antibiotics. Diphtheria antitoxin neutralizes circulating toxin but has no effect on the toxin that is bound to tissue. It should be administered as soon as possible after onset of disease and before the availability of culture results. Adjunctive treatment, including airway and cardiovascular supports, is indicated.

Diphtheria antitoxin is an equine serum; therefore, tests for sensitivity of the patient must be done before administration. If the patient has an immediate reaction, a desensitization procedure is indicated. The dosage of antitoxin is empiric and based on the extent of disease. The antiserum is administered intravenously. In addition, antimicrobial therapy, including penicillin or erythromycin, is indicated to render the patient noncontagious. After antibiotic therapy is completed, the throat and nasopharynx are cultured three times at least 24 hours apart to determine whether the pathogen has been eradicated. Respiratory isolation precautions are maintained until there is culture confirmation of eradication of the pathogen from the nasopharynx. If there is persistent nasopharyngeal carriage after the first course of therapy, a repeat course of antibiotics is indicated. Other adjunctive therapy may include the use of carnitine for protecting the cardiac muscles; however, its efficacy is not fully confirmed.

Household and other close contacts of an index patient with diphtheria are at increased risk of becoming asymptomatic carriers or of developing disease. Immunization provides antitoxic immunity but no immunity to infection with *C diphtheriae*. Thus, all exposed individuals should be examined and should receive prompt treatment. All close contacts should be kept under surveillance for 7 days. Previously immunized contacts should be given a booster dose of diphtheria toxoid if they have not received a booster within 5 years.

The fatality rate is about 10%, but the prognosis depends on type of disease, age and general condition of the patient, and the interval from onset of disease to antitoxin therapy. More than half the patients with bull neck diphtheria die of the infection in spite of aggressive intensive care. If myocarditis or renal failure occurs early in the course of disease, the prognosis is poor. If the patient is managed in an intensive care facility, death from airway obstruction is unlikely unless pseudomembrane extends into the bronchi. After recovering from the acute illness, patients remain at risk for late development of paralysis or myocarditis. There are no permanent sequelae of diphtheria unless anoxic damage of heart or other vital organs has occurred.

All infants should be routinely immunized with the schedules recommended by the Committee on Infectious Diseases of the American Academy of Pediatrics (see Chapter 1). Booster doses of diphtheria toxoid should be given every 10 years.

LOWER RESPIRATORY TRACT INFECTIONS

The child presenting with a cough and fever may have bronchial involvement, with cardinal signs of wheezing and crackles indicative of bronchial and lung parenchyma infection. Inflammation of the bronchi and parenchyma is often associated with upper-airway infection. Because of the potential aggressive nature of the disease, lower respiratory tract infections are common causes of morbidity and mortality in children. Viral infections, including RSV, parainfluenza, and influenza are the most common causes of infection. Common bacterial pathogens include *S pneumoniae, S aureus, H influenzae,* and *S pyogenes* for community acquired pneumonia. In addition, bacterial infections such as *B pertussis, C diphtheriae, M tuberculosis,* and *M mycoplasma* are found in the pediatric age group. In contrast, nosocomial infections found in chronically ill children are usually caused by gram-negative bacilli, including *E coli, Klebsiella,* and *Pseudomonas* species. For a child who presents with wheezing and lower airway disease, in addition to pneumonia, differential diagnosis must include reactive airway disease (asthma), environmental pollutants (eg, cigarette smoke), cystic fibrosis, foreign body aspiration, congenital malformations, and immotile cilia syndrome.

In newborns, bacterial causes of pneumonia are related to pathogens commonly found in neonatal sepsis, including group B *Streptococcus* and *E coli. S aureus* also can cause devastating disease in this age group. In addition, young infants may present with afebrile pneumonitis, a relatively benign infectious syndrome caused by different organisms, including *C trachomatis, P carinii,* and CMV.

PERTUSSIS SYNDROME

Pertussis syndrome can be caused by one of several etiologic agents, most commonly *B pertussis* and *Bordetella parapertussis.* Viruses such as adenovirus also can cause a similar clinical entity.

The syndrome is usually divided into three phases: catarrhal, paroxysmal cough, and convalescent. The prodromal catarrhal phase usually lasts 2 weeks, followed by 2–4 weeks of paroxysmal cough and 4–12 weeks of a convalescent stage; hence, its name the "hundred day cough" in ancient Chinese literature. Mild fever with URI symptoms is

typical of the catarrhal stage followed by the characteristic coughing, which usually brings the patient to the attention of the physician. This cough is of increasing severity and staccato in nature. It can be followed by a whooplike, high-pitched inspiratory noise, which lends the name "whooping cough." This characteristic noise is caused by deep inspiration through partially obstructed airways. Post-tussive emesis is another common finding in this syndrome.

The incidence of pertussis has declined steadily in the United States over the past 4 decades, associated with increases in nationwide immunization program with the use of pertussis vaccine. However, recurrent peaks of the disease caused by *B pertussis* and *B parapertussis* occur every 4 years. *B pertussis,* the cause of classic pertussis, is highly contagious, especially during the catarrhal prodrome. When exposed to a patient in this phase, as many as 90% of susceptible children acquire the disease. *B parapertussis* causes a less severe and protracted pertussis and is frequently diagnosed as bronchitis or URI unless paroxysmal symptoms develop. Both adults and children can serve as vectors for disease.

Common complications of pertussis include pneumonia and apnea (in infants). Other complications include seizures, atelectasis, intracerebral bleeding from tearing of small blood vessels during coughing, hypoglycemia, and neurologic deficits from hypoxia. Younger infants seem to be more susceptible to major complications. Long-term studies in a large British study demonstrated learning disabilities three times as often in children who had pertussis when compared with vaccinated children with no clinical history of the disease.

Laboratory findings often include peripheral leukocytosis with lymphocytosis, often up to 80% of total WBC count. Diagnosis is usually made by culture and/or immunofluorescent antibody (IFA) staining. IFA is often more sensitive than culture, with good specificity in experienced laboratories. Serologic tests are available, which are useful for epidemiologic studies but of limited value in clinical management.

Antimicrobial therapy is useful in reducing infectivity but does not change either severity nor duration of the disease. Erythromycin, the drug of choice, should be administered for 14 days to prevent relapse (Table 9–28). Trimethoprim-sulfamethoxazole is the alternative drug. Close contacts, regardless of age of immunization history, should be treated with erythromycin prophylactically to reduce secondary transmission.

BRONCHIOLITIS

Bronchiolitis is defined as inflammation of the bronchioles, usually the result of a viral illness. This clinical syndrome is characterized by rapid respiration, chest retractions, and wheezing. This clinical evidence of airway obstruction is caused by bronchiolar obstruction arising from inflammatory changes associated with thick, tenacious secretions and bronchiolar constriction. In infants

Table 9–28. Management of common lower respiratory tract infections.

Etiology	Treatment	Hospitalization
Pertussis syndrome	Erythromycin if causative agent is *Bordetella;* antibiotics reduce infectivity only	Warranted if patient < 1 year or if clinically indicated
Bronchiolitis	Possibly bronchodilator therapy; steroids probably not indicated; ribavirin may be indicated in certain high-risk situations; immunoglobulin therapy still controversial	Warranted in the young infant or if otherwise clinically indicated
Viral pneumonia/ pneumonitis	Usually no treatment, except in patients with underlying disease states, ie, immunosuppression; these children may benefit from specific antiviral agents, ie, ganciclovir for cytomegalovirus pneumonitis	When clinically indicated
Bacterial pneumonia	Empiric antibiotics based on age, history, physical examination, and laboratory studies	When clinically warranted

aged 2–6 months, bronchiolitis is a major cause of hospitalization. Epidemics occur in late fall and winter.

RSV is the most common etiologic agent, accounting for at least three quarters of all cases. Other viruses have been associated with bronchiolitis, including parainfluenza viruses 1 and 3, adenovirus, enterovirus, and influenza viruses. The infection is highly contagious; RSV infection develops in nearly half the infants of any given community during the first epidemic. RSV infections decrease in severity with age, suggesting that certain age-dependent anatomic determinants are important in the pathogenesis. In addition, there is a progressive reduction in severity after repeated infections, suggesting that immunity plays a role in mitigating the clinical course.

Clinically, the infant presents with rhinorrhea, cough, and a low-grade fever, followed within 1–2 days by the onset of rapid respirations, intercostal and subcostal retractions, and wheezing. The infant may be irritable, feed poorly, and vomit. Infants younger than 6 months may present with apnea before other signs of airway inflammation are present.

On physical examination, the hallmark is high respiratory rate, often greater than 50–60 breaths/min, associated with increased pulse rate, with or without fever. Other signs of URI include conjunctivitis, otitis media, and pharyngitis. Chest retractions are present, frequently with prolonged expiration. Often, wheezes or crackles are heard throughout the lungs. The respiratory distress may prevent adequate intake of fluids and may lead to dehydration. Cyanosis develops in a minority of patients, but severe gas-exchange abnormalities may be present without cyanosis. An increase in respiratory rate is a more sensitive indicator of impaired oxygenation: Respiratory rates of 60 or higher are frequently associated with reduction of partial pressure of arterial oxygen (Pao_2) and elevation of partial pressure of arterial carbon dioxide ($Paco_2$).

The radiographic appearance of bronchiolitis is nonspecific and includes diffuse hyperinflation of the lungs with flattening of the diaphragms, prominence of the retrosternal space, and bulging of the intercostal spaces. In most infants, patchy or peribronchial infiltrates are seen suggestive of interstitial pneumonia. Rarely, a small pleural effusion is observed.

Diagnosis of acute viral bronchiolitis is made by the clinical presentation, time of year, age of the child, and presence of epidemic of RSV in the community. Viral identification can be performed rapidly on nasal secretion using immunofluorescent techniques now available for RSV and most other respiratory viruses. This can be confirmed by viral culture of nasopharyngeal washings.

The treatment of bronchiolitis involves general supportive measure, such as IV hydration and administration of oxygen by air tent or cephalic hood. Aerosolized bronchodilators may provide transient improvement of the airway obstruction (see Table 9–28). Specific antiviral therapy is available, but its use is controversial and usually limited to severe cases of RSV bronchiolitis. Aerosolized ribavirin has been demonstrated to shorten the clinical course of the most severe cases. Its use also may be considered in patients with increased risk for serious infections, such as those with complex congenital heart disease, chronic lung disease, or multiple congenital anomalies. An additional concern regarding the use of ribavirin relates to possible toxic effects via environmental exposure by health care workers caring for patients receiving the medication. New delivery systems appear to be fairly effective in minimizing exposure to others.

Immunoglobulin therapy is currently a promising field of research. Its use both intravenously and aerosolized into the lower respiratory tract has been studied in both animal and human studies, and preliminary data look encouraging. Prophylaxis with IV γ-globulin for infants with significant risk factors for severe disease is also currently being studied.

ALVEOLAR INFECTIONS: PNEUMONIA

Infections of the alveoli are termed **pneumonitis** and **pneumonia.** Although most respiratory infections are mild or moderate in severity, some pathogens may be life-threatening. *S aureus* infection is aggressive and carries a high mortality rate in infants not treated promptly and properly.

Most bacterial pneumonias arise from invasion of the pathogen after an initial infection of the host with a respiratory virus. Consequent to the initial viral infection, the following factors enhance the risk of bacterial pneumonia development:

1. increases in the production of mucosal secretions, which are laden with bacteria
2. aspiration of the fluid into the lung
3. a decrease in ciliary activity resulting in diminished capacity to clear bacteria from the respiratory tract
4. a transient decrease in phagocytosis and bactericidal activity of alveolar macrophages.

Other predisposing factors include congenital anatomic defects, sequestration of a pulmonary lobe, tracheo-esophageal fistula, aspiration of fluid or foreign body, congenital or acquired immune defects, cystic fibrosis, and congestive heart failure.

Age is probably the single most important variable in determining the probable microorganisms involved. Because the URT is often colonized by human pathogens and normal flora, bacterial cultures obtained through the upper airway may not be conclusive. Detection of bacterial antigen in urine, serum, or nasopharyngeal secretions, or of viral antigen in nasopharyngeal secretions, may offer further diagnostic information. Usually, specific etiologic diagnosis can only be made if the bacterial pathogen is recovered from blood.

Viral Pneumonia

Influenza viruses cause disease predominantly in winter, and their incidence may vary yearly depending on the dominant strain. Death occurs predominantly in infants with underlying cardiorespiratory disease or from superimposed bacterial pneumonia. A protective role for passively acquired maternal antibody has been suggested but not proved.

Parainfluenza viruses also cause lower respiratory disease in young children. However, this infection more frequently presents as croup. Parainfluenza infection is not common in infants younger than 3 months; when it occurs, however, it is more prone to be associated with pneumonitis. Reinfections are less severe and often confined to the URT.

Bacterial Pneumonia

S Pneumoniae. Pneumonia due to *S pneumoniae* occurs most commonly in late winter and early spring, during the peak of viral respiratory infections. It presents typically with the abrupt onset of fever, restlessness, and respiratory distress, after an upper respiratory viral infection. Auscultation of the chest may reveal diminished breath sounds and fine crackles on the affected side, but these findings are less common in infants than in older children. Dullness on percussion may be caused by consolidation or by the presence of pleural effusion or empyema. Nuchal rigidity without meningeal infection may occur, with involvement of the right upper lobe. Laboratory studies usually reveal leukocytosis (15,000–40,000 WBC/mm); a WBC of less than 50,000/mm has been associated with a poor prognosis. A positive blood culture for *S pneumoniae* is diagnostic; however, bacteremia is found in fewer than 30% of cases. Lobar consolidation on chest radiograph is less common in infants than in older children. Parapneumonic effusion is relatively common.

Penicillin is the treatment of choice for pneumococcal pneumonia. Even with strains determined to have intermediate susceptibility to penicillin, drug levels in the lung are usually adequate. Erythromycin is an alternative choice if the patient is allergic to penicillin. With recent emergence of penicillin- and cephalosporin-resistant strains, vancomycin should be considered in a sick child until the sensitivity of the pathogen is determined.

H Influenzae. Before the introduction of HIB vaccine, the pathogen accounted for most cases of bacterial pneumonia in children younger than 5 years. On the basis of clinical findings and radiographs, it cannot be differentiated from pneumonia caused by other bacterial pathogens. It tends to produce a lobar pattern of consolidation, but disseminated pulmonary disease and bronchopneumonia have also been described. Empyema is often present in the young infant. Although it may be difficult to distinguish from pneumococcal pneumonia, it is more insidious in onset, and the course is usually prolonged over several weeks.

Diagnosis is established by isolation of the organism from blood, pleural fluid, lung aspirate, or bronchoscopic washings. Counter-immunoelectrophoresis or latex agglutination tests for *H influenzae* antigens on tracheal secretions, blood, urine, and pleural fluid may be helpful in making an early diagnosis. Suspected *H influenzae* pneumonia should be treated with IV cefuroxime; alternatively, third-generation cephalosporin (eg, cefotaxime), which offers excellent meningeal penetration if meningitis is a possible complication, can be used.

S Aureus. *S aureus* infection is common in children. It can cause a wide spectrum of diseases, ranging from mild furuncles to disseminated sepsis and toxic shock syndrome. *S aureus* infections are often difficult to treat because of antibiotic resistance of the organism, as well as its invasive nature and formation of sequestered sites of infection.

Because *S aureus* can colonize the respiratory tract, it can sometimes cause a primary pneumonia with a presentation similar to *S pneumoniae*. Alternatively, staphylococcal pneumonia can be a complication of bacteremia or septicemia arising from other sites. Clinically, it is important to be familiar with certain characteristic, ominous signs that distinguish staphylococci from other causes of pneumonia: (1) rapid progression of respiratory distress, (2) frequent formation of pneumatoceles, (3) empyema and pyopneumothorax due to rupture of pneumatoceles, and, most important of all, (4) toxic appearance of the patients with impending septic shock. Other sites of infection associated with staphylococcal pneumonia include otitis media, sinusitis, lymphadenitis, and periorbital cellulitis. Other complications include endocarditis, septic arthritis, and osteomyelitis. Thus, staphylococcal pneumonia is a serious infection that may evolve to become a medical emergency.

Diagnosis is established by isolation of the organism from blood, pleural fluid, lung aspirate, or bronchoscopic washings. Radiologic examination may show the various stages of the formation of pneumatoceles, empyema, and pyopneumothorax. In the presence of empyema, pleurocentesis should be performed, and the fluid should be sent for Gram stain and culture as well as measurement of total protein, glucose, and pH. If the pH is less than 7.2, it is usually suggestive of a pyogenic process.

The treatment of choice is IV administration of β-lactamase–resistant penicillin, such as nafcillin and cloxacillin, because most *S aureus* strains are capable of producing β-lactamase. Alternative drugs are first- and second-generation cephalosporins, such as cefazolin and cefuroxime. Cefixime, cefotaxime, and ceftriaxone are not recommended for treating staphylococcal infections. Other drugs, including clindamycin, erythromycin, and trimethoprim-sulfamethoxazole, may be useful. In the case of severe infections, combination therapy with nafcillin and an aminoglycoside or rifampin may be considered to provide synergistic effects. In recent years, it has been shown that certain strains adapt mutations that alter their penicillin-binding proteins, rendering the organisms resistant to all penicillin and cephalosporin products. These strains are known as methicillin-resistant *S aureus* (MRSA). The MRSA strains are sensitive to vancomycin. In the case of empyema, it is important to drain the pus, as an acidic and enclosed environment would inactivate β-lactam antibiotics, making them unable to exert their killing effects optimally. If indicated, a chest tube should be placed for continuous drainage.

Other Organisms: *Chlamydia, Mycoplasma, and Legionella.* As the incidence of bacterial and viral lower respiratory tract infections decreases with age, infections with other organisms, such as *C pneumoniae* and *M pneumoniae* represent an increasing percentage of disease in older children. *C pneumoniae* (TWAR) is more common in late childhood and in young adults and appears to exist worldwide. It is a distinct strain of *Chlamydia* that causes severe pharyngitis without exudate, laryngitis, fever, lymphadenopathy, and pneumonia. When pneumonia is present, usually only a single infiltrate is seen. The WBC usually is normal, and the ESR is elevated.

M pneumoniae is a major cause of respiratory infections in school-aged children and young adults. It is unusual before the age of 3–4 years, with a peak incidence at 10–15 years. Infection occurs through the respiratory route by large droplet spread, and the incubation period is thought to be 2–3 weeks. *M pneumoniae* accounts for

33% and 70%, respectively, of all pneumonias in children aged 5–9 years and 9–15 years. Previous infections, as demonstrated by the presence of circulating antibodies, prevent or ameliorate subsequent ones. Patients with immunodeficiency states or sickle-cell anemia have more severe mycoplasma infections than do normal hosts. *M pneumoniae* is the most common infectious cause of acute chest syndrome in patients with sickle-cell anemia.

In *M pneumoniae* infection, pneumonia, tracheobronchitis, and bronchopneumonia are the most commonly recognized clinical syndromes. Undifferentiated URT infections, pharyngitis, croup, bronchiolitis, otitis media, and bullous myringitis have been described. Patients with respiratory infections occasionally have multisystemic manifestations involving the skin, CNS (meningitis, encephalitis), heart (myocarditis or pericarditis), and joints (arthritis). Hematologic manifestations include mild degrees of hemolysis, as evidenced by a positive reaction to Coombs test, and minor reticulocytosis occurring 2–3 weeks after the onset of illness.

The onset of illness is gradual and is characterized by headache, malaise, and fever. Sore throat is frequent. Cough is prominent and usually worsens during the first 2 weeks of illness. All symptoms resolve gradually within 3–4 weeks. On physical examination, fine crackles are the most prominent sign.

Roentgenographic findings are nonspecific and are usually described as interstitial or bronchopneumonic; lower lobe involvement is the most common. Unilateral, centrally dense infiltrates are described in 75% of patients. Hilar lymphadenopathy may be seen in one third of patients. Pleural effusion is unusual but has been described. WBC and differential counts are usually normal.

A variety of serologic responses occur after *M pneumoniae* infection. Cold hemagglutinins develop late in the first or second week, appearing with titers of at least 1:32 in approximately 50% of patients. It increases by fourfold or more by the third week and lasts about 6 weeks. Specific IgG levels against *M pneumoniae* can be measured, and the diagnosis can be confirmed by a fourfold increase or decrease in the antibody level over 2–3 weeks (ie, acute and convalescent titers). Rapid diagnostic testing has not proved reliable, although a DNA probe assay is available that has shown good sensitivity and specificity. Cultures of the throat or sputum may demonstrate *M pneumoniae,* but these studies are not widely available.

Erythromycin and the tetracyclines are effective in shortening the course of mycoplasma illnesses. Erythromycin is the drug of choice in small children because of the risk of tetracycline toxicity in this age group. It should be given in full therapeutic doses for several days (usually 7–10) after defervescence. For patients older than 9 years, tetracycline is an alternate choice. Despite the efficacy of these drugs in ameliorating the clinical course, the organism may not be eradicated.

Legionella pneumonia is an entity that has been increasingly recognized in children over the past few years. Nosocomial cases are often linked to hospital water supplies. Children with underlying pulmonary disease or who are immunosuppressed seem to be at greatest risk. Increased incidence is probably reflective of improved methods of detection. Culture, direct fluorescent antibody testing, and urinary antigen detection systems currently are highly sensitive and specific. Clinical disease typically involves cough, fever, and often chest pain. Diarrhea and neurologic symptoms can also be seen. Therapy involves erythromycin or other macrolides. In the immunocompromised patient, a second drug may be beneficial. Nosocomial infections deserve careful investigation of water supplies and appropriate measures to decrease environmental reservoirs of the organism.

Afebrile Pneumonitis of Infancy

C trachomatis may cause up to one third of cases of pneumonia in infants aged 2–6 months. The illness is characterized by persistent cough, tachypnea, nonspecific abnormalities on chest radiograph, eosinophilia in the blood, and elevated specific immunoglobulin level. Clinical findings are often preceded by purulent conjunctivitis in the first 2 months after birth. Pneumonia usually is mild, but occasionally is severe.

Diagnosis can be made by staining a smear of nasopharyngeal specimen with fluorescein-conjugated monoclonal antibody against *C trachomatis,* which is available commercially. Infants with chlamydial pneumonia often have specific IgM antibodies, which is diagnostic. Specific IgG is only significant if found in levels at least fourfold greater than those of the mother, because of placental-fetal transfer.

Despite the absence of controlled clinical trials, therapy with erythromycin is believed to shorten the clinical illness significantly. For children who receive outpatient treatment, the combination of erythromycin and sulfisoxazole offers activity against *Chlamydia,* as well as other common bacterial pathogens.

P carinii infection may occur in infants younger than 1 year as an afebrile pneumonia, similar to *C trachomatis,* or in isolated patients with an underlying immunodeficiency. Infection is common and is acquired in early life, but most cases are subclinical.

Onset of symptoms in otherwise normal infants is slow and insidious. Nonspecific signs of restlessness, poor feeding, and diarrhea are common. Characteristically, fever is absent or low-grade. Cough, although not prominent, may appear later over 1–4 weeks. Eventually, patients exhibit increasingly severe tachypnea, dyspnea, and intercostal retractions and flaring of the nasal alae. Pulmonary physical findings consist primarily of fine crackles. Roentgenographic evidence of pulmonary infiltrates can be documented early in the course.

In most infants and older children with AIDS, *P carinii* pneumonia presents abruptly. High fever and nonproductive cough appear initially, followed by tachypnea and coryza. The course quickly progresses to full-blown disease with cyanosis and respiratory failure. Death may supervene if no treatment is given.

TUBERCULOSIS

M tuberculosis once was thought to be declining in incidence, with possibility of eradication. The past decade, however, has shown it to be a persistent and devious survivor. Tuberculosis in children remains an important cause of morbidity and mortality in the developing world. In the United States, tuberculosis is much less common; in certain populations, however, the disease is increasing in incidence and becoming increasingly drug resistant. Most cases occur in children younger than 1 year, with a median age of 3 years. The reservoir for infection in these children is adults with either newly acquired or reactivated disease. As with many infectious diseases, tuberculosis is closely associated with socioeconomic status and is most frequently found in areas of poverty and crowding.

Tuberculosis is transmitted by respiratory droplet from the cough or sneeze of an infected individual. This individual is usually an adult with numerous bacilli in a lung cavity. After inhalation by the host, the bacilli travel to the pulmonary alveoli and multiply. An inflammatory response is induced that involves mobilization of polymorphonuclear leukocytes and macrophages to surround the bacilli, forming the typical epithelioid cell tubercle. During the early stage of infection, some tubercle bacilli may enter the bloodstream and disseminate; this is especially more common in younger infants. Most bacilli are killed without establishing disease; others may progress or become quiescent. The first 12 months after primary infection is the time of greatest risk for dissemination. Children are especially susceptible to disseminated disease. Children younger than 5 years have a 4% chance of having meningitis or miliary tuberculosis; this risk then decreases but increases again at puberty. Bone infection with tuberculosis usually occurs 2–3 years after primary infection, and renal involvement occurs 2–3 years after that.

Four to six weeks after infection, delayed hypersensitivity to tuberculin develops, and skin testing with the PPD produces a positive reaction. Symptoms at this time usually are minimal, if any. Respiratory symptoms may be absent. The primary lesion becomes centrally necrotic (ie, the process of caseation), and the immune response walls off the area with collagen to form a capsule. At this point, the lesion either resolves completely, becomes fibrotic, or calcifies. On occasion the course of this primary complex is more acute, with progression to bronchopneumonia or lobar pneumonia. These patients frequently are febrile and have respiratory symptoms and night sweats.

Despite caseation or calcification of the parenchymal focus, viable tubercle bacilli may exist for years. The lymph nodes draining the primary lesion continue to enlarge, sometimes encroaching on adjacent structures, such as bronchi (5–20% in primary tuberculosis) or blood vessels. If the lymph node breaks though the wall of the bronchi or blood vessel, exuded infectious caseous material is then free to disseminate to other parts of the lungs or body. The infection may spread to involve the meninges, bones, superficial lymph nodes, and urinary tract.

Skin testing with 5 tuberculin units of PPD administered by the intradermal injection (Mantoux method) is helpful in establishing the presence of an infection but does not distinguish between past infection and active disease. The test should be read by trained medical personnel after 48–72 hours by measuring the induration but not the erythema at the test site. Interpretation of the skin test relies on knowledge of the individual's risk factors. An induration of 10 mm or more usually is considered to be a positive reaction. In the presence of suggestive history of exposure and symptoms and positive physical signs, even 5 mm or greater can be regarded as positive. These interpretation criteria were revised recently to reduce the high percentage of false-positive test results in populations with low disease prevalence. It must be emphasized that the Mantoux test is a screening test, and a negative reaction does not rule out the diagnosis of tuberculosis, especially in infants and in the immunocompromised host. Annual screening for tuberculosis is recommended in areas with high prevalence or in high-risk populations. Testing of low-risk individuals is dictated by local health departments.

Vaccination with bacillus Calmette-Guérin (BCG), an attenuated strain of *Mycobacterium bovis,* elicits immune response. Frequently in these children, a subsequent tuberculosis skin test will be reactive. A common situation arises when a child who has received BCG vaccine has a positive PPD reaction. The current recommendation is to ignore prior BCG administration and treat the individual on the basis of his or her risk group. Frequently, children who have received BCG are in a high-risk group because either they or their family members come from an area of high tuberculosis prevalence.

The diagnosis of tuberculosis is often difficult. Empiric therapy frequently is started on the basis of a reactive PPD or demonstration of acid fast bacilli from clinical specimens. *M tuberculosis* can be cultured from sputum, gastric aspirates, and other tissues. Cultures always should be performed to establish antimicrobial sensitivity patterns. *M tuberculosis* is a slow-growing organism, frequently requiring up to 6 weeks to grow in culture. Newer molecular biologic techniques, such as DNA probes and PCR assays, have allowed more rapid identification of *M tuberculosis* from clinical specimens such as sputum and CSF.

Central to the treatment of tuberculosis is the potential for the development of drug resistance in a heterogeneous population of bacilli. Traditional treatment for tuberculo-

sis includes three or four different antituberculosis medications for extended periods of time. Characteristic properties of select antimycobacterial drugs and the various therapeutic regimens are summarized in Tables 9–29 and 9–30. Individuals likely to be infected with drug-resistant strains initially should be treated with four antituberculosis medications. Immunocompromised individuals require longer and frequently lifetime treatment for tuberculosis.

The most commonly encountered clinical scenario is that of the immunocompetent child with a reactive Mantoux test result with unknown exposure. Frequently, such a child is the marker for an index case within the family, and contacts should be investigated aggressively. If a complete physical examination and chest radiograph fail to demonstrate active tuberculosis, the child should begin a 9-month course of isoniazid. Isoniazid prophylaxis in this setting has decreased the complication rate by 88% over a 10-year period and completely prevented tuberculous meningitis and miliary tuberculosis.

Effective prevention of tuberculosis relies on rapid identification and therapy of infected individuals. Currently, vaccination with BCG is used in Europe and in many developing countries. Immunization with BCG does not prevent primary infection with *M tuberculosis,* but has been shown to reduce the incidence of hematogenous spread and severe pulmonary disease by 20–80%; therefore, it does protect against tuberculous meningitis, miliary tuberculosis, and bone and joint infection.

In the United States, BCG has been used for PPD-negative children who have continued and unavoidable exposure to adults with active tuberculosis. Use of the vaccine is contraindicated in children and adults with underlying immunodeficiencies, including infection with HIV.

CENTRAL NERVOUS SYSTEM INFECTIONS

Infections of the CNS are more common in children than in adults. They pose two great potential dilemmas to pediatric practitioners because of the following issues:

Table 9–29. Antituberculosis chemotherapy.

Drug	Unique Features	Toxicity	Dose (mg/kg)
Isoniazid (INH)	CSF penetration	Hepatic, rare peripheral neuritis	10
Rifampicin (RIF)	CSF penetration	Hepatic, gastrointestinal tract	10
Pyrazinamide (PZA)	Intracellularly active; CSF penetration	Hepatic, gastrointestinal tract, rash	15–30
Streptomycin	Penetrates inflamed meninges; resistance develops rapidly; used in combination therapy; IM administration	Ototoxicity, rare nephrotoxicity	20–40
Ethambutol (EMB)	Bacteriostatic	Optic nerve toxicity	25

CSF = cerebrospinal fluid; IM = intramuscular.

Table 9–30. Recommended therapy for tuberculosis infection and exposure.

PPD (+) without disease	INH × 9 months
TB exposure	
PPD (−)	INH × 3 months; repeat PPD; if negative discontinue
PPD (+)	INH × 9 months if disease workup negative
Pulmonary TB	
Sensitive organism	INH, RIF, PZA × 2 months, followed by INH, RIF × 4 months
Suspect resistant organism	INH, RIF, EMB, PZA × 2 months, followed by INH, RIF, EMB × 6 months until sensitivities available
TB meningitis, bone/ joint disease	INH, RIF, PZA, streptomycin × 2 months, followed by INH, RIF × 10 months

INH = isoniazid; PPD = purified protein derivative; PZA = pyrazinamide; RIF = rifampin; TB = tuberculosis.

(1) the nonspecific nature of signs and symptoms often associated with these CNS infections, especially in infants, and (2) reluctance to perform invasive procedures in infants and children. These concerns, coupled with the serious nature of the processes, make CNS infections in the pediatric population a complex and challenging issue. The following discussion of common types of CNS infection seen in children is organized by etiologic agent and clinical syndrome.

Meningitis refers to inflammation of the meninges resulting in clinical presentation with neck stiffness, fever, headache, and irritability. CSF findings include abnormal number of leukocytes and, often, abnormalities in protein and glucose concentrations. Often meningitis is categorized as either septic or aseptic, implying a bacterial or nonbacterial etiology. This preliminary categorization is based on clinical presentation and the CSF findings and does not necessarily predict the actual pathogen accurately.

BACTERIAL MENINGITIS

Clinical Presentation

Usually a child or infant with septic or bacterial meningitis is acutely ill. This diagnosis is one of the most dreaded in pediatrics because it is potentially a rapidly fatal disease. Even with prompt, appropriate diagnosis and treatment, morbidity can be quite high. The risk for long-term CNS sequelae is related to many factors, including the specific pathogen, presence of underlying disease states, timeliness, age of the patient, and appropriateness of treatment.

In the neonate, signs can be variable and quite nonspecific. These include irritability, poor feeding, hyper- or hypothermia, lethargy, vomiting, seizures, bulging fontanelle, and poor tone. Because neonatal meningitis is often associated with generalized sepsis, other signs not related to the CNS, such as hypotension, jaundice, and respiratory distress, may be seen.

Neonates are at risk for development of meningitis partly because of intrinsic defects in their immune system, such as alterations in cytokine synthesis and impaired immune-cell function. These factors, together with perinatal exposure to bacteria colonized in the maternal gastrointestinal and genitourinary tract, help to explain why the highest incidence of meningitis is seen in the neonatal period.

Older children with meningitis may have similar signs, although fever is typically present. Symptoms may include headache. In older children, the Kernig and Brudzinski signs may be present, reflecting meningeal irritation and neck rigidity. The Kernig sign is performed by flexing the hip and knee, then extending the knee with the hip still flexed. Pain in the back and neck region with this maneuver represents a positive test result. The Brudzinski maneuver is considered positive if the hips flex when the neck is passively flexed. Other signs include altered consciousness, vomiting, and photophobia.

Progression of the disease can be quite variable, depending on such factors as age of the patient, specific organism, and therapy. Focal neurologic signs may develop with time or even be seen on presentation. Paresis, cranial nerve palsies, papilledema, and papillary abnormalities may result because of increased intracranial pressure or even vascular thrombosis.

Mechanisms of bacterial invasion remain similar for all age groups in septic meningitis. The disease usually begins with a viral infection of the URT with subsequent bacterial attachment to the mucosa and invasion of the bloodstream. Through hematogenous seeding of the meninges and CSF, the bacteria encounter a rich nutrient environment relatively deficient in host defense antibodies, phagocytes, and complement, where they multiply rapidly. Bacterial components, such as the lipopolysaccharides of gram-negative bacteria, lead to production of inflammatory cytokines. These substances, notably interleukin-1, platelet-activating factor, and tumor necrosis factor-α (TNF-α or cachectin) lead to chemotaxis and activation of granulocytes, stimulation of phagocytosis, activation of the complement cascade, and permeability changes in the blood-brain barrier. These developments result in brain edema, increased intracranial pressure, and decreased blood flow to the brain. Decreased transport of glucose across the blood-CSF barrier due to inflammation and increased use results in hypoglycorrhachia. Purulent exudate may cover the surface of the brain, spinal cord, and the ventricles.

Etiology & Epidemiology

Specific pathogens are associated with certain age groups as well as underlying conditions (Table 9–31). The most common pathogens in the neonatal period include group B *Streptococcus, E coli,* and *L monocytogenes.* Other less frequently seen bacteria include *Klebsiella, En-*

Table 9–31. Bacterial pathogens in meningitis and empiric therapy by age group.[1]

Age Group	Likely Organisms	Empiric Therapy
Neonate	Group B *Streptococcus, Escherichia coli* and other gram-negative organisms, *Listeria monocytogenes*	Ampicillin + gentamicin or ampicillin + cefotaxime
1–3 mo	Group B *Streptococcus* (late onset), *Streptococcus pneumoniae,* and rarely, *L monocytogenes*	Vancomycin with either ampicillin + gentamicin or ampicillin + cefotaxime
3 mo–3 y	*S pneumoniae, Haemophilus influenzae,* and *Neisseria meningitidis*	Vancomycin with either cefotaxime or ceftriaxone
3–12 y	*S pneumoniae, N meningitidis,* and occasionally, *H influenzae*	Vancomycin with either cefotaxime or ceftriaxone
12 y–adult	*S pneumoniae* and *N meningitidis*	Vancomycin with either cefotaxime or ceftriaxone

[1]Empiric use of vancomycin must be customized depending on the incidence of *S pneumoniae* resistance to penicillin and cephalosporins in the community.

terobacter, Serratia, and *Hemophilus* species. Occasionally, *S pneumoniae* and *Enterococcus* species are seen as pathogens in neonatal meningitis.

In infants aged 1–3 months, the primary pathogens are group B *Streptococcus* and *S pneumoniae.* Infection with group B *Streptococcus* at this time is termed "late-onset" and is somewhat different in its presentation than its neonatal counterpart. HIB, *N meningitides,* and *Salmonella* also are seen less commonly.

From 3 months to 3 years of age, HIB, *N meningitides,* and *S pneumoniae* are the most common agents of bacterial meningitis. The advent of *H influenzae* vaccines during the past decade has markedly decreased the incidence of HIB invasive diseases, including meningitis and epiglottitis.

From 3 to 12 years of age, the incidence of septic meningitis decreases significantly, with the most common pathogens being *S pneumoniae, N meningitides,* and, occasionally, *H influenzae.* In older children and adults, *S pneumoniae* and *N meningitides* predominate.

Certain conditions, both congenital and traumatically acquired, predispose children to specific types of bacterial meningitis. For example, children with galactosemia have an increased susceptibility to *E coli* infection and meningitis. Patients with asplenia, sickle-cell disease, nephrotic syndrome, and deficiencies of IgG2 and IgG4 have an increased incidence of septicemia and meningitis associated with the encapsulated organisms such as *S pneumoniae* and HIB. Recurrent *N meningitidis* infections are seen in children with C5–C8 complement system defects. Children with anatomic defects, such as congenital dermal sinus and traumatic CSF leaks, are at risk from a variety of gram-positive and gram-negative organisms. Staphylococcal meningitis is rare except in patients with ventriculoperitoneal shunts for the treatment of hydrocephalus. In most cases, the predominant organism is coagulase-negative *Staphylococcus.*

Specific Organisms

Several types of bacterial meningitis deserve a more de-

tailed description of both their clinical syndromes as well as their pathophysiology. Meningitis caused by group B *Streptococcus* (GBS), *S pneumoniae, H influenzae,* and *N meningitidis* will be discussed.

GBS is the most common cause of neonatal meningitis in the United States. Female gastrointestinal and genitourinary tract colonization occurs in up to one third of pregnant women. Unfortunately, colonization can be intermittent and, because it is usually asymptomatic, cultures performed on the mother are of little value unless obtained intra- or peripartum. Maternal prophylaxis with IV antibiotics in high-risk situations probably decreases the incidence of neonatal disease and is the standard of care. Despite these efforts, GBS infection continues to be a major cause of neonatal morbidity and mortality in developed countries. This organism is responsible for distinct clinical syndromes characterized by early and late onset of disease. Early-onset disease classically occurs within the first 72 hours postnatally. Presentation involves respiratory distress with pneumonia, sepsis, and meningitis in approximately 30% of cases. The profound shock and respiratory insufficiency are usually the most problematic aspects of this disease for the clinician. Late-onset GBS infections usually occur around 2–4 weeks of age and are less severe than early-onset disease. Presentation can occur up to 4 months of age. Meningitis is seen more often in late-onset disease, occurring in more than three quarters of infants with this clinical syndrome.

H influenzae meningitis is seen less and less in developed countries with improved immunization schedules. HIB is an encapsulated form that is associated with more invasive disease than other strains. This strain often is the pathogen seen in such childhood diseases as otitis media, sinusitis, epiglottis, pneumonia, and bacteremia. By age 5 years, most children have natural immunity to this strain and rarely manifest invasive HIB disease.

H influenzae meningitis is seen more frequently from October to November and from February to April. The incidence is increased in day-care centers and is greater among African-Americans, Alaskan Eskimos, Apaches, and Navajos. The increased incidence in African-Americans may be due to socioeconomic factors. The suboptimal living conditions and greater exposure of Navajos and Alaskan Eskimos, as well as decreased natural antibody titers and responsiveness to HIB vaccines, may be important factors in their higher rates of infection. Unvaccinated children in close contact with a household member in whom invasive disease has developed are at increased risk for infection. Prophylactic treatment with antibiotics (usually rifampin because of its nasopharyngeal mucosal penetration) is suggested for all members of households, including the patient, in which there is a child younger than 4 years. Alternatively, ceftriaxone can be used for prophylaxis. Children younger than 1 year who have had invasive disease are at risk for recurrence and should be vaccinated.

N meningitidis is a frequent cause of meningitis in children younger than 5 years, although it can be seen in any age group. There are at least 13 serogroups; A, B, C, and W135 are most prevalent in the United States. Disease can follow colonization of the URT after exposure to another colonized or infected person. This gram-negative diplococcus is capable of producing two distinct clinical entities, meningococcemia or meningitis, as well as a combination of both. Often, disseminated disease associated with meningococcemia is a much more fulminant, devastating process, even with prompt and appropriate therapy. With disseminating disease, the onset of sepsis is abrupt. Fever, chills, and prostration occur. Rash is common, usually initially pink colored and maculopapular. This initial form quickly changes into the more classic petechial or purpuric rash notoriously associated with this disease. Other focuses of infection include pericarditis, endocarditis, and pneumonia. In meningococcal meningitis without sepsis, the usual presenting signs and symptoms are fever, headache, malaise, meningismus, and altered mental status.

S pneumoniae is a gram-positive diplococcus that can be responsible for various diseases in pediatrics, including otitis media, pneumonia, sinusitis, and bacteremia. Meningitis caused by this pathogen can be quite severe, with a relatively high degree of associated morbidity and mortality. Predisposing host factors include hemoglobinopathy, status post-splenectomy, suppurative otitis media or sinusitis, and CSF leak. Transmission is via contact with respiratory secretions with incubation from 1 to 30 days. Presentation is similar to that of other types of non-neonatal septic meningitis.

L monocytogenes is a β-hemolytic gram-positive rod that can cause both neonatal sepsis and meningitis. Early-onset disease usually presents with pneumonia or sepsis and is acquired through transplacental or ascending intrauterine infection. Late-onset disease occurs after the first postnatal week and may result in meningitis. It is acquired during or after birth. Maternal infection may occur from ingestion of contaminated dairy products.

Diagnosis

Diagnosis of meningitis usually centers on evidence of inflammation in the CSF. A lumbar puncture must be performed when there is clinical suspicion of meningitis unless contraindicated by such factors as intracranial hypertension, an overlying infectious skin lesion, or severe clinical instability, making technical performance of spinal tap impossible. Because infants are at increased risk for meningitis associated with sepsis and because signs of meningitis in them can be nonspecific and variable, the clinician should maintain a very low threshold for performing a lumbar puncture in an infant.

The CSF findings for a child with bacterial meningitis usually include leukocytosis, increased protein concentration, and hypoglycorrhachia. In pediatrics, it is important to know that normal values for these parameters vary with age (Table 9–32). Other factors to be considered when evaluating CSF findings include history of previous antibiotic administration and prior traumatic lumbar punctures. A maternal history of antibiotic administration before delivery will affect the clinical course and laboratory findings in the newborn. Unfortunately, no hard and fast rules exist on how these factors influence the CSF. Various formulas that attempt to correct for these factors cannot be relied on.

Gram stain of the CSF may provide invaluable and immediate information that can aid the clinician in selecting an antibiotic before culture results are known. Occasionally, the Gram stain will reveal bacteria even before pleocytosis develops, especially in the case of pneumococcal or meningococcal meningitis.

Other diagnostic aids include latex agglutination testing, which detects bacterial antigen in the CSF. This test is most helpful in the setting of prior antibiotic therapy, which may interfere with culture results. Unfortunately, this test is neither very sensitive nor specific.

Blood culture should be obtained in the setting of suspected meningitis. Results may be positive in up to 90% of cases of *H influenzae* and meningococcal meningitis and 80% of pneumococcal meningitis. In neonates, there is a high correlation between positive blood cultures and CSF cultures in meningitis due to *H influenzae* and *S pneumoniae* and a lower correlation in meningitis due to GBS and *N meningitidis*. Initial investigations should also include peripheral WBC and differential count. Normal-appearing CSF does not completely rule out the possibility of meningitis. If cultures are sterile, causes of aseptic meningitis syndrome must be considered.

Table 9–32. Normal values of cerebrospinal fluid (CSF) in children.

	Neonates (< 1 mo)	Infants (> 1 mo)
White blood cell count	< 30	< 10
Percent neutrophils	60	0
Protein levels (mg/mL)	< 90	< 40
Glucose levels	70–80	50–60

Management

Empiric treatment for presumed bacterial meningitis includes antibiotics, fluid and electrolyte management, and, in specific cases, steroid therapy. In the setting of concurrent sepsis and/or significant neurologic compromise, other supportive measures may also be necessary. These may include the use of anticonvulsants, means to decrease cerebral hypertension or hydrocephalus, and ventilatory support.

Antibiotic therapy should be initiated promptly (see Table 9–31). In the neonate, appropriate coverage for GBS, coliforms, and *Listeria* should be instituted. Cefotaxime with ampicillin or gentamicin with ampicillin are appropriate choices. Cefotaxime is a better choice than other third-generation cephalosporins in that it does not displace bilirubin from serum proteins. Because *Listeria* is less of a concern in infants older than 3 months, most clinicians would discontinue using ampicillin in empiric therapy after this age.

Because of increasing resistance to penicillin and cephalosporins among *S pneumoniae* isolates, empiric therapy for infants and children older than 1 month with bacterial streptococcal meningitis should include vancomycin in addition to cefotaxime or ceftriaxone, as well as ampicillin if the patient is at risk for *Listeria*. Once the organism is identified and sensitivities determined, antibiotic therapy can be tailored appropriately.

Traditionally, the use of steroids in the management of meningitis has been considered controversial. More recently, several studies have demonstrated some benefit from the use of steroids in *H influenzae* meningitis. This benefit was demonstrated when steroids were given before or concomitantly with antibiotics. The rationale behind administration of steroids before or concurrent with antibiotic administration involves potential attenuation of the bacteriolytic inflammatory response associated with antibiotic administration. The benefit is probably most pronounced in infants and children with profound alterations in consciousness or cerebral hypertension. Different studies demonstrate different degrees of benefits. Although the decision on the use of steroids is not completely settled, many experts recommend their use under specific circumstances. The Costa Rica study demonstrated not only a statistically significant decrease in the incidence of one or more neurologic sequelae, but also a trend toward reduction of audiologic impairment in infants and children treated with dexamethasone before the initiation of antibiotic therapy versus antibiotic therapy alone. Of note, in most studies on the use of steroids, no differences were observed between mortality rates with or without adjunctive steroid therapy. Most experts would recommend the use of IV dexamethasone (0.15 mg/kg) given at the beginning of antimicrobial therapy and every 6 hours for 16 doses for suspected cases of bacterial meningitis and for proven *H influenzae* meningitis. On occasions, upper gastrointestinal bleeding has been reported as a complication with adjunctive steroid use in the management of patients with meningitis.

The patient must be monitored closely for the development of complications. Frequent physical and neurologic examinations, including daily measurement of head circumference in infants, should be performed. The status of electrolytes, body weight, and urine specific gravity should be followed to look for evidence of the syndrome of inappropriate secretion of antidiuretic hormone. This syndrome is usually transient and managed by fluid restriction if the patient is not hypovolemic or does not have decreased blood pressure. Other acute complications include toxic encephalopathy, cerebral edema, transtentorial herniation, cranial nerve palsies, deafness, seizures, subdural effusion, cerebral infarction, and cortical vein thrombosis. Subdural effusion is common and rarely lasts more than 3 months. Invasive therapy for subdural effusion is usually not required unless there are focal neurologic changes.

Long-term sequelae may include hearing deficit, seizures, language disorder, mental retardation, motor abnormalities, visual impairment, behavior disorders, learning disorders, attention deficits, and decreased intelligence quotients. Hearing loss, the most frequent complication, most often follows meningitis due to *S pneumoniae*, followed by meningitis due to *N meningitidis* and *H influenzae* (Table 9–33). Age of onset and duration of illness before treatment do not affect hearing loss. All children should undergo hearing evaluation after meningitis.

ASEPTIC MENINGITIS

Aseptic meningitis, a syndrome involving the CNS, is characterized by a mostly lymphocytic CSF pleocytosis, evidence of meningeal irritation on clinical examination, and history consistent with meningitis. However, there are no significant changes in level of consciousness, no growth on routine bacterial cultures, and no obvious etiologic agent on routine stains (Table 9–34). A wide variety of pathologic processes can cause this syndrome (Table 9–35).

Table 9–33. Complications of bacterial meningitis.

Complications
  Hearing loss—most common
  Visual impairment
  Neurologic deficits: hemiparesis, hypertonia, motor deficits, seizures, hydrocephalus
  Mental retardation, learning and behavioral disorders, attention deficits, language disorder
Follow-up evaluations
  Hearing tests
  Vision examinations
  Neurologic assessment: physical examination, electroencephalogram; when indicated, radiologic imaging including computed tomography and magnetic resonance imaging scans
  Psychological tests
  Language and learning assessment

Table 9–34. Characteristics of "septic" versus "aseptic" meningitis.

	"Septic"— Typically Bacterial	"Aseptic"— Usually Viral
Presentation	Usually acutely ill; no seasonal pattern	May be more insidious or chronic; often seasonal
CSF WBC	Pleocytosis usually > 1000 cells/mm^3	Pleocytosis usually hundreds to a few thousand cells/mm^3
CSF glucose concentration	Typically low, ie, < 40 mg/dL	May range from low to normal
CSF protein concentration	Elevated, usually 100–500 mg/dL	May range from normal to mildly elevated

CSF = cerebrospinal fluid; WBC = white blood cell count.

Viral Causes of Aseptic Meningitis

Viral causes for aseptic meningitis are very common, although outcomes and presentations can be quite variable depending on the specific virus (Table 9–36).

Enteroviruses. These RNA viruses belong to the picornavirus family and can cause a variety of illnesses, including gastroenteritis, URIs, conjunctivitis, rashes, hepatitis, myositis, myocarditis, and pericarditis. Enteroviruses commonly cause aseptic meningitis. Encephalitis also can occur, although this presentation of enteroviral disease is uncommon. However, in neonates with X-linked hypogammaglobulinemia, enterovirus can cause a chronic form of meningoencephalitis, which can be fatal.

Table 9–35. Aseptic meningitis: Etiology.

Infection	
Viral	
Bacterial	Mycobacterium tuberculosis
	Leptospira
	Syphilis
	Borrelia (Lyme disease)
	Nocardia
	Partially treated
Rickettsial	Rocky Mountain spotted fever
Mycoplasmal	Mycoplasma pneumoniae, Mycoplasma hominis
Fungal	Coccidioides, Blastomyces, Histoplasma, Cryptococcus
Protozoan	Toxoplasma, Malaria, Amebiasis, Cysticercosis
Post-vaccination	Influenza, rabies
Drugs	Trimethoprim-sulfamethoxazole, intrathecal drugs
Toxins	Heavy metals (eg, lead, mercury, and arsenic compounds)
Vascular	Collagen vascular diseases, hemorrhage, thrombosis
Neoplastic	Metastatic tumors, primary meningioma
Foreign bodies	Ventriculoperitoneal shunts, pressure monitors
Other	Kawasaki disease

Table 9–36. Viral meningitis: Etiology.

Enterovirus (most common)	Coxsackievirus, echovirus, poliovirus
Arbovirus	St. Louis encephalitis
	Eastern equine encephalitis
	Western equine encephalitis
	Venezuelan equine encephalitis
	Powassan and California encephalitis
Mumps, measles, rubella	
Herpes simplex virus	
Adenovirus	
Varicella, Epstein-Barr virus, cytomegalovirus	
Influenza, parainfluenza	

Otherwise, most enteroviral diseases, including meningitis, resolve spontaneously, leaving minimal, if any, sequelae. Transmission is by the fecal-oral route and is most prevalent during summer and fall.

Poliovirus. Poliovirus is an enteroviral infection that usually is asymptomatic but may present as aseptic meningitis with paralytic lower neuron disease. Given widespread immunization practices, poliomyelitis is rare in the United States, with most cases representing vaccine-related or imported diseases. Current vaccine schedules in the United States include the use of an attenuated live oral vaccine. However, a trend exists toward the use of the inactivated polio vaccine in the first year, primarily to control the occurrence of vaccine-related disease, which accounts for 10–20 cases a year in the United States. The virus is excreted in the feces for several weeks to months after vaccination with live virus. If the patient is known or suspected to be immunocompromised, or if the patient's close contacts are immunocompromised, inactivated poliovirus should be used.

Diagnosis of viral meningitis is often aided by negative routine bacterial cultures in the context of appropriate physical signs, season, and CSF findings. CSF viral cultures can be helpful, but sensitivity is often quite variable (50–75% for enteroviral CSF cultures). Stool viral culture by itself may provide additional evidence of enteroviral infection, but the result is not diagnostic of enteroviral meningitis. Typical CSF WBCs are lower than that of septic meningitis (ie, 100–1000/mm^3). Although a polymorphonuclear cell pleocytosis can be seen early in the disease, just as in bacterial meningitis, this usually changes over rapidly to a lymphocytic predominance within 12–48 hours. The hypoglycorrhachia seen in aseptic meningitis is usually much milder or absent. Elevations in CSF protein concentration are usually much milder than that seen in bacterial disease.

Mumps Virus. Mumps is a known cause of aseptic meningitis and encephalitis, which may be associated with neuritis or myelitis. CNS involvement may occur 1 week before or up to 3 weeks after the onset of parotitis. Lethargy, nuchal rigidity, photophobia, and vomiting are common manifestations. This form of meningitis is usually self-limiting and has an excellent prognosis.

Nonviral Causes of Aseptic Meningitis

Mycobacteria. *M tuberculosis* was once a very common cause of meningitis in young children. During the latter half of this century, screening, effective therapy, and general improvement in public health measures had drastically decreased the incidence of mycobacterial disease in this country. In the past decade or so, however, tuberculosis and mycobacterial disease have experienced a resurgence, particularly in patients with AIDS. Tubercular meningitis usually occurs within the first 12 months after a primary infection and is most commonly seen in children younger than 5 years. The onset is subacute, and symptoms are classically quite nonspecific. Fever, listlessness, headache, and anorexia are common during the first 1–2 weeks. These symptoms can progress to involve more significant changes in level of consciousness, cranial nerve deficits, evidence of meningismus, peripheral tremor, and deep tendon reflex abnormalities. Without treatment, opisthotonos, hemiplegia or paraplegia, and coma can develop, and the patient will ultimately die. CSF findings seen in tubercular meningitis typically have WBCs of 10–8500 cells/mm^3 with a lymphocyte predominance, although early in the disease one may see a large number of neutrophils. CSF glucose concentrations initially are normal, later becoming lower. Protein concentrations are characteristically elevated, becoming extremely high in advanced disease. Presumptive diagnosis is usually made on the basis of CSF findings and symptomatology. CT or MRI studies may show a basilar exudate. Definitive diagnosis involves CSF cultures, which traditionally are positive in 45–90% of cases and can take up to 8 weeks to grow. Acid fast stains of CSF are rarely positive, although using large volumes and multiple lumbar taps increases positivity. PPD testing or positive chest radiographs are seen in only about half the cases, although PPD results usually become positive later in the course of the disease. Therapy involves multiple antimycobacterials, usually including isoniazid, rifampin, and pyrazinamide. Adjunctive use of corticosteroids is recommended in the case of advanced disease. Mortality remains high at 20% in children younger than 5 years.

Spirochetes. Three spirochetes that can infect the CNS are *Leptospira, Borrelia burgdorferi,* and *T pallidum.* Leptospirosis is an uncommon zoonosis seen in the United States that is transmitted by contact with urine from infected animals, such as dogs, livestock, or rodents. Clinical disease can be quite mild to fulminant (Weil syndrome) and is usually biphasic in nature. Leptospiremia, fever, and headache are the most common findings during the first 4–7 days of the initial phase. The second phase occurs after 1–3 days of improvement and marks the beginning of the immunologic response to this disease, during which rash, uveitis, and meningitis are seen. The meningitis usually lasts for 2–3 days. CSF findings typi-

cally reveal fewer than 500 white blood cells/mm^3 of CSF with a mononuclear cell predominance. Usually, glucose concentration is normal and protein is normal to elevated. Leptospira usually cannot be cultured from the CSF during the period when the patient exhibits clinical meningitis, only during the initial phase of the disease. A more severe form of the disease (Weil syndrome) occurs in 10% of patients and is characterized by fever, jaundice, hemorrhage, altered states of consciousness, and renal insufficiency. Diagnosis is usually made by isolation of the leptospires from body fluid or tissues. Antibody test may be helpful in the second stage of the disease, when CSF and blood cultures are likely sterile. PCR techniques for detection of leptospire DNA currently are under development for clinical use. Treatment regimens are controversial, but penicillin G or ampicillin is usually recommended for moderate to severe disease.

B burgdorferi can cause a form of meningitis in Lyme disease. The diagnosis is made clinically by characteristic rash and history of tick bite. Meningitis is just one neurologic manifestation of Lyme disease. Others include facial palsy, encephalitis, chorea, and radiculoneuropathy. Diagnosis is primarily based on clinical presentation, history of tick exposure, and positive serology for *B burgdorferi.* Treatment depends on stage of the disease; for neuroborreliosis, however, treatment usually involves IV ceftriaxone, cefotaxime, or penicillin G.

Syphilis, caused by the spirochete *T pallidum,* is a disease that can involve many organ systems. It can affect the CNS in both congenital and acquired infection, causing an aseptic meningitis–like syndrome. In acquired syphilis, neurosyphilis appears decades after the initial infection. The CSF may show increased protein concentration, increased WBC, and a positive Venereal Disease Research Laboratory (VDRL) test result. A negative VDRL result does not exclude neurosyphilis. The result of the fluorescent treponemal antibody absorption test (FTA-ABS) in the newborn can be positive because of immunoglobulin being passively transferred from the mother. Patients with congenital neurosyphilis should have repeated evaluation of CSF every 6 months for 3 years or until CSF has returned to normal. Treatment for congenital neurosyphilis is penicillin. If the result of CSF VDRL testing is still reactive after 6 months, the child should again receive treatment.

Fungi. Fungal infections of the CNS are not common in children. The organisms most frequently seen are *C neoformans, C immitis,* and *H capsulatum.*

C neoformans infections of the CNS are seen most commonly in patients with immunologic defects involving T-cell–mediated functions. *C neoformans* is a common CNS pathogen in adult patients with AIDS but is much less common in the pediatric AIDS population. This encapsulated yeast is found in bird droppings and soil. It can cause a wide spectrum of disease involving lungs, myocardium, bone, and skin in addition to the CNS. Meningitis caused by *C neoformans* may be acute or chronic, often dependent on degree of immunosuppression seen in the host. Diagnosis can be made by identification of the or-

are similar to other types of viral encephalitis but may be more severe. Seizures and coma are common. The CSF often has an increased WBC with a predominance of polymorphonuclear leukocytes. Diagnosis is made by serologic studies or brain biopsy. Mortality rates are high, and survivors often are left with significant morbidity, especially neurologic sequelae.

St. Louis encephalitis, the most common arbovirus in the United States, occurs most frequently along states bordering the Ohio and Mississippi rivers. The virus is spread by mosquitoes that breed in irrigated farmland in rural areas and in stagnant sewage in cities. Birds are reservoirs. Morbidity and mortality rates are higher in the elderly. Death and sequelae in children are rare.

California encephalitis (La Crosse encephalitis) is caused by several California serogroup viruses and has a widespread distribution in the United States and Canada. The disease is most common in the upper Midwest. The virus is spread by mosquitoes living in hardwood forests. Animals such as squirrels are reservoirs. Encephalitis occurs mainly in children aged 5–10 years. The initial illness may be accompanied by seizures and stupor. Sequelae may include behavior changes and learning disability. There is no specific treatment.

Western equine encephalitis is a togavirus transmitted by mosquitoes from avian reservoirs. Equine outbreaks often precede human disease. The disease occurs in the central and western United States and Canada and in South America. Infants are at greatest risk for neurologic sequelae. There is no treatment.

Other Causes

Rabies. Rabies is caused by an RNA virus classified as a rhabdovirus. Transmission usually occurs as a result of an animal bite, with the virus present in saliva. Airborne infection also has been reported in bat caves. The disease has also been reported after corneal transplantation, when it was unknown that the donor died of rabies. Reservoirs of the disease in the United States are mainly wild animals.

After a bite from an infected animal, the virus is inoculated into subcutaneous tissue and muscle. The virus replicates slowly, and symptoms usually appear 1–3 months after the bite. Areas with greater nerve supply (fingers, genitalia, face) have shorter incubation periods than arm or leg bites. Children also have shorter incubation periods.

The virus ascends the infected peripheral nerve to the spinal cord, where it selectively infects the limbic system and then the rest of the brain. Patients may initially have pain and numbness at the inoculation site, with a prodrome of anxiety, malaise, and headache. This progresses to an encephalomyelitis with apprehension, delirium, meningismus, and mildly convulsive movements. Attempts to swallow or even the sight of water can result in painful laryngospasm (hydrophobia). A smaller percentage ·of patients may present with an ascending paralysis similar to the Guillain-Barré syndrome. Patients usually die of aspiration secondary to laryngospasm or of arrhythmias due to viral myocarditis.

Fluorescent antibody staining can detect virus in corneal epithelium and in skin samples. Antibodies to rabies can be detected in nonimmunized individuals about a week after onset of symptoms. Diagnosis of rabies in the biting animal can be made by fluorescent antibody staining of brain tissue. After a bite injury to a child, domestic animals should be observed for 10 days, as dogs and cats can shed the virus in saliva up to 12 days before they demonstrate symptoms. If no symptoms appear in the biting animal, immunotherapy for the child is not indicated.

Exposed individuals are treated by immunoprophylaxis. In the United States, skunks, raccoons, and bats are more likely to be infected, followed by foxes, coyotes, cattle, dogs, and cats. Rabies is rare in rodents, rabbits, and hares. When the decision to treat is made, all individuals must receive passive and active immunization. Passive immunity is achieved with rabies immunoglobulin; one half the dose is infiltrated in the wound, and the other half given intramuscularly. Active immunization is achieved by giving human diploid cell vaccine intramuscularly.

Cerebral Malaria. This is the most severe complication of *P falciparum* infections. It affects children almost exclusively and is a major cause of mortality in patients with malaria. It usually occurs in children younger than 6 years in endemic areas. In these patients, the plasmodia invade red blood cells, causing them to be "sticky" with respect to endothelial cells. Proinflammatory cytokines, including TNF-α, are produced, leading to upregulation of adhesion molecules on immune cells and other inflammatory processes and resulting in induction of fever. This adds to the tendency toward microvasculature sludging and thrombosis, ultimately leading to CNS damage. Consequently, the patient presents with fever, mental status changes, seizure, focal neurologic deficits, and even coma. Of these, mental status changes are the most common CNS presentation. A travel history can be crucial in making the diagnosis of this extremely serious but treatable disease. Diagnosis of cerebral malaria is made with the CNS presentation coupled with microscopic examination of thick and thin smears of blood samples from these patients. Giemsa or Wright stains can be used on the smears for parasite visualization. A fluorescent antibody test is available in some centers as a specific diagnostic test. DNA probes have been developed recently as additional diagnostic tools. Treatment of cerebral malaria is with IV quinidine gluconate in an intensive care setting. IV quinine is no longer readily available, and the use of IV quinidine for this disease is now well established. The patient must be monitored for arrhythmia and hypoglycemia during therapy. Once the clinical condition has improved and parasitemia reduced, oral quinine therapy can replace IV quinidine. Steroids are contraindicated in cerebral malaria because their use is associated with increased morbidity and mortality.

Postinfectious Encephalitis. This is a relatively common cause of encephalitis in which a current infectious agent cannot be isolated from the brain tissue but probably results from immunologic response to a previous infection. Agents known to trigger this response include measles, rubella, mumps, VZV, and *M pneumoniae* infections. It is also observed in patients after immunization with these vaccines.

APPROACH TO THE CHILD WITH DIARRHEA

Diarrhea is the second most common acute infection in pediatrics after URT infection. Worldwide, it is a leading cause of illness and death for millions of children with severe cases. The most serious complications of diarrhea are severe dehydration, electrolyte disturbances, and hypovolemic shock. Children younger than 4 years and those living in socioeconomically disadvantaged areas are most at risk.

Diarrhea is defined as an increase in water content of the stool associated with an increase in frequency. Many infectious agents lead to diarrhea in the host by several pathogenic mechanisms. After adherence to intestinal mucosa cells by use of projections such as flagella, pili, or fimbria, bacteria release mucinases and proteases. These enzymes result in gastrointestinal mucosal cell death with loss of digestive enzymes in the mucosal villi. Loss of these enzymes leads to malabsorption of specific substances, including lactose, resulting in the clinical appearance of an osmotic diarrhea. With bacterial invasion into the cells, direct enterocyte destruction ensues. Secretory diarrhea is a result of bacterial toxin production, eg, cholera toxin, which leads to huge losses of electrolytes and water.

Evaluation of patients with acute diarrhea first requires a detailed history and physical examination (Table 9–37). The ordering of diagnostic tests should be tailored to likely causes. Table 9–38 provides a summary of the characteristic features of each causative agent in childhood diarrhea (see also Chapter 13).

The stool should be tested for blood and fecal leukocytes. The presence of both erythrocytes and leukocytes indicates an invasive diarrhea from organisms such as *Campylobacter, Shigella, Salmonella, Yersinia,* and hemorrhagic *E coli.* Stool cultures and examination for ova and parasites should be reserved for patients with severe illness; suggestive histories, such as day-care outbreaks, foreign travel, or prolonged diarrhea; or stools positive for blood and leukocytes. Acid-fast staining may aid in the detection of *Cryptosporidium* oocysts and *Mycobacterium* strains. Most laboratories routinely test stools for *Salmonella, Shigella,* and *Campylobacter.* If less common organisms, such as *Yersinia* or *E coli,* are suspected, the laboratory should be notified and specific requests for pathogen identification should be made.

The mainstay of therapy for all patients with acute diarrhea is appropriate management of fluid and electrolyte abnormalities. Treatment with antimicrobial agents is rarely indicated and frequently results in prolonged shedding of the offending organism. Likewise, the use of antiperistaltic agents has not been shown to be of benefit in the treatment of children with infectious diarrhea.

Bacterial Diarrhea

Salmonella. *Salmonella* is a non–lactose-fermenting, motile, gram-negative rod with three pathogenic species: *Salmonella enteritidis, Salmonella choleraesuis,* and *Salmonella typhi. S enteritidis* and *S choleraesuis* cause acute gastroenteritis by enterocyte invasion in the small bowel. Leukocytes and blood may be found in the stools of an acutely infected patient, who may or may not have systemic symptoms. *Salmonella* can cause an asymptomatic carrier state. *Salmonella* also can cause bacteremia and focal infection, such as osteomyelitis. These complications appear to be more common in young infants and neonates.

Transmission is via the fecal-oral route and requires large inocula by contaminated food or water. Reptiles, such as domestic turtles, have long been known to be carriers of *Salmonella;* recently, other domestic reptiles, such as iguanas and snakes, have been implicated in *Salmonella* outbreaks. Eggs, poultry, and other meat products have high *Salmonella* infection rates and are frequently the source in reported outbreaks. The highest incidence of infection occurs in children younger than 5 years, especially in infants.

Treatment of gastroenteritis without bacteremia usually is contraindicated in *Salmonella* infections, as it can prolong the carrier state. In immunocompromised patients, patients with hemoglobinopathies, and in infants younger than 3 months, treatment is indicated, as these groups have a high incidence of *Salmonella* bacteremia.

S typhi is the cause of typhoid or enteric fever. It is transmitted by the fecal-oral route and by contaminated food or water. Humans are the only known carriers. Fewer than 500 cases are reported annually in the United States; most cases occur in individuals younger than 20 years. Bacteremia is universal, with invasion of the reticuloendothelial system. The bacterial cell wall contains a potent pyrogenic endotoxin, resulting in high fever with a paradoxical bradycardia. Emesis and constipation are followed

Table 9–37. Important questions for evaluating the patient with diarrhea.

Stool: frequency, color/consistency, odor, presence of blood or mucus
Travel
Antibiotic use
Contact with ill patients
Day-care attendance
Camping and exposure to wild animals
Pet and domestic animal exposure

Table 9–38. Childhood diarrhea: Characteristic features of each causative agent.

Pathogen	Site of Action	Season	Stool	Clinical	Laboratory Results
Bacterial (10–20%)					
Salmonella	Small and large bowel	Late summer, early fall	Foul-smelling, ± blood, soft, mucus	Gradual onset, extraintestinal, with cramps, chronic carrier	Neutrophil "left shift," no fever
Enteritis typhi	Ileum (bacteremia)				

Shigella
  sonnei
  flexneri
  boydii
  dysenteriae
	Large bowel (low inoculum)	Fall	Fruity smell (vinegar)
			
			Watery, mucus, bloody
				High temperature, toxic
				
				Seizures (infants)
					Low WBC, neutrophil "left shift"

Campylobacter
  jejuni
  fetus
	Large bowel	Summer	Foul smell, soft, mucus, ± blood	Most common; low-grade temperature, cramps; self-limited	

Yersinia entercolitica	Ileum	Winter	± Diarrhea, ± blood	Fever, abdominal pain, arthritis (Reiter syndrome), mesenteric lymphadenopathy (pseudoappendicitis; in older children)	
Vibrio cholerae	Small bowel	Epidemic	Large volume	Dehydration, crampy, watery diarrhea	
Aeromonas hydrophilia		Late summer–early fall	Chronic diarrhea (adults more than children) Acute diarrhea (children < 2 y)		
Escherichia coli					
ETEC ("turista")	Small bowel	Summer	Watery, no blood, large volume	Abrupt onset, no fever, cramps	Not helpful
EPEC	Small bowel	Fall	Musty odor; (–) blood, mucus; ± fever	Gradual onset, infants (< 3 mo)	
EIEC	Large bowel	Any	Small volume	Dysentery, (+) fever	
EHEC	Large bowel	Any	Bloody, no fever	Hemolytic uremic syndrome (0157:H7)	High WBC
Viral (70–90%)					
Rotavirus	Small bowel (upper)	Winter (October–May)	Large volume, foul-smelling; (–) blood, mucus	Dehydration, ± fever, (+) vomiting, mostly children 6–24 mo	
Adenovirus (types 40, 41)	Small bowel	Any	Watery	< 2 y, abdominal pain, fever, emesis	
Norwalk	Small bowel	Winter	Explosive	Abrupt onset: vomiting, no fever, adults/school-aged children	

EIEC = enteroinvasive *E coli*; EHEC = enterohemorrhagic *E coli*; EPEC = enteropathogenic *E coli*; ETEC = enterotoxigenic *E coli*; WBC = white blood cell count.

by diarrhea, hepatosplenomegaly, cholestatic jaundice, and the characteristic maculopapular rash called "rose spots." Complications include small-bowel perforation, glomerulonephritis, and numerous neurologic symptoms, such as encephalopathy, acute cerebellar ataxia, optic neuritis, aphasia, deafness, and cerebral thrombosis. The organism has become increasingly resistant to antibiotics, and many strains in the developing world have shown multiple resistance patterns. Empiric treatment should be with a third-generation cephalosporin until the susceptibility pattern is available. A vaccine is available and is recommended for intimate carrier contact, community outbreaks, or travel to an endemic area.

Shigella. *Shigella* is a non–lactose-fermenting, non-motile, gram-negative rod transmitted through fecal-oral contamination. Although most cases of shigellosis in the United States are caused by *Shigella sonnei* and *Shigella flexneri, Shigella dysenteriae* is more important in under-developed countries. Outbreaks are common in day-care centers and may follow ingestion of contaminated food and water. Only very small inocula are required for transmission. Its incubation period is about 2–4 days. Symptoms include fever, upper abdominal pain associated with tenesmus, headache, and profuse watery, mucoid stool containing blood and leukocytes. Additional features include seizures accompanying acute episodes and the occasional finding of lax anal sphincter tone, presumably due to release of a neurotoxin. Bacteremia is rare. WBC remains normal, but a marked increase in immature forms of granulocytes or leukopenia may occur. Complications are frequent and include toxic megacolon, cholestatic hepatitis, hemolytic uremic syndrome, and Reiter syndrome (arthritis, conjunctivitis, urethritis, and dermatitis). Previously, treatment consisted of trimethoprim-sulfamethoxazole or ampicillin; however, the organism, as with many intestinal pathogens, has shown increasing resistance to these traditional antibiotics. Most strains remain susceptible to parenteral third-generation cephalosporins, and these should be the empiric treatment of choice pending the susceptibility pattern of the pathogen. Ceftriaxone or cefixime, therefore, is used empirically as drugs of choice.

Campylobacter Jejuni. *C jejuni* is the most commonly isolated bacterial fecal pathogen. It is a curve-shaped, gram-negative organism causing grossly bloody diarrhea, fever, and abdominal pain that may mimic appendicitis. Bacteremia occurs with the other *Campylobacter* strains, including *Campylobacter fetus* and *Campylobacter abortus,* but rarely with *C jejuni.* Animals, including poultry, dogs, cats, and wild birds, serve as important reservoirs. Incubation is 1–7 days, and the diarrhea and abdominal pain continue for an average of 7 days. Erythromycin shortens the fecal excretion but does little to alleviate symptoms.

Yersinia Enterocolitica. *Y enterocolitica* is an aerobic, motile, non–lactose-fermenting, gram-negative coccobacillus. Rodents and swine serve as important reservoirs. Ingestion of large inocula from contaminated meats, dairy products, and seafood is required. After contaminated food products are ingested, an incubation period of 4–6 days occurs. Symptomatic patients typically present with fever, abdominal pain, and mucoid, bloody diarrhea with leukocytes. Complications are frequent and include erythema nodosum, reactive arthritis, terminal ileitis, mesenteric adenitis, meningitis, myocarditis, hepatitis, and glomerulonephritis. *Yersinia* infection is treated with gentamicin, chloramphenicol, or trimethoprim-sulfamethoxazole. In general, only infections outside the gastrointestinal tract are treated.

E Coli. *E coli* has four different subclasses, each named for its distinct mechanism of action on the intestinal mucosa. Enterotoxigenic *E coli* (ETEC) secretes one or more heat-labile or heat-stable toxins and can resemble infections with cholera. It is the only subclass that is not associated with fecal blood or leukocytes on stool examination. Enteropathogenic *E coli* (EPEC) can lead to chronic infection, malabsorption, and failure to thrive by a mechanism that is not well understood. In contrast, enteroinvasive *E coli* (EIEC) produces an acute illness that mimics shigellosis. In general, gastroenteritis due to *E coli* has an incubation period of less than 24 hours and rarely requires antimicrobial treatment. Because EPEC has a chronic nature, however, it may need to be treated in infants younger than 3 months; oral neomycin has been used successfully.

Enterohemorrhagic *E coli* (EHEC) is easily transmitted through the fecal-oral route. Strains of EHEC produce cytotoxic toxins. Among them, subclass 0157:H7 has been responsible for outbreaks in many day-care centers and for epidemic hemolytic uremic syndrome. Epidemics have been traced to undercooked contaminated meat. Treatment of EHEC is controversial; some studies indicate that antimicrobial therapy increases the incidence of hemolytic uremic syndrome.

Vibrio. *Vibrio* infections are important causes of diarrhea worldwide. Infection with these aerobic, motile, curved, gram-negative organisms results in crampy abdominal pain and explosive, watery diarrhea. Noncholera strains are common in sea water, especially in summer. A large inoculum is required, and incubation is less than 24 hours. Uncooked crustaceans and mollusks (eg, oysters, crabs, and shrimp) are well-known carriers. Once the flagella attaches to intestinal enterocytes, enterotoxin produced by cholera bacteria alters production of cellular cyclic adenosine monophosphate. Rapid and severe fluid loss resulting in death from hypovolemia is common. Cholera itself is more common in Asia, the Middle East, and southern Europe. Management includes meticulous fluid and electrolyte replacement and antimicrobial therapy, including tetracycline or trimethoprim-sulfamethoxazole.

Parasitic Diarrhea

G lamblia is a flagellated protozoan, with the cyst form being the infectious agent. After infestation, the trophozoites are found in the duodenum and are shed intermittently in stools. The protozoa are transmitted via the fecal-oral route; day-care outbreaks are common. Many patients remain asymptomatic, and symptoms vary greatly among patients. Flatulence and abdominal pain with diarrhea are most common, but malabsorption and failure to thrive are seen in children. Those with IgA deficiency and cystic fibrosis are at most risk for severe disease from *G lamblia.* Diagnosis can be made by examination of fresh stool, either by direct inspection or by ELISA. In adults, the preferred treatment is with quinacrine. In children, however, furazolidone is recommended; metronidazole is an alternative.

E histolytica results in loose, bloody, mucoid stools after ingestion of infectious cysts. Hepatic abscesses result from metastasis to the liver via the portal veins. Both stool examinations and immunoassays can aid in the diagnosis. Treatment consists of iodoquinol or metronidazole.

Viral Diarrhea

Viral diarrhea, the most commonly encountered type of diarrhea, is spread in children through close contact in families, day-care centers, hospitals, and residential institutions. Infections usually are self-limited, and the agents do not need to be routinely identified. Most can be identified by electron microscopic examination of the stool if specific diagnosis is necessary. In addition, enzyme immunoassays are available to test for rotavirus and adenovirus.

Rotavirus is an RNA virus with five known antigenic subtypes. Of all the gastrointestinal pathogens, it is the leading cause of infantile diarrhea and dehydration. Transmission is by the fecal-oral route with a 1- to 3-day incubation period. It is highly contagious, and outbreaks in day-care centers are common. Seasonal peaks occur in winter. Infection is characterized by the abrupt onset of vomiting, fever, and diarrhea. Blood, mucus, and leukocytes are not common in the stool. Premature infants are at increased risk of severe infection. Strict enteric precautions are essential for prevention of spread. Supportive therapy to maintain fluid and electrolyte balance is essential.

Adenovirus, subtypes 40 and 41, is also responsible for endemic diarrhea. It causes symptoms similar to rotavirus infection and spreads easily in close contact environments. Adenovirus typically affects older children, is more often associated with abdominal pain, and may have a more protracted course.

Norwalk agent, another RNA virus, causes diarrhea, usually accompanied by fever, abdominal cramps, and emesis. Fecal-oral transmission is common; outbreaks follow ingestion of contaminated shellfish and salads. The incubation period is 1–2 days.

Food and Waterborne Epidemic Diarrhea

Food and waterborne epidemic diarrhea refers to outbreaks occurring in many individuals after ingestion of contaminated substances. Inadequate storage and preparation of food lead to contamination. The most common causative organisms are *Salmonella, Clostridia,* and enterotoxin-producing *S aureus,* as listed above. Staphylococcal enterotoxin–mediated diarrhea typically produces vomiting and retching. The incubation period is short, usually 3–5 hours, and diarrhea usually is not prominent. Antimicrobials are of no help because the ingestion of heat-stable enterotoxins found in contaminated food, not the organism itself, is responsible for the symptoms. Proper food preparation and refrigeration are important control measures. Certain food sources are most likely to harbor specific organisms. Poultry, eggs, and unpasteurized milk are common sources of *Salmonella* outbreaks.

Antibiotic-Associated Diarrhea

Diarrhea is an adverse effect of many antibiotics that reduce the number of normal bowel flora, thus rendering permissive environment for overgrowth of other organisms. Some antibiotics can cause diarrhea by decreasing carbohydrate transport and intestinal lactase levels. Of particular importance is antibiotic-associated colitis (its most severe form is known as pseudomembranous colitis), usually the result of a toxin produced by *C difficile.* The use of broad-spectrum antibiotics allows for increased growth of this organism and subsequent toxin production. Ampicillin, clindamycin, and the cephalosporins are the commonly implicated antimicrobials. Symptoms may not appear for weeks after discontinuation of an antimicrobial. Blood, mucus, and leukorrhea are commonly found in the stool; on colonoscopy, the colon is typically lined with grayish plaquelike lesions. *C difficile* without the toxin may be found in the stool of normal, healthy infants without diarrhea. Thus, culture alone, without toxin along with the symptoms, is not indication for treatment. Severe cases may require treatment with oral vancomycin or metronidazole. In the very ill patient with pseudomembranous colitis who cannot tolerate oral medications, IV metronidazole can be used.

Endemic Diarrhea

Endemic diarrhea is the most common type of gastroenteritis encountered. By definition, it is spread in children through close-contact situations, as in families, day-care centers, and residential institutions. Viral causes predominate; rotavirus and Norwalk agent are the principal etiologic organisms. The viral infections are usually self-limited. Bacterial pathogens such as *Salmonella, Shigella,* and *Campylobacter* species, also are important causes of endemic diarrhea.

Diarrhea in the Immunocompromised Host

The immunocompromised host is susceptible to diarrhea-causing organisms that are of little or no consequence in the normal host. Examples include *Cryptosporidium* and *Mycobacterium avium-intracellulare.*

Cryptosporidium may cause outbreaks of frequent, watery stools in day-care settings. Although infection is self-limited in the normal host, significant chronic diarrhea occurs in the immunocompromised host, resulting in dehydration and malnutrition. There is no effective therapy. *Isospora belli* is another protozoan that causes severe diarrhea in AIDS patients but can be treated with trimethoprim-sulfamethoxazole or by combining pyrimethamine and sulfadiazine.

JAUNDICE

Pediatric jaundice is discussed in Chapter 14; however, infectious causes of jaundice are described below.

Hepatitis, or inflammation of the liver, is associated with a variety of causes but most frequently is the result of an infection. A viral pathogen most commonly is responsible, but bacterial, fungal, and parasitic causes exist as well (Table 9–39). Similar clinical features are seen with various viral causes of hepatitis, although there are some unique differences (Table 9–40). The clinical presentation of hepatitis can range from a mild, asymptomatic, anicteric illness to fulminant disease associated with liver failure leading to death. Alternatively, the patient may recover symptomatically and become a chronic carrier with persistent hepatitis leading to the development of liver cirrhosis and, ultimately, hepatocarcinoma.

Hepatitis A

Hepatitis A is a common cause of hepatitis in both developing and developed countries. This virus is a member of the picornavirus family. It is a nonenveloped single-stranded RNA virus and is transmitted by the fecal-oral route. Ingestion of contaminated food or water is a major source of infection. The incubation period is 15–40 days; 90% of children are asymptomatic. The virus is shed in feces 14–21 days before the onset of jaundice until approximately 1 week after. Therefore, most individuals are infectious for a long time before they realize that they have the disease. Because of this silent infectious period (late symptomatic period and frequent asymptomatic

cases), this disease is notoriously difficult to control. Large outbreaks frequently are associated with day-care centers. Diagnosis is best made by determination of IgM levels against the virus. Prophylaxis is recommended for household and other close contacts; immunoglobulin should be given within 2 weeks of exposure. Strict hand washing is the best prophylaxis. Preexposure prophylaxis is recommended for travel to developing countries. Recently, a killed-virus vaccine has become available that provides excellent immunity given in two doses 6–12 months apart.

Hepatitis B

Hepatitis B, a DNA virus belonging to the hepadna family, is double-shelled with several antigenically distinct parts. The outer lipoprotein envelope is the surface antigen (HBsAg). The inner core (HBcAg) contains three distinct parts: the genome of the partially stranded DNA, the DNA-dependent DNA polymerase, and the hepatitis B "e" antigen (HBeAg). Viral shedding occurs into blood, semen, and saliva, so transmission can be parenteral, sexual, mucosal, or perinatal, with an incubation period of 50–180 days.

A radioimmunoassay is available to measure serum concentrations of HBsAg. Antibodies to both HBsAg and HBcAg also can be measured. Response to the hepatitis B virus can be documented, and asymptomatic patients can be screened by determining the presence of antibody against HBsAg. A period of several weeks, called the "window phase," often elapses between the disappearance of HBsAg and the appearance of IgG anti-HBsAg antibody (Figure 9–3). IgM and anti-HBcAg antibody can be detected in the window phase; measurements of this antibody also help differentiate recent for past hepatitis B infection. The immunologic response is outlined in Figure 9–2. The e antigen (HBeAg) correlates with active viral replication and infectivity, and the presence of antibody against HBeAg implies less viral replication and chance of infecting others. The carrier state results when there is an ineffective immune response; these patients remain infectious to others. In adults, the carrier state occurs in about 5% of those infected, whereas in newborns, it may run as high as 90%.

Although the mortality rate associated with acute infection is less than 1%, complications and morbidity are very significant. Complications include fulminant hepatitis, cirrhosis, and hepatocellular carcinoma, especially in chronic carriers. Other extrahepatic manifestations are the result of immune complex vasculitis and manifest as glomerulonephritis, arthritis, serum sickness, polyarteritis nodosa, and urticaria. Therapies for chronic hepatitis B infection are now available. One example is interferon-α, which has been licensed in the United States for this indication. Response rates of 35% are seen in controlled trials after 4–6 months of therapy, as documented by normalization of liver enzyme levels and improved histologic appearance of the liver on the biopsy specimen. In addition, there is a delayed response to interferon therapy in another 10–15%

Table 9–39. Etiologic organisms for hepatitis.

Viruses	Fungi
Hepatitis A, B, C, D, E	*Candida albicans*
Herpes family	*Blastomyces dermatitidis*
CMV, EBV, HSV, VZV	*Histoplasma capsulatum*
Adenovirus	Parasites
Enterovirus	*Toxoplasma gondii*
Parvovirus B19	*Entameba histolytica*
Bacteria	*Schistosoma* species
Neisseria gonorrhoeae	*Toxocara canis*
Leptospira	
Mycobacterium tuberculosis	
Treponema pallidum	

CMV = cytomegalovirus; EBV = Epstein-Barr virus; HSV = herpes simplex virus; VZV = varicella zoster virus.

Table 9–40. Viral hepatitis: Types A, B, and C.

	Hepatitis A	Hepatitis B	Hepatitis C
Incubation period	15–40 d	50–180 d	1–5 mo
Transmission	Fecal-oral	Parenteral, sexual, mucosal, or perinatal	Parenteral, sexual, or perinatal (including breast-feeding)
Chronic infection	No	~ 5% of infected adults; if perinatally acquired, can approach 90%	50% of post-transfusion acquired cases
Treatment or post-exposure prophylaxis	Can give immunoglobulin if within 2 wk of exposure	Interferon-α, lamivudine, immunoglobulin post-exposure	Interferon-α
Vaccine available	Yes	Yes	No
Associated sequelae of chronic disease		Cirrhosis, hepatocellular carcinoma, immune complex manifestations	Cirrhosis, hepatocellular carcinoma

of treated patients. Different patient groups undergoing therapy have differences in response rates. It appears that patients who were infected shortly after birth by caretakers or the mother have a more recalcitrant disease and are less responsive to interferon therapy. Other promising antiviral therapies currently under investigation include lamivudine and thymosin.

Hepatitis C

Hepatitis C is a single-stranded RNA virus and is a member of the flavivirus family. This virus is the most common cause of non-A, non-B post-transfusion hepatitis. The incubation period is long, 1–5 months, and transmission is usually via parenteral, sexual, or perinatal exposure. Clinical disease usually is mild; most acute infections are anicteric but demonstrate mild and fluctuating elevations in alanine aminotransferase, aspartate aminotransferase, and bilirubin levels. Chronic carriage occurs

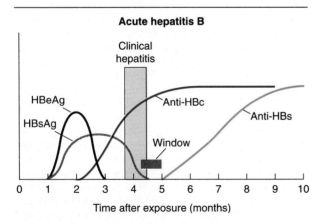

Figure 9–3. Schematic representation of viral markers in the blood throughout the course of self-limited, hepatitis B surface antigen (HBsAg)-positive primary hepatitis B virus infection. (Reproduced, with permission, from Mandell GL et al [editors]: Page 1209 in: *Principles and Practice of Infectious Diseases,* 3rd ed. Churchill Livingstone, 1990.)

in 50% of post-transfusion acquired infection. Hepatitis virus can be found in breast milk of infected mothers, but reliable data on risk of transmission from breast milk are not currently available. Both cirrhosis and hepatocellular carcinoma are reported complications. Interferon-α is used in treatment of chronic hepatitis C but unfortunately is associated with a high relapse rate after cessation of therapy.

Hepatitis D

This defective virus is really a coinfection or superinfection because it requires the presence of hepatitis B virus for replication. Also known as the delta virus, this small, circular, single-stranded RNA virus has an incubation period of 21–90 days. Transmission can be parenteral, sexual, or perinatal. Disease tends to be quite severe, with the highest mortality of all viral hepatitis (about 20%). Cirrhosis and portal hypertension often develop in survivors of the acute illness. Those who abuse IV drugs are at particular risk.

Hepatitis E

Hepatitis E is more common in adolescents and young adults and is similar to hepatitis A. This single-stranded RNA member of the calicivirus family was first identified in 1990. It has been called enterically transmitted non-A, non-B hepatitis. Transmission is by the fecal-oral route, and the incubation period is 2–9 weeks. The mortality rate is less than 1%; in pregnant women, however, the rate reaches 20%.

Approach to the Diagnosis of Viral Hepatitis

A history of exposure to a jaundiced individual or contaminated food or water may provide the initial clues leading to detection of hepatitis A. Potential parenteral exposures to hepatitis B should be sought. These include tattoos, transfusions, IV drug use, or inadvertent needlestick injuries, as well as exposures through sexual transmission. The definitive differentiation between hepatitis viruses cannot be made clinically and relies on serologic testing described previously.

Neonatal Hepatitis. Neonatal hepatitis is usually the result of an infection transmitted in utero or at the time of birth. It is often difficult to make definitive diagnosis of the causative agent. The microbial agent involved includes hepatitis A, B, and C, as well as CMV, rubella, syphilis, and toxoplasmosis. Among the cases in which the etiology is proved, hepatitis B is the most common cause. In the case of hepatitis B, transmission to the newborn is most frequent if the mother is positive for HBeAg; in such cases, transmission is as high as 90%. In contrast, if the mother is HBsAg-positive, but HBeAg-negative, transmission is less than 20%. Routes of transmission include viral invasion across the placenta during late pregnancy or labor (prenatal), ingestion of maternal blood or amniotic fluid (natal), and breast feeding with cracked and bleeding nipples (postnatal). To prevent perinatal infection, hepatitis B immunoglobulin and recombinant hepatitis B vaccine should be given to all newborns of infected mothers soon after birth.

Chronic Hepatitis. Chronic hepatitis is an ongoing inflammation of the liver that persists after the patient has recovered symptomatically from an acute infection. Usual causes of chronic hepatitis include infectious agents, as well as autoimmune or metabolic diseases. Infection with viral hepatitis B, C, and D, all of which are parenterally transmitted, can result in chronic disease. In contrast, the enterally transmitted forms (A and E) do not lead to chronic hepatitis. Historically, chronic hepatitis can be divided into two forms: chronic active hepatitis (CAH) and chronic persistent hepatitis (CPH). CAH features portal triad infiltration by immune cells, including lymphocytes and plasma cells, resulting in encroachment of the hepatocytes. This often leads to fibrosis, necrosis, and cirrhosis because of a chronic inflammatory process. In addition to hepatitis B, noninfectious causes include Wilson disease, autoimmune lupus hepatitis, α-1 antitrypsin deficiency, and adverse reactions to drugs. In CPH, the infiltrating immune cells are less extensive and are limited to the portal triad. Consequently, it carries a better prognosis and is not associated with cirrhosis. Whether there are two distinct forms of chronic hepatitis remains uncertain. Most likely, both represent a continuous spectrum of chronic hepatitis.

BONE OR JOINT INFECTIONS

Bacterial infections of the skeletal system can occur in any age group, but are most common in young children, in whom bone growth is rapid. Damage to the growth plate (physis) can have disastrous consequences to the skeletal system of a growing child. In the pre-antibiotic era, osteomyelitis and septic arthritis were crippling diseases. Now, with proper management, most children with these infections recover completely.

OSTEOMYELITIS

The pathogenesis, etiology, signs and symptoms, and management of osteomyelitis vary as a function of age and site of infection.

Pathogenesis

Bony infections in neonates, older infants, and children represent suppurative sequelae of bacteremia, penetrating trauma, or extension of infection from an adjacent foci. Osteomyelitis develops in the vast majority of immunologically normal children younger than 10 years as a late complication of bacteremia or septicemia. In children beyond the neonatal age group and without hemoglobinopathies, bony infections of hematogenous origin occur almost exclusively in metaphyses of long bones. In young children, it has been suggested that the unique vascular anatomy of immature bone is the basis for the pathologic process to start at this site. The terminal arterial ramifications of the nutrient artery form loops immediately adjacent to the epiphyseal plates and drain into a large venous sinusoidal system occupied in the intramedullary portion of the metaphyses. Consequently, decreased rates of blood flow through this region of bone predispose to osseous colonization and subsequent infection during bacteremia. Once the infection is established, it extends to the cortex causing periosteal elevation, through the intramedullary cavity or subperiosteum, and finally into the adjacent capsules of the joint beyond the epiphyseal growth plate. In children with sickle-cell disease, the diaphyseal portions of long bones typically are involved, probably as a consequence of prior bone infarction secondary to sludging from sickle hemoglobin in the erythrocyte under stress.

Osteomyelitis can follow direct bacterial inoculation of bone. Penetrating injury of the foot, such as stepping on a nail or repeated heel-sticks for blood sampling in a neonate, may introduce bacteria directly into bone. Premature infants often require indwelling venous or arterial catheters and repeated instrumentation and are at increased risk for bone infection. Osteomyelitis of the bones of the hand as a result of either human or animal bites may represent direct inoculation of bone or spread from an adjacent site of infection. Osteomyelitis of the facial bones typically follows extension from an infected sinus or from dental abscesses.

Clinical Presentation

Focal pain, tenderness, and limp or decreased use of an extremity are characteristics of bone infections regardless of age. Neonatal osteomyelitis usually presents 2–8 weeks after birth. Bone infections in this age group typically represent either late suppurative sequelae of bacteremia or direct inoculation of bone. Systemic signs and symptoms of infection, such as fever, irritability, and poor oral intake, are often absent. Unlike bony infections in older infants and children, osteomyelitis in the neonate is usually multifocal, with involvement of joints as well as bones. Lack of spontaneous movement of an extremity (pseudoparalysis) or evidence of joint space involvement (see below) are the usual clinical signs. Any bone may be involved in neonatal infections.

Beyond the neonatal period, infections of the femur, tibia, or humerus account for approximately two thirds of cases, whereas involvement of the hands and feet accounts for another 15% of infections. Infection of the skull, vertebrae, or pelvis is rare in childhood. Most infants and children present with the constellation of fever, focal tenderness to palpation of the affected bone, and pain on passive motion of the affected extremity. Concomitant joint infection and multiple foci of bony involvement are rare in children older than 3 years; however, osteomyelitis is a common complication of septic arthritis in children younger than 3 years, and up to 25% of these cases may be multifocal.

Soft-tissue swelling, local erythema, and drainage may not be present early in osteomyelitis of hematogenous origin but may accompany infections caused by penetrating trauma. In older children, osteomyelitis arising from penetrating injury is insidious in onset and lacks systemic signs of infection. Individuals with puncture wounds of the feet or bite injuries of the hands may experience persistent or episodic pain for several weeks to months before seeking medical attention. In these patients, focal tenderness, erythema, and drainage are often discovered on examination.

Etiology

The bacterial pathogens of neonatal osteomyelitis are similar to the etiology of neonatal sepsis. Group B *Streptococcus, E coli,* and *S aureus* are the most common bacterial pathogens. Most neonatal skeletal infections appear to accompany late-onset sepsis and represent horizontal rather than vertical acquisition of pathogens.

Beyond the newborn period, *S aureus* is the most common pathogen of bone in children. HIB, *S pneumoniae,* and *S aureus* are the predominant pathogens in hematogenously acquired skeletal infections in children younger than 3 years. HIB and *S pneumoniae* osteomyelitis usually are encountered as a complication of a joint infection. With the success of early *H influenzae* vaccination, the incidence of skeletal infection due to this pathogen has decreased dramatically.

In special circumstances, the causative agents are quite different from the conventional cases. These include hemoglobinopathies and foot infection from penetrating trauma, as well as human or animal bites. Although *S aureus* is still a significant bone pathogen among children with hemoglobinopathies, an increased percentage of these infections are due to *Salmonella* species and other gram-negative rods. *P aeruginosa* and *S aureus* are the most common causes of osteomyelitis after penetrating trauma of the foot. Oral streptococci, *Eikenella corrodens,* and facultative anaerobes may cause osteomyelitis after human bites. Osteomyelitis due to *Pasteurella multocida* follows dog or cat bites. Anaerobic bacteria and *M catarrhalis,* as well as aerobic streptococci and staphylococci, may be the cause of osteomyelitis accompanying sinusitis or dental infections.

Diagnosis

Osteomyelitis should be considered in any child with the following:

1. nonuse or decreased use of an extremity
2. a limp
3. focal, bony pain.

A good history is essential to evaluate any recent incidence of direct trauma, open wound, or infections associated with bacteremia. Further historical questions include underlying diseases, such as hemoglobinopathies or metabolic and immune disorders. Neonatal osseous infections must be distinguished from birth trauma and congenital neurologic defects. Beyond the neonatal age group, osteomyelitis complicating penetrating trauma, sinusitis, or dental infections must be distinguished from soft-tissue infections, bone cysts, malignant neoplasms, and chronic multifocal osteomyelitis (a syndrome of recurrent signs and symptoms of osteomyelitis without positive cultures). In older children with suspected osteomyelitis, the differential diagnosis includes septic arthritis, bacterial sepsis, leukemia, tumor (including osteosarcoma), collagen vascular diseases, and bone infarcts (Table 9–41).

Other special problems encountered in the diagnosis of osteomyelitis include pelvic osteomyelitis and hemoglobinopathies. Pelvic osteomyelitis is frequently confused with acute abdomen or other intrapelvic diseases. In patients with sickle-cell disease, aseptic bone infarct may have presentations similar to bone infection. In these cases, even technetium scan may not differentiate the two entities reliably.

Children with osteomyelitis from bacteremia usually have elevated peripheral WBCs, ESR, and serum C-reac-

Table 9–41. Differential diagnosis for bone and joint swellings.

Bacterial osteomyelitis
Septic arthritis
Other infections: viral (eg, rubella, hepatitis B), fungal, parasitic, rickettsial
Tumors: benign or malignant; bone cyst, histiocytosis, metastatic bone tumors
Collagen vascular diseases: juvenile rheumatoid arthritis
Acute rheumatic fever
Bone infarctions: sickle-cell crisis
Metabolic bone disorder; scurvy, rickets

tive protein concentrations. Results of blood cultures are positive in one half to two thirds of cases. Needle aspirates from infected bone yield pathogens in at least 70–80% of cases (Table 9–42).

Plain radiographs of the affected bone often do not show any changes for up to 2 weeks after symptoms first appear. Although the earliest radiographic finding is the loss of the periosteal fat line, focal bony destruction is the most common finding of osteomyelitis. Periosteal elevation and periosteal destruction are later findings as explained in the pathogenesis process above. The identification of a sequestrum (avascular, dead bone separated from adjacent bone) and involucrum (the thickened sheath around a sequestrum) are signs of chronic, long-standing infection.

Technetium-99m bone scans demonstrate increased bony uptake early in the course of osteomyelitis and can identify silent foci of infection in multifocal disease in both neonates and older infants and children. Results of these scans may be falsely negative in individuals with long-standing infections. Gallium or indium scans also may demonstrate areas of infected bone. These tests are indicative of inflammation with migration of white blood cells to the site of infection; thus, they are positive in soft-tissue infection and septic arthritis. CT and MRI are also useful for demonstrating the sites of infected bone.

Treatment

Successful management of bony infections in neonates and children requires close cooperation between the pediatrician and orthopedic surgeon. For proper treatment, bacterial culture of blood and closed bone aspirate should precede empiric initial antimicrobial therapy, because it is crucial for establishing the diagnosis and etiology. In borderline cases and in cases of chronic osteomyelitis, open surgical biopsy or debridement may be required to obtain the cultures. Empiric antibiotic therapy is based on the likelihood of specific pathogens for the given clinical situation.

Table 9–42. Laboratory investigations for evaluating osteomyelitis and septic arthritis.

Hematologic tests	
White blood cell counts, elevated	
Erythrocyte sedimentation rate, elevated in > 95%	
Bacterial cultures	
Sources	*Yield (%)*
Blood	50–60
Bone aspiration	70–80
Pus culture at surgery	80
Joint fluid	< 50
Radiologic imaging	
Bone plain films	
Technetium-99m scan[1]	
Gallium or indium scan[1]	
Computed tomographic scan	
Magnetic resonance imaging	

[1]Commonly used radiologic tests.

In neonates, because of the prevalence of group B *Streptococcus* and *E coli* in addition to *Staphylococcus,* a broad-spectrum, parenteral cephalosporin, such as ceftriaxone or cefotaxime, combined with an antistaphylococcal penicillin is recommended. Once the organism and its sensitivity are identified, the antibiotics can be adjusted.

For children younger than 5 years, the initial antibiotics coverage should include gram-positive cocci and *H influenzae.* Thus, cefuroxime, a second-generation cephalosporin, may be used. An alternative regimen is ceftriaxone or cefotaxime in combination with an antistaphylococcal penicillin.

Children older than 5 years with systemic signs and symptoms of infection should have therapy directed against *S aureus.* Cloxacillin or nafcillin are the drugs of choice in this setting, whereas parenterally administered clindamycin is recommended for patients allergic to penicillin. For patients with hemoglobinopathies and other immunocompromising conditions, a broader spectrum of antibiotics is essential. Clindamycin should be included in combination regimens developed for the empiric treatment of bites or dental abscesses.

Therapy for the treatment of osteomyelitis after puncture wounds of the foot may be delayed until culture results are known, as this type of infection is indolent and rarely life-threatening. If *P aeruginosa* is isolated from the wound, combined therapy with either an antipseudomonal penicillin or cephalosporin plus an aminoglycoside is suggested. Once the pathogen has been identified, therapy can be narrowed and directed against the specific organism.

Parenteral therapy should be continued until most of the initial clinical symptoms have resolved. The usual duration of IV therapy is at least 1 week. The remainder of the treatment can be given orally if the following criteria are met:

- The organism has been identified or the patient has shown improvement with antistaphylococcal therapy alone.

- An effective oral agent is available and is tolerated by the child.

- Adequate bactericidal titers have been achieved on oral therapy using the patient's own organism or a reference strain of *S aureus* (peak level 1:8; trough level 1:2); alternatively, serum antibiotics levels should be measured directly.

- Compliance with oral therapy is ensured.

- The patient is not a neonate.

For neonates, or in cases in which the criteria for oral therapy have not been met, the antibiotic course should be completed by the parenteral route. Parenteral therapy may be completed outside the hospital under the supervision of a home IV therapy team.

The optimal duration of the total course of antimicrobial therapy, parenteral plus oral, is controversial. In general, for uncomplicated cases due to staphylococci in a previously well patient, a minimum of 3–4 weeks of therapy is probably adequate. Furthermore, clinical findings should resolve rapidly, and the ESR and WBC count should return to normal 1 week before cessation of therapy. For *Pseudomonas* osteomyelitis in patients without other joint involvement, the infection can be treated with a short course of 10–14 days, especially when combined with adequate curettage. Chronic staphylococcal osteomyelitis is usually treated with 1 month of parenteral therapy, followed by at least 8–10 months of oral therapy.

Open drainage and debridement of necrotic bone are rarely required but are recommended in cases of chronic osteomyelitis or neonatal osteomyelitis, instances in which closed aspirate yields grossly purulent materials, patients with associated joint infection, patients who have nonfocal pain along the shaft of the infected bone or have persistent bacteremia in spite of adequate antimicrobial therapy, instances of failure of systemic symptoms and laboratory markers to normalize in a reasonable amount of time, and cases of *Pseudomonas* osteomyelitis.

Complications

Complications of osteomyelitis are rare, and, in general, most children recover without significant sequelae. The most common complications are the development of chronic infection and impaired function of the affected extremity. Symptoms of chronic infection, characterized by either constant or episodic pain at the site of the original infection, may not manifest for 8 weeks or more after completion of surgery. In some patients, a sinus tract with drainage may develop. In approximately 25% of these patients, the infection does not respond to extensive surgical debridement and prolonged antimicrobial therapy; these patients may require antimicrobial therapy for a longer period of time along with extensive surgical reconstruction and bone grafting.

Because the metaphyseal growth plate is the most common site of bony infection. a small percentage of children, particularly neonates, may experience loss of longitudinal bone growth. Without adequate treatment, this limb shortening is a well-known complication of childhood osseous infection.

INFECTIOUS ARTHRITIS

Infectious arthritis can be divided into three major categories: (1) acute pyogenic, (2) neonatal, and (3) reactive arthritis syndromes. Although there are similarities in the clinical appearance of arthritis in these entities, the etiologic agents, diagnoses, and management are different.

Clinical Presentation

Infectious arthritis in infants and children is characterized by fever and joint pain. The onset of illness usually is abrupt, with complaints of joint pain with passive and active motion. When lower extremities are involved, the child may limp or refuse to bear weight or walk. When the hip joint is involved, the affected limb usually is held in the position of greatest comfort, that is, flexed and externally rotated (the "frog-leg" position). On occasion, pain may be perceived at a site distal to the actual infection. For example, the child with a septic hip joint may point to the knee as the source of pain.

Examination of the affected joint reveals pain on motion, warmth, erythema, and swelling over the joint. Large joints are most commonly involved in childhood infections, such as knees, hips, and elbows, accounting for almost two thirds of cases. Small joints of the hands are often involved in post-traumatic infections, particularly after human or animal bites.

Diagnosis

The differential diagnosis of arthritis in children includes infectious diseases, malignant neoplasms, rheumatologic disorders, trauma, osteomyelitis, septic bursitis, fasciitis, myositis, cellulitis, and occult abscesses (see Table 9–41). Occult abscesses may mimic the clinical presentation of infectious arthritis. For instance, psoas muscle abscesses may present with fever and pain on hip movement. Antecedent events, such as gastroenteritis, urethritis, tick bite, pharyngitis, or sexually transmitted diseases (STDs), may precede the development of reactive arthritis.

In the neonate, prolonged ventilation, use of indwelling venous catheters, and hyperalimentation are risk factors for infectious arthritis. Because of the relative immaturity of the immune system, pyogenic arthritis in the neonate is frequently multifocal and associated with concomitant osteomyelitis.

Pyogenic arthritis in older children is typically monoarticular, unlike some forms of reactive and rheumatologic arthritis. Juvenile rheumatoid arthritis, Kawasaki syndrome, Henoch-Schönlein purpura, Crohn disease, and other rheumatologic disorders must be considered in children with multiple hot, swollen joints. In general, symmetric multiple joint involvement usually excludes infectious causes. However, Reiter syndrome must be considered in these cases, particularly with involvement of the eyes, skin, and mucous membranes (see below). A history of injury, penetrating trauma, or bleeding dyscrasia usually is elicited in cases of hemarthrosis.

Commonly available laboratory studies usually are nonspecific in patients with infectious arthritis. Elevations in peripheral WBC, ESR, and C-reactive protein are common in children with joint space infections. Arthrocentesis with synovial fluid analysis is the most useful study for establishing the presumptive diagnosis of infectious arthritis. The recovery of grossly purulent fluid with a high protein content and low glucose concentration is characteristic of infectious arthritis.

Definitive diagnosis of pyogenic arthritis requires the

recovery of a bacterial pathogen, either from purulent synovial fluid or from blood cultures. The bacterial recovery rate from infected synovial fluid is less than 50%; the result of blood culture is positive in approximately one third of cases (see Table 9–42).

Plain radiographs are not helpful in the early diagnosis of infectious arthritis. Radionuclide scans are useful in diagnosis, and technetium-99m bone scans may identify a coexisting osseous infection. The results from gallium scan are helpful to identify the infected joints but are not specific. Ultrasound study can confirm joint effusions and is particularly useful as a guide for diagnostic arthrocentesis in suspected hip infections. MRI can distinguish joint infections from cellulitis or suspected deep abscesses.

ACUTE PYOGENIC ARTHRITIS

Acute infectious arthritis of childhood is usually the result of hematogenous seeding of a large joint after an occult or overt episode of bacteremia. Systemic signs and symptoms of infection usually are present. Less commonly, a penetrating injury of the joint may lead to bacterial infection. Beyond the newborn period and up to 2 years of age, HIB, S aureus, and S pneumoniae are the usual causative pathogens. A recent national program in the vaccination of young children against HIB has reduced the incidence of acute pyogenic arthritis caused by this organism. In older children and young adolescents, S aureus, N gonorrhoeae, and S pyogenes are most common pathogens. Salmonella and other aerobic gram-negative bacteria usually are seen in patients with diarrheal illnesses or immunodeficiencies. The oral streptococci, Fusobacterium species, and E corrodens may cause pyogenic arthritis in children after a human bite. P multocida may cause pyogenic arthritis after dog or cat bites. The diagnosis of acute pyogenic arthritis is confirmed as described above by recovering bacteria from purulent joint fluid or blood.

Treatment of acute pyogenic arthritis consists of antimicrobial therapy and judicious surgical intervention. In cases suspected to be of hematogenous origin, an antistaphylococcal penicillin and either cefotaxime or ceftriaxone provide excellent antibiotic coverage for the typical pathogens. In patients with hypersensitivity to penicillins, clindamycin and aztreonam provide adequate coverage. Clindamycin or an antistaphylococcal penicillin can be used for the initial management of pyogenic arthritis after trauma or bites. Recent studies suggest that pneumococcal or H influenzae arthritis may be successfully treated for at least 10–14 days, whereas 21 days are required for staphylococcal infections. These shorter periods of therapy require prompt resolution of the initial signs and symptoms of infection. Joint infections caused by N gonorrhoeae are readily treated by a 7-day course of parenteral ceftriaxone as initial therapy.

The role of surgery in the management of acute pyogenic arthritis of childhood is largely empiric. All patients initially should undergo a closed arthrocentesis for diagnosis. Repeated arthrocentesis or closed drainage are recommended in cases in which the effusions reaccumulate rapidly. Open drainage and debridement are suggested in cases that fail to respond rapidly to conservative therapy and in those with concomitant osteomyelitis. Hip involvement requires emergent open drainage of the joint. This recommendation is based on the relatively high incidence of long-term sequelae after hip infections; necrosis of the femoral head is a significant concern because the blood supply to this area of the bone is tenuous and can be compromised in actively inflamed joint.

NEONATAL ARTHRITIS

Pyogenic arthritis and osteomyelitis are often associated infections in the neonate, and the bacterial pathogens are similar. Group B Streptococcus, Enterobacteriaceae, N gonorrhoeae, and S aureus are the most common organisms. Most infants with neonatal arthritis have a preceding episode of bacteremia. Typically, the infection presents 2–8 weeks after birth. As with osteomyelitis, the first clinical sign of neonatal skeletal infection may be pseudoparalysis, the absence of spontaneous movement of an affected extremity. Detailed examination often reveals an effusion and pain on passive motion of the affected joint.

Definitive diagnosis is made by recovery of purulent materials from the affected joint. The duration of treatment of neonatal joint infections is largely empiric. Initial antimicrobial therapy is based on the pathogens typically encountered in these infections. Antistaphylococcal penicillin (oxacillin or nafcillin), combined with a broad-spectrum cephalosporin (cefotaxime, ceftazidime), is appropriate for most bacterial pathogens. Amphotericin B should be used in cases of suspected fungal arthritis. Once the pathogen is identified, specific parenteral therapy is recommended for at least 3 weeks. Isolated neonatal infectious arthritis may be treated successfully with repeated arthrocenteses or closed drainage. However, if the underlying bone is involved, open drainage and bony debridement are usually performed.

REACTIVE ARTHRITIS SYNDROME

Reactive arthritis is defined as a sterile arthritis that occurs in the absence of bacteremia or sepsis and often accompanies or immediately follows an infectious illness. In general, the arthritis in these conditions is thought to be immune-mediated, but the inflammatory process is less aggressive than in pyogenic conditions.

ARTHRITIS & DIARRHEA

Gastrointestinal infections, particularly with *Shigella* and *Yersinia* species, must be considered in the differential diagnosis of arthritis. Although the knees are most commonly involved in both cases, the organism is usually recovered from the stool but not from the synovial fluid. In addition to using antimicrobial therapy for the elimination of pathogens from the gastrointestinal tract, nonsteroidal anti-inflammatory agents are required for treatment of the arthritis.

Reiter syndrome is a constellation of conjunctivitis, urethritis, reactive arthritis, rash, diarrhea, and stomatitis that may follow a number of infections, including bacterial gastroenteritis, chlamydiosis, or group A streptococcal infections.

GONOCOCCAL ARTHRITIS–DERMATITIS SYNDROME

The gonococcal arthritis–dermatitis syndrome is considered to be a complication of untreated primary infection caused by *N gonorrhoeae*. The syndrome represents a continuum of symptoms that include dermatitis and arthritis caused by disseminated gonococcal infection.

After an untreated primary infection, patients have a febrile, toxic illness characterized by a petechial rash, especially on the dorsum of the hands and feet, and periarthritis typically involving the tendon sheaths of the hands and feet. Cultures of joint fluid are almost always sterile, whereas cultures from the primary source of infection (genitourinary tract, throat, or rectum) and the blood are often positive. If left untreated, these symptoms initially resolve, only to return weeks later with arthritis of a large weight-bearing joint, usually the knee. At this later stage, the cultures of synovial fluid and primary infection sites are often positive. The arthritis-dermatitis syndrome may be treated readily with 7 days of parenteral ceftriaxone or oral amoxicillin. As with any gonococcal infection, these patients should be screened for other STDs.

LYME DISEASE

This arthropod-borne illness is caused by *B burgdorferi*, with the *Ixodes* species of ticks as the vector for Lyme borreliosis. *Ixodes dammini*, the eastern deer tick, is responsible for the disease in most parts of the northeastern and midwestern United States. *Ixodes pacificus* is the vector in the western United States, and other *Ixodes* species have been implicated in the southeast. All *Ixodes* vectors have multiple hosts. The white-footed mouse in the United States and the black mouse in Europe are the typical reservoirs of infection because these species tolerate intense spirochetemia. In general, the tick larvae feed on infected mice and then leave their hosts to develop into nymphs and infect new hosts the following year. The nymphs become adult ticks and seek larger mammals, such as deer and humans, in the late summer or early fall of the second year.

Human disease caused by *B burgdorferi* follows bites by infected ticks. The spectrum of disease caused by this agent is broad, with most cases being asymptomatic. In symptomatic cases, symptoms appear after an incubation period of 3–31 days. The classic early feature of infection is erythema chronicum migrans, a rash that appears in 50–75% of patients. It begins at the site of the bite, developing into an erythematous plaque that expands circularly and clears centrally. Later, the rash may progress into variable colors and forms, such as purpura or vesicles. The primary and secondary forms together typically last several weeks and may recur. The appearance of the rash may be accompanied by constitutional symptoms, including fatigue, fever, arthralgias, and arthritis, all of which resolve spontaneously.

Major concerns for Lyme disease are late manifestations, including arthritis, CNS, and cardiac complications, which occur several months after the primary infection. Approximately one half of children with untreated primary infections have episodes of arthritis, usually involving large joints such as the knees. Without treatment, these patients can have chronic synovitis and permanent joint disability. CNS disease may affect up to 15% of patients who do not receive treatment and has a variety of manifestations, including meningitis, encephalitis, cranial nerve palsies, radiculitis, and transverse myelitis. Cardiac disease is not a common complication of Lyme disease, with atrioventricular block of varying degrees being the most common manifestation. Myocarditis and pericarditis occur rarely.

Lyme disease is best diagnosed clinically. A history of travel to an endemic region and tick bite in an individual with erythema chronicum migrans is highly suggestive of the diagnosis. Although recovery of *B burgdorferi* from the skin lesion is diagnostic, this test is not widely available. Serologic testing is of limited value because the IgM response to a mixture of *Borrelia* antigens occurs as late as 4 weeks after the initial infection. In addition, the available ELISA assay for detection of antibody is highly nonspecific and poorly reproducible. Serologic testing is of value only in patients with a suggestive history or with suggestive signs of early or late infection.

The recommended treatment regimens for Lyme disease are shown in Table 9–43. A short course of oral therapy is recommended for children with erythema chronicum migrans and no systemic symptoms. Prophylaxis for children with tick bites is unproved but may be appropriate in highly endemic regions, such as New England. Parenteral therapy is recommended for established complications of late disease, such as cardiac diseases. In contrast, the efficacy of prolonged courses of antimicrobial therapy for chronic fatigue syndrome or other nonspecific CNS symptoms in seropositive individuals without recognized manifestations of early or late Lyme disease is unknown.

Table 9–43. Recommended treatment schedules for Lyme disease in children.[1]

Disease Category	Drug Dosage
Early disease (at the time of exanthem onset)	
≥ 9 years	Tetracycline 250 mg QID po or Doxycycline 100 mg BID po
< 9 years	Penicillin V 25–50 mg/kg/d TID po or Amoxicillin 25–50 mg/kg/d TID po
Late disease	
Arthritis	Same as early disease above
Mild carditis	Same as early disease above
Severe carditis, persistent arthritis meningitis/ encephalitis	Ceftriaxone 100 mg/kg/d IV or IM
	Penicillin 300,000 U/kg/d q4h IV or IM

[1]Reproduced, with permission, from American Academy of Pediatrics, Committee on Infectious Diseases: Treatment of Lyme borreliosis. Pediatrics 1991;88:176.
Oral regimen, 10–30 days; parenteral therapy, 14–21 days.

ACUTE RHEUMATIC FEVER

Acute rheumatic fever is a late, nonsuppurative sequela of group A streptococcal pharyngitis. This syndrome is the result of immune response against specific streptococcal strains that cross-react with cardiac and other tissues (see Chapter 8). Among the clinical manifestations, migratory polyarthritis is a unique feature of rheumatic fever. Patients have frank arthritis (joint effusion, pain, warmth, and tenderness), typically of the large joints including knees, ankles, wrists, and elbows, in a serial pattern. Arthritic presentations of the joints flare and resolve spontaneously, with each episode lasting several days. The frequent occurrences of cardiac valvar and myocardial involvement are important complications.

URINARY TRACT INFECTIONS: DYSURIA & FEVER

The term **urinary tract infection** encompasses a broad array of disease presentations, which have in common the presence of an infectious agent somewhere in the urinary system. Commonly, infections are separated into those that involve the renal parenchyma (upper tract) and those that are limited to the bladder (lower tract). Some terms used to describe specific infections are listed in Table 9–44.

UTIs present a challenge in detection, diagnosis, treatment, and follow-up. The goals of identification and management of UTIs are as follows:

Table 9–44. Urinary tract infection (UTI): Terms and definitions.

Bacteriuria	Isolation of bacteria from the urine; symptomatic or asymptomatic bacertiuria (see text)
Cystitis	Commonly implies an infection[1] limited to the bladder (lower-tract UTI)
Pyelonephritis	Involvement of the renal parenchyma (upper-tract UTI)
Pyuria	Presence of white blood cells in the urine; ≥ 5 white blood cell count/high-power field
Sterile pyuria	Presence of white blood cells in the urine with no identifiable infectious agent

[1]Noninfectious causes of bladder inflammation, such as hemorrhagic cystitis secondary to certain antineoplastic chemotherapy agents.

1. symptomatic relief
2. microbiologic cure
3. detection of predisposing conditions
4. detection of complications.

UTIs are not infrequently encountered by pediatricians in the clinical setting. They should be listed in the differential diagnosis of any young patient who presents with toxicity and fever. The incidence of infection is influenced by age and gender. In neonates, UTI is twice as common in boys as girls. However, in older children, the incidence of UTIs is greater in girls. From screening studies in school-aged children, the incidence of asymptomatic bacteriuria has been 0.03% in boys and 1–2% in girls. UTI has been reported in about 5% of boys and 10% of girls who were evaluated in studies of fever without localizing signs (see section on Fever).

Clinical Manifestations

Bacteria in the urinary tract may be asymptomatic or symptomatic. The occurrence of asymptomatic bacteriuria has been well described from large school-based screening studies. Infections with minimal or nonlocalizing symptoms may be detected during evaluation of febrile illnesses or secondary enuresis.

In infants and younger children, fever, irritability, abdominal pain, and/or vomiting may be the only signs of UTI. Older children and adolescents are more likely to exhibit signs and symptoms directed toward the urinary tract. These include the classic manifestations of dysuria, urinary frequency, urinary urgency, and cloudy or malodorous urine. In some cases, abdominal pain may be the presenting symptom. In the previously continent school-aged child, the development of secondary enuresis may implicate a recently acquired UTI.

Severe symptoms and constitutional signs (eg, fever) suggest upper urinary tract involvement. Costovertebral angle tenderness is a useful indicator of pyelonephritis in adolescents and adults but is infrequently elicited in infants and young children.

Pathogenesis

The urinary tract represents a normally sterile environment lined by uroepithelial cells. Infection may occur by (1) ascent of periurethral organisms through the urethra or (2) deposition of blood-borne organisms into the urinary tract. Ascending infection is the principal route of infection. In neonates, isolation of bacteria from both blood and urine cultures has provided evidence for hematogenous spread.

Both bacterial virulence factors and host susceptibility factors play a role in developing UTI. Some bacteria (eg, *E coli*) exhibit fimbriae or pili, which allow them to adhere to uroepithelial cells. Individuals vary in physiologic and anatomic characteristics that increase or decrease the likelihood of having a UTI. Factors that increase the likelihood of UTI include residual urine in the bladder, uroepithelial cell adhesiveness, presence of the penile foreskin, and congenital urogenital anomalies. Residual urine in the bladder can be secondary to neurogenic bladder, infrequent voiding, obstructive lesions, or vesicoureteral reflux (VUR). Uroepithelial cells may vary in how receptive they are to bacterial adhesion. In a study of almost 4000 infants by Wiswell et al, uncircumcised boys had a 10-fold greater incidence of UTI than did circumcised boys. In addition, other conditions, such as diabetes mellitus, renal calculi, constipation, and immunodeficiency, are associated with increased risk of UTI.

Microbiology

E coli is responsible for most acute UTIs in children. *Klebsiella-Enterobacter, Proteus mirabilis,* and *Streptococcus viridans* are other, less frequently isolated organisms. Bacteria other than *E coli* may be a more frequent cause of UTIs with frequent recurrence after instrumentation of the urinary tract, such as catheterization, or with underlying anatomic abnormality.

Diagnosis

Once a UTI is suspected on the basis of history and physical examination, a number of direct and indirect laboratory methods are available to document the presence of infection. At first glance, this would seem simply to require the isolation of bacteria from the urinary tract. Indeed, the urine culture remains the gold standard for diagnosing UTI. However, the interpretation of a positive urine culture is influenced by (1) the method of urine collection, (2) specific organism or organisms isolated, and (3) bacterial colony count.

Urine specimens can be collected for laboratory evaluation in several different ways:

1. midstream, "clean-catch" in children who are toilet-trained and can void on demand
2. bag specimens with sterile plastic bag taped to the perineal region
3. bladder catheterization
4. suprapubic aspiration with needle inserted directly across the abdominal wall into the bladder.

Each of these techniques has its respective advantages and disadvantages. For example, bag specimens are non-invasive but are more likely to become contaminated by perineal bacteria, whereas suprapubic aspiration is more invasive but is least likely to become contaminated.

Urine culture allows specific identification of organisms and the determination of their antibiotic sensitivities. Unusual organisms or multiple organisms may suggest improper collection and a contaminated specimen. In addition, urine culture provides quantitative colony counts. Bacterial colony counts of 100,000 or greater of a single organism are consistent with UTI regardless of the method of collection. Colony counts less than 100,000 require additional interpretation but may be acceptable from suprapubic aspiration or catheterization specimens or if multiple clean-catch yield the same results.

One disadvantage of the culture technique is the delay (usually 1–2 days) in getting the results. Urine microscopy and urinalysis can supplement urine culture by providing immediate results. Bacteria and white blood cells can be observed directly by urine microscopy. Dipstick urinalysis can detect the presence of bacteria or white blood cells indirectly; these strips are impregnated with reagents that change color in response to nitrite or leukocyte esterase. Certain bacteria (eg, *E coli*) have the ability to convert nitrate into nitrites, and white blood cells may release leukocyte esterase. The disadvantage of the conventional urinalysis is that it is less sensitive than the urine culture, with a 20% false-negative rate (higher in infants younger than 2 months). An enhanced urinalysis has been developed that may approach the sensitivity of culture.

Adjunctive tests have been used in an attempt to differentiate upper- from lower-tract disease. Elevation of ESR and C-reactive protein may suggest a more systemic infection, such as pyelonephritis. Nuclear medicine imaging with technetium-99m or gallium renal scan can be performed in the acute setting to demonstrate abnormal uptake in the renal parenchyma. Other tests have limited use in the clinical setting, such as urine tests for antibody-coated bacteria, increased urine concentrations of lactate dehydrogenase isoenzyme 5, and N-acetyl β-D-glucosaminidase. Likewise, bilateral ureteral catheterization and kidney biopsy are not commonly used to verify upper tract involvement.

Treatment

Decisions concerning therapy of UTIs include the following:

1. use of empiric therapy (versus waiting for culture results)
2. selection of appropriate antibiotics with respect to drug of choice, route of administration, and duration of therapy
3. setting for therapy as inpatient versus outpatient.

Once a UTI is suspected by initial evaluation, empiric therapy usually may be initiated. Choice of antibiotic would be based on the likely organism (eg, *E coli*) as well as on patterns of antibiotic resistance in the local area. In particular, *E coli* has demonstrated increasing frequency of ampicillin resistance. Adjustments in therapy can be made once the identity of the bacteria and antibiotic sensitivities are available from urine culture.

In addition to the age of the patient, the severity of infection and ability to maintain hydration are considerations in determining the setting and route of therapy. The degree of toxicity of the patient, which may interfere with compliance with oral medications, along with the degree of suspicion of upper tract disease, must be considered. In neonates and young infants (younger than 3–4 months), parenteral therapy with ampicillin and an aminoglycoside is a standard recommendation because very young infants with UTI are at much higher risk for bacteremia and sepsis.

Parenteral therapy is an important consideration, especially in neonates, because of the concern over a blood-borne infection with hematogenous spread to the urinary tract. In older infants and children, upper tract infection still could be treated with parenteral antibiotics, ampicillin, and an aminoglycoside or third-generation cephalosporin, or with intramuscular injection(s) of ceftriaxone.

Uncomplicated lower tract infections or cystitis can be treated with a variety of oral agents, including amoxicillin, trimethoprim-sulfamethoxazole, and cephalosporins. Duration of treatment of cystitis in children usually is still 7–10 days, although some support the utility of short-course therapy in children with uncomplicated infections. Duration of therapy depends on severity of initial illness, the rate of clinical improvement, evidence of microbiologic clearing on repeat culture, and presence or absence of underlying anatomic abnormality.

In select patients with defined anatomic abnormalities or at least three recurrent infections, the use of prophylactic antibiotics is warranted to limit recurrence and complications. Antimicrobial agents commonly used include sulfisoxazole, amoxicillin, nitrofurantoin, and trimethoprim-sulfamethoxazole. Patients with vesicourethral reflux should receive prophylaxis. The duration of prophylaxis can be guided by voiding cystourethrogram (VCUG) every year to determine the resolution of reflux. Such reflux usually resolves spontaneously in most pediatric patients and seldom requires surgical intervention.

Follow-up Investigations

UTI may be a marker for anatomic malformation or dysfunction of the urinary tract. In addition, infection of the kidney parenchyma may lead to renal scarring. Thus, adequate follow-up is crucial.

The clinician must decide whether additional investigation is indicated after a documented UTI. Because further testing may be invasive and expensive and may require exposure to radiation, patients are selected with careful consideration of the risks and benefits. The goals of further testing are (1) to identify host factors that may predispose to or increase risk of recurrent infection and (2) to detect or prevent possible sequelae of infection (eg, renal scarring). A reported 20–30% of children with UTI have an anatomic abnormality, most commonly VUR as well as obstructive lesions (eg, posterior urethral valves) and urolithiasis. VUR refers to the reflux of urine from bladder to ureter. Reflux may predispose to development of UTIs by causing residual urine in the bladder. Reflux of sterile or infected urine up to the kidneys may produce renal scarring. Both medical (eg, prophylactic antibiotics) and surgical (eg, surgical reimplantation of the ureters) options exist for severe reflux.

Recommendations from different experts differ on the basis of the patient's age, gender, and severity of illness. It is commonly recommended that all children with suspected upper tract infection and all boys with first documented UTI undergo further evaluation. Less clearly established is whether all girls with uncomplicated cystitis require testing for anatomic abnormalities and reflux. Recommendations vary with age, with younger girls being more commonly referred for evaluation. The age cutoff varies from preschool to adolescent.

A description of some studies available for evaluation of patients with documented UTIs is in included in Table 9–45. Currently, a renal ultrasound to evaluate the upper urinary tract is combined with a VCUG to evaluate the lower urinary tract. In general, renal ultrasound may be useful during the acute infection, especially for hospitalized patients with upper tract diseases, to rule out hydronephrosis and perirenal or renal parenchymal diseases. In contrast, the VCUG usually is performed a few weeks after successful completion of the treatment course because of the common occurrence of transient reflux secondary to hyperactivity of detrusor muscle, incompetent urinary sphincter, and decreased functional bladder capacity.

SEXUALLY TRANSMITTED DISEASES

STDs in pediatric patients, compared with adults, have a unique situation because of different presentations in different age groups. Some diseases are more common in neonates than in adults. Although adolescents and young adults are at greatest risk, newborns of infected mothers also may acquire many of these same infections. Because more than two dozen infectious agents are known to be acquired by genital, anal, and oral sexual contact, patients often are infected with more than one STD at a time. The identification of one STD should lead to investigation for others. Only the more common etiologies are discussed here. The STD syndromes are discussed further in Chapter 2, and HIV infection is discussed in Chapter 7.

Table 9–45. Imaging studies in urinary tract infection.

	Detects	Advantages	Disadvantages
Renal ultrasound	Renal size, shape, position Echogenicity Hydronephrosis, hydroureter, ureteroceles, bladder thickening	Little discomfort No radiation No IV contrast	Low sensitivity for renal scars No functional assessment Dependent on skill of sonographer
Intravenous (IV) pyelogram	Renal scarring Abnormal urinary tracts		Radiation Requires IV contrast (risk of contrast allergy)
VCUG[1]	Vesiculoureteral reflux (grading) Posterior ureteral valves Ureteroceles, bladder diverticula Bladder functions, emptying		Requires bladder catheterization Radiation
Radioisotope renal scans	Acute pyelonephritis Renal scars	Low radiation No contrast	
Nuclear VCUG	Vesicoureteral reflux	Low radiation	Requires bladder catheterization Difficult to grade reflux Less anatomic detail than VCUG

[1]The retrograde voiding cystourethrogram (VCUG) consists of instilling contrast material directly into the bladder via a small catheter inserted through the urethra.

CHLAMYDIA TRACHOMATIS

Chlamydiae are some of the most common bacterial pathogens found in the human host. However, chlamydia lacks the capability to produce its own adenosine triphosphate (ATP) and is therefore an obligate intracellular parasite, similar to viruses. Properties of chlamydiae resembling bacteria include possession of both DNA and RNA, replication through binary fission, presence of a cell wall, and, henceforth, their susceptibility to antimicrobials. The genus *Chlamydia* is divided into three species: *C psittaci,* which causes psittacosis and ornithosis; *C pneumoniae,* which causes pneumonia and bronchiolitis; and *C trachomatis,* which is the leading cause of nonspecific urethritis and the most common nonviral STD in the United States (Table 9–46).

C trachomatis has many different serotypes: types A–C are a leading cause of blindness worldwide. The types responsible for the common STDs include types D–K; types L1–L3 are the cause of lymphogranuloma venereum. The life cycle of chlamydiae is complex and involves attachment and then phagocytosis of the infectious elementary body by a host epithelial cell. The elementary bodies then reorganize into reticulate bodies, which take over the cellular machinery for reproduction while arresting cellular DNA and RNA replication. Once abundant in the cytoplasm, reticulate bodies condense and reorganize back into elementary bodies. Multiplication of *C trachomatis* deprives the host cell of its own cellular ATP, resulting in host cell death, lysis, and release of elementary bodies. Epithelial cell phagocytosis of the newly released chlamydial particles spreads the infection and perpetuates the cycle.

Chlamydial urethritis presents with dysuria, sterile pyuria, and urethral inflammation and discharge. It is estimated that 10–25% of infected men and 35–50% of infected women remain asymptomatic but are infectious to others. Disease may be localized to the initial point of sexual contact, resulting in urethritis, cervicitis, conjunctivitis, pharyngitis, or proctitis. It also may ascend the genitourinary tract, resulting in epididymitis and prostatitis in male patients and salpingitis in female patients. Secondary scarring of the fallopian tubes increases the risk of ectopic pregnancy and infertility.

This infection may also result in Reiter syndrome and a perihepatitis (Fitz-Hugh-Curtis) syndrome. The features of Reiter syndrome include arthritis, ocular inflammation, and urethritis. Although usually associated with *C trachomatis,* it may also be seen with other infections, notably with organisms responsible for gastrointestinal infections. The perihepatitis syndrome associated with *C trachomatis* may present with right upper quadrant pain, referred shoulder pain, pleuritic pain, and elevated liver transaminases. The liver may be tender to palpation with an audible hepatic friction rub.

Newborns of mothers infected with *C trachomatis* have a 30–50% chance of acquiring the infection through the birth canal. Ocular and nasal mucosa are the areas most likely to be infected. The resulting purulent discharge and red conjunctiva cannot be distinguished clinically from other causes of conjunctivitis, including gonococcus and

Table 9–46. Chlamydial infections.

Species	Serotypes	Clinical Manifestations
Chlamydia trachomatis	A, B, C	Trachoma
	D–K	Urethritis, epididymitis, cervicitis, pelvic inflammatory disease, conjunctivitis, infantile pneumonia
	L1–L3	Lymphogranuloma venereum
Chlamydia psittaci		Psittacosis, ornithosis
Chlamydia pneumoniae		Pharyngitis, pneumonia

viruses. Spread from the upper to the lower respiratory tract may result in interstitial pneumonitis by 1–6 months of age. These infants usually have a pertussis-like cough, hyperinflated chest, fever, and peripheral eosinophilia. The pneumonitis and conjunctivitis do not always occur simultaneously.

Testing for chlamydial disease remains difficult. A urethral Gram stain revealing granulocytes without intracellular gram-negative diplococci is suggestive. Other tests require proper collection of infected epithelial cells. In newborns, samples should be collected from nasal respiratory mucosa or the conjunctiva. Culture remains the gold standard but is labor intensive. Rapid testing is available with an ELISA-identifying antigen and immunofluorescent antibody staining to identify intracellular elementary bodies.

Doxycycline is the drug of choice; alternatives include tetracycline or erythromycin. In newborns, systemic therapy with erythromycin is recommended for both conjunctivitis and pneumonitis.

NEISSERIA GONORRHOEAE

Infection with *N gonorrhoeae,* a gram-negative diplococcus, is the most commonly reported STD in the United States, responsible for more than 1 million reported cases of STD per year. The organism's virulence is associated largely with its ability to use pili from its cell wall to adhere to mucoepithelial surfaces. Columnar epithelium is most susceptible to the infection.

Asymptomatic infection is less frequent than with chlamydial infection; however, it does occur and is most common in the female population and in pharyngeal infections. Most infections are symptomatic and localized to the site of direct contact. Symptoms are similar to those seen with chlamydial infection, such as urethritis, cervicitis, conjunctivitis, pharyngitis, and proctitis. Ascending infections of the genitourinary tract include prostatitis in male patients and salpingitis in female patients. Disseminated disease occurs in fewer than 2% of patients. Hematogenous spread of gonorrhea most frequently results in septic arthritis, tenosynovitis, and dermatitis (see section on Reactive Arthritis Syndrome). Skin lesions may be maculopapular, vesicular, or purpuric in appearance. Less frequent manifestations of disseminated disease include endocarditis and meningitis.

In newborns of infected mothers, gonococcal ophthalmia neonatorum may develop after a variable incubation period of several days to weeks. Copious purulent discharge from the infant's eyes is the presenting symptom. Without proper diagnosis and treatment, rapid progression of the infection results in corneal ulceration, opacification, and blindness. The use of prophylactic erythromycin ointment or 1% silver nitrate administered shortly after birth greatly reduces the rate of infection.

Diagnosis is confirmed by Gram stain and culture of purulent body fluids from the suspected site of infection.

Cultures require the use of Thayer-Martin medium, with increased carbon dioxide environment to enhance bacterial growth. Antimicrobial sensitivity testing is essential to guide therapy because of the rapid increase in numbers of penicillinase-producing organisms. Accepted treatments are outlined in Table 9–47. Concurrent therapy for chlamydial infection is recommended in all patients in whom gonorrhea is diagnosed.

SYPHILIS

Syphilis is caused by *T pallidum,* a prototypic spirochete bacterium. The organism is a thin, delicate spirochete 5–20 μm long with an appearance of a helical coil. It can be visualized with dark-field microscopy or immunofluorescence. Humans are the only hosts. Transmission is almost totally through sexual contacts, with the exception of congenital infections and very close physical contact between mucous membranes of the hosts. The treponemal organism attacks the human cells and multiplies actively during the initial phase. Fetal and neonatal cells are good targets because of relative immaturity of the mucosal barrier and the immune system.

The incidence of syphilis in the United States had been decreasing over the past few decades; however, there has been a recent resurgence in the incidence of both acquired and congenital syphilis. The number of congenital syphilis cases had increased from fewer than 200 in the early 1980s to approximately 3000 in 1991. This has become a major problem facing pediatric practitioners in many metropolitan centers. It is particularly challenging to identify a well-appearing infant born to a serologically positive mother and to manage appropriately. Beyond the neonatal group, for children in whom the infection is newly diagnosed, sexual abuse must be presumed, requiring a prompt report to children's protection services.

Acquired syphilis has three stages. The primary stage is characterized by chancre, which is a single, painless, ulcerated lesion with a raised border at the site of entry of the organism, eg, on the glans penis or labia, or within the vagina. The incubation period may last several weeks, and the primary lesion heals spontaneously in 1–2 months.

Table 9–47. Treatment for gonococcal infections.

Type of Infection	Drug of Choice	Alternative
Urethritis, cervicitis, proctitis	Ceftriaxone IM	Spectinomycin IM + doxycycline *or* ciprofloxacin
Pharyngeal	Ceftriaxone IM	Trimethoprim-sulfamethoxazole
Disseminated disease	Ceftriaxone IV	Cefotaxime *or* spectinomycin
Ophthalmia neonatorum	Cefotaxime IV	

IM = intramuscular; IV = intravenous.

The chancre lesion is often accompanied by regional lymphadenopathy. Several months later, the secondary stage begins with onset of symptoms, including fever, sore throat, headache, rhinitis, arthralgias, malaise, and anorexia. Signs include generalized lymphadenopathy, hepatosplenomegaly, and a copper-colored maculopapular rash that begins on the trunk and spreads rapidly to involve the extremities, including the palms and soles. Mucous patches are common. Other dermatologic manifestations include alopecia and condyloma. In some patients, complications, including meningitis, hepatitis, and glomerulonephritis, may develop. At this stage, patients are very infectious, and the lesions are often positive for *Treponema* by immunofluorescence. Serologic tests are invariably positive. If undiagnosed, symptoms resolve spontaneously after about 2 weeks. Tertiary or latent syphilis occurs months to years after untreated secondary syphilis. The lesions are gummatous in appearance and are probably the result of hypersensitivity reactions. Tertiary syphilis is primarily a disease of adults and can affect any organ. At this stage, the patient is no longer infectious to others. Gradual destruction of the nervous (neurosyphilis) and cardiovascular systems predominates in the third stage because of long-standing vascular disease and endarteritis.

Serologic testing is the diagnostic cornerstone. There are two general categories for these tests. Nontreponemal antigen tests use a component of normal tissue (eg, beef heart cardiolipin) as an antigen to assay for reagin, a nonspecific antibody formed by patients with syphilis. The most commonly used nontreponemal tests are Venereal Disease Research Laboratory (VDRL) and rapid plasma reagin (RPR) tests. Older tests that use complement fixation are seldom used today. Results of these surrogate markers become positive by 4 weeks after the initial infection and remain so through the second stage with high titers of more than 1:32. During the latent phase and after therapy, the VDRL and RPR titers often decrease gradually. False-positive test results are encountered frequently for a number of other disorders, such as collagen vascular diseases, malaria, EBV infections, and other nonvenereal treponemal infections as well as drug reactions. The RPR test is simpler than the traditional VDRL.

If VDRL or RPR results are positive, serum should be tested specifically for treponemal antibody with the FTA-ABS to confirm the diagnosis. The test is both sensitive and specific for treponemal antibody. This test is positive in most patients with primary syphilis and in virtually all secondary cases. In general, it remains permanently positive despite treatment. False-positive FTA-ABS results occur rarely in systemic lupus and other rare diseases with abnormal globulins. Diagnosis from primary chancres also can be made by darkfield microscopic examination for motile spirochetes. Current treatment recommendations are shown in Table 9–48.

Congenital Syphilis

Congenital syphilis develops by two different routes: (1) transplacental transmission of the spirochete, mostly in the first half of gestation, and (2) perinatal acquisition by direct contact with the organism through the vaginal canal. Many infants who are infected by the former mode are stillborn. Manifestations of the congenital infection in the survivors vary and may be nonspecific. The skin and bones are the most commonly affected sites. Bullous lesions on the skin, including the palms and soles, develop in most untreated cases. Profuse serous rhinorrhea, called "snuffles," is a characteristic mucous membrane lesion. Consequent to mucosal and cartilage infections in the nasal area, destruction of the nasal cartilage ensues, resulting in the classic saddle nose deformity. In addition, osteochondritis is diffuse and symmetric with involvement of the metaphyseal plates. Periosteal elevations in the humerus and tibia are most common. Involvement of the

Table 9–48. Management of syphilitic infections (children and adults).

Type of Infection	Drug of Choice	Alternative
Primary or secondary	Benzathine penicillin, IM 2.4 MU	Tetracycline or doxycycline po × 2 wk, or ceftriaxone
Tertiary or infection > 1 y	Benzathine penicillin G, IM 2.4 MU q wk × 3 wk	Tetracycline or doxycycline

Neurosyphilis	Penicillin G, 50 KU/kg, IV q 4 h, 10–14 d, followed
	   by benzathine pen G, 2.4 MU, IM, q wk × 3 wk
	or
	Procaine penicillin G, 2.4 MU, IM q d, + probenecid
	   500 mg QID, × 10–14 d, followed by benzathine
	   pen G, 2.4 MU, IM, q wk × 3 wk	

Congenital	Penicillin G IV × 10–14 d
	1st wk postnatally: 50 KU/kg IV q 12 h
	2nd wk: 50 KU/kg IV q 8 h
	or
	Procaine penicillin 50 KU/kg, IM, q D, 10–14 d
	Follow-up: development evaluation; visual, hearing
	   tests; serum VDRL or RPR at 3, 6, and 12 mo;
	   CSF VDRL at the end of therapy	

CSF = cerebrospinal fluid; IM = intramuscular; IV = intravenous; KU = 1000 units; MU = 1 million units; RPR = rapid plasma reagin test; VDRL = Venereal Disease Research Laboratory test.

reticuloendothelial system results in splenomegaly and generalized lymphadenopathy. Late congenital syphilis is characterized by the Hutchinson triad: Hutchinson teeth (peg-shaped, notched upper central incisors), interstitial keratitis, and cranial nerve VIII deafness.

HERPES SIMPLEX VIRUS

HSV is responsible for an increasing number of clinically significant infections each year. Two strains, HSV-1 and HSV-2, are identified by biologic and antigenic differences. They are among the most common infectious pathogens in the pediatric age group. HSV belongs to a family of DNA viruses that also includes CMV, VZV, EBV, and herpes virus 6 to 8. HSV has the capacity to persist, in active or dormant forms, throughout the life of the host. For primary infection, mucocutaneous epithelial cells provide the initial target for viral infection, whereas neural cells in trigeminal and sacral root ganglia constitute the sites of latent infection. In disseminated diseases, HSV-1 and HSV-2 can infect other tissue sites, such as brain, liver, and lung.

Because of the biologic differences, the two serotypes have different modes of transmission: HSV-1 is transmitted mainly via a nongenital route, whereas HSV-2 is most commonly transmitted venereally or from maternal genitalia to the newborn. As a general rule, HSV-1 infections occur most frequently during childhood and usually affect body mucosal sites above the waist, including mouth, lips, and eyes. In contrast, HSV-2 infections occur most often during adolescence and young adulthood and involve genital sites. HSV-2 produces vesicles similar to HSV-1 but occurs most often on the genitals and is sexually transmitted. Men have lesions on the glans, prepuce, or penile shaft. Women usually have lesions on the cervix but may have scattered involvement of the labia.

After a primary infection, the virus becomes latent in the ganglion cells of the nerves innervating the site of inoculation. Recurrence may be frequent and can be multifactorially precipitated by stress, trauma, or fever. Lesions are painful ulcerating vesicles and can be located on oral, rectal, or vaginal mucosa, as well as on the penis and labia. Regional lymphadenitis is common.

Neonatal Herpes

In neonates, most of the infection is caused by HSV-2 due to maternal genital infection transmitted to the infant during vaginal delivery. The incidence has been estimated to be in the range of 1:3000 to 1:30,000 deliveries, with higher incidence in premature than in term newborns. Transplacental transmission has been shown in a very small number of patients who present at birth with a congenital syndrome. The affected infants typically have CNS and ocular anomalies, accompanied by vesicular cutaneous lesions and scarring.

Neonatal herpes can manifest as localized or severe systemic disease complicated with meningoencephalitis. In the absence of effective antiviral therapy, disseminated HSV disease has a mortality rate of more than 70%. Almost all survivors have serious CNS sequelae. Without treatment, the initially localized disease will progress to the disseminated form after 1–2 weeks.

The disseminated form of HSV disease affects primarily the liver, adrenal gland, and CNS. The infant may present with hepatosplenomegaly, jaundice, bleeding diathesis, and seizures. In some cases, pneumonia has been described. Shock and disseminated intravascular coagulation may lead to death. Involvement of the eye may be manifested as conjunctivitis, keratitis, and chorioretinitis, leading to corneal scarring cataracts and blindness.

Management

A smear of cells scraped from the base of a vesicle stained with Wright stain (Tzanck preparation) demonstrating multinucleated giant cells is highly suggestive of the infection. The diagnosis can be confirmed by viral culture of vesicular fluid and confirmed by immunofluorescence.

Patients with overt herpetic lesions should have strict barrier isolation to avoid spread of the infectious fluid. Hospital personnel should wear protective gowns and gloves when caring for the patients. Immunocompromised hosts should avoid contact with individuals with overt HSV disease.

For adolescents and adults, the use of condoms and the practice of "safe sex" cannot be overemphasized. Treatment of primary herpes using orally administered acyclovir shortens the clinical course but does not prevent recurrent infections. Small daily doses of the drug may be helpful in preventing frequent recurrence after resolution of the acute infection.

With respect to perinatal situations, if a pregnant women is suspected of having active HSV-2 infection, the infant should be delivered by cesarean section before rupture of membranes or within 4 hours of membrane rupture. For neonates with HSV infection, systemic administration of acyclovir is indicated. Similarly, antiviral therapy should be instituted for patients with encephalitis and for immunocompromised hosts.

HUMAN PAPILLOMAVIRUS

Human papillomavirus (HPV) is the most common STD in the United States. The DNA papillomavirus causes a painless, firm, warty lesion at the site of infection. The incubation period may be several months. Diagnosis is made by inspection. The application of 3% acetic acid turns HPV lesions white. HPV-16 and HPV-18 are risk factors for cervical and anal carcinoma. Newborns exposed to HPV during birth may have laryngeal papillomatosis, leading to airway obstruction many months after birth. Treatment options are varied and include topical application of podophyllum in tincture of benzoin for nonmucosal lesions, application of trichloroacetic acid, cryosurgery, laser therapy, systemic interferon administration, and surgical excision.

OTHER INFECTIONS

Trichomonas vaginalis is a frequent cause of vaginitis in the female population and urethritis in the male population. The vaginal discharge often is foul-smelling, frothy, and yellow-green. The cervix usually is edematous and covered with punctate red lesions and a background of diffuse erythema. Wet mounts reveal live, motile organisms and numerous granulocytes. The infection can be treated with metronidazole.

Nonspecific vaginitis is most frequently associated with the facultative anaerobe *Gardnerella vaginalis.* Many patients have asymptomatic infections. The most common symptoms are profuse vaginal discharge with an offensive, fishy odor. No associated pelvic pain, dysuria, or dyspareunia is present unless accompanied by another STD. It is a diagnosis of exclusion; usually, three of the following four criteria should be met to make the diagnosis: (1) gray-white discharge adherent to vaginal mucosa; (2) vaginal pH greater than 4.5; (3) positive amine test, in which volatile amines are released on the addition of 10% KOH solution to vaginal secretions, enhancing the foul odors; and (4) presence of clue cells (vaginal epithelial cells speckled by the adherence of organisms) in addition to numerous leukocytes on a saline wet mount of vaginal fluids. Treatment is with a single dose of metronidazole.

Haemophilus ducreyi is a nonmotile, gram-negative rod that causes chancroid. At the site of inoculation, a painful ulcer with scalloped and irregular borders develops. There is also regional lymphadenopathy. The diagnosis is confirmed by bacterial culture of the exudate. Treatment consists of trimethoprim-sulfamethoxazole, erythromycin, or ceftriaxone.

RASH & FEVER: INFECTIOUS EXANTHEM

Rash and fever occur commonly during childhood. Classically, six infectious exanthems were described (Table 9–49). Although this classification scheme is somewhat antiquated, it is a marker for the progress we

Table 9–49. Historical nomenclature of infectious exanthems.

Disease	Infectious Agent
First	Rubeola or measles
Second	Streptococcal scarlet fever
Third	Rubella or German measles
Fourth	Filatov-Dukes disease
Fifth	Erythema infectiosum (parvovirus B19)
Sixth	Human herpes virus 6 (roseola)

have made in identifying the infectious etiologies for a variety of common childhood illnesses.

Although most childhood exanthems accompanied by fever are self-limited and benign, some are life-threatening and require urgent attention. For this reason, most ill children with rash should be examined promptly by medical personnel. The etiologies of what have been called "killer rashes," such as meningococcemia, Rocky Mountain spotted fever, toxic shock syndrome, and Stevens-Johnson syndrome, are discussed elsewhere. This section discusses the common early childhood infectious exanthems, as well as some other causes of rash and fever.

MEASLES

Rubeola, commonly referred to as the "10-day measles," is a highly contagious viral illness characterized by three stages: incubation, prodrome, and rash. Although the widespread use of the vaccine has decreased the incidence in children significantly, recent outbreaks in inadequately vaccinated children and adolescents remind us of the high morbidity and mortality associated with this disease.

Rubeola is an RNA virus of the Paramyxoviridae family. It spreads very efficiently through households with a greater than 90% infectious rate in susceptible individuals. Before the vaccine was available, measles occurred in epidemics during spring every 2–4 years.

The incubation period is typically 8–12 days after exposure. During the prodromal phase, the patient has low-grade fever and "the three C's": cough, coryza, and conjunctivitis, often with photophobia. This is followed by the appearance of the pathognomonic measles enanthem, Koplik spots. Koplik spots are gray, pinhead-sized dots surrounded by a ring of erythema, found on the buccal mucosa; they may last as briefly as 12 hours and are frequently missed on physical examination. The symptoms of the prodrome worsen until the fever spikes and the rash eruption. The rash usually starts as faint macules around the neck and ears and descends quickly. The maculopapular rash covers the face, arms, and chest within 24 hours. During the second day of rash, the lower torso and legs become involved. By the third day, the rash reaches the feet and has areas of confluence. The rash is centripetal in distribution, with the most dense confluences located proximally and superiorly. It appears that the severity of the disease is related directly to the severity of the rash. In severe cases, the rash may become hemorrhagic with petechiae and ecchymosis.

Measles is frequently associated with otitis media and bronchopneumonia. As many as one third of affected children have patchy infiltrates on chest radiograph. Infrequent but potentially serious complications include laryngotracheitis and encephalomyelitis. Subacute sclerosing panencephalitis (SSPE), a rare complication of persistent measles virus infection, is characterized by behavioral and intellectual deterioration and myoclonic seizures occurring several decades after the initial infection. The disease progresses to bulbar palsy, hyperthermia, and decerebrate posturing. Death occurs 1–2 years after onset of symptoms.

Measles is usually diagnosed clinically but can be confirmed by serology. Assays measuring both IgM and IgG are available commercially. In SSPE, high titers of measles antibody are found in the serum and CSF.

RUBELLA

Rubella, alternatively known as "German measles" or "3-day measles," continues to be a relatively common communicable disease despite reasonably effective vaccination program. Of major clinical significance is the risk for severe congenital anomalies associated with rubella infections during pregnancy in susceptible hosts.

Rubella is caused by the rubivirus, a pleomorphic RNA virus in the togavirus family. During clinical illness, the virus is present in nasopharyngeal secretions, blood, feces, and urine. The disease is spread by oral droplets or the transplacental route. Before the vaccine was available, the peak incidence was in children aged 5–14 years. Currently, most cases are seen in teenagers and young adults. In close quarters, the virus is highly contagious among susceptible individuals. Maternal antibody provides passive immunization for the first 6 months postnatally in infants. Active infection with rubella virus confers permanent immunity.

The incubation period is 14–21 days. Although similar to rubeola and scarlet fever, the exanthem associated with rubella may be distinguished by clinical criteria. Initially, there is a prodrome of mild catarrhal symptoms, which often go unnoticed. A characteristic sign of rubella is the markedly tender lymphadenopathy, which appears at least 24 hours before the rash and may last several days. Usually, the postauricular, posterior cervical, and postoccipital nodes are most remarkable. The exanthem is maculopapular and confluent, beginning on the face and spreading quickly to the trunk and extremities within the first 24 hours. The rash is nonpruritic and typically lacy in appearance. On the second day, the appearance becomes more pinpoint, resembling scarlet fever. The eruption usually clears by the third day; thus, its alternative name. Occasionally, mild desquamation ensues. The oropharynx and conjunctiva are usually inflamed, but there is no photophobia as occurs in rubeola. A slight fever may accompany the rash for up to 3 days. Polyarthritis may occur for several days to 2 weeks, especially in older girls and women.

After primary maternal infection during pregnancy, congenital rubella infection occurs in 25–90% of fetuses, depending on gestational stage. The highest rate of transmission is in the first trimester. Congenital anomalies can be seen in up to 30% of congenital rubella infections acquired before 12 weeks' gestation. With infection beyond 20 weeks' gestation, congenital anomalies are rare. The most common anomalies are congenital cataracts, patent ductus arteriosus, sensorineural hearing loss, and meningoencephalitis. In addition, infants with congenital rubella syndrome may have growth retardation, radiolucent bone disease, hepatosplenomegaly, thrombocytopenia, jaundice, and purpura. The appearance of the skin lesions gives the name "blueberry muffin syndrome." The clinical diagnosis of rubella can be confirmed by acute and convalescent IgG titers or by direct measurement of rubella IgM antibody. Viral culture of the urine is diagnostic in congenital infections. Except for cases of congenitally acquired infection, rubella is a self-limited illness. The vaccine is important to improve herd immunity and reduce the risk of infection in pregnant women. Young women should be vaccinated or tested for immunity to rubella before the onset of sexual activity. Therefore, the vaccine is currently given at 15 months of age and repeated at 11–12 years.

STREPTOCOCCAL SCARLET FEVER

Scarlet fever is an erythematous sandpaper-like rash with fever caused by one of the erythrogenic exotoxins produced by GAS, *S pyogenes*. It is associated most often with pharyngeal infection but can be seen with pyoderma and impetigo. Transmission occurs by contact with respiratory secretions from a person with active streptococcal infection, in particular in overcrowded environment including schools, military camps, and living quarters of the underprivileged. Infection can occur at any age but is most frequent in children older than 3 years.

The incubation period is 1–7 days, with an average of 3 days. Initially there is a rapid onset of fever and chills, vomiting, headache, and a toxic appearance. Examination of the posterior pharynx reveals erythematous tonsils, which frequently are covered with a white exudate. The tongue initially appears white with prominent edematous papillae ("white strawberry tongue"). After several days, the white coat desquamates, leaving the erythematous papillae ("red strawberry tongue"). The exanthem usually appears at the same time as the fever and is characterized by fine, mildly erythematous papules that first appear in the axilla, groin, and neck. Within 24 hours, the rash generalizes but spares the face. The cheeks and forehead are flushed, and there is circumoral pallor. The rash is most intense at pressure sites, and there may be some petechiae. Pastia lines are areas of linear hyperpigmentation in the deep creases, particularly the antecubital fossae. Miliary sudamina are small vesicular lesions that appear on the abdomen, hands, and feet in severe cases. The rash desquamates after approximately 1 week.

The diagnosis of scarlet fever is made clinically, and GAS can be cultured readily from the pharynx or wound. Patients with suspected scarlet fever should receive penicillin or erythromycin.

ERYTHEMA INFECTIOSUM
(Fifth Disease)

Erythema infectiosum is a common childhood illness caused by parvovirus B19, a single-stranded DNA virus. It is a relatively benign disease in the normal host but can cause aplastic anemia in patients with hemolytic anemias and HIV infection. Fetal hydrops occurs uncommonly in the fetuses of women with primary parvovirus B19 infection.

The disease is seen commonly in school-aged children, and community epidemics have been described. Outbreaks most frequently occur in the spring. Infection is common during the school years; approximately 50% of adults show serologic evidence of past infection. Infection is spread by contact with respiratory secretions or blood.

The most frequently seen clinical manifestation of infection with parvovirus B19 is erythema infectiosum. This is a mild systemic illness, with low-grade fever and distinctive rash. The cheeks show red flushing, with circumoral pallor, giving the appearance of "slapped cheeks." The rash on the torso and extremities is a pale maculopapular eruption, frequently lacy in appearance. This rash intensifies with fever and exposure to sunlight. The rash is frequently pruritic. The illness lasts 3–5 days, and there are no sequelae. A child is usually noninfectious once the rash appears. In older children and adults, especially women, there may be associated arthralgias and arthritis. Rarely, the rash will be limited to hands and feet, giving a "glove and stocking" appearance.

Parvovirus B19 affects the red-cell precursors in the bone marrow and reduces the number of circulating reticulocytes. This does not cause a significant anemia in healthy children, but severe anemia, termed transient aplastic crisis, can develop in children with a shortened red-blood-cell life span. This is seen most commonly in children with hemoglobinopathies and has been reported in patients infected with HIV. These patients have prolonged excretion of the virus and, if hospitalized, should be kept in respiratory isolation. The aplastic crises may be quite prolonged but have been successfully treated with IV immunoglobulin.

Diagnosis of erythema infectiosum is made clinically, but serologic tests measuring IgM and IgG are available. In addition, parvovirus B19 DNA can be detected in bone marrow from patients experiencing aplastic crises.

HUMAN HERPES VIRUS 6
(Roseola)

Roseola infantum is a common acute viral illness seen in infants and toddlers. The child with roseola typically will experience 3–4 days of high fever, followed by a diffuse erythematous maculopapular eruption when the fever subsides.

The etiology of roseola recently has been found to be human herpes virus 6. Epidemiologic studies also have implicated this virus in children with febrile seizures, leading to the expression "roseola without the rash."

Although patients may have a mild pharyngeal inflammation or coryza, the first symptom noted is the sudden onset of high fever. Temperatures as high as 39.5–41.0 °C are common. Within the first 24–36 hours of fever, the WBC is elevated, often with increased neutrophil counts. Over the second to third day of fever, the WBC decreases, sometimes resulting in neutropenia. With resolution of the fever on the third or fourth day, a diffuse maculopapular rash erupts, beginning over the trunk. The rash quickly spreads to the arms, neck, face, and legs. This eruption usually lasts less than 24 hours.

Roseola infantum usually is self-limited and requires no treatment. Antipyretics may be helpful in relieving the discomfort of the fever and reducing the risk of febrile seizure.

VARICELLA

Varicella zoster and herpes zoster are two clinical manifestations of the same virus. Varicella, or "chickenpox," is the primary infection with diffuse vesicular skin lesions. It is a disease of early childhood; 90% of individuals contract the disease and develop immunity during the first decade of life. In contrast, herpes zoster is a localized reactivation of the infection, characterized by distribution of lesions limited by dermatomes. A primary infection with varicella usually confers lifelong immunity against the systemic disease, but second episodes have been reported, particularly during periods of distress and in immunocompromised hosts. The viral agent that causes both varicella and herpes zoster is *Herpesvirus varicellae,* a DNA virus. It is indistinguishable by electron microscopy from *Herpesvirus hominis.* The skin lesions of both species are also identical histologically.

The virus is highly contagious and can be transmitted via direct contact, droplet, or airborne contact. Chickenpox usually is seen between January and May. Herpes zoster has no seasonal preference. The incubation period for varicella infection is 11–21 days. Viremia usually occurs 2 days before the onset of the exanthem. A mild prodrome of fever, malaise, and anorexia precedes the rash, usually by 24 hours. The rash consists of generalized, pruritic vesicular lesions that begin on the trunk and spread to the face and proximal extremities. A pertinent feature useful in distinguishing chickenpox from other vesicular exanthems is that the lesions are always at different stages of healing. At any time during the infection, one should find erythematous papules, "teardrop" vesicles on an erythematous base, ruptured vesicles, and crusted vesicles with scabs. In primary infection, the vesicular lesions are limited to the skin. Rarely, in severe infections, lesions may spread to the mouth, esophagus, trachea, and intestines. Varicella pneumonia and hepatitis are rare complications.

After primary infection, the virus remains dormant in a dorsal root ganglion in the normal host. Herpes zoster develops during periods of distress and in immunocompromised hosts, in whom reactivation of the virus replication causes pain in the corresponding dermatome. Within a few days, an eruption of vesicular lesions on an erythematous base occurs in the same painful dermatome. The lesions last 5–10 days, and regional lymphadenopathy may be seen. The dermatomes of the second thoracic to the second lumbar nerves are most commonly involved. In severe cases and in immunocompromised hosts, more than one dermatome may be involved. Rarely, herpes zoster may involve the ophthalmic branch of the trigeminal nerve, leading to a potentially serious ocular infection.

The fetus can be infected if primary varicella develops in a pregnant woman. Infection in the first half of pregnancy may result in congenital varicella syndrome, which is a constellation of malformations characterized by abnormalities in epidermal-tissue development of the fetus. Consequently, there is limb atrophy, cicatrized skin with severe scarring, CNS injury with cortical atrophy and microcephaly, and eye anomalies, including chorioretinitis and cataracts. Affected infants usually die in the first year after birth. The few survivors have profound neurologic abnormalities. In contrast, no malformations were observed in the offspring of 48 women with zoster during pregnancy in one study. This suggests that the risk of viremia and maternal-fetal infection is low in women with prior chickenpox infection.

Severe perinatal varicella is transmitted to the infant by a pregnant women who has the viral exanthem 5 days before and up to 2 days after delivery. This is due to the fact that it takes at least 5 days for the maternal antibodies to develop and be transferred to the fetus before delivery. As mentioned above, in primary infections, the infected mother is viremic 2 days before the onset of rash. Thus, maternal infection with primary varicella in this perinatal period could pose life-threatening consequences, with a significant mortality rate of 30–50%.

Diagnosis is usually clinical, but ELISA titers can confirm an acute infection. Varicella and herpes zoster infection are almost always self-limited in the otherwise healthy child. Patients with eczema can have an especially severe course of varicella (eczema herpeticum).

Immunocompromised patients, newborns younger than 10 days, or children with varicella pneumonia, varicella encephalitis, or hemorrhagic chicken-pox (black pox) should receive high-dose parenteral acyclovir for 7 days. Topical therapy is required for eye involvement. Oral acyclovir has been shown to decrease the duration of symptoms and the number of pox lesions when given to otherwise healthy children with chickenpox. However, the use of acyclovir in this setting is still controversial.

A live-attenuated varicella vaccine, first developed and tested in Japan, is now available in the United States. Studies show a 90% rate of antibody production and 80% efficacy in children who are subsequently exposed to varicella. Passive immunity can be induced by using varicella-zoster immunoglobulin (VZIG) in exposed, high-risk patients, including immunocompromised hosts and cancer patients, as well as neonates at risk for severe perinatal infections.

RICKETTSIAL INFECTIONS

Rocky Mountain spotted fever is a rickettsial disease associated with fever and a characteristic rash. It is caused by *R rickettsii*, an obligate intracellular pathogen. The disease is transmitted to humans by a tick bite (*Dermacentor americanus*); ticks are both the reservoir and vector for *R rickettsii*. The infection is widespread in the United States and is most common in the southeastern states. Of interest, sporadic cases have been reported in the northeast, including New York City. Spring and summer are the months of highest prevalence.

The incubation period for Rocky Mountain spotted fever is 1–14 days, depending on the size of inoculum. Patients present with a toxic appearance associated with fever, headache, delirium, myalgia, nausea, vomiting, and rash. An erythematous macular rash first appears on the wrists and ankles. The rash quickly becomes maculopapular or petechial as it spreads proximally to the trunk. The infection can be severe, lasting as long as 3 weeks and involving the CNS, heart, lungs, kidneys, and gastrointestinal system. In the most severe cases, disseminated intravascular coagulation, shock, and death can occur.

The diagnosis can be confirmed retrospectively by a fourfold increase in serum antibody titer to *R rickettsii* or by immunohistology of biopsy specimens obtained from skin lesions and is suspected in patients with Proteus OX-2 agglutinating antibodies. The clinical diagnosis must be suspected early to benefit from treatment. Chloramphenicol and tetracycline are the most effective antibiotics and should be administered until the patient is afebrile for at least 2 days. Side effects of tetracycline limit its use in children.

Epidemic typhus is a rickettsial disease transmitted by the body louse *Pediculus humanus,* which carries the infectious agent *R prowazekii* from human to human. The disease is seen most commonly in areas of overcrowding and unsanitary conditions, where lice spread quickly. Epidemic typhus is not transmitted between humans without the presence of the vector. The incubation period is 1–2 weeks. High fever, myalgias, headache, and malaise are the first symptoms and are often mistaken for influenza or other viral infections. Four to seven days later, a rash appears on the trunk and spreads to the limbs, leaving a concentrated eruption in the axillae. Initially, the rash is maculopapular but later becomes petechial or hemorrhagic. Mental changes are common, sometimes progressing to delirium or coma. Myocardial or renal failure may supervene. The illness is rarely fatal in children who do not receive treatment, but it is severe and usually lasts 2 weeks. In adults, however, the mortality rate is 10–41%.

The diagnosis is based on a high level of suspicion in the endemic area. A fourfold increase in antibody titers against *R prowazekii* confirms the disease; the disease can also be suspected in patients with positive Proteus OX-2 agglutinins, as above. To be effective, treatment should be instituted early, with chloramphenicol or tetracycline given parenterally or orally. Topical insecticides containing pyrethrins are most effective in controlling the spread of lice.

Endemic typhus resembles epidemic typhus clinically but runs a much milder course. Endemic typhus is caused by *R typhi,* which is transmitted to humans by the rat flea. The incubation period is 1–2 weeks. The patient has mild fever, headache, and myalgias, followed by a discrete maculopapular rash on days 3–5 of the illness, which lasts about 1 week. Because visceral involvement is unusual, the disease is rarely fatal. Once again, the diagnosis is confirmed by a fourfold increase in antibody to *R typhi.* Because of the benign nature of the infection, a single dose of tetracycline (5 mg/kg; maximum, 200 mg) is effective in eradicating the organism.

TOXIN-RELATED EXANTHEMS

Toxic shock syndrome is caused by an exotoxin of *S aureus* or, less commonly, *S pyogenes.* These toxins serve as superantigens that activate most T cells via direct binding to the β chain of T-cell receptors. Among the various homeostasis disturbances, dysregulation of the immune system results in uncontrolled expression of proinflammatory cytokines. Most notably, these cytokines include interleukins and TNF. Some of these factors are directly cytotoxic and induce a process similar to disseminated intracellular coagulation with massive fluid loss from the intravascular space.

The patient presents with rapid onset of high fever, myalgia, abdominal pain, vomiting, diarrhea, pharyngitis, and headache. Most notably, a diffuse, intensive sunburn-like rash appears within 24 hours, along with hyperemia of the pharynx, conjunctiva, and vaginal mucosal membranes. Petechiae may develop several days later. Severe cases can be complicated by hypotension, renal failure, hepatitis, thrombocytopenia, and encephalopathy with altered mental status. The disease can be fatal during the acute episodes of cardiovascular instability. Recovery occurs after 7–10 days and is heralded by desquamation of the rash, particularly of the palm and the sole.

In the past, most cases had been in women aged 15–25 years who used hyperabsorbent tampons in the presence of vaginal colonization with *S aureus.* With recognition of this syndrome and proper avoidance of these tampons, the syndrome is rather uncommon in this age group. Recently, colonization or infection with toxin-producing staphylococcal strains have occurred postoperatively as a complication of primary surgical infections. The diagnosis of toxic shock syndrome is made by fulfilling six major clinical criteria: (1) temperature greater than 39 °C, (2) diffuse macular erythroderma, (3) subsequent desquamation of the rash, (4) hypotension, (5) three or more organs involved (gastrointestinal system, muscle, mucous membrane, kidney, liver, hematologic, and CNS), and (6) negative findings on blood and CSF cultures (except for *S aureus*).

In the management of patients with toxic shock syndrome, cardiovascular support, together with vigorous fluid resuscitation, is essential. Multiorgan failure or dysfunction should be identified and managed conservatively. Tampons should be removed, and infected wounds should be explored and properly drained. In women with menstrual-related toxic shock syndrome, further use of tampons must be avoided. Antimicrobial agents should be used to eradicate the toxin-producing *S aureus.* However, this may not affect the course of the acute disease because of the pathogenetic mechanisms involved. Treatment, however, may reduce the risk of recurrence. In addition, the use IV immunoglobulin has been suggested with a varying but significant degree of success. This modality of therapy should be carefully considered in severe cases.

Staphylococcal scalded skin syndrome (SSSS) is characterized in children by the acute onset of fever, irritably, malaise, and a generalized fine erythematous rash. This is followed by exudative and crusty lesions around the mouth and eyes. Subsequently, the skin develops wrinkles and desquamates spontaneously, demonstrating the characteristic Nikolsky sign. This refers to exfoliation of the skin caused by gentle rubbing. The disease is caused by coagulase-positive *S aureus* bacteria, which secrete toxins. In the early phase of the disease presentation, differential diagnosis includes toxic shock syndrome, scarlet fever, drug-induced toxic epidermal necrolysis, and Kawasaki disease.

IMMIGRANTS & CHILDREN RETURNING FROM THE TROPICS

As recreational air travel and immigration increase, pediatricians encounter more patients who have spent time in the tropics. These patients most often harbor infectious diseases not frequently encountered in developed countries. Many of these infections are serious, and most require specific treatment (Table 9–50). Prompt recognition of some of these diseases, such as cerebral malaria, can be the difference between life and death. A thorough history is crucial; an interpreter should be used if necessary. The pediatrician should obtain details of the itinerary, exposures, vaccinations, prophylactic and treatment medicines taken, and a chronologic description of symptoms. In addition, a careful physical examination can reveal important clues to tropical diseases. In particular, the examination should focus on the detection of fever, lymphadenopathy, splenomegaly, alterations in consciousness, and abnormalities of the skin and mucous membranes.

Most of the diseases listed in Table 9–50 are contracted by prolonged exposure and, therefore, are far more common in immigrants than travelers. The most common dis-

Table 9–50. Some important pediatric infectious diseases among travelers and immigrants.

Disease/Agents	Exposures	Syndromes	Diagnosis	Treatment	Notes
Bacteria					
Acute diarrhea *Escherichia coli, non-typhi Salmonella, Shigella, Campylobacter jejuni*	Contaminated food and water	Bloody diarrhea, fever	Stool culture, toxin assay	Ciprofloxacin,[1] TMP/SMX, erythromycin (for *C jejuni*)	Loperamide[1] can decrease stool frequency
Brucellosis *Brucella* spp.	Contact with cattle, swine, goats, sheep; ingestion of unpasteurized milk or cheese	Chronic fever, arthritis, orchitis	Blood, bone marrow cultures; serology for IgG	Tetracycline[1] + AG, TMP/SMX	
Buruli ulcer *Mycobacterium ulcerans*	Direct inoculation, endemic in rural Australia and Africa	Painless chronic ulcers	Culture of skin lesions	INH + streptomycin	
Cholera *Vibrio cholerae*	Feco-oral, human cases	Severe "rice water" diarrhea, shock	Stool culture	Fluid and electrolytes, TMP/SMX	Without treatment, 50% mortality
Leprosy *Mycobacterium leprae*	Close contact with human cases	*Lepromatous:* diffuse, numerous nodules on skin, nose, ears (many bacilli, weak immunity) *Tuberculoid:* few anaesthetic hypopigmented macules, enlarged peripheral nerves (few bacilli, strong immunity)	Stain earlobe skin biopsy for acid fast bacilli Lepromin skin test	Rifampin + dapsone + clofazamine	Borderline leprosy shares clinical features with both lepromatous and tuberculoid forms
Melioidosis *Pseudomonas pseudomallei*	Endemic in Southeast Asia	Acute pneumonia with sepsis and disseminated abscesses	Culture of blood, sputum, or abscess	Third-generation cephalosporin, check sensitivities	Therapy lowers mortality from 95 to 30%
Oroya fever *Bartonella bacilliformis*	Sandfly bites in the Andes mountain valleys	Fever, hemolytic anemia, generalized lymphadenopathy After recovery, *Verruga peruanna*, hemangiomatous nodules on the skin, may develop	Blood smear for organisms in red blood cells	Ampicillin, chloramphenicol	Untreated mortality 40%
Plague *Yersinia pestis*	Flea bites, rodents	Septicemia, pneumonia, or buboes (regional suppurative lymphadenopathy)	Gram stain and culture from bubo or sputum	Streptomycin, tetracycline,[1] chloramphenicol	Untreated mortality > 50%
Relapsing fever *Borrelia* spp.	Tick bites (rural) Louse bites (epidemics during war, famine, disaster)	Febrile episodes lasting 2–9 d alternating with afebrile periods of 2–4 d; transient petechial rash	Blood smear to demonstrate organisms	Tetracycline,[1] penicillin	Untreated mortality 10–50%
Trachoma *Chlamydia trachomatis*	Contact with ocular discharges of human cases or flies	Follicular conjuctivitis → scarring of the cornea	Look for cytoplasmic inclusions in conjunctival epithelial cells	Erythromycin, tetracycline[1]; opthalmic surgery	Leading cause of blindness in the world
Typhoid fever *Salmonella typhi. paratyphi*	Feco-oral, human carriers	Chronic fever, encephalopathy, GI hemorrhage or perforation	Blood, stool, urine cultures	Third-generation cephalosporin, amoxicillin, ciprofloxacin[1]	Untreated mortality 10%

(continued)

Table 9–50 (cont'd). Some important pediatric infectious diseases among travelers and immigrants.

Disease/Agents	Exposures	Syndromes	Diagnosis	Treatment	Notes
Yaws *Treponema pertenue*	Direct contact with human cases; rural	Papilloma as primary lesions; multiple papillomata in second stage; destructive skin and bony lesions in third stage	False-positive syphilis serology result Darkfield examination of skin lesion	Penicillin	No organ involvement outside skin and bone
Viruses & rickettsiae Dengue	*Aedes* mosquito bites	Dengue fever: fever, petechial rash, retroorbital headache, thrombocytopenia Dengue hemorrhagic shock syndrome: shock, bleeding from gums, venipuncture sites	Serology for dengue IgG	Fluid and electrolytes for dengue hemorrhagic shock syndrome	Dengue hemorrhagic fever often occurs in children previously infected with a different dengue serotype; supportive care for shock reduces mortality from 40% to < 5%
Hepatitis A	Feco-oral, human cases	Jaundice, fever, malaise; occasionally fulminant hepatitis	Serology for hepatitis A IgM	Liver transplant in fulminant hepatitis	Travelers should receive vaccine before departure
Polio	Feco-oral and pharyngeal contact with human cases	Fever, myalgias, ± flaccid paralysis (usually legs, can involve muscles of respiration)	Stool or throat viral culture		Routinely vaccinated
Rabies	Bite of rabid animal (usually dogs in developing countries) or airborne exposure	Encephalitis, hydrophobia	Fluorescent antibody staining of brain, cornea, or skin Negri bodies in brain biopsy specimen	Vaccinate and give rabies immune globulin after exposure; no treatment available for encephalitis	Almost always fatal
Typhus *Rickettsia prowazekii* (louse-borne), *Rickettsia tsutsugamushi* (scrub typhus)	Louse bites (epidemics during war, famine, disaster; worldwide) Mite bites (scrub areas of Asia)	Louse-borne typhus: fever, severe toxicity, peripheral gangrene; recurrence (Brill-Zinsser) Scrub typhus: eschar at bite site, maculopapular rash, acute fever	Indirect fluorescent antibody, Weil-Felix test	Tetracycline[1]	Children usually have less severe illness, but mortality approaches 10%
Viral encephalitis: many agents, including Japanese B encephalitis	Bites of various arthropods in rural settings	Fever, delerium	IgM in CSF, serologic studies		More severe agents can lead to death or residual neurologic deficits
Yellow fever	*Aedes* mosquito bite	Fever, headache, jaundice, epistaxis, hematemesis	Isolation of virus from blood, serology	Ribavirin	Mortality 5–50% depending on immune status Vaccines required to enter many countries with *Aedes* vector

(continued)

Table 9–50 (cont'd). Some important pediatric infectious diseases among travelers and immigrants.

Disease/Agents	Exposures	Syndromes	Diagnosis	Treatment	Notes
Protozoa					
Amebiasis *Entamoeba his- tolytica*	Feco-oral	1. Prolonged dysentery with blood and mucus 2. Hepatic abscess; rarely abscesses elsewhere in the body 3. Ameboma, mass in intestine	For 1 and 3: Stool for ova and parasites For 2: Hepatic abscess; amebic precipitins serology	Iodoquinol and metronidazole	*Entamoeba hart- manni, E coli, Blastocystis hominis,* and *Endolimax nana* do not cause disease
Chagas disease *Trypanosoma cruzi*	Bite of the reduvid bug, which lives in thatched houses in Cen- tral and South America	1. Acute disease: includes unilateral eyelid swelling (Romana sign) 2. Chronic disease: sequelae include cardiac myopathy, megaesophagus, megacolon	For 1. Blood smear or culture For 2. Serology or xenodiagnosis	Nifurtimox	Infection rates in Central and South America 5–20%
Kala-azar *Leishmania donovani*	Sandfly bite on beach	Intermittent fever, splenomegaly, pancytopenia, darkening of skin	Bone-marrow biopsy for Giemsa stain and culture	Pentavalent anti- mony	
Malaria *Plasmodium falciparum, vivax, ovale, malariae*	Bite of female *Anopheles* mosquito at night	Periodic fever, hemolytic anemia Delerium and coma (cerebral malaria) especially in children *P vivax, ovale* can relapse years later	Thick and thin blood smears (thick more sen- sitive; thin allows speciation)	Chloroquine for non-*falciparum* and *P falciparum* from Mexico and Middle East *P vivax, ovale* re- quire primaquine to prevent re- lapses (check G6PD) *P falciparum:* quinine	Most common and most rapidly pro- gressive fatal tropical dis- ease, espe- cially *P falci- parum* All travelers re- quire prophy- laxis Malaria from Africa almost always *P falci- parum*
Cutaneous leishmania- sis: *Leishmania tropica, braziliensis, mexicana*	Sandfly bite on beach	Chronic ulcer with satellite lesion that spontaneously scars *L braziliensis*, if not treated properly, can recur as de- forming lesions on mucocutaneous membranes, eg, mouth and nose (espundia)	Smear and culture of biopsy speci- men from lead- ing edge of lesion	Pentavalent anti- mony	Mucocutaneous relapse occurs only in South America
Sleeping sickness *Trypanosoma brucei, gambiense, rhodesiense*	Bite of the tsetse fly in Africa	Acute: Intermittent fever and lymph- adenopathy (particularly posterior cervical node: Winterbottom sign) Later: CNS invasion → progressive mental deterioration, coma	Buffy coat, lymph node, and CSF smear serology	Without CSF in- volvement: suramin With CSF involve- ment: melarso- prol	*T rhodesiense* occurs in East and South Africa; more rapidly pro- gressive *T gambiense* occurs in West Africa; CNS invasion may take years to appear

(continued)

Table 9–50 (cont'd). Some important pediatric infectious diseases among travelers and immigrants.

Disease/Agents	Exposures	Syndromes	Diagnosis	Treatment	Notes
Helminths					
Cutaneous larva migrans: animal hookworms	Walking barefoot in soil contaminated by feces of infected dogs and other animals	Worms creeping underneath the skin Very itchy	Clinical diagnosis	Topical thiabendazole	Usually self-limited
Cysticercosis: *Taenia solium*	Feco-oral inoculation of pork tapeworm eggs	Calcified cysts in brain, spinal cord, muscle, and skin Seizures and focal neurologic signs	Serology, head CT, LP, muscle radiograph, stool for ova and parasites (proglottids), biopsy	Praziquantel, albendazole	Most common cause of seizures in Central America
Filariasis *Wuchereria bancrofti, Brugia malayi, Brugia timori*	Mosquito bites	Acute: Daily fevers and eosinophilia; recurrent lymphangitis Chronic: massive lymphedema of the legs and scrotum; chyluria	Stain of blood smears taken at midnight looking for microfilariae	DEC used but usually unsuccessful	
Guinea worm: *Dracunculus medinensis*	Drinking water infested with larvae	Multiple blisters, followed by worms spontaneously exiting body via skin surface	Clinical diagnosis	Pull worm out by winding it with a stick	
Hydatid cyst *Echinococcus granulosus*	Exposure to sheep dog feces	Large cysts in liver and other organs	CT scan, serology	Albendazole and surgery if symptomatic (cysts grow very slowly, so removal may not be needed)	Accidental spillage of cyst contents during surgery may cause anaphylaxis
Loiasis *Loa loa*	Mango fly bite in Central and West Africa	Episodes of hot, red swellings on extremities or around eyes (Calabar swellings) and occasional burning eye pain when worm migrates beneath conjunctiva	Stain blood smear for microfilariae Pluck visible adult worm from conjunctiva	DEC	
Liver flukes *Fasciola hepatica*	Eating watercress	Acute: Fever, hepatic tenderness Chronic: Obstruction of bile ducts	Stool for ova and parasites	Bithionol	Another liver fluke, *Clororchis sinensis,* rarely causes symptoms
Lung flukes *Paragonimus westermani*	Eating crabs and crayfish in Asia	Chronic cough and hemoptysis	Look for eggs in sputum	Praziquantel	
River blindness *Onchocerca volvulus*	Blackfly bite (fast streams of Africa and Latin America)	Itching and thickening of skin, subcutaneous nodules, enlarged lymph nodes Progressive scarring of the cornea and conjunctiva	Direct examination of skin snips for motile microfilariae Mazzotti test: Worsening of skin itch in response to test treatment dose	Ivermectin	Prolonged infection required before eyes involved

(continued)

Table 9–50 (cont'd). Some important pediatric infectious diseases among travelers and immigrants.

Disease/Agents	Exposures	Syndromes	Diagnosis	Treatment	Notes
Roundworms (intestinal): *Ascaris lumbricoides, Trichuris trichiura*	Feco-oral	*Ascaris*: Usually asymptomatic passage of long roundworm; intestinal obstruction in children *Trichuris*: Occasionally dysentery and rectal prolapse in children	Stool ova and parasites	Mebendazole	Occasionally, *Ascaris* can migrate to lungs, causing pneumonitis and eosinophilia
Schistosomiasis *Schistosoma mansoni, hematobium, japonica, mekongi*	Freshwater swimming *S hematobium* found in Middle East and Africa	Acute: Fever, generalized lymphadenopathy, eosinophilia (Katayama fever) Chronic: Portal vein obstruction leading to hepatomegaly and varices; *S hematobium* also causes hematuria and bladder cancer	Stool and urine (for *S hematobium*) for ova Serology	Praziquantel	Important to recognize and treat infection before chronic sequelae ensue A rare complication is transverse myelitis
Strongyloidosis *Strongyloides stercoralis*	Walking barefoot in soil contaminated by feces or reservoir hosts	Immunocompetent host: Diarrhea, pneumonitis, eosinophilia Immunocompromised host: Hyperinfection (often reactivation) causing shock, abdominal pain, gram-negative bacteremia, meningitis, and pneumonia	Stool and sputum for ova and parasites (larvae) Concentration techniques may be required	Thiabendazole	
Trichinosis *Trichinella spiralis*	Eating raw, infected pork	Fever, muscle pain` and tenderness, periorbital edema, petechial skin rash Occasionally, heart and CNS involvement	Muscle biopsy	Albendazole or high-dose mebendazole used, but not very effective	Muscle lesions eventually calcify

[1]Avoid in young children, if possible.
AG = aminoglycoside; CSF = cerebrospinal fluid; CT = computed tomography; CNS = central nervous system; DEC = diethycarbamazine; GI = gastrointestinal; INH = isoniazid; LP = lumbar puncture; TMP/SMX = trimethoprim-sulfamethoxazole.

eases in travelers are diarrhea, malaria, and dengue fever. In addition, many diseases that are not strictly tropical flourish in the developing world because of poverty, overcrowding, and inadequate preventative medicine. Such diseases include AIDS, tuberculosis, syphilis, meningococcus, impetigo, tetanus, leptospirosis, and the childhood exanthems; these should be considered in the differential diagnosis of an ill child arriving from the tropics.

Fever

Fever in a child coming from the tropics mandates blood smears and cultures for malaria and typhoid fever, respectively. These diseases have protean manifestations, such as cough, diarrhea, constipation, abdominal discomfort, and dizziness, and therefore are notoriously difficult to diagnose on clinical grounds. Classic fever patterns, such as the tertian fever of malaria, are not frequently seen. Both diseases can progress rapidly to death: malaria by coma or severe anemia, and typhoid fever by encephalopathy or gastrointestinal hemorrhage or perforation. Both diseases are relatively common and can be treated easily.

Another common cause of tropical fever is dengue virus, which can cause two separate syndromes. Dengue fever is a self-limiting infection characterized by a petechial rash, retro-orbital headache, saddle-back fever curve, and thrombocytopenia. Signs of spontaneous hemorrhage or shock indicate a different but more severe syndrome, dengue hemorrhagic shock, which mandates aggressive fluid replacement therapy. Dengue hemorrhagic shock is particularly common as a reinfection in children from Southeast Asia who have already experienced a previous episode of dengue fever.

Altered Consciousness

In addition to cerebral malaria and typhoid encephalopathy, the differential diagnosis of altered consciousness in a child from the tropics should include meningococcal meningitis, viral encephalitis (HSV and arthropod-borne viruses such as Japanese B encephalitis), rabies, and sleeping sickness. Appropriate diagnostic tests include a brain imaging study, blood smears and culture, and lumbar puncture. The child should be admitted expeditiously, probably to an intensive care unit.

Diarrhea

Enterotoxigenic *E coli* is the most common cause of traveler's diarrhea. Other common bacterial causes include non-typhi *Salmonella, Shigella,* and *C jejuni.* The infection usually is self-limiting, but fever, prolonged diarrhea, and blood in the stool could indicate the need for treatment. Although trimethoprim-sulfamethoxazole traditionally has been the antibiotic of choice, it is not effective against *C jejuni* and resistant strains of the other bacteria. All the pathogens remain susceptible to ciprofloxacin; unfortunately, this antibiotic is not recommended for children. Stool cultures sent before antibiotic treatment may be helpful.

The most important cause of diarrhea to recognize is cholera. *Vibrio cholerae* causes a profound watery diarrhea, which can cause hypovolemia and shock. If cholera is suspected, the child should be admitted for aggressive fluid and electrolyte replacement.

Diarrhea lasting several weeks is usually caused by parasites. Typically, *G lamblia* causes watery diarrhea, whereas *E histolytica* causes dysentery with mucus in the stool. Three separate sets of stool should be examined for ova and parasites. Because *Giardia* resides in the small intestine, diagnosis can be difficult. Options include serology, a duodenal string capsule test, or an empiric therapeutic trial.

Eosinophilia

Tropical eosinophilia usually is caused by a hypersensitivity reaction to helminths as they migrate though the human body. Protozoa and dormant intestinal helminths do not cause eosinophilia. The most common causes of parasitic eosinophilia are schistosomiasis, cysticercosis, and ascariasis.

Patients become infected with schistosomes by bathing in infected rivers and lakes. The schistosomes penetrate the skin and migrate to the hepatic portal veins or venous plexus of the bladder. During this migration, the patient typically experiences high fever (known as Katayama fever). If schistosomiasis is not treated, it leads to incurable chronic sequelae, such as cirrhosis of the liver and bladder cancer.

Consumption of improperly cooked, infested pork is the major risk factor for acquiring infection with the tapeworm *T solium.* The adult worm resides in the intestine, laying eggs that cause the disease cysticercosis in humans. These eggs can penetrate the intestinal wall and hatch into larvae, which migrate to various parts of the body, particularly the CNS, muscle, and skin. The larvae encyst, calcify, and cause symptoms through a mass effect. Cysticercosis is the most common cause of seizures in Latin America. Diagnosis of calcified cysts in the brains of immigrants from endemic areas can often be made without a brain biopsy.

One in four individuals in the world harbors the intestinal roundworm *Ascaris lumbricoides.* Usually, these individuals are asymptomatic and are shocked when a long, living roundworm comes out during a stool passage. In children, however, a very high worm burden can lead to intestinal obstruction. Ascaris does migrate though the lungs during its life cycle, so it can cause a transient pneumonitis with eosinophilia.

INFECTION OF THE IMMUNOCOMPROMISED HOST

The spectrum of infectious diseases prevalent in immunocompromised hosts is quite different from that of the normal host. In the normal host, invasion of infectious pathogens causes activation of different branches of the immune system, including cellular- and humoral-mediated responses. In the immunocompromised host, however, deficiency in different branches of the immune system results in defective responses and failure to protect the host from dissemination of the microbial agents. By studying these compromised patients, we can appreciate the importance of intact host defense mechanisms to maintain homeostasis.

In the immediate environment of the compromised host, the vast majority of organisms that are readily available to invade the host are the commensal or saprophytic microbes of the exogenous or endogenous flora. These opportunistic organisms account for most of the serious infections in immunosuppressed patients. In patients with specific diseases accompanied by distinctive immune defects, the infectious organism can be quite unique. These diseases include sickle-cell anemia, cystic fibrosis, diabetes mellitus, and absence spleen, as well as splenectomy.

Causative Agents

The organisms that account for more than 95% of serious infections in the immunosuppressed host are listed in Table 9–51. These originated predominantly from normal microbial flora of the intestinal tract, oral cavity, and skin. In the immunocompromised host, no organism isolated from sites including blood, bone marrow, CSF, or from biopsy specimens can be discounted as a contaminant without careful clinical evaluation.

Clinical Manifestations

Serious infection rarely occurs in the absence of any sign or symptom. Fever is usually the hallmark of infection and is seldom abated by immunosuppressive drugs. In

Table 9–51. Some common causative agents of serious infections in immunosuppressed patients.

Bacteria	Viruses
Pseudomonas aeruginosa	Varicella zoster
Escherichia coli	Cytomegalovirus
Klebsiella-Enterobacter species	Herpes simplex
Staphylococcus aureus	Epstein-Barr
Staphylococcus, coagulase-negative	Hepatitis A, B, and C
Mycobacterium avium-intracellulare	Protozoa
	Toxoplasma gondii
Fungi	*Pneumocystis carinii*
Candida albicans	*Cryptosporidium* species
Candida. non-*albicans* species	*Microsporida* species
Aspergillus species	*Isospora* species
Cryptococcus neoformans	
Mucor species	

these patients, fever always must be considered to be of infectious etiology until proved otherwise. Because of deficient immune response, the patient usually is unable to localize infection at the portal of entry. Thus, the expected signs and symptoms of a specific infection may not occur. For example, the neutropenic patient may have perianal abscess without signs of significant inflammation. Likewise, the patient with bacterial meningitis may not have obvious signs of meningeal irritation or neutrophils in the spinal fluid. As in normal hosts, bacterial sepsis in these immunocompromised hosts presents with fever, but jaundice, abdominal pain, lethargy, petechiae, and erythematous macules may occur. Careful physical examination must be performed to search for anal, oral, and infected IV sites and ulcerative skin lesions. In the febrile neutropenic host with an indwelling central venous catheter (eg, Hickman-Broviac), *S epidermidis* is the most frequent cause of bacteremia.

General Principles of Management

The following outlines some principles for the management of infections in the immunosuppressed host:

- Fever should be considered a sign of infection unless proved otherwise.

- Granulocytopenia with an absolute neutrophil count of 500/mm³ or less renders the host highly susceptible to bacterial infection.

- Any organism should be considered a potential pathogen.

- When the causative agent for an infection is identified, surveillance should be continued for mixed or sequential infections.

- Immunosuppressive therapy should be withheld or modified during infection if the status of the primary disease permits.

- Antibiotics, preferably bactericidal, should be administered when indicated with monitoring for toxicity.

- GM-CSF or G-CSF should be used when indicated for the prevention and treatment of certain conditions associated with granulocytopenia.

- Systemic fungal infection should be considered when the febrile granulocytopenic patient continues to be unresponsive to a course of broad-spectrum antibiotic treatment.

Preventing Infection

Parents and children should be instructed about increased susceptibility to infection. They should report early signs and symptoms of infection, follow basic principles of good hygiene, and avoid contact with individuals with even minor contagious infections. The patients should receive vaccination per the Centers for Disease Control and Prevention guidelines for the immunization of immunosuppressed infants and children. Diphtheria, tetanus, pertussis, *H influenzae,* and hepatitis B vaccines are recommended as routine immunizations. Live oral polio vaccine is contraindicated in the severely compromised patient, and close contacts of such patients should not receive the vaccine; the enhanced inactivated polio vaccine should be given instead. The live mumps, measles, and rubella vaccine is contraindicated in most severely immunocompromised patients, although it can be given to HIV-infected patients. Influenza and pneumococcal vaccines are suggested for those immunosuppressed patients who might have an immune response to the antigen. Prophylactic antibiotics, such as trimethoprim-sulfamethoxazole, should be used to prevent *P carinii* pneumonitis as well as certain bacterial infections. Alternatively, aerosolized pentamidine given once a month is equally effective in preventing the infection in children who do not tolerate trimethoprim-sulfamethoxazole. However, there has not been any generally accepted regimen for fungal prophylaxis.

REFERENCES

LABORATORY MEDICINE IN INFECTIOUS DISEASES

Dennehy PH: New tests for the rapid diagnosis of infection in children. Adv Pediatr Inf Dis 1993;8:91.

Washington JA (editor): *Laboratory Diagnosis of Infectious Diseases.* Vol 7 of: *Infectious Disease Clinics of North America.* Saunders, 1993.

ANTIMICROBIAL THERAPY

Grossman M: Bacterial and viral infections. Page 499 in: Rudolph AM et al (editors): *Rudolph's Pediatrics,* 20th ed. Appleton & Lange, 1996.

Lau AS et al: Biology and therapeutic uses of myeloid

hematopoietic growth factors and interferons. Pediatr Infect Dis J 1996;15:563.

Nelson JD: *Pocketbook of Pediatric Antimicrobial Therapy,* 11th ed. Williams & Wilkins, 1995.

APPROACH TO THE CHILD WITH FEVER

Baraff LJ et al: Practice guideline for the management of infants and children 0 to 36 months of age with fever without source. Agency for Health Care Policy and Research. Ann Emerg Med 1993;22:1198.

Feigin RD, Shearer WT: Fever of unknown origin in children. Curr Probl Pediatr 1976;6:3.

Gartner JC Jr: Fever of unknown origin. Adv Pediatr Infect Dis 1992;7:1.

Jaskiewicz JA et al: Febrile infants at low risk for serious bacterial infection: An appraisal of the Rochester criteria and implications for management. Febrile Infant Collaborative Study Group. Pediatrics 1994;94:390.

Steele RW et al: Usefulness of scanning procedures for diagnosis of fever of unknown origin in children. J Pediatr 1991;119:526.

Steele RW: Fever of unknown origin (FUO). Page 100 in: Steele RW (editor): *A Clinical Manual of Pediatric Infectious Disease.* Appleton & Lange, 1986.

EYE, MOUTH, & NECK INFECTIONS

Barnett ED, Klein JO: The problem of resistant bacteria for the management of acute otitis media. Pediatr Clin North Am 1995;42:509.

Bluestone CD, Klein JO: *Otitis Media in Infants and Children,* 2nd ed. Saunders, 1995.

Chow AW (editor): *Infectious Syndromes of the Head and Neck.* Vol 2 of: *Infectious Disease Clinics of North America.* Saunders, 1988.

Recent advances in otitis media treatment. Symposium proceedings, October 1, 1993, Minneapolis, Minn. Ann Otol Rhinol Laryngol (Suppl) 1994;163:1.

RESPIRATORY INFECTIONS

Denny FW, Clyde WA Jr: Acute lower respiratory tract infections in nonhospitalized children. J Pediatr 1986;108:635.

Stark JM: Lung infections in children. Curr Opinion Pediatr 1993;5:273.

Turner RB et al: Pneumonia in pediatric outpatients: Cause and clinical manifestations. J Pediatr 1987;111:194.

CENTRAL NERVOUS SYSTEM INFECTIONS

Bonadio WA: The cerebrospinal fluid: Physiologic aspects and alterations associated with bacterial meningitis. Pediatr Infect Dis J 1992;11:423.

Quagliarello V, Scheld WM: Bacterial meningitis: Pathogenesis, pathophysiology, and progress. N Engl J Med 1992; 327:864.

Saez-Llorens X, McCracken GH Jr: Bacterial meningitis in neonates and children. Infect Dis Clin North Am 1990;4: 623.

Toltzis P: Viral encephalitis. Adv Pediatr Infect Dis 1991;6: 111.

APPROACH TO THE CHILD WITH DIARRHEA

Guerrant RL, Bobak DA: Bacterial and protozoal gastroenteritis. N Engl J Med 1991;325:327.

Pickering LK: Therapy for acute infectious diarrhea in children. J Pediatr 1991;118:S118.

HEPATITIS

Hepatitis B virus: A comprehensive strategy for eliminating transmission in the United States through universal childhood vaccination. Recommendations of the Immunization Practices Advisory Committee (ACIP). MMWR 1991;40:1.

Hoofnagle JH, Di Bisceglie AM: Serologic diagnosis of acute and chronic viral hepatitis. Semin Liver Dis 1991;11:73.

Lemon SM: Type A viral hepatitis. New developments in an old disease. N Engl J Med 1985;313:1059.

Tabor E: Etiology, diagnosis, and treatment of viral hepatitis in children. Adv Pediatr Infect Dis 1988;3:19.

OSTEOMYELITIS

Faden H, Grossi M: Acute osteomyelitis in children. Reassessment of etiologic agents and their clinical characteristics. Am J Dis Child 1991;145:65.

Welkon CJ et al: Pyogenic arthritis in infants and children: A review of 95 cases. Pediatr Infect Dis 1986;5:669.

URINARY TRACT INFECTIONS

Durbin WA Jr, Peter G: Management of urinary tract infections in infants and children. Pediatr Infect Dis 1984;3:564.

Feld LG et al: Urinary tract infections in infants and children. Pediatr Rev 1989;11:71.

Ginsburg CM, McCracken GH Jr: Urinary tract infections in young infants. Pediatrics 1982;69:409.

Hellerstein S et al: Consensus: Roentgenographic evaluation of children with urinary tract infections. Pediatr Infect Dis 1984;4:291.

SEXUALLY TRANSMITTED DISEASES

Centers for Disease Control and Prevention: 1993 Sexually Transmitted Diseases Treatment Guidelines. MMWR 1993; 42:1.

Ikeda MK, Jenson HB: Evaluation and treatment of congenital syphilis. J Pediatr 1990;117:843.

Pelvic inflammatory disease: Guidelines for prevention and management. MMWR 1991;40:1.

Shafer MA, Sweet RL: Pelvic inflammatory disease in adolescent females. Epidemiology, pathogenesis, diagnosis, treatment, and sequelae. Pediatr Clin North Am 1989;36:513.

RASH & FEVER

Irving WL et al: Roseola infantum and other syndromes associated with acute HHV6 infection. Arch Dis Child 1990;65: 1297.

Kirk JL et al: Rocky Mountain spotted fever. A clinical review based on 48 confirmed cases, 1943–1986. Medicine 1990;69:35.

Ware R: Human parvovirus infection. J Pediatr 1989;114:343.

Williams CL et al: Lyme disease in childhood: Clinical and epidemiologic features of ninety cases. Pediatr Infect Dis J 1990;9:10.

10

Injuries & Emergencies

Joel A. Fein, MD, Dennis R. Durbin, MD, & Steven M. Selbst, MD

Each year, 90–100 million individuals are treated in emergency departments in the United States, and 25–30% of them are children. An estimated 10% of ambulance runs in this country involve individuals younger than 19 years of age. The emergency department has become the safety net for health care, treating those with life-threatening illness and injury, as well as those with minor problems who are either uninsured or poorly insured. Most children are treated in general emergency departments rather than in specialized pediatric emergency departments. Most are brought to the hospital because the caretaker or the patient perceives the problem to be serious and requiring urgent treatment. Only a small percentage of visits involve life-threatening emergencies, but most pediatric deaths are preventable or treatable if the problem is recognized early and managed appropriately.

The three leading causes of death in pediatric patients are injury, infection, and sequelae of prematurity and congenital malformations. Automobile-related injuries, including both occupants and pedestrians hit by cars, are the most common causes of death due to trauma. Other traumatic deaths involve drownings, poisonings, falls, fires, and smoke inhalation. Unfortunately, the number of deaths associated with firearms (used intentionally or unintentionally), homicide, and suicide has increased rapidly over the past few years. Deaths from infectious diseases usually involve the respiratory tract or the central nervous system (CNS).

Children require special attention because they are so different from adults. Children are less tolerant of blood loss, more likely to sustain serious respiratory problems, and more at risk for head injury. Therefore, the care of ill and injured children requires special training, special equipment of variable sizes, different medications, and unique diagnostic and procedural skills.

This chapter focuses on several important emergencies in pediatrics. First we discuss cardiopulmonary resuscitation (CPR). We then discuss sudden infant death syndrome (SIDS); shock; the injured child, including head injury; near-drowning; and burns and smoke inhalation. These discussions are followed by sections on child abuse, poisonings, and, finally, status epilepticus. A discussion on asthma, an important pediatric emergency, can be found in Chapter 18.

CARDIOPULMONARY RESUSCITATION IN INFANTS & CHILDREN

Cardiopulmonary arrest (the absence of a pulse and spontaneous respirations), fortunately, is rare in the pediatric age group. In children, cardiopulmonary arrest commonly results from a prolonged period of hypoxia secondary to a respiratory arrest. Hypoxia plays a central role in many events leading to cardiopulmonary arrest in children. The hypoxia may be acute or chronic and may result from either an acquired or a congenital illness. The primary goal of CPR is to reestablish cardiac output and tissue oxygen delivery through the use of artificial ventilation and chest compressions and the administration of pharmacologic agents.

The etiology of cardiopulmonary arrest in children differs greatly from that in adults. Adult arrests are typically sudden in onset and primarily cardiac in origin. On the contrary, children may go through a series of physiologic changes leading to cardiopulmonary arrest, typically after respiratory arrest. Table 10–1 lists the most common identifiable causes of cardiopulmonary arrest in children. Because respiratory arrest frequently precedes cardiac arrest in children, recognition of the child at risk of deterioration and intervention before full cardiopulmonary arrest occurs are of paramount importance. Resuscitation from respiratory arrest is successful in 75–90% of cases. Once cardiac arrest occurs, success rates for resuscitation are consistently less than 10%.

Most pediatric cardiopulmonary arrests occur in children younger than 1 year. This is due to the higher occur-

Table 10–1. Most common identifiable causes of cardiopulmonary arrest in children.

Respiratory
Pneumonia
Aspiration
Airway obstruction
Sudden infant death syndrome
Congenital heart disease
Central nervous system disease
Infection
Trauma (including child abuse)
Status epilepticus
Drowning
Smoke inhalation
Poisoning
Anaphylaxis

rence of congenital anomalies that predispose some children to cardiopulmonary arrest, as well as to unique differences in the anatomy and physiology of infants. The airway of a child differs from that of an adult. The trachea is more flexible, the tongue relatively larger, the glottic opening higher and more anteriorly placed in the neck, and the airway itself proportionately smaller, rendering infants more susceptible to airway compromise. Although the use of pediatric CPR is based on the adult model of resuscitation, important differences exist on the basis of these and other unique qualities of children.

MANAGEMENT

Cardiopulmonary resuscitation in the pediatric age group should be part of a community-wide effort that integrates basic life support (BLS), advanced life support (ALS), and postresuscitation care. BLS is the phase of emergency care that supports ventilation and circulation in the arrest victim without the use of adjuncts. It is typically used in the prehospital setting. ALS begins with BLS, with the additional use of adjunctive equipment, medications, and special techniques for establishing and maintaining effective ventilation and circulation.

The basic approach to pediatric CPR is the same as in adults with respect to the initial priorities: establishment of *A*irway, *B*reathing, and *C*irculation (the ABCs).

Establish Unresponsiveness. The first step in the sequence of CPR is to establish the unresponsiveness of patients by gently shaking, tapping, or shouting at them. Once unresponsiveness is established, help should be summoned, and the patient placed in a supine position on a firm, flat surface. Care should be taken in positioning the child at risk for head or neck injury. The child should be turned as a unit, with firm support of the head and neck so that the head does not twist or tilt forward or backward.

Airway. Once the patient is positioned properly, the first priority in management is evaluation and treatment of the airway. Most airway obstruction is related to the

tongue and the mandibular block of soft tissues lying against the posterior wall of the hypopharynx. This obstruction can be relieved by manual maneuvers, including the head tilt and chin lift or jaw thrust to pull the tissues forward physically. Because of the lack of firm cartilaginous support in the trachea of an infant or small child, hyperextension of the neck can lead to collapse of the trachea. Therefore, the head should be placed in a "sniffing position," with the occiput slightly higher than the shoulders.

If manual manipulation of the airway cannot maintain airway patency, artificial airways, such as oropharyngeal and nasopharyngeal airways, can be used. These function to stent or support the mandibular block of tissue off the posterior pharyngeal wall.

Breathing. Once a clear airway has been established, the patient should be reassessed for the presence and adequacy of spontaneous breathing. Movement of the chest and abdomen should be seen; movement of air during exhalation should be felt and heard. If no spontaneous breathing is detected, mouth-to-mouth or, in infants younger than 1 year, mouth-to-mouth and nose breathing is begun. Two slow breaths are given, with a pause between for the rescuer to take a breath. The volume should be sufficient to cause the chest to rise. If a mask with one-way valve or other infection control barrier is readily available, rescue breathing should be provided with such a device.

Once available, supplemental oxygen should always be administered to patients requiring resuscitation. If the patient has adequate spontaneous breathing, a variety of oxygen delivery devices can be used, including nasal cannulas, hoods, tents, and masks. If assisted ventilation is required, oxygen should be delivered via either a bag-valve-mask or bag-valve-endotracheal tube system.

Finally, endotracheal intubation during CPR may be performed for a variety of reasons. The endotracheal tube can maintain further patency of the airway, protect the airway from aspiration of gastric contents, and facilitate mechanical ventilation and delivery of high concentrations of oxygen to the lungs. For children older than 2 years of age, the correct endotracheal tube size can be approximated by using a simple formula based on the patient's age:

As this is an estimate, the next smaller and larger size endotracheal tubes should also be available. Only personnel skilled in the technique of endotracheal intubation of children should perform the procedure.

Circulation. Once a patent airway is established and adequate oxygenation and ventilation are ensured, many children reestablish cardiac output. Assessment of the adequacy of circulation includes palpating the brachial or femoral artery in children younger than 1 year of age, or the carotid artery in older children. One should also assess both the color of the skin and mucous membranes for cyanosis or pallor and capillary refill.

If no effective pulse is present, external chest compressions must begin. Adequate ventilation must be continued during chest compressions. A chest compression:ventilation ratio of 5:1 is considered optimal for children of all ages. The position of the hands for chest compressions varies depending on the age of the child. The depth and rate of compressions are likewise based on the child's age (Table 10–2). The compressions should be smooth, not jerky, and the hand should not be lifted off the chest between compressions.

DRUGS

If mechanical means fail to reestablish effective circulation, pharmacologic intervention is essential. The primary drugs used in pediatric CPR are oxygen, epinephrine, sodium bicarbonate, atropine, and glucose. Table 10–3 lists the doses and indications of the drugs commonly used during a pediatric resuscitation.

Placement of an intravenous (IV) line during CPR is often the most difficult and time-consuming aspect of resuscitation. During CPR, the preferred access site is the largest, most accessible vein that does not require interruption of resuscitation. Whenever possible, a central IV site should be obtained. Peripheral sites (antecubital, dorsum of the hand, saphenous vein) are a second choice and may be difficult to obtain owing to circulatory collapse. Frequently, the most rapid means of obtaining circulatory access is via intraosseous (into the bone) infusion into the anterior tibial bone marrow. Specific intraosseous needles are available, or a large spinal needle may be used. If IV access proves difficult, the endotracheal tube provides an effective route for administration of some drugs into the systemic circulation (Table 10–4). Doses of the resuscitation drugs given via an endotracheal tube probably should be greater than IV doses; however, optimal doses of drugs for endotracheal administration have not been determined because drug absorption may vary widely.

Oxygen

The most important agent delivered during CPR is oxygen. Because hypoxia plays such an important role in the development of cardiopulmonary arrest and irreversible organ injury, all children requiring CPR should receive 100% oxygen until resuscitation is achieved.

Epinephrine

Catecholamines are the primary class of drugs used to stimulate the cardiovascular system during resuscitation. Epinephrine, the primary agent used, has both α- and β-adrenergic stimulating effects. The α-adrenergic stimulation results in vasoconstriction with resultant elevation in systolic and diastolic blood pressure. This, in turn, improves coronary perfusion pressure, resulting in improved oxygen delivery to the heart. The β-adrenergic stimulation enhances spontaneous contractions and increases the contractile force of the heart. Controversy has arisen recently over the proper dose of epinephrine to be used during CPR. Clinical studies in animals and humans have demonstrated that a higher dose than traditionally recommended may improve the ability to obtain return of spontaneous circulation. Therefore, the currently recommended initial dose of epinephrine remains 0.01 mg/kg (0.1 mL/kg of a 1:10,000 solution) intravenously. Second and subsequent doses for unresponsive asystolic and pulseless arrest may be 10 times higher, or 0.1 mg/kg (0.1 mL/kg of a 1:1000 solution) given every 3–5 minutes. Indications for the use of epinephrine include asystole, electromechanical dissociation, hypotension, and conversion of a fine ventricular fibrillation to a coarse pattern, which is believed to be more easily converted to a sinus rhythm with electrical defibrillation.

Sodium Bicarbonate

Sodium bicarbonate is indicated for significant metabolic acidosis. It is important to recognize that with the onset of respiratory failure, respiratory acidosis can develop. The treatment for this type of acidosis is to provide adequate ventilation. With the onset of circulatory failure, lactic acid is produced and a concomitant metabolic acidosis develops. Sodium bicarbonate combines with hydrogen ions in the blood to produce carbon dioxide and water. This additional production of carbon dioxide must be eliminated through ventilation. In 1986, a consensus was reached to abandon the initial use of sodium bicarbonate until after 10 minutes of conventional CPR. Providing effective ventilation and chest compressions to generate adequate coronary perfusion pressures during CPR are most important. If arterial blood gases are

Table 10–2. Recommendations for external cardiac compressions in pediatric cardiopulmonary resuscitation.[1]

Age	Site	Procedure	Depth	Rate/Min
Infant	One finger below internipple line	2–3 fingers	0.5–1 in	At least 100
Child	One finger above xiphoid notch	Heel of one hand	1–1.5 in	80–100
Adult	Same as for child	Both hands	1.5–2 in	60–80

[1]Adapted and reproduced, with permission, from Bardossi K: Newest guidelines on pediatric CPR and first aid. Contemp Pediatr 1987;4:47.

Table 10–3. Drugs and procedures commonly used in pediatric cardiopulmonary resuscitation.

Drug	Dose	Indication
Oxygen	100%	Hypoxia (assumed in every resuscitation)
Fluids (0.9% NaCl solution)	20 mL/kg	Inadequate peripheral circulation
Epinephrine (1:10,000)	Initial: 0.01 mg/kg (0.1 mL/kg)	Asystole, hypotension, electromechanical dissociation, to convert
	Subsequent: 0.1 mg/kg (0.1 mL/kg of 1:1000)	from fine to coarse ventricular fibrillation
Atropine	0.02 mg/kg	Bradycardia with inadequate perfusion
	Minimum: 0.1 mg	Second- or third-degree atrioventricular block
	Maximum: 2 mg	
Bicarbonate	1 meq/kg	Metabolic acidosis
Glucose (D10W)	0.5–1 g/kg (5–10 mL/kg)	Hypoglycemia
Defibrillation	2 J/kg	Ventricular fibrillation or ventricular tachycardia without a pulse
Synchronized cardioversion	0.2–1 J/kg	Symptomatic supraventricular or ventricular tachycardias

known, sodium bicarbonate should be given according to the formula:

$$\text{meq NaHCO}_3 = \frac{\text{base deficit} \times \text{weight (kg)} \times 0.4}{2}$$

If blood gases are not available, the initial dose is 1 meq/kg given intravenously. Potential side effects of bicarbonate administration include hypernatremia, hyperosmolarity, impairment of oxygen delivery to the peripheral tissues due to a shift in the oxyhemoglobin dissociation curve to the left, and inactivation of catecholamines if given via the same IV line without interposed flushing of the line.

Atropine

Atropine is a parasympatholytic agent. It increases heart rate by increasing the rate of discharge from the sinus node, increases conduction through the atrioventricular node, and reverses vagally mediated hypotension. Indications for atropine are bradycardia associated with hypotension, ventricular ectopy, or symptoms of myocardial ischemia and the treatment of second- or third-degree heart block. A minimum dose of atropine (0.1 mg) is recommended to prevent a paradoxic bradycardia caused by the CNS action of atropine at low doses of the drug.

Glucose

Rapid assessment of blood glucose is a priority in the evaluation of any patient in need of resuscitation. If hypoglycemia is present, the initial dose of glucose is 0.5–1 g/kg given as either 5–10 mL/kg of 10% dextrose in water (D10W) or 2–4 mL/kg of D25W. The blood glucose level

Table 10–4. Drugs that can be given through an endotracheal tube during resuscitation.

Lidocaine
Atropine
Naloxone (Narcan)
Epinephrine
Diazepam (Valium)—**Caution:** may cause chemical pneumonitis

should then be monitored to determine the need for subsequent doses.

IV FLUIDS

During CPR, IV fluids are usually used to keep an IV line patent for drug administration. Ringer lactate or 5% dextrose in normal saline may be used for this purpose. Volume expansion in the patient with circulatory collapse is usually achieved with colloid solutions such as 5% albumin, crystalloid solutions such as Ringer lactate or normal saline, or blood products such as packed red blood cells or fresh-frozen plasma. The initial amount of volume is typically 20 mL/kg given as a bolus infusion. Subsequent fluid administration is determined by reassessment of the adequacy of cardiac output, as detailed above.

DEFIBRILLATION

Defibrillation is a relatively uncommon intervention in pediatric resuscitation. The most common arrhythmia seen in children presenting in cardiopulmonary arrest is asystole. Because it is unusual for a child's heart to fibrillate, the rhythm should be confirmed before defibrillation is attempted. Defibrillation produces a mass depolarization of the myocardium followed by the spontaneous return of sinus rhythm.

The larger adult defibrillator paddles are recommended for children weighing more than 10 kg. The smaller pediatric paddles should be used for infants weighing less than 10 kg. The paddles should rest firmly on the chest wall; one is placed over the right side of the upper chest and the other over the apex of the heart. The recommended dose of energy for ventricular fibrillation is 2 J/kg. If the first defibrillatory attempt is unsuccessful, second and third attempts are made with a dose of 4 J/kg. If these are also unsuccessful, lidocaine should be given and attention turned to correcting acidosis, hypoxemia, or hypothermia before proceeding with further attempts at defibrillation.

Synchronized cardioversion is distinguished from defibrillation. It is the timed depolarization of myocardial cells used when a patient is symptomatic with hypotension or poor perfusion from a rapid supraventricular or ventricular tachycardia. The depolarization must be synchronized with the existing rhythm. The energy dose is usually one tenth to one half the usual defibrillation dose (0.2–1 J/kg).

SUMMARY

Pediatric CPR requires effective integration of mechanical skills and pharmacotherapy used in both BLS and ALS paradigms. The immediate goal of CPR in children is to reestablish substrate delivery to preserve vital organ function and reverse ongoing tissue injury.

SUDDEN INFANT DEATH SYNDROME

Sudden infant death syndrome (SIDS) is defined as the sudden death of an infant younger than 1 year that remains unexplained after a complete postmortem examination. It should be emphasized that SIDS is a diagnosis of exclusion. The differential diagnosis of SIDS includes overwhelming infection (sepsis), congenital heart disease, cardiac arrhythmia, seizure, trauma (child abuse), poisoning, gastroesophageal reflux associated with apnea, infantile botulism, congenital CNS lesions associated with apnea, brain tumor, hypoglycemia, and inborn errors of metabolism. SIDS is the leading cause of death in infants between 1 month and 1 year of age. In the United States, the overall incidence of SIDS is approximately 1–2:1000 live births. The peak incidence is at 2–3 months after birth; it is rare before 1 month and after 9 months.

Several epidemiologic studies have demonstrated a number of factors significantly related to the risk of SIDS. Rates of SIDS are highest in poor and nonwhite infants, children of mothers who smoke or who have a history of substance abuse, preterm or small-for-gestational age infants, siblings of prior SIDS victims, and infants recovering from mild upper respiratory tract symptoms.

Infants who have experienced an **acute life-threatening event (ALTE),** such as prolonged apnea requiring resuscitation, may be at a higher risk for recurrence of such events. These infants, as well as others determined to be at a higher risk of SIDS (such as siblings of SIDS victims), may be offered home monitoring with an electronic cardiorespiratory monitor, and their caretakers should be instructed in BLS. Considerable controversy exists regarding the guidelines for instituting and terminating home monitoring.

Many theories have been offered to explain the mechanism of SIDS. One of the most actively studied areas is the **apnea hypothesis,** which speculates that apnea is the main mechanism and terminal event in SIDS. The apnea may be central, in which there is no respiratory effort; obstructive, in which there is an effort to breathe, but there is anatomic or functional obstruction to airflow; or a combination of the two. Although the apnea hypothesis has been one of the most active areas of SIDS research, it has not proved convincing. Most infants with prolonged apnea do not die of SIDS, and most SIDS victims did not have a known apnea event before death.

Other theories that have received attention include abnormal respiratory control response to hypoxia and hypercarbia; upper airway obstruction due to abnormal neuromuscular control; abnormalities in sleep patterns; cardiac arrhythmias, particularly the prolonged QT syndrome; and an imbalance of sympathetic innervation to the heart, rendering the heart more susceptible to life-threatening arrhythmias. Infantile botulism has been considered as the cause in some infants. Recently it has been reported that positioning infants in the prone position for sleeping is associated with an increased risk of SIDS. The mechanism responsible for this relationship between SIDS and sleep position has not been defined. Several studies have demonstrated a drastic reduction in the incidence of SIDS in regions where infants predominantly sleep on their sides or backs. The American Academy of Pediatrics now recommends that healthy infants be placed to sleep on their sides or backs.

Although no consensus exists as to the major determinant of SIDS, a single pathologic mechanism is clearly unlikely. Further research is needed to explore the interaction between sleep and other physiologic control systems in the developing infant.

SHOCK

Shock is a complex pathophysiologic state of circulatory dysfunction that results in the inability of the body to deliver adequate oxygen, glucose, and other nutrients to tissue beds. In **early or compensated shock,** blood flow is maintained by compensatory mechanisms but is uneven in the microcirculation. Cardiac output and most vital signs may be normal. However, if untreated, compensated shock progresses to **late or uncompensated shock.** Unless this process is corrected, **irreversible shock** occurs, with permanent damage to important organs such as the brain and heart.

The etiology of shock has been divided into three categories: hypovolemic, distributive, and cardiogenic. Table 10–5 summarizes the etiology of shock in children. Hypovolemic shock is the most common category. When the circulating blood volume is reduced, cardiac output falls. The body compensates for the decrease in cardiac output by increasing heart rate, systemic vascular resistance, and myocardial contractility. This response maintains the

Table 10–5. Differential diagnosis of shock.

Hypovolemic shock
Hemorrhage
Internal bleeding
External bleeding
Gastroenteritis
Diabetes mellitus or insipidus
Severe burns
Distributive shock
Septic shock
Toxic shock syndrome
Anaphylaxis
Drug intoxication
Neurogenic shock (spinal cord transection)
Cardiogenic shock
Cardiomyopathy
Congenital heart disease
Congestive heart failure
Arrhythmia
Tension pneumothorax
Pericardial effusion or tamponade
Hypoxia (near-drowning, smoke inhalation)

child's blood pressure until almost 40% of blood volume is lost. However, the systemic vasoconstriction leads to ischemia in many tissues, and thus cell metabolism and function suffer. As cells die, they release enzymes that may cause vasodilation and pooling of blood in capillary beds. "Toxic" substances are released, which depresses myocardial function and affects the coagulation system, resulting in disseminated intravascular coagulopathy.

In distributive shock, peripheral vascular resistance is severely reduced. While this is most often triggered by gram-negative infection (septic shock), it can also be due to gram-positive organisms or viruses. Distributive shock also can result from anaphylaxis due to an allergic reaction to medications, insect bite, or snake bite. Transection of the spinal cord is rare in children but may lead to vasodilation and shock. However, this should not be considered the source of shock in the initial evaluation of the trauma patient because hypovolemic shock is much more common. Toxic shock syndrome is another example of distributive shock; it is triggered by toxin-producing *Staphylococcus aureus* either colonizing the vagina after the use of heavy-absorbency tampons or invading injured skin. Frequently, diarrhea, vomiting, or diffuse erythematous rash are the first symptoms, followed by shock. Overdoses of some medications can also cause hypotension and shock. Distributive shock results in increased venous capacitance, shunting past some capillary beds, and ischemia in many underperfused tissues. The result is release of other vasoactive substances such as serotonin, endorphins, prostaglandins, leukotrienes, and histamine, which cause further capillary leakage and inadequate tissue oxygenation. Cardiac function is affected by poor perfusion and release of toxic myocardial depressant factors.

In cardiogenic shock, abnormal heart function results in failure to meet the metabolic demands of the body. Although this is the least common cause of shock in children, it can result from arrhythmias (such as supraventric-

ular tachycardia), cardiomyopathies (such as viral myocarditis), drug intoxication, or tension pneumothorax and pericardial tamponade, which inhibit the heart's ability to fill and pump adequately. The body compensates for decreased stroke volume by increasing systemic vascular resistance to maintain blood pressure and increasing sodium and water retention to increase central blood volume. However, this increased afterload and preload only further increases the metabolic demands on the heart and may result in myocardial ischemia and decreased ventricular function. Figure 10–1 summarizes the pathophysiology of shock in children.

DIAGNOSIS & CLINICAL MANIFESTATIONS

The diagnosis of shock is made by an abbreviated physical examination (Table 10–6). When evaluating a child who may be in shock, complete vital signs should be obtained. Initially the child is anxious or irritable, with cool extremities and tachycardia, and may appear gray or ashen due to poor perfusion. Pulses may be weak and thready, and capillary refill may be delayed beyond 2–3 seconds. (Capillary refill cannot be determined accurately in hypothermic patients.) At this point, blood pressure may be normal due to compensatory mechanisms; hypotension is a late finding with shock in the pediatric patient. Later, as shock progresses and decompensation occurs, tachypnea, somnolence, and oliguria may develop. Eventually, obtundation, periodic breathing, apnea, and hypotension ensue. Cardiopulmonary arrest may result.

Additional **physical findings** may be present, depending on the cause of the shock. For instance, there may be evidence of trauma or burns. Fever or hypothermia may occur in patients with septic shock. Petechiae may be noticed if a coagulopathy has developed, or a fine, erythematous, sandpaper-like rash may be present in toxic shock syndrome. Hepatomegaly may be present, with muffled heart sounds or a gallop rhythm, if cardiac failure is the cause of shock. However, distended neck veins may be absent when shock is present.

A brief, relevant **history** should be obtained while the child is being examined to help determine the etiology. It is important to learn whether there has been trauma or burns, whether the child has had fever or other signs of infection, or whether allergies are present, as well as whether the child could have taken any medications, or has had evidence of diabetes. If the patient in shock is a teenage girl, it should be noted whether she is menstruating and using tampons.

The diagnosis of shock is made clinically before any laboratory tests are obtained. However, several **laboratory studies** may help to determine the cause or guide management. Because of poor perfusion, an arterial or venous blood gas will always show some degree of metabolic acidosis. Hypoxia and hypercarbia may also be noted. A complete blood count may show leukocytosis

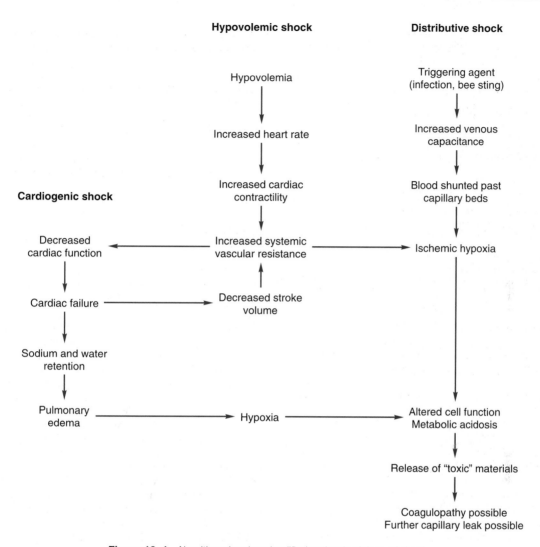

Figure 10–1. Algorithm showing simplified pathophysiology of shock.

with a left shift as a nonspecific response to stress or a sign of infection. A blood glucose level should be determined, including a bedside rapid dextrose strip to rule out hypoglycemia. Hepatic enzyme and blood urea nitrogen (BUN) and creatinine concentrations may be elevated be-

Table 10–6. Recognition of shock.

Gray, ashen color
Tachycardia
Delayed capillary refill
Altered mental status—irritable, lethargic
Decreased urine output
Cool, clammy skin
Weak pulses
Hypotension

cause liver and renal function are impaired owing to poor perfusion. A coagulopathy may be present. A chest radiograph may show evidence of pulmonary venous congestion (shock lung), and the heart size may be normal or enlarged. This radiographic picture is often seen after fluid resuscitation has begun. A blood culture should be obtained if sepsis is suspected; a vaginal culture should also be obtained, and a tampon, if present, should be removed if toxic shock is suspected.

MANAGEMENT

Shock must be recognized and treated immediately; the initial management is the same regardless of the cause. Figure 10–2 summarizes the management of shock in pe-

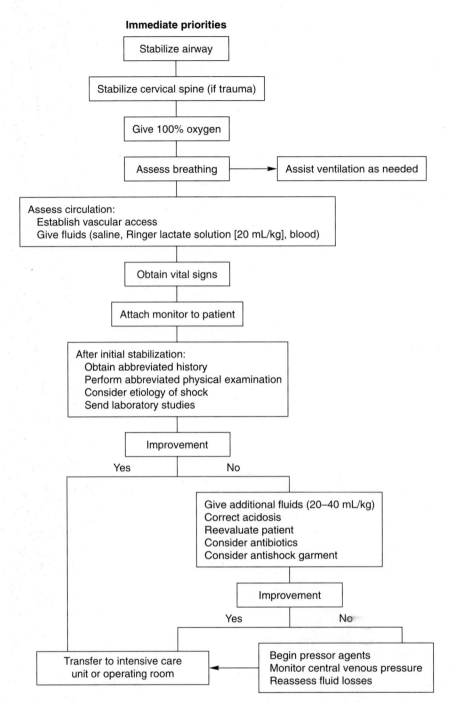

Figure 10–2. Algorithm showing the initial management of shock in the pediatric patient. (Adapted and reproduced, with permission, from Olson KR et al: Physical assessment and differential diagnosis of the poisoned patient. Med Toxicol 1987;2:52.)

diatric patients. The first intervention is to assess the child's airway and ensure that it is not obstructed. The child's breathing effort should be assessed by looking at the chest wall and auscultating the lungs.

Oxygen (fractional inspired oxygen [FiO_2] 100%) should be delivered even if the child is not obviously cyanotic. It is desirable to maintain a partial pressure of oxygen (PaO_2) of at least 100 mm Hg. Once the airway and breathing have been assessed, the circulation should be evaluated. Vascular access must be obtained quickly. It is preferable to place two large-bore, short-length catheters into peripheral veins. Hand veins and those in the antecubital fossae may offer the best opportunities for success. However, even these may be difficult to cannulate in a child who is in shock. If unsuccessful after a brief search for peripheral access, the physician should consider alternative routes. The femoral vein may be cannulated by passing a guidewire through a needle and then inserting a catheter over the wire (Seldinger technique). When venous access is accomplished, blood can be sent for laboratory studies, including type and cross-match. Besides the femoral vein, the internal jugular and subclavian veins can be accessed in a similar manner. These are technically more difficult to reach and have a higher complication rate; thus, access should be attempted only by those with experience. In addition, a saphenous vein cutdown can be used as an alternative means of securing vascular access, but this procedure may require additional time and surgical skills. If venous access is not possible, the intraosseous route should be attempted in children younger than 6 years. Specific intraosseous needles, an 18- or 20-gauge spinal needle with a stylet, or a bone marrow needle may be used. Using aseptic technique, the needle is inserted into the flat medial surface of the proximal tibia 2 cm below the tibial tuberosity; this provides an effective route for delivery of fluids and medications during resuscitation.

Once vascular access is achieved, fluid resuscitation must begin promptly. Saline (0.9%) or Ringer lactate solution are the initial fluids, given in a dose of 20 mL/kg very quickly, over about 10 minutes. Although controversy persists, there is no evidence that colloid solutions (albumin, plasma) are more valuable than crystalloid solutions in the initial management. Packed red blood cells should be given to maintain a hematocrit of 33%, at a rate of 10 mL/kg over 1–2 hours. Saline or Ringer lactate solution is given until this is available. In extreme emergencies, type O-negative blood may be used.

The child should be attached to a cardiac monitor to record heart rate, respirations, and blood pressure continuously. An abbreviated history is obtained, and a physical examination is performed. If hypoglycemia is noted by rapid blood glucose screening, an infusion of 25% dextrose (2–4 mL/kg) should be given quickly, followed by a 10% dextrose continuous infusion. Temperature control is important; an overhead warmer may be needed to prevent hypothermia.

A urinary catheter should be placed to monitor the child's response to fluid resuscitation. The child must be reevaluated constantly. If the patient remains poorly perfused (ie, with persistent metabolic acidosis, prolonged capillary refill, tachycardia, weak pulses, oliguria, or hypotension), additional fluids are indicated. Another bolus of saline or Ringer lactate solution (20 mL/kg) should be infused rapidly. Most children in shock require at least 40–60 mL/kg in the first hour before improvement is noted; more is needed if ongoing losses occur.

If the circulation remains poor despite adequate fluid resuscitation, pressor agents may be needed. Dopamine is usually the preferred drug. It has different effects depending on the dosage. When infused at 1–3 µg/kg/min, it causes renal and splanchnic vasodilation with a slight decrease in systemic vascular resistance. Thus, renal blood flow increases with little or no change in blood pressure, and cardiac output may increase. When infused at 3–8 µg/kg/min, dopamine increases the blood pressure and may increase cardiac output. These changes may result in warmer extremities with improved capillary refill. At higher doses, more severe vasoconstriction often occurs; this may be undesirable because it interferes with perfusion. Another useful agent for circulatory failure is dobutamine; it is an effective inotropic agent that improves cardiac output and blood pressure and is purported to have less effect on heart rate or rhythm than other catecholamines. It is therefore a useful agent for cardiogenic shock. Other catecholamines include epinephrine infusions, which are used to treat endotoxemia and anaphylaxis, and norepinephrine infusions, which may be helpful when there is low diastolic blood pressure and coronary perfusion is threatened. Both of these agents cause peripheral vasoconstriction. Amrinone is a newer, nonadrenergic inotropic agent that may be useful when there is severe myocardial failure that is resistant to adrenergic agents.

Other agents used in the management of shock include sodium bicarbonate, given intravenously for severe metabolic acidosis (pH < 7.25) that does not respond to fluid therapy alone. Adequate ventilation should be ensured if bicarbonate is used. Further doses are guided by the child's acid-base status as determined by blood gas analysis. Half-strength sodium bicarbonate should be used for infants in the first few months after birth. Bicarbonate therapy is not a substitute for attempts to improve blood flow and ventilation.

Broad-spectrum antibiotics should be given if septic shock is suspected. Calcium chloride is rarely used but may be of value if the ionized serum calcium concentration is low; in addition, it sometimes is given empirically if massive amounts of blood, albumin, or plasma are used in resuscitation. Calcium chloride must be given through a central line (5–7 mg/kg). Alternatively, calcium gluconate may be infused peripherally (10 mg/kg). Although corticosteroids have been recommended in the past by some centers in the management of shock, studies with adult patients have shown that they have little value in improving the outcome of patients with septic shock.

Diuretic agents are occasionally used with caution to

improve pulmonary congestion, which is usually due to capillary leakage and responds best to mechanical ventilation with positive end-expiratory pressure (PEEP).

Afterload reduction may be helpful when the child is more stable and central venous pressure can be monitored. Nitroprusside and other drugs are used to improve peripheral circulation, but this form of treatment is administered optimally in the setting of the intensive care unit (ICU) rather than the emergency department. Table 10–7 summarizes the medications useful in managing the child in shock.

Continuous monitoring of pulse, respirations, blood pressure, and pulse oximetry is essential. Frequent reassessment of mental status, skin perfusion, and urine output is also necessary.

Once the child in shock is stabilized, plans should be made to transfer the patient to an ICU. It is very important to maintain constant surveillance of the child's vital signs, urine output, skin perfusion, and mental status.

SEIZURE DISORDERS

STATUS EPILEPTICUS

Status epilepticus is a common medical emergency in children. A patient who is experiencing a seizure or series of seizures for 30 minutes or longer without a return to baseline mental state is in status epilepticus (see Chapter 21). Status epilepticus occurs in 60,000–160,000 persons annually, and the majority of these are in the pediatric age group. The mean age of onset is 5 years, with 64% of the episodes occurring earlier. It is estimated that 1% of the US population will experience an episode of status epilepticus in their lifetime, with an overall 1% mortality rate. Morbidity and mortality in these patients are usually related to the specific cause of the seizure rather than the seizure activity itself.

The etiology of status epilepticus is summarized in Table 10–8. In some cases, such as hypoglycemia, hyponatremia, and CNS hemorrhage, treatment of the cause should help considerably in treatment of the seizure. In other cases, seizure activity must be controlled until the cause is discovered. The cause of seizures in children is also age related.

Status epilepticus can be classified as either generalized or partial. The most clinically apparent and potentially compromising are the generalized convulsive types of status epilepticus: tonic, clonic, tonic-clonic (**grand mal**), and myoclonic. **Tonic seizures** ("with tone") are manifested as either flexion or extension of the extremities. **Clonic seizures** manifest as jerking of the extremities, without an initial tonic phase. These movements are usually asymmetric and arrhythmic. **Tonic-clonic** seizures are the most common presentation of status epilepticus; they begin with a short tonic phase and progress to a longer, more dramatic clonic phase of seizure activity. The seizures are typically discontinuous and can begin as either a generalized seizure or a partial convulsion that generalizes secondarily.

Seizures can affect the maintenance of adequate ventilation, oxygenation, and perfusion. There is also evidence that prolonged seizure activity can cause irreversible neuronal cell damage despite optimal correction of oxygenation, ventilation, and metabolic derangements. This is likely a result of cellular hypoxia, due to increased cellular demand and decreased availability of oxygen. The end-organ dysfunction seen in status epilepticus results initially from sympathetic and parasympathetic activation. Complications include tachycardia, hypertension, diaphoresis, salivary and tracheobronchial hypersecretion, hyperpyrexia, and hyperglycemia. Later in the course of the seizure, metabolic complications result from high energy expenditure and muscular fatigue; these include

Table 10–7. Medications useful in treating shock.

Drug	Recommended Dose	Actions/Remarks
Dopamine	1–3 µg/kg/min	Renal, splanchnic vasodilation
	3–8 µg/kg/min	Cardiac output ↑, BP ↑
	> 10 µg/kg/min	Peripheral vasoconstriction
Dobutamine	7–10 µg/kg/min	Potent inotropic agent, cardiac output ↑, BP ↑, minimal change heart rate or rhythm
Epinephrine	0.05–2 µg/kg/min	Peripheral vasoconstriction, cardiac output ↑, BP ↑
Norepinephrine	2–10 µg/kg/min	Peripheral vasoconstriction, cardiac output ↑, BP ↑
Isoproterenol	0.05–2 µg/kg/min	Heart rate ↑, BP ↑, cardiac output ↑, causes peripheral vasodilation
Sodium bicarbonate	0.5–1 meq/kg	For metabolic acidosis unresponsive to fluids and electrolytes
Antibiotics	Variable	Broad-spectrum drugs if sepsis considered
Calcium chloride	5–7 mg/kg	If ionized calcium is low
Nitroprusside	1–10 µg/kg/min	Peripheral vasodilation, to improve peripheral circulation when BP stable
Amrinone	0.75 mg/kg over 2–3 min Maintenance rate 5–10 µg/kg/min	For low cardiac output states

BP = blood pressure.

Table 10–8. Etiology of status epilepticus in children.

Mnemonic: "in status"
*I*nsufficient medications
*N*eoplasm/masses
*S*pinal infection
*T*oxins
*A*noxia
*T*rauma
*U*nknown/febrile
*S*ugar/sodium

metabolic acidosis, hyperkalemia, hypoglycemia, hyperazotemia (increased BUN), and hyponatremia (Table 10–9). Respiratory compromise may result from hypoventilation, aspiration or blockage of the airways by secretions, or glossopharyngeal dystonia. This eventually can lead to cardiopulmonary arrest. In addition to the organ system and cellular dysfunction, trauma to the head and extremities may occur during the severe tonic-clonic movements.

DIAGNOSIS & CLINICAL MANIFESTATIONS

In most cases, the diagnosis of generalized convulsive status epilepticus is not subtle. However, recognition of other forms of status epilepticus, such as myoclonic status epilepticus or infantile spasms, can be more difficult. In general, a complete history should be obtained but can wait until the patient is stabilized and the seizure treated. However, some important historical points can be helpful initially in determining both the presence and cause of a seizure. A history of prior seizures leads one to question the inappropriate use of anticonvulsants, whereas a history of diabetes, head trauma, ingestion, or febrile illness suggests other etiologies.

Physical examination begins with vital signs and mental status examination. All generalized convulsive seizures result in the patient's unresponsiveness to voice or command. Most clonic movements are difficult to miss. However, some other motor activity might be difficult to differentiate from spontaneous movements or rigors. In general, one cannot alter or stop the clonic movements of status epilepticus by holding the extremity down. Close observation of mental status and movement patterns may

Table 10–9. Systemic effects of status epilepticus.

Early Findings	Late Findings
Tachycardia	Metabolic acidosis
Hypertension	Hyperkalemia
Diaphoresis	Hyperazotemia
Salivary/tracheobronchial hypersecretion	Hypoglycemia
Hyperpyrexia	Hyponatremia
Hyperglycemia	

provide diagnosis of very subtle presentations of status epilepticus.

During the postictal period, patients might appear lethargic, confused, and even comatose. The diagnosis of a seizure at this point is based on the history obtained from witnesses. Although this period may still correlate with abnormal CNS neuronal discharges, muscle tone is no longer increased, but rather normal or hypotonic. The patient may experience glossopharyngeal hypotonia and increased secretions, which obstruct the airway despite the cessation of seizure activity.

Laboratory values are not as helpful in diagnosing the presence of a seizure. Laboratory evaluation should focus on two issues: guiding management of ABCs and identifying correctable causes of seizures, such as hypoglycemia, hyponatremia, and hypoxia. Rarely, and only if the history is suggestive, is it necessary to evaluate immediately for uremia, hypocalcemia, and hypomagnesemia. Anticonvulsant levels and toxicologic evaluation may be ordered as well, but these results are rarely ready in time to alter the initial management.

MANAGEMENT

Stabilization

As mentioned previously, the management of status epilepticus begins as all pediatric emergencies do: with the ABCs (see this chapter, Cardiopulmonary Resuscitation). However, certain problems associated with status epilepticus deserve special consideration. The establishment of an adequate airway takes priority over all other management issues. The patient's airway may be compromised during the seizure from increased muscular tone in the pharynx and hypopharynx, increased secretions, and decreased level of consciousness with concomitant loss of the gag reflex. An adequate airway must be established, and both the quality of air entry and the success of repositioning and jaw thrust should be determined. If these maneuvers are insufficient to provide adequate ventilation, bag-valve-mask manual ventilation or endotracheal intubation should be performed. It should be remembered that although patients might withstand up to 30 minutes of seizure activity without neurologic sequelae, they can tolerate only a few minutes of apnea before cardiorespiratory arrest ensues.

Oxygen should always be administered to patients in status epilepticus regardless of the adequacy of ventilation or pulse oximeter reading. In status epilepticus, IV access is helpful for the rapid administration of antiepileptic medications. The need for IV hydration is variable and often determined by the underlying cause of the seizure. Abnormalities of circulation are rarely due to hypovolemia or distributive shock in patients with status epilepticus. Nevertheless, the children in status epilepticus appear to have poor circulation secondary to the increased catecholamine levels and subsequent shunting of blood away from peripheral areas.

A blood sugar concentration should be determined to evaluate the presence of early hyperglycemia or late hypoglycemia seen in status epilepticus. This can easily be done at the bedside. In addition, antipyretics can be administered rectally in an attempt to counteract the effects of elevated body temperature on the seizure threshold.

Antiepileptic Medications

Seizures lasting longer than 10–15 minutes are usually treated with anticonvulsant medications. In addition, rapidly reversible causes of seizures, such as metabolic disturbances or expanding cerebral mass lesions, should be dealt with. Many anticonvulsant medications can be administered by alternative routes, eg, endotracheal, intramuscular (IM), or rectal, which should be considered if IV access is not rapidly attained. Medications commonly used for status epilepticus are presented in Table 10–10.

Benzodiazepines. The two most common medications used initially in the management of seizures are lorazepam (Ativan) and diazepam (Valium). Both have a rapid onset of action (within 2–3 minutes) and are effective in stopping seizures 80–85% of the time. Diazepam can be given by the endotracheal or rectal route. Its relatively short duration of action, however, necessitates either repeated dosages or the use of a second, longer-acting medication, such as phenobarbital or phenytoin. The anticonvulsant activity of lorazepam can last 24–48 hours, and it has been shown to be equally as effective in controlling status epilepticus as diazepam. Midazolam (Versed), a third benzodiazepine, is infrequently used but theoretically effective in controlling status epilepticus. Its main advantage is that it can be given intramuscularly because of its aqueous solubility. When used in conjunction with a barbiturate such as phenobarbital, the benzodiazepines can potentiate respiratory depression.

Phenytoin. Because of its slower onset of action, phenytoin (Dilantin) is frequently used as a second medication in the management of status epilepticus. The incidence of bradycardia and hypotension resulting from its use can be reduced by administering the drug slowly, at a rate no greater than 0.5–1 mg/kg/min or 50 mg/min maximum. Because of the slow rate of drug administration, phenytoin concentrations might not reach therapeutic levels until 30–50 minutes after onset of infusion. Despite these caveats, phenytoin is used frequently because of its high efficacy and its lack of effect on mental status. Therapeutic levels of 10–20 meq/mL are commonly required, and toxic effects include nystagmus and ataxia.

Phenobarbital. Phenobarbital also has a relatively delayed onset of action (20 minutes), as well as an extremely long half-life and duration of action. Its other advantages include the potential for IM administration when IV access is difficult and its wide therapeutic range. Disadvantages include a significant risk of respiratory depression, especially when administered in conjunction with a benzodiazepine. Phenobarbital also causes significant depression of mental status. Children who have received phenobarbital may be sedated and appear ataxic for days after their initial dose.

If seizure activity continues for 30–60 minutes after administration of maximum doses of anticonvulsant medications, general anesthesia can be induced to control status epilepticus. This is rarely needed but can be performed intravenously using barbiturates such as pentobarbital, thiopental, or high-dose phenobarbital. General anesthesia can be induced with the use of inhaled anesthetics such as

Table 10–10. Anticonvulsant medications used in the acute management of status epilepticus.

Drug	Dosage	Route[1]	Onset of Action	Duration of Action	More Common Side Effects[3]
Diazepam (Valium)	0.1–0.2 mg/kg Maximum: 10 mg/dose Repeat q 5 min 0.5 mg/kg	IV, ET PR[2] in saline PR	2–3 min	10–15 min	1, 2
Lorazepam (Ativan)	0.05–0.10 mg/kg Maximum: 4 mg/dose Repeat q 5 min	IV, PR[2]	2–3 min	24–48 h	1, 2
Midazolam (Versed)	0.05–0.20 mg/kg Maximum: 5 mg/dose	IV, IM	2–5 min	1–5 h	1, 2, 4
Phenytoin (Dilantin)	18–20 mg/kg Maximum: 1 g/dose	IV slowly (0.5–1 mg/kg/min in saline)	20–40 min	24 h	3
Phenobarbital (Luminal)	20 mg/kg Maximum: 300 mg/dose	IV, IM	20 min (24 h IM)	24–72 h	1 (especially in conjunction with benzodiazepines), 2

[1]All IV medications can be administered by intraosseous route if necessary.
[2]Per rectum (PR) administration, inserted 4–6 cm into rectum with 1 mL syringe or rectal tube.
[3]1 = respiratory depression; 2 = alters mental status; 3 = hypotension/bradycardia if administered too quickly—monitor electrocardiogram and blood pressure continuously; 4 = amnesia.
IV = intravenous; ET = endotracheal; IM = intramuscular.

halothane or isoflurane. These medications are titrated until the electroencephalogram (EEG) reveals a "burst-suppression" pattern—suppression of seizures with occasional flurries of activity. Close cardiorespiratory monitoring must be implemented, and patients are almost always intubated for airway protection and mechanical ventilation.

SUMMARY: GENERAL APPROACH

The decision to administer anticonvulsant medications is based on the child's clinical status, oxygenation, and duration of seizure. If the decision is made to treat the seizure, a benzodiazepine (preferably lorazepam) should be administered upon obtaining IV access. This drug can be repeated 2–3 times over the subsequent 15 minutes before initiating phenytoin therapy. If IV access cannot be achieved, diazepam (0.5 mg/kg) may be administered rectally, or midazolam (0.2 mg/kg) may be administered intramuscularly. These drugs may be repeated 2–3 times.

If status epilepticus continues despite benzodiazepine and phenytoin therapy, barbiturate therapy or inhalational general anesthetic should be considered. When these treatments are instituted, the child should have continuous evaluation by physical examination, pulse oximetry, and cardiorespiratory monitoring. Once seizure activity has ceased, clinical assessment should continue to focus on the child's respiratory pattern, mental status, and neurologic examination.

Frequently during the postictal phase, the child will require supplementary ventilatory support in the form of bag-valve-mask positive-pressure ventilation. The duration of this phase may range from a few minutes to a few hours. The patient should be expeditiously transferred to the appropriate inpatient unit for further management.

FEBRILE CONVULSIONS

Febrile convulsions occur in 3–4% of children younger than 5 years of age and account for approximately 50% of all seizures in this age group. Because of their relatively benign nature and good prognosis, it is important to be able to differentiate febrile convulsions from seizures secondary to acute CNS disease or epilepsy. The criteria for diagnosis of simple febrile seizures are listed in Table 10–11.

Boys are affected more often than girls, and there is frequently a strong family predisposition to this type of seizure. Because the rate of rise of the fever is thought to be more of an instigating factor than the actual height of the fever, the typical clinical picture is one in which the child's caretakers had not noticed a fever before the event. The convulsion is usually completed before the child arrives in the emergency department, but the child may be in the lethargic or sleepy postictal state. Postictal EEG recordings are normal in 85–95% of cases.

Table 10–11. Diagnostic criteria for simple febrile convulsions.

Age 6 mo to 6 y
Fever > 38.4 °C
Generalized tonic-clonic seizure
Duration < 15 min
No known underlying cerebral disease
No neurologic sequelae

Approximately 0.2% of children with febrile convulsions have permanent neurologic sequelae. The benign nature of this entity significantly affects the patient's evaluation in the emergency department. The physician who initially screens the patient should be suspicious of other potential causes for the child's seizure. In children younger than 18 months who have a febrile seizure, many physicians consider performing a lumbar puncture to rule out meningitis. It is unlikely, however, that a pleocytosis will be found on examination of the CNS in a well-appearing child who has no other findings of meningitis. In addition, further episodes of seizure activity within 24 hours of the first episode should raise the suspicion of other diagnoses.

The management of febrile convulsions is similar to the management of seizures mentioned previously. If a febrile child is actively seizing, support of ABCs should be instituted. Antiepileptic medications could be withheld if the total duration of seizure has been short. In many cases, the seizure stops after a few minutes, and the child awakens after a short postictal period. Because most children with this entity are not actively seizing in the emergency department, a detailed history must be undertaken. Physical examination should be directed toward finding a source for the child's fever and ruling out any possibility of cerebral infection. If the child appears well, many physicians do not perform any laboratory analysis. Discharge instructions should include the proper use of antipyretic medications as well as anticipatory guidance regarding the chances of further seizures. The parents should be instructed to call their physician or return to the emergency department if a second seizure occurs. In the case of "atypical" febrile convulsions, referral to a pediatric neurologist is warranted.

More than 90% of children with febrile convulsions have an excellent prognosis. Approximately one third of these experience another febrile convulsion, and another one third have a third seizure. Only about 2–6% of children in whom febrile convulsions are initially diagnosed go on to have spontaneous afebrile seizures and a diagnosis of epilepsy. This risk increases, however, as the number of febrile convulsion episodes increases and if the initial convulsion is unusually long.

HYPONATREMIA

A sodium level below 120 meq/L may precipitate epileptic seizures in children. In these cases, the history is usually suggestive of water intoxication. A typical history is of a small, ill child who is given hyposmolar solutions, such as weak tea or plain water. Electrolytes such as sodium and potassium are lost in the urine, stool, and sweat and are not replaced. The serum concentrations of these electrolytes may decrease and precipitate seizures or cardiac conduction abnormalities. If there is a strong history of water intoxication in a seizing child, it is appropriate to administer enough sodium chloride to increase the serum level by 10 meq/L. This can be accomplished using 15 mL/kg of 0.9% sodium chloride (normal saline) or 2–4 mL/kg of 3% normal saline for children in whom a larger fluid bolus is not advisable. Seizures due to hyponatremia alone usually stop when a sufficient amount of sodium is administered intravenously. Hyponatremia can be caused by other underlying problems, such as syndrome of inappropriate antidiuretic hormone in a patient with meningitis. In these cases, the cause of the seizure is still unclear, and rapid sodium administration might not be as effective.

CHILDHOOD POISONING

Accidental ingestions are common in pediatrics. Children younger than 19 years of age constituted nearly 70% of the 1.9 million human exposures reported to the American Association of Poison Control Centers in 1994. In pediatrics, two fairly distinct age groups are involved in poisonings. Children younger than 5 years account for the vast majority of pediatric poisonings, virtually all of which (99.4%) are considered accidental. The natural inquisitiveness and impulsivity of toddlers make them vulnerable "hosts" for toxic ingestions. The home environment in which the poisoning typically occurs is often disrupted and under some stress. Factors such as a recent move, new pregnancy, or the absence of one parent all have been associated with an increased risk of poisoning in this age group.

Teenagers are the second distinct age group involved in pediatric poisonings. Approximately half the poisonings in this age group are considered intentional, and half, accidental. Drug experimentation and suicidal gestures are commonly associated with poisonings in adolescents.

There are five basic routes of exposure for accidental poisonings. Ingestion accounts for approximately 75% of all poisonings, followed, in decreasing frequency, by dermal exposure, ophthalmic exposure, inhalation, and envenomation (bites and stings).

A wide range of substances is involved in poisonings. Children younger than 6 years are more likely to be poisoned by nonpharmaceutical products. Table 10–12 represents the categories of substances most frequently involved in accidental poisonings in this age group.

Table 10–12. Categories of the substances most frequently involved in poisonings for children younger than 6 years of age in 1994.[1]

Type of Substance	% of All Exposures
Cosmetics/personal care items	11.6
Cleaning substances	10.8
Plants	7.2
Analgesics	7.2
Cough/cold preparations	6.4
Topicals	5.0
Foreign bodies/toys	4.9
Antimicrobials	3.5
Vitamins	3.4
Gastrointestinal preparations	3.1

[1]Adapted and reproduced, with permission, from Litovitz TL et al: 1994 annual report of the American Association of Poison Control Centers National Data Collection System. Am J Emerg Med 1995;13:551.

Despite the fact that children younger than 12 years of age account for almost 90% of all pediatric poisonings, the same group accounts for only 40% of all poisoning fatalities in children. In contrast, teenagers account for only 10% of pediatric poisonings but for 60% of deaths due to poisoning in children. The more favorable outcome in the younger group is explained by the less dangerous type and smaller amount of substances ingested, and the fact that the younger children are brought for medical care more promptly after ingestions than are teenagers or adults. Substances causing the largest number of deaths are analgesics and antidepressants, sedatives, hypnotics, stimulants, and cardiovascular drugs, and somewhat less frequently, alcohol, gases, asthma remedies, hydrocarbons, and other chemicals.

DIAGNOSIS & CLINICAL ASSESSMENT

Most childhood poisonings can be assessed and managed at home by telephone, as demonstrated by the success of Regional Poison Control Centers. These centers are staffed 24 hours a day by specialists highly trained in poison information who have access to computerized information on virtually every potentially poisonous substance available. A child with a potentially serious or an unknown ingestion is referred to a hospital emergency department for medical evaluation.

The approach to the poisoned patient should begin with a brief history of the exposure. Basic historical information to obtain includes confirmation that a poisoning has occurred or is suspected, identification of the potential toxic substance(s), route and dose of the exposure, time of the exposure, any symptoms occurring before arrival at the hospital, any preexisting medical conditions, and the use of therapeutic medications. Although information obtained during the initial history may be inaccurate, it is often possible to make a judgment regarding the potential severity of the exposure and the level of treatment that may be required.

Frequently, children present to the emergency department after a poisoning without a specific history of a toxic exposure. For this reason, poisoning is often a diagnosis of exclusion and must be considered in the differential diagnosis of any child in the high-risk age groups (younger than 5 years or teenagers) who presents with an acute unexplained illness or altered consciousness.

As with any potentially critically ill patient, the physical examination of the poisoning victim begins with an evaluation of the patient's ABCs. Specific attention should be paid to the heart rate; respiratory effort and pattern; blood pressure; CNS function, as manifested by the level of consciousness and pupillary size and reactivity; and hemodynamic status of the patient. Assessment of skin temperature, color, and perfusion, the presence or absence of sweating, and bowel and bladder function can provide clues to the type of poison involved. Smelling the patient's breath can also be of value in establishing the type of poisoning, as some substances have characteristic odors (Table 10–13).

Many drugs have a characteristic constellation of physical findings because of their effects on the autonomic nervous system. Table 10–14 lists the four most common autonomic toxic syndromes. By performing a directed "toxicologic" physical examination, the physician may be able to make a tentative clinical diagnosis, allowing for the empiric use of specific antidotes or selective toxicologic tests. Because there are frequent exceptions to these guidelines, and because ingestion of multiple agents can demonstrate overlapping or divergent effects, the categorization of physical findings into specific syndromes can be very difficult.

One approach to this dilemma is to consider five major acute clinical signs with which poisoned patients may present: coma, cardiac arrhythmias, metabolic acidosis, seizures, and gastrointestinal symptoms.

Coma

A decreased level of consciousness is a common manifestation of poisoning by a variety of drugs and chemicals. Table 10–15 lists several drugs that characteristically cause stupor or coma. The mechanism by which the ma-

Table 10–13. Substances with characteristic odors.

Odor	Substance
Sweet	Chloroform
	Acetone
	Ether
Pear	Chloral hydrate
Bitter almond	Cyanide
Garlic	Arsenic
	Phosphorus
Violet	Turpentine
Wintergreen	Methyl salicylate

Table 10–14. Most common autonomic toxic syndromes.[1]

Anticholinergic	
Signs	Delirium; tachycardia; dry, flushed skin; dilated pupils; urinary retention; decreased bowel sounds; hyperthermia.
Common causes:	Atropine, scopolamine, tricyclic antidepressants, skeletal muscle relaxants, antihistamines, antipsychotics, many plants (eg, jimson weed and *Amanita muscaria*).
Cholinergic	
Signs	Confusion, central nervous system depression, salivation, lacrimation, urinary and fecal incontinence, bradycardia or tachycardia, miosis, diaphoresis, seizures, muscle fasciculations, pulmonary edema, emesis.
Common causes	Organophosphate and carbamate insecticides, physostigmine, edrophonium, and some mushrooms.
Sympathomimetic	
Signs	Tachycardia (or reflex bradycardia if agent is a pure α-agonist), hypertension, hyperpyrexia, diaphoresis, mydriasis, delusions, seizures. Hypotension and arrhythmias may also occur.
Common causes	Cocaine, amphetamines, methamphetamines, over-the-counter decongestants (phenylpropanolamine, ephedrine, pseudoephedrine), caffeine, and theophylline.
Opiate or sedative	
Signs	Coma, respiratory depression, miosis, hypotension, bradycardia, hypothermia, pulmonary edema, hyporeflexia. Seizures may occur after propoxyphene overdose.
Common causes	Narcotics, barbiturates, benzodiazepines, ethanol, clonidine.

[1]Adapted and reproduced, with permission, from Kulig G: Initial management of ingestion of toxic substances. N Engl J Med 1992;326:1677.

jority of toxins cause coma is via a diffuse encephalopathy, which results in global depression of the CNS.

Pulmonary aspiration of gastric contents and progressive respiratory failure are constant concerns in the comatose patient. The most common cause of death in comatose patients is respiratory arrest, which may occur abruptly. Therefore, protection of the airway, assisted ventilation, and supplemental oxygen are the most important interventions in comatose patients.

When evaluating a comatose patient for possible poisoning, it is important to look carefully for other serious conditions that cause coma, including intracranial trauma, hypoglycemia, hypothermia, meningitis, and encephalitis.

Cardiac Arrhythmias

A full 12-lead electrocardiogram (ECG) should be part of the initial evaluation in all patients with suspected toxic ingestion. Sinus tachycardia is a nonspecific finding in a variety of poisonings and is usually not helpful in identifying a specific toxin. Drugs with characteristic ECG find-

Table 10–15. Drugs associated with major symptoms at presentation.[1]

Toxic causes of coma	Toxic causes of anion gap acidosis
Antihistamines	
Atropine	Carbon monoxide
Barbiturates	Cyanide
Benzodiazepines	Ethanol
Carbon monoxide	Ethylene glycol
Clonidine	Iron
Cyanide	Isoniazid
Ethanol	Methanol
Narcotics	Salicylates
Organophosphates	**Toxic causes of arrhythmia**
Phenothiazines	β-Blockers
Tricyclic antidepressants	Calcium channel blockers
Toxic causes of seizures	Digoxin
Anticholinergics	Tricyclic antidepressants
Camphor	Amphetamines
Carbon monoxide	Cocaine
Cocaine	Chloral hydrate
Phencyclidine (PCP)	Phenothiazines
Phenothiazines	Theophylline
Propoxyphene	**Toxic causes of gastrointestinal symptoms**
Theophylline	
Tricyclic antidepressants	Arsenic
β-Blockers	Iron
Type Ia antiarrhythmic agents	Lithium
	Mercury
Quinidine	Poisonous mushrooms
Procainamide	
Phenothiazines	

[1]Adapted and reproduced, with permission, from Olson KR, et al: Physical assessment and differential diagnosis of the poisoned patient. Med Toxicol 1987;2:52.

ings are listed in Table 10–15. Treatment depends on the specific rhythm present and the hemodynamic status of the patient. Sinus bradycardia is characteristic of digoxin, β-blockers, and cyanide, or as a reflex response to hypertension induced by α-adrenergic agonists like phenylpropanolamine. Prolonged QT intervals suggest phenothiazines or type Ia antiarrhythmics (quinidine or procainamide). Widened QRS complexes are seen with tricyclic antidepressants and propoxyphene (a synthetic narcotic). Patients with these findings are at risk for the development of life-threatening ventricular arrhythmias.

Metabolic Acidosis

Persistent, unexplained metabolic acidosis may be the only initial clue to a toxic ingestion. Evaluation of metabolic acidosis should include measurement of arterial blood gases, serum electrolyte, BUN, glucose concentrations, and serum osmolality. Calculation of the anion gap can be helpful in the differential diagnosis of metabolic acidosis:

$$\text{Anion gap} = \text{Na (meq/L)} - \text{Cl (meq/L)} - \text{HCO}_3 \text{ (meq/L)}$$
$$\text{(Normal is 8–12 meq/L)}$$

As listed in Table 10–15, poisonings that may lead to an elevated anion gap acidosis include methanol, paraldehyde, iron, ethylene glycol, and salicylates. Likewise, the

calculation of the expected serum osmolality with the following formula:

Calculated serum osmolality =

$$2 \text{ (Na [meq/L])} + \frac{\text{Urea (mg/dL)}}{2.8} + \frac{\text{Glucose (mg/dL)}}{18}$$

can be compared with the measured serum osmolality for the presence of an osmolal gap. A measured osmolality that is more than 10 mOsm greater than the calculated value suggests the presence of osmotically active substances that are not accounted for by the calculation. The family of alcohols including ethanol, methanol, isopropyl alcohol, ethylene glycol, or glycerol can produce an osmolar gap metabolic acidosis, the presence of which can provide a tentative diagnosis pending results of specific toxicologic testing.

Seizures

Like coma, seizures are a feature of many drug and chemical poisonings (Table 10–15). Because poisoning is a relatively uncommon cause of seizures in children, other causes must be considered, including hypoxia, hypoglycemia, hyponatremia, intracranial injury, CNS infections, and febrile seizures. In most cases of drug-induced seizures, immediate identification of the specific toxin is not necessary because the treatment of most toxin-induced seizures is generally similar to that of seizures resulting from other causes. However, seizures caused by toxins are often more difficult to control. Prolonged seizures, with the development of both respiratory and metabolic acidosis, may also aggravate the potential effects of a toxin on the cardiovascular system.

Gastrointestinal Symptoms

Gastrointestinal (GI) symptoms of poisoning include emesis, nausea, abdominal cramps, and diarrhea. These may be because of direct toxic effects on the intestinal mucosa or systemic toxicity subsequent to absorption. A single, self-limited episode of vomiting may accompany almost any ingestion. However, iron, lithium, mercury, arsenic, or poisonous mushrooms characteristically cause severe vomiting, diarrhea, or both (see Table 10–15). GI hemorrhage may also accompany iron ingestion. Persistent vomiting or diarrhea may result in hypovolemia and shock. Therefore, the adequacy of the patient's circulation must be assessed.

LABORATORY EVALUATION

Every patient with a potentially significant poisoning should have some routine laboratory evaluation. Studies that should be considered for all patients include a complete blood count (CBC), serum electrolyte, BUN and glucose concentrations, arterial blood gas, and serum osmolality. As mentioned previously, a 12-lead ECG can reveal arrhythmias or conduction delays that may aid in diagnosis or management. A chest radiograph looking for evidence of aspiration or noncardiogenic pulmonary edema may help to guide management. A plain radiograph of the abdomen may reveal radiopaque pills (eg, iron, chloral hydrate, some phenothiazines, and heavy metals).

A differential diagnosis can usually be constructed on the basis of the history, physical examination, and some routine laboratory tests. Even though the majority of drugs and chemicals commonly ingested today can be measured in serum, urine, or gastric aspirates, the routine toxicology screen is of minimal value in the initial care of the poisoned patient in the emergency department. Toxicology screening is expensive, time-consuming, and subject to false-positive and false-negative results. On the other hand, specific quantitative levels of certain drugs may be useful in determining the need for a specific intervention or antidote. Specific drug levels are most useful when the patient has ingested an overdose of acetaminophen, salicylates, anticonvulsants, digoxin, ethanol, iron, or theophylline. The use of toxicologic screening should be reserved for patients with signs of major toxicity with an unknown substance and for those cases in which there is direct communication with the laboratory about the suspected agents. Many hospitals now use abbreviated qualitative screening of urine for common drugs of abuse as an alternative to comprehensive toxicologic screening.

MANAGEMENT

Initial management of seriously poisoned patients is similar to that of other critically ill patients. An approach to the management of poisoned patients is outlined in Table 10–16. General supportive management according to the principles of BLS and ALS should always be initiated. Priority is given to ensuring a patent airway, adequate ventilation, and the administration of oxygen. If altered mental status or the threat of seizures or life-threatening cardiac arrhythmias is present, endotracheal intubation and mechanical ventilation may be required. Placement of at least one, and preferably two, IV catheters is indicated in all potentially significant poisonings. Hemodynamic instability should be managed promptly with bolus infusions of normal saline as needed to improve peripheral perfusion and to stabilize the vital signs. The evaluation of a bedside test for blood glucose and the administration of dextrose (0.5–1 g/kg intravenously) for hypoglycemia is the next priority. A rapid assessment of the patient's neurologic examination should be performed with attention to the level of consciousness and the pupillary light reflexes. Patients with depressed levels of consciousness should receive 2 mg of naloxone (Narcan) regardless of their age or size. Repeated doses may be required to reverse the effects of some synthetic narcotics such as propoxyphene or dextromethorphan.

Toxin-induced seizures can be difficult to control. In general, diazepam or lorazepam can be administered ini-

Table 10–16. Initial approach to the management of a poisoned patient.[1]

A	Airway	Positioning
		Suctioning
		Consider endotracheal intubation
B	Breathing	Oxygen
		Assisted ventilation
C	Circulation	Establish intravenous access
		Fluid boluses (20 mL/kg) as needed
D	1. Dextrose	Check bedside glucose
		Administer dextrose (0.5 g/kg as needed)
	2. Disability	Assess level of consciousness, consider naloxone
		Pupillary examination
		Treat seizures with benzodiazepines and phenytoin if necessary
	3. Decontamination	Irrigation of affected skin or eyes
		Induced emesis
		Gastric lavage
		Activated charcoal
		Whole-bowel irrigation

[1]See text for specific recommendations regarding poison management.

tially with consideration for subsequent use of phenytoin (Dilantin) if further seizures are noted. Seizures caused by toxin-induced hypoglycemia must be recognized and treated promptly with dextrose.

Decontamination should begin as soon as possible after initial stabilization to limit the systemic absorption of the toxin from the skin or GI tract. For respiratory exposure, removal of the patient from the toxic environment is usually all that is necessary, with careful observation for latent pulmonary effects of the toxin. If a patient's skin or eyes have been exposed to an irritating or corrosive substance, the affected areas should be irrigated with copious amounts of water after contaminated clothing is removed.

GI decontamination of ingested toxins can be accomplished through a variety of means. Considerable controversy exists as to the efficacy and appropriateness of the primary methods of removing a toxin from the GI tract. Options include induced emesis, gastric lavage, the use of activated charcoal, and, most recently, whole-bowel irrigation.

Emesis

Emesis may occur spontaneously after the ingestion of many substances. If spontaneous emesis has not occurred or has resulted in the evacuation of only a small amount of the ingested agent, the induction of emesis may be considered. Induced emesis can be effective when performed within 30–60 minutes of an ingestion. It is typically used at home by a parent after phone consultation with a physician or Regional Poison Control Center. Syrup of ipecac is the method of choice for inducing emesis. The following doses should be used depending on the child's age: 6–12 months, 10 mL; 1–10 years, 15 mL; older than 10 years, 30 mL. More than 90% of patients vomit within 20–30 minutes after a single dose of ipecac. Emesis is contraindicated in the following situations: if the patient has a decreased level of consciousness; if the toxin may abruptly lead to seizures or coma; after ingestion of a caustic agent; after ingestion of some hydrocarbons; and in children younger than 6 months.

The amount of gastric contents recovered by ipecac-induced emesis is highly variable and generally less than 50%. Because efficacy decreases substantially with longer delays after an ingestion, and because protracted emesis delays the institution of further GI decontamination, the use of ipecac in the emergency department has fallen out of favor.

Like induced emesis, the efficacy of **gastric lavage** is highly variable and dependent on its institution within 1–2 hours after the ingestion. Its role may be limited to patients who arrive in the emergency department soon after a potentially life-threatening ingestion. In particular, if the patient is comatose or seizing and tracheal intubation is being considered for airway protection, gastric lavage can be performed after securing the artificial airway. To carry out the most effective lavage, a large-bore orogastric tube should be inserted. After confirming its location in the stomach, aliquots of normal saline are used until the return is clear. Potential complications of gastric lavage include mechanical injury to the airway, esophagus, or stomach and an increased risk of aspiration pneumonia.

Because neither induced emesis nor gastric lavage completely removes an ingested substance, the administration of **activated charcoal,** either with or without initial gastric emptying, is recommended in most cases of poisoning. Activated charcoal functions by binding a wide variety of drugs and chemicals, preventing their subsequent absorption from the GI tract. The dose of activated charcoal is 1 g/kg given either orally or via a nasogastric tube. Like the gastric-emptying procedures, it is most effective when given as soon as possible after the ingestion. Activated charcoal has been demonstrated to act as a reservoir to adsorb some drugs directly from the blood perfusing the GI tract in a process referred to as GI dialysis. Repeated doses of charcoal may benefit children who have ingested drugs that undergo enterohepatic circulation or active secretion into the intestinal lumen.

Gastric-emptying procedures (emesis or lavage) before the use of activated charcoal have not been demonstrated consistently to provide any additional benefit. Therefore, most authorities recognize activated charcoal as the decontamination procedure of choice in the majority of pediatric poisonings, provided the ingested agent is known to be adsorbed by charcoal. Activated charcoal does not bind well to a few notable substances (Table 10–17).

Several charcoal preparations are packaged in a slurry with 70% sorbitol. Repeated doses of the charcoal-sorbitol combination may result in significant diarrhea with fluid and electrolyte losses. In contrast, activated charcoal alone may cause constipation. If repeated doses of charcoal are to be administered, it is preferable to alternate between preparations with and without sorbitol, titrating the

Table 10–17. Substances not effectively bound by activated charcoal.

Acids	Hydrocarbons
Alcohols	Iron
Alkali	Lead
Cyanide	Lithium

relative amounts of each to achieve the desired effect without unwarranted side effects.

Whole-Bowel Irrigation

Whole-bowel irrigation (WBI) describes the technique of administering large volumes of a polyethylene glycol electrolyte lavage solution into the GI tract to produce diarrhea. It effectively prevents the absorption of potential toxins by mechanically flushing the agent out of the GI tract. WBI has been used extensively as a bowel preparation before surgery or colonoscopy. It has recently gained attention in the management of poisonings in the following situations: (1) ingestion of a drug that is not adsorbed by charcoal (eg, iron); (2) late presentation after ingestion because the drug may have entered the small intestine, rendering it unavailable for charcoal binding; or (3) ingestion of very large amounts of a substance that may result in persistently toxic amounts of drug even after other initial decontamination procedures.

The solution is delivered either orally or through a nasogastric tube at a rate of 0.5 L/h for children up to 5 years of age and 2 L/h for adolescents and adults. The procedure should be continued until the rectal effluent clears, typically in 6–12 hours. The most common adverse effects of the procedure are nausea or vomiting. Contraindications to the use of WBI include evidence of major GI dysfunction, such as ileus, obstruction, perforation, or severe GI hemorrhage.

ANTIDOTAL THERAPY

The number of ingestions for which a specific antidote is necessary or available is small. With rare exceptions, stabilization of the patient through general supportive care takes precedence over trying to determine which, if any, antidote should be given. The antidotes most commonly used within the first hour of management are listed in Table 10–18. Some of the antidotes may be harmful if used inappropriately, as when multiple drugs have been ingested, resulting in a confusing clinical picture. Even when available, antidotes do not diminish the need for meticulous supportive care with primary attention directed to the support of the patient's vital functions.

PREVENTION

Poison prevention strategies have resulted in lower morbidity and mortality from poisoning in children. Edu-

[handwritten margin notes:]
Lead
Iron
Arsenic/Mercury
cyanide
Heparin
MetHgb

EDTA
deferoxamine
dimercaprol (BAL)
Lilly cyanide kit
Protamine
methylene blue

Table 10–18. Antidotes commonly used in the first hour of management after an overdose.[1]

Toxin	Antidote
Opiates	Naloxone
Methanol, ethylene glycol	Ethanol
Anticholinergics	Physostigmine *(Antilirium)*
Organophosphate or carbamate insecticides	Atropine *or pralidoxime (Protopam)*
β-blockers	Glucagon
Tricyclic antidepressants	Bicarbonate
Digitalis	Digoxin-specific antibody fragments *Digoxin Fab*
Benzodiazepines	Flumazenil
Calcium channel blockers	Calcium

[1]Adapted and reproduced, with permission, from Kulig G: Initial management of ingestion of toxic substances. N Engl J Med 1992;326:1677.

cational activities in the form of anticipatory guidance by the pediatrician can be effective when continually reinforced. These efforts can be aimed both at the parents and, in a developmentally appropriate way, at the child. "Poison-proofing" the environment by storing potentially poisonous household products and medications in proper containers and in places inaccessible to curious toddlers should be expected of every family. One of the most effective methods of prevention from accidental poisoning was the introduction of child-resistant packaging through the Poison Prevention Packaging Act of 1970. Child-resistant closures have significantly reduced the morbidity and mortality from poisoning in children younger than 6 years of age.

ACETAMINOPHEN

Acetaminophen is one of the most widely used analgesics and antipyretics; it is among the most common medications involved in overdose in children. In therapeutic doses, acetaminophen has few side effects; however, toxic doses may be associated with hepatic necrosis and, rarely, renal failure.

Acetaminophen is absorbed rapidly after an oral dose, reaching a peak plasma level within 30–60 minutes. Absorption may be delayed in an overdose, with peak levels occurring up to 4 hours after ingestion. Acetaminophen is metabolized in the liver predominantly by two mechanisms. The vast majority (up to 94%) of the drug is converted to glucuronide or sulfate conjugates, which are then excreted in the urine. Another 4% is metabolized by the cytochrome P-450 mixed-function oxidase system to a toxic intermediate, which is rapidly inactivated by conjugation with glutathione. This pathway is of primary interest in the overdosed patient. A large dose of acetaminophen may deplete the stores of glutathione available to detoxify the intermediate. This highly reactive intermediate may then bind to hepatic macromolecules, producing

a centrilobular hepatic necrosis. The lower incidence of hepatotoxicity in children younger than 6 years may relate to a relatively smaller amount of metabolism via the P-450 pathway. Antidotal therapy for acetaminophen overdose is based on replacement or substitution of glutathione stores to prevent the production of the toxic intermediate.

DIAGNOSIS & CLINICAL PRESENTATION

Evaluation of a patient after a known or suspected acetaminophen overdose should begin with a determination of the amount ingested. The history is notably unreliable in adolescents who have intentionally ingested acetaminophen. All adolescents should be managed as if they ingested a potentially toxic amount, with initial evaluation in an emergency department. For children younger than 6 years of age, if a reliable history indicates ingestion of less than 100 mg/kg, no treatment is required. Most ingestions of 100–140 mg/kg can be managed at home with ipecac-induced emesis. Ingestions of greater than 140 mg/kg are considered potentially toxic, and all children with this or an unknown amount of ingestion should be evaluated in an emergency department.

The clinical course of an acute acetaminophen overdose follows four stages (Table 10–19). Early symptoms, such as coma, seizures, or cardiac arrhythmias, within the first 24 hours are associated with acetaminophen but are likely related to coingestants. A high index of suspicion of acetaminophen ingestion must be maintained, however, so that an acetaminophen level may be determined to guide possible antidotal therapy.

MANAGEMENT

Management of acetaminophen overdose begins with good supportive care followed by GI decontamination. Activated charcoal should be administered to all patients

Table 10–19. Clinical course of acetaminophen overdose.

Stage 1	12–24 h after ingestion
	Nausea, vomiting, diaphoresis, anorexia
Stage 2	24–48 h after ingestion
	Clinically asymptomatic
	ALT (SGPT), AST (SGOT), bilirubin, and PT begin to rise
Stage 3	72–96 h after ingestion
	In patients who are untreated or treated late:
	Peak hepatotoxicity (AST [SGOT] > 1000 IU/L)
Stage 4	7–8 days after ingestion
	Recovery

ALT (SGPT) = alanine aminotransferase (serum glutamic pyruvic transaminase); AST (SGOT) = aspartate aminotransferase (serum glutamic oxaloacetic transaminase); PT = prothrombin time.

with an intentional or significant accidental overdose to prevent the occurrence of a potentially toxic acetaminophen level. This is also useful in case there are significant coingestants, which may also be bound to charcoal. A specific serum acetaminophen level should be obtained no sooner than 4 hours after ingestion. This level is then plotted on the Rumack-Matthew nomogram (Figure 10–3) to predict the likelihood of hepatic injury. Baseline alanine aminotransferase (serum glutamic pyruvic transaminase (ALT [SGPT]) and aspartate aminotransferase (serum glutamic oxaloacetic transaminase (AST [SGOT]), bilirubin and glucose concentrations, and prothrombin time are also indicated in significant ingestions.

If the 4-hour acetaminophen level is on or above the nomogram line, indicating possible hepatotoxicity, specific antidotal therapy with oral *N*-acetylcysteine (NAC) is indicated. Because NAC is adsorbed to activated charcoal, its use in patients who have received charcoal has been the subject of recent controversy. Current recommendations are either to wait 2 hours after a dose of charcoal before administering NAC, or to increase the dose of NAC by 40% to account for part of it being bound by the charcoal. NAC increases glutathione synthesis and, as a glutathione substitute, inactivates the toxic acetaminophen metabolite. Its efficacy has been proved when given within the first 16 hours after an acute ingestion. NAC has maximum efficacy when given within 8 hours of inges-

tion, when it is protective against hepatotoxicity regardless of the initial plasma acetaminophen level. However, it should be used even up to 24 hours after an ingestion and can be stopped if the acetaminophen level is subsequently found to be nontoxic according to the nomogram.

With prompt recognition of patients at risk of acetaminophen toxicity, good supportive care, and timely institution of antidotal therapy with NAC, outcome should be excellent with little risk of severe hepatic necrosis.

TRICYCLIC ANTIDEPRESSANTS

Tricyclic antidepressants are among the most widely prescribed drugs in the United States. They are used not only in the treatment of depression, but also for enuresis, hyperkinesis, sleep disorders, and a number of atypical pain syndromes, such as trigeminal neuralgia. Tricyclic antidepressants have the highest case-fatality ratio of any class of drugs and consistently are a leading cause of death from poisoning.

Tricyclic antidepressants have a variety of pharmacologic effects, four of which are of primary concern with overdose. These effects include blockage of reuptake of norepinephrine and serotonin at presynaptic sites in the CNS (the primary mechanism for their antidepressant effects), anticholinergic effects, membrane depressant or "quinidine-like" effects on the myocardium, and α-adrenergic receptor blockade. These four effects may result in a characteristic "toxic syndrome" of signs and symptoms, as listed in Table 10–20.

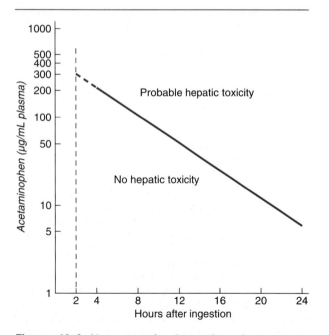

Figure 10–3. Nomogram for interpreting plasma acetaminophen showing semilogarithmic plot of plasma acetaminophen concentrations versus time. (Adapted and reproduced, with permission, from Rumack BH, Matthew H: Pediatrics 1975;55:873.)

Table 10–20. Signs and symptoms of tricyclic poisoning by their mechanism of action.

Blockage of reuptake of nor- epinephrine and serotonin in the central nervous system Central nervous system agitation followed by de- pression Coma	"Quinidine-like" effects Widened QRS com- plexes Prolonged PR, QT$_c$ inter- vals Second- or third-degree atrioventricular block Atrial and ventricular ar- rhythmias Hypotension
Anticholinergic effects Seizures Coma Tachycardia Warm, flushed skin Dry skin and mucous membranes Dilated pupils Decreased or absent bowel sounds Urinary retention	**Peripheral α-adrenergic receptor blockade** Hypotension

DIAGNOSIS & CLINICAL PRESENTATION

The tricyclic antidepressants are generally well absorbed from the GI tract. With acute overdose, however, absorption is unpredictable because of the anticholinergic effects on GI motility. Onset of life-threatening symptoms may be abrupt, usually within 6 hours of the overdose. Tricyclic overdose should be suspected in any patient who presents with seizures, coma, cardiac arrhythmia, or signs of anticholinergic poisoning. Primary attention must be paid to the patient's vital signs and level of consciousness. After this, the physical examination should specifically seek to identify signs of anticholinergic effects, such as dry skin or mucous membranes, dilated pupils, flushing, decreased or absent bowel sounds, and urinary retention. Most of the important effects of tricyclics are on the cardiovascular system and CNS.

The most common causes of death in fatal tricyclic overdoses are hypotension and cardiac arrhythmias. Hypotension can occur secondary to direct myocardial depression, an arrhythmia, or from peripheral α-adrenergic receptor blockade. The "quinidine-like" effects of tricyclics on the cardiac conduction system may result in a widened QRS complex (> 100 msec), which is the best clinical predictor of the severity of a tricyclic poisoning. Patients with a widened QRS complex are at increased risk for the development of life-threatening ventricular arrhythmias and sudden death.

CNS effects are usually prominent in tricyclic overdose. An initial phase of agitation or excitement is followed by sedation, which may progress to coma or seizures. Seizures occur in 10–20% of patients, usually after the onset of coma.

MANAGEMENT

As with all critically ill patients, initial priorities in management should focus on the patient's ABCs. Because the onset of coma, seizures, or significant cardiac arrhythmias may be abrupt, a decision to protect the airway with endotracheal intubation must be made early in the assessment of the severity of the ingestion.

Continued monitoring of the patient's respiratory, cardiovascular, and neurologic status is essential. Respiratory failure can occur from CNS depression, seizures, upper airway obstruction, or pulmonary aspiration. Hypoxia and acidosis aggravate the effects of tricyclics on the cardiovascular system and must be treated aggressively.

As soon as the patient's vital functions are stabilized, efforts at GI decontamination are begun. Even in the home setting, induced emesis with syrup of ipecac is contraindicated because of the potential for seizures or an abrupt deterioration in the patient's level of consciousness. Gastric lavage with a large-bore orogastric tube is ideally performed after protection of the airway with an endotracheal tube. Activated charcoal therapy effectively binds tricyclic antidepressants and should be instituted as soon as possible.

Seizures induced by tricyclics are treated with IV diazepam. Recurrent seizures can be managed by loading the patient with a longer-acting anticonvulsant, such as phenobarbital or phenytoin.

Cardiac conduction abnormalities (prolonged QRS, bradyarrhythmias) are treated by producing an alkalemia (pH 7.4–7.5) with either hyperventilation or the use of bicarbonate. When this fails to prevent the onset of malignant ventricular arrhythmias, lidocaine, phenytoin, or ventricular pacing can be tried. Hypotension is initially managed with bolus infusions of isotonic saline (20 mL/kg). If there is no response to repeated fluid boluses, pressor agents should be used.

As soon as possible, all symptomatic patients should be transferred to an ICU for continued monitoring and supportive care. Signs of toxicity usually resolve within 24–36 hours.

IRON

Accidental iron poisoning is among the more common serious ingestions in children younger than 6 years of age. Factors contributing to the incidence of iron poisoning include its widespread availability as well as the fact that most people do not consider iron potentially dangerous. A typical scenario of acute iron poisoning involves a toddler who ingests his mother's iron supplement during or just after her new pregnancy.

The toxicity of iron stems from both direct corrosive effects on the GI mucosa, as well as systemic effects related to the presence of free iron in the circulation. Systemic toxicity may include cardiovascular, metabolic, and CNS derangements, and, infrequently, hepatic failure.

DIAGNOSIS & CLINICAL PRESENTATION

The severity of acute iron poisoning should be assessed by estimating the amount of elemental iron ingested. Different iron preparations have different concentrations of elemental iron; therefore, the exact name of the preparation, as well as the estimated number of tablets ingested, is necessary to make the best determination.

Ingestion of less than 40 mg/kg of elemental iron is considered nontoxic; these children can usually be managed safely at home. Accidental ingestions of more than 40 mg/kg, as well as all intentional ingestions, should be evaluated in an emergency department. A proposed strategy for the evaluation and management of iron ingestions is presented in Figure 10–4. As with the evaluation of any potentially ill child, initial emphasis is placed on the overall appearance of the child, the level of consciousness, and

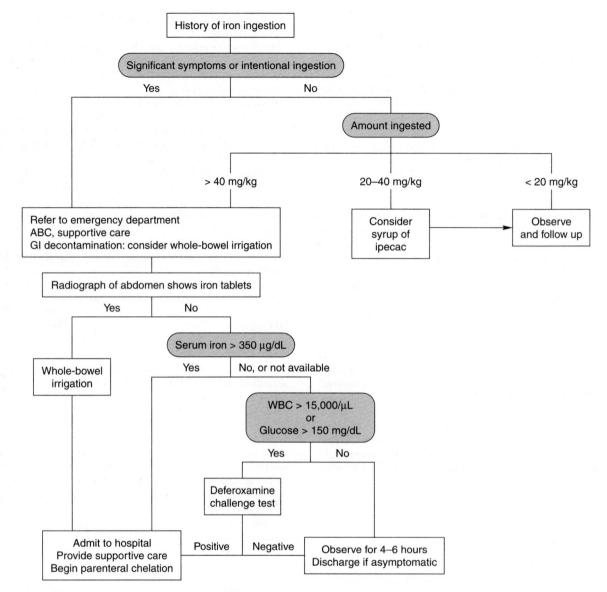

Figure 10–4. Algorithm showing a proposed strategy for the evaluation and management of iron ingestions. ABC = airway, breathing, and circulation; GI = gastrointestinal; WBC = white blood count.

the vital signs. Significant vomiting, diarrhea, or GI hemorrhage may result in hypovolemia. Therefore, the adequacy of the patient's circulation should be monitored continuously, with institution of fluid replacement as indicated. Laboratory evaluation after a potentially serious iron ingestion should include a determination of blood glucose and electrolyte concentrations and a CBC. An arterial blood gas, blood type, and cross-match may be indicated in patients who manifest signs of serious toxicity. Because many iron preparations are radiopaque, an abdominal roentgenogram is an easy, noninvasive way of es-

timating the potential for toxicity. The presence of visible iron tablets on an abdominal roentgenogram correlates with more serious symptoms and may guide management decisions about further GI decontamination.

Determination of a serum iron concentration 2–4 hours after an acute iron ingestion provides the most reliable laboratory evidence of the severity of an ingestion. If serum iron levels are not available on an emergency basis, clinical assessment coupled with some simple laboratory tests can be used to assess the severity of an ingestion. Patients with protracted vomiting or diarrhea for 6 hours, a serum glucose level greater than 150 mg/dL, or a white blood cell count greater than 15,000/μL, coupled with the presence of radiopaque tablets on a plain roentgenogram of the abdomen, all correlate highly with toxic serum iron levels. A "challenge" dose of deferoxamine, 50 mg/kg given intramuscularly, will chelate any free unbound iron in the circulation, producing a characteristic reddish-brown *vin rose* appearance of the patient's urine. This signifies the need for further chelation.

The clinical effects of acute iron poisoning have been classically divided into four phases (Table 10–21). **Phase 1,** which occurs up to 6 hours after an acute ingestion, represents the direct corrosive effects of iron on the GI tract. Most patients with mild to moderate ingestions do not progress beyond this phase. **Phase 2,** classically described as lasting 6–24 hours after ingestion, is characterized by recovery from GI symptoms. This phase may be transient or completely missed in severe iron poisonings that progress rapidly to phase 3. **Phase 3,** which occurs up to 48 hours after ingestion, is characterized by recurrence of GI symptoms and the onset of metabolic acidosis, severe lethargy or coma, and cardiovascular collapse. Circulating free iron is a potent vasodilator and may also increase capillary permeability, resulting in hypovolemia and the development of shock. Iron-induced mitochondrial dysfunction interferes with the normal mechanisms of cellular respiration, resulting in the development of metabolic acidosis. The development of jaundice, hypoglycemia, and coagulopathy secondary to hepatic damage may also occur during this phase. Finally, **phase 4,** which occurs 4–6 weeks after ingestion, is usually seen only after a severe poisoning with marked early GI corrosive effects, resulting in the development of pyloric or small-bowel strictures. Children typically present with symptoms of GI obstruction.

MANAGEMENT

As outlined in Figure 10–4, management of serious iron ingestions begins with good supportive care. Once vital signs have been stabilized, attention is turned to efforts at GI decontamination. Because iron is not bound to activated charcoal, GI decontamination can be complicated. If the patient is seen soon after the ingestion, an attempt at gastric lavage should be made via a large-bore orogastric or nasogastric tube. If radiopaque material is seen on a postlavage abdominal roentgenogram, or if the patient exhibits signs of moderate to severe toxicity, WBI may be attempted. WBI has been demonstrated to remove iron tablets safely and effectively from the GI tract, thereby preventing further absorption.

When the patient has been stabilized and GI decontamination has been instituted, a decision must be made concerning the use of the specific chelator, deferoxamine. A serum iron concentration, available within the stabilization phase of management, provides the most reliable method to indicate the need for specific chelation therapy. Serum iron concentrations of 150–350 μg/dL may produce mild phase 1 symptoms but usually do not produce systemic toxicity requiring chelation. Concentrations greater than 350 μg/dL signify the appearance of free iron in the circulation, necessitating a short course of chelation. Concentrations greater than 500 μg/dL are associated with signs of serious systemic toxicity, necessitating aggressive efforts at GI decontamination, general supportive care, and specific chelation.

Upon chelation with iron, the deferoxamine-iron complex is excreted in the urine. Deferoxamine can be given either by intermittent IM injection or by continuous IV infusion at a rate of 10–15 mg/kg/h.

The vast majority of children with iron poisoning survive without significant sequelae. Fatality is correlated with the early onset of coma or shock. Both good supportive care and specific chelation therapy are required to improve the outcome of seriously poisoned patients.

ETHANOL

Ethanol is widely available in a variety of beverages, as well as in a large number of other products, including decongestants, cough medicines, mouthwashes, perfumes, and colognes. The American Association of Poison Control Centers reported more than 7000 cases of ethanol exposure in the pediatric age group in 1994. One quarter of all ethanol exposures in children are from nonbeverage sources of ethanol, some of which contain ethanol concentrations as high as 80%. Among exposures in all age groups, ethanol, either alone or in combination with other substances, was involved in almost 10% of all poisoning fatalities.

Ethanol is rapidly absorbed from the GI tract; peak blood concentrations are reached within 1 hour of ingestion. Ethanol is metabolized primarily in the liver by the hepatic enzyme alcohol dehydrogenase. In spite of the fact that this enzyme does not reach adult levels in children

Table 10–21. Clinical phases of acute iron poisoning.

Phase 1	0–6 h after ingestion
	Nausea, vomiting, hematemesis, diarrhea, melena, abdominal pain
	Lethargy or coma in severe ingestions
	Tachycardia
	Hyperglycemia, leukocytosis
Phase 2	6–24 h after ingestion
	Resolution of gastrointestinal symptoms
	Intermittent lethargy
Phase 3	12–48 h after ingestion
	Recurrence of gastrointestinal symptoms
	Lethargy, coma
	Cyanosis, tachycardia, cardiovascular collapse
	Metabolic acidosis, coagulopathy
Phase 4	4–6 wk after ingestion
	Gastrointestinal scarring and obstruction

until they are 5 years of age, young children metabolize ethanol at a rate twice that of adults. Alcohol dehydrogenase uses nicotinamide adenine dinucleotide (NAD) as a cofactor, resulting in increased levels of reduced nicotinamide adenine dinucleotide (NADH). The increased hepatic cell NADH-NAD ratio inhibits gluconeogenesis. Children younger than 7 years of age who have limited glycogen stores may become hypoglycemic after an ethanol ingestion because of the inhibition of gluconeogenesis. This hypoglycemia, as well as the global depressant effects of ethanol on the nervous system, account for the major mechanisms of ethanol toxicity.

DIAGNOSIS & CLINICAL PRESENTATION

Ethanol poisoning should be considered in any child presenting with the acute onset of seizures or altered mental status. Information obtained from the history should include not only the availability of alcoholic beverages, but also access to mouthwash, perfumes, and over-the-counter liquid cough or cold medications. The physical examination is directed toward a rapid assessment of the patient's ABCs and level of consciousness, as outlined in the section on Diagnosis and Assessment of the poisoned patient. Laboratory evaluation of patients with known or suspected ethanol ingestion should include a rapid evaluation of blood glucose concentration in addition to a blood ethanol level, serum electrolyte and BUN concentrations, and osmolality. Significant ethanol poisoning may result in metabolic acidosis, primarily because of the increased production of lactic acid. A characteristic anion gap and osmolal gap metabolic acidosis is often the first clue to ethanol poisoning in a child with no history of ingestion.

The initial clinical effects of acute ethanol ingestion include nausea and vomiting because of direct gastric irritation. A characteristic odor may be detected on the patient's breath. Early CNS effects include emotional lability, mild ataxia, muscular incoordination, and decreased reaction time. Severe ethanol intoxication may result in coma, hypothermia, respiratory failure, and, rarely, shock. The severity of systemic symptoms and signs correlates with the blood ethanol concentration (Table 10–22). Hypoglycemia, which may be present at blood ethanol concentrations less than 100 mg/dL, may result in lethargy, coma, or convulsions.

MANAGEMENT

The initial priority in management of known or suspected significant ethanol ingestion is the rapid evaluation and management of the patient's airway and breathing. As soon as possible, a rapid bedside test of a blood glucose concentration should be performed to determine the presence of hypoglycemia. Patients with documented or symptomatic hypoglycemia should be given 0.5 g/kg of dextrose (2 mL/kg D25W) followed by a dextrose-containing continuous IV infusion, with frequent monitoring of the blood glucose level. If hypoglycemia is not recognized and treated in a timely fashion, significant illness or death may result despite peak ethanol concentrations in a range not typically considered dangerous.

Efforts at GI decontamination are usually of limited value. Because ethanol is rapidly absorbed from the stomach and produces alteration of mental status relatively quickly, ipecac-induced emesis and gastric lavage are usually not used if there is a delay in seeking medical attention. Ethanol is not significantly bound to activated charcoal. Unless there is a known or suspected history of coingestion with other substances adsorbed by charcoal, it too, is of little value.

Any child with hypoglycemia or significant alteration in mental status should be admitted to the hospital for prolonged observation until awake enough to eat and drink. Good general supportive care is usually all that is required in the management of mild to moderate ethanol intoxications. Hemodialysis removes ethanol from the body and may be considered in patients with blood ethanol concentrations greater than 500 mg/dL who are deteriorating despite good supportive care.

CAUSTIC AGENTS

Cleaning products are the second leading category of substances (after cosmetics and personal care items) involved in poisonings in children younger than 6 years of age. Many of these cleaning products (eg, bleaches and detergents) contain caustic agents that are available in both crystalline and liquid forms. In many households, they are frequently stored in inappropriate containers without child-resistant seals, giving them an attractive appearance for inquisitive toddlers.

Caustic agents include both acids and alkalis. Their mechanism of toxicity stems from their potential to produce tissue damage on contact. Acids account for approximately 15% of caustic ingestions in children. They produce tissue damage by coagulation necrosis, a process that

Table 10–22. Correlation of clinical effects to blood ethanol levels.

Ethanol Concentration (mg/dL)	Common Signs and Symptoms
< 25	Usually asymptomatic
25–100	Mild behavioral changes
100–150	Mild incoordination, slowed reactions, visual impairment
150–300	Moderate incoordination, slurred speech
300–500	Severe incoordination, stupor
> 500	Coma, depressed respirations, potentially lethal

usually limits the penetration of the acid into deeper tissue levels. In contrast, alkalis, which are responsible for most significant caustic ingestions in children, produce a liquefaction necrosis. They can penetrate tissues, producing further extensive damage. The extent of injury is dependent on the pH of the substance (serious damage is seen with pH > 12.5), its concentration, and the amount of time it is in contact with the tissue.

All corrosive acids and alkalis produce inflammation on contact with the skin or mucous membranes. Because acidic solutions are bitter-tasting and cause immediate pain on contact, their exposure is usually limited by the patient unless the ingestion is intentional. In contrast, alkaline solutions are often tasteless and odorless, and large quantities can be ingested before the onset of pain. Granular agents are more likely to cause focal injuries to the oropharynx and proximal esophagus, whereas liquid agents typically can produce extensive, continuous damage throughout the entire length of the esophagus and into the stomach.

DIAGNOSIS & CLINICAL PRESENTATION

Information obtained from the history should include the specific product name, approximate amount ingested, time of ingestion, and the presence and onset of any symptoms before arrival in the emergency department. Common initial signs and symptoms after a caustic ingestion include drooling, vomiting, stridor, or, in older patients, dysphagia. Nausea, abdominal pain, and abdominal tenderness may also be seen. Physical examination may reveal erythema of the mucous membranes of the mouth, lips, and perioral skin. Erythema may also be seen in characteristic patterns on the trunk from drooling with contaminated saliva. Oropharyngeal ulcerations, edema, or grayish-white membranes on the mucosa may also be seen. The presence or absence of oropharyngeal findings does not reliably predict the presence or extent of esophageal injury. Up to one third of children with significant esophageal or gastric burns have no oropharyngeal burns.

MANAGEMENT

As with all other potentially serious poisonings, management should begin with an evaluation of the patient's ABCs. Of note, the presence of stridor suggests the presence of significant laryngeal edema, and strict attention should be paid to the continued patency of the patient's airway. Efforts at decontamination should include irrigation of the eyes or skin if continued contact with the corrosive substance is suspected. Ipecac-induced emesis is contraindicated with caustic substances so as to limit their contact with the esophagus and oropharynx. Benefits of gastric lavage have not been clearly demonstrated, and the risk of further injury to a damaged esophagus usually pre-

cludes its use after caustic ingestions. Patients should be admitted to the hospital for further management. Appropriate supportive care includes withholding oral feedings, judicious use of parenteral nutrition, and careful observation for the development of complications, such as hemorrhage, perforation, or sepsis.

Significant esophageal or gastric burns are the most feared complication of caustic ingestions. Therefore, most physicians agree that esophagoscopy is indicated in the evaluation of any patient after a significant caustic ingestion. As mentioned previously, the absence of oropharyngeal lesions cannot reliably exclude the presence of esophageal burns. The presence of fewer than two serious signs or symptoms (vomiting, drooling, or stridor) has been correlated with the absence of esophageal injury. However, esophagoscopy is still recommended in the evaluation of caustic ingestions.

Of even greater controversy is the management of significant esophageal burns after they are diagnosed. The greatest area of controversy involves the early use of steroids to prevent extensive inflammation with subsequent stricture formation. A recent long-term prospective evaluation of the use of steroids after caustic injury to the esophagus demonstrated no benefit from steroids in the prevention of stricture formation. The severity of the initial burn was highly predictive of the development of strictures, regardless of whether steroids were used.

As soon as the child is able to swallow, liquids should be provided by mouth. Parenteral nutrition may be required if the child cannot eat after an extensive injury. Patients with second-degree (limited to the mucosa) or third-degree (deep ulceration into the muscle) burns of the esophagus should be reevaluated by esophagoscopy 2–3 weeks after the initial injury for the development of strictures. Barium swallow radiographs can also be used to diagnose the presence of strictures. The treatment of strictures includes repeated mechanical dilations, placement of stents to limit the extent of scarring, or, in severe cases, replacement of a segment of esophagus with a colonic or jejunal interposition.

CHILD ABUSE & NEGLECT

The syndrome of child abuse was first formally described by radiologist Dr. John Caffey in 1940. He noted a group of children with fractures as well as subdural hematomas. In 1962, Henry Kemp coined the term **battered child syndrome** to describe children who were beaten by their parents or parental figures. Then, in 1963, Fontana discussed the **maltreatment syndrome in children,** which introduced the concept that besides physical abuse, children can be emotionally abused or neglected by depriving them of food, clothing, or medical attention or by leaving them alone and unsupervised.

Child abuse has been defined as any interaction, or lack of interaction, between family members that results in nonaccidental harm to the child's physical or developmental well-being. This includes actions that result in obvious bruises, lacerations, or fractures, as well as more unusual forms of abuse, such as intentional poisonings, hypernatremic dehydration because of water deprivation, and subarachnoid hemorrhage from vigorous shaking of infants. Child neglect encompasses a spectrum of parental omissions, including starvation, abandonment, and improper care. A particularly serious form of neglect involves prolonged emotional deprivation of a child by a parent. This may involve failure to meet the emotional needs of a child or constant criticism, and it can result in poor growth of the child, or **failure to thrive.**

Child abuse differs from ordinary punishment; all parents discipline their children, and some use corporal punishment, despite the fact that it may not be the most effective way to change behavior. However, even corporal punishment is not considered child abuse unless significant force is used, resulting in injury to the child. Legally, the child has been abused if discipline results in injury. Unfortunately, many parents believe they can discipline their child by any means they choose.

Child abuse is common in the United States. It is estimated that each year more than 1 million children are physically abused, and 1000 deaths result.

The most severe physical injuries are inflicted on children younger than 6 years because they are less able to flee or defend themselves. Many of these children are more vulnerable or somehow "different" from other siblings; they may be handicapped, chronically ill, or hyperactive or may have had a difficult neonatal course that limited the parents' ability to bond with them. Other high-risk children are twins or siblings of twins, who may be abused because of the stress created by inadequate spacing between children. Likewise, children of an unwanted pregnancy may be at risk because a new burden has been placed on the family.

Child abuse occurs in all countries, races, and socioeconomic groups. The abusive parent may have been abused as a child and is depressed and emotionally immature, with poor impulse control. Some of these parents also have unrealistic expectations for their child's growth and development. For example, a child may be abused because a parent is frustrated that the young toddler is not yet toilet trained. Children of young (teenage) mothers are at increased risk of maltreatment. Undoubtedly, many abuse cases in some way involve the use of illicit drugs by caretakers.

DIAGNOSIS & CLINICAL MANIFESTATIONS

A witness to the abuse may bring the child for medical attention, in which case the diagnosis of child abuse is ob-

vious. Often, however, the physician is presented with an injured child and must determine whether the injury resulted from intentional harm. Although unintentional injuries do happen, the physician must investigate every injury in a child for evidence of abuse.

The history is important in determining the presence of abuse. A history of significant stress in the family should increase one's suspicion about the injury. One should also be concerned if the cause of the injury is unknown, if the caretakers are reluctant to give information, if they change the story of how the injury occurred, or if they seem inappropriately concerned or tardy in bringing the child for care. Abuse should also be considered if the account of how the injury occurred seems incompatible with the child's developmental abilities. For instance, if the caretakers claim the child climbed and fell from a height, the infant must be old enough or adept enough to accomplish this feat. The past history may contribute important information. If the child's records reveal inadequate medical care in the past, eg, the child was never brought for immunizations or has had frequent "accidents" with injuries, one should have increased concerns about the current injury.

Physical examination should be conducted after completely undressing the child. Child abuse must be considered if the injury does not fit the story. For instance, bruises should not appear on both sides of the head if the story describes the child falling only once; a child cannot get linear bruises from falling down steps. Bruises noted to be in different stages of healing suggest recurrent battering rather than a single episode of trauma; Table 10–23 describes the color of skin bruises at various healing stages. However, "dating" of bruises is not an exact science, and the estimated age of the bruise should not be the sole criterion for a diagnosis of child abuse. Injuries that conform to a particular pattern are usually diagnostic of abuse. For instance, loop-shaped bruises are characteristic of an injury inflicted by a belt or a cord. A circumferential burn of the feet and lower legs or buttocks is characteristic of a child forced or dipped into hot water. Children would not voluntarily put their entire leg into a bathtub if the water were scalding hot, and children never get into a tub with both feet at the same time, or with their buttocks first. Injuries to certain anatomic areas often are because of abuse. For instance, the hand is commonly injured as a form of punishment, and genitalia may be injured intentionally out of frustration over toilet training. Likewise, frenulum injuries may result from forcibly stuffing an object like a bottle into an infant's mouth.

Table 10–23. Estimated dating of healing bruises.

Color of Bruise	Days Since Injury
Red	0–1
Bluish-purple	1–4
Greenish-yellow	5–7
Yellowish-brown	> 8

An injury that otherwise does not seem unusual may take on more importance in the face of signs of general neglect, failure to thrive, malnutrition, poor hygiene, or withdrawn personality. Many serious injuries can occur without obvious bruises; thus, abdominal trauma can result in duodenal hematoma or lacerated liver or spleen without external evidence of injury. Similarly, the "shaken baby syndrome" can present without skin bruising. This syndrome deserves special consideration as it is one of the most common causes of death from child abuse. The typical victim is an infant younger than 1 year of age who is violently shaken and, in many cases, thrown against a soft surface such as a bed or carpeted floor. The young infant comes to the emergency department in respiratory distress of sudden onset. The parents usually relate no other history. The baby may be found comatose or may experience seizures. Respiratory arrest may occur in the presence of respiratory distress, yet there is no evidence of upper airway obstruction or lower airway disease. The respiratory distress occurs because of CNS injury, such as a subdural hematoma. Careful physical examination reveals a full fontanelle, and retinal hemorrhages occur in 80–90% of cases. Radiographic imaging of the brain will confirm the injury.

Laboratory tests, including radiographs, are often helpful in confirming the diagnosis of child abuse. Fractures are found frequently in abused infants and young children. Half the skeletal injuries in abused children occur in children younger than 1 year of age, and 90% in children younger than 5 years. Extremities are most commonly fractured, followed by the skull and ribs. Transverse fractures of the diaphysis of long bones are common and are because of direct force against the bone. Spiral or oblique fractures are caused by twisting of the bone. These fractures can occur unintentionally if the foot gets caught between fixed objects and twists as the child falls, but such fractures of the upper extremities are more suspicious. Metaphyseal chip fractures are characteristic of abuse because the forces necessary to produce these are rarely generated by accidental falls in young children. They are caused by vigorous "yanking," or jiggling of extremities left dangling while the child is shaken. Furthermore, skull fractures in young infants should arouse suspicion of abuse; studies have shown that these rarely occur from minor trauma, such as a fall from a bed or down stairs. Also, rib fractures in children younger than 2 years are rarely because of unintentional trauma. Such fractures are because of squeezing the infant's thorax rather than a direct blow, and they cannot occur with chest compressions during resuscitation. Old fractures need an explanation, and multiple fractures, or fractures in various stages of healing, are usually indicative of child abuse.

Because fractures are so common among abused infants, it is recommended that a "skeletal survey" be obtained if abuse is suspected. This survey, which includes radiographs of the chest, skull, and long bones, has the highest yield in infants younger than 2 years; it is rarely worthwhile in children older than 5 years. These radiographs are preferred over a nuclear bone scan, which will not identify metaphyseal fractures or allow determination of the age of the injury. However, a bone scan may help to identify subtle fractures missed by conventional radiography. A computed tomography (CT) scan is important if head injury is suspected or the shaken baby syndrome is considered. Magnetic resonance imaging may be more useful in identifying small intracranial bleeding.

Other conditions should be considered in the differential diagnosis. For instance, platelet disorders and leukemia can lead to unusual bruising. Furthermore, rickets or osteogenesis imperfecta could lead to unusual or unexplained fractures. The history, physical examination, and some laboratory studies or radiographs should distinguish these conditions from abuse.

MANAGEMENT

Once the diagnosis of child abuse is suspected, the physician is responsible for protecting the child. Ideally, a multidisciplinary team of caregivers, including a pediatrician, nurse, psychologist, and social worker, should be available to participate in the child's care. It is often helpful for members of the care-giving team to interview the child in a quiet, nonthreatening setting. It is important to document the history as thoroughly as possible and to record children's exact words if they are old enough to speak. Color photographs of any significant injury are useful, but a good written description of the injury with diagrams will suffice. Hospitalization may be necessary if the injury is serious or if a satisfactory disposition that guarantees the child's safety cannot be arranged. The child should not be sent home to an unsafe environment! Physicians should know how to obtain a court order for custody, if needed, and should know where to refer the child if they are unable to provide necessary care for the child and family. Physicians are obligated to report suspected abuse to the local agency that has responsibility for the child's welfare. This reporting must take place regardless of the time of day and regardless of the physician's relationship with the family or desire to avoid court action. The physician need not be certain, but rather only suspicious of abuse, to file a report. If the injury proves to be unintentional, the physician is protected against legal action related to the report. However, failure to report suspected abuse is considered a misdemeanor and may result in fines, civil suits, loss of license, and possible imprisonment. More importantly, there is a 50% chance of repeated abuse and a 10% chance of fatal injury if children are returned to the abusers without proper precautions.

It is best for the examining physician to confront the caretakers with the suspected diagnosis and the need to report this to local authorities. However, the physician must remain nonjudgmental, not accusatory or punitive. It is not the role of the physician to prove that child abuse occurred or to find out who inflicted the injury. The physician can be helpful in arranging for needed follow-up care, counseling, and psychotherapy for the child and family.

Because all but 5–10% of abused children remain with their families, one goal of treatment must be to prevent further child abuse. Ideally, high-risk situations for potential abuse will be noticed before a child is actually harmed. Thus, many centers have set up telephone hotlines for stressed parents to call for advice or crisis nurseries where children can be left temporarily until parents can work out their problems. Primary care physicians can help by scheduling more frequent visits to the office for families at high risk for abuse and by arranging for available community services. The physician can also help by providing information about child rearing and development so that parents can have realistic expectations. The community needs to provide self-help groups, parent education groups, and early intervention programs for high-risk families.

SEXUAL ABUSE

Sexual abuse is defined as any sexual act performed by an adult with a minor younger than 18 years of age, including indecent exposure, digital manipulation of the genitals, masturbation, fellatio, sodomy, and coitus. Others define sexual abuse as exposure of children to sexual stimulation that is inappropriate for their age, level of psychosocial development, and role in the family.

Because of recent media exposure and parental awareness, reporting of sexual abuse is increasing. It is estimated that more than 300,000, or about 1%, of children are sexually abused each year in the United States.

Girls are six times more likely to be abused than boys. The abuser is usually a family member (35–45%), such as a father, stepfather, uncle, or a trusted friend. Only about 20% are assaulted by strangers, and this usually involves older boys and girls assaulted in the street or other public places.

Sexual abuse is unlike criminal rape in that violence is rarely associated. Usually there is disorganization or stress in the family, such as alcoholism, mental illness, or drug abuse. Abusers usually have weak egos and low self-esteem and are often impotent. They expect failure in adult heterosexual acts and, therefore, seduce children.

The child may become a victim for a variety of reasons. Infants and toddlers cannot verbalize their feelings of fright or confusion and so have no choice but to participate. The young, school-aged child has no concept of real sexuality and does not know to refuse compliance. Also, these young children trust the adult to do nothing wrong. The adult is not hurting the child physically and may instead offer reassurances or bribes. An older child may enjoy the special attention given by the adult, especially if another family member has been physically abusive. Adolescents may pity the adult or feel guilty about reporting the incidents. They may also fear punishment for reporting and are often threatened with harm if they do. When the father is the sexual abuser, the mother may be aware of the abuse but may allow it to continue out of fear of breaking up the family or of imprisonment of the father with loss of financial support for the family.

DIAGNOSIS & CLINICAL MANIFESTATIONS

The diagnosis of sexual abuse depends primarily on the history from the child or caretaker. Some events are witnessed by the adult who brings the child for care, but more often suspicion exists without definite evidence that abuse has taken place. Some children who are sexually abused have behavioral problems, depression, or anger, but it is difficult to relate these problems to sexual abuse in the emergency department setting. Some may have nonspecific complaints of dysuria, vaginal itch, or discharge. Although some young children can be "coached" to say anything (ie, in the midst of a custody battle), the physician should be quite concerned about sexual abuse when young children can vividly describe a sexual incident that they experienced. A child's account of the abuse is the most important factor in determining what occurred. A recent review of criminal court cases found that 75% resulted in conviction, yet only 23% had physical evidence of injury, sexually transmitted disease, or seminal fluid.

The physical examination of a child with suspected sexual abuse usually results in normal findings. Signs of trauma are rare, especially as most cases involve fondling or exposure rather than penetration. Even when penetration has occurred, nonspecific or normal findings are noted in about 40% of cases. The size of the hymenal orifice cannot be used reliably to determine whether abuse has occurred because it can vary with the degree of relaxation at the time of examination, the position of measurement, presence of estrogenization, and age of the child. Instead, genital findings consistent with sexual abuse (acute cases) include bruising, tears, and lacerations of the hymen, perihymen, and posterior fourchette. In chronic cases, the genitalia may show disruption, scarring, and attenuation or loss of hymenal tissue to indicate prior penetrating trauma. Presence of semen or evidence of sexually transmitted disease indicates sexual abuse until proved otherwise. The perianal area may also show evidence of trauma or infection.

MANAGEMENT

The physician plays a key role in diagnosing sexual abuse. A sensitive interview with the child is of the utmost importance; this should be done in a quiet, nonthreatening environment. If the alleged abuse occurred more than 72 hours before medical attention was sought, it is best to manage the case in a relaxed setting outside the emergency department. The interview questions should be open-ended and nonleading and should take into consideration the age and developmental level of the child. Allowing a child to draw or to use anatomic dolls may be helpful if he or she has difficulty verbalizing. The physician must carefully document the questions asked and the child's responses using the child's exact words and adding a description of the child's affect. Next, a gentle physical examination should be performed; this can be done with the child in the frog-leg position on the mother's lap. The child can also be supine on the examining table in the frog-leg position to allow easy visibility of the genitalia. An alternative is the knee-chest position for genital examination. Diagrams and photographs may be helpful to record abnormal findings. Sedation is rarely needed if reassurance is given frequently. An internal pelvic examination is not indicated in prepubertal children. If significant trauma is suspected, examination under general anesthesia may be necessary but is rarely needed.

Some acute infections, such as syphilis or gonorrhea, are almost certainly indicative of sexual abuse; others, such as chlamydiosis, trichomoniasis, herpes simplex virus type 2, and condylomatosis, indicate probable sexual abuse, whereas herpes simplex virus type 1 is possibly related to sexual abuse. It may not be necessary to collect specimens from all children with alleged sexual abuse, but approximately one half of children with sexually transmitted diseases because of abuse have no symptoms at the time of evaluation. Thus, it is prudent to obtain cultures for sexually transmitted diseases if there is significant concern that the child was abused. This includes cultures of the oropharynx for gonorrhea and of the vagina/urethra and rectum for gonorrhea and *Chlamydia*. Rapid tests for *Chlamydia* should not be used, as false-positive results may occur. If a discharge is present, it should be examined for *Trichomonas*. Serology and testing for HIV infection should be considered. A urine pregnancy test should be obtained in the child who is postmenarche. If there was a recent assault, a "rape kit" should be used to collect evidence of the perpetrator's secretions or hair that would likely be found on the victim. This collection includes two saline swabs of the ejaculation site (vagina, rectum, or skin) and two cotton swabs of the throat and gum line if oral-genital contact occurred. Saliva should be obtained from the victim to determine antigen status; the procedure involves placing a sterile 2×2 gauze pad in the victim's mouth and then placing the gauze in a sterile tube. Blood (2–3 mL) must also be obtained from the victim for serologic testing and blood typing. Pubic hairs, if present, should be collected in an envelope, and clothing should be placed in brown paper bags. All evidence must be carefully documented and turned over to police.

Antibiotic therapy for possible sexually transmitted disease can be withheld pending cultures. The alleged abuse must be reported to the local child protective services agency, and the safe disposition of the child must be arranged. The physician should arrange for follow-up evaluation of the child, including counseling for the child and family if needed.

THE INJURED CHILD

Accidents, the leading cause of morbidity and mortality during childhood, account for more than 14 million physician visits, 600,000 hospitalizations, and 22,000 deaths per year. Motor vehicle accidents are the most common cause of death in children. Although the number of deaths caused by motor vehicle accidents in the United States has decreased over the past decade, the incidence of homicide has increased tremendously. Homicide is the second leading cause of death in children younger than 4 years of age and the most common cause of death for all African-American children.

Although the overall approach to the pediatric trauma patient is the same as for the adult, the higher incidence of multisystem injury and the relatively limited communication skills in children necessitate an ordered and comprehensive approach to these patients.

The next section addresses the initial evaluation and management of the pediatric trauma patient, following protocols suggested in the Advanced Trauma Life Support (ATLS) course designed by the American College of Surgeons and focusing on the common pediatric entities of head trauma, near-drowning, and fire-related injuries.

FEATURES UNIQUE TO PEDIATRIC TRAUMA PATIENTS

The anatomic differences between children and adults transcend the obvious size discrepancy. Until the age of 11–12 years, children's heads constitute a relatively greater proportion of their total body mass. When they fall, children are more likely to land on their heads. The larger head also contributes to higher level cervical spine injuries (C2–3) in children than in adults. A child's large body surface area-mass ratio allows more rapid loss of heat and fluids, necessitating close attention to these issues. Because of their small size, children sustain multiple organ system injuries more frequently than adults. Their immature skeletons sustain less frequent bone injuries but more frequent soft tissue and internal organ damage. When bone injury does occur, however, it may be subtle because of the presence of open growth plates at the epiphyses. These growth plates often are not as strong as the tendons connected to them and therefore can be damaged despite a normal radiographic appearance. Finally, children require age-specific equipment and weight-specific drug dosages during resuscitation. Knowledge of age-specific vital signs and developmentally appropriate examinations of neurologic and mental status also help in assessing pediatric trauma patients.

Optimal care of these patients requires a team approach involving personnel trained in surgery, anesthesia, pediatric care, respiratory therapy, and specialty nursing. The identification of one person, usually a trauma surgeon or pediatric surgeon, as the "team leader" helps to ensure proper delegation of duties and facilitates efficient, thorough evaluation and resuscitation.

MANAGEMENT

The assessment and management of the trauma patient begin with the basic principles of CPR: the ABCs (see this chapter, Cardiopulmonary Resuscitation). This is quickly followed by the assessment of neurologic status (*Disability*) and then the *Exposure* of the entire body for evaluation. This approach, known as the **primary survey** of the trauma patient, is summarized in Table 10–24. Although many activities are happening at once during the resuscitation, one must adhere to the order of these priorities. For instance, focus should never be diverted from the airway

Table 10–24. Trauma: overall priorities.[1]

I. Primary survey
Airway/cervical spine
Breathing
Circulation
Disability (neurologic)
Exposure
II. Resuscitation phase
Control hemorrhage
Supplemental oxygen administration
Fluid administration
Electrocardiogram monitoring
III. Secondary survey
"A finger or tube in every orifice"
Foley/gastric decompression
Blood tests
Head and maxillofacial trauma—check for signs of basilar skull fracture
Cervical spine—continue immobilization until clinically and radiographically cleared
Chest—continuous reevaluation; palpate for fractures
Abdomen—distention; tenderness. Obtain computed tomography scan
Rectum—check prostate in males; bleeding
Pelvis—check stability
Extremities—deformity, tenderness, crepitus
Neurologic—Glasgow Coma Scale; frequent reassessment
Laboratory studies/radiographs
IV. Definitive care phase
History
A—Allergies
M—Medications
P—Past illnesses
L—Last meal
E—Events surrounding the injury
Determine disposition
Operating suite
Intensive care unit
Regular inpatient care area
Specialized care facility

[1]Adapted and reproduced, with permission, from American College of Surgeons, Committee on Trauma: Advanced Trauma Life Support Student Manual, 1993.

to correct a circulation problem. Some special considerations in performing the primary survey on children subjected to trauma are presented in Table 10–25.

Even if the child is breathing spontaneously and no supplemental airway maneuvers are deemed necessary, 100% oxygen should be administered to all victims of major trauma. Ensuring cervical spine stabilization while an adequate airway is secured is paramount in all unconscious or head- and neck-injured trauma patients. This is accomplished either by putting the patient in a rigid cervical collar with sandbags or by placing one's fingers on the mastoid and mandible to impede lateral movement as well as flexion-extension.

Once cervical spine stabilization has been achieved, attention is focused on the adequacy of respiration. Certain traumatic injuries may compromise the child's ability to expand the lungs. Pneumothorax or hemopneumothorax may need to be evacuated by needle aspiration and subsequent chest-tube catheter placement. In addition, flail chest may occur when two or more adjacent ribs are broken in multiple locations, thereby impeding the development of negative pressure inside of the thoracic cavity. If the patient requires endotracheal intubation, a rapid-sequence technique should be used. Pressure should be placed on the cricoid ring to move it posteriorly, thereby compressing the esophagus and preventing aspiration of gastric contents (Sellick maneuver). In the acute setting, nasotracheal intubation should be avoided because it is difficult to perform in the young child, and the danger exists of entering the cranial vault if there is a cribriform plate fracture.

While the airway and breathing problems are being addressed, vascular access should be obtained. In patients suffering from major trauma (determined by patient condition and mechanism of injury), two large-bore IV catheters should be inserted. If peripheral IV access is not

Table 10–25. Special considerations of the primary survey for pediatric trauma patients.

Airway	**Circulation**
Cervical spine immobilization	Intraosseous infusion or peripheral vein cutdown if needed
Rapid-sequence intubation	Normal vital signs different for children, ie, systolic BP = 80 + (2 × age in years)
Cricoid pressure	
Lidocaine (1 mg/kg) in head trauma	
Ketamine contraindicated as sedative in head trauma	**Disability**
	Pupillary response
	AVPU (see Table 10–26)
Avoid nasotracheal intubation	Treat seizures.
Breathing	**Exposure**
Pneumothorax/hemopneumothorax	Get patient completely exposed.
Flail chest not well tolerated	Beware of hypothermia in infants and small children.
Pulmonary contusions more common	

BP = blood pressure.

obtained within a few minutes, then either a peripheral vein cutdown, central venous access, or an intraosseous infusion should be considered. The techniques for these procedures are discussed previously (see Shock).

Fluid resuscitation is based on the assessment of four organ systems: cardiac, renal, CNS, and skin. Tachycardia is often the first sign of hypovolemia. Low blood pressure is a late finding; up to 40% of the blood volume may be lost before hypotension is manifest. More subtle signs, such as weak pulses; confusion; cool, clammy skin; or decreased urine output, may suggest that large amounts of fluids are still needed. Hemoglobin concentrations and hematocrit may not immediately reflect acute blood loss until sufficient time has elapsed for the blood volume to reequilibrate.

It is prudent to begin fluid resuscitation with the administration of 20 mL/kg of lactated Ringer solution and then observe for improvement of the patient's condition. If necessary, this bolus may be repeated several times while waiting to administer 10 mL/kg of packed red blood cells or whole blood. Children requiring further volume support are likely to require operative management of their injuries. The insertion of a Foley catheter to measure urine output will help to determine the adequacy of the fluid resuscitation. However, the presence of blood at the urethral meatus or the presence of a high-riding prostate on rectal examination signify a possible urethral tear and are, therefore, contraindications to this procedure.

During the primary survey, the evaluation of neurologic disability is brief and consists of checking pupillary size and response and assessing mental status (using the AVPU system presented in Table 10–26). The patient is then exposed to complete the initial assessment.

The next part of evaluation is the secondary survey. The goal of the secondary survey is to discover any injuries that were not apparent on initial evaluation (Table 10–24). The catchphrase for this portion of the evaluation used in the ATLS protocols is: "tubes and fingers in every orifice," which emphasizes its thorough nature. One begins the survey at the head, neck, and face and proceeds caudally to inspect and palpate each and every portion of the body. The patient should be "log-rolled" to permit examination of the back and rectum for injury. The back is palpated for tenderness or step-offs. The Glasgow Coma Scale (GCS) is used at this point to assess neurologic status in more detail (Table 10–27). Intra-abdominal or retroperitoneal bleeding may be difficult to assess; suspicion of internal injuries must be high in patients with abdominal tenderness, guarding, or distention. In children, peritoneal lavage is more difficult to perform than in

adults, and many trauma centers instead perform abdominal CT scans in the initial evaluation for intra-abdominal pathology.

Fractures suspected because of deformity, crepitus, or tenderness should be immobilized with a splint. Blood loss from femur or pelvic fractures can be extensive, and the patient with isolated orthopedic injuries might require substantial fluid resuscitation. Cervical spine evaluation is best done radiographically with lateral, anteroposterior, and open-mouth (odontoid) views. The immobilization process should continue until the patient is cleared both radiographically and clinically. This means that the comatose patient with negative cervical spine radiographs should remain immobilized while in the emergency department. Radiographs of the chest and pelvis are also obtained routinely soon after the secondary survey is complete.

The delineation of the patient's injuries by primary and secondary survey helps to determine their eventual disposition: operating suite, ICU, regular inpatient care unit, or specialized care facility (see Table 10–24). Included in this decision is the patient's past medical history, present medical illnesses, and the mechanism of injury.

HEAD TRAUMA

One in 10 school-aged children experiences an episode of head trauma with a change in level of consciousness. One third of these children require hospitalization, accounting for almost 250,000 admissions annually. The mortality rate is 2%; many die within hours of the injury. Severe neurologic sequelae occur in 2–5% of head-injured children. In view of these figures, methods of injury prevention and prompt medical management must be emphasized to parents, caretakers, and medical professionals.

Although motor vehicle accidents account for the majority of head injuries in children, falls down staircases (especially in child walkers), falls from standard beds and bunk beds, and violence-related injuries, such as child abuse, play a role. In addition, penetrating injuries are being encountered more frequently in urban pediatric emergency departments.

DIAGNOSIS & CLINICAL MANIFESTATIONS

The primary injury to the CNS is the shearing of the white matter tracts caused by the acceleration and deceleration of the brain within the skull. The neuronal cell death and vascular disruption that occurs within the first few milliseconds of impact cannot be reversed. Management therefore is guided toward prevention of secondary injury to the brain and blood vessels. Head injuries can be divided into focal injuries, such as fractures or hematomas,

Table 10–26. Rapid neurologic evaluation.

A—*Alert*
V—responds to *Vocal* stimuli
P—responds to *Painful* stimuli
U—*Unresponsive*

Table 10–27. Glasgow Coma Scale for assessing neurologic status.

	Adults/Older Children	Numerical Score[1]	Modified Score (Infants)
Eye opening	Spontaneous	4	Spontaneous
	To verbal stimuli	3	To speech
	To pain	2	To pain
	None	1	None
Best verbal response	Oriented	5	Coos and babbles
	Confused	4	Irritable cries
	Inappropriate words	3	Cries to pain
	Nonspecific sounds	2	Moans to pain
	None	1	None
Best motor response	Follows command	6	Normal spontaneous movements
	Localizes pain	5	Withdraws to touch
	Withdraws to pain	4	Withdraws to pain
	Flexes to pain	3	Abnormal flexion
	Extends to pain	2	Abnormal extension
	None	1	None

[1]The numerical scores of each of the three categories are added:
A score of 12–15 is found in children who are awake and alert; it is usually considered unnecessary to obtain a computed tomography scan or to hospitalize such children.
A score below 12 is usually considered an indication to admit the child for careful observation, preferably in an intensive care unit.
A score below 8 indicates a severe head injury, usually with considerable cerebral edema and considerable risk of intracranial hypertension.

and diffuse injuries, such as concussion, increased intracranial pressure, and diffuse axonal injury (DAI).

Focal Injuries

Scalp lacerations and contusions are common in head injuries. Because of the high degree of vascularity of the scalp, blood loss from a moderately sized laceration can be extensive. Careful exploration of these wounds must include evaluation for retained foreign bodies, such as glass, as well as assessment of the depth of the wound and underlying skull fractures. The galea aponeurotica, a strong tendinous sheath located just above the periosteal layer of the skull, is occasionally traversed and may need to be sutured separately to control bleeding.

Even after a child sustains minor head trauma, the first change that the parents notice is often a "lump" on the child's head. Because the galea is very loosely attached to the pericranium in toddlers and older children, this finding usually represents a subgaleal hematoma. In infants, however, there is a chance that the collection of blood occurs on a deeper level, between the periosteum and the table of the skull. The cephalhematoma is more common in traumatic newborn deliveries (see Chapter 4).

Collections of blood beneath the limits of the skull can be either epidural or subdural in origin. Table 10–28 summarizes the differences between these entities. Subdural hematomas are the result of acceleration/deceleration injuries that cause disruption of the veins that bridge the subarachnoid space to the dural venous sinuses. Subdural hematomas can be acute, subacute, or chronic. **Acute sub-**

Table 10–28. Supratentorial epidural versus subdural hematoma.

	Epidural	Acute Subdural
Etiology	Arterial (middle meningeal)	Venous
		Bridging veins below dura
Incidence	Uncommon	Common
Peak age	Usually > 2 y	6 mo (usually < 1 y)
Location	Unilateral	75% bilateral
	Usually parietal	Diffuse, over cerebral hemispheres
Skull fracture	Common	Uncommon
Associated seizures	Uncommon	Common
Retinal hemorrhages	Rare	Common
Decreased level of consciousness	Common	Very common
Mortality rate	Low	Moderate
Morbidity in survivors	Low	High
Clinical findings	Dilated ipsilateral pupil	Decreased level of consciousness
	Contralateral hemiparesis	
Radiographic findings (computed tomography)	Convex "lens-shaped" enhancement	Diffuse, concave enhancement surrounding cerebral hemisphere

dural hematomas become symptomatic within 24 hours of injury. The most common finding in these patients is a change in level of consciousness, ranging from irritability or lethargy to a comatose state. Subacute subdural hematomas present with similar symptoms between 24 hours and 2 weeks after the injury. **Chronic subdural hematomas,** on the other hand, present with more subtle neurologic findings 2 weeks or more after injury, when the blood clot slowly expands as it liquefies.

Epidural hematomas are less often associated with underlying brain injury than are subdural hematomas. Commonly, a blow or penetrating injury to the parietotemporal region results in a skull fracture with underlying disruption of the middle meningeal artery. In children, however, epidural hematomas are commonly venous in origin. Subsequent extravasation of blood between the dura and the inner table of the skull is limited by the dural reflections and results in a convex, lenticular (lens shaped) appearance on CT scan. Because of the unilateral nature of these lesions, unilateral uncal herniation is seen more commonly in epidural hematomas than in subdural hematomas. Physical examination may reveal ipsilateral pupillary dilatation secondary to compression of the parasympathetic fibers of the oculomotor nerve and contralateral motor deficits from disruption of motor tracts. The overall mortality of epidural hematoma is extremely low, and severe neurologic sequelae are rare in survivors.

Cerebral contusions can occur on the area of the brain initially contacting the cranium (coup injury) or on the portion "rebounding" into the opposite side of the cranium (contracoup injury). If disruption of intracerebral vessels results in cerebral hemorrhage along with cerebral contusion, uncal herniation may follow. Nevertheless, the most common manifestation of cerebral contusion is post-traumatic epilepsy. Cerebral lacerations usually result from penetrating injury to the brain, or a depressed skull fracture.

Skull Fractures. Although the possibility of skull fractures after minor head trauma often brings children to medical attention, it is usually more important to investigate the underlying pathology and neurologic ramifications of the blow that created the fracture. Controversy exists regarding the appropriateness of obtaining a radiograph of the skull. Many physicians believe that if sufficient force was generated to create a fracture, a CT scan of the head is necessary to investigate possible intracranial lesions as well. Therefore, the decision to obtain skull radiographs is based on the patient's age, the mechanism of injury, and the need for other radiologic evaluation.

There are several types of skull fractures. **Linear fractures** account for 75–90% of all skull fractures. Although no treatment is usually necessary, the presence of a fracture indicates that a large amount of force was endured during the event. If the fracture is located over a vascular structure, such as the middle meningeal artery, the incidence of epidural hemorrhage increases.

Basilar skull fractures typically occur in the petrous portion of the temporal bone. Although the diagnosis is difficult to make using only a skull radiograph, the clinical picture is helpful. The four potential findings in patients with basilar skull fractures are (1) pooling of blood in the soft tissues below the eyes ("raccoon eyes"), (2) ecchymoses located at the mastoid bones behind the ears (Battle sign), (3) cerebrospinal fluid (CSF) leak from the nose **(rhinorrhea)** or ears **(otorrhea)**, and (4) blood behind the eardrum **(hemotympanum)**. CT scan of the brain might reveal pneumocephali (air inside the cranial vault), usually originating from the sinuses. The communication between the paranasal sinuses and the intracranial contents subjects the child to increased risk for bacterial meningitis. In addition, damage to the first, sixth, seventh, and eighth cranial nerves can result in anosmia (loss of the sense of smell), ocular and facial palsy, and sensorineural hearing loss.

Depressed skull fractures sometimes can be diagnosed by palpation of the depression underneath a hematoma or by radiographic evaluation using tangential views of the skull or CT scan. In older children, depression of the skull can be associated with laceration and bruising of the dura, and the fractures require surgical elevation if they extend past the inner table of the skull.

Diffuse Lesions

Concussion syndromes, the most common form of diffuse brain injury, are diagnosed when blunt head injury results in a transient impairment of consciousness with loss of awareness and responsiveness. The duration of the loss of consciousness can range from seconds to hours and is caused by damage to the reticular activating system. The presence of anterograde or retrograde amnesia might help to diagnose concussion if the history of unconsciousness is unclear. Although almost all children with a concussion syndrome experience a period of lucidity lasting minutes to hours, drowsiness and vomiting may develop. Symptoms usually resolve over the next 6–8 hours; however, a few will complain of persistent headaches, dizziness, and subtle differences in memory, anxiety level, and sleep patterns for days to weeks after the injury.

Diffuse axonal injury is characterized by persistent functional or physiologic brain abnormalities unassociated with gross anatomic abnormalities. It is thought to be because of the shearing of nerve fibers on initial impact. DAI can result in a prolonged comatose state (> 6 hours) and is subsequently associated with a high morbidity and mortality.

The volume of the cranial vault is normally constant and contains three compartments: CSF (10%), blood (10%), and brain tissue (80%). An increase in one component necessitates a decrease in another, or the intracranial pressure (ICP) will increase. If the ICP continues to rise, brain tissue and blood vessels are increasingly compressed, with resulting displacement of brain contents inside and outside the cranial vault **(herniation)** and disruption of cerebral blood flow.

The exact location of brain herniation differs depending on the mechanism of ICP. If increased pressure causes displacement of the uncal portion of the temporal lobe through the tentorium, the portion of the brain stem that normally lies below the tentorium is compressed. This can disrupt the parasympathetic fibers of the third cranial nerve and result in an unreactive and dilated pupil on the side ipsilateral to the lesion. Motor deficits are usually contralateral to the lesion. If the uncal herniation is bilateral, as occurs in a diffuse injury, the pupillary and motor deficits will be noted bilaterally as well.

Two less common forms of brain herniation involve the cerebellum and the brain stem. **Cerebellar herniation** is usually a result of a posterior fossa lesion, whereas **brain stem herniation** can occur with almost any severe brain injury. Both of these entities involve compression of medullary autonomic structures, thereby affecting heart rate, respirations, and level of consciousness. The classic "Cushing triad" is a late finding of increased ICP. The triad consists of hypertension, bradycardia, and irregular respirations. With brain stem compression, decerebrate posturing can also be noted.

MANAGEMENT

The initial priorities in a child with severe head injury involve protection of the airway, maintenance of adequate tissue perfusion, and rapid assessment of neurologic status (Figure 10–5). Although the primary injury to the brain is irreversible, the secondary injury due to hypoxia, hypercarbia, or increased ICP must be minimized in the acute care setting.

The indications for establishing an artificial airway in a child with head trauma are listed in Table 10–29. In view of the 5% incidence of cervical spine fracture in patients with severe head injury, it is prudent to obtain cervical spine radiographs in all but the most minor head trauma patients (see this chapter, Trauma). Hyperventilation using an artificial airway should be instituted in any child with signs of increased ICP. It is most effective when the partial pressure of carbon dioxide ($Paco_2$) is kept at 25–30 mm Hg, which minimizes cerebral blood flow and reduces cerebral blood volume without causing ischemic damage.

Attention should then be focused on the adequacy of circulation. Neurogenic shock secondary to spinal cord injury is a diagnosis of exclusion and should not be considered until hypovolemic shock has been ruled out. Shock should be dealt with aggressively in the trauma patient, regardless of concern for increased ICP. The perfusion of the brain depends on an adequate mean arterial pressure; lack of perfusion leads to irreversible neuronal cell damage.

After the patient's cardiopulmonary status is stabilized, the secondary survey should be performed. First, a brief history of the events preceding and subsequent to the trauma episode may be obtained. This history should focus on the time and mechanism of injury, duration of unconsciousness, presence of amnesia, neurologic assessment at the scene, and any preexisting medical conditions.

At this point, a more detailed neurologic assessment, including the GCS, should be performed (see Table 10–27). The eyes are examined for abnormal pupillary reflexes or abnormal eye movements that might indicate increased ICP, cranial nerve dysfunction, or seizure activity. The gag reflex should be checked relatively early in the evaluation process to determine the need for intubation. The secondary survey should also include a close inspection of the head for lacerations, depressions, contusions, or signs of basilar skull fracture. Examination of the chest, torso, abdomen, genitalia, and extremities should follow soon after the primary survey.

Evaluation of brain stem function using the oculocephalic ("doll's eye") reflex should be deferred until the cervical spine is evaluated radiographically and clinically. A normal response implies that the cranial nerve pathways most proximal to the brain stem (third, sixth, and eighth cranial nerves) are intact and that, by association, the brain stem is functional. If necessary, the oculovestibular reflexes ("cold caloric") may be implemented if there is no evidence of a perforation of the tympanic membranes. The "normal" reflex is noted as a slow eye deviation toward the cold side and a rapid nystagmus away from the cold side. In general, however, this test can be delayed until after the secondary survey is completed.

Specific Further Management

If there are signs of increased ICP or of a deteriorating or persistently abnormal neurologic examination, a CT scan of the head is helpful in differentiating focal neurosurgical lesions from more diffuse injury. A head CT scan is also indicated if there is evidence of a skull fracture.

Emergency management of the patient with increased ICP is aimed at reducing the cerebral blood volume to prevent the herniation of brain tissue while maintaining cerebral perfusion pressure. In addition to hyperventilation, other immediate measures can help with this task. The patient's head should be elevated to a 30 degree angle, and adequate arterial blood pressure must be maintained to compensate for the effects of increased ICP. Seizure activity, if present, should be treated. IV mannitol acts as an osmotic diuretic to draw water out of the brain and thereby reduce the "tissue" portion of the intracranial vault. The presence of hypotension or hypovolemia is a relative contraindication to its administration.

Further management of increased ICP may include barbiturate coma, muscle paralysis, and ventriculostomy for CSF drainage. These therapies are usually instituted in an ICU setting.

Post-traumatic Epilepsy

The incidence of seizures occurring after head trauma is 5–10%. The majority are classified as early post-traumatic seizures, ie, within 1 week of the initial injury. Twenty percent of these patients go on to experience late seizures more than 1 week after the injury. Post-traumatic seizures are correlated with depressed skull fractures. Early seizures are usually associated with cerebral lacerations

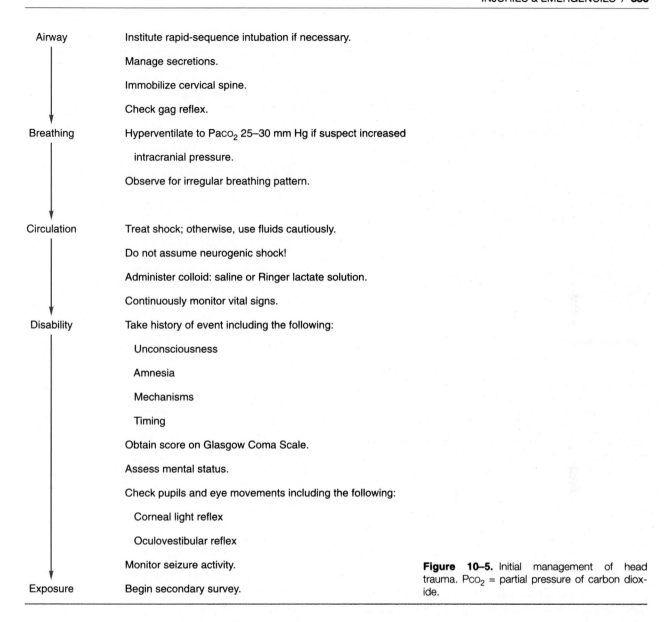

Airway	Institute rapid-sequence intubation if necessary.
	Manage secretions.
	Immobilize cervical spine.
	Check gag reflex.
Breathing	Hyperventilate to Paco$_2$ 25–30 mm Hg if suspect increased
	intracranial pressure.
	Observe for irregular breathing pattern.
Circulation	Treat shock; otherwise, use fluids cautiously.
	Do not assume neurogenic shock!
	Administer colloid: saline or Ringer lactate solution.
	Continuously monitor vital signs.
Disability	Take history of event including the following:
	Unconsciousness
	Amnesia
	Mechanisms
	Timing
	Obtain score on Glasgow Coma Scale.
	Assess mental status.
	Check pupils and eye movements including the following:
	Corneal light reflex
	Oculovestibular reflex
	Monitor seizure activity.
Exposure	Begin secondary survey.

Figure 10–5. Initial management of head trauma. Pco$_2$ = partial pressure of carbon dioxide.

and contusions but do not frequently progress to epilepsy. About 50% of patients with late-onset seizures will continue to have seizures for the next few years. The drug of choice for such seizures is phenytoin, although in the acute setting, a benzodiazepine should be used because of its rapid onset of action.

DISPOSITION OF PATIENTS WITH HEAD TRAUMA

The patient who has experienced severe head trauma is almost always admitted to the hospital for aggressive therapy and invasive monitoring. However, patients with less

severe injury present a more difficult decision. In general, patients with no history of amnesia and a short duration (< 5 minutes) of unconsciousness may be observed without treatment if results of the neurologic examination are normal. This observation can usually occur at home, provided there is a reliable caretaker. Caretakers are instructed to awaken the patient every 3–4 hours and allow the patient to walk and talk. In addition, they are instructed to bring the patient back to the emergency department if any signs develop of increased ICP, focal expanding mass, or CNS infection (Table 10–30). In contrast, patients with a prolonged episode of unconsciousness, significant amnesia, post-traumatic seizure, persistent neurologic deficit, or evidence of a depressed or basilar skull

Table 10–29. Indications for endotracheal intubation in the patient with head trauma.

Upper airway obstruction
Abnormal respiratory rate or rhythm
Loss of protective airway reflexes
Concomitant trauma
Chest wall instability
Pulmonary contusion
Signs of increased intracranial pressure

Table 10–31. Factors associated with a poor outcome in head trauma.

Age < 2 y
Glasgow Coma Scale score < 5
Subdural hematoma
Decerebrate or flaccid posture
Coma > 24 h

fracture should be admitted to the hospital and receive a CT scan of the head. Suspected child abuse victims should also be admitted for evaluation.

PROGNOSIS

There is a 3% mortality rate for all head trauma patients, and a 2–5% incidence of severe handicap. Nevertheless, complete recovery is the rule for mild to moderate head trauma victims. The GCS is a reliable prognostic indicator in patients with moderate to severe head trauma. Patients with a GCS score of 5 or less and a subdural hematoma have a 75% mortality rate, and surviving children become severely disabled. Factors associated with a worse outcome are listed in Table 10–31. Of all children with severe head trauma, 20% have permanent neurologic deficits, and almost 50% will have some behavioral or emotional problem.

NEAR-DROWNING

Drowning is the third most common cause of death in children aged 1–14 years and a cause of significant neurologic sequelae in near-drowning survivors. **Drowning** is defined as submersion in water resulting in death. **Near-drowning** is defined as survival after asphyxia because of submersion.

Children of all ages are at risk for drowning. However,

Table 10–30. Reasons for immediate medical follow-up of discharged head trauma patients.

Headache worsening or unrelieved by acetaminophen
Frequent vomiting
Change in behavior or gait or difficulty seeing
Fever or stiff neck
Evidence of clear or bloody fluid draining from nose or ear
Difficult to awaken from sleep
Seizure
Bleeding from scalp wound that is unrelieved by 5 min of constant pressure

two age groups are particularly at risk: toddlers and adolescents. Toddlers are most likely to encounter the unknown dangers of ambulating near an open body of water without adequate supervision. Approximately 40% of drowning deaths occur in children younger than 4 years; more than half of these occur in freshwater swimming pools. Adolescent drowning incidents are commonly secondary to unsafe swimming or diving practices or boating accidents; as many as 50% of these deaths are related to alcohol consumption. Most drowning incidents occur during the summer months. An exception is in infants younger than 1 year, in whom bathtub drowning incidents constitute a large percentage. Children with epilepsy have a risk four times greater than that of other children. Child abuse or neglect should be considered in cases of drowning or near-drowning in children who are not ambulatory. Most drowning deaths are preventable; public health measures and legislation are needed to require complete enclosure of all outdoor pools and strict limits on alcohol consumption near boating and swimming areas. In addition, efforts are needed to supply rescue equipment and CPR instruction to responsible individuals at waterside.

DIAGNOSIS & CLINICAL MANIFESTATIONS

The initial course of events in submersion injury varies according to the child's age and swimming ability and the mechanism of encounter with the body of water. The common denominator of these events is asphyxia because of respiratory failure, as shown in Figure 10–6. Initially, voluntary breath-holding and voluntary closure of the glottis is accompanied by ingestion of various amounts of water into the GI tract. Ten percent of near-drowning injuries reveal no evidence of pulmonary aspiration and are termed "dry drowning" injuries. In most cases, however, profound hypercarbia leads to an involuntary gasp and aspiration of water into the airway. The contact of water with the larynx causes reflex laryngospasm and bronchospasm that lead to a marked decrease in ventilation. If water has been aspirated, secondary apnea can occur, thereby adding to the ventilation and oxygenation difficulties. Persistent hypoxemia results from alveolar injury and an intrapulmonary shunt, as the child's airways are perfused but not ventilated. In addition, the denaturation (freshwater) or washout (saltwater) of surfactant adds to the alveolar collapse and hypoxemia. Prolonged hypox-

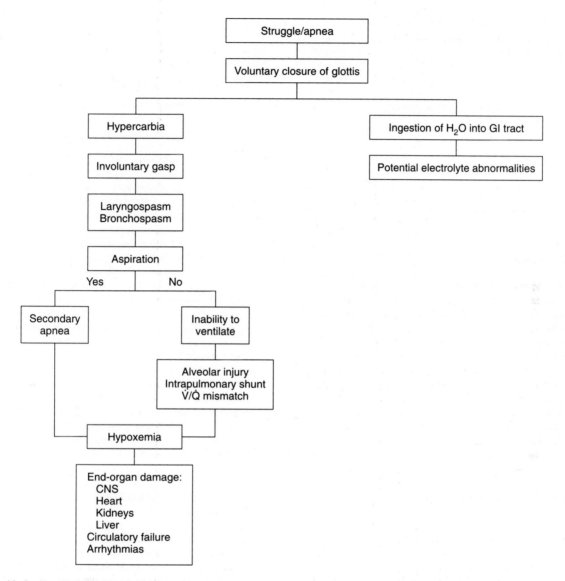

Figure 10–6. Algorithm showing pathophysiology of near-drowning or drowning. CNS = central nervous system; GI = gastrointestinal; V̇/Q̇ = ventilation-perfusion.

emia results in arrhythmias, pulmonary edema, circulatory failure, and death.

The near-drowning victim's prognosis depends on when the above events were interrupted and the duration of hypoxemia. Neuronal cell damage begins approximately 6 minutes after submersion, becoming irreversible at approximately 9 minutes.

Hypothermia is an invariable sequela of almost all near-drownings. The temperature of the water in which a child is submerged is a double-edged sword. On one hand, body temperature less than 32 °C is likely to result in loss of consciousness and subsequent drowning. The cold heart is more prone to cardiac conduction abnormalities, such as ventricular fibrillation. In addition, the involuntary gasp that leads to fluid aspiration occurs earlier in cold water, and tissue oxygen delivery is impaired in hypothermic states. On the other hand, some evidence indicates that severe hypothermia relates a protective effect to the near-drowning victim by reducing brain metabolism and overall oxygen consumption during a time of severe hypoxemia. Overall, survival has been noted to be better in cases of cold-water submersion than with warm-water submersion. The physical examination of the hypothermic patient may reveal dilated pupils, increased muscle tone, bradycardia, slow and shallow respirations, and CNS depression. Patients may appear dead. However, the saying "a patient is not dead until he is warm and dead" provides impetus to continue resuscitation efforts accordingly.

Electrolyte abnormalities are rare in near-drowning victims unless a large amount of water is swallowed, in which case dilutional hyponatremia and hypokalemia may occur.

MANAGEMENT

The goals of management of the near-drowning patient are to improve oxygenation and to maintain sufficient cardiac output to reverse hypoxic injury to the end organs and prevent further injury to the brain.

On the Scene

Even if the child is still in the water, mouth-to-mouth resuscitation should be initiated immediately. External chest compressions are deferred until the patient is on solid ground and pulses are checked. Once on land, CPR is continued and cricoid pressure is applied to prevent vomiting by compressing the esophagus between the cricoid and the vertebral column. Foreign bodies should be removed from the oropharynx, but the Heimlich maneuver is indicated only if there is a high suspicion of tracheal foreign body. Cervical spine immobilization should be strongly considered if there is any potential mechanism for neck injury. Stabilization for transport to a medical facility should include rewarming by removing wet clothing and covering the child with dry blankets or towels.

Hospital Management

The need for endotracheal intubation is based initially on the presence of apnea or respiratory distress. If the child's trachea was intubated in the prehospital setting, endotracheal tube placement should be evaluated by listening for bilateral and symmetrical breath sounds. Cervical spine immobilization should be considered again unless the history from witnesses absolutely rules out any chance of head trauma or cervical-spine injury. If the child is not already intubated, rapid-sequence intubation should be performed for the following reasons: apnea, severe respiratory distress, hypoventilation, or decreased level of consciousness. In addition, if further evaluation of breathing reveals evidence of pulmonary edema or severe hypoxia, endotracheal intubation should be performed. Severe hypoxia in this scenario is defined as a PaO_2 less than 60 mm Hg despite the administration of an FiO_2 greater than 0.5. Regardless of the condition of the child or need for intubation, 100% oxygen should be provided in the initial resuscitation, and oxygen saturation should be monitored by pulse oximetry. If positive pressure ventilation is required, a high PEEP and respiratory rate may be required to combat pulmonary edema and hypercarbia. Vigorous suctioning of secretions should be applied in all cases.

After airway and breathing issues are managed, attention must be turned to the circulation to ensure substrate delivery to the tissues. Two competing factors in near-drowning must be considered: hypovolemia and head trauma with increased ICP. Many near-drowning victims are hypovolemic because of capillary leak into the pulmonary parenchyma. Regardless of the ICP considerations, this hypovolemia must be corrected. IV crystalloid fluids should be administered in aliquots of 20 mL/kg to maintain adequate circulation on the basis of heart rate, capillary refill, blood pressure, and urine output. Sodium bicarbonate (1–2 meq/kg) can be administered once adequate ventilation is established.

Most patients with a GCS below 8 require endotracheal intubation and hyperventilation. After an adequate airway has been secured, a nasogastric tube can be inserted to remove any ingested water from the stomach and help prevent dilutional electrolyte disturbances. A Foley catheter can help to assess adequate hydration.

The patient's temperature should be obtained rectally with a thermometer capable of reading temperatures as low as 25 °C. Hypothermia should be managed aggressively in the emergency department. If not already done at the scene, the child's wet clothing should be removed, and the child should be dried and wrapped in warm blankets. If the patient's core temperature is 32–35 °C, external rewarming methods, such as a radiant warmer and heating blanket, should be used to raise the core temperature. If body temperature is less than 32 °C, active internal rewarming is accomplished with warmed, humidified oxygen, warmed IV fluids, and warm gastric lavage. Because of the increased incidence of ventricular dysrhythmias in the hypothermic patient, care should be taken not to move the patient too abruptly. In severe cases and when available, extracorporeal blood rewarming can be used for cases of hypothermia with refractory ventricular fibrillation. In patients with severe hypothermia (< 32 °C) but no apparent cardiac abnormalities, slow rewarming can be accomplished using both internal and external rewarming methods. Remember, resuscitation efforts should not be halted in patients with a core temperature less than 32 °C.

DISPOSITION

Transfer to an appropriate inpatient setting should be done quickly to maximize the monitoring status of near-drowning victims. All near-drowning victims require at least 4–6 hours of observation in the emergency department, regardless of how trivial the history or physical examination. Children with a significant history of submersion, a history of apnea or cyanosis, or loss of consciousness, or those who have required CPR, must be admitted to the hospital for observation. Patients with abnormal physical findings, abnormal chest x-ray findings, acidosis, or hypoxemia require admission as well. In some cases, the respiratory symptoms may not be apparent until 12–24 hours after the incident, when significant pulmonary edema or pneumonitis requires medical intervention. Patients with a change in mental status, respiratory compromise requiring prolonged resuscitation, mechanical ventilation, or high inspired oxygen concentrations should be observed and treated in an intensive care setting (Table 10–32).

PROGNOSIS

The outcome of the near-drowning victim is related to the amount of irreversible brain injury from hypoxia that occurs during submersion. Poor prognostic factors for survival are listed in Table 10–33. Observation of a stable or improving mental status while in the hospital is a good prognostic sign. A few studies have demonstrated that moderately lower body temperatures may confer some protection against anoxic injury and improve recovery after rewarming and resuscitation.

BURNS

More than 10% of accidental deaths among children between the ages of 1 and 14 years are caused by thermal injury. The nature of these injuries includes scalding, contact with flames or hot solids, and electrical and chemical burns. Although only 3–5% of burn injuries are life-threatening, the pain and psychological ramifications from these injuries argue for efforts to be focused on prevention as well as optimal treatment. Prevention efforts can be helped by informing parents of the benefits of keeping the tap-water temperature below 54.4 °C (130 °F) and by encouraging the use of smoke alarms.

Approximately 80% of burn injuries occur in the home; most injuries in the pediatric population are caused by scalds from hot liquids. However, most deaths in burn patients are caused by direct contact with flames. As children become ambulatory and can gain access to matches or lighters, flame injury becomes the most common form of thermal injury in the 5- to 13-year-old age group. Although a small percentage of thermal injuries are the result of child abuse, 10% of all battered children suffer burns. The typical pattern of these lesions is immersion scald injuries in either a stocking-glove appearance or on

Table 10–33. Poor prognostic factors in near-drowning.

Prolonged submersion > 10 min
Need for cardiopulmonary resuscitation (CPR)
Delay in necessary CPR efforts in first 10 minutes
Arrival to emergency department in coma
Initial temperature < 30 °C
Initial pH ≤ 7.10

the buttocks. It is difficult for children by themselves to suffer a scald burn to the buttocks or symmetric scald burns to extremities. Similarly, few children will intentionally place the full palms of both hands flatly on a hot surface. A high index of suspicion of child abuse needs to be maintained for all cases of burn injury.

DIAGNOSIS & CLINICAL MANIFESTATIONS

Burns can be categorized as either partial thickness (first- and second-degree burns) or full thickness (third- and fourth-degree burns) (Table 10–34). **First-degree burns** involve little tissue destruction and, clinically, appear erythematous and possibly edematous but without blistering (eg, sunburn). These usually heal within 3–6 days without permanent scarring.

Second-degree burns involve some or all of the dermis; new skin may be regenerated from this level of burn injury, thereby reducing the need for skin grafting. However, a second-degree burn may progress to full thickness if it becomes infected or is subject to further trauma. The appearance of second-degree burns varies with the extent of damage to the dermal layer. Shallow lesions result in an exquisitely sensitive blister with underlying erythema. Deeper lesions become white and are painful only to pressure stimulation. This wound is more difficult to distinguish from third-degree burns, especially if a significant amount of edema is present. Second-degree burns usually heal in 10–21 days.

Third-degree burns transcend the depth of the dermis, destroying entire hair follicles and sweat glands. The burn usually appears white and is insensitive to painful stimuli. The edges of a third-degree burn are often more shallow and therefore may be painful to touch. Third-degree burns can also be charred or parchment-like in appearance. It is

Table 10–32. Disposition of near-drowning patients.

Observation for 4–6 h	Hospitalization for at Least 24 h	Admission to Intensive Care Unit
All children with history of submersion injury	Apnea/cyanosis	Prolonged cardiopulmonary resuscitation
	Loss of consciousness	Persistent change in mental status
	Required cardiopulmonary resuscitation	Mechanical ventilation
	Findings suggesting anoxia or pulmonary damage	Frequent arterial blood gas monitoring

Table 10–34. Degrees of burn injury.

Type	Degree	Depth	Appearance	Sensitivity
Partial thickness	First	Epidermis	Red	Painful
	Second	Shallow: portion of dermis	Blisters	Exquisitely painful
		Deep	Red/white	May be anesthetic or painful only to pressure
Full thickness	Third	Entire dermis; no remaining adnexal structures	White, parchment-like, ± blisters, thrombosed veins	Insensitive to stimuli
	Fourth	Muscle, fascia, bone	Black, charred	Insensitive to stimuli

sometimes possible to see thrombosed superficial vessels through the eschar.

Fourth-degree burn is a term sometimes used when the injury extends into the subcutaneous tissue, muscle, fascia, or bone. The area is anesthetic and appears charred. There is a danger of systemic toxicity resulting from absorption of toxic products, as well as from unrecognized deep infection. Severe scaldings, molten metal burns, and electrical burns result in fourth-degree injury with greater frequency.

Aside from the skin and adnexal structures, other organ systems can be affected by a major burn injury (Table 10–35). In large thermal injuries, circulating blood volume can be diminished because of increased water loss from the external surface as well as increased capillary permeability in the involved areas. This hypovolemia, in conjunction with direct depression of cardiac output in patients with large burns, may result in "burn shock." These cardiovascular sequelae usually occur only in burn patients with involvement of 30% or more of the body surface area (BSA).

Besides extensive fluid losses, the other most life-threatening complication of thermal injury is infection. The majority of these infections originate from the patient's own GI tract rather than those present on the burn unit. Although the bacterium most frequently implicated is *Pseudomonas aeruginosa,* the most serious infections result from invasion by other gram-negative organisms. These organisms are more likely to thrive on wounds that are treated with topical therapy. Conversely, when broad-spectrum antibiotics are used, the incidence of infections with *Candida* increases dramatically.

MANAGEMENT

At the scene, the patient's ABCs, sensorium, and potential for smoke inhalation should be addressed. Smaller burn areas may be doused with cold, wet compresses, whereas larger burns or those encountered more than 10–15 minutes after the injury are covered with clean, dry sheets to minimize heat loss.

Continued assessment of the ABCs should occur in the emergency department. Special attention should be given to the presence of stridor, carbonaceous sputum, edema of the laryngeal structures, or singed nares as evidence of potential burn injury to the upper or lower airways. If these are present, direct laryngoscopy should be performed. Consideration should be given to prophylactic intubation of the trachea if upper airway obstruction appears likely.

The initial approach to the management of fluids in the burn patient begins with a rapid estimation of the wound depth and percentage of BSA involved. The depth of injury should be evaluated, and clinical signs of first-, second-, third-, and fourth-degree burns should be determined (see Table 10–34). The BSA of the injury can be estimated from published diagrams of BSA. Notice that the main difference between infants and older children is the relative surface area of the head. If this type of figure is not available, the size of the child's palm can be used as an estimate of 1% of the BSA. The "rule of 9's" can be applied to adults and children older than 10 years, with a BSA of 9% assigned to the head and each upper extremity, and 18% to each side of the torso and each lower extremity.

Patients with burns exceeding 10% of total BSA should have an IV catheter placed for fluid administration. The estimation of the fluid requirements of burn patients should rely on assessing the patient's pulse, capillary refill, mental status, and urine output. Initially, the patient should receive lactated Ringer solution to maintain adequate tissue perfusion. Lactated Ringer solution most closely approximates the extracellular fluid lost through the skin. Therapy begins with administration of 3–4 mL/kg per percentage of burn injury for the first 24 hours of replacement. One half of the required fluid is adminis-

Table 10–35. Common sequelae of major burns.

Skin (see text)	**Infectious**
Cardiovascular	Bacterial
Hypovolemia	Pseudomonas
Myocardial depression	Other gram-negative
Renal	organisms
Acute tubular necrosis	Yeast
Acute renal failure	*Candida* species
Hematologic	Viral
Neutropenia	**Nutrition/gastrointestinal**
Thrombocytopenia	Increased nutritional re-
Anemia	quirements
Microangiopathic hemo-	
lytic anemia	
Acute erythrocyte hemolysis	

tered over the first 8 hours, and the remainder, over the following 16 hours.

After the first 24 hours of burn injury, capillary permeability returns to normal and sodium losses decrease. Therefore, patients are administered either D5 1/4 normal saline or D5 1/3 normal saline with maintenance concentrations of potassium. In addition, serum protein previously lost may be replaced to restore normal plasma oncotic pressure. Children who are able may be allowed to drink hypotonic fluids (Table 10–36). Continued monitoring of serum electrolytes, acid-base status, and urine output cannot be overemphasized.

All persons coming into contact with a burn patient should wear sterile gloves and gowns. Procedures such as IV catheter placement and phlebotomy should be performed using sterile technique. An IV should be placed through an area of burn injury as a last resort. Routine use of parenteral antibiotics is not recommended. The initial wound management involves cleaning, debriding, and covering the wound with a topical antibiotic agent. If the patient needs to be transferred to another institution, the wound is covered only with sterile, dry gauze or sheets to facilitate reassessment of the wound by the receiving physicians. Because burn injuries are considered "dirty" wounds, tetanus prophylaxis should be considered for all burn patients.

A stepwise approach to burn wound management is presented in Table 10–37. Depending on the severity of the burn and the comfort of the parents, this can be accomplished on an inpatient or outpatient basis. The patient may require analgesia during the initial stage of burn wound healing, especially during dressing changes. Frequent reassessment of the wound is necessary, and systemic antibiotic therapy is indicated only if signs of infection are present. After epithelialization begins to occur, local wound care may be needed less frequently; however, close observation of the wound is still needed.

The decision of whether to admit a patient to the hospital for burn injury depends on many factors, ranging from the presence of associated injuries to the relative safety of the home environment (Table 10–38). If adequate outpatient management cannot be ensured, hospitalization is necessary. Children should also be admitted who require IV fluid resuscitation or who are at risk for infection or neurovascular compromise. Because of the potential for disfigurement or impaired function, children with significant facial or perineal injury are also admitted for care and observation. Transfer to a regional burn center should be considered for children with severe injury or for those who will require long-term management of their injuries.

ELECTRICAL & CHEMICAL BURNS

Two categories of burn injury requiring special consideration are electrical and chemical burns. Injuries from electrical burns are not always immediately recognizable. There may be deep tissue destruction despite the relatively benign appearance of the entry and exit lesions. Electricity tends to travel along blood vessels. Therefore, thrombosis of these blood vessels may occur, as well as injury to muscle, nerves, and bone. This is particularly ominous when the cardiac muscle is involved. Assessment of these patients should include a thorough evaluation of capillary refill, distal sensory and motor neurologic function, and ECG (if there is a chance that the electrical current passed through the heart). Fluid requirements might be higher than originally assumed owing to the aforementioned hidden injuries. One type of electrical burn injury that is unique to young children occurs in the corner of the mouth after the child chews through an electrical cord. In these cases, the usual treatment is "masterful observation." The necrotic facial tissue should be left alone until 2–4 weeks later. There is a chance of severe bleeding as the eschar begins to separate after 5–9 days, revealing the underlying labial artery. Parents can be warned about this possibility and should be instructed to apply direct pressure near the point of bleeding and to bring the child to an emergency department.

Chemical injuries in children usually involve household cleaners. Because alkali burns are more severe than those caused by acids, it is important to determine which agent caused the injury. After removal of all involved clothing, the treatment of these wounds includes copious irrigation with water or saline, generous fluid replacement, and application of a topical antibiotic agent.

SMOKE INHALATION

Inhalational injury is a significant contributor to the morbidity and mortality rates of fire-related injuries.

Table 10–36. Fluid management of burn patients.[1]

	Type of Fluid	Amount
First 24 h	Lactated Ringer solution	3–4 mL/kg per % BSA plus maintenance
Second 24 h	Maintenance fluid—dextrose 5% in 0.25% or 0.33% normal saline	3750 mL/m^2 of burned BSA + 1500 mL/m^2 of total BSA or to maintain adequate urine output
	Colloid (5% albumin in 0.9% NaCl)	0.5 mL/kg per % BSA

[1]Maintain urine output > 1 mL/kg/h or 30–60 mL/h; assess tissue perfusion continuously.
BSA = body surface area.

Table 10–37. Burns: Wound management.

Procedure	Materials	Comments
Cleaning	Sterile saline + antibacterial soap	Avoid vigorous scrubbing
Debriding	Sterile scissors/forceps	Sterile technique
		Remove debris and charred epithelium
		Remove broken blisters
Rinsing	Sterile saline	Copious irrigation
Applying topical cream (lightly over burn area)	Silver sulfadiazine 0.5% (Silvadene)	Poor penetration of infected burns
	Polysporin on face	
	Alternatives	
	Silver nitrate 0.5%	
	Mafenide acetate	
Dressing	Nonadherent gauze	
	Loose bulky external gauze	

DIAGNOSIS & CLINICAL MANIFESTATIONS

A common result of the derangements caused by smoke inhalation is cellular hypoxia. Patients who are trapped in a closed space during a fire are at highest risk for immediate asphyxia and frequently do not survive the initial resuscitation efforts. Thermal injury because of inhalation of gases greater than 500 °C primarily causes damage to the larynx, supraglottic, and epiglottic regions; thermal injury to the lower airway is rarely seen after inhalation of dry gases. This is mostly because of the efficient cooling function of the respiratory mucosa, which can exponentially lower the heat of dry inspired gases. The resulting upper airway edema can cause early airway obstruction in these patients. Steam, on the other hand, can cause significant damage to the lung parenchyma. Chemical injury to the lungs is due mostly to the inhalation of the toxic products of combustion, such as plastics, cotton, polyvinyl chloride, and polyurethane. These irritants can facilitate bronchoconstriction, increase mucosal edema, and impair mucociliary transport. In almost all survivors of severe smoke inhalation, bronchopneumonia develops after 2–3 days.

Some of the inhaled products of combustion, eg, carbon monoxide and cyanide, can severely hinder oxygen transport and delivery.

Carbon Monoxide Poisoning

Carbon monoxide contributes to cellular hypoxia in three ways: (1) preferential binding to hemoglobin, thereby leaving fewer sites for oxygen binding; (2) shifting the oxygen-hemoglobin dissociation curve to the left, allowing hemoglobin to "hold on" to oxygen more tightly and thereby decreasing the oxygen delivery to the tissues; and (3) binding to cytochrome oxidase, thereby poisoning the intracellular oxygen transport system.

Aside from the cellular anoxia caused by carbon monoxide poisoning, specific organ system damage may also occur. Pulmonary damage because of mucociliary dysfunction, bronchoconstriction, and pulmonary edema can result in severe respiratory distress. The CNS is most commonly affected by carbon monoxide toxicity. The most frequent neurologic findings in patients with carbon monoxide poisoning are memory loss and personality changes. Other early symptoms include slurred speech, dizziness, and headache. Neurologic symptoms, such as seizures, cerebral edema, and hearing or vision loss, may follow later. Cardiac effects, such as focal myocardial necrosis, leukocyte infiltration, and punctate hemorrhages, are manifested as ECG changes ranging from ST segment abnormalities to atrial fibrillation. The muscle, skin, and subcutaneous tissue are particularly susceptible to necrosis, which can lead to myoglobinuria and acute renal failure. Cutaneous findings of carbon monoxide poisoning include blistering, edema, and, infrequently, a "cherry red" discoloration.

Carbon monoxide poisoning is quantified by measure-

Table 10–38. Criteria for hospital admission of patients with burn injuries.

Absolute criteria
Second-degree burns > 10% BSA or third-degree burn > 2% BSA
Burn of entire hand or foot, or potential for vascular compromise of extremity
Severe burns of face or perineum
Inadequate patient compliance
Major electrical burn
Child abuse or neglect
Relative criteria
Young age (< 2 years)
Burns crossing a major joint
Electrical burn of mouth
Underlying illness or concomitant injury
Consider transfer to a regional burn center
Second-degree burns > 20% BSA
Second and third-degree burns > 10% BSA
Third-degree burns > 5% BSA
Major concomitant injury
Systemic effects of electrical burn
Involvement of respiratory tract
Burn of extremity or chest with neurovascular or respiratory compromise

BSA = body surface area.

ment of the carboxyhemoglobin (COHb) level, with normal ranges less than 5% for nonsmokers and less than 10% for smokers. Note that because of the short half-life of COHb in the presence of oxygen, the levels obtained in the emergency department do not reflect the level at the scene of the fire.

Cyanide Poisoning

The contribution of cyanide toxicity to the morbidity of smoke inhalation has been recently substantiated in the literature. Cyanide is inhaled as a product of the combustion of substances such as polyurethane. The half-life of cyanide is approximately 1 hour. Cyanide causes cellular anoxia by binding to the heme ion in the cytochrome complex A-a3, thereby shutting off the last step of oxidative metabolism. Cellular hypoxia results in CNS effects such as headaches, dizziness, seizures, coma, and death. Cardiac effects include tachycardia and hypertension, followed by bradycardia and hypotension. Determination of cyanide concentrations usually is not helpful in the acute care setting because of the length of time required for values to be returned. However, there is some evidence that serum lactate concentrations can estimate cyanide levels with some accuracy. Antidotes to cyanide toxicity are available and are recommended as early adjuncts in the treatment of smoke inhalation.

MANAGEMENT

Before or upon the patient's arrival in the emergency department, certain historical points should be elicited. These include the duration and severity of smoke exposure (open versus closed space), the types of burning material present, and the presence of unconsciousness at the scene. The physical examination should focus initially on the potential for airway compromise and the presence of respiratory symptoms. For patients exposed to smoke and fire, the initial threats to the airway are from laryngeal or supraglottic burns and edema and from failure to protect the airway from secretions. The indications for endotracheal intubation of these patients are listed in Table 10–39. In cases of unknown mechanism of injury, cervical

spine stabilization should be maintained until properly evaluated. Although the presence of respiratory symptoms is a poor prognostic indicator, the absence of such symptoms does not eliminate the possibility of pulmonary injury. Initial assessment should also include the extent and severity of burns on the body. Again, the absence of cutaneous burns does not rule out significant inhalational injury.

Oxygen administration is the mainstay of therapy for smoke inhalation. The half-life of carbon monoxide is approximately 5 hours in room air, approximately 1 hour in 100% Fio_2, and less than 0.5 hour in 100% Fio_2 at two atmospheres of pressure (hyperbaric oxygen therapy). Hyperbaric oxygen requires a special hyperbaric chamber, and, despite its potential advantages, the patient must be stabilized before transfer for this type of treatment. In the emergency setting, the highest possible concentration of oxygen should be administered once adequate ventilation has been established. The patient's circulatory status should then be addressed, and symptoms of shock should be treated accordingly. If the patient does not exhibit signs of shock, an estimate of the extent and depth of burn injury helps in arriving at a plan for fluid management. Because of the potential for pulmonary edema, overhydration should be avoided if possible. A Foley catheter for measurement of urine output should be placed to aid in fluid management.

The assessment of neurologic dysfunction follows. As mentioned in Table 10–39, the presence of coma or an absent gag reflex are indications for endotracheal intubation. Seizures should be treated expeditiously to prevent further respiratory compromise. Po_2 and COHb concentrations should be measured by arterial blood gas analysis, and a cyanide antidote administered if available. A cyanide antidote is most helpful when administered early and may require repetitive dosing. The safest and most commonly used antidote is 25% sodium thiosulfate, which binds to CN to form an easily excretable sodium thiocyanate. Hyperbaric oxygen therapy should be considered.

Even patients who have not suffered severe sequelae initially from smoke inhalation must be observed carefully for evidence of late injury. Indications for admission of these patients are listed in Table 10–40.

Table 10–39. Smoke inhalation: Indications for endotracheal intubation.

Stridor or hoarseness
Upper airway edema
Profuse tracheal secretions
Severe burns of face, mouth, or nares
Coma
Absent gag reflex
Severe hypoxia or hypercarbia
Carboxyhemoglobin level > 50%

Table 10–40. Indications for admission of smoke inhalation patients.

Closed space exposure
Facial or mucosal burns
Loss of consciousness or change in mental status
Increased secretions or carbonaceous sputum
Abnormal arterial blood gases, chest radiograph, or electrocardiogram
Abnormal respiratory examination
Carboxyhemoglobin level > 15%

REFERENCES

CARDIOPULMONARY RESUSCITATION IN INFANTS & CHILDREN

American Heart Association, Emergency Cardiac Care Committee and Subcommittees: Guidelines for cardiopulmonary resuscitation and emergency cardiac care. JAMA 1992;268:2171.

Goetting MG: Mastering pediatric cardiopulmonary resuscitation. Pediatr Clin North Am 1994;41:1147.

Goetting MG: Progress in pediatric cardiopulmonary resuscitation. Emerg Med Clin North Am 1995;13:291.

Von Planta M et al: Pathophysiologic and therapeutic implications of acid-base changes during CPR. Ann Emerg Med 1993;22:404.

Zaritsky A: Pediatric resuscitation pharmacology. Ann Emerg Med 1993;22:445.

SUDDEN INFANT DEATH SYNDROME

American Academy of Pediatrics Task Force on Infant Positioning and SIDS: Positioning and SIDS. Pediatrics 1992;89:1120.

Dwyer T et al: The contribution of changes in the prevalence of prone sleeping position to the decline in sudden infant death syndrome in Tasmania. JAMA 1995;273:783.

Freed GE et al: Sudden infant death syndrome prevention and an understanding of selected clinical issues. Pediatr Clin North Am 1994;41:967.

Klonoff-Cohen HS, Edelstein SL: A case-control study of routine and death scene sleep position and sudden infant death syndrome in southern California. JAMA 1995;273:790.

Spiers PS, Guntheroth WG: Recommendations to avoid the prone sleeping position and recent statistics for sudden infant death syndrome in the United States. Arch Pediatr Adolesc Med 1994;148:141.

SHOCK

Astiz ME et al: Pathophysiology and treatment of circulatory shock. Crit Care Clin 1993;2:183.

Saez-LLorens X, McCracken GH: Sepsis syndrome and septic shock in pediatrics: Current concepts, terminology, pathophysiology, and management. J Pediatr 1993;123:497.

Tobias JD: Shock in children: The first 60 minutes. Pediatr Ann 1996;25:330.

SEIZURE DISORDERS

Mizrahi EM: Seizure disorders in children. Curr Opin Pediatr 1994;6:642.

Working Group on Status Epilepticus: Treatment of convulsive status epilepticus. JAMA 1993;270:854.

CHILDHOOD POISONING

Gaar GG: Gastrointestinal decontamination for acute poisoning by ingestion: Prevention of absorption of toxic compounds. J Fla Med Assoc 1994;81:747.

Henretig FM et al: Toxicologic emergencies. Pages 745–801 in: Fleisher G, Ludwig S (editors): *Textbook of Pediatric Emergency Medicine,* 3rd ed. Williams & Wilkins, 1993.

Kulig K: Initial management of ingestions of toxic substances. N Engl J Med 1992;326:1677.

Litovitz TL et al: 1994 Annual Report of the American Association of Poison Control Centers. A toxic exposure surveillance system. Am J Emerg Med 1995;13:551.

Lovejoy FH et al: Common etiologies and new approaches to management of poisoning in pediatric practice. Curr Opin Pediatr 1993;5:524.

Acetaminophen

Anker AL, Smilkstein MJ: Acetaminophen: Concepts and controversies. Emerg Med Clin North Am 1994;12:335.

Smilkstein MJ et al: Efficacy of oral N-acetylcysteine in the treatment of acetaminophen overdose. N Engl J Med 1988;319:1557.

Tricyclic Antidepressants

Berkovitch M et al: Assessment of the terminal 40 millisecond QRS vector in children with a history of tricyclic antidepressant ingestion. Pediatr Emerg Care 1995;11:75.

Goodwin DA et al: Extracorporeal membrane oxygenation support for cardiac dysfunction from tricyclic antidepressant overdose. Crit Care Med 1993;21:625.

Haddad LM: Managing tricyclic antidepressant overdose. Am Fam Physician 1992;46:153.

Iron

Anderson AL: Iron poisoning in children. Curr Opin Pediatr 1994;6:289.

Mills KC, Curry SC: Acute iron poisoning. Emerg Med Clin North Am 1994;12:397.

Tenenbein M, Rodgers GC: The four A's of decreasing the toll of childhood non-poisoning deaths. Arch Fam Med 1994;3:754.

Ethanol

Bleich HL, Boro ES: Metabolic and hepatic effects of alcohol. N Engl J Med 1977;296:612.

Leung AKC: Ethyl alcohol ingestion in children, a 15-year review. Clin Pediatr 1986;25:617.

Olson KR, McGuigan MA: Childhood poisoning. Page 801 in: Rudolph AM (editor): *Rudolph's Pediatrics,* 19th ed. Appleton & Lange, 1991.

Caustic Agents

Gorman RL et al: Initial symptoms as predictors of esophageal injury in alkaline corrosive ingestions. Am J Emerg Med 1992;10:189.

Howell JM et al: Steroids for the treatment of corrosive esophageal injury: A statistical analysis of past studies. Am J Emerg Med 1992;10:421.

Lahoti D, Broor SL: Corrosive injury to the upper gastrointestinal tract. Indian J Gastroenterol 1993;12:135.

CHILD ABUSE

Adams JA et al: Examination findings in legally confirmed child sexual abuse: It's normal to be normal. Pediatrics 1994;94:310.

Leventhal JM et al: Fractures in young children: Distinguishing child abuse from unintentional injuries. Am J Dis Child 1993;147:87.

Schwartz AJ, Ricci LR: How accurately can bruises be aged in abused children? Literature review and synthesis. Pediatrics 1996;97:254.

Stier DM et al: Are children born to young mothers at increased risk of maltreatment? Pediatrics 1993;91:642.

THE INJURED CHILD

Schwarz DF: Violence. Pediatr Rev 1996;17:197.

Head Trauma

Goldstein B, Powers KS: Head trauma in children. Pediatr Rev 1994;15:213.

Near-Drowning

Levin DL et al: Drowning and near drownings. Pediatr Clin North Am 1993;40:321.

Burns

Carvajal HF: Fluid resuscitation of pediatric burn victims: A critical appraisal. Pediatr Nephrol 1994;8:357.

Deaths resulting from residential fires—United States, 1991. MMWR 1994;43:901.

Smoke Inhalation

Ruddy RM: Smoke inhalation injury. Pediatr Clin North Am 1994;41:317.

Drug Disposition & Therapy

Robert H. Levin, PharmD

GENERAL PHARMACOKINETIC PRINCIPLES

Drug disposition in children varies with the maturity of the child's organ systems. When a drug is given to a child, it must reach the plasma in a therapeutic concentration to be effective. It must be absorbed from the administration site, eg, the gastrointestinal (GI) tract, muscle, or skin; distributed into the plasma; and carried to tissues and receptors. It is then removed from the tissues and receptors, usually by metabolism, and finally eliminated from the body. Metabolic enzymes in the liver and other tissues alter many drugs to more water-soluble inactive metabolites for easier elimination. Drugs and their metabolites are then usually eliminated by the kidney but may also be excreted by the GI or biliary tracts.

DRUG ABSORPTION

GI Route

Oral administration of drugs is the most common method used in children. Neonates, compared with infants and older children, have less acid secretion in the stomach for the first few weeks after birth; this allows acid-labile drugs, like the penicillins, to be better absorbed (Table 11–1). Other drugs, not dependent on GI acidity, are not affected; drugs that are better absorbed in acid media have decreased absorption in neonates (Table 11–1). GI transit time is more rapid for the first 5 years of childhood, and this especially affects absorption of drugs administered in a sustained-release preparation. Thus, Theodur Sprinkles are only about 50% absorbed.

The rectal route can also be used in neonates and children. Absorption in the rectum is usually adequate but may be erratic when aminophylline suppositories are used. Glycerin, acetaminophen, and aspirin are commonly administered in suppositories and usually achieve adequate absorption.

Parenteral Route

When the oral and rectal routes cannot be used, the parenteral route is often used. Drugs administered intravenously achieve the highest serum concentrations because they are already in solution. Drugs given intramuscularly achieve serum concentrations that are dependent on perfusion of the muscle and the type of vehicle used to solubilize the drug. Drugs in solution (eg, gentamicin) are absorbed best, followed by those in aqueous suspension (eg, procaine penicillin). Neonates requiring parenteral medication should receive it intravenously and not by the subcutaneous or intramuscular (IM) route. The subcutaneous tissue and limited musculature of neonates are poorly perfused and therefore are subject to the development of sterile abscesses at the injection site. If IM injection is required in an infant 2 months of age or older (eg, for diphtheria, pertussis, and tetanus vaccine), the lateral thigh muscle should be used.

Topical Application

Neonates have a relatively high surface area of skin to body weight, and the skin is much thinner and more hydrated than in children and adults. Because percutaneous absorption of drugs is inversely proportionate to skin thickness and proportionate to skin hydration, neonates absorb much more through their skin than do older children. In fact, some drugs are administered topically because they absorb well in neonates (eg, a specially formulated theophylline gel). Others have caused toxicity when applied in excess amounts (eg, hexachlorophene and lindane).

DRUG DISTRIBUTION

Drugs are distributed from the plasma to different organs largely on the basis of their affinity for tissues with high water or lipid content. Drugs that are more water-sol-

Table 11–1. Comparing oral drug absorption in neonates and older infants and children.[1]

Drug	Oral Absorption in Neonates
Ampicillin	Increased
Nafcillin	Increased
Penicillin G	Increased
Diazepam	Normal
Digoxin	Normal
Sulfonamides	Normal
Acetaminophen	Decreased
Iron	Decreased
Phenobarbital	Decreased
Phenytoin	Decreased

[1]Modified and reproduced, with permission, from Levin RH: Principles of drug disposition and therapy in neonates, infants, and children. In: Rudolph AM et al (editors): *Rudolph's Pediatrics,* 20th ed. Appleton & Lange, 1996.

uble or more polar in nature (eg, gentamicin) reach higher concentrations in body organs with high water content (kidneys, heart, liver, muscle, bone, and GI tract) compared with drugs (eg, diazepam) that are more soluble in tissues with high lipid content (adipose tissue and the central nervous system). However, the amount of body water changes with development (Table 11–2). In premature infants, water represents 85% of body weight (60% as extracellular), whereas in the 1-year-old child it represents only 60% (40% extracellular water). When the percentage of extracellular water is high, as in the neonate, a drug must be given in a larger dose on a milligram per kilogram basis to achieve the same serum concentration (eg, tobramycin is given in a dose of 7.5 mg/kg/d in a 2-month-old infant and 6 mg/kg/d in an adolescent. The changing percentages of extracellular versus intracellular water during the first year of life also account for the changing volumes of distribution of a number of drugs. The volumes of distribution for the following drugs illustrate this point: phenytoin, 1 L in children younger than 1 year and 0.65 L in those older than 2 years; theophylline, 1 L in children younger than 1 year and 0.48 L in those older than 1 year; and aminoglycosides, 0.5 L in those younger than 5 years and 0.25 L in those older than 5 years.

Table 11–2. Percentages of body water in children.[1]

Age	Extracellular H_2O (%)	Total Body H_2O (%)
Premature infant	60	85
Full-term infant	55	75
5-month-old child	50	60
1-year-old child	40	60
Adolescent	40	60

[1]Modified and reproduced, with permission, from Levin RH: Principles of drug disposition and therapy in neonates, infants, and children. In: Rudolph AM et al (editors): *Rudolph's Pediatrics,* 20th ed. Appleton & Lange, 1996.

Protein binding also may affect the distribution of drugs. Acidic drugs (aspirin, phenytoin, and sulfonamides) bind to serum albumin, whereas basic drugs (lidocaine and quinidine) bind to serum globulins. Acidic drugs displace bilirubin from albumin binding sites, and sulfonamides can cause kernicterus in neonates who are unable to metabolize the displaced bilirubin. Neonates also have low albumin concentrations and cannot bind drugs like phenytoin as well as adults can. In neonates, 70% of phenytoin binds to albumin, compared with 90% in adults. Because the unbound fraction of phenytoin is the active portion, neonates with a serum level of 10 μg/mL have 3 μg/mL of active drug, compared with adults, who have only 1 μg/mL of active drug. In other words, a therapeutic phenytoin total serum concentration of 15 μg/mL in adults is equivalent to a serum level of about 5 μg/mL in neonates.

DRUG METABOLISM

The predominant pathway for drug metabolism is the liver. There are two major metabolic pathways: phase 1 and phase 2 reactions. Phase 1 reactions metabolize endogenous substances or drugs and consist of the mixed function oxidase system, the cytochrome P-450 system, and the *N*-demethylation pathways. Premature and full-term neonates have 50–75% of these enzymes compared with the levels in infants, so that drugs metabolized by these systems (phenytoin, phenobarbital, diazepam, caffeine, theophylline, meperidine) may have higher serum concentrations for the same relative dose in neonates than in older infants. Phase 2 reactions conjugate endogenous compounds or specific drugs and their metabolites into water-soluble entities by glucuronidation (acetaminophen, chloramphenicol, steroids, morphine, and bilirubin), sulfation (steroids and acetaminophen), or acetylation (sulfonamides and isoniazid [INH]). The phase 2 reactions are usually adequate to metabolize most drugs and endogenous compounds by 1–2 weeks after birth in full-term infants. The doses of the drugs mentioned above must be adjusted in the first few weeks of neonatal life because the longer half-lives may predispose the infant to drug toxicity (Table 11–3). Other drugs have caused serious problems in neonates when their dosage has not been adjusted, eg, chloramphenicol can cause gray baby syndrome.

DRUG ELIMINATION

The primary route of elimination of drugs is via the kidney. Drugs are also eliminated via the biliary, GI, and respiratory tracts, but to a much lesser degree. Renal excretion of drugs depends on maturation of the kidney. Compared with adults, full-term neonates have only about 30% of glomerular filtration rate (GFR) and 25% of maximal tubular secretion (MTS) (Table 11–4). Because of this decreased renal elimination, the doses of drugs dependent

Table 11–3. Changing half-lives of drugs in neonates and adults.[1]

Drug	Neonatal Age	Neonates $(t_{1/2})$ (hours)	Adults $(t_{1/2})$ (hours)
Acetaminophen		2.2–5	1.9–2.2
Diazepam		25–100	15–25
Digoxin		60–107	30–60
Phenobarbital	0–5 days	200	64–140
	5–15 days	100	
	1–30 mo	50	
Phenytoin	0–2 days	80	12–18
	3–14 days	18	
	14–50 days	6	
Salicylate		4.5–11	2–4
Theophylline	Neonate	20–30	5–6
	Child	3–4	

[1]Reproduced, with permission, from Levin RH: Principles of drug disposition and therapy in neonates, infants, and children. In: Rudolph AM et al (editors): *Rudolph's Pediatrics*, 20th ed. Appleton & Lange, 1996.

on renal excretion (penicillins, cephalosporins, aminoglycosides, probenecid, furosemide, thiazide diuretics, and aspirin) must be adjusted in neonates on the basis of both gestational age and weight. By 1 month of age, the normal infant has 50% adult values for both GFR and MTS and therefore does not require drug dose to be corrected for decreased renal elimination. If, however, the infant or older child has decreased renal function, it is necessary to measure and calculate creatinine clearance (ClCr) to adjust properly the doses of drugs excreted by the kidney.

Several formulas are available to predict ClCr in children aged 1–18 years; one of the more accurate ones is depicted in equation 1:

$$\text{ClCr (mL/min)} = \left[\frac{(0.48)\,(\text{Height [cm]})}{\text{SrCr}}\right] \times \left[\frac{\text{wt (kg)}}{70}\right]^{0.73} \quad (1)$$

In this equation, the actual ClCr is determined using the measured serum creatinine (SrCr), adjusted by the child's body surface area. Accurate calculation of ClCr in infants younger than 1 year has been difficult. Winter and Wong have developed equation 2 to use for preterm and term neonates and infants up to 1 year of age:

$$\text{ClCr (mL/min)} = 120\ \text{mL/min} \times \left[\frac{\text{wt (kg)}}{70}\right]^{0.73}$$
$$\times \frac{0.4\ \text{mg/dL}}{\text{SrCr}} \times \text{Factor} \quad (2)$$

Correction factors:
GA < 36 wk and < 10 day old: 0.18
GA ≥ 36 wk and < 10 day old: 0.25
GA < 36 wk and > 10 day old: 0.36
GA ≥ 36 wk and > 10 day old: 0.50
Age > 1 month but < 1 year: 0.5 + age in months/24

Table 11–4. Development of the kidney in children.

Age	Glomerular Filtration Rate (mL/min/1.73 M²)	Maximal Tubular Secretion (mg/min/1.73 M²)
Full-term neonate	33	16
1 mo	50	30
2 mo	70	50
6 mo	110	60
3 y	130	75

Table 11–5. Usual therapeutic serum drug concentrations.

Drug	Therapeutic Level	Toxic Level
Antibiotics		
Amikacin	Peak: 20–35 µg/mL	> 35 µg/mL
	Trough: 1–10 µg/mL	> 10 µg/mL
Chloramphenicol	Peak: 10–20 µg/mL	> 25 µg/mL
Gentamicin	Peak: 4–8 µg/mL	> 12 µg/mL
	Trough: < 2 µg/mL	> 2 µg/mL
Netilmicin	Peak: 4–10 µg/mL	> 10 µg/mL
	Trough: < 2 µg/mL	> 2 µg/mL
Tobramycin	Peak: 4–8 µg/mL	> 12 µg/mL
	Trough: < 2 µg/mL	> 2 µg/mL
Vancomycin	Peak: 20–50 µg/mL	> 80 µg/mL
	Trough: 5–10 µg/mL	
Anticonvulsants		
Carbamazepine	4–12 µg/mL	> 12 µg/mL
Ethosuximide	40–80 µg/mL	> 100 µg/mL
Phenytoin	< 12 weeks old:	> 20 µg/mL
	6–14 µg/mL	> 20 µg/mL
	> 12 weeks old:	
	10–20 µg/mL	
Phenobarbital	15–30 µg/mL	> 40 µg/mL
Primidone	5–15 µg/mL	> 15 µg/mL
	15–30 µg/mL	> 40 µg/mL
	(phenobarbital)	
Valproic acid	50–125 µg/mL	> 150 µg/mL
Antifungals		
Flucytosine	40–80 µg/mL	> 125 µg/mL
Antineoplastic agents		
Cyclosporin	100–400 µg/mL	> 400 µg/mL
Methotrexate	24 h: 10 mol/L	> 50 mol/L
	48 h: 1 mol/L	> 5 mol/L
	72 h: < 0.2 mol/L	> 0.2 mol/L
Antipsychotic agents		
Lithium	0.8–1.5 meq/L	> 1.5 meq/L
Antipyretic/analgesic		
Aspirin	15–30 mg/dL	> 50 mg/dL
Bronchodilators		
Theophylline	Asthma: 10–20 µg/mL	> 20 µg/mL
	Neonatal apnea:	> 20 µg/mL
	5–10 µg/mL	
Cardiovascular agents		
Digoxin	0.5–2 ng/mL	> 3 ng/mL
Lidocaine	2–5 µg/mL	> 6 µg/mL
Quinidine	1–5 µg/mL	> 7 µg/mL
Procainamide	4–10 µg/mL	> 10 µg/mL
	10–30 µg/mL (+ NAPA)	> 30 µg/mL

NAPA = *N*-acetyl-*p*-aminophenol.

Table 11–6. Autonomic clinical symptoms occurring with drug overdoses.

Systems Affected	Sympathetic or Sympatholytic Effects				Parasympathetic or Parasympatholytic Effects			
	Sympatholytic (α- or β-Blockers)	α-Agonist	β-Agonist	Mixed α- & β-Agonist	Nicotinic	Muscarinic	Mixed Muscarinic & Nicotinic	Antimuscarinic (Anticholinergic)
Examples of drugs	Clonidine Methyldopa Propranolol Phentolamine Sedative hypnotics (alcohol, narcotics, barbiturates)	Phenylephrine Methoxamine Phenylpropanolamine	Albuterol (β₂) Terbutaline (β₂) Caffeine Theophylline	Amphetamine Cocaine LSD, THC PCP	Nicotine	Bethanechol Pilocarpine	Organophosphates	Atropine Antidepressants Antihistamines Antipsychotics
Pupils	Constrict	Dilate	↔ or dilate	Dilate[5]	Constrict or dilate	Constrict	Constrict then dilate	Dilate[2]
Blood pressure	↓[6]	↑	↓ due to vasodilation	↑	↑ or ↓	↓	↓ then ↑	↑
Heart rate	↓[6,7]	↓ due to reflex	↑ due to chronotropic effect	↑ even with hypertension	↑ or ↓	↓	↓ then ↑	↑
GI motility	↓	↓	↓	↓	↑	↑	↑ then ↓	↓
Mucous membrane	↔	Dry	Moist	Dry[5]	↑ salivation	Excess moisture	Excess moisture	Dry
Sweating	↔	Yes	Excess unlikely	Marked	Yes	Excessive	Excessive	Absent
Respiration	↓	↔	↑	↑	Weakness	Excessive Bronchorrhea, wheeze	Excessive Bronchorrhea	↑ or ↓
CNS effects	↓[6]	↔	↑ seizures[1]	↑ seizures[5]	↑ seizures	↔	↑ seizures	Delirium, agitation, seizures, coma[3]
Striated muscles	↓	↔	Tremor	Tremor	Fasciculations	↔	Fasciculations	
Temperature	↓	↔	↔	↑	↔	↓	↓	↑ or ↓[4]

[1] Seizures with overdoses are probably not β₂ mediated.
[2] Phenothiazine antipsychotics cause small pupils because of adrenergic blockade.
[3] Seizures are not specifically caused by anticholinergic effects.
[4] Phenothiazines decrease temperature secondary to vasodilation.
[5] PCP usually does not change pupil size (it may cause miosis in 30% of children); it causes vertical nystagmus, increased mucous membrane secretion, waxing and waning CNS symptoms, seizures, and catatonia.
[6] β-Blockers can cause seizures with overdoses, and those with intrinsic sympathomimetic activity, eg, carteolol, penbutolol, and pindolol, may cause tachycardia and hypertension.
[7] Phentolamine causes tachycardia secondary to a direct stimulation of the heart.

LSD = lysergic acid diethylamide; PCP = phencyclidine; THC= tetrahydrocannabinol; GI = gastrointestinal; CNS = central nervous system; ↓ = decreased effect; ↑ = increased effect; ↔ = little or no effect.

The factors used in equation 2 are gestational age (GA), chronologic age, SrCr, and the child's body surface area. For comparison, the formula usually used to calculate adult ClCr is shown in equation 3 (predicting ClCr in adults):

$$\text{ClCr (mL/min)} = \frac{(140 - \text{age}) \times \text{wt (kg)}}{72 \times \text{SrCr}} \quad (3)$$

For females, multiply the above equation by a factor of 0.8

DRUG MONITORING

Drug Concentrations

Serum concentrations can be very useful for monitoring therapy, ensuring compliance, and avoiding toxicity. Except for antibiotics, peak serum concentrations are not often used to measure clinical efficacy against the minimum inhibitory concentration (MIC) of known organisms. Peak serum concentrations are drawn as early as 30 minutes after an infusion of aminoglycosides to as long as 4–6 hours after an IV or oral dose of digoxin. For most drugs, therapeutic serum concentrations should be measured at trough concentration, or just before the next dose. Trough levels for aminoglycosides are the exception to this recommendation. With these drugs, trough levels are used only to monitor toxicity; thus, a level of less than 2 μg/mL is desired to prevent renal toxicity. If the trough concentration is within the therapeutic range and the patient is responding to therapy as desired, without drug side effects, no dosage adjustment is necessary. If the patient is not responding to therapy and has no drug side effects, an increase in dosage is warranted even if the drug serum level is in the therapeutic range. If the drug level is in the therapeutic range and the patient is experiencing side effects but not therapeutic effects, an increase in dosage is not warranted. In this case, the addition of another drug to the therapy may be required. Although it is not necessary to measure serum concentrations of most drugs routinely, it is very useful with some drugs (eg, aminoglycosides, chloramphenicol, theophylline, and anticonvulsants). Table 11–5 lists some drugs commonly used in children and their usual therapeutic serum and toxic levels. Therapy maintained in the therapeutic range usually will not cause side effects. If, however, excessive doses of drugs are administered, or if an accidental ingestion occurs and toxic drug levels are reached, symptoms of overdosage may appear.

Drug Interactions

Whenever a new drug is added to a patient's therapy regimen, a drug interaction could occur. One drug may interfere with another by affecting its absorption, distribution, metabolism, or excretion. Antacids containing aluminum, calcium, or magnesium decrease the absorption of tetracyclines by forming insoluble complexes. The absorption of digoxin is decreased by kaolin-pectin mixtures used for diarrheal illnesses or metoclopramide. Drugs that are highly protein bound in serum can have their systemic distribution enhanced and possibly lead to toxicity when they are displaced from their binding sites; for example, phenytoin can be displaced by valproic acid, and warfarin can be displaced by chloral hydrate or sulfonamides. The metabolism of many drugs is inhibited, which causes an increase in their serum concentrations and possible toxicity, eg, theophylline inhibited by erythromycin or cimetidine, digoxin inhibited by amiodarone, or phenytoin inhibited by cimetidine. The metabolism of other drugs is enhanced, causing a decreased serum level and lack of efficacy, eg, theophylline metabolism enhanced by phenytoin or phenobarbital, or corticosteroids enhanced by carbamazepine. Finally, increased serum levels can occur when one drug interferes with the renal elimination of another drug; for example, probenecid affects penicillins, and sodium bicarbonate (causing alkalinized urine) affects quinidine or amphetamines.

Miscellaneous Dosage Considerations

The particular characteristics of the different dosage forms of drugs must be considered. Sustained-release tablets should not be crushed or chewed, as this destroys their sustained action. However, sustained-release capsules may be opened and the beads taken with liquids or applesauce without affecting the sustained-release proper-

Table 11–7. Drugs excreted in breast milk.[1]

Drugs contraindicated during breast-feeding
Amethopterin
Bromocriptine
Cimetidine
Clemastine
Cyclophosphamide
Other antineoplastic agents
Ergotamine
Gold salts
Methimazole
Phenindione
Thiouracil
Abuse drugs in large doses
Stimulants (eg, cocaine, amphetamines)
Narcotics (eg, heroin)
Barbiturates (eg, pentobarbital, phencyclidine, marijuana, nicotine)
Breast-feeding may resume after these drugs are effectively eliminated from the body
Cascara
Lithium
Metronidazole
Radiopharmaceuticals
Gallium-69
Iodine-125
Iodine-131
Radioactive sodium
Technetium-99m

[1]Data modified and reproduced, with permission, from American Academy of Pediatrics Committee on Drugs: Transfer of drugs and other chemicals into human milk. Pediatrics 1989;84:924.

ties. Low-sodium and sugar-free preparations are also available. Most oral liquid preparations can be mixed together before ingestion to facilitate a child's acceptance of the drug. However, many parenteral medications are incompatible when mixed together, eg, calcium preparations and sodium bicarbonate or diazepam with any other drug.

Toxicity From Drug Overdosage

Many drugs taken by children affect the autonomic nervous system and cause predictable side effects (Table 11–6). When using the information on this chart, the most useful changes on which to concentrate are those affecting the GI tract, pupils, sweating, and cardiovascular system.

Toxic effects from drugs can also mimic symptoms from a number of disease states. Certain drugs can cause changes in the respiratory rate, central nervous system, or muscular system and may affect temperature. Drugs can also change the color of urine and feces, eg, red urine from rifampin or phenytoin or black stools from iron or antacids. This change, especially when the color becomes red, may be mistaken for bleeding.

DRUGS IN BREAST MILK

All drugs taken by the mother that achieve a maternal serum level will partition into breast milk. Most of these drugs are present in such small quantities that they pose no threat to the infant. Several publications provide detailed information about excretion of drugs in breast milk. Several drugs are absolutely contraindicated during the whole course of breast-feeding. With others, breast-feeding should be discontinued until the drug has been excreted by the mother (Table 11–7).

REFERENCES

American Academy of Pediatrics Committee on Drugs: Transfer of drugs and other chemicals into human milk. Pediatrics 1994;93:137.

Atkinson HC et al: Drugs in human milk. Clinical pharmacokinetic considerations. Clin Pharmacokinet 1988;14:217.

Bolinger AM: Drug interactions. Page 791 in: Rudolph AM et al (editors): *Rudolph's Pediatrics,* 20th ed. Appleton & Lange, 1996.

Levin RH: Principles of drug disposition and therapy in neonates, infants, and children. Page 787 in: Rudolph AM et al (editors): *Rudolph's Pediatrics,* 20th ed. Appleton & Lange, 1996.

Taketomo CK et al: Page 854 in: *Pediatric Dosage Handbook,* 3rd ed. Lexi-Comp, 1996–1997.

Wong AF: Pharmacokinetics. Page 794 in: Rudolph AM et al (editors): *Rudolph's Pediatrics,* 20th ed. Appleton & Lange, 1996.

12

Skin

Sheila Fallon Friedlander, MD, & Lawrence F. Eichenfield, MD

CLINICAL EVALUATION OF THE SKIN

Skin-related disorders account for approximately 30% of all pediatric visits. The skin is the most accessible body organ and thus provides the first visible clues to many underlying infectious, metabolic, and neurologic disorders. Therefore, understanding the basic terminology and principles of dermatologic diagnosis is important for all pediatric practitioners. Although there are thousands of skin disorders, a much smaller number account for the vast majority of patient visits. This chapter presents the more common entities and reviews an approach to dermatologic diagnosis.

PRINCIPLES OF DIAGNOSIS

Successful evaluation of the patient depends on obtaining an accurate history, performing an appropriate examination, collecting necessary laboratory data, and generating a differential diagnosis. When evaluating patients with skin disorders, it is often appropriate to perform a cursory examination of the skin lesion while simultaneously obtaining a focused history of present illness. Certain basic historical facts must always be elicited: location of the problem; duration of the lesion or rash; associated symptoms, such as itch or pain; and previous treatment. One must also inquire whether the patient has underlying illnesses or any allergies or takes any medications. With this information, one can perform a directed physical examination and then expand history-taking and examination as appropriate. Although focused histories and examinations are often adequate for diagnosis, a complete mucocutaneous examination is appropriate in most patients.

Basic Approach

Evaluation begins with assessment of the characteristics of the individual lesions. The color is noted first, then the morphology or shape of the lesion. Primary lesions may be macules (flat), papules or nodules (raised, palpable lesions), flat-topped plaques, edematous wheals, or blisters of varying size (vesicles and bullae) (See definitions, Table 12–1). Identification of secondary changes is important for diagnosis. Often the primary lesions take on secondary or superimposed changes that can either complicate or assist in diagnosis. Scaling or crusting may be late signs of dermatitis. Lichenification is a change secondary to chronic rubbing, and, along with excoriations, reveals a pruritic skin disease, such as atopic dermatitis. Erosions, fissures, and ulcerations are skin disruptions of various depths. Table 12–2 lists the most commonly encountered secondary changes of skin lesions.

The examiner should next note the configurations, ie, how the individual lesions are arranged. Skin lesions in a linear pattern may be from congenital anomalies (epidermal nervus) or from skin diseases that localize in areas of trauma or scratching (Koebner phenomenon). Annular lesions may be caused by tinea infection (ringworm) or a variety of other noninfectious disorders (eg, nummular eczema and granuloma annulare). Table 12–3 lists the most common configurations and examples of each. Finally, identifying that distribution (Table 12–4) will usually limit the diagnostic possibilities. Does the rash involve the entire body or is it limited to the hands and feet? For instance, if a rash presents in a single dermatomal area, it is unlikely to be measles and most probably is herpes zoster.

Two other morphologic descriptions are commonly used to categorize a series of diseases: the papulosquamous and eczematous disorders. Papulosquamous (scaling papules) disease refers to the group that shares the common characteristics of discrete scaling papules, usually of an erythematous or violaceous color. Eczema, on the other hand, refers to less–well-defined papules or plaques that usually show some disruption of the epidermis, with either oozing, fissuring, or scale crusting present. With time, eczematous lesions often become lichenified, or thickened, because of chronic rubbing.

Patient age, personal and family history, and knowledge of infectious diseases that might be prevalent in the

Table 12–1. Terminology: Primary skin lesions and morphologic patterns.

Macule: Flat area of circumscribed color change; the lesion is not palpable
Patch: Nonspecific term generally referring to larger macules
Papule: Raised palpable lesion < 0.5 cm
Nodule: Papule that has enlarged in all three dimensions: length, width, and depth
Plaque: Flat-topped lesion > 1 cm in diameter horizontally but lacking significant depth or height
Wheal: Edematous or fluid-filled area of dermal edema without epidermal changes; classic lesion of urticaria
Vesicle: Blister containing clear fluid
Bulla: Vesicle > 0.5 cm
Pustule: Vesicle containing milky or purulent fluid
Papulosquamous: Sharply marginated scaly violaceous papules or plaques
Eczematous: Inflammatory lesions with oozing, crusting, or thickening (lichenification)

community should also be considered in arriving at a diagnosis. Careful clinical inspection of primary and secondary lesion morphology, configuration, and distribution, along with patient age and history, will help with diagnosis. The skin conditions presenting in infants and children are listed in Tables 12–5 and 12–6 on the basis of the description of the lesion.

Physical Signs & Laboratory Evaluation

Several physical signs and laboratory evaluations are of particular use in the diagnosis of skin disease. **Dermatographism** refers to a change that occurs when the skin is stroked lightly with an item such as the blunt end of a pen. The normal response is mild erythema at the stroked site. In patients with underlying urticaria, a linear wheal also develops at the stroked site; this is referred to as **red dermatographism.** In some patients with atopic dermatitis, a white wheal develops and is therefore referred to as **white dermatographism.** Although these signs are not pathognomonic, they can provide supportive evidence of the appropriate diagnosis.

Table 12–2. Terminology: Secondary skin changes.

Erosion: Disruption of the skin lacking part or all of the epidermis, which is usually moist and red; lesions are sometimes covered by a crust
Ulcer: Lesion deeper than an erosion in which part or all of the dermis (as well as the epidermis) is missing
Fissure: Linear, wedge-shaped erosion or ulcer
Scale: Visible flake of stratum corneum on the skin surface
Crust: Yellowish, firm covering on the skin surface consisting of dried plasma or exudate
Excoriation: Scratch mark, usually linear or oval depression in the skin
Lichenification: Thickening of the epidermis due to chronic rubbing
Atrophy: Area of depressed or thin skin
Sclerosis: Firm, smooth induration or thickening of the skin

The **Darier sign** refers to the elicitation of a hive or blister when one repeatedly strokes a lesion of mastocytosis. This results from the release of histamine from an excess number of mast cells present at the site. The **Auspitz sign** occurs when the adherent scale from a lesion of psoriasis is picked off, revealing multiple pinpoint areas of bleeding. It represents trauma induced to the increased numbers of dilated vessels found in the dermal papillae of a psoriatic lesion. The **Nikolsky sign** refers to the ability to spread or enlarge a blister by applying pressure over the center of the lesion. This occurs in diseases such as staphylococcal scalded skin syndrome or in pemphigus.

Potassium Hydroxide Preparation (KOH). This is probably the single most useful laboratory examination in dermatology. It can be used when searching for dermatophytes; yeasts, such as *Candida* and tinea versicolor; and parasites, such as scabies. A superficial cutaneous scraping is performed to obtain as much scale as is reasonably possible. In the case of scabies, one should always scrape the areas of highest yield (burrows, hands, feet, and, in teenagers, genitalia). It is often necessary to draw a bit of blood at the site, and it is always necessary to sample more than one lesion. The scrapings should be placed on a slide, a few drops of potassium hydroxide 10% solution applied, and a coverslip placed over the specimen. It is often advisable to do this immediately after obtaining the specimen, because scales may blow off the slide. One should firmly press the coverslip against the sample, then gently heat the specimen. The slide is then examined under the microscope at low to medium power with the light source damped. Focusing up and down in the plane of the specimen is helpful, as the walls of dermatophytes appear birefringent. Dermatophytes appear as septate hyphae, whereas yeasts appear as budding spores with short nonseptate hyphae. Scabies eggs and feces (scybala) are seen more often than the mite itself.

Skin Biopsy. A skin biopsy specimen is particularly useful to identify inflammatory lesions and possible neoplasias. The involved area is carefully cleaned and anesthetized. An appropriate-sized incision or punch is made and the tissue gently removed, taking care never to squeeze the sample. The wound edges are then brought together and closed with suture material. In this manner, material can be obtained for routine histology (hematoxylin and eosin stain), immunofluorescence microscopy, or electron microscopy.

SKIN DISEASES OF THE NEONATE

Neonates possess distinct characteristics that must be considered when evaluating and treating dermatologic diseases. In addition, some disorders occur only or more

Table 12–3. Terminology: Configuration (pattern of arrangement of lesion).

Name	Characteristics	Example
Linear	In a straight line	Linear epidermal nevus
Grouped	Clustered	Herpes simplex virus
Annular	Ringlike, oval with central clearing	Tinea corporis
Discrete	Having well-defined distinct borders	Guttate psoriasis
Confluent	Individual lesions that are ill-defined and tend to merge	Urticaria, measles
Target	Having a bull's-eye appearance; concentric rings	Erythema multiforme
Zosteriform	Grouped in a dermatomal pattern	Zoster
		Urticaria
Polycyclic	Oval lesions with multiple ringlike coalescent borders	Tinea cruris
Serpiginous	Twisted, spiral, or snakelike	Erythema marginatum

commonly in the neonatal period. The newborn infant has less–well-developed adnexal structures, no protective endogenous flora, and an increased susceptibility to external irritants. Of importance is the increased relative absorption of any topical agents. The neonate also differs in ability to bind, metabolize, and excrete drugs.

PHYSIOLOGIC & TRANSIENT CHANGES

Newborns are subjected to a number of conditions that can lead to drying and damage. Skin irritation and subsequent breakdown can result from frequent manipulation, application of adhesive tapes and monitors, and exposure to phototherapy. Small breaks in the skin can then serve as portals of entry for bacteria or other organisms. Application of moisturizers can rehydrate the skin and may help decrease the incidence of skin-related infections in premature infants.

A number of "normal" changes occur in the first weeks of life. The most common are briefly discussed below. The following discussion reviews these disorders, as well as other serious conditions with which they can be confused.

Vascular Changes

Acrocyanosis. A purplish-blue discoloration of the lips, hands, and feet is quite common in newborn infants. This is most noticeable during periods of chilling or crying and does not indicate any underlying pathology.

Cutis Marmorata. A bluish-purple mottling of the trunk and extremities, which is reticulated, often occurs when newborns are chilled. It probably results from vasodilation of peripheral small vessels. This condition usually resolves after 2–3 weeks and usually is not serious. Persistence of this condition may occasionally be associated with an underlying condition, such as Cornelia de Lange, Down syndrome, or trisomy 18.

Cutis Marmorata Telangiectatica Congenita. This consists of a persistent bluish mottling that extends during the first few weeks of life and is present on the trunk, extremities, and, occasionally, the face. Atrophy and ulcerations can occur; these tend to improve or resolve with time. This disorder has been associated with other vascular abnormalities, glaucoma, and a variety of other congenital abnormalities, such as cleft lip, syndactyly of the toes, and mental retardation.

Salmon Patches. These vascular stains are frequently noted at birth and commonly occur on the nape of the neck, glabella, and eyelids. In contrast to port-wine stains, these lesions are usually centrally located and fade with time. → smooth prominence of the frontal bone above the root of the nose.

Port-wine Stains. These stains are red, flat, and often unilateral (Figure 12–1). They are most responsive to therapy early in life; if left untreated, they persist and deepen in color over time. If located on the face, the current therapy of choice is the pulsed dye laser, which is usually initiated in early infancy. The possibility of Sturge-Weber syndrome must be considered if such facial vascular stains involve the area of distribution of the trigeminal nerve. This disorder can include cerebral angiomatosis, seizures, and glaucoma, all of which should be considered when a port-wine stain occurs in the distribution of the first branch of the trigeminal nerve. Only a minority of children with port-wine stains in this area will actually have

Table 12–4. Terminology: Distribution (area of the body surface involved).

Name	Characteristics	Example
Generalized	Involving the entire body	Varicella, measles
Localized	Dermatomal, segmental, or limited to a specific area	Zoster
Acral	Favoring face, distal extremities, hands, feet	Erythema multiforme minor, Rocky Mountain spotted fever
Photodistribution	Light-exposed areas	Lupus, photosensitivity eruption
Intertriginous	Where skin rubs against skin (ie, groin, axillae, inframammary)	Seborrheic dermatitis, candidal dermatitis

Table 12–5. Pediatric cutaneous disorders: Neonates.

Generalized vesicopustules	**Flat lesions**
Erythema toxicum	White
Miliaria rubra, crystallina, profunda	Ash-leaf macules
	Hypomelanosis of Ito
Staphylococcal impetigo	Piebaldism
Bacterial sepsis	Nevoid (anemicus,
Congenital cutaneous candidiasis	depigmentosus)
	Brown
Congenital HSV	Mongolian spots
Scabies	Café-au-lait
Transient neonatal pustular	Freckles
melanosis	Lentigo
Incontinentia pigmenti	Transient neonatal pustular
Congenital syphilis	melanosis
Acne	Linear and whorled
Acropustolosis of infancy	hypermelanosis
	Incontinentia pigmenti
Bullae	
Sucking blister	**Eczematous disorders**
Epidermolysis bullosa	Diaper dermatitis
Bullous impetigo	Seborrheic dermatitis
Mastocytosis	Atopic dermatitis
Burns	Scabies
Acrodermatitis enteropathica	Leiner disease
	Acrodermatitis enteropathica
Papules	Severe combined
Red	immunodeficiency syndrome
Erythema toxicum	Histocytosis X
Acne	
Candidiasis	**Vascular lesions**
Insect bites	Purpuric
Epidermal nevus	Congenital infections:
Furuncles	STORCH (syphilis, toxoplasmosis, rubella, cytomegalovirus, HSV)
Brown	
Congenital nevi	
Epidermal nevi	
Mastocytoma	Autoimmune disorders
Yellow	Coagulation defects, disseminated intravascular coagulation
Nevus sebaceous	
Juvenile xanthogranuloma	
Epidermal nevi	Vasculitis
Flesh-colored or white	Blanching
Milia	Nevus simplex ("angel's
Molloscum	kiss," "stork bite")
	Hemangioma
Papulosquamous lesions	Port-wine stain
Tinea	Cutis marmorata
Ichthyosis	
Neonatal lupus	
Candidiasis	
Epidermal nevi	
Psoriasis	

HSV = herpes simplex virus.

Table 12–6. Pediatric cutaneous disorders: Infants and children.

Papulosquamous	**Papules**
Psoriasis	Red
Lichen planus	Acne
Pityriasis rosea	Viral exanthems
Tinea	Arthropod/bug bites
Lupus	Drug reactions
Parapsoriasis, mycosis	Urticaria
fungoides	Erythema multiforme
Secondary syphilis	Furuncles
Keratosis pilaris	Secondary syphilis
Pityriasis rubra pilaris	Cherry angiomas
Pityriasis lichenoides (Mucha-Habermann diagnosis)	Pyogenic granuloma
	White/flesh-colored
	Milia
Eczematous	Keratosis pilaris
Atopic	Molluscum contagiosum
Contact	Verrucae
Nummular	Angiofibroma
Scabies	Granuloma annulare
Polymorphous light eruption	Sarcoidosis
HIV	Epidermal nevus
Dermatitis herpetiformis	Basal cell carcinoma
Histocytosis X	Yellow
Seborrheic dermatitis	Juvenile xanthogranuloma
	Urticaria pigmentosa
Pustular	Nevus sebaceous
Folliculitis	Xanthomas
Bacteremia	Nevus lipomatosis
Acne rosacea	Necrobiosis lipoidica
Pustular psoriasis	diabeticorum
Deep fungal infections	Brown
Impetigo	Nevi
Acropustulosis of infancy	Urticaria pigmentosa
Scabies	Dermatofibroma
Bug bites	Melanoma
Vesicular	**Nodules**
Impetigo	Red
Contact dermatitis	Furuncles
Herpes simplex virus	Abscesses
Varicella zoster virus	Erythema nodosum
Other viral infection (eg, Coxsackievirus)	White/flesh-colored
	Keloid
Panniculitis (lupus, others)	Epidermal inclusion cyst
Burns	Lipoma
Arthropod bites	Pilomatricoma
Erythema multiforme	Corn
Toxic epidermal necrolysis	Brown
Staphylococcal scalded skin	Burns
syndrome	Dermatofibroma
Polymorphous light eruption	
Bullous fixed drug	**Flat Lesions**
Linear IgA disease	White
Dyshidrotic eczema	Pityriasis alba
Epidermolysis bullosa	Vitiligo
	Tinea versicolor
Bullous	Ash-leaf macule
Contact dermatitis	Lichen sclerosus et
Impetigo	atrophicus
Erythema multiforme	Postinflammatory
Arthropod/bug bites	hypopigmentation
Burns	Scleroderma
Pemphigus	Brown
Pemphigoid	Freckle
	Lentigines
Vascular reactions	Nevi (junctional, other)
Telangiectasias	Café-au-lait spot
Hemangiomas	Postinflammatory
Purpura	hyperpigmentation
Venous lake	Tinea versicolor
	Becker nevus
	Incontinentia pigmenti

Sturge-Weber syndrome. All children with suspicious facial lesions must be evaluated for glaucoma because early treatment is crucial for this ophthalmologic complication (Table 12–7).

Hemangiomas. These vascular lesions develop within the first 2–4 weeks of life. They initially appear as flat red patches and subsequently darken and thicken over time. Occasionally they are surrounded by an area of pallor. (See section on Proliferative Vascular Lesions.)

Benign Papular Lesions

Milia. These small (1–2 mm) discrete smooth white

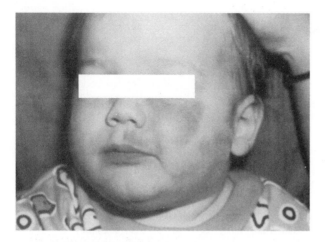

Figure 12–1. Port-wine stain.

papules are most frequently located on the face. They represent small inclusion cysts and require no therapy. They usually resolve within the first few months of life. Persistent or extensive involvement raises the possibility of an underlying disorder, such as oral-facial-digital syndrome.

Sebaceous Gland Hyperplasia. This condition presents as multiple small yellow papules on the nose, cheeks, and upper lip. It may be related to prenatal maternal hormonal stimulation and resolves spontaneously within the first months of life.

Infantile Acne. Little is understood regarding the pathophysiology of "baby acne." It is thought to be the result of maternal hormonal stimulation of infantile sebaceous glands. Neonatal acne usually appears at 2–4 weeks of age and resolves by 6–8 months. Reassurance is the best therapy; in severe cases, however, a weak keratolytic agent, such as 2.5% benzoyl peroxide, may be used. Infantile acne is a more severe eruption that presents later (3–4 months of age) and may persist until 2–3 years of age. In this condition, other topical agents, such as topical or systemic antibiotics and topical retinoids, may be used if the severity warrants such therapy.

Table 12–7. Differences in port-wine stains and hemangiomas.

Port-wine Stains	Hemangiomas
Present at birth	Usually first 2 months of life
Relatively rare (0.1–0.3%)	Common (10% of children)
Macular (flat)	Palpable
Growth proportionate with child	Rapid growth phase (1–6 mo) Plateau phase (6 to 12–18 mo)
No involution: Hypertrophy, nodules in adulthood	Natural involution (30%, 3 years; 50%, 5 years; 80–90%, 9 years)
Pathology: Dilated dermal capillaries; nonproliferative	Pathology: Proliferating angioblastic endothelial cells
Treatment: Laser ablation (pulsed-dye vascular laser)	Treatment: Generally allow natural involution

Subcutaneous Fat Necrosis. The etiology of these lesions is unknown but may relate to trauma in the neonatal period. Such lesions most often present as well-defined firm subcutaneous nodules on exposed surfaces and bony prominences. These lesions usually resolve spontaneously. Extensive calcification of the lesions can occur with liquification, spontaneous drainage, and, occasionally, scarring. Incision and drainage of persistent nodules are recommended. Hypercalcemia is a rare complication; therefore, evaluation of calcium levels is recommended, particularly in extensive cases.

Iatrogenic Lesions

Neonatal skin lesions can result from procedures performed either ante- or postpartum.

Amniocentesis Puncture Marks. Approximately 1% of fetuses undergoing the procedure will have such lesions, which present as pits or depressions. They can occur anywhere, and multiple lesions may be apparent. Digital reductions or losses can occur after chorionic villus sampling undertaken before 10 weeks' gestation.

Fetal Scalp Monitor Trauma. Erythema, bleeding, abscesses, and hair loss can occur at the site of fetal scalp monitor placement. Application of a topical antibiotic may help prevent the development of some of these complications.

Noninvasive Monitor Lesions. Transcutaneous oxygen monitors and pulse oximeters can cause erythema and even blistering burns with necrosis at the site of placement. Careful observation and frequent rotation of the monitored site are important to avoid such complications.

Calcinosis Cutis. These irregular, rock-hard subcutaneous nodules can present at any site of prior trauma but are noted most frequently at the sites of prior heel sticks. The calcium in these lesions usually migrates to the skin surface and extrudes over time.

VESICOPUSTULAR OR BULLOUS/ EROSIVE LESIONS

This category is extensive and best divided on the basis of benign, infectious, or mechanobullous disorders.

Benign Vesicopustular Lesions

These lesions constitute the vast majority of vesicopustular neonatal skin lesions encountered (Table 12–8).

Erythema Toxicum Neonatorum. This condition presents within the first 2 weeks of life. During the first few days of life, a blotchy macular red eruption is noted; in time, papular or papulopustular centers appear in the eruption. The disorder requires no therapy. Palms and soles are usually spared. This condition is occasionally confused with more serious pustular disorders, such as congenital candidiasis or bacterial lesions; in such cases, evaluation of a pustule with Gram stain, KOH, or Wright or Giemsa stain will help differentiate among these disorders. A smear of erythema toxicum will reveal numerous eosinophils.

Table 12–8. Differential diagnosis: Vesicopustules in the neonate.

Type	Findings	Laboratory Tests
Infectious		
Herpes simplex virus	Blisters and erosions, often of the head	+ Tzanck stain + Wright stain } Multinucleate giant cells + Viral culture
Candidal (congenital = present first day after birth)	Morbilliform papulovesicles Pustules (often generalized, often involve palms and soles)	+ KOH + Gram stain } Pseudohyphae + Culture
Bacterial (eg, staphylococcal, streptococcal, *Escherichia coli*)	Vesicles, pustules	+ Gram stain + Culture
Syphilis	Erosions, hemorrhagic bullae, mucous patches, petechiae, pustules, erosions	+ Serology + Darkfield examination: spirochetes
Scabies	Papules, nodules, acral and periumbilical predilection	+ Scabies preparation (mineral oil or KOH): mites, eggs or scybala
Transient		
Erythema toxicum	Erythematous, blotchy macules ± central pustular component	+ Wright stain + Gram stain } Perifollicular eosinophils
Incontinentia pigmenti	Streaky, linear, clustered aggregates, ± verrucous or linear pigmentary changes	+ Wright and Gram stain for eosinophils + Eosinophilic pustules on biopsy specimen
Transient neonatal pustular melanosis	Pustules, vesicles, hyperpigmented macules with collarette of scale	+ Wright stain + Gram stain } PMNs
Miliaria	Nonfollicular papules and papulopustules	– Culture and gram-stain negative (usually no organisms, few cells)
Acropustulosis of infancy	Pruritic papules and vesicopustules favor acral sites	+ Gram stain for PMNs
Epidermolysis bullosa	Generalized blisters, bullae, erosions	+ Nikolsky sign – Gram stain

KOH = potassium hydroxide preparation; PMN = polymorphonuclear neutrophils.

Transient Neonatal Pustular Melanosis. This benign condition consists of very small and superficial vesicles present at birth or shortly thereafter. It is more common in African-Americans. Lesions rupture quite easily, leaving a collarette of scale. Hyperpigmented macules often develop at these sites. Occasionally only hyperpigmented macules will be noted at the time of birth. The lesions resolve spontaneously. The main difficulty with this disorder is in distinguishing it from more serious vesicopustular disorders. Evaluations of a smear will reveal a predominance of neutrophils without organisms.

Miliaria. "Prickly heat" is the result of destruction of the eccrine sweat ducts. The rash of this disorder can be vesicular, papular, or nodular, depending on the depth of involvement of the affected eccrine sweat ducts. The lesions are often small erythematous papules or vesicles present on the trunk. Treatment consists of decreasing sweating and relieving obstruction by airing out the skin and avoiding overheating in affected children. Cool baths are often useful therapeutic interventions.

Sucking Blisters. These result from vigorous sucking of the affected site in utero. They are most common on the fingers, forearms, or wrists. The lesions may be vesicles, bullae, or erosions at the time of birth and usually resolve without need for treatment.

Infectious Causes of Neonatal Vesicopustules

The list of possible infections in the newborn period is extensive and includes bacterial pathogens such as *Liste-* *ria, Staphylococcus aureus,* and *Streptococcus.* Viral infections, including herpes simplex and varicella, are possible pathogens, as are fungal etiologies, including *Candida.* As most of these conditions are extensively addressed elsewhere, we will limit our discussion to candidiasis.

Congenital Candidiasis. This infection is contracted in utero, and lesions may be present at birth. Small erythematous papules or papulopustules may be present on the trunk, extremities, palms, and soles. Microscopic examination of a skin scraping of a pustule will reveal budding yeast and pseudohyphae. In full-term healthy children the infection usually poses no risk, and treatment involves local topical antifungal therapy or no intervention at all. In debilitated or premature infants, however, systemic antifungal therapy is usually recommended, as severe systemic illness may result from congenital infection.

Mechanobullous Disorders

Epidermolysis Bullosa. This disorder consists of a number of inherited disorders of the skin that result from defective structures in the epidermis or dermis. The skin's normal barrier function is compromised; therefore, friction or trauma to the skin leads to "lifting" of the epidermis from the underlying dermis. The level of separation depends on the type of epidermolysis bullosa present and the site of the defective structure (keratinocyte, hemidesmosome, or anchoring fibril). Blisters and erosions develop at the sites of trauma. Severely affected patients may also have nail, mucous membrane, and gastrointestinal complications. Newborns with erosions or blisters suspicious for epidermolysis bullosa should first be examined for the possibility of an infectious etiology for their blisters. A dermatology consultation should be procured so that biopsy specimens (which should include electron micrographic evaluation) can be obtained. In addition, these children require careful handling of the skin, surveillance for infectious complications, and monitoring of fluid and electrolyte status.

Other Blistering Disorders in the Neonatal Period

Mastocytosis. This disorder of mast cells can present in the neonatal period with solitary lesions or a diffuse blistering eruption. Mast cells possess histamine and, when traumatized, release this cytokine with subsequent erythema, vasodilation, and edema. Severe reactions consist of blisters and erosions. When blistering and erosion are prominent, the disorder may be mistaken for an infectious process. Isolated lesions of mastocytosis may be flesh-colored, tan, pink, or hyperpigmented. They almost always possess the ability to swell or blister when stroked or rubbed vigorously (the Darier sign). Wheezing and gastrointestinal symptoms may result if enough histamine is released from such lesions. (For addition information, see section on Raised [Papular] Pigmented Lesions.)

Aplasia Cutis Congenita. This condition can appear as an oval or angular scar present on the vertex of the scalp. It is a congenital defect in the epidermis and dermis and occasionally also involves the subcutis. It is commonly seen on or near the midline. The appearance of the lesions, which may be multiple, is variable. At times, the surface may look eroded and red; at other times, however, a thin blister or bulla will be present over the lesion. This condition usually will heal without complication, although alopecia commonly results at the involved site. Rarely, defect may occur over the sagittal sinus and be complicated by bleeding and infection. A hydrocolloid dressing may be used when erosion is a major problem. These dressings expedite wound healing.

PAPULOSQUAMOUS DISORDERS IN THE NEONATAL PERIOD

Papulosquamous disorders (scaling red rashes) in the neonatal period are common and usually do not signify severe pathology. Occasionally, however, a scaling papular disorder in the neonatal period is a marker for severe systemic illness or a chronic cutaneous condition.

Benign Papulosquamous Disorder

Seborrheic Dermatitis. This greasy, red, scaly eruption is the most common scaling disorder of infancy. It presents shortly after birth and involves the scalp (cradle cap), post auricular areas, and groin. It can be confused with diaper dermatitis when it affects the groin area. Other sites of involvement include the intertriginous areas (neck, axillary, groin, and leg creases).

Well-circumscribed discrete and confluent erythematous patches with superimposed greasy or dry scale are the hallmark of seborrheic dermatitis. The rash can be bright red and, if severe enough, may ooze or become eroded. Adherent yellow scales may be present on the scalp, brows, and face. The condition usually resolves by 3–6 months of age.

Treatment consists of weak topical corticosteroids if necessary. Hydrocortisone lotion 1 or 1½% to the scalp twice a day for a short period is helpful, as is the use of a steroid cream, such as hydrocortisone, to the involved body surfaces twice a day. Secondary candidal infection is common. Simultaneous use of an antifungal agent, such as nystatin or clotrimazole cream, may help prevent this secondary fungal infection.

The scalp frequently responds to shampoos, such as zinc pyrithione or selenium sulfide. The use of mineral oil to soften the scales before shampooing will often expedite removal of the scale and hasten response to therapy.

Children with severe findings should be evaluated for evidence of failure to thrive and gastrointestinal symptoms, such as diarrhea. Hepatosplenomegaly and lymphadenopathy should also be ruled out. The presence of such findings raises the possibility of more serious papulosquamous erythemas (caused by systemic diseases such as Leiner disease, Langerhans cell histocytosis, and immunologic and nutritional deficiencies), which are discussed below.

Psoriasis. This disorder can occasionally present in the neonatal period and may lead to a diffuse erythrodermic condition. Family history, chronicity, and severity of the condition raise the suspicion of psoriasis. Treatment is similar to that for seborrheic dermatitis; however, stronger topical corticosteroids and other agents, such as tars and topical calcipotriene, may be required. The frequent use of emollients and avoidance of drying and irritation are crucial in patients with psoriasis. Patients may become secondarily infected with bacterial pathogens as a result of scratching, and antibiotic therapy will then be required.

Atopic Dermatitis (Eczema). Eczema does not usually present until 4–6 weeks of life. Discrimination between this disorder and seborrheic dermatitis in the first few months of life may be difficult; however, atopic dermatitis tends to be less well defined with finer white scales. Atopic dermatitis more commonly involves the cheeks, trunk, and flexor surfaces, whereas seborrheic dermatitis favors the scalp and creases. Irritants and drying should be avoided. Moisturizers and weak topical corticosteroids are the mainstay of therapy.

Ichthyotic Disorders. Ichthyotic refers to fishlike scale and is usually used to describe four major categories of abnormal generalized scaling that can present at birth. Table 12–9 further describes these diseases.

More Serious Causes of Red, Scaly Eruptions in the Neonate

Red, scaling rashes in childhood occasionally signal a serious underlying illness.

Table 12–9. Ichthyoses.

Type	Inheritance	Characteristics	Defect
Ichthyosis vulgaris	AD 1:250	Fine white scales on legs, face, back, extensor surfaces—flexural sparing, increased palmoplantar skin markings, keratosis pilaris, xerosis and atopy	Unknown; histology—increased granular layer
X-Linked ichthyosis	X-Linked recessive 1:6000 male	Collodion membrane at birth; scales are dark and large, generalized; palms and soles spared; + corneal opacities	Steroid sulfatase deficiency
Lamellar ichthyosis	AR 1:300,000	Collodion membrane or erythema at birth, then thick, large, dark plate-like brown scales, then plaques. Nails absent; thick palms and soles; accentuated markings; severe ectropion and eclabion	Unknown; histology—hyperkeratosis acanthosis and mild inflammatory infiltrate
NBCIE (nonbullous congenital ichthyosiform erythroderma)	AR < 1:100,000	Often collodion membrane at birth; persistent erythroderma, finer, whiter scales, also nail and palmar changes; less severe eye involvement	Probable increased n-alkanes; increased epidermal turnover
Epidermolytic hyperkeratosis (bullous congenital ichthyosiform erythroderma)	AD 1:300,000	Early childhood: Recurrent episodes of bullae formation; generalized erythroderma followed by large, thick, dark scales, often verrucous malodorous flexural involvement	Mutations of keratin genes; histology—giant, coarse, keratohyalin granules and vacuolation of the granular layer

AD = autosomal dominant; AR = autosomal recessive.

Immunologic Disorders.

HIV Infections (AIDS). Infants with HIV may often have thrush and severe diaper rash. Severe generalized seborrheic atopic dermatitis or recurrent bacterial skin infections should also raise a suspicion for HIV.

Any child with severe seborrheic, atopic, or diaper dermatitis should be evaluated for the presence of oral thrush, lymphadenopathy, and hepatosplenomegaly. Failure to thrive should also be ruled out. If indicated by history and clinical findings, appropriate laboratory evaluation should be performed to rule out HIV infection.

Severe Combined Immunodeficiency and Leiner Disease. A number of immunodeficiency disorders can present with red scaling skin. Patients with severe combined immunodeficiency disorder often have recurrent infections as well as failure to thrive. Leiner disease was once thought to be a specific disorder of complement function that led to a severe generalized rash, infections, and diarrhea. It is no longer clear whether this is a specific disorder. Any infant with such symptoms should be examined for an underlying immunologic abnormality.

Graft-Versus-Host Disease (GVH). Maternal lymphocytes will occasionally engraft in neonates, leading to a GVH reaction. A scaling red rash, hepatosplenomegaly, and diarrhea can result. This can also occur if neonates receive transfusions of blood products that have not been irradiated.

Omman Disease. This is another neonatal immunodeficiency disorder that can present with a red, scaly rash and hepatosplenomegaly. The patient may also have alopecia and massive lymphadenopathy. In both GVH and Omman disease, skin biopsy specimens can help make the diagnosis, as satellite cell necrosis within the epidermis will be present.

Metabolic Deficiencies. These disorders often present with scaling red rashes and failure to thrive. Zinc deficiency causes a red and sometimes eroded rash that commonly occurs in the perioral, diaper, and acral areas. Diarrhea and failure to thrive are also common in this condition. Rarely, cystic fibrosis may have as its first obvious manifestation a red, scaly rash secondary to zinc malabsorption. Essential fatty acid, biotin, and multiple carboxylase deficiencies can also present in a similar fashion, although the erythema and scaling are usually more diffuse in these conditions.

Histiocytosis X (Langerhans Cell Histiocytosis). This histiocytic malignancy can present in infancy with a seborrheic dermatitis-like picture. The presence of infiltrated brown-yellow papules within the rash, purpuric lesions, and systemic findings of lymphadenopathy and hepatosplenomegaly point toward this diagnosis. A biopsy specimen must be obtained if this neoplastic disorder is suspected.

DIAPER DERMATITIS

The most common dermatologic condition occurring in infancy is diaper rash. Under this general category are a number of distinct types of eruptions caused by a variety of agents.

Irritant Contact Dermatitis. If skin is directly irritated by an agent such as stool or urine, an irritant reaction will develop. This does not require an immunologic response. The occlusion offered by diapers and the humid environment provided by sweat and urine, combined with friction, lead to maceration and breakdown of the skin. This is the most common cause of diaper dermatitis.

Allergic Contact Dermatitis. This involves an allergic reaction to a contactant and can occur when a patient is exposed to cleansing wipes, perfumed talc, or an agent in the diapers. Occasionally, a medication being applied is the culprit.

Candidiasis. Yeast are found as normal residents in the oral cavity and stool and are not always pathogens. When skin is damaged, however, the yeast can become invasive and lead to the development of papular, erythematous, and, sometimes, erosive rashes.

It is usually fairly easy to distinguish between contact and candidal dermatitis. Contact rashes more commonly involve convex surfaces or areas rubbing against the diaper. The creases will often by spared. Candidiasis, in contrast, will involve the creases and scrotum and often manifests satellite papules and pustules; a beefy red appearance is not uncommon.

Initial therapy consists of the following: frequent diaper changes, gentle cleansing with plain water or a mild soap (cleansing wipes should be avoided, as a contact dermatitis to their components may develop), exposure to air of the affected area when possible, and application of zinc oxide or other protective agents after diaper changes.

Severe cases may benefit from mild topical corticosteroids, such as hydrocortisone cream and topical antifungal agents. Potent steroid-antifungal combination agents are not recommended, as they may lead to atrophy, striae, and telangiectasis. The use of Mycostatin drops four times a day orally will help decrease the concentration of candidal infection in the gastrointestinal tract and may expedite improvement. Occasionally, the mother may need treatment of candidal infection of the nipples or genial tract, which may be contributing to the infant's disorder. Rarely, the infection may be severe enough to necessitate the use of a systemic fungal agent, such as fluconazole. This is reserved only for refractory cases.

Secondary infection with *Streptococcus* or *S aureus* may occur in the affected areas. Group A β-hemolytic streptococcus can cause a severe red erosive condition, particularly in the intertriginous areas. Culture and systemic antibiotic therapy should be carried out in such cases.

The possibility of another diagnosis must be considered if a diaper rash does not improve despite appropriate therapy in a compliant family. Metabolic, infectious, and immunodeficiency disorders are major categories that must be ruled out in such cases (Table 12–10).

VASCULAR LESIONS

Vascular lesions are composed of blood vessels, including capillaries, veins, arteries, and lymphatics. Vascular lesions are usually red or blue; deeper lesions may be skin

Table 12–10. Differential diagnosis of diaper dermatitis.

- Candidiasis
- Irritant contact dermatitis
- Seborrheic dermatitis
- Atopic dermatitis
- Allergic contact dermatitis
- Bullous impetigo, streptococcal infection
- Psoriasis
- Histiocytosis X
- Zinc deficiency
- Scabies
- Granuloma gluteale infantum
- Tinea corporis
- Essential fatty acid and biotin deficiency
- Severe combined immunodeficiency
- Graft-versus-host disease

colored. These lesions are quite common, ranging from innocuous lesions, such as "stork bites," to those of significant medical consequence. A useful categorization is based on whether lesions are nonproliferative malformations or proliferative tumors.

VASCULAR MALFORMATIONS (Nonproliferative)

Most nonproliferative vascular malformations are salmon patches (nevus simplex) or port-wine stains (nevus flammeus). These are described in the previous section, Skin Diseases of the Neonate.

Klippel-Trenaunay Syndrome. This disorder is the association of a port-wine stain with hypertrophy of underlying soft tissue or bone. It usually occurs on an extremity or portion of the trunk and may have associated varicosities or phlebectasias. Lymphangiomatous components may be present as well. Leg-length discrepancy may be functionally significant in lower-extremity lesions.

Lymphangiomas

Lymphangiomas are malformations of lymphatic origin; 70–90% are present at birth or develop within the first 2 years. Lesions may be flesh-colored dermal or subcutaneous tumors, or thick-walled vesicles with a "frog-spawn" appearance. Lesions may have a hemangiomatous component or deep cavernous component with large cystic areas of lymphatic tissue. There is no spontaneous regression. Surgical excision is difficult, as multiple channels are often present, which leads to difficulty with complete excision and a high recurrence rate.

PROLIFERATIVE VASCULAR LESIONS

Hemangiomas

Hemangiomas, also known as "strawberry marks," are benign proliferative tumors of capillaries seen in 10% of infants (Figure 12–2). They may be present at birth but more

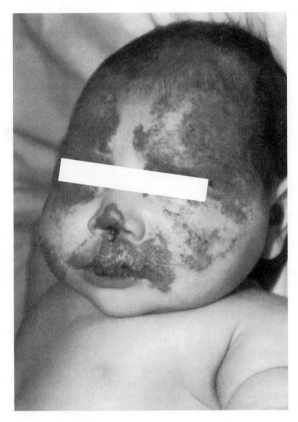

Figure 12–2. Hemangiomas.

commonly appear in the first few weeks. Classically, hemangiomas appear as raised, bright red, lobulated tumors with well-defined borders and prominent capillaries. Hemangiomas located superficially in the dermis have a "strawberry" appearance, whereas lesions deeper in the dermis (**cavernous hemangiomas**) may be skin-colored or bluish with indistinct borders. Lesions undergo a rapid growth phase in the first 6 months after birth, plateau usually from 6 to 12 months, and begin to involute between 12 and 18 months. Spontaneous regression occurs over several years. After year 3, approximately 10% of lesions clear per year (30% at 3 years, 50% at 5 years, 80% at 8 years).

Complications from hemangiomas are rare. They include ulceration and cutaneous infection, bleeding, functional organ compromise (eg, periocular lesions), platelet trapping (Kasabach-Merritt syndrome), and high-output congestive heart failure from arteriovenous shunting. Owing to a low rate of complications and natural involution, conservative observation is the most reasonable plan of management. Therapy is appropriate for lesions that compromise function, such as vision, or cause airway obstruction or other complications. Oral prednisone, α-interferon 2a, embolization, and pulsed-dye laser therapy may be used to treat these problematic hemangiomas.

Pyogenic Granulomas

Pyogenic granulomas are vascular, red, pedunculated papules and nodules that may appear anywhere on the skin or mucous membranes. Lesions most commonly occur on the head and neck. They usually occur in childhood (unlike hemangiomas), with sudden onset and rapid growth over a period of several weeks. The surface of pyogenic granulomas is friable, causing bleeding with minimal trauma. Children often present with a "Band-Aid sign" from application of multiple adhesive bandages to stop hemorrhage. Despite the label "pyogenic," lesions are not thought to have an infectious origin and may be post-traumatic. Although benign, pyogenic granulomas usually persist, unlike capillary hemangiomas. Treatment consists of curettage, electrodesiccation, pulsed-dye laser, or full-thickness excision.

Adenoma Sebaceum (Angiofibromas)

Adenoma sebaceum is a term used to describe multiple red-brown papules commonly seen on the central face or cheeks in patients with tuberous sclerosis. These lesions are angiofibromas and histologically show an increased number of fibroblasts and capillaries in the dermis. Lesions may begin in the first few years of life and are commonly misdiagnosed as "early acne." Isolated angiofibromas are benign growths of no medical significance.

FLAT PIGMENTED LESIONS & OTHER CUTANEOUS TUMORS

Most pigmented lesions that are light tan, blue-brown, or deep brown contain melanin. Increased concentrations of melanin may occur in the epidermis, as in freckles and lentigines; nests of melanocytes may be present in the epidermis or dermis, as in melanocytic nevi and melanoma; and melanin and/or melanocytes may be present deep in dermis, as in mongolian spots and nevus of Ota or Ito (Table 12–11).

Café-au-Lait Spots

Café-au-lait spots are even-colored, tan to brown, flat, pigmented lesions seen in 10–20% of children (Figure 12–3). Lesions may be present anywhere on the body and range in size from a few millimeters to more than 20 cm. Lesions may be present at birth and may increase in size and number with age. Although most individuals with café-au-lait spots are healthy, multiple lesions may be seen with neurofibromatosis type 1 (NF-1) and other neurocutaneous disorders. The presence of six or more café-au-lait spots larger than 1.5 cm in adolescents or adults, or

Table 12–11. Differential diagnosis of flat pigmented lesions.

Lesion	Clinical Appearance
Mongolian spots	Blue-gray macules; commonly lumbosacral area
Café-au-lait spots	Even-colored tan-brown macules with normal skin markings; multiple lesions seen in neurofibromatosis and other phakomatoses
Freckles/lentigines	Small light-tan to brown macules on sun-exposed skin
Nevus spilus	Circumscribed tan macule with darkly pigmented flat or raised spots; color is generally lighter than congenital nevi
Becker nevus	Gray-brown hyperpigmented area with hypertrichosis, commonly unilateral on shoulder, anterior chest, scapula; usually appears during early adolescence or adulthood
Nevus of Ota	Blue-gray macule of the face surrounding the eye, often involving sclerae and conjunctivae
Nevus of Ito	Blue-gray macule of the shoulder, clavicular area

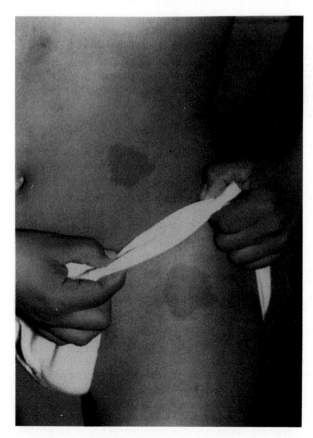

Figure 12–3. Café-au-lait spots.

0.5 cm in prepubertal children, raises a high degree of suspicion for NF-1. Multiple small (1–4 mm) café-au-lait spots in the axillary and inguinal area, termed "freckling," may also be a sign of NF-1 in children. Café-au-lait spots may also be seen with other syndromes, including tuberous sclerosis, polyostotic fibrous dysplasia (McCune-Albright syndrome), and Russell-Silver syndrome. Café-au-lait spots themselves are benign, and treatment is unnecessary. For lesions of cosmetic importance, pigmented lesion laser therapy is effective.

Mongolian Spots

Mongolian spots are blue-gray, flat, macular lesions usually located on the lumbosacral areas, buttocks, and, occasionally, limbs or trunk of normal infants. Lesions are present at birth and usually fade by late childhood. The lesions are composed of melanocytes in the dermis (**dermal melanocytosis**), presumed to be the result of embryonal failure of melanocytes to migrate from the neural crest to the epidermis. Occasionally, they may be mistaken for bruising associated with child abuse.

Freckles & Lentigines

"Freckles" (**ephelides**) are small (usually 2–4 mm), light tan to brown pigmented lesions that appear on sun-exposed skin. They are more common in early childhood, vary seasonally with sun exposure, and usually fade during winter months. They are more commonly seen in children who have fair skin and red hair. Although lesions themselves are of cosmetic significance only, some studies have reported freckles to be a risk factor for melanoma. The best treatment is prevention, with avoidance of the sun. **Lentigines** are usually darker tan, brown, or black, flat lesions seen in childhood and adult life. Lentigines acquired in early childhood may fade with time, whereas those acquired in later life tend to persist. Lentigines may be seen in several syndromes, including Peutz-Jeghers syndrome, Leopard (*L*entigenes, *E*CG conduction defects, *O*cular hypertelorism, *P*ulmonary stenoses, *A*bnormalities of genitalia, *R*etardation of growth, and *D*eafness) syndrome, and Lamb (*L*entigenes, *A*trial myxomas, *M*ucocutaneous myxomas, and *B*lue nevi) syndrome.

Nevus of Ota & Ito

Large blue-gray discoloration of the face surrounding the eye is seen with the nevus of Ota. Ipsilateral bluish coloration of the sclera is common. Nevus of Ito displays the same clinical features located over the shoulder, neck, and clavicular area. Although both lesions have histology (dermal melanocytosis) and color similar to mongolian spots, nevus of Ota and Ito usually persist throughout life. Lesions are usually benign, with rare cases of malignant transformation recorded. Laser treatment may lighten or remove these lesions if desired.

RAISED (PAPULAR) PIGMENTED LESIONS

Pigmented nevi may appear light tan, brown, or brown-black. They are formed by collections of melanocytes, termed nevus cells. Although these lesions are usually benign in childhood, malignancy can occur. Nonmelanocytic cell collections may mimic pigmented lesions, such as urticaria pigmentosa, which is composed of mast cell skin infiltrates.

Congenital Melanocytic Nevi

Pigmented melanocytic nevi present at birth or in the first few months are termed **congenital nevi** (Figure 12–4). They appear in 1–2% of newborns as light tan, brown, or black plaques. Lesions are usually solitary but can appear in groups or clusters; they vary in size, ranging from 1 mm to many centimeters ("giant nevi"). The vast majority are smaller than 3 cm. Nevi may be differentiated from other "dark spots" by shining a light from the side of the lesion; nevi have more prominent skin lines, a distorted surface, and speckling. These lesions may be classified on the basis of size: small congenital nevi, 1.5 cm; intermediate nevi, 1.5–20 cm; giant nevi, greater than 20 cm. However, this classification is of limited usefulness because the lesions may grow over time.

Other names for giant nevi include "garment nevi," "bathing trunk nevi," or "giant hairy nevi." Classically, congenital nevi differ from acquired nevi histologically by involving deeper portions of the dermis, with nevus cells streaming around collagen bundles, nerves, vessels, and skin appendages.

The natural history of most congenital nevi is benign; they grow proportionately throughout the patient's life. Lesions may be flat, papular, nodular, with or without hair, firm, or warty. The risk of melanoma is dependent on the size of the congenital nevus. The lifetime risk of melanoma in giant congenital nevi is estimated to be 6% (with ranges of 2–42% documented in published studies). The risk of intermediate and small congenital nevi is uncertain. Lesions overlying the skull or spine may be associated with leptomeningeal melanosis or underlying spinal defects.

The management of congenital nevi is quite controversial. Giant nevi pose a significant health hazard but are difficult or, at times, impossible to excise prophylactically owing to involvement of vital structures and technical complexity. Many authorities recommend early excision, whereas others suggest serial observation for changes in morphology or color. The risk of complications from multiple surgical procedures should be balanced with the risk of development of melanoma. The risk of melanoma developing in intermediate and small congenital nevi is not known; malignant transformation in childhood is quite rare. Routine prophylactic excision, although recommended by some experts, is considered impractical and unnecessary by most. Clinical observation over time is reasonable, with consideration of elective excision when the child is old enough to cooperate with local anesthesia. Families should be taught how to recognize changing nevi (Table 12–12) of clinical importance.

Acquired Melanocytic Nevi

Acquired melanocytic nevi, or "common moles," usually appear from early childhood to early adulthood. There is a large range in the number of lesions, with white adults having 10–40 nevi on average. Nevi are composed of melanocytic "nests" of cells and are classified by the predominant location of the cells. **Junctional nevi** are composed of nevus cells predominantly in the epidermis and clinically are smooth or minimally elevated, even-colored, tan to black macules. **Compound nevi** have melanocytic nests at both the dermoepidermal junction and within the dermis. These lesions are similar in color to junctional nevi, with more prominent elevation. **Intradermal nevi** are formed by melanocytic nests fully within the dermis. These lesions are dome-shaped, raised, or pedunculated; they may be pigmented or flesh-colored. It is believed that melanocytic nevi may progress from junctional nevi to compound nevi, and then to intradermal nevi as part of their normal biology. Nevi are predominantly seen in sun-exposed areas of the body, and evidence has linked sun exposure to subsequent development of an increased mole burden.

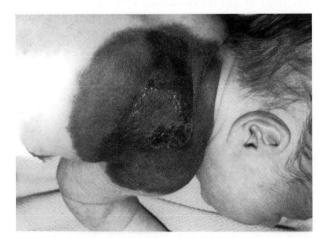

Figure 12–4. Congenital nevi.

Table 12–12. ABCs of worrisome changes in congenital nevi.

A	=	Asymmetry
B	=	Border irregularity
C	=	Color: Localized color variation to red, dark brown, blue, or black
D	=	Diameter: Changing size of atypical area
E	=	Elevation: Elevated, firm nodules

The clinical appearance of acquired moles is quite variable. Routine excision of acquired nevi is not necessary unless lesions have unusual characteristics. The characteristics of normal acquired nevi are listed in Table 12–13. Lesions with pruritus, pain, rapid change in size or color, or bleeding should be excised and evaluated histologically.

Atypical (Dysplastic) Nevi

Atypical nevi are clinically unusual moles that may connote an increased risk of malignant melanoma. Clinical characteristics are outlined in Table 12–14. Atypical nevi may be seen in families with a propensity for large numbers of atypical moles and malignant melanoma. This entity, the familial atypical mole syndrome (FAMS), is also known as **familial dysplastic nevus syndrome** or **"BK mole syndrome."** Individuals with FAMS demonstrate multiple dysplastic nevi and have two first-degree relatives with malignant melanoma; lifetime risk of melanoma approaches 90–100%.

Melanoma

Melanoma is quite uncommon in children, with only 2% of melanomas occurring in patients younger than 20 years. However, melanoma must be considered in unusual congenital and acquired melanocytic nevi. Pediatricians should also be aware of the risk factors of melanoma (Table 12–15) and that childhood sun exposure is a key risk factor for development of melanoma in adulthood.

Spitz Nevi
(Spindle & Epithelioid Cell Nevi)

Spitz nevi are dome-shaped, pink to reddish-brown nodules. Lesions are usually solitary but may be multiple or grouped. They usually appear in early childhood to adolescence, commonly on the face. Despite their original name "juvenile melanoma," Spitz nevi are benign, with characteristic histopathologic features (spindle and epithelial cell nests). Lesions may be difficult to distinguish from true melanoma, and expert dermatopathologic review may be necessary. Recommended treatment is surgical excision.

Urticaria Pigmentosa
(Mastocytosis)

Mast cell infiltration of the skin and other organs is the hallmark of mastocytosis. Urticaria pigmentosa is the common form in childhood, presenting as solitary or multiple red-brown macules, papules, or nodules, usually 1–3

Table 12–13. Characteristics of normal acquired nevi.

Size: ≤ 5 mm
Symmetric pigmentation
Round or oval shape
Smooth border and sharply demarcated
Symmetrically or uniformly pigmented, typically tan or brown (may be mottled or stippled)

Table 12–14. Clinical characteristics of atypical (dysplastic) nevi.

Moles are large (6–15 mm)
Occur in usual sites plus scalp, buttocks, other sun-protected sites
Irregular borders, mixed colors (tan, brown, dark brown, pink)
Indistinct margins
Macular component very common; may have "pebbly" or "fried-egg" appearance

cm in size, and often found on the trunk. Lesions become hivelike when firmly stroked; this phenomenon is a positive Darier sign, a result of the release of histamines from the increased number of mast cells in these lesions. In the first few months after birth, lesions may become vesicular or bullous with vigorous contact. Repeated blistering at the same site or a nonhealing sore may be a clue to this diagnosis.

Lesions develop in more than 75% of patients by 2 years of age; most of these legions clear spontaneously by puberty. Systemic involvement is more common in older children and adults. Symptoms and signs include flushing, headaches, tachycardia, hypotension, cramps, and coagulation abnormalities. Fewer than 5% of children with onset of urticaria pigmentosa before age 10 years have systemic involvement, compared with 10–30% of older children. Mast cells may infiltrate bone marrow, liver, spleen, and gastrointestinal tract in the systemic form. Occasional familial forms of diffuse cutaneous, bullous mastocytosis have been reported.

An increased number of mast cells in the dermis and subcutaneous tissue on skin biopsy specimens can confirm the diagnosis. Toluidine blue or Giemsa stains will show metachromatic staining.

No effective therapy exists for mastocytosis. Patients should avoid mast cell degranulators, such as aspirin, codeine, opiates, procaine, polymixin B, and radiographic dyes (Table 12–16). Scopolamine and pancuronium may also lead to exacerbation of symptoms. Hot baths and vigorous rubbing of the skin can lead to mast cell degranulation. Both H1 and H2 antihistamines have been used with some success, as have oral cromolyn sodium and ketotifen. Psoralen and ultraviolet A therapy are reserved for severe cases. Topical fluorinated steroids may be beneficial for treatment of a small number of isolated cutaneous lesions.

Table 12–15. Risk factors for development of melanoma.

Fair skin
Blond/red hair
Freckling
Skin types I and II (easily burns, tans poorly)
History of sun exposure
Childhood
Cumulative
Intermittent
Local environment (in sunbelt states, rate of increase of melanoma at 34% per year versus 10% per year for other states)

Table 12–16. Precipitants of mast cell degranulation in urticaria pigmentosa.

Drugs	Physical Agents
Salicylates	Very hot or cold water
Alcohol	
Opiates (morphine, codeine)	
Polymyxin B	
Scopolamine	

RAISED NONPIGMENTED LESIONS

Nonpigmented raised papules and nodules may be skin-colored, tan, brown, or orange-yellow. Nonpigmented lesions in infants and children are associated with numerous differential conditions, several of which are discussed below.

Epidermal Nevi

Epidermal nevi are benign growths that may occur anywhere on the skin. Lesions are usually present at birth but may appear during childhood and adolescence as well. Lesions may be minimally elevated at birth but usually become more papular with a verrucous surface in later years. Color may range from skin color to dark brown or black. Lesions grow proportionately with the child and often take on a linear appearance (**linear epidermal nevi).** Epidermal nevi may be mistaken for verrucae; persistence, proportionate growth, and linear configuration are useful differentiating features. Lesions may be large and expansive and arranged as spiral streaks, especially on the trunk. Extensive epidermal nevi may be associated with a congenitally acquired syndrome termed the **epidermal nevus syndrome.** Associated anomalies include central nervous system involvement (including seizures, mental retardation, and focal deficits), skeletal defects, and hemihypertrophy, as well as renal and ocular anomalies.

Nevus Sebaceous

Nevus sebaceous (nevus sebaceous of Jadassohn) is a benign epidermal tumor present at birth. Initially it appears as a flat or minimally raised, hairless plaque. The tumor has a characteristic waxy texture and yellow-orange or pink color and is most commonly present on the scalp or face. Nevus sebaceous lesions thicken with puberty, as the sebaceous glands that constitute much of the tumor are hormonally stimulated. Extensive nevus sebaceous may be associated with central nervous system disease and skeletal anomalies, as a variant of the epidermal nevus syndrome. Secondary neoplasia may occur in 15–20% of lesions, usually in adolescence or adulthood. Basal cell carcinoma and syringocystadenoma papilliferum (a tumor of apocrine sweat glands) are the common tumors; rare squamous cell carcinomas and appendage tumors have also been reported. Because of the neoplastic risks, elective excision is recommended before or at puberty.

Juvenile Xanthogranulomas

Juvenile xanthogranulomas are 2–10 mm, yellow, brown, or red-brown papules and nodules that typically occur in the first few months after birth. Lesions may be solitary or multiple; occasionally, hundreds of lesions are present. These histiocytic tumors usually are self-limited, and two thirds of lesions resolve spontaneously within 1 year. Associated iris xanthogranulomas may cause ocular hemorrhage or glaucoma. Xanthogranulomas are also associated with juvenile chronic myeloid leukemia; children with neurofibromatosis and juvenile xanthogranulomas seem to be at much greater risk. Xanthogranulomas do not require treatment, as lesions spontaneously regress.

Pilomatricomas

Pilomatricomas (calcifying epitheliomas) are benign, firm, calcifying lesions that most often occur on the head and neck in the first two decades of life. Lesions may be skin-colored but often have a bluish color and stonelike consistency. Although these lesions are benign, surgical excision is recommended for prevention of discomfort and periodic inflammation and for cosmetic reasons. Multiple pilomatricomas have been associated with myotonic dystrophy.

Connective Tissue Nevi

Connective tissue nevi are benign collections of dermal collagen or elastic tissue. These slightly elevated, firm or rubbery plaques are commonly seen on the trunk, buttocks, or extremities. Connective tissue nevus plaques may be seen in patients with tuberous sclerosis; these are termed **shagreen patches.** Connective tissue nevi are also associated with Buschke-Ollendorf syndrome, which consists of osteopoikilosis with bony dysplasia. Lesions may be hereditary without associated anomalies or sporadic. They are benign and require no treatment other than biopsy for diagnostic purposes.

Dermatofibromas

Dermatofibromas, which are firm, flesh-colored to tan, brown, or black papules or nodules often occurring on the extremities, are seen occasionally in children, although more often in adolescents and adults. They are fixed firmly to the skin but move freely above the subcutaneous fat.

Neurofibromas may be isolated growths or seen as a major finding of NF-1 (von Recklinghausen disease). Tumors vary greatly in size and consistency, ranging from smooth and soft to firm and polyploid. Although large, plaquelike, plexiform neurofibromas associated with neurofibromatosis may be present at birth, the vast majority of NF-1–associated fibromas present after age 10 years. Excision is recommended for lesions that enlarge rapidly, cause marked pain, are functionally significant, or are disfiguring.

HYPERSENSITIVITY REACTIONS

Urticaria & Angioedema

Urticaria is common in infancy and childhood. Often referred to as "hives," these lesions consist of erythematous, raised wheals, which may be present anywhere on the body. Lesions may range from a few millimeters to giant edematous plaques and typically have a pale or whitish center. These may be mistaken for lesions of erythema multiforme. Urticarial lesions occur suddenly, are quite pruritic, and persist for 1–12 hours. Although lesions shift or new lesions develop, individual lesions usually do not remain fixed. In contrast, lesions of erythema multiforme persist for a minimum of 1 week.

Extension of urticaria to deeper cutaneous tissue is termed **angioedema.** This may be associated with marked swelling of the face, hands, and feet. Laryngeal or bronchial edema can lead to life-threatening airway obstruction.

Urticaria is due to vasodilatation and increased permeability of capillaries and small blood vessels, with transudation of fluid into the upper dermis. This occurs when mast cells (often through antigenic stimulation) release a number of vasoactive substances, such as histamines, kinins, and prostaglandins. Urticaria results from a variety of causes, including foods, drugs, infections, bites and stings, physical agents, genetic diseases, and systemic diseases (Table 12–17).

Most urticarial reactions resolve spontaneously. Urticarial lesions that persist for more than 24 hours may represent urticarial vasculitis; skin biopsy is diagnostic. The term chronic urticaria is restricted to urticaria present for at least 6 weeks. Uncovering the instigating agent in these cases is often quite difficult. Physical urticarias should be considered (cholinergic, cold, and pressure urticaria). Unfortunately, an underlying cause can be found in only 20% of cases.

Treatment of urticaria depends on the severity of the condition and the presence or absence of airway involvement. Extensive skin or airway involvement should be treated with epinephrine as well as antihistamines. Oral antihistamines are effective in the treatment of urticaria. Systemic glucocorticoids are rarely necessary to manage urticaria or angioedema. It is appropriate to identify and alleviate any precipitating agent.

Drug Eruptions

Drug-induced rashes commonly occur in the pediatric age group. The morphologic diversity of these eruptions, as well as their resemblance to other exanthems, often leads to difficulty in diagnosis and management. Frequently, a patient with fever is treated with an antibiotic and subsequently has a rash; in such cases, it is difficult to discern whether the rash is infectious or drug induced. A variety of drug-related eruptions occur, ranging from be-

nign macular or morbilliform eruptions to life-threatening entities, such as toxic epidermal necrolysis (Table 12–18). The time course for drug eruptions is typically 7–14 days into the course of initial exposure, with eruptions within a few days if there has been prior sensitization. However, there is great variability; some eruptions occur immediately on administration, whereas others develop weeks after discontinuation of the agent.

Morphologic features, although not diagnostic, may offer clues to both diagnosis and prognosis. Acneiform eruptions more commonly follow the ingestion of steroids, phenytoin (Dilantin), lithium, isoniazid (INH), or halogens and resolve after discontinuation of the offending agent. In contrast, toxic epidermal necrolysis (TEN) consists of severe sheetlike erosions of the skin and mucous membranes and have a more serious prognosis, with a significant mortality rate resulting from superinfection and sepsis. The most common agents associated with TEN are sulfonamides, anticonvulsants, and nonsteroidal anti-inflammatory drugs. The most frequently seen drug reaction is much less specific as to etiology and consists of a generalized erythematous morbilliform (macular and papular) eruption. Penicillins and cephalosporins are the most likely offenders, although a variety of other drugs and blood products also can induce these cutaneous findings. The eruption typically lasts 1–2 weeks and may be associated with moderate to severe pruritus.

Table 12–17. Causes of urticaria.[1]

Infections
Bacterial: streptococcal
Viral: Epstein-Barr, hepatitis, adenovirus, enterovirus
Parasites
Other: Sinusitis
Foods
Eggs, nuts, milk, shellfish, berries, others
Drugs
Penicillins, cephalosporins, opiates, salicylates, nonsteroidal anti-inflammatory agents, blood products
Bites/stings
Hymenoptera (bees, wasps, hornets), spiders
Systemic diseases
Juvenile rheumatoid arthritis, systemic lupus erythematosus, dermatomyositis, Sjögren syndrome, Behçet syndrome, rheumatic fever

[1]Adapted and reproduced, with permission, from Weston W, Lane A: *Color Textbook of Pediatric Dermatology.* Mosby–Year Book, 1991.

Table 12–18. Drug eruptions.

Urticaria	Exfoliative
Serum sickness–like	Erythema multiforme
Morbilliform	Erythema nodosum
Maculopapular	Toxic epidermal necrolysis
Macular	Fixed drug eruption
Scarlatiniform	Photosensitivity dermatitis vasculitis
Vesicobullous	Eczematous contact dermatitis

Mild drug eruptions can progress to more severe processes, such as erythema multiforme, toxic epidermal necrolysis, or vasculitis. Drug hypersensitivity may involve multiple organs, including liver, kidneys, gastrointestinal tract, and central nervous system. Peculiar and life-threatening hypersensitivity reactions may be seen with phenytoin, phenobarbital, or carbamazepine. These reactions usually present 1–4 weeks after exposure to the drug and are characterized by fever, morbilliform eruptions, lymphadenopathy, and hepatitis. Drugs must be discontinued promptly. These medications appear to be cross-allergic; if anticonvulsants are needed, no agents of these three classes should be used. There is evidence of a possible enzymatic predisposition to this anticonvulsant hypersensitivity reaction.

Erythema Multiforme

Erythema multiforme (EM) is an acute hypersensitivity reaction characterized by distinctive skin lesions with or without mucosal involvement. There is a spectrum of disease, with EM minor and major as distinct syndromes; TEN may be a severe form of EM major. EM minor presents with symmetric erythematous macules or papules, often with superimposed vesicles, which evolve into annular target or iris lesions. Lesions occur primarily on the upper extremities and trunk. EM major, or Stevens-Johnson syndrome, is characterized by blistering of at least two mucosal surfaces accompanying typical cutaneous EM lesions. TEN presents with widespread erythema and necrosis of full-thickness epidermis that resembles deep scalding injury. TEN is complicated by fluid and electrolyte imbalance, severe mucosal injury, and sepsis and has an estimated mortality rate of 20–70%.

Lesions of EM may have central dusky areas from profound inflammation, termed "target" or "iris" lesions. Individual lesions persist for a minimum of 1 week, in sharp contrast to urticaria. Although urticarial wheals may appear "target-like" because of central clearing or bluish color, they resolve within hours.

Erythema multiforme has been associated with a variety of infections and drugs. EM minor, especially when recurrent, is almost always associated with preceding herpes simplex virus (HSV) infection. Herpes virus antigens and DNA have been found in cutaneous lesions. Other precipitants of EM include *Mycoplasma pneumoniae* infections and drugs, especially sulfonamides, penicillins, anticonvulsants, and nonsteroidal anti-inflammatory agents.

The management of EM in children is controversial. Clearly, any instigating agent, such as a drug or infection, should be identified and eliminated if possible. Further treatment of EM is dictated by the type and extent of disease. EM minor is usually self-limited; it typically evolves over 1–2 weeks and completely heals by 3–4 weeks. Patients may be treated conservatively with cool compresses to lesions and oral antihistamines. Oral lesions may be painful, and patients may benefit from soothing mouthwashes (eg, viscous lidocaine-diphenhydramine elixir-

antacid combination). Acyclovir is not efficacious for treating established EM but may be effective prophylactically for those patients with HSV-associated EM minor. The use of steroids in EM is controversial. If they are to be used, they should be given early in the course of the disease, within the first 1–2 days of the rash. Mildly affected patients usually do well with supportive care only. For patients with extensive EM (> 20% denudation) or TEN, the risks of steroids seem to outweigh any potential (and unproved) benefit.

Erythema Nodosum

Erythema nodosum (**erythema contusiformis**) presents with distinctive tender erythematous nodules, classically on the pretibial surfaces. These nodules represent a hypersensitivity reaction to a variety of infections, drugs, and disease states (Table 12–19). These warm nodules are intensely painful and may be seen on any body surface, including the face and upper extremities. Lesions may evolve from pink-red to purple or yellow-brown and may appear bruiselike.

Lesions of erythema nodosum may be mistaken for cellulitis, bruises, bug bites, or other inflammatory diseases of subcutaneous tissue. Arthralgias and arthritis are commonly associated with erythema nodosum and do not necessarily suggest underlying rheumatic disease. A lesional biopsy specimen displays distinctive pathologic findings of inflammation of fatty tissue, primarily of the connective tissue surrounding fat lobules (**septal panniculitis**).

Erythema nodosum is usually self-limited, resolving in 2–3 weeks. Ibuprofen, salicylates, or other nonsteroidal anti-inflammatory agents may minimize the discomfort.

INFECTIOUS DISEASES

Many infectious diseases have cutaneous manifestations. This discussion is limited to important cutaneous diseases not discussed in Chapter 9.

Table 12–19. Erythema nodosum: Precipitating factors.

Infections:	Streptococcus, tuberculosis, histoplasmosis, coccidiomycosis, blastomycosis, cat-scratch disease, leptospirosis
Drugs:	Oral contraceptives, sulfonamides, penicillin, tetracycline, halogens
Systemic diseases:	Inflammatory bowel disease, sarcoidosis, connective tissue diseases, malignancies

BACTERIAL INFECTIONS

The skin serves as a common portal of entry for bacterial invaders. Excessive moisture or drying, friction, or trauma can damage the structural integrity of the epithelium or appendageal structures and predispose to infection.

Impetigo is the term for superficial bacterial infection of the epithelium (Figure 12–5). It occurs most commonly in young children, particularly in those exposed to conditions of crowding and poor hygiene. The lesions favor the periorificial areas and are initially erythematous macules that evolve into thin-roofed vesicles or pustules, which quickly rupture. The erythematous erosion that results is often covered by a honey-colored crust. **Bullous impetigo,** another variant, is characterized by inflamed bullae that also eventually rupture, leaving a rim of epithelial roof and an eroded surface.

Ecthyma is the term for lesions with deeper bacterial penetration through the epidermis. Although these lesions initially consist of vesiculopustules, a firm, dark crust subsequently develops beneath which usually can be found a small amount of purulent exudate. **Cellulitis** is a bacterial infection that predominantly involves the dermis; it is characteristically a raised warm, erythematous plaque that can expand rapidly. **Necrotizing fasciitis** occurs if infection extends to the subcutaneous fat and fascia. This is a life-threatening process and is more common in patients with diabetes and other immunocompromised patients.

Folliculitis occurs when bacteria superficially invade the hair follicle. Multiple erythematous follicular papules or papulopustules usually are noted. **Furuncles** are deeper infections of the follicles, with tender erythematous follicular nodules. **Carbuncles** are formed by multiple coalescent furuncles, which, if fluctuant, are referred to as **abscesses. Ecthyma gangrenosum** is a rare deep cutaneous infection caused by *Pseudomonas aeruginosa.* This may look similar to streptococcal-induced ecthyma, although it is usually more necrotic and occurs in debilitated or immunocompromised patients.

Etiology & Therapy

S aureus and group A β-hemolytic streptococci are the most commonly isolated organisms in skin infections. Impetigo, ecthyma, and cellulitis often harbor streptococcus, whereas furunculosis is almost always secondary to staphylococcus infection. Impetigo frequently harbors both organisms. Special mention should be made of *Haemophilus influenzae* cellulitis, which usually occurs in early childhood and may be accompanied by sinusitis or bacteremia. These tender, bluish-red plaques typically occur on the face; therefore, any cellulitis in the younger age group, particularly involving the face, necessitates evaluation and antibiotic coverage for *H influenzae.* In neonates, colonization and infection with flora endogenous to the maternal perineum (eg, group B streptococci and *Escherichia coli*) can occur. Therapy is directed toward the appropriate bacterial pathogens. Because im-

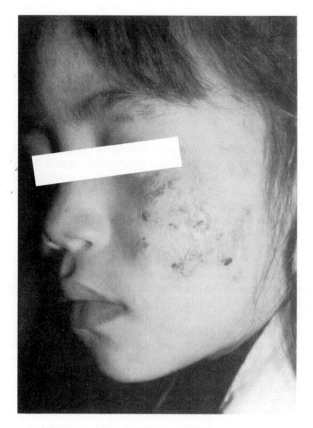

Figure 12–5. Impetigo.

petigo is commonly found to harbor both streptococcus and staphylococcus, antibiotic therapy covering both organisms (eg, a semisynthetic penicillin) is recommended. Although dicloxacillin would be a reasonable choice, most young children find its flavor offensive, and a cephalosporin is often substituted for improved treatment compliance. Topical mupirocin ointment may be used for treatment of localized lesions, eliminating the need for oral therapy.

VIRAL INFECTIONS

Molluscum Contagiosum

Molluscum contagiosum is a relatively common cutaneous infection caused by the DNA pox virus. Lesions are single or multiple, white, opalescent, flesh-colored, or pink papules (Figure 12–6). They are often dome-shaped with a central pinpoint core. Although usually 1–3 mm in size, they can occasionally be larger than 1 cm and are then referred to as "giant molluscum." Lesions favor the face, neck, and trunk but can also involve the genitals. Genital lesions are not necessarily the result of abuse and may occur secondary to autoinoculation from other affected sites. In addition, an eczematous eruption may occur around afflicted areas. Treatment is not necessarily required, as the disease follows a natural course of spontaneous resolution. However, lesions often persist for months to years, and familial, school, and swimming pool transmission can occur. In addition, parents often become anxious concerning the cosmetic aspects of prolonged involvement. For these reasons treatment is often prescribed. Because no uniformly efficacious treatment exists, multiple applications, and often multiple agents, are required. Needle extraction or curettage is often curative but is difficult to perform on multiple lesions. Cryotherapy and topical cantharidin can be effective treatments. Some authors report a response to less invasive treatment, which involves nightly application of surgical or other thick tape to each lesion, with removal or stripping of the tape the following morning.

Verrucae (Warts)

Verrucae are epidermal and mucocutaneous growths caused by human papillomavirus (HPV) (Figure 12–7). They are categorized predominantly on the basis of their most common locations.

Verruca vulgaris lesions, also referred to as "common warts," usually involve the hands and fingers. They are flesh-colored to brown, discrete, rough-surfaced papules and are particularly persistent when they involve the periungual or subungual area. **Digitate warts,** a variant seen more commonly on the face, tend to be filiform or finger-like with a narrow base. **Verrucae plantaris ("plantar warts")** refer to those lesions present on the sole of the foot. These are often quite painful and difficult to eradicate. They can be single papules or may consist of multiple coalescent hyperkeratotic lesions. **Verruca plana (flat warts)** are flatter, often barely perceptible, 1–4 mm, flesh-colored to brown lesions that usually involve the face and legs. They are often spread by trauma, such as scratching or shaving. *Condylomata acuminata (genital warts)* most commonly involve the mucous membranes or perigenital area. They can be sexually transmitted or occur as a result of transmission via an infected birth canal.

Etiology & Therapy. All warts are the result of infection with HPV. This viral agent is ubiquitous, and more than 30 types currently have been identified. Most types show a predilection for a particular body surface: HPV-1 affects the palmar and plantar surfaces, whereas HPV-6 and -11 commonly cause condylomata acuminata. HPV-16, -18, -31, -33, and -35 have also been isolated from genital warts and have been associated with cervical dysplasia and neoplasia. HPV typing can be performed from tissue specimens if necessary. Not all warts require treatment, and no completely effective therapy exists for any form of verrucae. As 60–70% of common warts resolve spontaneously within 2 years, reassurance is often the best form of therapy. However, indications for treatment include discomfort, extensive spread on the digits or face, and genital involvement. Multiple therapies exist, but no ideal agent is available. Verrucae plana often respond to topical tretinoin, light electrodesiccation, or cryotherapy (freezing with liquid nitrogen). Genital warts may respond to topical therapies, such as podophyllin resin or trichloroacetic acid. Treatment of common and plantar warts often initially consists of less invasive therapies, such as topical acetic or salicylic acid with or without occlusion. If required, paring of the lesion, cryotherapy, or curettage can be used subsequently. Multiple and repeated treatments are often required.

FUNGAL INFECTIONS

Superficial fungal infections may involve the scalp, nails, or skin. These dermatophyte infections use keratin as a metabolic substrate and can be quite difficult to eradicate. They are mildly infectious; many individuals can be exposed to the same inoculum (eg, in locker room show-

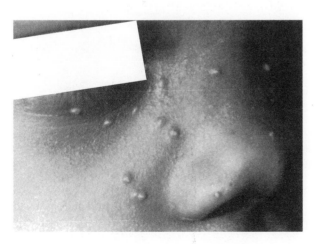

Figure 12–6. Molluscum contagiosum.

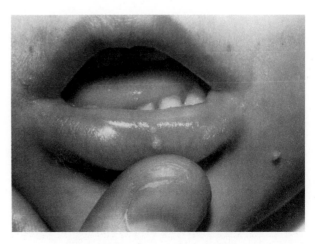

Figure 12–7. Warts, or verruca vulgaris.

ers), yet only a few will be infected. Tinea infections are named by location (eg, capitis, head; corporis, body; manuum, hand; and pedis, foot). Evaluation of possible tinea infections should include KOH preparations of scale, and culture on appropriate media.

Tinea Capitis

Tinea capitis may take several forms: (1) a dry, scaling, dandruff-like involvement with mild or no hair loss; (2) discrete areas of scarring alopecia with broken-off hairs and some element of scale; and (3) single or multiple erythematous, boggy masses, with overlying hair loss, known as **kerions** (Figure 12–8). The most common causative agent is *Trichophyton tonsurans,* which may be epidemic in communities. Both *Microsporum* and *Trichophyton* species can be the causative agents in infections of the scalp. Family pets are sometimes the vehicle of transmission for *Microsporum* infections. Kerions reflect a more extensive inflammatory reaction. All forms of tinea capitis require systemic therapy. Griseofulvin is most commonly used, and concurrent topical selenium sulfide 2.5% shampoo therapy is recommended to decrease spore counts and expedite response to therapy.

Tinea Corporis, Pedis, & Manuum

Tinea corporis, pedis, and manuum represent infections of the skin, usually by a *Trichophyton* or *Microsporum* species. The lesions are annular, gyrate, and discrete or coalescent scaling papules or plaques (Figure 12–9). Lesions can be indolent or actively inflammatory with erythema and erosions. Secondary bacterial infection is commonly seen in the interdigital web spaces of the feet. Treatment consists of topical antifungal therapy such as the imidazoles. Systemic griseofulvin therapy may be required for recalcitrant cases.

Onychomycosis

Onychomycosis is a fungal invasion of the nails. Toenail involvement is most frequent and most difficult to

eradicate. Afflicted areas commonly exhibit distortion of the nail with whitening and subungual debris. The differential diagnosis for such findings includes psoriasis and lichen planus. The most common causative agent is *Trichophyton rubrum.* Whitening of the dorsal aspect of the toenail is seen in nail infections caused by *Trichophyton mentagrophytes.* Although superficial forms of onychomycosis may clear with topical antifungals, onychomycosis most often requires systemic therapy. Both griseofulvin and ketoconazole have shown limited efficacy in this disease.

ACNE

Acne vulgaris is the most common skin disease of adolescence, with more than 90% of the population affected. Although not a life-threatening disease, acne may have substantial psychological effects on those afflicted. Acne lesions include closed comedones (whiteheads), open comedones (blackheads), papules, pustules, and nodules. Open comedones appear as pale, slightly raised skin-colored or white papules. Closed comedones are flat or slightly elevated lesions with a brown or black central opening. The dark color of "blackheads" is not due to dirt but to compact keratin and melanin pigment. Acne "cysts" are large suppurative nodular lesions that resemble inflamed epidermal cysts. Acne lesions may be followed by postinflammatory hyperpigmentation or a fibrous response causing pitted, hypertrophic, or papular scars. In severe cases, scarring can be substantial.

Pathogenesis

Acne pathogenesis is multifactorial. It is primarily a

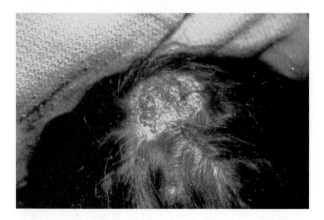

Figure 12–8. Tinea capitis.

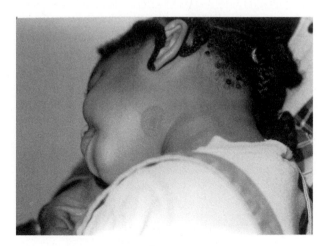

Figure 12–9. Tinea corporis.

disease of the sebaceous follicle. Sebaceous follicles are cell-lined units with large sebaceous glands and a fine vellus hair that rarely extends out of the follicular lumen. The follicles are most common in acne-prone areas (cheeks, nose, forehead, midline chest, and back). Sebaceous glands are responsive to androgenic hormones, which increase in early puberty. These hormones increase the mass and activity of sebaceous glands. Acne severity usually correlates with sebum production.

Cells lining the follicle canal are cornified keratinocytes. These cells normally slough into the follicular canal and are normally carried out to the skin surface with sebum secretion. The normal epithelium is altered in active acne, and sloughed cells plug the follicle, forming a "microcomedone." Subsequent dilation results in a thin-walled structure known as a "comedo." In addition to sebum and shed follicular cells, the canal normally contains a population of organisms, including *Propionibacterium acnes,* an anaerobic diphtheroid. Follicular plugging facilitates a hospitable environment for bacterial proliferation. Chemotactic factors and cellular response to bacteria result in inflammatory lesions.

Genetic factors, as well as the hormonal milieu, may influence the tendency to form microcomedones. There is no evidence that chocolate, fatty foods, or other dietary indiscretions affect the development of acne.

Treatment

The ideal drug would correct abnormal keratinization, decrease sebaceous gland activity (sebum secretion), inhibit the growth of *P acnes,* have anti-inflammatory effect, and promote drainage of closed comedones and resolution of established inflamed lesions. It would be entirely topical to limit systemic effects and toxicities. It should have no adverse effects and cause no irritation or sensitization. Unfortunately, no such agent exists. On the basis of acne pathogenesis, treatment is directed at microcomedone formation, bacterial proliferation, inflammation, and hormonal or sebaceous gland activity. Therapy of acne begins with educating the patient about good skin care and attempting to dispel myths about acne being a disease of improper cleansing or poor diet. Vigorous scrubbing is to be avoided, as it may aggravate acne, and does not prevent further lesion formation.

Topical therapies are the mainstay of acne therapy for the vast majority of patients. Topical preparations include antibiotics, benzoyl peroxide, tretinoin, and tretinoin-like agents. Erythromycin, clindamycin, benzoyl peroxide, benzoyl peroxide–erythromycin combination, and sulfacetamide are effective topical agents. Formulations include lotions, cremes, and gels. Topical antibiotics effectively decrease inflammatory papules and pustules.

Tretinoin (Retin A). This topical vitamin A analogue normalizes keratinization of the sebaceous follicle and decreases horny cell adhesion. It effectively promotes deplugging of comedones and prevents new microcomedone formation. Tretinoin requires appropriate patient education, counseling concerning the possibility of irritation

and photosensitivity, and consistent use over several weeks for optimal tolerance and response to therapy. Non-tretinoin retinoids and retinoid-like agents (eg, adapalene gel and azelaic acid) work similarly to diminish comedone production.

Antibiotics. Papulopustular, nodular, and nodulocystic acne may be treated with systemic antibiotics with activity against *P acnes.* Tetracycline, minocycline, dioxyline, and erythromycin are effective agents with anti-inflammatory effects as well. Treatment over many months is standard.

Isotretinoin (Accutane). This systemic vitamin A analogue is useful for severe papular, nodulocystic, scarring acne unresponsive to topical and systemic treatments described above. Isotretinoin is associated with serious side effects and potential toxicities and is a teratogen. It should be prescribed only by physicians skilled in its use. Use in women of child-bearing age requires mandatory contraception.

An algorithm delineating the use of topical, systemic, or combination treatments, depending on type of acne, is presented in Figure 12–10.

ECZEMATOUS DISORDERS

Eczema is a term that is commonly misused and often confusing to the medical student. The term actually means "to boil over" and is most correctly used to describe a reaction pattern rather than a particular disease. This pattern consists of inflammation of the skin with the presence of intercellular edema (**spongiosis**), pruritus, erythematous papules, vesiculation, and oozing. The pattern can be seen in many disorders, including atopic dermatitis, contact dermatitis, seborrheic dermatitis, and dyshidrotic and nummular eczema. Although "eczema" is frequently used to denote atopic dermatitis, one must keep in mind that the reaction pattern it signifies can be noted in any of the diseases mentioned above. Table 12–20 lists the differential diagnoses for eczematous eruptions and their distinguishing characteristics.

Atopic Dermatitis

Atopic dermatitis is an inherited skin disorder often found in association with asthma or hay fever. These three conditions or atopic states are characterized by an enhanced capacity to form IgE in response to a variety of antigens. There is a strong genetic predisposition: A child with one atopic parent has a 60% chance of being affected; if both parents are afflicted, the odds increase to 80%. Atopic dermatitis affects approximately 30% of the childhood population and, because of its chronic nature, accounts for almost one third of pediatric dermatology visits.

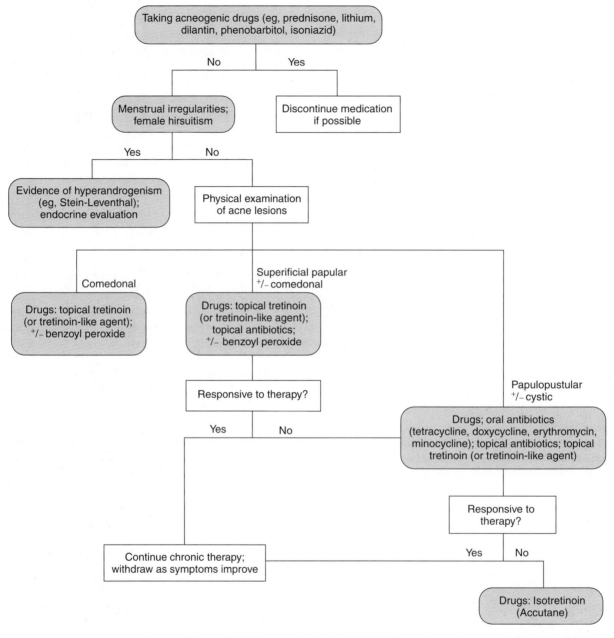

Figure 12–10. Approaches to the patient with acne.

The distribution of atopic dermatitis is age dependent. It usually presents in children before the age of 5 years and frequently 3–4 months after birth. In infancy, it favors the face and extensor extremities; in later childhood, it predominantly involves the antecubital and popliteal fossae. At all ages, the atopic skin tends to be dry and easily irritated. Acutely, the lesions are erythematous, vesicular, and oozing with superimposed scale crust. With time, however, these lesions tend to become dry and thick from chronic rubbing (Figure 12–11). It is customary to separate the disease into acute, subacute, and chronic states, depending on the degree of vesiculation and lichenification present. At all stages, pruritus is a cardinal finding; however, many have questioned whether pruritus is in fact the primary finding and whether the associated skin lesions are merely secondary changes caused by scratching ("an itch that rashes, rather than a rash that itches").

Associated findings include facial and especially peri-

Table 12–20. Differential diagnosis: Eczematous disorders.

Disorder	Clinical Appearance
Atopic dermatitis	Lesions ill defined, distribution age dependent, + xerosis/lichenification (see text)
Contact dermatitis (diaper dermatitis)	Localized, usually with discrete margins
Tinea corporis	Usually annular, discrete borders, less pruritic, scale significant
Seborrheic dermatitis	Most common in infants and teens; greasy scale favors scalp, face, groin
Scabies	Severely pruritic, favors hands and feet; burrows, nodules, papules
Nummular eczema	Coin-shaped lesions, favor lower extremities, severely pruritic
Rare:	Ataxia-telangiectasia (see Chapter 7)
	Wiskott-Aldrich syndrome (see Chapter 7)
	Acrodermatitis enteropathica
	Leiner disease
	Cystic fibrosis (see Chapter 18)

oral pallor, infraorbital folds (Dennie-Morgan lines), xerosis, increased linear markings of the palms, and keratosis pilaris. The differential diagnosis includes other eczematous disorders (see Table 12–20), scabies, histiocytosis X, and a variety of immunodeficiency disorders including Wiskott-Aldrich syndrome and ataxia-telangiectasia.

Although it has long been recognized that some immunologic abnormalities occur in patients with atopic dermatitis, the pathogenesis of the disease is still not clear. Current speculation rests on the presence of an immunologic maturational defect involving T-suppressor cells that allows for relatively unopposed IgE synthesis. This is the basis for the experimental use of both evening primrose oil (which contains high levels of γ-linoleic acid) and thymopoietin, which are thought to act as maturational factors for T cells. Although both modalities have shown some promise, neither has led to clear-cut, significant improvement in patients; thus, the pathogenesis and optimal treatment of the disease remain in question.

Fortunately, the course of the disease in most cases is one of progressive improvement and eventual resolution. Parents must be informed that, although there is no cure, it is possible to control disease manifestations and that the disease resolves with time in most patients. Treatment rests on educating the patient and family regarding dry-skin care, as in many cases change in bathing habits and emollients improve the patient's condition markedly. Other therapies include the use of low or moderate-potency steroids and, occasionally, tar or oatmeal baths.

One must also watch vigilantly for secondary bacterial infections, as *S aureus* colonization is common in patients with atopic dermatitis. If a patient does not respond to emollients and steroids, empiric treatment with a short course of antistaphylococcal therapy is sometimes appropriate. A semisynthetic penicillin or the more pleasant-tasting cephalosporins are the drugs of choice (Table 12–21). Elimination diets usually are not helpful, although the occasional patient responds to the elimination of egg, milk, or nut products. Although uncommon, secondary infection of atopic lesions with HSV can occur and lead to generalized, erosive lesions (**eczema herpeticum**). When appropriate, Tzanck preparation should be performed and acyclovir administered.

PAPULOSQUAMOUS ERUPTIONS

Papulosquamous eruptions denote a group of diverse diseases unified by the physical characteristics of discrete papules or plaques with superimposed scale. Papulosqua-

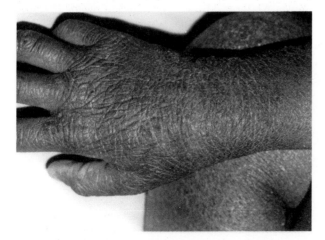

Figure 12–11. Chronic atopic dermatitis.

Table 12–21. Approach to treatment of atopic eczema.

- Break the itch-scratch cycle: Wear long-sleeve clothes, cotton mittens at night, trim fingernails, use antihistamines liberally.
- Decrease inflammation: Avoid irritating substances (eg, wool, polyester) and friction, apply topical steroids and emollients, tepid soaks.
- Moisturize the skin: Take short, infrequent baths with tepid water; use moisturizers (eg, petroleum creams and lotions) frequently.
- Treat secondary bacterial or fungal infection: Consider empiric antistaphylococcal therapy when a patient's condition proves resistant to conventional therapy; use mupirocin ointment for localized, secondarily infected sites or treatment; culture for yeast and fungi in intertriginous areas when appropriate.
- Educate the family regarding the chronic (but gradually improving) nature of the disease and the need to avoid drying and irritation.

mous lesions, in contrast to eczema, are almost always well marginated and lack epidermal changes, such as oozing, fissuring, and scale crust. The differential diagnosis includes pityriasis rosea, seborrheic dermatitis, psoriasis, parapsoriasis, and secondary syphilis. KOH preparation and the Venereal Disease Research Laboratory (VDRL) test for syphilis should be performed when doubt exists as to the diagnosis. Two disorders, psoriasis and pityriasis rosea, are briefly discussed.

Psoriasis

Psoriasis is a chronic inflammatory disease with a strong genetic predisposition that afflicts 1–3% of the population. The disease can present in four distinct forms: (1) discrete scaling papules and plaques that favor the scalp, sebum-producing areas, knees, and elbows; (2) small ovoid or guttate lesions, which tend to generalize and frequently occur after infection, particularly streptococcal pharyngitis; (3) groups of pustules that favor the palms and soles but can occur elsewhere; and (4) a diffuse erythematous or erythrodermic eruption, often with pustules. Nail findings are also common and include discrete pitting, onycholysis, yellow discoloration, and distortion with subungual debris. Psoriasis is thought to be a T cell–mediated disorder; recent research has focused on the role of calcium in the control of cell proliferation and adhesion in this disease. It is evident that the disorder leads to hyperproliferation of keratinocytes, with impaired differentiation and a relative increase in certain forms of keratin. Genetics certainly plays a significant role in the development of the disorder, but stress, trauma, and infection clearly can exacerbate the course of the disease.

Treatment is less than optimal and consists of emollients, topical steroids, tars, and phototherapy. Fortunately, many patients respond to sunlight and a decrease in stressful conditions. If a patient does not respond to therapy, one must look for evidence of secondary bacterial or fungal infection and treat the infection appropriately.

Pityriasis Rosea

Pityriasis rosea, a self-limited inflammatory disorder of probable infectious origin, most commonly occurs in winter. The first lesion often consists of a red scaling plaque known as the "herald patch." Although pityriasis rosea is usually asymptomatic, some patients report a preceding "flulike" illness, and the skin lesions are sometimes pruritic. The lesions initially tend to involve the upper trunk, then gradually extend to the abdomen and legs. They are ovoid, erythematous, and scaly and follow the lines of cleavage in what is referred to as a "Christmas tree" pattern. The palms and soles are not involved, but oral lesions consisting of white or hemorrhagic patches may be seen. Resolution may take 6–12 weeks. Treatment is not required, but ultraviolet light sometimes shortens the course, and topical steroids and antipruritics may be used for pruritic cases.

REFERENCES

Hurwitz S: *Clinical Pediatric Dermatology: A Textbook of Skin Disorders of Childhood and Adolescence.* Saunders, 1981.

Hurwitz S: Skin lesions in the first year of life. Contemp Pediatr 1993;10:110.

Leyden JJ: Therapy for acne vulgaris. N Engl J Med 1997;336:1156.

Lynch PA: *Dermatology for the House Officer,* 2nd ed. Williams & Wilkins, 1987.

Schachner LA, Hansen RC (editors): *Pediatric Dermatology.* Churchill Livingstone, 1988.

Singalavanija S, Frieden IJ: Diaper dermatitis. Pediatr Rev 1995;16:142.

Thornton CM, Eichenfield LF: Treatment of common cutaneous vascular disorders of childhood. Dermatol Ther 1997;2:68.

Tucker MA et al: Clinically recognized dysplastic nevi: A central risk factor for cutaneous melanoma. JAMA 1997;277:1439.

Weston WL, Lane AT: *Color Textbook of Pediatric Dermatology.* Mosby-Year Book, 1991.

Williams ML, Pennella R: Melanoma, nelanocytic nevi, and other melanoma risk factors in children. J Pediatr 1994;124:833.

13

The Gastrointestinal Tract & Liver

Donald Wayne Laney, Jr, MD, & William F. Balistreri, MD

VOMITING

Vomiting is a common occurrence among pediatric patients; yet, despite the frequency with which episodes of vomiting occur, they tend to provoke anxiety and apprehension on the part of the caregivers. This emphasis on the importance of vomiting is often justified, as vomiting may be the cardinal manifestation of one of several serious and potentially life-threatening disorders.

PHYSIOLOGY

Vomiting is a highly complex event involving the coordinated responses of the abdominal and respiratory musculature to a variety of stimuli delivered through the nervous system. The first phase in an episode of vomiting is the sensation of nausea. This feeling of the need to vomit may be brought on by emotional stimuli, by labyrinthine stimuli (eg, motion sickness), by unpleasant tastes or odors, or through stimulation of mechanoreceptors or chemoreceptors in the gastrointestinal (GI) tract. If vomiting is due to a cause that does not involve any of these pathways (eg, increased intracranial pressure [ICP]), nausea may be absent. Nausea is not always followed by vomiting, but when it is, the second phase in the process is retching.

Retching consists of increasingly forceful movements of the chest and abdominal musculature. Inspiratory efforts are made by the respiratory muscles while the abdominal muscles contract, causing negative intrathoracic pressure. As these events are occurring, the gastric fundus dilates and the pylorus and distal stomach contract. Retching may or may not culminate in emesis.

Emesis occurs as a combined result of sustained contraction of the abdominal muscles and contraction (downward movement) of most of the diaphragm. The central portion of the diaphragm, which normally serves to aid the lower esophageal sphincter in preventing gastroesophageal reflux (GER), must relax for emesis to occur.

A much less violent retrograde passage of gastric contents into the esophagus occurs in regurgitation. Regurgitation occurs without the forceful muscular contractions that characterize emesis. The symptoms of nausea and retching are also usually absent. Typically, regurgitation appears to be relatively effortless and painless, causing only minimal distress. Because occasional regurgitation is almost universal among normal infants and decreases in frequency with maturation, it is more properly viewed as a physiologic, rather than a pathologic, process. It becomes pathologic when it occurs with excessive frequency, as with GER.

CLINICAL EVALUATION

A crucial first step in the evaluation of a patient with vomiting is to determine the relative severity of the problem, ie, whether there is truly forceful emesis or whether the symptom is instead more accurately described as regurgitation or spitting. A careful and thorough history often serves to make this distinction. In an infant who appears to be otherwise normal and who is growing and developing normally, regurgitation is present more often than is frank emesis.

The age at onset of symptoms is important in determining the etiology. Vomiting in the first few days after birth may be caused by obstructive lesions in the GI tract. Vomiting in early infancy may also be caused by several metabolic diseases. In an older infant, acute gastroenteritis becomes more likely. The coexistence of fever and diarrhea adds further support to this diagnosis. Food allergies or intolerances may also present in children during the first year, as the composition of their diet becomes more varied.

Older children are often able to describe other symptoms that they experience coexistent with their vomiting. These may include vomiting associated with ingestion of a particular food item, raising the question of contamination or food allergies. Complaints of abdominal pain in addition to vomiting necessitate investigation to rule out appendicitis or other abdominal emergencies.

A description of the vomitus may also prove useful in evaluation. Bile staining of the emesis often indicates the existence of intestinal obstruction. The presence of blood in the vomitus (hematemesis) may be due to esophagitis, esophageal varices, gastritis, or peptic ulcer disease. Hematemesis may also occur after ingestion of blood from nasopharyngeal sources. The evaluation of patients with these and other causes of upper GI bleeding is discussed below. Vomitus may also be noted to contain "curdled milk" or food particles recognizable from a previous meal. Also important in the description of the vomitus is the manner of its delivery. A description of emesis that exits the mouth with unusual force (projectile vomiting) is classically associated with hypertrophic pyloric stenosis.

Physical examination of a patient with vomiting should begin with an assessment of the state of hydration. This is especially important in the neonate and young infant, in whom vomiting can rapidly lead to dehydration. Palpation of the abdomen may reveal abdominal distention or the presence of masses or organomegaly. The existence and site of tenderness or guarding should be noted. Jaundice may be noted in patients whose vomiting is due to hepatitis or to metabolic diseases involving the liver. Non-GI causes of vomiting often present with other characteristic physical findings.

Several laboratory investigations may be useful in the evaluation of a patient with vomiting. Evaluation of serum electrolytes is often beneficial. In hypertrophic pyloric stenosis, for example, a frequent characteristic finding is hypochloremic metabolic alkalosis. Metabolic acidosis may be due to one of the many metabolic diseases associated with vomiting. Urine and serum evaluations for organic acids and amino acids are indicated.

In patients in whom intestinal obstruction is suspected, abdominal radiographs may be useful. Contrast studies (barium swallow, upper GI series) and ultrasonography are two other potentially useful sources of information. Endoscopic visualization of the upper GI tract allows for direct mucosal visualization and the obtaining of biopsy specimens. Such studies may be helpful in the diagnosis of esophagitis, gastritis, or peptic ulcer disease. Esophageal pH monitoring may be used to document the reflux of acidic GI contents into the normally alkaline environment of the esophagus, as occurs in GER.

DIFFERENTIAL DIAGNOSIS

Vomiting may be the sole or major manifestation of a disease, as with GER, or may exist as one of a constellation of symptoms, as exemplified in several metabolic diseases. Table 13–1 lists many of the diseases known to cause vomiting. A thorough discussion of most of these entities may be found elsewhere in this text. In this chapter, we concentrate on those disorders in which vomiting is the predominant symptom, and the GI tract is the site of the causative lesion.

Hypertrophic Pyloric Stenosis

Hypertrophy of the circular muscle of the pylorus, which results in stenosis and gastric outlet obstruction, is a relatively common cause of vomiting, occurring in approximately 1:500 births. Male infants are more commonly affected than are female infants, and the incidence is far greater in full-term infants than in premature infants. The etiology of pyloric stenosis remains unknown, although recent evidence indicates the involvement of defective enteric innervation. Recently, endothelium-derived relaxing factor (EDRF), a vasodilator of vascular smooth muscle, has been implicated as a possible factor in pyloric stenosis. EDRF has been shown to be nitric oxide, and its deficiency in smooth muscle of the pyloric sphincter may cause contraction. The disorder is not congenital but develops during the first few weeks after birth.

Patients with hypertrophic pyloric stenosis typically experience the onset of nonbilious vomiting during the first few weeks after birth. The frequency of the episodes of vomiting increases, as does the force with which the vomitus is delivered, culminating in the projectile vomiting characteristic of this disorder. Affected infants are apparently hungry and initially take feedings eagerly. As the obstructed stomach is filled, reverse peristalsis begins; the rhythmic muscular contractions sometimes may be apparent on abdominal observation. As the disease progresses, emesis increases and dehydration develops.

In addition to these findings, the diagnosis of hypertrophic pyloric stenosis is supported by the palpation of the hypertrophied muscle itself, which has been described as an "olive" owing to similarities in size and shape. Hypochloremic hypokalemic metabolic alkalosis sometimes occurs. If the diagnosis is in doubt, radiologic studies may provide further information. Plain radiographs may demonstrate absence of air distal to the pylorus; barium contrast studies may reveal the movement of a small amount of barium through the narrowed pylorus (the "string sign"), as shown in Figure 13–1. Ultrasound studies are useful in demonstrating the thickened and elongated pylorus typical of this disorder.

Management of patients with pyloric stenosis should begin with the correction of dehydration and electrolyte imbalances. Once this goal is accomplished, definitive treatment of the problem is achieved through a pyloromyotomy. After surgery, most patients recover without complications and have no further signs or symptoms of obstruction.

Other Anatomic Malformations

Several other anatomic malformations of the GI tract may cause vomiting. **Hiatal hernias** occur when the abdominal esophagus and a portion of the gastric fundus protrude above the diaphragm into the thoracic cavity. This may lead to a decrease in the competence of the

Table 13–1. Differential diagnosis: Vomiting.

Anatomic causes	**Metabolic diseases**
Malformations	Urea cycle defects
Hypertrophic pyloric stenosis	Aminoacidopathies
Hiatal hernia	Organic acidurias
Intestinal duplications	Galactosemia
Intestinal atresias	Hypercalcemia
Malrotation	Uremia
Webs	
Obstructions	**Endocrinologic disorders**
Acquired gastric outlet obstruction	Diabetes mellitus (especially with diabetic ketoacidosis)
Chronic granulomatous disease	Diabetes insipidus
Prostaglandin infusion	Congenital adrenal hyperplasia
Intussusception	
Volvulus	**Dietary causes**
Meconium ileus	Feeding problems
Distal intestinal obstruction syndrome	Overfeeding
Bezoars	Maternal anxiety or inexperience
Hirschsprung disease	Contaminated food or water
Other	Food allergies and intolerances
Gastroesophageal reflux	Milk–soy protein intolerance
Peptic ulcer disease	Celiac disease
Testicular torsion	
Ménétrier disease	**Toxin-induced**
	Poisons
Infectious causes	Pharmacologic and chemotherapeutic agents
Acute gastroenteritis	Radiation
Meningitis	
Sepsis	**Psychological**
Urinary tract infections	Cyclic (periodic) vomiting
Hepatitis	Anorexia nervosa
Appendicitis	Bulimia
Pneumonia	
Otitis media	
Oral candidiasis	
Neurologic causes	
Intracranial neoplasms	
Chronic subdural hematoma	
Hydrocephalus	
Migraine	
Motion sickness	

lower esophageal sphincter mechanism and be associated with vomiting or GER (see below, Gastroesophageal Reflux). In many patients, however, these hernias are asymptomatic.

Atresias are malformations in which the lumen normally present in an organ is not developed. **Stenoses** are similar disorders involving lumenal narrowing. Atresias occur in the esophagus and throughout the small and large intestine. Duodenal atresia is associated with Down syndrome and several other congenital malformations, including intestinal malrotation, annular pancreas, and imperforate anus. Duodenal atresia is recognizable radiographically as the "double bubble" sign, consisting of air in the stomach and in the distended first portion of the duodenum. There is absence of intraluminal gas distal to the duodenum (Figure 13–2). Atresia is more common in the jejunum and ileum than in the duodenum.

Patients with intestinal atresias present with bilious vomiting and abdominal distention, sometimes with palpable loops of bowel. In neonates, there may be failure to pass meconium. Treatment begins with the restoration of fluid and electrolyte balance and relief of the obstructive symptoms through nasogastric suction. Definitive treatment is then accomplished surgically.

Malrotation & Volvulus

During normal fetal development, the intestines undergo counterclockwise rotation and are then affixed to the posterior abdominal wall. When this process is not properly accomplished, malrotation results. The cecum lies in the right upper quadrant, and the duodenal-jejunal region is on the right side of the abdomen. Although malrotation itself may not cause symptoms, it allows for the occurrence of a volvulus, in which a segment of intestine twists on itself and causes obstruction. This may present in a manner similar to intestinal atresias, with bilious vomiting and abdominal distention. Radiographic studies may reveal the "double bubble" sign of duodenal obstruction, as well as the underlying anatomic abnormality. This disorder is treated with surgical correction.

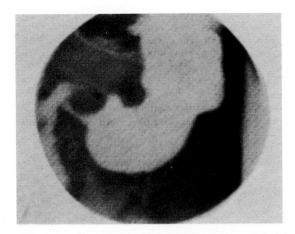

Figure 13–1. Characteristic radiographic findings in hypertrophic pyloric stenosis. The narrow, elongated pyloric channel causes the barium to appear as a thin "string," a finding often referred to as the "string sign." (Reproduced, with permission, from Rudolph AM [editor]: *Pediatrics,* 18th ed. Appleton & Lange, 1987.)

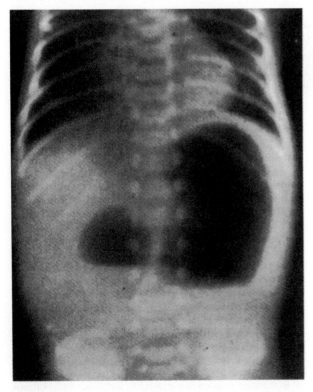

Figure 13–2. Abdominal radiograph demonstrating the "double bubble" characteristic of duodenal obstruction. (Reproduced, with permission, from Rudolph AM [editor]: *Pediatrics,* 18th ed. Appleton & Lange, 1987.)

Gastrointestinal Obstructions

In patients with meconium ileus, the normally soft meconium is abnormally viscid and causes intestinal obstruction. This condition is seen almost exclusively in patients with cystic fibrosis (see Chapters 4 and 8). Patients demonstrate signs and symptoms typical of intestinal obstruction, including abdominal distention. Rectal examination usually reveals a narrow rectum empty of stool. When this diagnosis is suspected, a sweat test for cystic fibrosis is indicated. Barium enema studies may be useful in revealing the presence of microcolon and simultaneously accomplishing removal of the meconium obstruction. If the obstruction is not relieved by barium enema, surgical removal is required. The **meconium ileus equivalent syndrome,** also known as **distal intestinal obstruction syndrome,** occurs in older patients with cystic fibrosis. In these patients, abdominal distention and pain are more common presenting symptoms than is vomiting.

Bezoars are collections of indigestible material found in the GI tract, usually the stomach. Bezoars may be composed of undigested milk solids **(lactobezoars),** hair **(trichobezoars),** or undigested vegetable matter **(phytobezoars).** Typically these masses cause gastric outlet obstruction and produce symptoms of vomiting with abdominal pain and distention, often accompanied by anorexia and weight loss. Examination may reveal the presence of an abdominal mass; halitosis is also often noted. Lactobezoars are often digested if the stomach is kept otherwise empty for a few days and the patient nourished intravenously. Other bezoars may require surgical removal.

Gastroesophageal Reflux

GER is a commonly diagnosed disorder characterized by effortless and painless regurgitation. It occurs when gastric contents move past the lower esophageal sphincter and enter the esophagus. Reflux may vary in severity from an occasional burp (probably similar to an adult's heartburn), to persistent emesis and its consequences. GER is thought to be physiologic in infancy, resulting from immaturity of the lower esophageal sphincter mechanism. In these infants, reflux has no significant consequences.

In other patients, however, reflux may be much more severe. Failure to thrive may result from inadequate retention of feedings. If the esophagus is exposed to the acidic gastric contents for prolonged periods of time, esophagitis develops, leading to blood loss and anemia, and there is potential for development of esophageal strictures.

GER may be diagnosed by using one of several combinations of diagnostic modalities. A barium swallow may be useful to document retrograde passage of a swallowed bolus of contrast material. More important, it may be used to rule out the presence of an anatomic abnormality as the cause of the regurgitation. Monitoring of the intraesophageal pH with an electronic probe may be used to document the frequency of regurgitation of acidic gastric contents into the esophagus as well as the duration of the episodes, giving a measure of the severity of the problem.

Esophageal manometry allows for the measurement of esophageal sphincter pressure and may aid in the diagnosis. Direct visualization of the esophageal mucosa with endoscopy is useful in the diagnosis of esophagitis and permits biopsy specimens to be obtained. Radionuclide scans may also be useful in providing an evaluation of the rate of gastric emptying.

The selection of treatment for GER should take into account the severity of the symptoms and their possible consequences. When reflux is so mild that normal growth and development are not impaired, minimal intervention is appropriate. Intervention may include changing the infant's sleeping position from supine (the position recommended by the American Academy of Pediatrics because of a decreased incidence of sudden infant death syndrome among infants sleeping in that position) to prone with the head of the crib slightly elevated. In the prone position, aspiration is less likely; elevation of the head of the crib makes reflux mechanically more difficult and consequently less likely. Changes in feedings may also be beneficial; this includes the use of smaller volumes, offered at more frequent intervals, and the use of cereals and other foods to thicken the feedings.

In patients with more severe symptoms, pharmacotherapy is sometimes helpful. Both antacids and histamine H_2-receptor antagonists may be used to decrease the acidity of gastric contents, thus decreasing the risk of esophageal damage secondary to reflux. Metoclopramide has also been commonly used in treating GER because it increases lower esophageal sphincter pressure and hastens gastric emptying. Cisapride, a pro-motility agent, is gaining widespread use in the treatment of significant GER in children despite an absence of data documenting efficacy. Cisapride is associated with fewer serious side effects than is metoclopramide; mild to moderate diarrhea is the most common complaint. Caution should be used, however, in the concomitant use of cisapride with ketoconazole and other similar antifungal agents and with erythromycin, as cardiac arrhythmias have been reported under those circumstances. In some patients who do not benefit from the drugs, surgical procedures aimed at improving the competence of the lower esophageal sphincter may be helpful. The Nissen fundoplication is the procedure most commonly used.

DIAGNOSTIC EVALUATION

An approach to the evaluation of a patient with vomiting is outlined in Figure 13–3. Note that evaluation of the patient's hydration status is a crucial first step in this schema. Also important initially is the uncovering of any possible historical or physical clues that might narrow the differential diagnosis.

Description of the emesis itself provides further clues as to the most likely causes and focuses the diagnostic evaluation. Bloody vomiting (hematemesis), for example, is caused by a separate group of diseases; its evaluation is

discussed later in this chapter (see Upper Gastrointestinal Tract Hemorrhage, Clinical Evaluation). Bilious emesis usually indicates an obstructive lesion. Another possibility is that the emesis is not truly vomiting, but rather regurgitation, which is usually caused by GER.

MANAGEMENT

Specific therapies have been mentioned in conjunction with the previously discussed disease entities. Regardless of the etiology of vomiting, however, several general management techniques are important.

Because of the possibility of dehydration resulting from vomiting, initial management should include restoration of adequate hydration. In patients with acute infectious gastroenteritis associated with vomiting, rehydration may be successfully achieved orally, as discussed later in this chapter (see Oral Rehydration). However, if the severity of the emesis precludes adequate fluid delivery orally, intravenous administration is necessary. Having addressed the patient's fluid status, and simultaneously corrected any electrolyte abnormalities, further diagnostic studies may be performed.

With long-standing vomiting complicated by malnutrition and failure to thrive, nutritional replenishment is also important. In many instances, this requires parenteral delivery of nutrients.

Pharmacologic agents should be used with great caution to stop vomiting in children. This is especially true in children who cannot adequately communicate symptoms to their caregivers. In these children, antiemetic agents may mask the outward signs of disease even as the problem progresses. An exception to such limited use of antiemetics is in patients receiving chemotherapeutic agents and radiation therapy. In these situations, and in others in which the cause of vomiting is apparent, the use of antiemetics is indicated.

CONSTIPATION

Constipation is frequently encountered in children, especially in more developed countries where a diet composed largely of highly refined foods is the norm. Effective evaluation of constipation requires an understanding of normal defecation physiology and normal stooling patterns. This allows the clinician to determine whether a situation perceived to be a problem is truly abnormal or whether the patient's stooling pattern merely is not meeting the parents' expectations for normalcy.

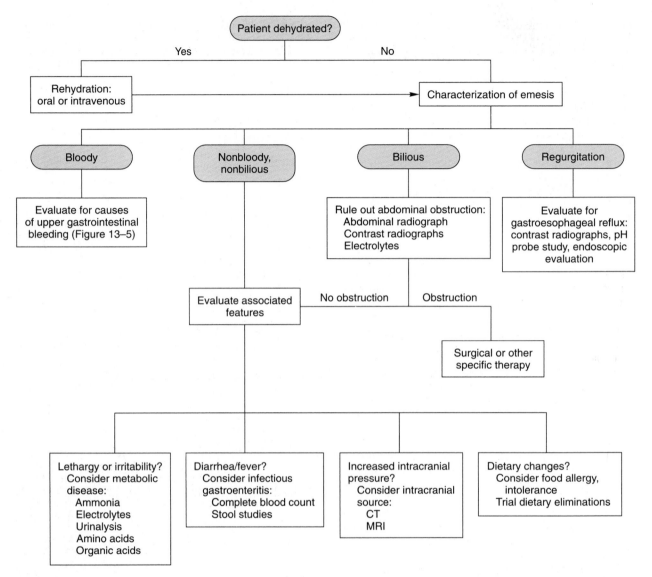

Figure 13–3. Algorithm presenting an approach to the evaluation of a patient with vomiting. CT = computed tomography; MRI = magnetic resonance imaging.

ANATOMY & PHYSIOLOGY

The colon terminates in the rectum, which, in turn, passes through the levator ani muscles and becomes the anal canal. The anal canal is circled by two groups of muscles, the internal and external anal sphincters. The internal sphincter, composed of smooth muscle, is under involuntary (reflex) control. The external sphincter provides a means of voluntary control over defecation. Also important in the control of defecation is the near 90-degree angle formed at the junction of the rectum and the anal canal. This junction straightens with flexion of the hips, which explains the physiologic advantage of squatting for defecation.

The fecal mass is propelled distally through the intestine by peristalsis. In the colon, water is passively reabsorbed, making the feces more solid. Stools eventually reach the rectal ampulla, where they distend the rectum and activate a neuromuscular pathway resulting in relaxation of the internal anal sphincter and contraction of the external anal sphincter. Relaxation of the internal sphincter allows the rectal contents to come in contact with the sensory epithelium of the anal canal where their nature (ie, solid, liquid, or gas) is discernible. To defecate, the external sphincter and the puborectalis sling are voluntarily relaxed, allowing stool to pass the anus. A voluntary increase in intra-abdominal pressure (Valsalva maneuver) assists the process.

A definition of "normal" stooling patterns involves several parameters, including stool size, consistency, and frequency. For more than 90% of adults, stooling occurs from three times per day to three times per week. For children, however, more frequent stooling may be normal. In infants, stooling is normally much more frequent, occurring from one to seven times per day in the first week. Stooling may continue at this frequency in breast-fed infants, but in formula-fed infants, stool frequency tends to decrease over subsequent weeks. In the toddler years, stooling typically decreases further in frequency, so that preschool children usually have bowel patterns more similar to those of adults.

Stool size and consistency are much more difficult to measure objectively than is stool frequency, yet even subjective information is useful in determining whether a patient has constipation. Stools that cause extreme discomfort in passing, because of either excessive size or extreme firmness, are abnormal. Constipation, then, is present when stools are excessively large, uncomfortably large, or abnormally infrequent. It is important to keep in mind, however, that this definition allows for a broad range of "normal" and that which is perceived by a parent as abnormal in fact may be physiologic for a particular patient.

CLINICAL EVALUATION

Several points are of special importance in the history of a patient with constipation. The child's age at the onset of symptoms may be significant. Patients with Hirschsprung disease, for example, often have had symptoms since birth. Constipation due to other causes may present after a period of normal stooling. The history of the child's toilet training and subsequent fecal control is useful. Also important is the association of pain with defecation (**tenesmus**) or the passage of blood (**hematochezia**). The child's psychosocial situation may also be useful in making a diagnosis.

The dietary history may provide helpful information. Breast-fed infants, at least in the first few weeks after birth, tend to have looser and more frequent stools than do formula-fed infants. Children who drink excessive amounts of cow's milk may be more prone to constipation. Diets low in fiber may also predispose the patient to constipation. Numerous pharmacologic agents, such as narcotics and anticholinergics, are known to cause constipation.

The physical examination should begin with a thorough general examination. Inspection of the lower back, for example, may reveal the presence of a sacral dimple, possibly indicating the involvement of a spinal cord lesion. Examination of the abdomen should include palpation, as large fecal masses often can be detected in the descending colon.

The rectal examination should begin with visual inspection of the anal skin, noting the presence of any skin tags, fissures, or other abnormalities. Evaluation of the neuromuscular integrity of the anus may be grossly gauged by attempting to elicit the reflex anal "wink" by lightly stroking the perianal skin with a cotton swab. Digital examination provides a means of evaluating the resting tone of the external sphincter and the relative capacity of the anal vault. Any stool present on the examining glove should be tested for the presence of occult blood.

DIFFERENTIAL DIAGNOSIS

A partial listing of the causes of constipation is given in Table 13–2. Despite this broad range of differential diagnosis, the vast majority of patients are found to have no discernible cause for their symptoms and thus are labeled as having chronic functional (or idiopathic) constipation.

Functional Constipation

Patients with functional constipation may present with complaints of abdominal distention or recurrent abdominal pain in addition to a history of infrequent, often large stools. The results of the physical examination are usually entirely normal, with the exception of palpable fecal masses in the lower colon and an enlarged, stool-filled rectal vault.

Some patients with functional constipation may also have a lack of voluntary control over defecation (**encopresis**). Encopresis develops as a result of long-standing constipation with progressive enlargement of the rectal vault. Eventually, the sensation prompting an urge to defecate is lost. Large fecal masses accumulate in the rectum, allowing only liquid stool to pass. Soiling of the underclothing occurs commonly. When the large stool is finally passed, it is often associated with great discomfort. The association of pain with defecation discourages the patient from voluntarily passing stools, leading to continued stooling infrequency and perpetuation of the cycle.

In addition to the physical unpleasantness of their condition, patients with encopresis are subject to social and behavioral problems. Understandably, other children often avoid them, making them social outcasts. The physical aspects of this problem are almost always resolved using therapy beginning with bowel evacuation, followed by use of stool softeners and implementation of behavioral modification techniques (see below, Management). Treatment of the psychosocial aspects of the disease may require the involvement of experienced mental health care personnel.

Although patients with encopresis are typically of early school age, the stool-withholding behavior that is often the initial cause of their problem may be seen in much younger children. This often occurs in 2- to 3-year-old children and may develop in response to attempts at toilet training. Symptoms such as grimacing and grunting are

Table 13–2. Differential diagnosis: Constipation.

Anatomic defects	**Neurologic defects**
Localized to the anus, rectum, or colon	Central nervous system defects (eg, cerebral palsy)
Aganglionosis	Spinal cord trauma
Congenital (Hirschsprung disease)	Infectious polyneuritis
Acquired (Chagas disease)	Amyotonia congenita
Anal stenosis	Neurofibromatosis
Imperforate anus (postsurgical correction)	Down syndrome
Anterior ectopic anus	Hypotonia
Anteriorly located anus	
Anal fissures	**Neuromuscular/motility disorders**
Dermatitis	Idiopathic slow transit constipation
Colonic stricture	Pseudo-obstruction syndromes
Primary	Infant botulism
Secondary (eg, secondary to inflammatory bowel disease	
or necrotizing enterocolitis)	**Connective tissue disorders**
Localized to the gastrointestinal tract	Lupus erythematosus
Malrotation	Scleroderma
Congenital intestinal bands	
Stenosis	**Psychological disorders**
Gastric emptying defects (eg, pyloric stenosis)	Depression
Generalized	Anorexia nervosa
Abnormal abdominal musculature	Denial of bowel action
Eagle-Barrett syndrome	Stool withholding
Gastroschisis, postrepair	Sexual abuse
Postabdominal surgery	
Neurologic	**Dietary causes**
Spina bifida	Inadequate dietary fiber
Meningomyelocele	Excessive cow's milk intake
Spinal cord trauma	
Paraplegia	**Pharmacologic causes**
Sacral teratoma	Antacids (especially those containing calcium and aluminum)
	Anticholinergics
Endocrinologic or metabolic defects	Bismuth
Hypothyroidism	Iron preparations
Hyperparathyroidism	Opiates
Pregnancy	
Diabetes insipidus	**Idiopathic constipation**
Infantile renal acidosis	
Hypokalemia, hyponatremia	
Uremia	

often erroneously interpreted by the parents as signs of difficulty with defecation. In fact, these signs may accompany a child's voluntary withholding of stool. Appropriate treatment of stool withholding with agents such as fiber or simple laxatives (nonabsorbable carbohydrates or salts) may prevent the problems from progressing to chronic constipation.

Hirschsprung Disease

In young children with constipation, especially those younger than 1 year, the diagnosis of Hirschsprung disease must always be considered. This congenital disorder is characterized by an absence of ganglion cells from the myenteric (Auerbach) and submucosal (Meissner) plexuses of the rectum. The aganglionic segment includes the internal anal sphincter as its most caudal point and extends proximally for a variable distance. In most patients with Hirschsprung disease, the aganglionic segment is limited to the sigmoid colon, but it may extend throughout the colon and has been known to extend as far as the duodenum. If the aganglionic segment involves 5 cm or less

of the rectum, it is referred to as ultrashort segment disease.

The absence of ganglion cells causes the affected segment constantly to be contracted and without peristalsis. This creates a functional obstruction, which causes proximal intestinal dilatation and hypertrophy, manifested clinically as constipation, abdominal distention, and bilious vomiting. Hirschsprung disease is often diagnosed soon after an infant is born because of the delayed passage of meconium (later than 48 hours after birth). When the disease is not diagnosed in the neonatal period, clinical features typically include failure to thrive in addition to the previously listed symptoms.

Fecal soiling is uncommon in patients with aganglionosis, except in those in whom only a very short segment of the colon is affected. Older patients with Hirschsprung disease may report absence of sensation of the need to defecate, because fecal contents do not come in contact with the sensory epithelium of the anal mucosa where this sensation is triggered. Rectal examination usually is remarkable for increased sphincter tone, often described as a "sleeve effect." Frequently, withdrawal of the examining finger is followed by a sudden expulsion of stool.

The most severe complication of untreated Hirschsprung disease is the development of enterocolitis. This condition, characterized by fever, heme-positive and watery stools, and abdominal distention, occurs in approximately one third of patients with Hirschsprung disease. In some cases, the enterocolitis is mild and not detected until the time of surgical resection of the aganglionic segment. Typically, however, patients with enterocolitis are extremely ill, and about one third do not survive, making this the most likely cause of death in patients with Hirschsprung disease. Enterocolitis associated with aganglionosis does not occur in patients older than 2 years.

Diagnosis of Hirschsprung disease may be confirmed by information obtained from several studies. A plain radiograph of the abdomen, taken in the prone position, that reveals the absence of intraintestinal air in the pelvis is suggestive of Hirschsprung disease and necessitates further studies. A barium enema is often effective in delineating the location of the transition zone between the normal and aganglionic segments. It may also reveal a rectal diameter narrower than that of the sigmoid colon, which is typical of Hirschsprung disease. To provide useful information in making this diagnosis, barium enemas should be done without prior evacuation of the colon by enemas or cathartics.

Manometric studies of the anus are also useful in the diagnosis of aganglionosis. Distention of a balloon-tipped catheter in normal patients stimulates reflex relaxation of the internal anal sphincter. In patients with Hirschsprung disease, however, the internal sphincter contracts. This study is especially useful in the diagnosis of patients whose aganglionic segment is 5 cm or less in length.

Tissue obtained from rectal biopsy allows for a definitive diagnosis. Although this tissue may be obtained surgically, a more usual method is through the use of suction-assisted biopsy forceps. Histologic examination reveals the absence of ganglion cells. Staining for acetylcholinesterase, an enzyme present in parasympathetic nerve fibers, reveals abnormally prominent nerve fibers in the rectal mucosa of patients with Hirschsprung disease.

Management should begin with stabilization of acutely ill patients, including restoration of fluid and electrolyte balance, administration of broad-spectrum antibiotics, and evacuation of the colon with enemas. Definitive treatment requires surgical intervention with the creation of a colostomy to provide relief of the obstruction followed by reanastomosis of the normal portion of the colon with the rectum. In older patients, it is sometimes possible to remove the abnormal segment and perform the reanastomosis without the creation of a colostomy. In patients with short-segment and ultrashort-segment disease, an anorectal myomectomy may provide effective relief of the obstruction.

Other Causes of Constipation

Several congenital anatomic defects of the anorectal region have been associated with constipation. **Anal stenosis** may cause stools to be of abnormally small caliber and

thus lead to chronic stool retention. In mild cases, this may be corrected by progressive dilation of the anus with the examining finger. **Anterior ectopic anus** and **anteriorly located anus** are conditions that cause constipation, most often in females, beginning in early infancy. With an anterior ectopic anus, the anal canal and internal sphincter exit anterior to the normally located external sphincter. Rectal examination of patients with this disorder may reveal a "rectal shelf" posterior to the anal opening. With an anteriorly located anus, both the anal canal and the external sphincter are located anterior to their normal position. In either disorder, the anal wink may be present in its normal location. Both conditions may require surgical repair for symptomatic relief. **Anal fissures** and dermatitis of the anorectal region may cause discomfort during defecation and lead to constipation.

Strictures of the colon may also cause obstruction and consequent constipation. These may be congenital anatomic defects or may occur later in life secondary to other disorders. In the neonate, strictures may arise secondary to necrotizing enterocolitis. In older children, inflammatory bowel disease (IBD) may be the cause. Correction usually entails surgical resection of the affected portion of the bowel. Constipation may occur in hypothyroidism and, in fact, is often the presenting manifestation of hypothyroidism. Feeding difficulties, prolonged jaundice, and hypotonia are also commonly present.

Disorders of GI motility may also produce constipation. **Intestinal pseudo-obstruction** is a condition in which motility of all or portions of the intestine are abnormal. Patients experience symptoms of obstruction, including dysphagia and vomiting, in addition to constipation, in the absence of any anatomic obstruction. Management of patients with these disorders may require dietary modifications and the use of stool softeners and laxatives to prevent constipation. Prokinetic agents, including cisapride, are often used in the treatment of pseudo-obstruction.

DIAGNOSTIC EVALUATION

An approach to the evaluation of a patient with constipation is outlined in Figure 13–4. The initial history and physical examination may reveal abnormalities or arouse suspicion of specific organic problems known to cause constipation. These possibilities should be evaluated using the appropriate diagnostic tests. In most patients with constipation, the initial history and physical examination reveal no other problems. In patients younger than 1 year, the possibility of Hirschsprung disease should specifically be considered. However, in older patients with constipation, "functional" constipation is the most likely diagnosis. It is therefore appropriate initially to treat these patients with a therapeutic regimen designed for those with functional constipation (see below, Management). Patients who improve with therapy may be presumed to have functional constipation and should continue to receive therapy until the problem is resolved. Those not respond-

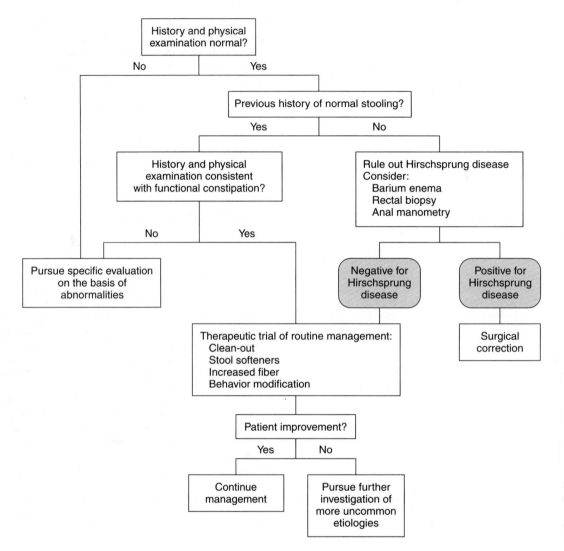

Figure 13–4. Algorithm presenting an approach to the diagnosis and management of the patient with constipation.

ing to therapy should be reevaluated in an attempt to find the cause of their problem.

MANAGEMENT

Management of constipation should be directed toward resolution of the underlying problem. In patients with idiopathic or functional constipation and in those with constipation secondary to causes that cannot be corrected (eg, cerebral palsy), therapy must be directed toward lessening the symptom.

The first step in treating a patient with constipation is to remove fecal material from the colon. In many of these patients, the rectal vault has been stretched far beyond its normal capacity by the accumulation of stool. Removal of this material may rarely require manual disimpaction but

is usually accomplished through the use of enemas. A variety of enema solutions have been used for this purpose. Plain water enemas have been associated with the development of water intoxication and are not recommended. Sodium biphosphate enemas are commercially available in both adult and pediatric sizes; although these products are commonly used, caution is necessary because hyperphosphatemia and hypernatremia have occurred secondary to their administration. A preparation of equal parts of milk and molasses has long been used successfully in treating patients at Children's Hospital Medical Center in Cincinnati, Ohio, with no known side effects. Regardless of the preparation used, enemas should be continued on a twice-daily basis until the colon is evacuated (usually less than 3 days). Colonic clean-out may also be achieved through the use of oral laxatives or cathartics (magnesium citrate) or by the oral or nasogastric administration of polyethylene glycol-electrolyte solutions. The subsequent use of enemas or cathartics is usually not needed after the initial cleansing.

The second step in the management of constipation is aimed toward the production of smaller, softer stools so that frequent defecation is unavoidable. This more frequent stooling eventually leads to the return of the rectal vault to normal size and, consequently, to the return of sensation of the need to defecate. Multiple pharmacologic agents, including stool lubricants (mineral oil), osmotic agents (lactulose), and stimulants (senna, bisacodyl), have been shown to be effective in this stage of therapy. Mineral oil is an inexpensive and safe agent widely used for this purpose; however, because of the risks of aspiration, it should be used cautiously in the young child. The dose should be titrated so that the patient has bowel movements twice daily to every other day. Once stooling patterns have returned to normal, the medications should be tapered and eventually discontinued. Patients typically require these medications for several months. Increasing the dietary fiber content, either with commercially available supplements or through dietary modification, is also beneficial in alleviating the symptoms of constipation.

Behavioral modification also plays an important role in the management of constipation. Patients should be encouraged to have established, routine periods of sitting on the toilet once or twice each day. Preferably, these times should be soon after meals to take advantage of the increased colonic motility induced by gastric activity (the gastrocolic reflex). For younger children, praise for the successful elimination of stool may be helpful. For all patients, the use of criticism or other negative approaches should be avoided. As part of behavior modification, the patient and family can be encouraged to improve their dietary habits by decreasing intake of highly refined foods and by increasing intake of foods high in fiber.

Probably the most important facet of the treatment of constipation is education of the patient and family. Most are pleasantly surprised to learn that constipation is a common problem that can almost always be treated successfully. Involvement in support groups with other patients assists in the education process and may further help to lessen these children's feelings of being abnormal. Patient education and encouragement should be an important part of the follow-up care of these patients.

GASTROINTESTINAL TRACT HEMORRHAGE

Bleeding from the GI tract is usually classified as either "upper" or "lower" tract, on the basis of the location of the bleeding site either proximal or distal to the ligament of Treitz (near the duodenojejunal junction). Bleeding from upper-tract lesions usually results in hematemesis, whereas bleeding from lower-tract lesions is more apt to present as loss of blood per rectum. These two groups of disorders are sufficiently distinct that they are discussed as separate entities. We first consider the diagnosis and management of upper GI bleeding.

UPPER GASTROINTESTINAL TRACT HEMORRHAGE

CLINICAL EVALUATION

Hematemesis, or the vomiting of blood, can be associated with the rapid loss of relatively large amounts of blood. The initial evaluation of patients experiencing hematemesis includes assessment of hemodynamic status: blood pressure decreases, and pulse rate increases with acute blood loss. The hematocrit, by contrast, serves as a better measure of **chronic** blood loss and may not accurately reflect the patient's status during or soon after an acute bleed. Hemodynamic instability, if present, should be addressed immediately through administration of appropriate intravenous fluids and blood products.

The next important step is to determine the **site** of bleeding. Placement of a nasogastric tube to aspirate gastric contents is useful in this step of the evaluation. Absence of blood in the gastric aspirate may indicate that the source of bleeding is in the nasopharynx; however, an aspirate that tests positive for hemoglobin does not rule out the nasopharynx as the source, because blood may have been swallowed. The presence of apparently fresh, bright red blood in the gastric aspirate is evidence of an actively bleeding lesion. Blood that has been partially altered by the gastric contents may have the appearance of "coffee grounds."

Another potential explanation for a negative gastric aspirate is that the substance perceived to be blood is actually some other red substance. Food colorings found in beverages and gelatin products may impart a red color to the vomitus and be mistaken for blood.

The passage of blood from the mouth without vomiting may also occur with upper GI bleeding. If the amount of blood is small, an oral lesion may be the cause. Far more serious, though, is the effortless passage of large amounts of fresh blood from the mouth, as may occur with bleeding esophageal varices. Blood from varices also passes into the stomach and comes to the physician's attention as hematemesis.

DIFFERENTIAL DIAGNOSIS

A variety of diseases are known to cause bleeding localized to the upper GI tract (Table 13–3). Diseases that

Table 13–3. Differential diagnosis: Upper gastrointestinal tract bleeding.

Mucosal lesions	Vascular lesions
Esophagitis	Esophageal varices
Mallory-Weiss tear	Hereditary hemorrhagic telangiectasia (Osler-Weber-Rendu
Gastritis	syndrome)
Primary gastritis	
Secondary gastritis	**Coagulopathies**
Peptic ulcer disease	Hemophilia A or B
Duplications	Pharmacologically induced
Mucosal erosion	Vitamin K deficiency, including hemorrhagic disease of the newborn
Foreign body	Secondary to chronic liver disease
Caustic ingestion	
Stress-related ulceration	**Miscellaneous**
Central nervous system lesion (Cushing ulcers)	Swallowed maternal blood
Burn lesion (Curling ulcers)	Nasopharyngeal bleeding
Intramural hematoma (secondary to trauma,	Rumination
including physical abuse)	
Milk–soy protein intolerance	

cause vascular lesions and coagulopathies may present with bleeding in either the upper or lower GI tract and, with the exception of esophageal varices, are not specifically discussed here. The remaining causes of upper GI bleeding are attributable to mucosal damage in the duodenum, stomach, or esophagus.

Esophageal Mucosal Disorders

Esophagitis describes a nonspecific inflammatory response of the esophageal mucosa to a variety of noxious stimuli. The diagnosis of esophagitis may be made through the endoscopic observation of erythematous, possibly eroded or ulcerated mucosa. Biopsy specimens characteristically show the presence of increased numbers of intraepithelial eosinophils. Esophagitis varies in severity, and only the more severe cases present with upper GI bleeding.

Most cases of esophagitis in pediatric patients are secondary to the prolonged and recurrent exposure of the esophageal mucosa to acidic gastric contents that occurs with GER. In its most severe manifestation, this form of esophagitis not only results in upper GI bleeding, but also potentiates the development of esophageal stricture.

Infectious microorganisms may also cause esophagitis. Most frequently these infections occur in patients whose immune mechanisms are suppressed, either pathologically or pharmacologically. *Candida* is the most common agent identified in immunocompromised patients. In patients with intact immune-response mechanisms, infectious esophagitis usually develops as a secondary phenomenon, following esophageal mucosal damage due to another cause. Infectious esophagitis in and of itself is more likely to present as pain on swallowing than as upper GI bleeding. The presence of a foreign body in the esophagus and the ingestion of caustic substances are also possible causes of esophagitis.

Treatment of esophagitis relies on the diagnosis and management of the underlying condition responsible for the irritation. Antacids, histamine-receptor antagonists, and proton-pump inhibitors all decrease the acidity of gastric secretions and, consequently, decrease the amount of acid to which the esophageal mucosa is subjected. Sucralfate, a minimally absorbed disaccharide, serves as a cytoprotective agent and may provide symptomatic relief for esophageal discomfort secondary to esophagitis.

Mallory-Weiss syndrome involves the spontaneous laceration of the esophagus secondary to prolonged or forceful vomiting. The severity of bleeding associated with this lesion depends on both the location and the depth of the mucosal tear. Diagnosis is made with upper GI endoscopy. The lacerations usually heal spontaneously, and only the most severe require surgical repair.

Gastric Mucosal Disorders

Gastritis describes nonspecific inflammatory changes in the gastric mucosa. These changes are usually manifested as abdominal pain and upper GI bleeding. When gastritis is attributable to one of the several known causes of gastric inflammation, it is referred to as **secondary gastritis.** When the cause is uncertain, it is considered to be **primary gastritis.** Primary gastritis may be associated with peptic ulcer disease (see subsequent discussion).

Secondary gastritis has several causes. Stress-related gastritis may occur in patients with severe illnesses or injuries, including sepsis, severe burn injury, and head trauma, and in those who have undergone major surgical procedures. Many ingested agents are also known causes of gastritis. Alcohol is among the more common causes, but medications, including corticosteroids and nonsteroidal anti-inflammatory agents, and corrosive substances, may also produce gastric inflammation. Secondary gastritis may occur in patients with other inflammatory disease, such as Crohn disease, and in patients with allergic disease, as is seen in eosinophilic gastritis.

Primary gastritis has traditionally denoted cases in which no cause could be determined. In recent years, evidence has accumulated that a significant portion of these cases are actually due to infection with *Helicobacter py-*

lori. This organism has been implicated in the pathogenesis of peptic ulcer disease as well.

Diagnosis of gastritis is based on histologic criteria and therefore necessitates obtaining mucosal biopsy specimens endoscopically. Cultures for *H pylori* should be included in the evaluation. Pharmacologic treatment of gastritis with antacids, histamine H$_2$-receptor antagonists, or proton-pump inhibitors provides some benefit by reducing gastric acidity. Sucralfate and other agents designed to "coat" the gastric mucosa may also be useful. When *H pylori* is present, specific antimicrobial therapy, including metronidazole, bismuth subsalicylate, and amoxicillin, should be added to the treatment regimen. In older children and adults, tetracycline is usually substituted for amoxicillin.

Peptic ulcer disease occurs when the normal balance between acidic gastric secretions and the mucosal protective elements is disrupted. The ulcers themselves are well-circumscribed regions of tissue damage, with loss of mucosa, submucosa, and muscularis. The lesions are described as either primary or secondary; the causes of secondary ulcers are similar to those of secondary gastritis. Important among these is the use of nonsteroidal anti-inflammatory agents. The Zollinger-Ellison syndrome of excessive gastrin secretion from a gastrinoma and consequent peptic ulcer disease, another cause of secondary ulcers, is rare in children. There is increasing evidence that *H pylori* also may cause peptic ulcer disease in the pediatric population.

Peptic ulcers may be found in the stomach or duodenum. In children younger than 6 years, the majority of ulcers are located in the gastric antrum. These may present clinically with abdominal pain or GI bleeding. In older children, ulcers are more commonly located in the duodenum. Older boys are affected approximately four times as often as are older girls. Dramatic episodes of hematemesis are less likely to occur in these patients than in children younger than 6 years with peptic ulcer disease.

Diagnosis of peptic ulcer is best made through direct visualization of the lesions by upper GI endoscopy. Treatment involves the use of antacids, histamine H$_2$-receptor antagonists, and mucosal coating agents. Surgical intervention is sometimes required in the management of severe hemorrhage or perforation occurring as a complication of peptic ulcer disease. Once healed, gastric ulcers are not likely to recur. Children with duodenal ulcers may experience recurrences throughout their life, possibly as a result of persistent or recurrent infection with *H pylori.*

Variceal Bleeding

Varices are submucosal veins that become engorged as a result of obstructed outflow; they commonly develop in patients with portal hypertension, which in turn may be secondary to a variety of causes (Table 13–4). Veins in the esophagus and stomach are possible sites of varix formation, as are the internal hemorrhoidal veins and venous channels around the umbilicus (which when engorged are called the **caput medusae**).

Bleeding from esophageal varices is often massive and sudden in onset. Therefore, the restoration of hemodynamic stability through appropriate use of intravenous fluids and blood products is of utmost importance in managing these patients. The second priority is to stop the bleeding. Placement of a nasogastric tube allows aspiration of gastric contents and provides some gross measure of ongoing blood losses. The nasogastric tube is also useful therapeutically for gastric lavage. The administration of vasopressin is often used to decrease blood pressure and portal blood flow. Although usually effective, this medication should be used with great caution because of its many side effects, mainly related to ischemia. Mechanical tamponade of the bleeding varices may be accomplished through a special balloon catheter (Sengstaken-Blakemore tube). This tube should be placed only by those experienced in its use.

Patients with conditions known to be associated with the development of portal hypertension, and those who have previously experienced variceal bleeding, are often monitored endoscopically for the development and progression of esophageal varices. Injection of the varices with sclerosing agents (sodium tetradecyl sulfate or sodium morrhuate) is often effective in preventing recurrent episodes of variceal bleeding. Surgical procedures aimed at shunting the blood flow away from the portal cir-

Table 13–4. Etiology of portal hypertension.

Prehepatic	Posthepatic
Portal vein obstruction (eg, thrombosis)	Hepatic vein obstruction
Congenital (cavernous transformation or portal vein thrombosis)	(Budd-Chiari syndrome)
Acquired	Inferior vena cava obstruction
Omphalitis	Congenital
Umbilical vein catheterization	Acquired
Coagulopathies	Trauma
Protein C deficiency	Tumor
Protein S deficiency	Clotting dysfunction
Paroxysmal nocturnal hemoglobinuria	Congestive heart failure
	Constrictive pericarditis
Intrahepatic	
(Secondary to cirrhosis of any cause)	

culation are seldom required in the management of pediatric patients.

DIAGNOSTIC EVALUATION & MANAGEMENT

Figure 13–5 presents an approach to be used in the evaluation of patients with upper GI bleeding. Many present with substantial blood loss, hemodynamic instability, or shock. Intervention should begin with administration of intravenous fluids. An assessment of the need for transfusion therapy should also be included in the initial evaluation. Excessive administration of fluids and blood products, especially in patients whose bleeding is secondary to esophageal varices, may actually increase bleeding and forestall efforts at hemostasis. In situations of less rapid blood loss, hemostasis is usually spontaneous.

Once the patient has been stabilized, diagnostic evaluation may proceed. In most disorders causing upper GI bleeding, endoscopic examination is the procedure of choice. Radiologic studies, especially when done with the addition of a contrast agent, may provide evidence of ulcers and other gross mucosal lesions but do not permit biopsy specimens necessary for the diagnosis of gastritis and esophagitis to be obtained. The absence of evidence of mucosal lesions with contrast-enhanced radiographic studies, however, does not rule out the presence of lesions, because lesions that are small or out of the plane of the film will not be detectable. Another advantage of endoscopy is that it allows for sclerosis of esophageal varices, if present.

LOWER GASTROINTESTINAL TRACT HEMORRHAGE

The passage of blood from the rectum may be caused by a variety of disorders, some localized to specific sites along the GI tract and others more generalized in distribution. This section addresses those disorders that affect the lower (ie, distal to the ligament of Treitz) GI tract.

CLINICAL EVALUATION

Loss of blood from the rectum is not necessarily caused by a bleeding source in the distal intestine or colon but may be due to bleeding in the upper GI tract that, because of either chronicity or location, is not associated with he-

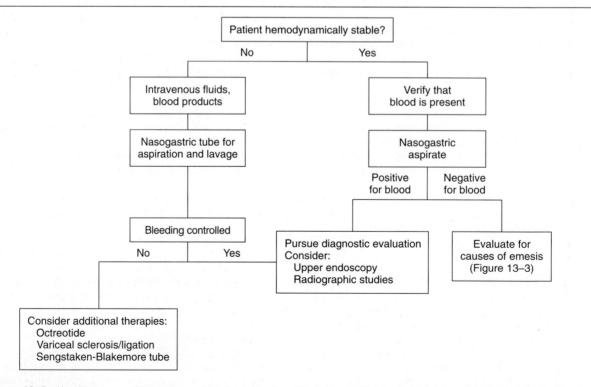

Figure 13–5. Algorithm presenting an approach to the evaluation of the patient with bleeding from the upper gastrointestinal tract.

matemesis. If there is any question as to the upper tract being the source of the bleeding, a nasogastric tube should be inserted to aspirate gastric contents. Bleeding from lesions in the upper GI tract, especially varices, is more likely to be associated with the sudden loss of significant amounts of blood and hemodynamic instability. Assessment of the patient's intravascular volume is an important initial step in the evaluation of a patient with rectal bleeding.

Information regarding the location of the bleeding site may be obtained from the history. The passage of bright red blood (hematochezia) is more likely to be due to a bleeding site in the colon or rectum. Streaks of blood on the outside of the stool are more likely to be caused by lesions in the rectum and anus. Blood noted on the toilet paper suggests the possibility of an anal source. When the bleeding source is in the upper GI tract, the blood is more likely to be mixed with the feces. Blood that has been partially degraded by the action of bacterial and digestive enzymes may cause the stool to appear black and tarry (melena) or dark red. Blood in the stool from an upper GI tract source does not always appear dark or black and may even remain bright red, especially when the bleeding is occurring rapidly or when there is rapid GI transit.

Characterization of the stool is also important. Loose, watery stools occurring in a previously healthy patient may be caused by infectious gastroenteritis. Several organisms that cause acute gastroenteritis may also cause bleeding, including *Salmonella, Shigella, Campylobacter,* and rotavirus. By contrast, the passage of extremely hard stools associated with bleeding suggests an external lesion (eg, anal fissure) as a likely source. Mucus or white blood cells may be present in the stool as a result of intestinal inflammation. Mucus is often present in the stools of patients with IBD, but this finding is not specific for IBD and also may be present in patients with bacterial or amebic infections.

Coexistence of other symptoms should be evaluated. Abdominal pain may be present when the bleeding is secondary to IBD. These patients may also report a feeling of urgency accompanying the need to defecate (tenesmus), especially when the disease affects the rectum. Acute abdominal pain may also accompany rectal bleeding because of an obstructive intestinal lesion; episodic abdominal pain is often described with intussusception. Painless rectal bleeding may occur with rectal polyps. A history of recent use of medications is important because several drugs, notably aspirin, may be associated with bleeding disorders that present as blood in the stool.

The physical examination should first assess the patient's hemodynamic status. A complete examination should be done to detect any abnormalities or unusual features, such as dermatologic manifestations of Henoch-Schönlein purpura or the extraintestinal manifestations of Crohn disease. The abdomen should be examined for signs of obstruction (eg, rigidity, absence of bowel sounds), tenderness, or organomegaly. Rectal skin tags, fissures, or other abnormalities should be noted. If no gross blood is present on digital examination of the rectum, the fecal material should be tested for the presence of occult blood to verify that the apparent blood is not merely pigmentation caused by the ingestion of colored foods or beverages or medications (eg, iron preparations, ampicillin, and bismuth preparations).

DIFFERENTIAL DIAGNOSIS

Table 13–5 outlines the more common causes of rectal bleeding.

Anal/Rectal Disorders

Anal fissures are the most common cause of rectal bleeding in young children beyond the age of infancy. There is usually a history of constipation, with passage of excessively large or hard stools before development of the fissure. The amount of bleeding with a fissure is usually small, coating the outside of the stool or appearing as small amounts of bright red blood in the diaper or on the toilet tissue. The fissure often causes severe pain during defecation. This may lead to avoidance of defecation, worsening of constipation, and eventually the painful passage of yet another large, hard stool with further irritation of the fissure.

In patients with anal fissure not related to constipation, the possibility of perianal cellulitis, usually caused by either *Candida albicans* or streptococci, should be considered. Patients with Crohn disease (see Inflammatory Bowel Disease) may also have anal fissures, which may be accompanied by edema and purulent discharge. The possibility of sexual abuse must also be considered in the patient with an anal fissure.

The diagnosis of a fissure can be made by inspection. Digital examination causes great pain and usually is not necessary. Treatment of uncomplicated anal fissures includes maintenance of good anal hygiene by washing or sitz baths and correction of constipation. Patients with perianal cellulitis should receive appropriate antimicrobial therapy. Persistence of painful defecation may indicate sphincter spasm, which is often alleviated by gentle digital dilation. Surgical repair is rarely necessary, usually with chronic fissures.

In **rectal prolapse,** the rectal mucosa intermittently protrudes through the anus for brief or, less often, more protracted periods of time. It is most commonly associated with constipation, but prolapse also occurs in patients with cystic fibrosis or parasitic infestations. Rectal bleeding is not a prominent feature of prolapse and is typically slight. Diagnosis must rely on the history, as the physical findings are rarely persistent. Successful management is usually accomplished through treatment of the underlying disorder.

Hemorrhoids are also a potential cause of rectal bleeding. They are usually **exterior** to the anus, associated with infection and edema related to an anal fissure. Minor rectal bleeding may occur; no treatment is required. **Internal**

Table 13–5. Differential diagnosis: Lower gastrointestinal tract bleeding.

Anorectal origin 　Anal fissure 　Rectal prolapse 　Skin tags 　Hemorrhoids 　Foreign body 　Trauma/sexual abuse **Colonic origin** 　Colitis 　　Infectious 　　Antibiotic associated 　　　(pseudomembranous colitis) 　　Allergic 　　Ulcerative colitis 　　Necrotizing enterocolitis 　　Secondary to Hirschsprung disease 　　Polyposis **Small intestinal origin** 　Meckel diverticulum 　Intussusception 　Malrotation and volvulus	**Generalized gastrointestinal origin** 　Crohn disease 　Transient ischemia related to vigorous exercise 　Upper gastrointestinal bleeding 　　Varices 　　Peptic ulcer disease 　　Gastritis 　　Foreign body and other ingestions 　　Duplications 　Pharmacologically induced **Hematologic and vascular diseases** 　Coagulopathies 　Hemangiomas and telangiectasias 　Henoch-Schönlein purpura 　Hemolytic-uremic syndrome

hemorrhoids are dilations of the rectal venous system; in children, they are most often secondary to portal hypertension. Although uncommon, bleeding from rectal varices may be substantial. Treatment of internal hemorrhoids may necessitate ligation.

Colonic Disorders

Colitis is a general term used to describe inflammation in the colon; it may be associated with varying degrees of rectal bleeding. In **infectious colitis,** the causative agents include *Salmonella, Shigella, Campylobacter, Yersinia,* enterohemorrhagic *Escherichia coli,* and rotavirus. (For further information, see Chapter 9.) With colitis of bacterial etiology, the stool typically shows polymorphonuclear leukocytes in addition to the presence of gross or microscopic amounts of blood. Diagnosis may usually be made from stool cultures. Treatment is by appropriate antibiotics. Rotavirus may be diagnosed with the use of a specific enzyme-linked immunoassay.

Pseudomembranous colitis is caused by the toxin produced by *Clostridium difficile.* It differs from the other infectious colitides in that its pathogenesis depends on colonization of the colon by *C difficile* after eradication of the normal microflora by a course of antibiotics. Virtually all antibiotics have been implicated in this process.

Patients with pseudomembranous colitis present with symptoms ranging from mild, watery diarrhea to severe, bloody diarrhea, possibly associated with tenesmus and abdominal pain. In its most severe form, a fulminant colitis may develop, resulting in progressive loss of muscular tone in the colon. This condition, referred to as **toxic megacolon,** may progress to colonic perforation and peritonitis.

Diagnosis of pseudomembranous colitis may be made sigmoidoscopically by the identification of accumulations of inflammatory exudate, the pseudomembrane, on the colonic mucosa. Stool culture for the detection of *C difficile* or assays for its toxin are useful in the diagnosis of older children and adults, as these markers may be positive in patients in whom pseudomembranes cannot be found. In infants, however, these studies are not useful because as many as 70% of patients in this age group have been shown to be asymptomatic carriers of *C difficile.*

Allergic colitis may be associated with loss of blood in the stool; the most commonly implicated allergens are milk and soy proteins. Mucosal biopsy specimens in these patients may reveal increased numbers of eosinophils. Treatment is accomplished through elimination of the offending protein. Malabsorption, which may accompany allergic colitis, is discussed below.

Ulcerative colitis is a chronic IBD primarily affecting the colon. Because of its similarities to Crohn disease, these two disorders are discussed together (see below, Inflammatory Bowel Disease).

Mucosal polyps commonly cause rectal bleeding. Polyps are defined as gross protrusions of intestinal mucosa into the lumen and, in children, occur most commonly in the colon. They occur less frequently in the small bowel and stomach. Polyps may cause abdominal pain, either by serving as the lead point for an intussusception or, less commonly, through luminal obstruction. More often, however, polyps are the source of painless rectal bleeding, which results from either mucosal trauma from contact with passing stool or from ischemic necrosis as the polyp outgrows its blood supply.

Although they may be neoplastic, more than 90% of polyps in children are inflammatory (juvenile polyps) and are thought to carry little if any malignant potential. If left untreated, most polyps undergo self-amputation as they outgrow their blood supply. Diagnosis is best made through colonoscopy; this allows for definitive treatment by polypectomy. During examination, about half the patients with polyps are found to have more than one lesion.

Juvenile polyposis coli is a condition of multiple (more than 10) colonic polyps that occurs in both a familial and a sporadic form. In both conditions, the potential for malignant change is thought to be greater than that associated with isolated juvenile polyps. Generalized juvenile polyposis is a similar condition, with polyps not limited to the colon. **Familial polyposis coli** is an autosomal-dominant disorder in which patients have hundreds to thousands of adenomatous polyps, usually not recognized until after puberty. In **Gardner syndrome,** these polyps may occur throughout the small intestine and colon and are associated with tumors of bone and soft tissues as well as hypertrophy of the retinal pigment epithelium. In the **Peutz-Jeghers syndrome,** multiple hamartomatous polyps are associated with abnormal pigmentation of the lips and buccal mucosa.

Disorders of the Small Intestine

Meckel diverticulum is a vestigial remnant of the omphalomesenteric duct that, in the fetus, connects the gut to the yolk sac (Figure 13–6). It is the most common congenital malformation of the GI tract, occurring in approximately 1.5% of the population, most of whom experience no symptoms.

The diverticulum is typically located on the antimesenteric side of the ileum, within 100 cm of the ileocecal valve, and is approximately 2 cm in length. Symptomatic diverticula occur in boys twice as often as in girls and usually present before 2 years of age. These features have been described as the "rule of 2's."

Ectopic mucosa, most often gastric, is found in approximately one third of Meckel diverticula. The acid secreted by this mucosa may cause ulceration and bleeding. In young children, bleeding is usually painless, but pain is a prominent feature in older children, especially when the diverticulum causes intestinal obstruction through intussusception or volvulus. Diagnosis of a Meckel diverticulum is made via radionuclide scanning in which radiolabeled technetium, concentrated by gastric mucosa, is visualized in an ectopic location. Treatment is by surgical resection.

Intussusception is the invagination of a segment of bowel into itself, sometimes described as "telescoping" (Figure 13–7). Although intussusception may occur in any segment of the small intestine or colon, most often it is near or includes the ileocecal junction. Most cases are idiopathic, but in some, an identifiable "lead point" causes the intussusception. Polyps, Meckel diverticula, parasites, and tumors are known to act as lead points.

Intussusception typically occurs in children older than 2 years and presents with acute onset of episodic, crampy abdominal pain. In infants, pain is much less prominent. In time, the mucosa of the involved segments of bowel becomes edematous, and intestinal obstruction develops. Vomiting may occur, and an abdominal mass may be pal-

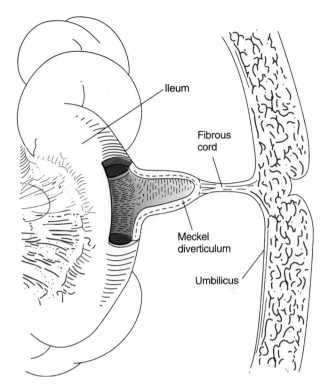

Figure 13–6. An illustration of a Meckel diverticulum, a persistent remnant of the omphalomesenteric duct, and its relationship to the normal gastrointestinal anatomy. (Reproduced, with permission, from Milov DE, Andres JM: Sorting out the causes of rectal bleeding. Contemp Pediatr 1988;5:80.)

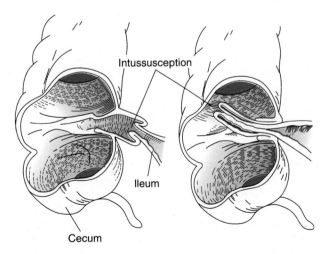

Figure 13–7. An illustration of the "telescoping" movement of one part of the bowel into another, which constitutes intussusception. (Reproduced, with permission, from Milov DE, Andres JM: Sorting out the causes of rectal bleeding. Contemp Pediatr 1988;5:80.)

pable. The classically described passage of maroon stools mixed with mucus ("currant-jelly" stool) occurs in only two thirds of patients.

Enema, using either air or barium as the contrast agent, is the diagnostic modality of choice, and when positive, reveals the so-called coiled spring appearance. Reduction of the intussusception can be accomplished in approximately 75% of cases through the use of hydrostatic or pneumatic pressure delivered through the enema catheter. These techniques carry a slight risk of intestinal perforation and a 10% risk of recurrence. When reduction is unsuccessful, surgical correction is indicated.

Inflammatory Bowel Disease

Idiopathic IBD is a term that encompasses both ulcerative colitis and Crohn disease. These disorders are similar in that they tend to produce symptoms of diarrhea, often mixed with blood, and abdominal pain. Other features are sufficiently distinct to allow for the differentiation of the two diseases, as shown in Table 13–6.

Crohn disease causes transmural inflammation of the GI mucosa at any point from the mouth to the anus, with the ileocecal region most commonly affected. Within a diseased segment of mucosa, areas of normal tissue ("skip lesions") may be interspersed. Noncaseating granulomas are often present, as are longitudinal ulcers, which create the characteristic cobblestone appearance. Progression of the inflammatory lesions may lead to bowel wall thickening, causing stenosis and obstruction, and to the formation of fistulae.

The onset of Crohn disease is often insidious. Patients may experience diarrhea, weight loss, or abdominal pain and tenderness. With ileal disease, rectal bleeding is often present. Signs of growth failure, delayed sexual maturation, arthritis, and unexplained fevers may also be among the initial manifestations.

The diagnosis may entail the use of multiple modalities. Contrast radiographic studies may reveal mucosal thickening, cobblestone features, and ulcer formation, as well as the presence of areas of stenosis. Endoscopy provides direct mucosal visualization as well as the opportunity to obtain biopsy specimens for histologic diagnosis.

Medical therapy for Crohn disease usually includes corticosteroids in an effort to reduce inflammation. When pos-

sible, steroid doses are gradually tapered to a dose sufficiently low to cause few side effects (hirsutism, fat deposition, cataract formation). In patients unresponsive to steroids or in those who are steroid dependent, 6-mercaptopurine and azathioprine are sometimes beneficial therapeutic alternatives. Despite effective medical therapy, many children with Crohn disease eventually require surgical intervention to relieve an obstruction secondary to stenosis, to remove an inflammatory mass, or to repair a fistula. In addition to pharmacologic and surgical therapy, meticulous attention to the patient's nutritional status and dietary supplementation, when needed, have been shown to have a significant impact on the patient's overall condition.

Ulcerative colitis causes inflammatory changes limited to the colon. The rectum is almost always involved, and varying portions of the more proximal colon are often affected. In only about 15% of patients is disease confined to the rectum. The disease is recognized histologically by the presence of superficial ulcerations associated with increased numbers of polymorphonuclear leukocytes. Crypt abscesses may also be present.

Patients with ulcerative colitis often experience rectal bleeding and abdominal pain, which is relieved on defecation. Fever, anemia, and hypoalbuminemia are typical associated features. As in Crohn disease, weight loss and growth failure may also be noted. Occasionally, ulcerative colitis may present acutely as toxic megacolon.

Diagnosis of ulcerative colitis is sometimes made by barium enema, which may reveal the loss of normal haustral markings, but no abnormalities may be evident. Sigmoidoscopy or colonoscopy with biopsy is a preferable means of diagnosis. Endoscopically the mucosa appears inflamed and friable. In contrast to Crohn disease, the lesion is continuous, without intervening areas of normal mucosa. Both barium enema and colonoscopy should be delayed in patients with severe disease because of the risk of precipitating toxic megacolon. Because the histologic changes of ulcerative colitis are similar to those seen in acute infectious colitis, appropriate bacterial cultures should also be part of the diagnostic regimen.

Pharmacotherapy of ulcerative colitis usually includes sulfasalazine or 5-amino salicylic acid, which acts as an anti-inflammatory agent affecting the colonic mucosa. Corticosteroids, administered either orally or topically (as

Table 13–6. Comparison of characteristics of Crohn disease and ulcerative colitis.

	Crohn Disease	Ulcerative Colitis
Histology	Transmural involvement; noncaseating granulomas	Involvement of mucosa and submucosa only; crypt abscesses
Gross appearance	Longitudinal ulcerations; cobblestone features	Friable mucosa; pseudopolyps
Radiologic findings	Ulcers; "thumbprinting"; areas of stenosis	Loss of haustral markings
Location	Throughout the gastrointestinal tract; diseased areas interposed with areas of normal tissue	Rectum ± variable colonic involvement
Fistula formation	Possible	Not typical
Toxic megacolon	Not typical	Possible
Extraintestinal disease	Delayed maturation; arthralgias and arthritis; erythema nodosum; conjunctivitis and uveitis	Delayed maturation; erythema multiforme

enemas), may be necessary in more severe disease. Nutritional supplementation is also frequently required.

Despite optimal medical therapy, approximately 25% of children with ulcerative colitis do not respond adequately and require surgical intervention, with colonic resection and construction of an ileostomy. Because of the increased risks of colon cancer in patients with ulcerative colitis, surveillance with colonic biopsies every 1–2 years is recommended beginning 8 years after the initial diagnosis. Colectomy is recommended when mucosal dysplasia is found. Patients with disease limited to the rectum or rectosigmoid are thought not to have an increased risk for colon cancer.

Other Causes of Lower Gastrointestinal Bleeding

Henoch-Schönlein purpura is a vasculitic syndrome of unknown cause, characterized by arthritis, purpuric skin lesions, abdominal pain, and hematochezia. Skin lesions, which are typically the initial manifestation, often precede GI manifestations by several days. GI symptoms are provoked by edema and hemorrhage in the GI mucosa, which may be apparent endoscopically. Purpuric lesions may also be seen in the gastric, duodenal, and colonic mucosae. Treatment of the GI manifestations of Henoch-Schönlein purpura includes supportive measures beginning with nasogastric suction and the administration of intravenous fluids. The use of corticosteroids is thought by some to be beneficial in lessening abdominal pain and rectal bleeding and may also decrease the risk of intussusception occurring as a complication.

The **hemolytic uremic syndrome** is characterized by microangiopathic hemolytic anemia, uremia, and thrombocytopenia after enteric infection with one of several microorganisms including enterohemorrhagic *E coli*, especially those of the serotype O157:H7. These *E coli* may be carried in contaminated and insufficiently cooked hamburger and other food sources and have been implicated in multiple outbreaks of bloody diarrhea in which the hemolytic syndrome subsequently developed in some patients. Bloody diarrhea is often the presenting symptom and may be accompanied by abdominal pain and vomiting. Diagnosis is made by recognition of the characteristic combination of clinical symptoms. Treatment of the GI symptoms is largely supportive. The use of ampicillin, to which the often-implicated *E coli* strains are susceptible, is also frequently advocated even before a positive culture is obtained. There is no convincing evidence, however, that the use of antibiotics is effective either in lessening the severity of the initial infection or in decreasing the risk of developing the hemolytic-uremic syndrome or other sequelae (see Chapter 16).

DIAGNOSTIC EVALUATION & MANAGEMENT

An approach to the evaluation of patients with rectal blood loss is presented in Figure 13–8. Evaluation should begin with testing of the stool to determine whether the observed pigmentation is actually blood. If blood is present, a decision must be made as to whether the source of the blood is in the lower or upper GI tract. If an upper-tract source is suspected, nasogastric intubation for aspiration of gastric contents should follow. If the result is positive, evaluation may proceed as described in the previous section (see Figure 13–5). If the aspirate is negative for blood, a lower-tract source is likely responsible.

In patients with rectal bleeding who are ill, evidence of obstruction, including abdominal distention, tenderness to palpation, and vomiting, should be sought, and abdominal radiographs obtained. If obstruction is ruled out, investigation may continue with endoscopy and other studies. In those who are not acutely ill, the evaluation may progress with less urgency. With passage of bright red blood per rectum, anal pathology, such as a fissure, is most likely. Rectal polyps may also cause painless passage of bright red blood. With a Meckel diverticulum the blood may appear somewhat darker.

Conditions causing colonic inflammation, including the colitides and IBD, may present with mild bleeding associated with little or no pain. Evaluation of these disorders may require colonoscopy in addition to laboratory investigations.

Determination of the hematocrit is helpful in ascertaining the extent of blood loss in chronic disorders; patients who are anemic may benefit from iron supplementation. In those with acute loss of larger amounts of blood, blood products may be required.

ABDOMINAL PAIN

Abdominal pain is frequently encountered in pediatric practice and often presents challenges both in diagnosis and management. A wide variety of disorders may be associated with abdominal pain, ranging from acute, potentially life-threatening obstructions and infections to chronic functional disorders, which, although difficult to tolerate, are not typically associated with dire consequences. An approach to the evaluation of patients with abdominal pain is presented in Figure 13–9.

ACUTE ABDOMINAL PAIN

CLINICAL EVALUATION

In the patient suffering from an acute episode of abdominal pain, a description of the pain itself is most im-

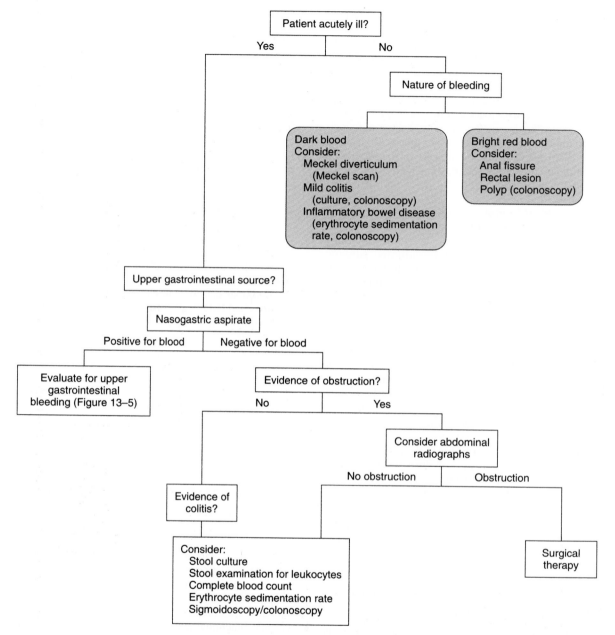

Figure 13–8. Algorithm presenting an approach to the evaluation of the patient with bleeding from the lower gastrointestinal tract.

portant. The time of onset and duration of the pain and its relationship to any possible initiating event, especially trauma, should be determined. Also important is the character of the pain (eg, burning or cramping) and any change in that character over time. In appendicitis, for example, pain is first vague and poorly localized and then gradually becomes more localized as the inflammation progresses to involve the visceral peritoneum. Pain may also be perceived to radiate to other sites.

The relationship of the pain to other symptoms should also be clarified. Vomiting that precedes pain, for example, may occur with acute gastroenteritis. With intestinal obstruction, pain typically precedes other symptoms. Bilious emesis should be considered to be due to intestinal obstruction until proved otherwise. Diarrhea, constipation, and fever commonly accompany abdominal pain. The past medical history, especially in regard to surgical procedures, should be noted.

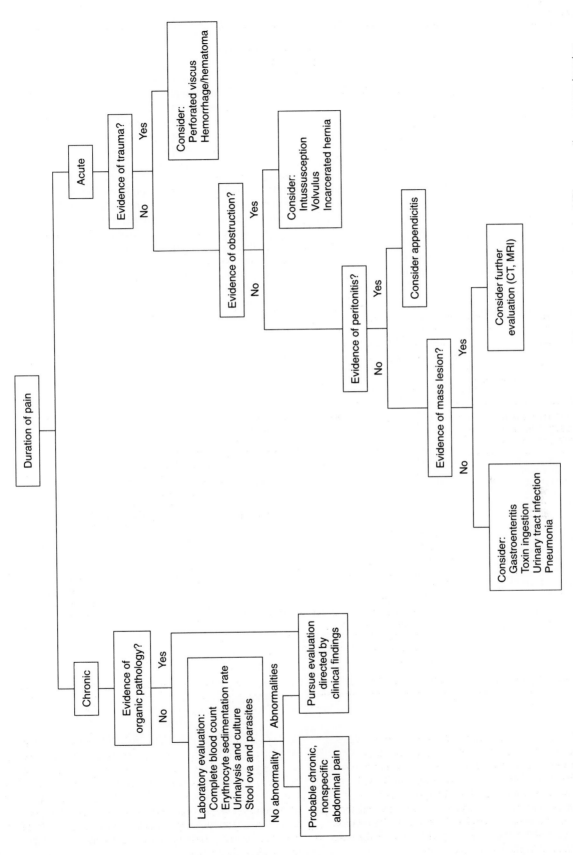

Figure 13–9. Algorithm presenting an approach to the evaluation of the patient with abdominal pain. CT = computed tomography; MRI = magnetic resonance imaging.

Physical examination of patients with acute abdominal pain is often difficult because they frequently are in too much distress to cooperate. One should note whether the child prefers to lie motionless or writhes about. If children are not too ill, asking them to jump up and down may reproduce pain related to peritoneal inflammation.

Distention, gross asymmetry, or associated skin lesions should be noted on abdominal examination. Bowel sounds should be characterized on auscultation. Early in intestinal obstruction, sounds may be high-pitched, but with longstanding obstruction, as well as with ileus (ie, nonmechanical obstruction), sounds are typically absent. Gentle palpation of the abdomen will localize areas of tenderness, reproduce the pain, and determine the presence of involuntary guarding. Deeper palpation may lead to the discovery of mass lesions. Digital rectal examination should also be performed to localize possible areas of peritoneal irritation.

DIFFERENTIAL DIAGNOSIS

Diseases that may cause acute abdominal pain are presented in Table 13–7.

Appendicitis

Inflammation of the appendix results from obstruction of the appendiceal lumen by factors such as fecaliths, foreign bodies, and lymphoid hyperplasia. Dilatation of the appendix follows, compromising the organ's blood supply and decreasing resistance to bacterial invasion. Untreated, this most often leads to appendiceal perforation and subsequent peritonitis. Appendicitis is approximately twice as frequent in males and more common in the adolescent-young adult age group.

The initial symptom is usually vague abdominal pain, which is poorly localized, but with a periumbilical focus. With progression of appendiceal distention, the pain may become crampy and be associated with nausea and vomiting. When the inflammatory process in the appendix becomes transmural, the parietal peritoneum becomes involved, and the pain becomes sharper in character and localized to the site of the appendix (usually in the right lower quadrant but potentially at any location in the abdomen or pelvis). With peritoneal inflammation, patients may also experience fever and chills.

The physical findings vary with the stage of the inflammation. Initially, when pain is poorly localized, findings

Table 13–7. Differential diagnosis: Acute abdominal pain.

Infectious causes	**Hematologic disease**
Gastrointestinal	Leukemia/lymphoma
Appendicitis	Hemolytic crisis
Mesenteric adenitis	Spinal cord tumors
Infectious gastroenteritis	
Food poisoning	**Endocrine disease**
Peritonitis	Hypoglycemia
Hepatitis	Diabetes mellitus
Pancreatitis	(especially with diabetic ketoacidosis)
Nongastrointestinal	
Pharyngitis (especially streptococcal)	**Vasculitic disease**
Pneumonia (especially right lower lobe)	Henoch-Schönlein purpura
Pyelonephritis/glomerulonephritis	Periarteritis nodosa
Pelvic inflammatory disease	Mucocutaneous lymph node syndrome
Abdominal abscess	(Kawasaki disease)
Pericarditis	
Serositis	**Renal disease**
Epididymitis	Nephrotic syndrome
Generalized	Renal colic
Herpes zoster	
Mononucleosis	**Miscellaneous**
Acute rheumatic fever	Ascites
	Colic
Intestinal obstruction	Toxin ingestion
Intussusception	Testicular torsion
Volvulus	Ovarian torsion
Adhesions	Mesenteric artery occlusion
Hernia with incarceration	Hypokalemia (causing paralytic ileus)
	Black widow spider bite
Gallbladder	
Cholecystitis	
Cholelithiasis	
Hydrops	
Abdominal trauma	
Abdominal wall muscle bruise/strain	
Splenic rupture/hematoma	
Liver laceration or hematoma	
Pancreatic pseudocyst	

may be equally nonspecific. When the parietal peritoneum is involved, the child usually prefers to lie fairly motionless in a supine position. There is localized tenderness over the site of the appendix, most commonly at the McBurney point (about 2 inches from the anterior superior iliac spine on a line to the umbilicus). Voluntary guarding is also common. Rectal examination often reveals tenderness.

With perforation of the appendix, peritoneal signs (involuntary guarding and rebound tenderness) are usually present. If the inflammation is confined to the immediate area of the appendix, an abscess may develop. If uncontained, generalized peritonitis occurs.

Laboratory evaluation of patients suspected to have appendicitis includes a complete blood count (CBC) and differential count. Typically, there is a neutrophil leukocytosis, although the white cell count may be normal. Urinalysis is useful to exclude urinary tract infection. Evaluation of the serum electrolytes may be useful, especially if vomiting has been a prominent feature.

Radiologic studies, although not usually helpful, may reveal a calcified fecalith, suggesting appendicitis, and may help to exclude intestinal obstruction. Abdominal ultrasound occasionally may be useful in demonstrating dilatation of the appendix, a finding highly suggestive of appendicitis.

Treatment of appendicitis is by appendectomy. In patients who have experienced significant vomiting, rehydration and correction of associated electrolyte abnormalities should precede surgery. Many surgeons also advocate the use of preoperative antibiotics. If perforation and abscess formation have already occurred, operative incision and drainage may be instituted, or the infection may be treated with antibiotics, followed by elective appendectomy a few weeks later.

Pancreatitis

Although pancreatitis is not commonly encountered in children, it should be considered in the differential diagnosis of acute abdominal pain. **Pancreatitis** is a nonspecific inflammatory response of the pancreas to a variety of causes. In adults, biliary tract disease, especially gallstones, and ethanol toxicity are the most common precipitating factors. In children, the usual causes are systemic infections, notably mumps; abdominal trauma; pancreatic disease, including cystic fibrosis and diabetes mellitus; and pharmacologic agents.

Regardless of the etiology, the pathogenesis of pancreatitis involves the premature activation of trypsinogen to trypsin, which in turn catalyzes the activation of other proteolytic enzymes within the ductal lumen. The quantity of proteolytic enzymes generated is sufficient to overwhelm the protease inhibitors that are also normally present, and autodigestion of the pancreatic tissue ensues.

Patients with acute pancreatitis usually experience abdominal pain, which may vary from mild to severe. Classically the pain is sudden in onset, gradually increases in severity, and is localized to the right upper quadrant with radiation to the back. Many patients, however, describe their pain as periumbilical and may or may not experience radiation to other sites. Vomiting frequently accompanies the pain and sometimes may be bilious. Physical examination typically reveals epigastric tenderness and absent or decreased bowel sounds. Fever, if present, is usually mild. Rarely, hypotension and shock may occur in severe cases of acute pancreatitis.

The laboratory evaluation of patients suspected to have pancreatitis usually includes measurement of serum amylase concentrations; in pancreatitis, values are three to four times normal or greater. Increased amylase concentrations are not specific for pancreatitis, and a normal value does not preclude the diagnosis. A more sophisticated test quantitates the various isoforms of amylase. In acute pancreatitis, the predominant pancreatic isoamylase is elevated. Measurement of the urinary amylase-creatinine clearance ratio is not helpful in differentiating elevated amylase levels due to pancreatitis from those due to other causes. Serum lipase levels may also be elevated in pancreatitis.

Radiologic studies of the abdomen may be helpful to exclude other causes of acute abdominal pain. They may also show areas of calcification within the pancreas, although this finding is more typical of chronic pancreatitis. Ultrasound studies are more helpful in detecting areas of abnormal density, cystic areas, or ductal dilatations. Computed tomography (CT) is sometimes useful to define pancreatic structure further. Endoscopic retrograde cholangiopancreatography allows precise visualization of the pancreatic ducts, but experience with this technique is limited in children.

Treatment of pancreatitis in children is primarily directed at eradicating the underlying disorder. Often the cause is not known or specific treatment is not available; consequently, only supportive measures can be provided. Withholding of enteral nutrition to "rest" the GI tract is presumably a beneficial means of decreasing pancreatic secretions and controlling the autodigestive process. Nasogastric suction to achieve gastric decompression is probably of no benefit unless persistent vomiting or ileus is also present. Analgesic agents may be necessary for severe pain. Morphine and codeine preparations should be avoided, because they may cause spasm of the sphincter of Oddi with consequent worsening of the pancreatitis. Surgery may be necessary in some patients, especially those whose pancreatitis is secondary to an obstruction.

The prognosis of patients with pancreatitis is variable, depending on the severity. Usually, symptoms resolve with no long-term effects. With more severe disease, especially with accompanying hemodynamic instability and renal failure, pancreatitis may be fatal. In patients who survive the acute episode, inflammatory lesions, such as phlegmon (an area of pancreatic tissue with swelling, inflammation, and possible necrosis), abscess, or pseudocyst, could develop. Recurrent pancreatitis is rare in children, but it can lead to chronic pancreatitis and, ultimately, pancreatic insufficiency.

Gallbladder Disease

Diseases of the gallbladder are uncommon in children, but, when present, tend to produce abdominal pain. **Cholecystitis,** an acute inflammation of the gallbladder, is usually accompanied by vague abdominal pain, which gradually localizes to the right upper quadrant. Obstruction of the cystic or common bile duct by stones, the most common inciting factor in adults with cholecystitis, is unusual in children. More commonly, cholecystitis is attributed to an intercurrent infectious illness. Ultrasound studies are useful in making the diagnosis of cholecystitis. Treatment is surgical.

Cholelithiasis, or gallstone disease, is far less common in children than in adults. Hemolytic diseases and conditions that lead to a low concentration of bile acids are the usual predisposing factors in children. Jaundice is often present, in addition to abdominal pain. Diagnosis is usually possible radiologically, and treatment of symptomatic patients is accomplished through cholecystectomy.

CHRONIC ABDOMINAL PAIN

CLINICAL EVALUATION

Persistence or recurrence of abdominal pain over a period of 3 months or longer defines the condition as chronic abdominal pain. In contrast to acute abdominal pain, which demands rapid diagnosis and expeditious institution of therapy, evaluation of the patient with chronic pain requires patience, and treatment may consist largely of consolation and reassurance.

The history should be directed at differentiating between organic and functional pain. Inquiries should be made regarding changes in weight, appetite, or energy level or other symptoms, such as vomiting or fever, which may accompany the episodes of abdominal pain. The character of the pain and its duration, severity, location, and quality should be determined, as well as factors that alleviate or exacerbate it. The relationship to other events may be important; thus, pain that awakens the child from sleep is usually of organic origin, whereas pain that occurs only near school time is more likely to be functional.

An important aspect of the history is to assess the patient's personality. Children who are especially tense, who are "worriers," or who are described as "overachievers" may experience abdominal pain as a manifestation of stress. Despite the relationship of chronic abdominal pain to stress, however, it should be appreciated that the pain is real and not simply imagined.

On physical examination, the general behavior of the child, such as facial expression, presence or absence of eye contact with the examiner, and other manifestations of "body language," should be observed. This could be helpful in determining whether psychological factors are contributing to the child's problems. On abdominal examina-

tion, the precise location of the pain should be noted. Apley and others have noted that functional pain is almost always localized to the umbilicus or central abdomen. Attention should be given to maneuvers that may elicit the symptoms. Abnormalities on physical examination increase the likelihood of an organic cause of the symptoms. With functional pain, the results of the physical examination are almost always entirely normal.

DIFFERENTIAL DIAGNOSIS

Table 13–8 presents a differential diagnosis of chronic abdominal pain. Many of these disorders are of non-GI origin and are discussed elsewhere in this test. Of the GI causes of chronic abdominal pain, most may also be present with acute symptoms and are covered elsewhere in this chapter. Not covered elsewhere are lactose intolerance, non-ulcer dyspepsia, irritable bowel syndrome, and chronic nonspecific abdominal pain.

Lactose Intolerance

Lactose intolerance, a commonly recognized cause of chronic abdominal pain in adults, may occur in pediatric patients as well. Lactose, a disaccharide found in the milk of cows and other mammals, is broken down in the intestine by the action of the brush-border enzyme lactase. In most of the world's population, lactase levels decline with maturation corresponding to the natural process of weaning from mother's milk. As lactase levels decline, more and more lactose passes undigested to the colon. There it is digested by colonic bacteria, releasing hydrogen and carbon dioxide and giving rise to the abdominal discomfort, bloating, and "gassiness" often described in these patients. Diarrhea often accompanies these symptoms.

Diagnosis of lactose intolerance may be made presumptively by eliminating lactose-containing foods from the diet and monitoring the patient for symptomatic improvement. A more definitive diagnosis may be made by using a lactose breath hydrogen test. After an overnight fast, patients are given a solution containing a known quantity of lactose. The amount of hydrogen expired in the patient's breath is measured. In patients who digest lactose poorly, expired hydrogen concentrations increase within 2–3 hours. Hydrogen in the expired air is the product of colonic bacterial fermentation of lactose not digested in the small bowel.

In older children and adults, treatment of lactose intolerance is accomplished by eliminating lactose from the diet. In children for whom such elimination is undesirable or impractical, the addition of commercially available lactase enzymes to dairy products is often beneficial.

Non-ulcer Dyspepsia

Another subgroup of pediatric patients with chronic abdominal pain has symptoms that are predominantly peptic in nature. These symptoms include nausea, heartburn, and regurgitation. Excessive belching, bloating, and hiccups

Table 13–8. Differential diagnosis: Chronic abdominal pain.

Gastrointestinal causes	**Hematologic disease**
Anatomic abnormalities	Sickle cell anemia
Hiatus hernia	Porphyrias
Linea alba hernia	Abdominal neoplasms
Duplications	Wilms tumor
Choledochal cyst	Neuroblastoma
Mass lesions	
Hepatomegaly/splenomegaly	**Gynecologic disease**
Bezoars	Dysmenorrhea
Constipation	Mittelschmerz
Irritable bowel syndrome	Ovarian cyst
Peptic ulcer disease	Hematocolpos
Inflammatory bowel disease	Endometriosis
Parasitic infection	
Lactose intolerance	**Neurologic disease**
Heavy metal ingestion	Migraine
Recurrent pancreatitis	Familial dysautonomia
Cystic fibrosis with meconium ileus equivalent	Abdominal migraine
	Abdominal epilepsy
Collagen vascular disease	
Juvenile rheumatoid arthritis	**Miscellaneous**
Systemic lupus erythematosus	Chronic nonspecific abdominal pain of childhood
	Aerophagia
Endocrine disease	Familial Mediterranean fever
Hyperparathyroidism	Hereditary angioneurotic edema
Addison disease	Diskitis
Cardiovascular disease	
Superior mesenteric artery syndrome	
Arrhythmias	
Coarctation of the aorta	

are also commonly described. When such symptoms are present and organic etiologies that may cause similar symptoms (eg, esophagitis, gastritis, and peptic ulcer) have been excluded, the diagnosis of non-ulcer dyspepsia may be made.

The pathogenesis of non-ulcer dyspepsia remains elusive; consequently, treatment is symptomatic. Some patients note improvement with gastric acid reduction or neutralization agents, but this may be, at least in part, a placebo effect.

Irritable Bowel Syndrome

The irritable bowel syndrome (IBS), also known as spastic colon, is a common cause of chronic abdominal pain in children and adults. Patients with IBS often complain of episodic pain, typically cramping in nature, that occurs with varying intensity and duration. The pain is frequently localized to the lower abdomen but may be perceived in any part of the abdomen, including the upper mid-abdomen. Some patients with IBS experience the onset of symptoms when eating and may feel the need to defecate soon after a meal. In many patients, diarrheal stools are passed on these occasions. After the passage of stool, patients frequently report alleviation or resolution of their pain.

The etiology of IBS is not thoroughly understood, but it is generally believed that the pain of IBS results from a disruption in peristalsis. Rather than normal, smooth, wavelike movements, peristalsis in patients with IBS is thought to be uncoordinated or spastic. This may account for the cramping nature of the pain that often occurs in IBS. Some speculate that IBS may be physiologically similar to infantile colic; a history of colic is not uncommon in patients with IBS.

The speed of intestinal transit is also apparently affected in IBS. Frequently, transit is rapid, giving rise to episodes of diarrhea with urgency. Transit time is not always rapid, however, and in some patients it may be slower than usual, giving rise to constipation.

Many patients with IBS note the clear relationship between stressful situations and episodes of pain. Often the recognition of this connection by the physician, patient, and family relieves some anxiety associated with episodes of pain. Decreased anxiety, in turn, may be associated with a decrease in the severity and duration of painful episodes. It is also reassuring to the patient and family to be informed of the lack of any known association between IBS and subsequent development of another, more serious medical problem.

In addition to reassurance, treatment of IBS should include counseling on the importance of a high-fiber diet. Dietary fiber, in fact, is the only intervention that has been proved consistently to be beneficial in the treatment of IBS. Fiber is equally efficacious whether provided through dietary sources or through commercially available supplements. Other dietary modifications, including the elimination of caffeine, may be associated with lessening of symptoms in some patients.

Pharmacotherapy for IBS is controversial. Multiple antispasmodic agents, including hycosamine, dicyclomine, and clidinium, are commonly used, and varying degrees of efficacy in relieving symptoms have been reported. In limited amounts, these agents are probably safe and may have a role in the treatment of IBS.

Chronic Nonspecific Abdominal Pain

Chronic, nonspecific abdominal pain (also referred to as **recurrent abdominal pain**) is thought to be caused by the interaction of physical or psychosocial stressors and the autonomically controlled motor activity of the intestinal tract. The child may complain of various types of abdominal pain but typically presents with gradual development of paroxysmal pain, often periumbilical in location, unrelated to meals or any other specific event but severe enough to interrupt normal activities. Some patients may describe their pain as upper abdominal in location, in association with features similar to non-ulcer dyspepsia often described in adults as previously discussed. Excluding patients with IBS symptoms, those remaining may appropriately be said to have chronic nonspecific abdominal pain.

Some features of the history are characteristic of chronic nonspecific abdominal pain. Stressful events in the child's family or school environment often predate the onset of pain; the family is often unaware of the relationship to these events. Often the family is noted to be "enmeshed" and overly involved in minute details of the child's life. A family history of similar functional disturbances is also common.

The diagnosis of chronic nonspecific abdominal pain is difficult because the symptoms may vary in severity and character, the physical findings are elusive or absent, and no specific tests can establish the diagnosis. On the other hand, the differential diagnosis of chronic abdominal pain is too extensive to attempt to exclude all possible causes before making the diagnosis of functional pain. A more reasonable approach is to conduct a thorough history and physical examination. If there are no indications for the presence of organic disease, and if the results of routine laboratory studies (including CBC, erythrocyte sedimentation rate, urinalysis and culture, and stool specimen for ova and parasites) are normal, the diagnosis of functional pain may be considered. It is important to establish a definite diagnostic plan and adhere to it. Otherwise, the evaluation may readily be prolonged with multiple tests and procedures. In addition to possible discomfort and high costs, continuing diagnostic studies may also convey to the patient and family the message that the physician is concerned about the presence of occult organic disease.

Treatment of chronic nonspecific abdominal pain in a child should begin with a discussion of the problem with the patient and the parents, including affirmation that the pain is "real." The presumed relationship of stressors and GI motility in the etiology of the pain should be explained. This information will make it easier for the diagnosis to be accepted as "legitimate."

If specific physical or psychosocial stressors have been identified, eliminating these factors may help to decrease the frequency and severity of the pain. When these stressors are psychosocial in nature, the assistance of mental health professionals may be beneficial both to identify the stressors and to alleviate them (see Chapter 3). Every attempt should be made to have the child reestablish a "normal" life. The child should go to school, despite the presence of pain. As little attention as possible should be given to the pain itself, and patients encouraged to deal with it on their own.

A high-fiber diet may be beneficial in treating functional abdominal pain. Excessive fiber, however, may cause colonic distention, increased gas, and increased pain. There is little evidence that antispasmodic agents are effective in the treatment of functional pain, but individual patients may report diminution or cessation of pain.

DIARRHEA

In less developed countries, diarrheal diseases contribute to problems of malnutrition and delayed growth and are responsible for several million deaths each year. In countries with better developed sanitation and more widely available health care, diarrheal diseases cause far fewer deaths but do cause significant morbidity. Among young children in the United States, approximately 20% of acute-care medical visits and 10–15% of hospitalizations are prompted by diarrheal illnesses.

Diarrheal diseases, especially those of infectious etiology, are much more frequent in children than in adults. The reasons for this difference include a relatively immature immune system, greater likelihood of spread of organisms by the fecal-oral route, and clustering of children in day-care centers. In addition to the high incidence of diarrhea, children are more prone to have dehydration. Children have a greater fecal water loss due to incomplete reabsorption of water in the colon; this loss is increased during diarrhea. Fever, which often accompanies infectious diarrhea in children, also contributes to dehydration through an increase in evaporative fluid losses. An understanding of the physiology of fluid and electrolyte processing is important in the diagnosis and management of diarrheal diseases.

PHYSIOLOGY

The small intestine selectively absorbs required nutrients, electrolytes, and water and secretes and eliminates

nonessential or indigestible substances. These complex processes are accomplished by the specialized functions of the various intestinal segments.

In the **duodenum,** partially digested foodstuffs are further mixed and their pH and osmotic pressure adjusted to achieve optimal conditions for nutrient and electrolyte absorption. The **jejunum** is the site of sodium-coupled active transport of amino acids and sugars accompanied by the passive absorption of water. Small peptides, which are the result of protein hydrolysis, are also absorbed in the jejunum, as are many vitamins and trace elements. In the **ileum,** additional sodium chloride is absorbed as are bile acids and vitamin B_{12}. The colon is equipped to absorb sodium and chloride despite their relatively low concentrations in colonic fluid. Residual carbohydrates are metabolized by bacteria in the colon to absorbable short-chain fatty acids. The colon is also an important site of further absorption of water.

At each of these intestinal sites, the selective absorption of fluid and electrolytes depends on the intact functioning of cellular transport processes. Sodium-potassium adenosine triphosphatase (ATPase), located on the basolateral membrane of enterocytes, "pumps" sodium out of the cells, creating a concentration gradient. Sodium enters the cells from luminal fluid, causing passive movement of water intracellularly. Other active transport processes important in normal intestinal functioning include sodium-coupled glucose transport, sodium-coupled amino acid transport, and the sodium-hydrogen exchange pump. Intestinal fluid **secretion** is achieved primarily by active transport of chloride ions.

On a macroscopic level, normal intestinal fluid and electrolyte processing rely on the existence of an adequate intestinal surface area. This is normally achieved through the microvillous and villous structure of the intestinal mucosa. If the villi are damaged or decreased in number, a decrease in effective absorptive surface area results. Normal intestinal motility is also necessary for optimal intestinal functioning. If intestinal motility is increased, fluid passage may be too rapid to allow for adequate absorption; if decreased, fluid stasis facilitates bacterial overgrowth and its consequent problems.

Normal intestinal function allows the body to process ingested fluid and foodstuffs as well as the significant volume of endogenously secreted fluids that accompany the digestive process. Diarrhea results when one or more components of the normal absorptive processes malfunction. Thus, from a physiologic basis, it is logical to define diarrhea as an excessive amount of water loss in the stool. This is easier to quantitate than is frequency, number, or liquidity of stools, and, indirectly, this definition encompasses each of those parameters. Under normal conditions, an infant produces approximately 5–10 g stool/kg body weight/d. Adults typically produce 100–200 g/d. Amounts in excess of these are usually abnormal and may have serious physiologic consequences.

Given the complex nature of normal intestinal fluid and electrolyte functioning, it is not surprising that disruption of any one of a number of parameters may upset fluid homeostasis, resulting in diarrhea. To simplify the study of these parameters, however, the abnormalities that cause diarrheal diseases traditionally have been classified as either malabsorptive or secretory in nature, on the basis of the predominant mechanism of action. In malabsorptive disorders, luminal fluid osmotic concentration is greater than normal because of the presence of nonabsorbable substances. These substances may be unabsorbed owing to a variety of causes: decreased absorptive surface area, absence or impaired functioning of mucosal enzymes, or presence of normally nonabsorbable substances in increased amounts (eg, sorbitol). Increased luminal osmotic pressure causes more water to be retained in the lumen, which results in diarrhea.

In secretory disorders, the presence of certain substances within the intestinal lumen provokes an increase in chloride secretion by the intestinal crypt cells, resulting in increased luminal fluid. Certain bacterial enterotoxins (eg, those of *E coli* and *Vibrio cholerae*) and certain chemicals (laxatives, long-chain fatty acids) are known to be potent intestinal secretagogues. Secretory hormones, namely vasoactive intestinal peptide, have also been demonstrated to provoke secretory diarrhea when excessively secreted, as occurs with some tumors.

From a clinical point of view, the physiologic mechanisms directly responsible for diarrhea may be less important—and are certainly less readily accessible for investigation—than its physical manifestations. These physical and historical characteristics of diarrheal diseases are the major means through which etiologies may be determined and management strategies formulated.

CLINICAL EVALUATION

In examining a patient with diarrhea, assessment of the status of hydration is of primary importance. Among the most reliable measures of changes in a patient's state of hydration are changes in weight. Comparison of a child's normal weight and "dehydrated" weight reveals the apparent "fluid deficit." Replacement of this fluid deficit can be accurately achieved through various techniques of rehydration (see below and Chapter 16). If a comparison of weights is not possible, the fluid deficit may be estimated on the basis of a variety of clinical signs and symptoms, many of which are listed in Table 13–9. Measurement of the urine specific gravity is also useful, as it is increased with dehydration.

Examination of the stool is also potentially useful. If blood is suspected to be present, this should be evaluated by using an indicator for occult blood. This will exclude the possibility that the abnormal color is from ingested dyes or foods. Whether the blood is from the upper or lower GI tract should also be determined (see earlier in this chapter, Gastrointestinal Tract Hemorrhage). The stool should also be examined for undigested vegetable matter, a finding characteristic of chronic, nonspecific di-

Table 13–9. Method of estimating degree of dehydration on the basis of clinical findings.

5%	5–10%	> 10%
Normal fontanelle	Sunken fontanelle	Deeply sunken fontanelle
Normal skin turgor	Normal or mildly reduced skin turgor	Reduced skin turgor
Moist mucous membranes	Tacky to dry mucous membranes	Very dry mucous membranes
Eyes with tears	Dry eyes; slightly sunken	Dry, sunken eyes
Normal urine output	Decreased urine output	No urine output
Normal peripheral circulation	Delayed capillary refill	Extremities cool and mottled
Normal mental status	Increased irritability or lethargy	Obtunded
Normal heart rate	Normal to increased heart rate	Rapid heart rate
Normal blood pressure	Orthostatic hypotension	Severe hypotension or shock

arrhea of childhood (see later in this chapter, Chronic Nonspecific Diarrhea of Infancy).

Microscopic examination of stool may provide useful information. The presence of leukocytes in the stool, which can be made more easily visible by the addition of a drop of methylene blue stain, is an indicator of colitis, caused by either bacterial infection or inflammation. Lymphocytes may be seen in the stool of patients with diarrhea due to chronic inflammatory causes, and eosinophils may be seen in patients with diarrhea due to food sensitivities. Fat in the stool, visualized with the assistance of a fat-specific stain such as Sudan red or black, suggests malabsorption or insufficiency of pancreatic enzymes. Microscopic examination may reveal the presence of parasites.

The presence of reducing substances (carbohydrates) in the stool is an indicator of malabsorption; this is usually assessed by use of the Clinitest reagent. This test underestimates the amount of carbohydrate present and does not recognize the presence of sucrose and other nonreducing sugars. Stool pH less than 5.5 also suggests the existence of carbohydrate malabsorption.

Evaluation of the electrolyte composition of stool has also been used to differentiate malabsorptive from secretory causes of diarrhea. A stool sodium concentration greater than 70 meq/L is usually indicative of a secretory etiology, whereas a concentration less than 50 meq/L is more typical of malabsorptive diarrhea. The stool osmotic gap

$$\text{stool mOsm} - 2 \times ([\text{Na}] + [\text{K}])$$

provides another method of differentiating malabsorptive from secretory diarrheas; an osmotic gap less than 100 mOsm/L indicates a secretory etiology, and an osmotic gap greater than 100 mOsm/L indicates a malabsorptive cause. All these measurements are merely estimates, however, and must be interpreted with caution.

A history of diarrhea in other members of the family is important. Any change in diet or use of medications or nutritional supplements before onset of diarrhea should be determined. Exposure to infectious causes of diarrhea should be evaluated, particularly regarding recent travel history of the patient or close contacts, or exposure to other children, as in day-care centers. The patient's gen-

eral health, including growth and development, should also be assessed.

In evaluating the diarrheal illness, any change in the child's normal bowel habits should be determined. Also, as diarrhea may be a manifestation of many childhood diseases (eg, otitis media, urinary tract infections), these should be considered.

The duration of the diarrhea is often used to classify various causes of diarrhea. Diarrhea that lasts less than 2 weeks is said to be acute in nature, whereas if symptoms persist longer, it is considered to be chronic.

DIFFERENTIAL DIAGNOSIS

Causes of diarrhea in children are listed in Table 13–10. From a physiologic standpoint, it is logical to group these disorders, as they are in this table, on the basis of the organ or organ system that is primarily affected. For the purpose of diagnostic evaluation, however, it is convenient to consider them as acute or chronic in nature.

Acute Diarrhea

Infectious Gastroenteritis. Acute diarrhea in children most frequently is caused by infection with viral, bacterial, or parasitic agents. Rotavirus is the single most common cause. Although several enteric viral pathogens can now be detected, no specific antiviral therapies are available. Treatment of diarrhea is limited to supportive measures, including the effective use of rehydration techniques (see later in this chapter, Oral Rehydration). With bacterial infection, antibiotics may be beneficial, in addition to rehydration. Viral and bacterial enteric pathogens and their treatment are discussed in Chapter 9.

Food Poisoning Syndromes. Acute diarrhea may also result from food poisoning. Foods may be infected with bacteria or parasites or may contain preformed bacterial toxins. *Staphylococcus aureus* is frequently implicated in the contamination of custards and cream-filled pastries that are either insufficiently cooked or not properly refrigerated. Symptoms of staphylococcal poisoning, which include nausea, vomiting, and abdominal cramps in addition to diarrhea, develop within 4–6 hours of ingesting contaminated food. This short incubation period is

Table 13–10. Differential diagnosis: Diarrhea.

Gastrointestinal infections
Viruses
Rotavirus
Norwalk agent
Enteric adenovirus
Bacteria
Salmonella
Shigella
Campylobacter
Yersinia
Escherichia coli
Clostridium difficile
Vibrio cholerae
Parasites
Giardia lamblia
Amoeba
Fungi
Candida
Cryptosporidium
Disorders probably of infectious etiology
Necrotizing enterocolitis
Inflammatory bowel disease

Dietary causes
Contaminated food/water
Malnutrition
Overfeeding
Inadequate dietary fat
Sorbitol, fructose, or other poorly absorbed carbohydrates
Nutrient deficiencies
Niacin deficiency (pellagra)
Zinc deficiency
(acrodermatitis enteropathica)
Folic acid deficiency
Food allergies/intolerances

Extraintestinal infections
Urinary tract infections
Otitis media
Pneumonia
Sepsis
Pancreatitis

Toxins
Boric acid
Naphthalene (moth balls)
Organophosphates
Carbamates
Iron overdosage
Arsenic
Lithium
Mercury
Poisonous mushrooms
Acquired immunodeficiency syndrome (AIDS)

Pharmacologic agents
Antibiotics
Decongestants
Theophylline
Chemotherapeutic agents
(including irradiation)
Liquid medications
(containing poorly absorbed sugars)

Anatomic defects
Malrotation
Intestinal duplications
Hirschsprung disease
Intestinal lymphangiectasia
Postoperative
Short-bowel syndrome
Blind-loop syndrome

Nutrient absorption disorders
Pancreatic defects
Cystic fibrosis
Schwachman syndrome
Chronic pancreatitis
Lipolytic defects
Congenital lipase deficiency
Congenital colipase deficiency
Bile acid malabsorption
Proteolytic defects
Congenital trypsinogen deficiency
Congenital enterokinase deficiency
Hydrolytic defects
Sucrase-isomaltase deficiency
Lactase deficiency
Transport defects
Glucose-galactose malabsorption
Familial chloride diarrhea
Disorders causing villous atrophy
Celiac disease
Protein intolerances
(milk, soya, rice, wheat)
Autoimmune enteropathy
Lymphatic obstruction
Abetalipoproteinemia
Intestinal lymphangiectasia
Whipple disease

Metabolic defects
Galactosemia
Hartnup disease

Endocrine defects
Thyrotoxicosis
Addison disease
Adrenogenital syndrome and hypoadrenalism
Hypoparathyroidism
Hyperparathyroidism
Wolman disease

Neoplastic disease
Neuroblastoma
Ganglioneuroma
Pheochromocytoma
Carcinoid syndrome

Immunologic defects
IgA deficiency
Hypogammaglobulinemia/agammaglobulinemia
Combined immunodeficiency syndrome
Wiskott-Aldrich syndrome
Ataxia-telangiectasia
Defective cellular immunity

Neurologic disorders
Familial dysautonomia
Neurofibromatosis

Miscellaneous etiologies
Stress
Overflow diarrhea secondary to encopresis

characteristic enough that it is used to make a presumptive diagnosis. Symptoms usually resolve spontaneously within 24 hours.

Clostridium botulinum produces toxins that are among the most potent poisons known. Despite their potency, however, they are readily destroyed by boiling or thorough cooking of foods. Botulism is often acquired through home-canned foods or raw or commercially processed seafood. Nausea, vomiting, and diarrhea usually develop 12 hours to 3 days after ingestion of contaminated food. Symptoms associated with the central nervous system include dry mouth, dysphagia, blurred vision, and possibly paralysis of the respiratory muscles. Treatment includes administration of specific antitoxin and supportive measures, including ventilatory assistance when indicated. *C botulinum* infection in infants may be contracted through ingestion of contaminated foodstuffs. Of interest, in this age group, botulism tends to cause constipation rather than diarrhea (see Chapter 21).

Clostridium perfringens, typically carried by contaminated meat and poultry products, causes a diarrheal illness within 8–15 hours of ingestion. *Vibrio parahaemolyticus* produces illness 8–22 hours after ingesting uncooked fish or shellfish. *Salmonellae, Shigellae, Yersinia,* and many other enteric pathogens may cause diarrhea.

Toxin Ingestions. Ingestion of toxic substances is common in children. Because many of these agents provoke GI symptoms, toxins should always be considered in the differential diagnosis of acute diarrhea. The specific diagnosis and treatment of toxin ingestion is discussed in Chapter 10.

Pharmacologic Agents. Pharmacologic agents are also frequently responsible for acute diarrhea. The temporal relationship between administration of the medication and the onset of diarrhea suggests the drug's involvement. Discontinuation of the suspected medication may be sufficient treatment.

Medications may be given surreptitiously by a parent to provoke symptoms and make a child appear to be ill. This situation has been described as Münchausen syndrome by proxy. Laxatives and stool softeners may be given to the child to induce diarrhea. The possibility of Münchausen syndrome by proxy should be considered in a patient with diarrhea—either acute or chronic—that cannot be explained.

Chronic Diarrhea

Diarrhea that persists for longer than 2 weeks is defined as chronic. Chronic diarrhea may result from the same enteric infectious agents that cause acute diarrhea. If the child's resistance is decreased by other concurrent illnesses, the diarrhea may become chronic. There is also a risk for prolonged infectious diarrhea in patients with congenital or acquired immunodeficiencies. Coinfection with more than one enteric pathogen may also cause a more chronic diarrhea than would be expected with either organism alone.

Another related cause of chronic diarrhea is postenteritis enteropathy, in which transient mucosal damage is sustained secondary to an enteric infection. This mucosal damage often includes the loss of digestive enzymes, namely lactase. These patients experience transient carbohydrate intolerance and its accompanying diarrhea. Treatment with lactose-free or elemental formulas is often adequate, and symptoms resolve in 4–8 weeks.

Various causes of chronic diarrhea are presented in Table 13–10.

Short-Bowel Syndrome. The "short-bowel syndrome" results from resection of significant portions of the intestine. The clinical features are mainly attributable to malabsorption and its consequences: diarrhea and growth failure. Conditions in which bowel resection is significant enough to cause symptoms of malabsorption are (1) congenital anomalies of the GI tract, including atresias, omphaloceles, gastroschisis, and vascular anomalies of the superior mesenteric artery; and (2) inflammatory or ischemic disorders, especially necrotizing enterocolitis (in neonates) and Crohn disease.

After resection, the remaining intestine undergoes adaptation to maintain adequate absorption. Mucosal hyperplasia may be so great as to increase the effective surface area fourfold. This adaptive response appears not to occur, however, in the absence of enteral nutrition. It is therefore important to initiate enteral nutrition as soon as possible after the fluid and electrolyte status has been stabilized in the initial postoperative period. As the patient's tolerance of enteral nutrition increases, the proportion of calories supplied by this method may be decreased. The gradual change from parenteral to enteral nutrition may require months to years, depending on the amount and location of the initial bowel segment resection. Although many of these patients require extended hospitalizations, the increasing availability of nursing services that assist in the administration of home parenteral and enteral nutrition make earlier discharge possible. Intestinal transplantation is being explored as a means of therapy for patients with the short-bowel syndrome.

Bacterial overgrowth is a common complication of the short-bowel syndrome. Disruption of the normal anatomy and changes in normal motility allow for intestinal fluid stasis and increased colonization by bacteria normally present in the intestine. The bacteria cause deconjugation of bile acids and mucosal inflammation, both of which cause malabsorption. This problem may be diagnosed by aspiration and culture of the intestinal fluid or by use of breath hydrogen testing. Treatment with broad-spectrum antibiotics is recommended.

Chronic Nonspecific Diarrhea of Infancy. Chronic, nonspecific diarrhea of infancy describes an entity characterized by chronic diarrhea with no definitive cause in an otherwise healthy baby who is well nourished and who has grown normally. This condition, also called "toddler's diarrhea," and the "sloppy stool syndrome," typically affects children aged 6–24 months. The parents often note that stools contain particles of undigested food. Several factors have been implicated in the etiology of this disor-

der, including dietary fat restriction, excessive intake of fluids, excessive intake of poorly absorbed carbohydrates contained in fruit juice or sorbitol (a nonabsorbed sweetening agent), and abnormal small intestinal motility. Treatment may begin with the removal of any of these potential provocative agents. The mainstay of treatment, however, is reassurance to the parents that the problem usually resolves, spontaneously and without sequelae, when the child is 2–4 years old.

Protracted Diarrhea of Infancy. Protracted diarrhea of infancy is defined as diarrhea of greater than 2 weeks' duration in an infant younger than 3 months of age, in which 3 or more stools have had no ova or parasites and the cultures are negative. Unlike children with chronic, nonspecific diarrhea, these babies experience significant malabsorption and often fail to thrive. Protracted diarrhea may have its onset with an episode of acute infectious diarrhea; this emphasizes the importance of appropriate management and follow-up of infants with acute diarrhea. Bile-acid malabsorption and the existence of antienterocyte antibodies have also been proposed as possible mechanisms for protracted diarrhea. These infants are managed by administering elemental formulas enterally and by providing parenteral nutrition when warranted.

Diarrhea due to Malabsorption. Chronic diarrhea may be caused by one or more defects in processing of nutrients. These disorders are characterized by the symptoms of chronic diarrhea, abdominal distention, and failure to thrive.

The normal digestion and absorption of nutrients is a complex process, involving separate mechanisms for carbohydrate, protein, and fat. It would be logical to classify problems of malabsorption on the basis of the affected nutrient. Unfortunately, isolated defects affecting the absorption of only one class of nutrients are the exception rather than the rule. An alternative method of classification, which considers the site of the defect itself, has therefore been devised: intraluminal, at the intestinal mucosal surface, or at a site encountered after absorption into the enterocyte. Both models are presented schematically in Figure 13–10.

Intraluminal Defects. Disorders of intraluminal digestion with malabsorption are most commonly caused by pancreatic insufficiency, which may affect all three classes of nutrients. **Cystic fibrosis,** an autosomal-recessive inherited defect of chloride secretion, causes exocrine pancreatic insufficiency. This process apparently begins in utero with decreased rate of fluid flow through the pancreatic ducts with consequent plugging, leading to a loss of exocrine function. In addition to severe malabsorption, GI manifestations include meconium ileus and meconium ileus equivalent, focal biliary cirrhosis, and hypofunctioning of the gallbladder with the possible development of gallstones. Once recognized, these symptoms may be remedied through the use of pharmacologic supplements. Rectal prolapse also occurs at increased frequency in patients with cystic fibrosis and may be the presenting symptom.

The diagnosis of cystic fibrosis is usually confirmed by use of the sweat chloride test. Pancreatic function tests and measurements of pancreatic enzymes in the stool are much more difficult to perform and are also of more limited utility. The pulmonary manifestations and other aspects of this disease are discussed in Chapter 18.

Schwachman syndrome is also a disorder of exocrine pancreatic function. Pancreatic function is not as severely affected as in cystic fibrosis, and significant fat malabsorption may not be present. The results of sweat chloride tests in these patients are normal. In addition to GI manifestations, patients with Shwachman syndrome also typically have short stature, skeletal abnormalities, bone marrow dysfunction, neutropenia, and, consequently, recurrent infections. Those with significant fat malabsorption benefit from pancreatic enzyme replacement. Of interest, the need for these supplements may decrease with age.

Isolated pancreatic enzyme deficiencies, which result in the malabsorption of only one class of nutrient, are rare. Intraluminal fat malabsorption may result from congenital lipase or colipase deficiency, disorders of bile acid synthesis and absorption, and disorders of bile acid excretion (eg, biliary atresia). Selective protein malabsorption is rare but occurs with congenital enterokinase deficiency.

Mucosal Surface Defects. Malabsorption may also be caused by defects in the intestinal mucosae. The most common group of these disorders is associated with intestinal villous atrophy and includes celiac disease, milk-soy protein intolerance, *Giardia lamblia* infection, and postenteritis enteropathy.

Patients with **celiac disease** are intolerant of gluten, a protein found in wheat and rye but not in corn and rice. Exposure to gluten-containing foods leads to small intestinal mucosal damage and eventually to villous atrophy and malabsorption. The nature of the disorder leading to this protein intolerance is not yet known. Preliminary evaluation in patients suspected to have this disorder may include testing for antiendomesial antibodies. Presence of these antibodies is suggestive of celiac disease and usually warrants further diagnostic testing. A presumptive diagnosis of celiac disease may be made on the basis of a small intestinal mucosal biopsy specimen demonstrating characteristic villous atrophy. Patients are then treated with a gluten-free diet. Resolution of symptoms of malabsorption and the return of normal villous morphology on a subsequent biopsy specimen add further evidence to the diagnosis.

Cow's-milk protein allergy, the most common food allergy in children, may also induce villous atrophy and malabsorption. Patients may exhibit other allergic symptoms including rhinorrhea, cough, and eczema. Treatment necessitates removal of the offending allergen; soy-based formulas have been tried in most infants. However, as many as 25% of infants with cow's-milk allergy are also allergic to soy-based products. These patients may be fed formulas containing hydrolyzed proteins. Milk protein allergy should be differentiated from milk intolerance,

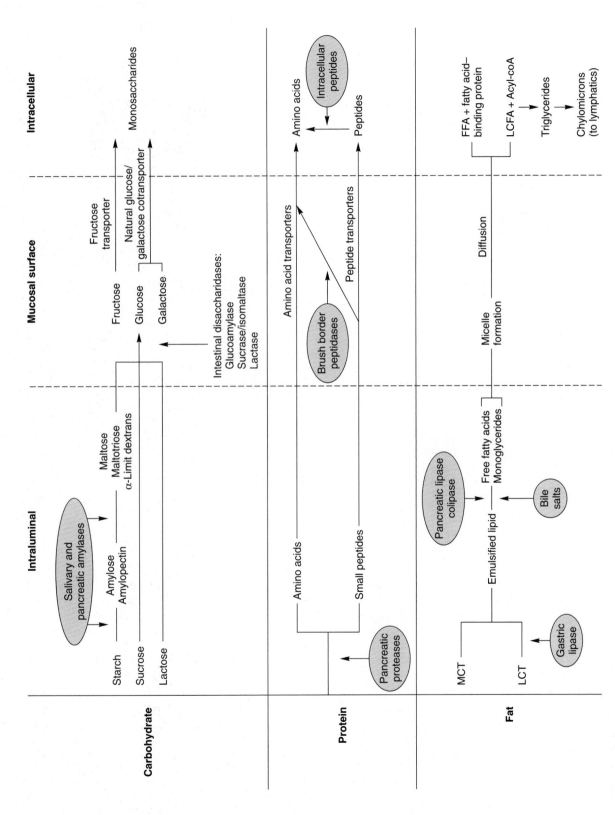

Figure 13–10. Chart representing the major components involved in the digestion of carbohydrates, proteins, and fats. FFA = free fatty acids; LCFA = long-chain fatty acids; LCT = long-chain triglycerides; MCT = medium-chain triglycerides.

which may be due to lactase deficiency (see below), fat intolerance, and other causes.

Intracellular Defects. The third group of malabsorptive disorders is associated with defects at the cellular level, with no frank morphologic changes. Patients with **sucrase-isomaltase deficiency** have complete or almost complete absence of sucrase activity accompanied by a variable decrease in maltase and isomaltase activities. The disease, inherited in an autosomal-recessive manner, leads to the onset of watery diarrhea when affected individuals are exposed to sucrose or starch-containing foods. Diagnosis is made presumptively with a sucrose hydrogen breath test and definitively by assay for the specific enzymes in intestinal mucosal biopsy specimens. Treatment involves elimination of sucrose and starch from the diet. Dietary restriction is usually necessary only during the first few years after birth. **Congenital lactase deficiency,** a similar but even rarer disorder, causes malabsorption of lactose, the major sugar in milk. **Hypolactasia,** which refers to the normal decline in lactase activity occurring with maturation, is much more common.

Malabsorption may be due to defective nutrient transport in the mucosa. **Glucose-galactose malabsorption** occurs when the sodium-coupled transport protein for those sugars is absent. Typically, these patients present with profuse, watery diarrhea in the first few days after birth; if untreated, severe dehydration and acidosis develop. Treatment is based on the elimination of the malabsorbed sugars from the diet by use of commercially available formulas designed especially for patients with this defect.

Another mechanism for malabsorption involves abnormal nutrient passage away from the absorptive cells. In **intestinal lymphangiectasia,** the lymphatics that drain the intestinal villi are dilated, because of either a congenital structural defect or an obstructed lymphatic drainage. These dilated lymphatics are evident in intestinal biopsy specimens of affected individuals. As dilatation progresses, lymphatic rupture occurs, with ensuing loss of serum proteins and possible development of edema and ascites. This condition may be mitigated by the use of diets enriched in medium-chain triglycerides.

Abetalipoproteinemia, another defect of nutrient transport, may lead to malabsorption. Congenital inability to synthesize apoprotein B leads to defective chylomicron synthesis and subsequent transport from the absorptive cells into the lymphatics. Intestinal biopsy specimens show accumulated lipid droplets. Non-GI manifestations of this disease include ataxia and progressive neuromuscular degeneration, ocular disease including retinitis pigmentosa, and acanthocytosis, all of which are related to vitamin E deficiency. Relief of the symptoms of malabsorption may be accomplished through dietary restriction of long-chain fatty acids. Supplementation with medium-chain triglycerides, as well as fat-soluble vitamins, may also be beneficial.

Algorithms for an approach to the evaluation of a patient with diarrhea are shown in Figure 13–11.

MANAGEMENT

Oral Rehydration

In almost all cases of diarrheal illness, the most crucial facet of management is the timely determination of the patient's degree of dehydration (see Diarrhea, Clinical Evaluation) and the restoration of normal hydration. Rehydration may be accomplished either orally or intravenously; for a variety of reasons, however, the oral route is usually preferable. Oral rehydration solutions are widely available and may be safely administered at home. It is less invasive than intravenous therapy and, consequently, less painful to the patient. The simplicity and safety of oral rehydration make it far more economical as well.

The selection of appropriate fluids is of crucial importance in oral rehydration. Home remedies, including carbonated beverages and liquid gelatin, do not provide the appropriate concentrations of glucose and electrolytes necessary for the most efficient and safe restoration of fluid balance. It is recommended that commercially available oral rehydration solutions be used. Much attention has been given to the development of optimal oral rehydration solutions. Acceptable oral rehydration solutions are formulated to provide an isotonic combination of sodium and glucose to which potassium and bicarbonate are added. Glucose, in concentrations of 110–140 mmol/L (yielding 2–2.5% glucose), takes advantage of glucose-coupled sodium transport mechanisms, maximizing sodium absorption. The concentration of sodium in currently available oral rehydration solutions ranges from 30 to 90 mEq/L. These products, regardless of their sodium concentration, have been shown to be effective and safe in the reestablishment of hydration. Because of concern regarding the possibility of iatrogenic hypernatremia, however, the American Academy of Pediatrics recommends that solutions with sodium concentrations in the range of 70–90 mEq/L be used only for initial replacement of the water and sodium deficit. Solutions with lower sodium concentrations (40–60 mEq/L) are then recommended as maintenance fluids until the patient resumes a normal diet. For most patients in developed countries, however, solutions that have a sodium concentration in the 40–60 mEq/L range may be used safely for both rehydration and maintenance. Contraindications to oral rehydration therapy are (1) severe dehydration (> 10%) and hemodynamic instability, (2) stool output greater than 10 mL/kg/h, and (3) the coexistence of ileus. Vomiting is not a contraindication to the use of oral rehydration therapy. Complications in the use of oral rehydration solution are uncommon.

Once it has been determined that a patient is an appropriate candidate for oral rehydration, an estimate of the fluid deficit is needed. This may be determined either from documented weight loss since onset of illness or from the estimated degree of dehydration. For example, in a patient weighing 7.0 kg with 5% dehydration, the deficit is $(0.05)(7.0) = 0.35$ L or 350 mL. The deficit amount, in addition to the normal maintenance requirement, should

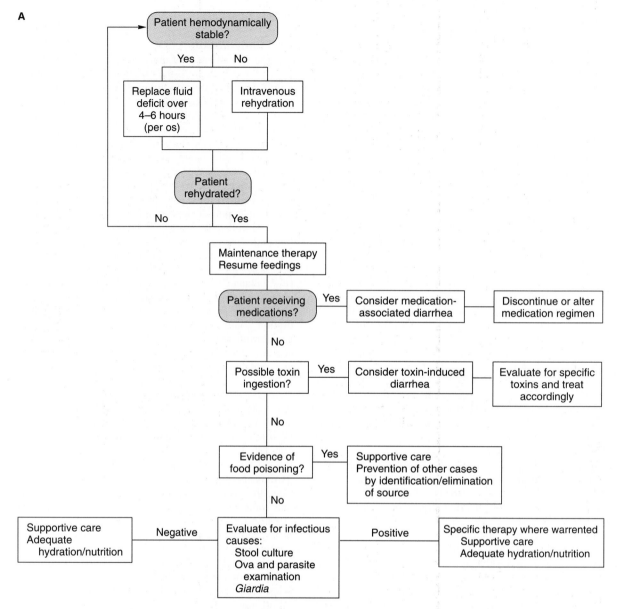

Figure 13–11. *A:* Algorithm presenting an approach to the evaluation of the patient with acute diarrhea. ***B:*** Algorithm presenting an approach to the evaluation of the patient with chronic diarrhea. RAST = radioallergosorbent test. (Adapted and reproduced, with permission, from Laney DW, Cohen MB: Approach to the pediatric patient with diarrhea. Gastroenterol Clin North Am 1993;22:499.)

be replaced over 4–6 hours by offering the patient frequent small amounts from a spoon, bottle, or cup. After the initial deficit is replaced, the patient's hydration status should be reevaluated. If the patient is appropriately hydrated, maintenance therapy only should be continued. If significant dehydration persists, the deficit amount should again be determined and replaced. Only if the patient's clinical status deteriorates should the oral route be abandoned and intravenous therapy substituted.

Refeeding

After restoration of a normal state of hydration, it is necessary to restore normal diet. Common practice has been to withhold feedings in the early phases of treatment of acute diarrhea. This offers some benefit by shortening the severity and duration of diarrhea. The benefits of more rapid reintroduction of foods, however, seem to outweigh those of withholding. These include stimulation of intestinal digestive enzymes and increased mucosal cell growth.

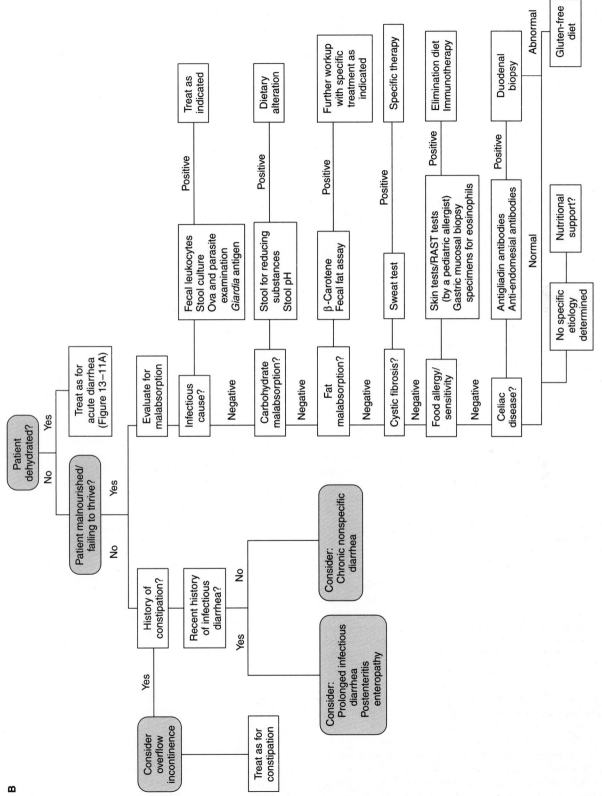

Patient dehydrated?

Yes → Treat as for acute diarrhea (Figure 13–11A)

No → Patient malnourished/failing to thrive?

Yes → Evaluate for malabsorption

Infectious cause?

Fecal leukocytes
Stool culture
Ova and parasite examination
Giardia antigen

Positive → Treat as indicated

Negative → Carbohydrate malabsorption?

Stool for reducing substances
Stool pH

Positive → Dietary alteration

Negative → Fat malabsorption?

β-Carotene
Fecal fat assay

Positive → Further workup with specific treatment as indicated

Negative → Cystic fibrosis?

Sweat test

Positive → Specific therapy

Negative → Food allergy/sensitivity

Skin tests/RAST tests
(by a pediatric allergist)
Gastric mucosal biopsy
specimens for eosinophils

Positive → Elimination diet
Immunotherapy

Negative → Celiac disease?

Antigliadin antibodies
Anti-endomesial antibodies

Positive → Duodenal biopsy

Abnormal → Gluten-free diet

Normal → Nutritional support?

No specific etiology determined

No → History of constipation?

Yes → Consider overflow incontinence

Treat as for constipation

Recent history of infectious diarrhea?

Yes → Consider:
Prolonged infectious diarrhea
Postenteritis enteropathy

No → Consider:
Chronic nonspecific diarrhea

B

429

In the breast-fed infant, it is also advantageous to resume nursing as soon as possible. In light of these advantages, many recommend resumption of feedings as soon as rehydration has been achieved. In the formula-fed infant, use of lactose-free formula in the first 48 hours of feeding may be of some advantage. In the nursing infant, breast milk is normally well tolerated. In older children, reintroduction of solid foods may begin with complex carbohydrates, adding other foods as the patient returns to normalcy. Feedings initially should be in small amounts, offered at frequent intervals.

Other Therapies

The techniques of oral rehydration and reintroduction of a normal diet are applicable to all patients with diarrhea and dehydration, regardless of the cause. In patients with chronic diarrhea, management may be more difficult. This may involve dietary modifications and the use of specific or general nutritional supplementation. Efforts should focus on achieving as nearly normal growth and development as is possible.

JAUNDICE IN THE NEONATE

Jaundice may be associated with benign, self-limiting conditions, or with progressive disorders that lead to cirrhosis and end-stage liver disease. Many of these disorders become apparent in the neonatal period and discussed in this section. Causes of jaundice more often presenting in childhood or adolescence are discussed in the next section.

PHYSIOLOGY

Bilirubin is the major product of the breakdown of heme. Heme is first converted to biliverdin, which is then reduced to bilirubin. This "free," or unconjugated, bilirubin is released into the plasma, where it combines with albumin, making it water soluble and facilitating transport to the liver. Unconjugated bilirubin is taken up by the hepatocytes, where it is conjugated with glucuronic acid by the action of enzymes in the microsomal and canalicular membranes. Most of this conjugated, lipid-soluble bilirubin is then excreted as a component of bile into the intestine. A small portion of the conjugated bilirubin reenters the blood.

In the intestine, bilirubin is catabolized to urobilinogen by the action of the indigenous bacterial flora. A portion of this water-soluble urobilinogen is reabsorbed from the intestine and returns to the liver (the enterohepatic circulation). A small percentage of the reabsorbed urobilinogen

is excreted by the kidneys as urobilin. The urobilinogen remaining in the intestine is converted to stercobilin and excreted in the feces. Urobilin and stercobilin, respectively, are largely responsible for the pigmentation of the urine and stool, therefore explaining the association of acholic (**unpigmented**) stool and dark urine with disorders that impair bilirubin metabolism or excretion.

Several aspects of bilirubin metabolism are not fully developed in the newborn infant. The shorter life span of erythrocytes and the higher red-cell mass are responsible for an increased bilirubin load in the neonate. Binding of albumin to unconjugated bilirubin is less efficient in the neonate, as are the mechanisms of conjugation. Bile flow is decreased owing to a combination of factors, including inefficient bile acid uptake and conjugation and decreased hepatocellular excretion. The structure of the neonatal liver may also add to the decreased efficiency of bile excretion. The enterohepatic recirculation of unconjugated bilirubin may be increased in the neonate, in part because of the relative sparseness of bacterial colonization of the neonatal intestine and consequent decreased conversion of bilirubin to urobilinogen.

CLINICAL EVALUATION

The history may provide important clues regarding the cause of jaundice in the neonate. Prenatal course, gestational age, and delivery history should be noted. The infant's behavior should be evaluated, because irritability, vomiting, or poor feeding often accompany metabolic disturbances. The appearance of the stools is important; acholic stools often indicate extrahepatic biliary obstruction. The family history should be explored for possible genetic or inherited defects.

In addition to a detailed physical examination, certain specific features should be noted, such as the degree of jaundice in the skin and sclera, the presence of distinctive or unusual facial appearance, and presence of abdominal organomegaly or masses. The chest should be examined for murmurs; peripheral pulmonic stenosis may be associated with arteriohepatic dysplasia.

In evaluating the neonate with jaundice, it is crucial to differentiate jaundice due to increased **unconjugated** bilirubin (indirect hyperbilirubinemia) from that due to increased **conjugated** bilirubin (direct hyperbilirubinemia). This is important not only for diagnostic purposes, but also because there is some urgency in recognizing direct hyperbilirubinemia and cholestasis (reduction of bile flow).

DIFFERENTIAL DIAGNOSIS

The differential diagnosis of neonatal jaundice is presented in Table 13–11; the more important disorders are discussed below.

Table 13–11. Differential diagnosis: Neonatal jaundice.

Unconjugated hyperbilirubinemia	
Increased bilirubin production	Decreased bilirubin uptake or storage
Hemolytic disease	Crigler-Najjar syndrome, type I
Isoimmune hemolysis (Rh, ABO, or other incompatibility)	Crigler-Najjar syndrome, type II (Arias syndrome)
Erythrocyte defects	Gilbert syndrome
Congenital spherocytosis	Lucey-Driscoll syndrome
Hereditary elliptocytosis	Drug inhibition
Infantile pyknocytosis	Hypothyroidism/hypopituitarism
Erythrocyte enzyme defects	Congestive heart failure
Glucose 6-phosphatase dehydrogenase	Portacaval shunt
Pyruvate kinase	Hypoxia
Hexokinase	Acidosis
Infection	Sepsis
Enclosed hematoma	Altered enterohepatic circulation
Polycythemia	Breast milk jaundice
Drugs (eg, vitamin K)	Intestinal obstruction
	Antibiotic administration
Conjugated hyperbilirubinemia	
Intrahepatic disorders	Hepatitis
Idiopathic neonatal hepatitis	Infectious (including cytomegalovirus, ECHO virus, rubella)
Intrahepatic persistent cholestasis	Toxic (secondary to total parenteral nutrition or sepsis)
Arteriohepatic dysplasia (Alagille syndrome)	Genetic/chromosomal (trisomy E, Down syndrome, Donahue
Byler disease (persistent familial intrahepatic cholestasis)	syndrome)
Zellweger syndrome	Miscellaneous disorders
Anatomic disorders	Histiocytosis X
Congenital hepatic fibrosis/infantile polycystic disease	Shock/hypoperfusion
Caroli disease	Intestinal obstruction
Metabolic disorders	Polysplenia syndrome
Disorders of amino acid metabolism (eg, tyrosinemia)	Extrahepatic disorders
Disorders of lipid metabolism (eg, Wolman disease,	Biliary atresia
Niemann-Pick disease, Gaucher disease)	Bile duct stenosis
Disorders of carbohydrate metabolism (eg, galactosemia,	Anomalies of the choledochopancreaticoductal junction
fructosemia, glycogen storage disease type IV)	Mass (neoplasia, stone)
Disorders in which the defect is uncharacterized	Bile/mucous plug
α_1-Antitrypsin deficiency	
Cystic fibrosis	
Neonatal iron storage disease	

ECHO = enteric cytopathogenic human orphan (virus).

Unconjugated Hyperbilirubinemia

Physiologic Jaundice. As mentioned above, inefficient bilirubin metabolism and increased bilirubin production combine to make unconjugated hyperbilirubinemia a physiologic phenomenon of the newborn. Bilirubin concentrations are somewhat elevated in newborn infants and continue to increase to maximal levels of 8–9 mg/dL by 3–5 days postnatally. The concentrations then gradually decrease, reaching normal values (approximately 2 mg/dL) by the end of the second week. In premature infants, the peak value may be somewhat higher, and hyperbilirubinemia may persist somewhat longer than 2 weeks.

In the absence of any evidence of an underlying disorder, normal term infants with unconjugated bilirubin concentrations of 10–12 mg/dL or less do not usually require further evaluation or treatment. If the bilirubin concentration is higher or remains elevated for more than 2 weeks, the possibility of hemolytic disease, impaired bilirubin conjugation, or other causes of indirect hyperbilirubinemia, including breast-feeding, must be investigated.

With physiologic jaundice, as well as with indirect hyperbilirubinemia due to other causes, the major concern is the development of kernicterus. **Kernicterus** is the staining of the basal ganglia, pons, or cerebellum caused by the accumulation of unconjugated bilirubin. This condition may manifest clinically with a variety of neurologic symptoms, ranging from lethargy and hypotonia to severe encephalopathy. Kernicterus is often fatal; in survivors, some degree of neurologic insult is usually present. Kernicterus apparently does not develop unless the serum concentration of unconjugated bilirubin exceeds 20 mg/dL. Therapy should be instituted when levels are in this range. Unconjugated bilirubin is subjected to photochemical reduction by light with a wavelength of 450 nm. Phototherapy is useful in decreasing the levels of unconjugated bilirubin, regardless of the cause.

Breast Milk Jaundice. Breast-fed infants commonly have higher plasma concentrations of unconjugated bilirubin than do bottle-fed infants. Typically, these infants show a slow progression of jaundice, with peak bilirubin values of 10–20 mg/dL occurring 2–3 weeks after birth. In some breast-fed infants, especially those with poor caloric intake or inadequate hydration, jaundice may be noted somewhat earlier.

The mechanism of breast milk–associated jaundice is not well understood but may involve increased intestinal bilirubin reabsorption. Treatment of breast milk jaundice usually is not necessary. If levels of unconjugated bilirubin are increasing rapidly and nearing 20 mg/dL, therapy is often instituted, even though kernicterus has not been documented to occur in association with breast milk jaundice. Brief interruption of breast-feeding is often sufficient to allow for reduction in serum bilirubin levels. When nursing is resumed, bilirubin levels typically increase, but with a peak value lower than previously.

Other Causes of Unconjugated Hyperbilirubinemia. Several enzymatic defects cause hyperbilirubinemia as a result of alterations in uptake, storage, or conjugation of bilirubin. **Crigler-Najjar syndrome** is characterized by absent (type I) or deficient (type II) hepatic glucuronyl transferase activity and consequent hyperbilirubinemia with levels of unconjugated bilirubin in the 20–40 mg/dL range. Kernicterus develops unless the disorder is treated aggressively, usually with bilirubin binding agents, phenobarbital, or phototherapy. Orthotopic liver transplantation may be necessary in patients with type I Crigler-Najjar syndrome.

Patients with **Gilbert syndrome** have **mildly** elevated levels of unconjugated bilirubin secondary to decreased hepatic bilirubin uptake, the exact mechanism of which remains poorly understood. These patients will be found to have bilirubin diglucuronide in their bile, which helps to differentiate them from those with Crigler-Najjar syndrome. Typically, patients with Gilbert syndrome experience fluctuating levels of bilirubin, with increases noted secondary to stressors including illness and fasting. Often the disorder is so mild that it is not diagnosed until puberty or later; the sole physical finding may be the presence of scleral icterus. No treatment is necessary.

Lucey-Driscoll syndrome (transient familial neonatal hyperbilirubinemia) is a rare disorder characterized by the presence of marked (> 60 mg/dL) hyperbilirubinemia, usually beginning on the first day after birth. This condition is thought to be caused by the transient presence of a glucuronyl transferase inhibitory factor. Kernicterus commonly develops if the disorder is not treated. With the use of exchange transfusions, however, most infants recover and have no permanent sequelae.

Conjugated Hyperbilirubinemia

Unlike conditions associated with elevations of unconjugated bilirubin, which are often transient, elevations of conjugated bilirubin concentrations tend to be prolonged. These conditions are referred to collectively as **neonatal cholestasis.** Both the extent of possible differential diagnoses of neonatal cholestasis and the similarity of the clinical presentations of many of the disorders make diagnosis a challenge. Furthermore, arriving at the correct diagnosis should be undertaken with urgency, to identify diseases for which there are effective therapies and to institute treatment in a timely manner.

Idiopathic Infantile Cholangiopathies. After the known causes of cholestasis have been ruled out, most patients are found to have one of the idiopathic infantile cholangiopathies: biliary atresia or neonatal hepatitis. Neither of these terms denotes a specific etiology. Rather, they describe recognizable groups of signs and symptoms.

Neonatal hepatitis, the most common cause of neonatal cholestasis, tends to be more frequent in low-birth-weight infants. Jaundice usually develops within the first week and is always present before 2 months of age. Acholic stools are uncommon, but hepatomegaly may be present. Vitamin K malabsorption and deficiency may lead to a bleeding diathesis.

The diagnosis of neonatal hepatitis can be made only after excluding metabolic and infectious causes of cholestasis. Once this has been done, a liver biopsy may be performed. The histologic features necessary for diagnosis include disturbance of the normal hepatic architecture, increased presence of inflammatory cells in the portal areas, and evidence of increased extramedullary hematopoiesis. Multinucleated giant cells are also often present (Figure 13–12). However, these features are not pathognomonic.

There is no specific therapy for neonatal hepatitis; general measures used in treatment of cholestasis are applied (see Management below). The condition is heterogeneous, making it difficult to define the prognosis. However, the prognosis is worse in the familial, as compared with the sporadic, form.

Approximately one third of cases of neonatal cholestasis are due to **extrahepatic biliary atresia.** The defect involves obliteration of all or part of the extrahepatic biliary ductular system. In the early stages of disease, hepatic architecture may be relatively normal; with progression, however, there is bile stasis and proliferation of the intrahepatic bile ducts. These findings and the presence of bile plugs in the portal ducts are characteristically noted in biopsy specimens (Figure 13–13). The progression of hepatic lesions associated with this disorder has suggested that an inflammatory process may be involved, which leads to fibrosis and eventual ductal obliteration.

Biliary atresia, unlike neonatal hepatitis, occurs almost exclusively in full-term infants. Jaundice may be present from birth or may develop in the first few weeks. Stools are often acholic. Hepatomegaly is common and may be associated with splenomegaly as a result of portal hypertension. Progression of disease is associated with the development of cirrhosis and the consequent problems of failure to thrive and nutritional deficiencies.

When extrahepatic biliary atresia is suspected, radioisotope scanning may be performed. With biliary atresia, uptake of isotope by the liver is usually normal, but no excretion into the intestine is visualized, confirming the presence of an obstructive lesion. This is in contrast to neonatal hepatitis, in which isotope uptake is delayed because of parenchymal disease, but excretion is normal (Figure 13–14). Characteristic findings on radionuclide scanning and liver biopsy specimens necessitate confirmation of the diagnosis by exploratory laparotomy with in-

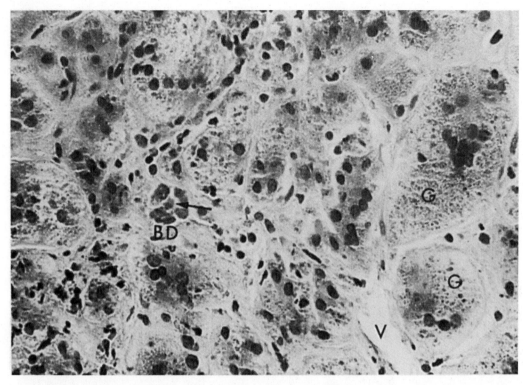

Figure 13–12. Photomicrograph illustrating characteristic histologic findings of the liver with idiopathic neonatal hepatitis. Note the presence of giant cells (G) containing deposits of bile components near a terminal (central) vein (V). The bile ductule (BD) contains a bile plug (arrow). (Hematoxylin & eosin, × 250.) (Reproduced, with permission, from Page 1140 in: Rudolph AM et al [editors]: *Rudolph's Pediatrics,* 20th ed. Appleton & Lange, 1996.)

traoperative cholangiography. With cholangiography, the gallbladder is filled with contrast material; if no reflux into the proximal ductular system is apparent, the diagnosis is confirmed. This procedure is performed intraoperatively so that if the diagnosis is confirmed, the appropriate surgical procedure can be performed. In approximately one fifth of patients, the proximal extrahepatic duct is patent to the level of the porta hepatis and the obstruction is distal. In these patients, surgical correction allows resumption of adequate bile drainage. In most patients, however, the obstruction is proximal and not correctable. For these patients, the Kasai procedure (hepatoportoenterostomy with Roux-en-Y enteroanastomosis) is performed in an attempt to allow some biliary drainage. The success of this procedure is directly related to the patient's age at the time of surgery, with patients younger than 2 months experiencing the best results. After this procedure, ascending cholangitis is the most common complication.

Even in those patients in whom the Kasai procedure is successful in relieving extrahepatic obstruction, progression of intrahepatic disease may lead to cirrhosis and portal hypertension. The availability of orthotopic liver transplantation for patients with end-stage liver disease has improved their prognosis remarkably.

α_1-Antitrypsin Deficiency. α_1-Antitrypsin is a protease inhibitor, synthesized in the liver, which acts as the major inhibitor of potentially destructive enzymes such as trypsin. When deficient, hepatic disease (neonatal cholestasis or cirrhosis) or pulmonary disease (emphysema) may result. Clinically, patients with hepatic disease secondary to α_1-antitrypsin deficiency may be indistinguishable from those with idiopathic neonatal hepatitis; they present with jaundice, acholic stools, and hepatomegaly. The histologic findings of the two disorders are also similar, with giant-cell transformation, bile stasis, inflammation, and portal fibrosis often present.

Phenotyping should be performed to confirm the diagnosis. The protease inhibitor (*Pi*) phenotype *PiMM* is present in most individuals and is therefore considered to be "normal." Patients with the phenotype *PiZZ* are much more likely to have low serum concentrations of the enzyme and clinically apparent symptoms. Individuals with the heterozygous phenotype (*PiMZ*) may or may not have a clinically significant enzyme deficiency. The presence of either the *ZZ* or *MZ* phenotype in an infant with cholestasis is diagnostic of this disorder. Another test that may be helpful is periodic acid-Schiff staining of liver biopsy tissue, which with α_1-antitrypsin deficiency, may show intrahepatic

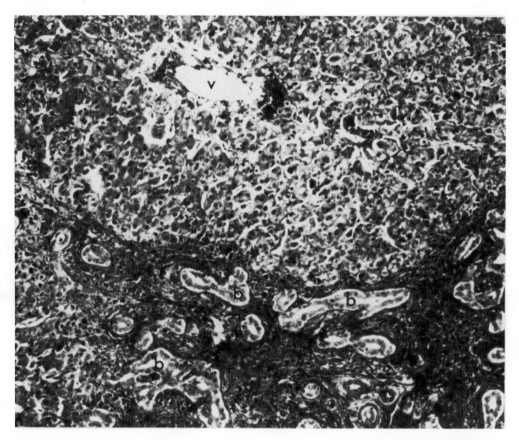

Figure 13–13. Photomicrograph of hepatic tissue from a patient with extrahepatic biliary atresia. Characteristic features include proliferation of interlobular bile ducts (b) and the presence of copious amounts of fibrous tissue. Biliary deposits are near the central vein (v). (Masson trichrome stain, × 100.) (Reproduced, with permission, from Page 1145 in: Rudolph AM et al [editors]: *Rudolph's Pediatrics,* 20th ed. Appleton & Lange, 1996.)

globules that are resistant to the effects of diastase. α_1-Antitrypsin concentrations can be measured, but these must be interpreted with caution because α_1-antitrypsin is an acute-phase reactant, and concentrations may be increased by various stressors, including inflammation.

Treatment of patients with α_1-antitrypsin deficiency is supportive and consists of measures aimed at minimizing cholestasis and its complications (see Management), but gene therapy for the disease is an area of active investigation. If the condition progresses to end-stage liver disease, orthotopic liver transplantation is a therapeutic option and converts the recipient to the *Pi* phenotype of the donor liver.

Alagille Syndrome. Alagille syndrome, or arteriohepatic dysplasia, describes a constellation of symptoms associated with paucity of intralobular bile ducts and, consequently, neonatal cholestasis. In addition to having liver abnormality, these patients may have some or all of the following characteristic manifestations: (1) unusual facies (Figure 13–15); (2) ocular abnormalities, such as posterior embryotoxon; (3) cardiovascular abnormalities, including peripheral pulmonic stenosis; and (4) vertebral arch defects, including anterior vertebral arch fusion and the presence of butterfly vertebrae.

Because the paucity of bile ducts is progressive and because other findings may be subtle or not present, the diagnosis of Alagille syndrome in early infancy may be difficult. It is crucial, however, that this disorder be differentiated from extrahepatic causes of cholestasis, such as biliary atresia, so that unnecessary portoenterostomy is avoided. Treatment of these patients is limited to efforts to minimize the effects of cholestasis.

Byler Disease. This progressive familial disorder causing intrahepatic cholestasis is differentiated from Alagille syndrome by the absence of extrahepatic manifestations and by the less frequent occurrence of bile duct paucity. These patients experience progressive cholestasis, which eventually reaches end-stage liver disease.

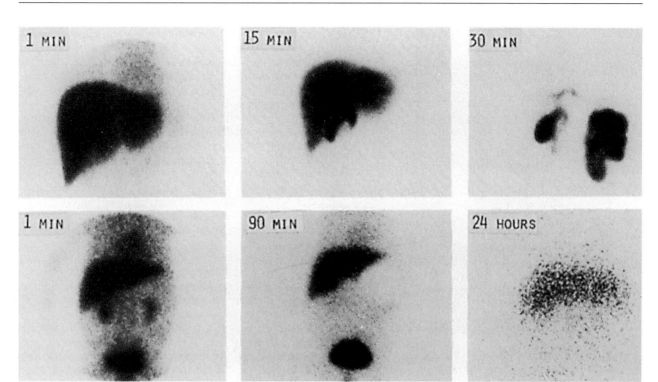

Figure 13–14. Typical scintigraphic findings of patients with idiopathic neonatal hepatitis *(upper panel)* and extrahepatic biliary atresia *(lower panel)*. In the upper panel, note that the uptake of radionuclide into the intrahepatic bile ducts and gallbladder was delayed (15 minutes), whereas excretion into the extrahepatic bile ducts and intestine occurred normally (30 minutes). This is consistent with a diagnosis of idiopathic neonatal hepatitis. In the lower panel, uptake of the radionuclide occurred normally, but excretion into the extrahepatic ducts and intestine was not demonstrated even after 24 hours. Such a pattern is typical of patients with extrahepatic biliary atresia. (Reproduced, with permission, from Rudolph AM [editor]: *Rudolph's Pediatrics,* 19th ed. Appleton & Lange, 1991.)

DIAGNOSTIC EVALUATION

Figure 13–16 presents an algorithm outlining an approach to the diagnosis of neonatal jaundice. Serum bilirubin concentrations, including conjugated and unconjugated fractions, should first be measured. When the conjugated bilirubin concentration is 2 mg/dL, or 20% or more of total bilirubin, the child should be evaluated for disorders of conjugated hyperbilirubinemia.

Examination of the peripheral blood smear is useful in determining whether hemolysis is a causative factor. In the absence of hemolysis or infection, unconjugated hyperbilirubinemia is most likely physiologic or related to intake of breast milk. For patients whose jaundice does not fit the typical pattern of physiologic or breast milk jaundice, enzyme defects that lead to alterations in bilirubin uptake and storage should be considered.

A far more complex evaluation is usually necessary to determine the etiology of conjugated hyperbilirubinemia. Because of the importance of early intervention in some of these disorders, this evaluation should be accomplished as expeditiously as possible. Initially, a group of studies

should be undertaken to look for evidence of one of the several known causes of neonatal cholestasis. These studies may include cultures of blood and urine, viral titers, thyroid hormone levels, sweat chloride concentrations, and α_1-antitrypsin phenotype. A urine Clinitest should also be done to check for reducing substances; a positive test may suggest galactosemia, the diagnosis of which can be confirmed by finding reduced levels of galactose-1-phosphate uridyl transferase activity in erythrocytes. Positive findings may then be confirmed with additional studies, as indicated. Specific therapy can then be initiated.

In most patients, the initial screening studies fail to reveal the etiology. Evaluation should then proceed to determine the patency of the bile ducts. This includes observation of the presence or absence of stool pigmentation, examination of duodenal fluid pigmentation, and investigation of biliary uptake and excretion with scintigraphy. In patients with evidence of decreased or absent excretory function, biliary atresia is likely and evaluation should proceed accordingly. Ultrasound is useful to investigate the possibility of choledochal cyst or cholelithiasis as a cause of extrahepatic biliary obstruction.

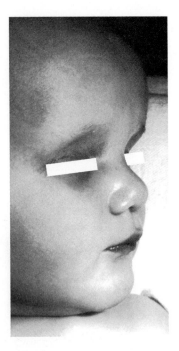

Figure 13–15. Patient with Alagille syndrome exhibiting the characteristic facies. Note the prominent forehead, flat, wide nasal bridge, antimongoloid ocular slant, and the relatively small, forward-jutting chin. (Reproduced, with permission, from Page 1147 in: Rudolph AM et al [editors]: *Rudolph's Pediatrics,* 20th ed. Appleton & Lange, 1996.)

In patients in whom extrahepatic causes of cholestasis have been ruled out, liver biopsy should be performed. Histologic findings in many of these patients will be consistent with the diagnosis of idiopathic neonatal hepatitis. Alternatively, biopsy findings may reveal a cause of cholestasis.

MANAGEMENT

For most patients with **unconjugated** hyperbilirubinemia, no specific therapy is necessary, as the bilirubin level will gradually return to normal without intervention. In patients with hemolytic disease, exchange transfusions may be required. For those with erythrocyte enzyme defects, transfusion may be necessary to correct anemia.

Because of the association of kernicterus with plasma concentrations of unconjugated bilirubin in excess of 20 mg/dL, patients with unconjugated hyperbilirubinemia of any etiology are often treated with phototherapy. This process involves the photoisomerization of bilirubin to forms that are less lipophilic and thus more readily excreted, even without conjugation. During phototherapy, dehydration due to the accompanying increase in insensible water losses must be avoided. The eyes must also be protected to avoid retinal injury. The use of phototherapy in infants with conjugated or mixed hyperbilirubinemia may result in the "bronze baby syndrome," in which the skin assumes a bronze discoloration because of the retention of photo-oxidation products of bilirubin; this may last for several months.

In patients with **conjugated** hyperbilirubinemia, treatment is directed to the cause, if known. Symptomatic treatment should also be provided. Malnutrition may occur in patients with cholestasis because of poor caloric intake and malabsorption of fat. Nutritional deficiencies should be treated appropriately. Fat-soluble vitamin deficiencies may also result from malabsorption due to diminished intestinal bile acid concentration. Vitamin D deficiency may present as rickets, and progressive neuromuscular disease, including areflexia and peripheral neuropathy, may occur with vitamin E deficiency. Deficiency of vitamin K, with hypoprothrombinemia, and of vitamin A, with visual impairment, may also be present. Supplementation of the fat-soluble vitamins should thus be routine in the management of patients with cholestasis.

Pruritus is another common complication of cholestasis. Medications intended to increase choleresis (eg, phenobarbital) and those designed to bind bile acids (eg, cholestyramine) may be useful in treating pruritus. More recently, ursodeoxycholic acid has been found to be useful in diminishing pruritus.

Hepatic cirrhosis and portal hypertension often develop in patients with cholestatic disorders. Ascites, which may accompany portal hypertension, may be diminished by sodium restriction and diuretic administration. The development of esophageal varices may necessitate the use of sclerotherapy. Despite these temporizing measures, patients typically progress to end-stage liver disease. In these patients, the possibility of orthotopic liver transplantation should be strongly considered.

THE CHILD WITH JAUNDICE

CLINICAL EVALUATION

The evaluation of jaundice in childhood or adolescence should be directed at determining the time of onset, duration, and changes in severity of the jaundice. Other important aspects of the history are exposure to infections, use of prescription or nonprescription medications, and exposure to toxins. The relationship of jaundice to dietary changes may be important, particularly in patients with hereditary fructose intolerance in whom jaundice develops after fructose ingestion. The family history may indicate the possibility of genetic or inherited disorders.

Distribution of the skin discoloration should be noted.

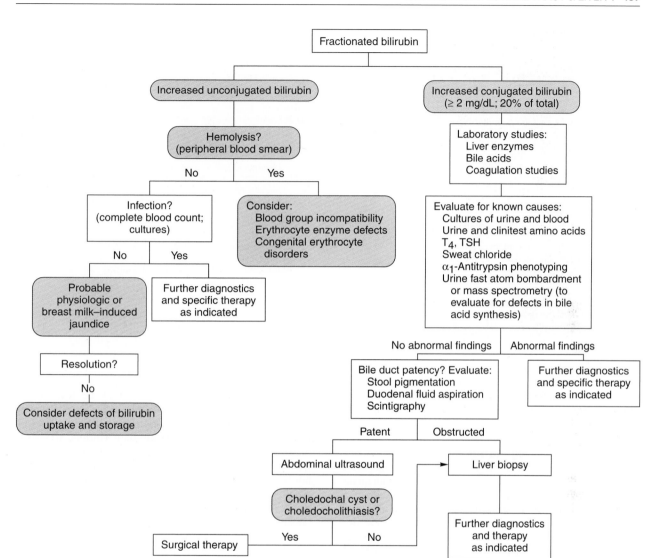

Figure 13–16. Algorithm presenting an approach to the evaluation of the neonate with jaundice. TSH = thyroid-stimulating hormone.

In patients with Gilbert syndrome, for example, icterus may be limited to the sclerae. Children with carotenemia have yellow-orange skin pigmentation resulting from absorption of pigments from carrots and other yellow vegetables; this may be differentiated from bilirubin pigmentation by its absence from the sclerae. Abdominal examination should include an assessment of the size and texture of the liver and determination of the presence of abdominal masses.

DIFFERENTIAL DIAGNOSIS

Table 13–12 provides a partial list of disorders that may cause jaundice in childhood; many are similar to those that cause jaundice in the neonate (see Table 13–11). Furthermore, in older children with a previously unremarkable medical history and evidence of normal growth and development, the likelihood of diagnosing a previously undetected congenital disorder as the cause of jaundice is low. Congenital disorders that are undetected and asymptomatic during the neonatal period are included in the differential diagnosis outlined in Table 13–12. Most disorders that cause jaundice in children and adolescents are discussed elsewhere in this chapter.

Infectious Hepatitis

Infection with the hepatotropic viruses (hepatitis A, B, C, etc) causes a variety of clinical presentations, depending on both the specific virus and the age of the patient.

Table 13–12. Differential diagnosis: The child with jaundice.

Disorders causing increased bilirubin production	
Hemolytic diseases	Reabsorption of hematoma
Erythrocyte enzyme defects	Transfusion
Hemaglobinopathies	

Disorders causing decreased bilirubin clearance	
Hereditary defects of bilirubin metabolism	Hepatocellular disease
Gilbert syndrome	Infectious hepatitis
Crigler-Najjar syndrome	Toxin-induced liver disease
Dubin-Johnson syndrome	Total parenteral nutrition
Rotor syndrome	Pharmacologic agents (acetaminophen, phenytoin)
Disorders causing cholestasis	Intrahepatic persistent cholestasis
Metabolic diseases	Alagille syndrome
Tyrosinemia	Byler disease (Persistent familial intrahepatic cholestasis)
Wilson disease	Sepsis
Disorders of carbohydrate metabolism	Biliary tract obstruction
Galactosemia	Congenital hepatic fibrosis/infantile polycystic disease
Hereditary fructose intolerance	Caroli disease
Glycogen storage disease (types I, III, and IV)	Bile duct stenosis
Disorders of lipid metabolism	Anomalies of the choledochopancreaticoductal junction
Wolman disease	Choledocholithiasis
Niemann-Pick disease	Tumors
Disorders in which the defect is uncharacterized	Sclerosing cholangitis
α_1-Antitrypsin deficiency	Pancreatitis
Cystic fibrosis	

Serum transaminase concentrations are often increased, and jaundice and hepatomegaly may be associated. Viral hepatitis is discussed in Chapter 9.

Hepatolenticular Degeneration

Hepatolenticular degeneration, or **Wilson disease,** is an autosomal-recessive disorder associated with inadequate biliary excretion of copper. The metabolic defect remains unknown but may involve impaired synthesis of the copper-binding protein ceruloplasmin. Regardless of the defect, the result is the accumulation of copper in the liver leading to hepatocyte necrosis. Copper is then released into the circulation and may be deposited in the eyes, central nervous system, and kidneys.

Patients with Wilson disease rarely manifest symptoms in early childhood. More commonly, they are well throughout childhood and begin to experience hepatomegaly, jaundice, and other symptoms commonly associated with acute infectious hepatitis in early adolescence. If these are untreated, cirrhosis and portal hypertension gradually develop. Occasionally patients may present with acute hepatic failure associated with hemolytic anemia.

Diagnosis of Wilson disease requires evidence of abnormal copper metabolism. Slit-lamp examination may show copper deposition in the eye (Kayser-Fleischer rings). A neurologic evaluation should be done to determine the presence of subtle neurologic findings, including changes in school performance. More severe neurologic disease is typically seen in older patients. Serum transaminase levels may be low, especially with the fulminant form of the disease. Decreased plasma ceruloplasmin levels are present in most patients homozygous for Wilson disease. Ceruloplasmin levels also may be low in heterozygotes and in patients with other liver diseases or with malnutrition. Measurement of urinary copper excretion from a 24-hour collection should be performed if Wilson disease is suspected. Although urinary copper excretion typically is low in patients with Wilson disease, this may not be a consistent finding. A more reliable test in those in whom the diagnosis is uncertain involves measurement of urinary copper both before and after treatment with chelating agents. An increase in copper excretion after treatment is typical of Wilson disease. The finding of elevated copper content in liver tissue obtained by biopsy is diagnostic.

Treatment of Wilson disease relies on the use of D-penicillamine, a copper-chelating agent, to increase urinary copper excretion. Dietary restriction of copper to less than 1 mg/d should also be instituted. These therapies usually lead to resolution of symptoms as the extrahepatic sites of copper deposition are gradually cleared. In patients with fulminant disease, plasmapheresis, and possibly liver transplantation, are indicated. If untreated, Wilson disease is always fatal.

DIAGNOSTIC EVALUATION & MANAGEMENT

An approach to the diagnosis of the child with jaundice is presented in Figure 13–17. Specific use of imaging and other diagnostic studies are discussed in the section Jaundice in the Neonate, as are general techniques of managing the patient with cholestasis.

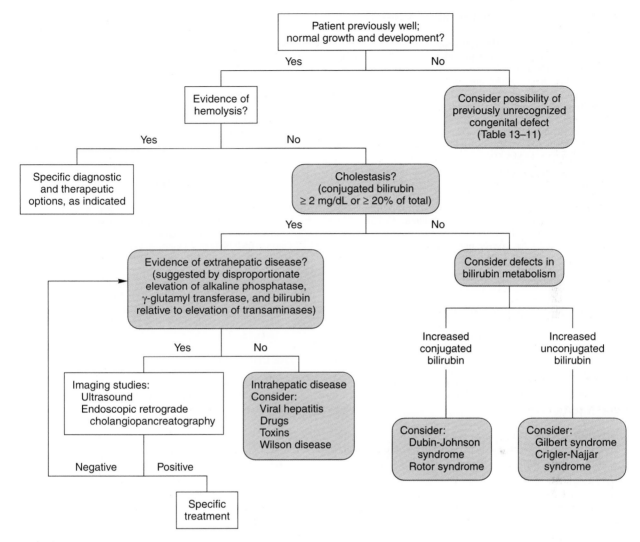

Figure 13–17. Algorithm presenting an approach to the evaluation of the patient in whom jaundice develops after the neonatal period.

REFERENCES

VOMITING

Fonkalsrud EW, Ament ME: Gastroesophageal reflux in childhood. Curr Probl Surg 1996;33:1.

Garcia VF, Randolph JG: Pyloric stenosis: Diagnosis and management. Pediatr Rev 1990;11:292.

Glassman M et al: Gastroesophageal reflux in children. Clinical manifestations, diagnosis, and therapy. Gastroenterol Clin North Am 1995;24:71.

Hillemeier AC: Gastroesophageal reflux. Diagnostic and therapeutic approaches. Pediatr Clin North Am 1996;43:197.

CONSTIPATION

Loening-Baucke V: Encopresis and soiling. Pediatr Clin North Am 1996;43:279.

Rudolph C, Benaroch L: Hirschsprung disease. Pediatr Rev 1995;16:5.

Seth R, Heyman MB: Management of constipation and encopresis in infants and children. Gastroenterol Clin North Am 1994;23:621.

GASTROINTESTINAL TRACT HEMORRHAGE

Upper Gastrointestinal Hemorrhage
Mezoff AM, Balistreri WF: Peptic ulcer disease in children. Pediatr Rev 1995;16:257.

Sherman PM: Peptic ulcer disease in children. Diagnosis, treatment, and the implication of *Helicobacter pylori.* Gastroenterol Clin North Am 1994;23:707.

Lower Gastrointestinal Hemorrhage
Fekety R, Shah AB: Disgnosis and treatment of *Clostridium difficile* colitis. JAMA 1993;269:71.

Grand RJ et al: Inflammatory bowel disease in the pediatric patient. Gastroenterol Clin North Am 1995;24:613.

Hyams JS: Crohn's disease in children. Pediatr Clin North Am 1996;43:255.

Kirschner BS: Ulcerative colitis in children. Pediatr Clin North Am 1996;4:235.

Milov DE, Andres JM: Sorting out the causes of rectal bleeding. Contemp Pediatr 1988;5:80.

ABDOMINAL PAIN

Apley J: *The Child with Abdominal Pains,* 2nd ed. Oxford, Blackwell, 1975.

Boyle JT: Abdominal pain. Chapter 17 in: Walker WA et al (editors): *Pediatric Gastrointestinal Disease: Pathophysiology, Diagnosis, Management.* Decker, 1991.

Buchert GS: Abdominal pain in children: An emergency practitioner's guide. Emerg Med Clin North Am 1989;7:497.

DIARRHEA

Dellert SF, Cohen MB: Diarrheal disease. Established pathogens, new pathogens, and progress in vaccine development. Gastroenterol Clin North Am 1994;23:637.

Laney DW, Cohen MB: An approach to the pediatric patient with diarrhea. Gastroenterol Clin North Am 1993;22:499.

Northrup RS, Flanigan TPL: Gastroenteritis. Pediatr Rev 1994;15:461.

Sherman PM et al: Infectious gastroenterocolitides in children: An update on emerging pathogens. Pediatr Clin North Am 1996;43:391.

Troncone R et al: Gluten-sensitive enteropathy. Pediatr Clin North Am 1996;43:355.

Vanderhoof JA et al: Short bowel syndrome in children and small intestinal transplantation. Pediatr Clin North Am 1996;43:533.

JAUNDICE IN THE NEONATE

Balistreri WF, Schubert WK: Liver disease in infancy and childhood. In Schiff L, Schiff E (editors): *Diseases of the Liver,* 7th ed. Lippincott, 1993.

Gartner LM: Neonatal jaundice. Pediatr Rev 1994;15:422.

Hicks BA, Altman RP: The jaundiced newborn. Pediatr Clin North Am 1993;40:1161.

Lasker MR, Holzman IR: Neonatal jaundice: When to treat, when to watch and wait. Postgrad Med 1996;99:187.

Schwarzenberg SJ, Sharp HL: Pediatric gastroenterology. Update on metabolic liver disease. Pediatr Clin North Am 1996;43:27.

THE CHILD WITH JAUNDICE

Brewer GJ: Practical recommendations and new therapies for Wilson's disease. Drugs 1995;50:240.

14

Blood

Caroline A. Hastings, MD, & Bertram H. Lubin, MD

The diagnosis of hematologic problems in the pediatric age group poses several challenges to health care practitioners. One must not only take into account variation in normal hematologic values for different age groups, but be able to decide which of the many paths of testing to follow from basic examination results. To facilitate this process, careful attention must be given to the family history, history of the current illness, and physical examination. Similarly, the blood smear should be evaluated before ordering more specific laboratory tests or obtaining a consultation with a pediatric hematologist. This chapter discusses courses of diagnosis and care of the more common hematologic problems in the pediatric age group.

RED CELLS: ANEMIA

Mature red cells are derived from the stem cells, which exist within bone marrow. Erythrocytosis is regulated by erythropoietin, cytokines, and growth factors. During the maturation of red cell progenitors, hemoglobin (Hb) synthesis increases, the nucleus is extruded from the cell, membrane remodeling occurs, and cell volume decreases.

Anemia, the most common hematologic problem diagnosed in children, is a condition in which tissue hypoxia occurs because of inadequate oxygen-carrying capacity of the blood. Failure to produce red cells or an imbalance between red cell production and red cell destruction causes anemia. The diagnosis is most often made by comparing the patient's Hb or hematocrit value with age-matched normal values. Although practical and effective in most cases, this approach does not take into consideration the physiologic, and more accurate, definition of anemia. This point is exemplified by studies of patients with cyanotic heart disease or of patients with Hb variants characterized by a high oxygen affinity, in which the Hb level may be elevated or within the normal range, although tissue hypoxia exists.

History & Physical Examination

Important clues about the underlying cause of anemia can be obtained by obtaining a careful medical history, including age, sex, race, ethnicity, neonatal history, diet, drug exposure, infections, inheritance, and history of gastrointestinal dysfunction. The obstetric, perinatal, and birth history should be reviewed carefully, and questions should be asked regarding perinatal blood loss, maternal illness or risk factors, and maternal history of transfusion. Information regarding a family history of splenectomy, red cell transfusions, jaundice, and cholecystectomy are useful in evaluating patients suspected of having a hemolytic anemia (Table 14–1).

The symptoms of anemia depend on the degree of reduction in the oxygen-carrying capacity of the blood, the change in blood volume, the rate at which these changes occur, and the ability of the cardiovascular and hematopoietic systems to compensate. General signs of anemia in childhood can include poor feeding or dyspnea, irritability, inactivity, faintness, change in behavior, and poor school performance. Pallor and jaundice, in association with dark urine, suggest hemolytic anemia (Table 14–2).

Cardiac enlargement and signs of congestive heart failure may be present with either acute blood loss or chronic anemia. Tachycardia, prominent arterial pulses, bruits, tachypnea, dyspnea, and postural hypotension can be detected in patients with modest to severe anemia. Hemic murmurs reflect an increase in cardiac output, stroke volume, and heart rate associated with decreased peripheral resistance and decreased blood viscosity. Gallop rhythm may also be present in a hemodynamically compromised state. These abnormalities disappear after blood transfusion or treatment of the anemia.

Patients in whom marrow hyperplasia develops to compensate for their hemolytic anemia may have frontal bossing and prominent malar eminences. Specific dysmorphic features can be seen with certain inherited anemias, such

Table 14–1. Important historical points in evaluation of anemia.

History	Consider
Prematurity	Anemia of prematurity (erythropoietin-responsive) Iatrogenic blood loss
Perinatal risk factors	
Maternal illness (autoimmune)	Hemolytic anemia
Drug ingestion	
Infections (TORCHES, hepatitis)	
Mechanical problems at delivery	Acute blood loss Fetal-maternal hemorrhage
Ethnicity	
African-American	HbS, C; G6PD deficiency
Mediterannean	α, β-Thalassemia; G6PD deficiency
Southeast Asian	α, β-Thalassemia; HbE
Family history	
Gallstones, cholecystectomy	Inherited hemolytic anemia
Splenectomy, jaundice	Spherocytosis, elliptocytosis
Isoimmunization (Rh or ABO)	Hemolytic disease of newborn Predisposed to iron deficiency
Male sex	X-linked enzymopathies (G6PD)
Early jaundice (< 24 h)	Isoimmune, infectious
Persistent jaundice	Hemolytic anemia
Diet (usually > 6 mo)	
Pica (ice, dirt)	Lead toxicity, iron deficiency
Excessive milk intake	Iron deficiency
Macrobiotic diets	Vitamin B$_{12}$ deficiency
Goat's milk	Folic acid deficiency
Drugs	
Sulfa, anticonvulsants	Hemolytic anemia (G6PD deficiency)
Chloramphenicol	Aplastic anemia
Low socioeconomic status	Pica (lead, iron deficiency) Iron deficiency
Malnutrition	
Malabsorption	Anemia of chronic disease
Environmental	Iron, vitamin B$_{12}$ deficiency Vitamin E, K deficiency
Liver disease	Shortened red cell survival
Renal disease	Shortened red cell survival Decreased red cell production (decreased erythropoietin)
Infectious diseases	
Inflammation, acute gastroenteritis, otitis media, pharyngitis	Transient mild decreased Hb
Bacterial, viral, mycoplasma	Hemolytic anemia

G6PD = glucose-6-phosphate dehydrogenase; Hb = hemogloblin; TORCHES = *toxoplasmosis, rubella, cytomegalovirus,* and *herpes simplex.*

as radial limb abnormalities in Diamond-Blackfan anemia and Fanconi anemia.

Splenomegaly may be a prominent finding in infants and children with hemolytic anemia, storage diseases, infections, and malignancies. The spleen is occasionally enlarged in patients with iron deficiency anemia or megaloblastic anemia of infancy. In pathologic states, the edge of the spleen is hard and occasionally tender. In contrast,

if the spleen is palpable in a normal child, it has a soft edge and is nontender. If lymphadenopathy is detected, infection or leukemia should be excluded.

The liver may be enlarged in patients with anemia because of acute or chronic congestive heart failure. Hepatomegaly is also noted in patients who have received frequent blood transfusions for diseases such as aplastic anemia, sickle cell anemia, and β-thalassemia as a consequence of iron overload.

Laboratory Procedures

Normal hematologic values reported from birth to adolescence are shown in Table 14–3. Changes occur dramatically during the first few weeks after birth and then more gradually over the next 5–7 years. Use of automated electronic cell counters provides information on Hb, hematocrit, red cell count, red cell indices (mean corpuscular volume [MCV], mean corpuscular Hb [MCH], and mean corpuscular Hb concentration [MCHC]), and red cell distribution width (RDW).

An examination of the peripheral blood smear is perhaps the simplest, and most often overlooked, laboratory procedure in the evaluation of the anemic patient. The morphology of the red cells can serve to identify children with nutritional anemias, red cell membrane defects, and hemoglobinopathies. Figure 14–1 demonstrates several of these characteristic morphologic changes in the more common forms of anemia in childhood.

The reticulocyte count is useful in determining the rate of red cell destruction and in monitoring response to treatment. The normal value in the newborn is 3.2 ± 1.4% and in children 1.2 ± 0.7%. Anemia is classified as hemolytic if red cell survival is less than 120 days. In these cases, the reticulocyte count is elevated and the Hb concentration is normal, in the case of compensated hemolytic anemia, or low.

Additional laboratory tests that can be used to document hemolysis include serum haptoglobin and hemopexin concentrations. These proteins bind Hb and heme released from red cells after their destruction. The complexed proteins that are formed after intravascular hemolysis are removed from the circulation. As a consequence, haptoglobin and hemopexin levels are low in patients who have hemolytic anemia. When haptoglobin is saturated, free plasma Hb can be detected. The indirect bilirubin level frequently is determined to provide evidence for a hemolytic process; however, it is an insensitive measurement of hemolysis and is elevated only when liver function is impaired or when hemolysis is extensive. Another means of detecting hemolysis is by measuring endogenous carbon monoxide production. When Hb is degraded, the α-methyl group of heme becomes carbon monoxide. Determination of endogenous production of carbon monoxide may be useful to detect hemolysis in the neonatal period but is of limited value in older children owing to the background levels of carbon monoxide in the environment.

When nutritional anemias are suspected, measurements

Table 14–2. Physical examination of the anemic child.

General signs		
Skin	Pallor	Severe anemia
	Jaundice	Hemolytic anemia, acute and chronic
		Hepatitis, aplastic anemia
	Petechiae, purpura	Autoimmune hemolytic anemia with thrombocytopenia
		Hemolytic uremic syndrome
		Bone marrow aplasia or infiltration
	Cavernous hemangioma	Microangiopathic hemolytic anemia
Head and neck	Frontal bossing, prominent malar and maxillary bones	Extramedullary hematopoiesis (thalassemia major, sickle cell anemia, other congenital hemolytic anemias)
	Icteric sclerae	Congenital hemolytic anemia and hyperhemolytic crisis associated with infection (Red cell enzyme deficiencies, red cell membrane defects, thalassemias, hemoglobinopathies)
	Angular stomatitis	Iron deficiency
	Glossitis	Vitamin B_{12} or iron deficiency
Chest	Rales, gallop rhythm, tachycardia	Congestive heart failure, acute or severe anemia
Extremities	Radial limb dysplasia	Fanconi anemia
	Spoon nails	Iron deficiency
	Triphalangeal thumbs	Red cell aplasia
Spleen	Splenomegaly	Congenital hemolytic anemia, infection, hematologic malignancies, portal hypertension

of iron status, vitamin B_{12}, and folic acid may be indicated. The red cell indices, free erythrocyte protoporphyrin (FEP), and RDW can be used efficiently to diagnose iron deficiency with minimal cost to the patient.

The osmotic fragility test is used to measure the osmotic resistance of red cells. Red cells are incubated under hypotonic conditions, and their ability to swell before lysis is determined. The osmotic fragility of red cells is increased when the surface area–volume ratio of the cell is decreased, as in hereditary spherocytosis, in which

membrane instability results in membrane loss and decreased surface area. Conversely, it is decreased in liver disease and in iron deficiency, in which the surface area–volume ratio of the red cell is increased. A recently developed test performed on an Ektacytometer measures the deformability of red cells subjected simultaneously to shear stress and osmotic stress.

In patients in whom hemolytic anemia is suspected, immunologic tests, such as the direct and indirect Coombs tests, are required to exclude antibody-mediated red cell

Table 14–3. Red blood cell values at various ages: Mean and lower limit or normal.[1]

Age	Hemoglobin (g/dL) Mean	–2 SD	Hematocrit (%) Mean	–2 SD	Red Cell Count (10^{12}/L) Mean	–2 SD	MCV (fL) Mean	–2 SD	MCH (pg) Mean	–2 SD	MCHC (g/dL) Mean	–2 SD
Birth (cord blood)	16.5	13.5	51	42	4.7	3.9	108	98	34	31	33	30
1–3 d (capillary)	18.5	14.5	56	45	5.3	4.0	108	95	34	31	33	29
1 wk	17.5	13.5	54	42	5.1	3.9	107	88	34	28	33	28
2 wk	16.5	12.5	51	39	4.9	3.6	105	86	34	28	33	28
1 mo	14.0	10.0	43	31	4.2	3.0	104	85	34	28	33	29
2 mo	11.5	9.0	35	28	3.8	2.7	96	77	30	26	33	29
3–6 mo	11.5	9.5	35	29	3.8	3.1	91	74	30	25	33	30
0.5–2 y	12.0	10.5	36	33	4.5	3.7	78	70	27	23	33	30
2–6 y	12.5	11.5	37	34	4.6	3.9	81	75	27	24	34	31
6–12 y	13.5	11.5	40	35	4.6	4.0	86	77	29	25	34	31
12–18 y—female	14.0	12.0	41	36	4.6	4.1	90	78	30	25	34	31
male	14.5	13.0	43	37	4.9	4.5	88	78	30	25	34	31
18–49 y—female	14.0	12.0	41	36	4.6	4.0	90	80	30	26	34	31
male	15.5	13.5	47	41	5.2	4.5	90	80	30	26	34	31

[1]Compiled from the following sources: Dutcher: Lab Med 1971;2:32; Koerper et al: J Pediatr 1976;89:580; Marner: Acta Paediatr Scand 1969;58:363; Matoth et al: Acta Paediatr Scand 1971;60:317; Moe: Acta Paediatr Scand 1965;54:69; Okuno: J Clin Pathol 1972;25:599; Oski, Naiman: *Hematological Problems in the Newborn.* Saunders, 1972, p 11; Penttilä et al: Suomen Lääkärilehti 1973;26:2173; and Viteri et al: Br J Haematol 1972;23:189. Emphasis is given to recent studies using electronic counters and to the selection of populations that are likely to exclude individuals with iron deficiency. The mean ± 2 SD can be expected to include 95% of the observations in a normal population. Cited in: Rudolph AM (editor): *Rudolph's Pediatrics,* 16th ed. Appleton & Lange, 1977.
MCH = mean corpuscular hemoglobin; MCHC = mean corpuscular hemoglobin concentration; MCV = mean corpuscular volume.

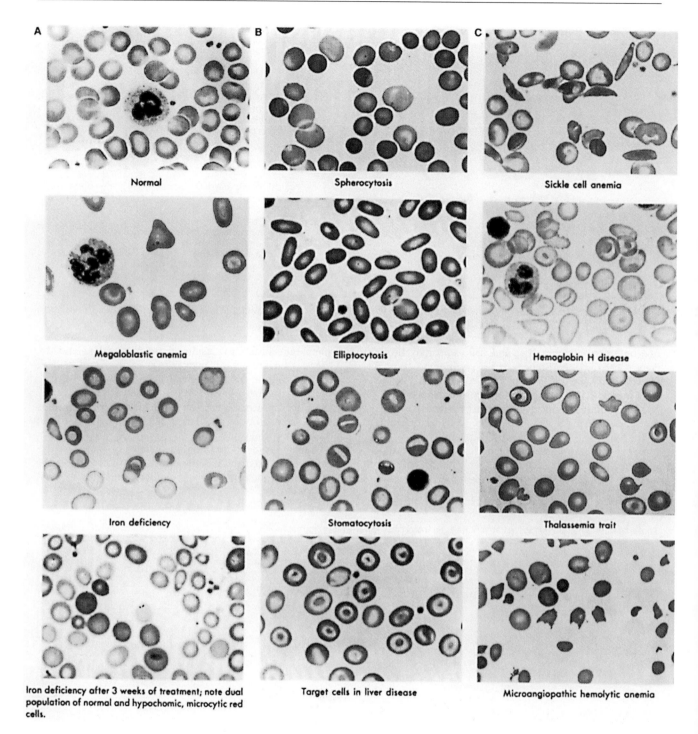

Figure 14–1. Red cell appearance in various diseases. **A:** Peripheral blood morphology—various anemias. **B:** Membrane abnormalities. **C:** Hemoglobinopathies and other conditions.

destruction. Intrinsic defects in the red cell can be assessed by analysis of red cell membrane proteins, Hb electrophoretic tests, and specific enzyme or cations and water determinations. Details of these disorders are presented in the section Extracorpuscular Defects.

Examination of bone marrow is useful in the assessment of anemia associated with reticulocytopenia, neutropenia, or thrombocytopenia. Histologic examination of the stained bone marrow aspirate allows one to identify red cell precursors as well as myeloid and megakaryocytic precursors, and to detect malignant or infiltrating cells. The bone marrow sample also can be used to determine iron stores by using a Prussian blue stain. In certain cases of familial anemias, cytogenetic analysis of bone marrow samples can be useful.

Age-Related Causes of Anemia

The causes of anemia in children vary with age. Understanding the age-related causes can simplify diagnosis by quickly excluding factors not generally associated with each age group.

Figure 14–2 demonstrates a useful diagnostic approach to the diagnosis of anemia in the newborn. An Hb concentration less than 13.5 g/dL during the first week after birth is 2 SD below the norm for that age and requires investi-

gation. If the reticulocyte count is elevated, a hemolytic anemia or blood loss should be suspected. Performance of a Coombs test is necessary to exclude immune hemolytic anemia. With a negative Coombs test result, blood loss, an intrinsic red cell disorder, or an infection must be excluded. If the reticulocyte count is low, either a defect in erythropoiesis or a congenital infection must be considered. The MCV is also useful to categorize the cause of anemia. Low values are seen with iron deficiency owing to intrauterine hemorrhage or to α-thalassemia. Note that infection can produce hemolysis (elevated reticulocyte count) or inhibit erythropoiesis (decreased reticulocyte count). When associated with hemolysis, the peripheral smear is abnormal, showing microangiopathic changes. Laboratory diagnosis in patients with congenital hemolytic anemias should include procedures to identify defects in membrane structure or function, abnormal cell metabolism, or defects in Hb structure and function. The specific laboratory tests are described in the sections dealing with these disorders.

Blood loss can occur before delivery in association with abruptio placentae or twin-to-twin transfusion, or can occur through the gastrointestinal tract. Internal bleeding can occur within the cranium or within organs, such as the liver or lung. If extensive blood loss has occurred in utero,

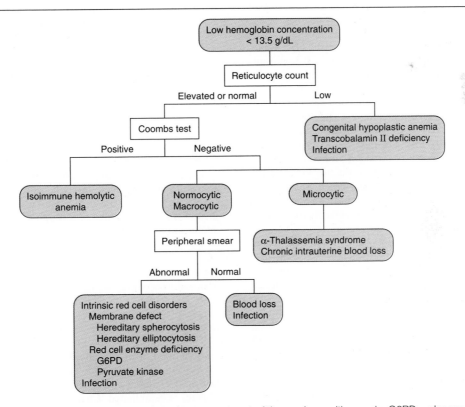

Figure 14–2. Algorithm diagramming an approach to the management of the newborn with anemia. G6PD = glucose-6-phosphate dehydrogenase.

as might be the case with fetal-maternal transfusion or partial placental abruption, the infant may be in congestive heart failure at birth. When fetal-to-maternal hemorrhage is suspected, a prompt search for fetal cells in the maternal circulation is indicated, using the Kliehauer-Betke staining technique.

When the Coombs test produces a positive result, the various causes of immune hemolysis should be pursued. Although the Coombs test result is positive in cases of Rh incompatibility, some cases of ABO incompatibility may not give a positive test result. If the reticulocyte count is elevated and the Coombs test result is negative, hereditary red cell membrane defects (eg, spherocytosis, pyropoikilocytosis, or elliptocytosis) or enzyme deficiencies (eg, glucose-6-phosphate dehydrogenase [G6PD] deficiency or pyruvate kinase [PK] deficiency) should be considered. Intrauterine or acquired infections may produce either hemolytic anemia or hypoplastic anemia. Infants with either of these conditions often have splenomegaly, may have petechiae, and are jaundiced.

A physiologic decrease in the Hb concentration is reached by approximately 2 months after birth. The decrease in Hb concentration is most dramatic in the premature infant, in whom this condition has been called anemia of prematurity. Although the relative reticulocyte count may be elevated, if corrected for anemia, the absolute reticulocyte count is often low. Most infants tolerate this anemia and recover without intervention. However, with cardiorespiratory distress, red cell transfusion may be required. Recovery is heralded by an increase in the reticulocyte count and a subsequent increase in the Hb value. Red cell transfusion may delay this process. It is not unusual to confuse the recovery period, associated with reticulocytosis, with a hemolytic anemia. When one observes the patient over the following 6–8 weeks, the Hb will increase and the reticulocyte count decrease. In contrast, children with congenital hemolytic anemia have persistent reticulocytosis and anemia. Some groups have recommended that premature infants be treated with therapeutic doses of recombinant erythropoietin to minimize this physiologic anemia; such therapy could decrease the need for red cell transfusions. Studies of this approach are currently under investigation, as the precise treatment regimen has not been established.

Nutritional anemias, particularly due to iron deficiency, peak between ages 6 months and 2 years. Because the premature infant has limited iron stores at birth, iron deficiency likely will occur unless the diet contains sufficient iron. A similar situation is noted in full-term infants who are neither breast-fed nor fed iron-fortified formulas. Although most often related to nutritional inadequacy, iron deficiency anemia in childhood can also occur as a result of gastrointestinal blood loss, as with Meckel diverticulum or gastroenteritis due to milk protein intolerance.

Pure red cell aplasia (Diamond-Blackfan syndrome) is usually detected by 3 months of age. Although initially it may be confused with physiologic anemia, in Diamond-Blackfan syndrome, the reticulocyte count does not in-

crease over time, nor does the anemia resolve without therapeutic interventions. Examination of the bone marrow in children with pure red cell aplasia reveals few, if any, erythroid progenitors. Megaloblastic anemia of infancy occurs chiefly between 2 and 18 months of age. Macrocytic red cells are seen in the peripheral blood, and megaloblastic red cell precursors are found in the bone marrow. Fanconi anemia, an inherited form of progressive pancytopenia, can present with anemia early in life, but usually not until 3–4 years of age. Transient erythroblastopenia of childhood usually occurs in the first few years after birth. Clinical and hematologic features of the hemoglobinopathies, such as β-thalassemia and sickle cell anemia, are usually evident by 6 months, when the switch from fetal Hb to adult Hb synthesis is complete.

By early adolescence, the causes of anemia are similar to those in adulthood, with the exception of the high incidence of iron deficiency. This is usually related to the pubertal growth spurt or to a diet lacking in essential nutrients. Pregnant adolescents are at particular risk for nutritional deficiencies because of greater nutritional requirements during pregnancy.

Classification of Anemia

Anemias are classified on either a physiologic or a morphologic basis. The physiologic classification includes anemias due to increased red cell loss, increased red cell destruction, and impaired red cell production. Table 14–4 illustrates the types of anemias grouped according to these approaches. The morphologic classification schema is based on red cell size, red cell indices, and red cell morphology.

BLOOD LOSS

The symptoms associated with blood loss are related to its acute or chronic pattern. Acute blood loss may follow trauma or surgery. Chronic blood loss may be due to gastrointestinal tract bleeding, as is seen with inflammation, ulcers, or recurrent nose bleeds. Chronic blood loss can also occur into the lungs or through the kidney in diseases such as idiopathic pulmonary hemosiderosis and nephritis.

The medical history often provides important clues to the site of blood loss. Examination of the stool and urine for occult blood is essential. Specialized radiographic tests and endoscopy may be required. An underlying bleeding disorder, such as von Willebrand disease (VWD) or a defect in platelet function, should be considered, especially in patients with recurrent, severe epistaxis.

The degree of anemia after blood loss depends on the amount and rate of loss and the ability of the bone marrow erythroid pool to respond. The Hb concentration may not fall until 24 hours *after* acute blood loss, when fluid equilibrium is established. Changes in vital signs, such as increased pulse rate, tachypnea, and decreased blood pressure, occur when blood loss is significant. In cases of

Table 14–4. Physiologic classification of anemia.

Increased Red Cell Loss	Increased Red Cell Destruction	Inadequate Red Cell Production
Blood loss	Inherited intracorpuscular defects	Abnormalities of cytoplasmic maturation
Acute	Defective red cell membrane	Iron deficiency
Chronic	Hereditary spherocytosis	Lead poisoning
Milk protein intolerance	Hereditary pyropoikilocytosis	Sideroblastic anemias
Ulcers	Hereditary stomatocytosis	Abnormalities of nuclear maturation
Iatrogenic (blood sampling)	Hereditary xerocytosis	Vitamin B_{12} deficiency
	Abnormal glycolysis	Folic acid deficiency
	Red cell enzyme deficiencies	Orotic aciduria
	Hexose monophosphate shunt	Dyserythropoietic anemias
	Embden-Myerhof pathway	Hereditary erythrocytic multinuclearity
	Glucose-6-phosphate dehydrogenase	with a positive acidified serum test,
	Pyruvate kinase	types I, II, III
	Others	Impaired erythropoietin production
	Hemoglobinopathies	Renal disease
	Sickle cell disease and other structural variants	Chronic infection
	Unstable hemoglobins	Hypothyroidism, hypopituitarism
	Thalassemias	Protein malnutrition
	Thalassemia syndromes	Liver disease
	Thalassemia	Defective marrow response
	Extracorpuscular defects	Aplastic anemia
	Isoimmune hemolytic anemia	Congenital (Fanconi anemia)
	Autoimmune hemolytic anemia	Acquired
		Pure red cell aplasia
		Congenital (Diamond-Blackfan, Ase
		syndromes)
		Acquired (transient erythroblastopenia
		of childhood)
		Marrow replacement
		Malignancies
		Myelofibrosis

anemia secondary to acute blood loss, the red cell indices are normal. Within 3–5 days after the bleed, erythrocyte production can be detected, as evidenced by an elevated reticulocyte count. Leukocytosis and thrombocytosis may also occur. With chronic blood loss, iron deficiency may develop, and red cells may become microcytic and hypochromic.

INCREASED RED CELL DESTRUCTION

The normal life span of the erythrocyte is 120 days. In the newborn, normal survival rates for red cells are reduced to 80–100 days, and survival rates as low as 45–60 days have been reported in the literature. Any anemia in which the life span of the red cell is shortened is classified as a hemolytic anemia. A useful approach in considering these types of anemia is shown in Figure 14–3. Each of these disorders is reviewed briefly.

INHERITED INTRACORPUSCULAR DEFECTS

Red Cell Membrane Disorders

Hereditary Spherocytosis. Hereditary spherocytosis (HS) is the most common congenital red blood cell membrane disorder. Patients with HS are often of northern European descent. The usual patient with HS has intermittent jaundice, as well as hemolytic and/or red cell aplastic episodes associated with viral infection, splenomegaly, and cholelithiasis. However, the clinical presentation is quite variable, with the most severe cases presenting in the newborn period or early childhood and milder cases presenting in adulthood. The family history is positive in only 20% of cases, and autosomal-dominant and autosomal-recessive inheritance patterns have been reported.

Several membrane protein defects are responsible for HS. Most result in instability of spectrin, one of the major skeletal membrane proteins. This skeletal defect is classified as a vertical defect in membrane stability because the attachment of the extrinsic (cytosolic skeleton) to the intrinsic membrane proteins is altered. There is a good correlation between the extent of spectrin deficiency and the degree of hemolysis. Structural changes that result as a consequence of protein deficiency lead to membrane instability, loss of surface area, abnormal membrane permeability, and decreased red cell deformability. Metabolic depletion accentuates the defect in HS cells, which accounts for an increase in osmotic fragility after a 24-hour incubation of whole blood at 37 °C. The splenic sinusoids prevent passage of nondeformable spherocytic red cells. This explains the occurrence of splenomegaly in HS and the therapeutic effect of splenectomy.

Patients with HS have a mild to moderate chronic he-

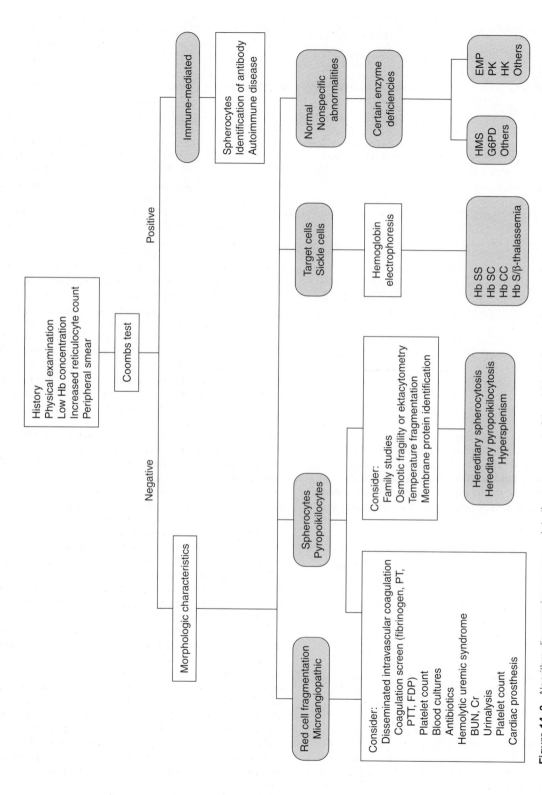

Figure 14–3. Algorithm diagramming an approach to the management of the child with hemolytic anemia. BUN = blood urea nitrogen; Cr = creatinine; EMP = Embden-Meyerhof pathway; FDP = fibrin degradation products; G6PD = glucose-6-phosphate dehydrogenase; Hb = hemoglobin; HK = hexokinase; HMS = hexose monophosphate shunt; PK = pyruvate kinase; PT = prothrombin time; PTT = partial prothrombin time.

molytic anemia. Red cell indices reveal a decreased MCV. Cellular dehydration increases the MCHC (characteristically > 36%). The RDW is elevated because of the variable presence of microspherocytes, and the reticulocyte count is increased in proportion to the degree of hemolysis. Osmotic fragility tests and Ektacytometry studies are characteristic for HS, with increased fragility in hypotonic environments. In unusual cases, in which patients have bile stones related to obstructive liver disease, the red cell surface area may increase because of the accumulation of unesterified cholesterol in the membrane. This clinical point must be considered, as such patients have normal osmotic fragility curves. When the obstructive jaundice clears, the osmotic fragility again becomes abnormal.

As with other hemolytic anemias, affected individuals are susceptible to hypoplastic crises during viral infections. Human parvovirus B19, a frequent pathogen and the organism responsible for erythema infectiosum, selectively invades erythroid progenitor cells and may result in a transient arrest in red cell proliferation. Recovery begins within 7–10 days after infection and is usually complete within 4–6 weeks. If the initial presentation of a patient with HS is during an aplastic crisis, a diagnosis of HS might not be considered because the reticulocyte count will be low and the peripheral blood smear may be undiagnostic. The family history of HS should be explored; if it is positive, the patient should be evaluated for HS after recovery from the aplastic episode.

Splenectomy is often considered for patients who have had severe hemolysis requiring transfusions or repeated hospitalization. In patients with mild hemolysis, the decision to perform splenectomy should be delayed; in many cases, it is not required. For pediatric patients who have excessive splenic size, an additional consideration for splenectomy is to diminish the risk of traumatic splenic rupture. The risk of splenectomy must be considered before any clinical decision is made regarding this procedure.

Red cell survival returns to normal values after splenectomy unless an accessory spleen develops. Although an increased number of spherocytes can be seen in the peripheral blood smear after splenectomy and the osmotic fragility is worse, the Hb value is normal. Platelet counts frequently increase to more than 1,000,000/μL immediately after splenectomy but return to normal levels over several weeks. No therapeutic interventions are required for postsplenectomy thrombocytosis in patients with HS.

To minimize the risk of sepsis due to *Haemophilus influenzae* and *Streptococcus pneumoniae,* the splenectomy procedure (when necessary) is often postponed until after the child's fifth or sixth birthday. Patients should be immunized against streptococcal pneumonia and *H influenzae* with a pneumococcal vaccine (pneumovax) and *H influenzae* type B vaccines, and prophylaxis with penicillin is often recommended after splenectomy. The duration of penicillin prophylaxis depends on evaluation of the patient's and family's ability to recognize and promptly seek medical attention for febrile episodes. In some cases, penicillin prophylaxis is continued for several years, and the patient is then advised to take penicillin at the first sign of fever. The increase in penicillin-resistant strains of *S pneumoniae* has raised questions regarding the use of prophylactic penicillin. No studies have determined the frequency of this problem in children receiving prophylactic penicillin after splenectomy.

Hereditary Elliptocytosis. Hereditary elliptocytosis (HE) is a congenital red cell disorder in which the red cells appear elliptical on peripheral blood smears (see Figure 14–1). The membrane protein abnormalities that cause these disorders result in lateral defects in membrane stability. These refer to side-to-side protein interactions that stabilize the membrane cytoskeleton; the abnormalities involve primarily the α and β chains of spectrin. Considerable clinical heterogeneity exists depending on the effect of the structural spectrin defect on membrane stability.

In autosomal-dominant HE, elliptocytes can be detected in the peripheral blood smear, but the patient is not anemic, the reticulocyte count is normal, and red cell indices are normal. Although the osmotic fragility may be normal, the membrane abnormality in HE can be detected by the fragmentation patterns of red cell membrane preparations using an Ektacytometer. Elliptocytes also can be seen in the blood smear of patients with thalassemia, iron deficiency anemia, and megaloblastic anemia. In these cases, the abnormal red cell morphology is secondary to an acquired membrane defect. Protein electrophoresis patterns of spectrin show abnormalities, and functional studies reveal defects in tetramer formation.

In cases in which HE is coinherited with another skeletal protein defect, the red cell morphology may show elliptocytes and poikilocytes. These patients have a moderate to severe hemolytic anemia, and their red cells fragment in vitro as the incubation temperature is increased above 37 °C. As a consequence, this disorder is called **hereditary pyropoikilocytosis (HPP).**

Depending on the precise molecular defect, the newborn with HE may have a transient, moderate to severe hemolytic anemia similar to that seen in patients with HPP. This anemia corrects in 4–6 months, at which time elliptocytes are seen on the peripheral blood smear and the Hb and reticulocyte counts are normal. An interesting mechanism has been proposed to explain this transition. Because fetal Hb does not bind 2,3-diphosphoglycerate (2,3-DPG), the concentration of unbound 2,3-DPG inside the neonatal red cell is increased. Because 2,3-DPG can weaken skeletal protein interactions, it is possible that the combination of a hereditary protein defect with a weakened skeletal network results in the poikilocytes noted in the peripheral blood smear. As adult Hb increases, the unbound 2,3-DPG associates with the Hb and no longer weakens the membrane. This hypothesis might also explain why some patients with hereditary spherocytosis have problems in the newborn period, whereas most do not.

Other Inherited Membrane Defects. Several other less common forms of inherited membrane defects include **hereditary stomatocytosis** and **hereditary xerocytosis.** These rare congenital hemolytic anemias are associated with permeability defects in the membrane leading to abnormalities in red cell water and cation content. The stomatocyte is characterized by a "stoma" fish mouth-like appearance, excess water, and a marked cation permeability defect that lowers intracellular K^+ and increases intracellular Na^+. The MCV is greater than 110 fL. Patients with hereditary xerocytosis have dense, dehydrated red cells and a mild to moderate hemolytic anemia. The MCHC is greater than 36%, the MCV is low, and the cells are depleted of intracellular cations. Both of these disorders result in severe hemolytic anemia that is only partially corrected by splenectomy.

Abnormalities in Red Cell Glycolysis

Glucose is the primary metabolic substrate for the red cell. Because the mature red cell does not contain mitochondria, it can metabolize glucose only by anaerobic mechanisms. The two major metabolic pathways within the red cell are the Embden-Meyerhof pathway (EMP) and the hexose monophosphate shunt (HMS). Other minor metabolic pathways involve the reduction of oxidized Hb, the methemoglobin reductive pathway, and the reutilization of purines, the purine salvage pathway. A flow diagram of red cell metabolism is shown in Figure 14–4.

In the EMP, which accounts for 90% of the glucose used by the red cell, two molecules of adenosine triphosphate (ATP) are generated for each molecule of glucose

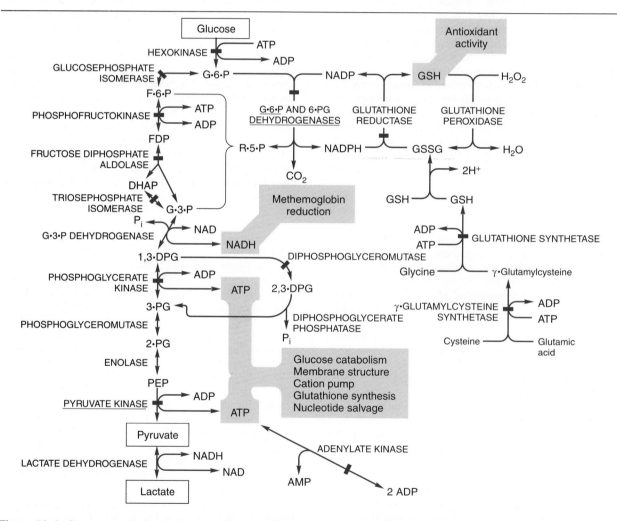

Figure 14–4. Glucose metabolism in mature erythrocytes. The hexose monophosphate shunt and glutathione metabolism are shown within the shaded area. Reactions involved in the synthesis of glutathione are indicated at the lower right. Solid bars indicate enzymatic deficiencies the association of which with hereditary hemolytic disorders is well established. ADP = adenosine diphosphate; AMP = adenosine monophosphate; ATP = adenosine triphosphate; DHAP = dihydroxyacetone phosphate; DPG = diphosphoglycerate; FDP = fructose diphosphate; F-6-P = fructose-6-phosphatase; G-3-P = glucose-3-phosphate; G-6-P = glucose-6-phosphate; GSH = glutathione (reduced); GSSG = glutathione (oxidized); NAD = nicotinamide-adenine dinucleotide; NADH = reduced NAD; NADP = nicotinamide adenine nucleotide (oxidized); NADPH = nicotinamide adenine nucleotide (reduced); PEP = phosphoenolpyruvate; PG = phosphoglycerate; P_i = inorganic phosphate; R-5-P = ribose-5-phosphatase.

consumed. ATP is the high-energy phosphate required for phosphorylation reactions in cellular functions such as deformability, membrane permeability, membrane lipid turnover, and protein phosphorylation. The inability to maintain ATP results in shortened red cell survival. In the HMS, where the remaining 10% of the red cell glucose is metabolized, substrates required to protect against red cell oxidation are generated. Defects in this pathway render the cell susceptible to oxidative injury. As a consequence, oxidized Hb (Heinz bodies), lipids, and membrane proteins accumulate in the red cell, resulting in hemolysis.

Genotypic and phenotypic variations have been reported for almost every red cell enzyme. The clinical manifestations associated with these disorders are determined by the net effect of the enzyme abnormality on ATP production, 2,3-DPG content, or red cell antioxidant capacity. Several of the enzyme deficiencies affect tissues in addition to the erythrocyte and have associated symptoms (Table 14–5).

In cases in which the enzyme abnormality is distal to the synthesis of 2,3-DPG, 2,3-DPG accumulates in the red cell, and its interaction with Hb facilitates oxygen delivery. This explains why patients with pyruvate kinase deficiency, who have elevated red cell 2,3-DPG, can tolerate anemia much better than patients with hexokinase deficiency, who, although they exhibit a similar inability to maintain normal levels of red cell ATP, have lower levels of 2,3-DPG.

Red cell morphologic changes are minimal in patients with red cell enzyme deficiency involving the EMP. Red cell indices are usually normochromic and normocytic. The reticulocyte count is elevated in proportion to the extent of hemolysis. The diagnosis may require measurement of multiple red cell enzyme activities, as well as determination of the concentration of glycolytic intermediates. The latter is important, as certain enzyme deficiencies are more likely to be detected by the accumulation of a particular intermediate than by a dramatic change in enzyme activity. Because many enzyme activities are normally increased in young red cells, a mild deficiency in one of these may be obscured by the reticulocytosis. Under these circumstances, techniques to eliminate the effects of red cell age must be used, and a relative deficiency in the enzyme of interest signifies that this enzyme is responsible. Family studies can facilitate diagnosis. As many of the enzyme deficiencies have been characterized at the molecular level, molecular techniques can be used to establish a diagnosis and provide the option of intrauterine diagnosis. Except in the case of pyruvate kinase or G6PD deficiency, the two most common enzyme deficiencies responsible for hemolytic anemia, reference laboratories should be used to measure the panel of red cell enzymes and glycolytic intermediates.

Pyruvate Kinase Deficiency. This is the most common enzyme deficiency in the EMP. The inheritance pattern of this disorder is autosomal recessive. Homozygotes

Table 14–5. Enzyme deficiencies of the Embden-Meyerhof pathway.[1]

Enzyme		Tissues Involved	Clinical Features	Red Cell Metabolites		Other Remarks
				ATP	2,3-DPG	
Hexokinase	AR	RBC	CNSHA	↓	↓	Increased hemoglobin O_2 affinity, decreased exercise tolerance for degree of anemia
Glucose phosphate isomerase	AR	RBC, WBC, skin fibroblasts	CNSHA	↓, N	N	Spiculated microspherocytes sometimes observed
Phosphofructokinase	AR	RBC, muscle	CNSHA, myopathy (muscle glycogen storage disease)	↓	↓	
Aldolase	AR	RBC	CNSHA	N	↑	Fructose-1,6-diphosphate accumulates in RBC
Triosephosphate isomerase	AR	RBC, WBC, muscle, serum, CSF	CNSHA, severe progressive neurologic disorder	↓	—	Dihydroxyacetone phosphate accumulates in RBC, increased susceptibility to infection
Phosphoglycerate kinase	Sex-linked	RBC, WBC	CNSHA, mental retardation, myopathy	N	N,↑	
2,3-DPG mutase	AR, AD	RBC	?CNSHA or polycythemia	N,↑	↓	Increased hemoglobin O_2 affinity
Pyruvate kinase	AR	RBC, liver	CNSHA	N,↓	↑	Decreased hemoglobin O_2 affinity, increased exercise tolerance for degree of anemia

[1]Reproduced, with permission, from Mentzer WC: Abnormalities of erythrocyte metabolism. In: Rudolph AM (editor): *Rudolph's Pediatrics,* 19th ed. Appleton & Lange, 1991.
AR = autosomal recessive; AD = autosomal dominant; ATP = adenosine triphosphate; CNSHA = congenital nonspherocytic hemolytic anemia; CSF = cerebrospinal fluid; 2,3-DPG = 2,3-diphosphoglycerate; N = normal; RBC = red blood cell; WBC = white blood cell.

usually have hemolytic anemia with splenomegaly, whereas heterozygotes are usually asymptomatic. The disorder is found worldwide, although it is most common in whites of northern European descent. The range of clinical expression is variable, from severe neonatal jaundice to a fully compensated hemolytic anemia. Anemia is usually normochromic and normocytic, but macrocytes may be present shortly after a hemolytic crisis, reflecting erythroid hyperplasia and early release of red cells from the marrow. In severe cases, the morphologic examination of the peripheral smear shows polychromasia, anisocytosis, poikilocytosis, and nucleated red cells. The osmotic fragility of red cells is normal or slightly reduced. Diagnosis is confirmed by a quantitative assay for pyruvate kinase, by the measurement of enzyme kinetics and glycolytic intermediates, and by family studies. It may be necessary to measure enzyme kinetics using several substrates, because in some PK-deficient patients with unusual forms of the disease, the enzyme defect cannot be identified using one substrate.

Splenectomy is a therapeutic option for PK-deficient patients. As with HS, the decision should be made on the basis of the patient's clinical course. Unlike HS patients, PK-deficient patients, although they improve after splenectomy, do not have complete correction of their hemolytic anemia. Because reticulocytes contain mitochondria, they are capable of oxidative metabolism and have a selective survival in patients with PK deficiency. The spleen, with its hypoxic and acidotic environment, results in destruction of reticulocytes as well as mature red cells in PK deficiency. When the spleen is removed, the Hb count increases slightly, but the reticulocyte count increases dramatically. Thus, it is not uncommon to have a reticulocyte count greater than 50% in a PK-deficient patient after splenectomy. In contrast to HS, Kupffer cells in the liver are also capable of destroying PK-deficient cells, partially explaining why splenectomy is not as effective in PK deficiency as in HS. As with all hemolytic anemias, these patients should have dietary supplementation with folic acid (5 mg/d) to prevent megaloblastic complications associated with relative folate deficiency and immunization against *S pneumoniae* and *H influenzae,* as well as consideration for lifelong prophylactic penicillin for the splenectomized patient.

Glucose-6-Phosphate Dehydrogenase Deficiency.
G6PD, the most common red cell enzyme deficiency, is sex-linked, with partial expression in the female population and full expression in the affected male population. The distribution of G6PD deficiency is worldwide, with the highest incidence in Africans and African-Americans. Mediterraneans, American Indians, Southeast Asians, and Sephardic Jews are also affected. In African-Americans, 12% of the male population have the deficiency, 18% of the female population are heterozygous, and 2% of female population are homozygous. In Southeast Asians, G6PD deficiency is found in approximately 6% of the male population. One hypothesis for the prevalence of this enzyme abnormality is that it confers resistance to malaria. Once

the malaria parasite invades a red cell, it generates oxidants during metabolism. The inability of G6PD-deficient cells to detoxify these oxidants may result in red cell death and, along with it, death of the parasite.

Many variants of G6PD deficiency are known and have been characterized at the biochemical and molecular levels. Depending on the molecular defect and the ability of the mutant enzyme to stabilize cellular enzymes required for antioxidant defense, some of the enzyme deficiencies result in extreme depletion of enzyme and auto-oxidant reserve (reduced glutathione, in particular) and are associated with chronic hemolytic anemia. These are often found in Mediterraneans. Other variants are associated with an unstable enzyme that has normal levels in young red cells. These result in hemolysis only in association with an oxidant challenge; this is the type found in African-Americans. In some cases of G6PD deficiency, the defect can be identified in both granulocytes and erythrocytes. In addition to having chronic hemolytic anemia, such patients may be susceptible to bacterial infections.

In the African-American type of G6PD deficiency, hemolysis may be triggered by the oxidant intermediates generated during viral or bacterial infections or after ingestion of oxidant compounds (Table 14–6). Shortly after exposure to the oxidant, Hb is oxidized to methemoglobin and eventually denatured, forming intracellular inclusions called Heinz bodies. **Heinz bodies** attach to the red cell membrane and aggregate certain intrinsic membrane proteins, in particular band 3. The reticuloendothelial cells recognize this perturbation in the membrane as a new antigenic site and ingest this portion of the cell. The resulting cell, often called a "bite" cell as a consequence of this unusual phagocytic process, has a shortened survival owing to its loss of membrane components. To compensate for hemolysis, red cell production is increased and the reticulocyte count is elevated.

In normal red cells, G6PD is an age-dependent enzyme. Because the molecular basis of G6PD deficiency in African-Americans is due to enzyme instability and not enzyme deficiency, as is the case of Mediterranean variants of the enzyme, levels of G6PD are normal in the reticulocyte but decreased in older red cells. Therefore, after an oxidant exposure, only the older cell is destroyed and hemolysis is limited. This can cause a diagnostic problem, as cells not destroyed by the oxidant are reticulocytes in G6PD-deficient African-Americans and have normal or elevated enzyme levels. However, methods are available to sort out the older red cells so that they can be analyzed for enzyme activity. Once the patient has been removed from the oxidant challenge, the hemolytic anemia will resolve, at which time the enzyme assay can readily be performed.

Individuals with the Mediterranean or Asian forms of G6PD deficiency, in addition to being sensitive to infections and certain drugs, often have a chronic, moderately severe anemia, with nonspherocytic red cells and jaundice. Hemolysis usually starts in early childhood. Reticulocytosis is present and can increase the MCV. This se-

Table 14–6. Some agents reported to produce hemolysis in patients with glucose-6-phosphate dehydrogenase (G6PD) deficiency.[1]

Drugs and chemicals clearly shown to cause clinically significant hemolytic anemia in G6PD deficiency:	
Acetanilid	Pentaquine
Methylene blue	Sulfanilamide
Nalidixic acid (NegGram)	Sulfacetamide
Naphthalene	Sulfapyridine
Niridazole (Ambilhar)	Sulfamethoxazole
Nitrofurantoin (Furadantin)	(Gantanol)
Phenylhydrazine	Thiazolesulfone
Primaquine	Toluidine blue
Pamaquine	Trinitrotoluene

Drugs probably safe in normal therapeutic doses for G6PD-deficient individuals (without nonspherocytic hemolytic anemia):	
Acetaminophen (Paracetamol Tylenol, Tralgon Hydroxyacetanilid)	Menaphtone
	para-Aminobenzoic acid
Acetophenetidine (Phenacetin)	Phenylbutazone
	Phenytoin
Acetylsalicylic acid (aspirin)	Probenecid (Benemid)
	Procaine amide hydrochloride (Pronestyl)
Aminopyrine (Pyramidone, Amidopyrine)	Pyrimethamine (Daraprim)
Antazoline (Antistine)	Quinidine
Antipyrine	Quinine
Ascorbic acid (vitamin C)	Streptomycin
Benzhexol (Artane)	Sulfacytine
Chloramphenicol	Sulfadiazine
Chlorguanidine (Proguanil, Paludrine)	Sulfaguanidine
	Sulfamerazine
Chloroquine	Sulfamethoxypyriazine (Kynex)
Colchicine	Sulfisoxazole (Gantrisin)
Diphenhydramine (Benadryl)	Trimethoprim
L-Dopa	Tripelennamine (Pyribenzamine)
Menadione sodium bisulfite (Hykinone)	Vitamin K

[1]From Beutler: *Hemolytic Anemia in Disorders of Red Cell Metabolism.* Plenum, 1978. Cited by Mentzer WC: Abnormalities of erythrocyte metabolism. Page 1138 in: Rudolph AM (editor): *Rudolph's Pediatrics,* 19th ed. Appleton & Lange, 1991.

vere variant is most common in the Greek population. Molecular studies of these variants may show complete absence of the enzyme in all red cells.

In Asian newborns with G6PD deficiency, stress related to delivery, infection, or antibiotics can precipitate hemolysis. Indeed, G6PD deficiency can be a cause of hemolytic jaundice and kernicterus in the newborn period, and many hospitals where susceptible populations are born (eg, in Hawaii) have instituted newborn screening programs for this enzyme deficiency. Jaundice is particularly common in premature infants who are G6PD deficient.

Favism, a severe form of G6PD deficiency, occurs after ingestion or inhalation of materials released from the fava bean. It has been reported in Asians and Mediterraneans but not in African-Americans. After exposure to the bean, acute, life-threatening hemolysis can appear within 24 hours. The pathophysiology of favism appears to involve both G6PD deficiency and an undefined susceptibility of the red cell membrane to damage secondary to a toxin released by the fava bean. Although hemolysis may be sufficient to cause severe anemia, requiring transfusion to prevent cardiorespiratory distress, most cases resolve spontaneously and will not recur if the patient is not exposed to the fava bean.

When a hemolytic crisis occurs in G6PD deficiency or favism, pallor, scleral icterus, hemoglobinemia, hemoglobinuria, and splenomegaly may be noted. Plasma haptoglobin and hemopexin concentrations are low. The peripheral smear shows the fragmented bite cells and polychromatophilic cells. Red cell indices may be normal. Special stains can detect Heinz bodies in the cells during the first few days of hemolysis.

A diagnosis of G6PD deficiency should be based on family history, ethnicity, laboratory features, physical findings, recent exposure to oxidants, and an acute hemolytic event. It can be confirmed by a quantitative enzyme assay or by molecular analysis of the gene. Treatment is directed toward supportive care for the acute event and counseling regarding prevention of future hemolytic crises. In patients with chronic hemolysis, dietary supplements with folic acid, 1–5 mg/d, are recommended. Use of vitamin E, 500 mg/d, may improve red cell survival in patients with chronic hemolysis.

Hemoglobinopathies

Disorders in Hb structure and synthesis, collectively called the hemoglobinopathies, are due to molecular defects that result in changes in the structure or synthesis of a particular globin chain. The clinical manifestations of the structurally abnormal Hb depend on the charge and location of the amino acid substitution. Alterations in oxygen transport or Hb stability or physical changes in the Hb molecule can occur. Hemoglobinopathies due to defective synthesis of either α or β globin chains are called **thalassemia.** Partial or complete absence of globin synthesis results in an imbalance of globin chain synthesis. The excess globin chains, either α or β, that accumulate within the developing red cell interact with the red cell membrane, alter cellular properties, and ultimately shorten red cell survival. Depending on the degree of imbalance, red cell destruction can occur within the bone marrow.

The structure of the predominant Hbs is shown in Table 14–7. Adult Hb (HbA) is composed of two α-globin chains and two β-globin chains. Fetal Hb (HbF), the predominant Hb in the newborn, contains two α-globin chains and two γ-globin chains. HbA$_2$, which represents no more than 3.6% of the total Hb in adults, consists of two α-globin chains and two δ-globin chains. HbH (β^4) and Bart Hb (γ^4) are found in α-thalassemia.

The chromosomal location and organization of the genes responsible for globin-chain synthesis are shown in Figure 14–5. The two genes responsible for β-globin production are located on chromosome 11, whereas the genes responsible for α-globin production are located on chro-

Table 14–7. Hemoglobin composition.

Hemoglobin	Structure	Percentage of Total Hemoglobin	Increased	Decreased
A	$\alpha_2\beta_2$	Adult 98 Newborn 10–40		
A$_2$	$\alpha_2\delta_2$	Adult 1.6–3.5 Newborn < 1	β-Thalassemia	α-Thalassemia Iron deficiency
F	$\alpha_2\gamma_2$	Adult < 1 Newborn 60–90	β-Thalassemia Hereditary persistence of fetal hemoglobin Stress erythropoiesis	
H	β^4	20	Hemoglobin H disease Hydrops fetalis due to homozygous thalassemia	
Bart	γ^4	10 5–30	Hydrops fetalis α-Thalassemia syndromes	

mosome 16. Because there are four genes for α-glo-bin–chain production, the clinical manifestations and laboratory diagnosis of disorders involving the α-globin genes are quite variable. If one gene is structurally abnormal, approximately 25% of the Hb will be altered. Because there are only two β-globin genes, a defect in one will affect approximately 50% of the Hb.

The molecular mechanisms responsible for the switch from HbF to HbA begin during the second to third trimester of pregnancy; at birth, the predominant Hb is HbF. Rare, structural defects in γ-globin have been reported, although most of these are benign. However, they can result in hemolysis if the γ-chain variant is unstable. Therefore, an Hb disorder should be considered in the workup of a newborn with a hemolytic anemia. When the switch from fetal to adult Hb is complete, the clinical manifestations associated with these γ-chain variants disappear.

Defects in α-globin are much more common than defects in γ-globin in the newborn. These can result in a structurally abnormal Hb or in an α-thalassemia–like pattern. The structural defects are usually benign, as they are caused by mutations affecting only one of the four α-globin genes. In contrast, the consequences of synthetic defects in α-globin chains (α-thalassemia) can be quite significant.

Sickle Cell Disease. Structural defects involving the β-globin genes are the most frequent types of hemoglo-binopathies affecting children in the United States. Sickle cell disease is the most common of these. Sickle cell anemia (homozygous inheritance of the sickle gene), sickle cell–HbC disease (doubly heterozygous for sickle cell Hb [HbS] and HbC), and sickle cell–β-thalassemia (either β+ or β⁰) are classified as the sickle cell diseases. In the United States, the sickle cell diseases primarily affect African-Americans. However, as distribution of the sickle gene is worldwide because of the selective advantage that individuals with sickle cell trait have when infected by malaria, sickle cell disease quite possibly will be detected in a number of white or Hispanic newborns as experience is gained with newborn screening.

The sickle cell diseases are inherited in an autosomal, codominant manner. The molecular defect in HbS is due to the substitution of valine for glutamic acid in the sixth position of the β-globin chain. The charge and location of this substitution cause HbS to be converted from a soluble state into a polymer when it undergoes the structural changes that accompany release of oxygen. Hypoxia, acidosis, and hypertonicity facilitate polymer formation. The polymerization of Hb causes the red cell to transform from a deformable, biconcave disk into a rigid, sickle-shaped cell. The process of sickling and loss of cell deformability is reversible to a point, at which time the cell is permanently damaged. At this point, it is called an **irreversibly sickled cell (ISC).** Even under completely oxygenated conditions, ISCs remain sickled. The sickled red

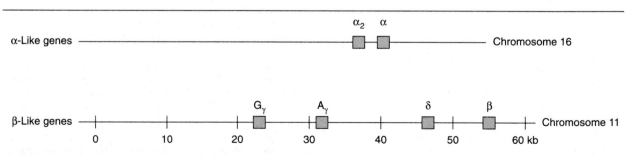

Figure 14–5. Chromosomal organizations of the globin genes. The β-like gene clusters are located on chromosome 11, and the α-like gene clusters on chromosome 16.

cells seen on examination of the peripheral blood smear are examples of ISCs.

Clinical Manifestations. The clinical manifestations of sickle cell disease are due to anemia and vascular occlusion. Sickled cells are rigid and fragile, and these properties contribute to the moderate to severe hemolytic anemia characteristic of this disease. The life span of the erythrocyte may be as short as 20 days. For unexplained reasons, these cells are very sticky. This abnormal adhesive property causes them to stick to endothelial surfaces, as well as to other cells, and contributes to the vascular occlusive events, pain, and organ damage characteristic of this disease. Vascular obstruction within the spleen results in loss of splenic function and increases the susceptibility of patients to bacterial sepsis. Vascular obstruction in cerebral vessels can lead to stroke, and all organs can be damaged by vascular obstruction.

In African-Americans, the frequency of the sickle cell gene is 8%; the HbC gene, 4%; and β-thalassemia gene, approximately 1%. Approximately 1:600 African-American infants has sickle cell anemia.

The clinical severity of sickle cell diseases is quite variable. Although several factors have been recognized that contribute to variations in clinical severity (Table 14–8), many additional factors likely remain to be identified. The most important of these is the type of the sickle cell disease. The frequency and severity of both anemic and vaso-occlusive complications is highest in patients with homozygous sickle cell anemia (HbSS), whereas patients with sickle cell–β+ and sickle cell–HbC disease have the least severe forms of disease. These variations have been explained on the basis of the ease with which Hb polymerization and sickling occur in these disorders.

In sickle cell anemia, the level of HbF within each red cell affects the polymerization of HbS: Pain crises as well as life span have an inverse correlation with the level of HbF. A genetic polymorphism, determined by analysis of the DNA in proximity to the sickle globin gene, has identified four categories of patients, whose genetic origins are Bantu, Benin, Indian, and Senegalese. HbF levels are highest in the India and Senegal haplotypes.

The polymerization of HbS is logarithmically proportional to the MCHC. Thus, if the MCHC is reduced, the chance that polymers will form as the red cell releases oxygen in the capillary bed is reduced. When α-thal-

assemia is coinherited with sickle cell trait or disease, the MCHC and MCV of the red cell are decreased. The frequency of α-thalassemia trait is 1–3% in African-Americans. Patients who have both α-thalassemia and sickle cell anemia are less anemic than those who have sickle cell anemia alone. However, α-thalassemia trait does not appear to prevent the frequency or severity of vaso-occlusive complications or organ damage.

The coinheritance of both HbC and HbS results in a mild form of sickle cell disease. Nevertheless, patients with sickle cell–HbC disease can have all of the complications found in patients with sickle cell anemia. This includes vascular as well as infectious complications.

When the sickle cell gene is coinherited with a β-thalassemia–trait gene, the patient has sickle cell–β-thalassemia. Clinical severity depends on the type of β-thalassemic gene, either β0-thalassemia, in which no HbA is synthesized, or β+-thalassemia, in which a variable amount of HbA is made. In sickle cell–β+-thalassemia, due to the thalassemic gene, the Hb electrophoresis shows more HbS than HbA. This contrasts with sickle cell trait, in which the amount of HbA is greater than that of HbS. This distinction is extremely important as individuals with sickle cell trait do not have a disease, whereas those with sickle cell–β+-thalassemia have sickle cell disease. Patients with sickle cell–β0-thalassemia have only HbS on electrophoresis and can have symptoms identical to those in patients with sickle cell anemia. Analysis of Hb in the parents of these patients should show sickle cell trait in one parent and normal Hb in the other. Rather than consider nonpaternity, it is important to exclude β-thalassemia trait in the parent who has only HbA. This can be done by determining the MCV and by measuring the level of HbA$_2$.

As a result of early diagnosis, comprehensive medical care, and education of families and health care providers, the mortality in the first decade of life from sickle cell disease has decreased dramatically over the past several years, from approximately 25% to less than 3%. Most states have instituted newborn screening for hemoglobinopathies. Because HbF is the predominant Hb in newborns, the electrophoretic pattern in a newborn with sickle cell disease is FS. A similar FS pattern is seen in newborns with sickle cell–β0-thalassemia, sickle cell–hereditary persistence of fetal Hb (HPFH), or sickle cell–HbD or HbG. Family studies or repeated testing at 4–6 months of age may be necessary to confirm the diagnosis. Molecular biology techniques can also be used to distinguish these disorders at birth.

Hematologic values for each of the sickle cell diseases are shown in Table 14–9. In sickle cell anemia, the hematocrits can vary from 18% to 28%. The reticulocyte count is elevated (12–25%), reflecting the rate of hemolysis. The MCV is elevated as the result of the young red cell population. If the MCV is low, coinheritance of α- or β-thalassemia trait or iron deficiency should be suspected. The coinheritance of α-thalassemia trait with sickle cell disease increases the hematocrit, lowers the reticulocyte

Table 14–8. Factors that affect clinical severity of sickle cell disease.

Type of sickle cell disease:
SS > S β0-thalassemia > SC > S β+-thalassemia
Fetal hemoglobin concentration
β-Globin gene cluster haplotype
α-Thalassemia
Nonerythroid factors
Adhesive molecules and their interaction with plasma proteins
Regulators of microcapillary tone
Psychosocial

Table 14–9. Hematologic values in sickle cell disease.[1]

Syndrome	Hematocrit (%)	Reticulocyte (%)	MCV (mm³)	Electrophoresis
SS	18–28	12–25	86	80–100% S 0–20% F
SC	30–36	5–10	77	50% S 50% C
S β⁰-thalassemia	20–30	10–15	66	75–100% S 0–20% F 3–6% A₂
S β⁺-thalassemia	30–36	3–6	70	50–80% S 0–20% F 10–30% A 3–6% A₂
SS α-thalassemia	25–30	5–10	70	80–100% S 0–20% F

[1]Reproduced, with permission, from Platt OS, Nathan DG: Disorders of hemoglobin: Sickle cell disease. In: Nathan DG, Oski FA (editors): *Hematology of Infancy and Childhood,* 3rd ed. Saunders, 1987.
MCV = mean corpuscular volume.

count, and lowers the MCV. The amount of HbS, A, or C is shown for each of the sickle cell diseases. Note the similar levels of HbS in sickle cell anemia and sickle cell–β⁰-thalassemia.

The white cell count is elevated (12,000–18,000/µL), but the differential count remains normal. Platelet counts are also elevated. Leukocytosis and thrombocytosis represent the products of a hyperplastic marrow in an asplenic person who has a persistent chronic hemolytic process. HbF levels vary among the different disorders and between patients.

The clinical manifestations of sickle cell disease are related to the degree of hemolytic anemia and to the frequency and location of vaso-occlusive events. Almost every organ of the body can be affected. Susceptibility to infection is increased primarily because of splenic infarction, but also because of other acquired immunologic abnormalities. This can result in life-threatening episodes of sepsis. Recognition of this susceptibility and aggressive medical management have resulted in an increased life span for most patients.

Complications in sickle cell disease are characterized by sudden, unexpected onset, including vascular occlusion (pain), splenic sequestration, hyperhemolysis, and infections. Associated chronic medical complications due to organ damage increase with age. The kidney is frequently affected, and many adult patients require dialysis or renal transplantation. Cerebrovascular occlusion is a devastating complication and can present as clinically manifest strokes or silent cerebral infarctions in children and as cerebral hemorrhage in adults. Acute medical complications in young children can occur because of splenic sequestration. A major cause of morbidity and mortality in sickle cell disease is the acute chest syndrome, a complication in which pulmonary function is rapidly compromised owing to vascular obstruction, changes in ventilation-perfusion ratios, atelectasis, infection, and pulmonary fat embolism secondary to sickling-related bone marrow infections.

Management. Although details of appropriate treatment for complications of sickle cell disease are beyond the scope of this chapter, general guidelines are described briefly. A recent National Institutes of Health monograph, available from the Sickle Cell Disease Branch of the National Heart, Lung & Blood Institute, records an excellent description of treatment in sickle cell disease. First, it is important to deliver comprehensive care. Prophylactic penicillin, immunizations, attention to growth and development, and concern regarding psychosocial issues are necessary. One must always consider the patient with sickle cell disease as a compromised host, and, if the patient is febrile, the disease should be aggressively diagnosed and treated with antibiotics. The possibility of penicillin-resistant *S pneumoniae* should be considered. Underlying causes must be sought for vaso-occlusive complications. Prompt attention should be given to changes in hematologic status, such as a decrease in Hb (aplastic crisis), as seen with parvovirus infections. In addition, parents and family members should be taught to palpate the spleen and recognize early signs of splenic sequestration. Any pulmonary complication requires careful monitoring and aggressive intervention if progressive pulmonary dysfunction is detected.

Adequate hydration is an important component of therapy for many complications of sickle cell disease. Dehydration occurs frequently in these patients because of inadequate fluid intake and sickle cell hyposthenia. Because renal function is altered, urine specific gravity measurements cannot be used to assess hydration. Comparison of the patient's weight with baseline values is the best method to assess fluid requirements. Except for pulmonary complications, in which excess hydration should be avoided as it can lead to pulmonary edema, 1.5 times maintenance fluid therapy is generally used. Red cell transfusions should be given for conditions recognized to benefit from this treatment. Abuse of transfusion therapy can lead to iron overload and alloimmunization. Pain management should be aggressive; combinations of narcotic with non-narcotic drugs may be beneficial. Concerns regarding potential for drug addiction can result in inadequate therapy for painful complications and lead to secondary "chronic pain" behavior patterns while having no impact on the incidence of drug addiction. Current trials with agents to stimulate Hb production, such as hydroxyurea, are encouraging. This drug should be used only in a setting that provides appropriate monitoring for drug toxicity. Bone marrow transplantation may have a role for selected patients when appropriate donors can be identified. The future holds the promise of gene therapy as methods have become available to target genes to erythroid progenitors.

Sickle Cell Trait. Individuals who have sickle cell trait do not have a disease. They are not anemic, their red cell indices and reticulocyte counts are normal, and they do not have painful vaso-occlusive complications. However, hyposthenuria and hematuria may occur in individuals with sickle cell trait because of the harsh metabolic conditions within the kidney, which induce polymer formation even in conditions in which the intracellular concentration of HbS is less than 50%. Other rare complications have been reported in individuals with sickle cell trait, primarily as a consequence of these persons exposing themselves to conditions in which oxygen tension is low, eg, at high altitudes (skiing, mountain climbing) or high pressures (diving), and during extreme exertion associated with dehydration during basic training in the military.

Homozygous HbC Disease. HbC is due to a different mutation at the same site as seen in HbS, with lysine, rather than valine, substituted for glutamic acid. The inheritance of two genes for HbC is associated with a mild hemolytic anemia and splenomegaly. Oxyhemoglobin C can crystallize within red cells when they are dehydrated. Typical red cell morphology includes a few fragmented red cells, a few microspherocytes, and target cells. Patients with homozygous HbC disease usually do not require therapy for their hemolytic anemia, nor do they have evidence of vascular obstruction as do patients with sickle cell disease. Individuals with HbC trait have normal hematologic laboratory parameters except for high numbers of target cells, which can be seen in the peripheral blood smear.

HbE Disease. HbE, the second most common Hb variant worldwide, is the result of an amino acid substitution of glutamic acid for lysine at the 26th position of the β-globin chain. Besides the charge difference in HbE, the synthesis of HbE is decreased compared with HbA. This results in a β-thalassemia minor-like phenotype with mild anemia and microcytosis in individuals with HbE trait. Because of its charge, the electrophoretic pattern of HbE is similar to that of HbC. HbC is rarely seen in Asians; therefore, a laboratory report of HbC in a person of Asian background should be repeated, and a specific request made to identify HbE. In homozygous HbE, patients have mild hemolytic anemia (Hb concentrations, 11–14 g/dL) with moderate to severe microcytosis (MCV, 50–65 fL).

The reticulocyte count is not particularly abnormal (approximately 2%), and target cells, microcytes, and hypochromic cells are seen on the peripheral blood smear. The RDW is normal.

In contrast to these mild disorders, the coinheritance of HbE (which has a mild defect in β-globin synthesis) with β-thalassemia trait (a more severe defect in β-globin synthesis) results in significant hematologic problems. These HbE–β-thalassemia patients are phenotypically similar to those with β-thalassemia intermedia and have ineffective erythropoiesis and anemia. They often become transfusion dependent and require chelation therapy. The degree of anemia depends on the type of β-thalassemia globin gene (β^0 or β^+). The distinction between homozygous HbE and HbE–β^0-thalassemia is important, as the former requires no specific medical attention, whereas the latter is a disease associated with complications. This distinction can be made on the basis of hematologic changes in patients by 1 year of age. Moderate to severe anemia (Hb levels > 3 g/dL below normal) is noted in HbE–β-thalassemia, and mild anemia is noted in homozygous HbE. Family studies, as well as molecular techniques, can help to establish a diagnosis. Molecular techniques are of particular value if both parents are not available for study. Furthermore, molecular techniques can be used to distinguish readily homozygous HbE from HbE–β-thalassemia in the newborn and to facilitate subsequent counseling and medical care.

Other Structural Hb Variants. In addition to the common Hb variants described above, several rare, structural heterozygote Hb defects are associated with clinical findings. In one group, the oxygen affinity (P_{50}) of whole blood is increased. The electrophoretic mobility of the Hb may be affected on the basis of the charge conferred by the amino acid substitution. In cases in which the oxygen affinity is increased, the Hb concentration is above normal because of erythrocytosis. The differential diagnosis of erythrocytosis should include hypoxia (pulmonary or cardiac related) or hereditary erythrocytosis. Patients with low oxygen-affinity Hb variants have Hb levels below normal. However, they are not anemic from a physiologic standpoint because the Hb can deliver more oxygen to the tissue at a given partial pressure of oxygen (Po_2) than normal Hb. Measurements of arterial blood gas, serum erythropoietin levels, and Hb oxygen affinity are required to establish a diagnosis in patients with high or low oxygen-affinity variants. Familial erythrocytosis due to an abnormality in the erythropoietin receptor on erythroid progenitors has been reported.

Another structural group of Hb variants that can give rise to hemolysis is the unstable Hb variants. In these disorders, the amino acid substitution in the globin chain weakens the Hb tetramer and causes it to dissociate and oxidize, resulting in intracellular methemoglobin and Heinz bodies. This process is accelerated by exposure of the red cell to oxidant stress. Unstable Hb variants can be detected by their charge, instability in the presence of isopropanol, and the presence of intracellular Heinz bodies after oxidant stress. The interaction between Heinz bodies and the cell membrane is believed to result in perturbations in membrane structure and function and to lead to both intravascular and extravascular cell destruction.

Patients with unstable Hb variants display a wide range of clinical severity, ranging from no symptoms to severe hemolytic anemia. This is determined by the site of the mutation, its charge, and its location on an α- or β-globin gene. The inheritance pattern is autosomal-dominant, and symptoms occur in the heterozygote state. β-Globin variants are associated with more symptoms than are α-globin variants, as a greater proportion of Hb is affected when one of the two β-globin genes, rather than one of the four α-globin genes, is involved. When the disease is severe, it usually presents with hemolytic anemia in childhood. Severe intravascular hemolysis, jaundice, extensive reticulocytosis, and hemoglobinuria can occur. In some patients, the oxygen affinity of the Hb is also affected.

Normal Hb transports oxygen without becoming oxidized by maintaining its iron in the reduced state. However, 3% of Hb is oxidized to methemoglobin each day. Methemoglobin reductase, an intracellular enzyme, reduces this methemoglobin to oxyhemoglobin. Methemoglobin can be formed when there is a deficiency in methemoglobin reductase or when the red cell's antioxidant capacity is overwhelmed, as noted in G6PD deficiency, favism, and unstable Hb disorders. Hb can also undergo oxidation to methemoglobin if there is an amino acid substitution in α- or β-globin chains in the vicinity of the heme pocket.

Methemoglobinemia. Methemoglobinemia can be hereditary or acquired. The hereditary disorders are associated with a deficiency of the cytoplasmic enzyme, NADPH-methemoglobin reductase, or a structural defect in Hb that facilitates oxidation of the iron molecule. These Hb variants are called HbM, and several types have been identified. Methemoglobin reductase deficiency is rare and is inherited in an autosomal-recessive mode. There are few associated physical findings, other than cyanosis and erythrocytosis. Methemoglobin levels are usually 15–30%; methemoglobin cannot transport oxygen, and when the level exceeds 15%, erythrocytosis and cyanosis result. In HbM disorders, mild hemolysis may be present because of the unstable nature of the Hb. Specific electrophoretic techniques can be used to identify HbM, and structural characterization will establish a diagnosis.

In acquired cases of methemoglobinemia, exposure to certain chemicals, such as nitrates (found in well water, certain foods, hemodialysis), aniline dyes, and sulfonamides, causes the rate of Hb oxidation to exceed the reductive capability of methemoglobin reductase. The clinical features are usually mild and include cyanosis, fatigue, and tachycardia. Newborns in whom methemoglobinemia develops often are considered to have pulmonary or cardiac disease and are extensively examined for these conditions. A diagnosis can be made by quantitation of methemoglobin using spectrophotometric methods. Treatment involves identification and avoidance of the toxic agent.

Reducing compounds, such as ascorbic acid or methylene blue, can be used if clinically indicated.

Disorders of Hemoglobin Synthesis

The thalassemias are a heterogeneous group of inherited disorders characterized by a defect in synthesis of normal globin chains that leads to an intracellular imbalance in the α:β chain ratio. The excess globin chains bind to the cell membrane and cause significant damage, resulting in ineffective erythropoiesis and shortened red cell survival. The geographic distribution of the thalassemia gene includes areas near the Mediterranean, Southeast Asia, the Middle East, and the Orient. This distribution suggests a selective advantage and resistance to malaria has been the underlying factor.

α-Thalassemia. In α-thalassemia, there may be a deletion or defect in the regulation of 1–4 α-globin genes. The spectrum of clinical manifestations depends on the nature and number of affected genes. The genetic basis for the spectrum of α-thalassemias is shown in Figure 14–6.

The most severe form of α-thalassemia, in which there is complete suppression of α-globin synthesis, causes hydrops fetalis. Although intrauterine transfusion has been successful in a few cases, and could provide benefit if the fetus survives and is placed on chronic transfusion or has bone marrow transplantation, this condition is usually incompatible with extrauterine life and results in a stillbirth.

The clinical picture is that of a pale, premature, edematous (hydropic) baby with massive splenomegaly and severe anemia. Hb electrophoresis reveals no HbF, no HbA, and approximately 90–100% Hbγ^4, which is called Hb Bart. Hbγ^4 has a high oxygen affinity and lacks the Bohr effect; although it readily picks up oxygen, it cannot release it to the tissues under physiologic conditions.

The Asian parents of infants born with homozygous α-thalassemia have the type of α-thalassemia trait with two α-globin gene deletions on the same chromosome. Because Hb electrophoresis is normal in α-thalassemia trait, the microcytic anemia associated with α-thalassemia trait can be confirmed only by gene mapping techniques. Because of the high frequency of α-thalassemia among Southeast Asians, prenatal programs have been encouraged to screen pregnant women for α-thalassemia trait. If the trait is detected, the male partner should be tested, and, if the test result is positive, the option for intrauterine diagnosis should be reviewed with the family. In contrast to Asians, African-Americans who have α-thalassemia trait (6%) have the two gene deletions on separate chromosomes. This might explain why homozygous α-thalassemia does not occur in African-Americans.

HbH Disease. This disease is due to deletion of three α-globin genes. Family studies reveal that one parent has α-thalassemia trait, whereas the other has completely normal hematologic findings (silent carrier). Using molecular techniques, a variety of defects in the α-globin genes can be detected. The most common is a two-gene deletion in one parent and a one-gene deletion in the other. Occasionally, an Hb called **constant spring** can be detected in as-

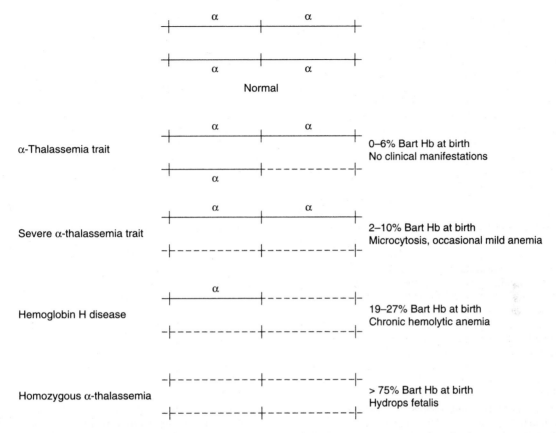

α

α

α

α

Normal

α-Thalassemia trait

α

α

α

0–6% Bart Hb at birth
No clinical manifestations

Severe α-thalassemia trait

α

α

2–10% Bart Hb at birth
Microcytosis, occasional mild anemia

Hemoglobin H disease

α

19–27% Bart Hb at birth
Chronic hemolytic anemia

Homozygous α-thalassemia

> 75% Bart Hb at birth
Hydrops fetalis

Figure 14–6. Genetic origins of the "classic" α-thalassemia syndromes due to gene deletion, with associated Bart hemoglobin (Hb) expression and clinical manifestations. (Reproduced and modified, with permission, from Schwartz E, Benze EJ: The thalassemia syndromes. Page 385 in: Hoffman B [editor]: *Hematology: Basic Principles and Practice.* Churchill Livingstone, 1991.)

sociation with HbH disease, as this structural abnormality is associated with a decrease in α-globin synthesis similar to that seen in individuals who are silent carriers.

The pathophysiology of HbH disease is due to the accumulation of excess β chains within the red cell. These β^4 tetramers are very unstable and readily oxidized. When this occurs, the red cell membrane is damaged, and the survival of the red cell is shortened. The clinical picture is quite similar to that of a patient with mild to moderate HS. Significant variation exists among patients. Recent reports suggest that patients with HbH disease who have constant spring have more severe hemolysis than do those with HbH caused by the three α-globin gene deletion alone. The identification of constant spring requires molecular techniques in most patients, as the amount of the variant may be too small to detect by electrophoretic methods. In some cases, splenectomy is useful to diminish hemolysis.

Infants who have HbH disease are anemic at birth. The Hb electrophoresis shows Hbγ^4 (Hb Bart) and some HbH (β^4). Over the first few months after birth, Hbγ^4 disappears, and HbH (approximately 20%) and HbA are seen.

Hb concentration ranges from 9 to 12 g/dL, and the red cell morphology is abnormal. Evident on the smear are hypochromia, microcytosis, target cells, and polychromasia. The reticulocyte count is slightly elevated except during a hemolytic crisis, during which it increases in response to the worsening anemia.

α-Thalassemia minor is characterized by deletions of two of the four α-globin genes and is fairly benign, with little or no anemia. Red cell morphology shows microcytosis, and, as with β-thalassemia trait, the RDW is normal. The reticulocyte count is normal to slightly increased. HbA$_2$ levels are low (1–2%). α-Thalassemia minor can be diagnosed in infancy (Hbγ^4, 3–10%). After the first few months of life, the diagnosis can be established by the use of gene mapping or α:β globin chain ratios. Figure 14–7 illustrates the use of laboratory tests to distinguish the most common forms of microcytosis, including α- and β-thalassemia trait.

The silent carrier state (heterozygous α-thalassemia-2) is a variant that does not produce any clinical or hematologic abnormalities. Suspected carriers are the parents or

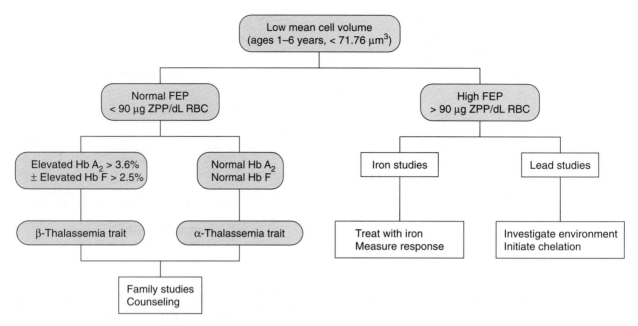

Figure 14–7. Algorithm diagramming the evaluation of microcytosis. FEP = free erythrocyte protophyrin; RBC = red blood cell; ZPP = zinc protoporphyrin.

siblings of children affected with HbH disease, and confirmation is made by gene mapping. In the newborn, $Hb\gamma^4$ levels may be as high as 3%. By 3 months of age, $Hb\gamma^4$ can no longer be detected.

β-Thalassemia. The clinical manifestations of the β-thalassemia disorders vary, and classification into thalassemia major, intermedia, and minor has been made. Laboratory measurements, age of onset of anemia, the course of the disease, and the severity of the clinical manifestations make it possible to distinguish between these forms.

Many of the molecular defects are well characterized and include more than 100 recognized abnormalities of the globin genes or their regulatory sequences. There are two genes for β-globin production, and the location of the mutation(s) within the β-globin gene or in regulatory sequences on chromosome 11 determines the clinical pictures. In the β^0-thalassemias, β-chain synthesis is lacking, often despite the presence of intact β genes. In the β^+-thalassemias, β-chain synthesis is present but reduced. In thalassemia trait, one β-globin gene has normal function and the other is affected.

The β-thalassemias, like the α-thalassemias, produce a wide range of clinical and hematologic findings. These disorders are characterized by decreased rates of β-chain synthesis and, consequently, reduced amounts of HbA in the red cells. Individuals with homozygous β-thalassemia require lifelong transfusion therapy and iron chelation to prevent iron overload. If iron accumulation from chronic transfusion exceeds iron loss because of chelation,

parenchymal damage can be detected, most notably in cardiac, liver, and endocrine organs. Skeletal deformities occur as a consequence of massive ineffective erythroid hyperplasia in patients who do not receive adequate transfusions. Splenomegaly occurs because of extramedullary hematopoiesis and entrapment of abnormal cells not destroyed in the marrow.

β-Thalassemia major, or homozygous β-thalassemia, is not clinically expressed in the first few months after birth because of the protective effects of γ-globin synthesis, which is able to balance α-globin synthesis. Within 2–3 months, however, progressive pallor associated with anemia develops, and, in the patient who has not received transfusion therapy, growth retardation may become a prominent feature. Hepatosplenomegaly occurs as a consequence of extramedullary hematopoiesis and transfusion-related organ damage. Infections are frequent owing to iron overload (*Yersinia enterocolitica*) and acquired splenic dysfunction.

The laboratory features of β-thalassemia major include severe, microcytic anemia with marked anisocytosis, poikilocytosis, and hypochromia and numerous target cells. There is a paucity of reticulocytes, although nucleated red cells are common. A slight leukocytosis and thrombocytosis can be seen, related to bone marrow stimulation. Serum iron and the free plasma Hb concentrations are elevated. Serum transferrin is often fully saturated. Ferritin levels are elevated as a consequence of transfusion therapy and must be monitored to adjust chelation therapy. Haptoglobin concentrations and red cell survival are decreased. The bone marrow aspirate shows a normoblastic, erythroid hyperplasia and increased iron stores, especially in patients who have received transfusion therapy. Ringed sideroblasts occasionally can be seen as a consequence of disordered globin synthesis. Iron kinetics reflect ineffective erythropoiesis with rapid uptake into the marrow and minimal return to the peripheral blood. HbF is the predominant Hb, and HbA_2 concentrations are elevated (typically 3.5–8.0%).

In the heterozygous form of β-thalassemia, or thalassemia minor, mild anemia with slight reticulocytosis is present. The peripheral blood smear shows microcytosis, hypochromia, poikilocytosis, basophilic stippling, and target cells. The degree of microcytosis is disproportionate to the degree of anemia. The marrow is normal or may show mild erythroid hyperplasia from a slight degree of ineffective erythropoiesis. The Hb electrophoresis shows elevations of HbA_2 (> 3.6%) and HbF. Figure 14–7, which shows the diagnostic approach to microcytosis, demonstrates the laboratory procedures that can distinguish β-thalassemia trait from iron deficiency or α-thalassemia trait.

Thalassemia intermedia is characterized by an intermediate depression in β-globin chain synthesis when compared with thalassemia major and thalassemia trait; as a consequence, hematologic and clinical parameters are relatively mild compared with β-thalassemia major. Transfusion therapy usually is not required. The genetic defect does not result in elevated HbA_2 in heterozygotes. The degree of anemia and the hematologic characteristics are determined by the molecular defects causing the disorder. Treatment of thalassemia includes transfusions at 3 to 4–week intervals with leukocyte-depleted packed red cells and aggressive iron chelation. Comprehensive treatment guidelines are followed in established thalassemia treatment centers. Hydroxyurea and other agents to increase fetal hemoglobin are currently being evaluated. In addition, studies are being conducted with oral iron-depleting agents. These agents will be especially important in view of the difficulty related to compliance with subcutaneous deferoxamine chelation.

Hereditary Persistence of Fetal Hb. This disorder, found principally in the African-American and Mediterranean populations, is characterized by persistence of HbF throughout adult life in the absence of any clinical stigmata. HPFH is classified by the type of HbF present (γA, fetal, or γG, adult) and frequently is a result of large deletions of the β-globin gene on chromosome 11. It does not result in unbalanced globin chain synthesis, a fact that sets it apart from α- and β-thalassemia. The association of HPFH trait with other β-globin chain structural variants, such as HbS, results in a benign disorder, with no anemia or vascular obstruction. The benign nature of this disorder is most likely related to the fact that the HbF is homogeneously distributed in the red cells, inhibiting the polymerization and sickling of the cells. Proper identification of newborns with sickle cell trait–HPFH is important, as these infants do not have a disease. Family studies, lon-

gitudinal evaluation, and molecular biology studies can be used to confirm the diagnosis.

EXTRACORPUSCULAR DEFECTS

Plasma and vascular factors can cause premature destruction of red cells. Immune hemolytic anemias result in early red cell destruction by the interaction of antibodies with the red cell. Mechanical trauma, such as that induced by prosthetic heart valves, and vasculitis secondary to inflammation can also cause premature red cell destruction. The clinical severity of these disorders is determined by the type and amount of antibody that binds to the red cell.

Isoimmune Hemolytic Anemia

Although transfusion reactions are rare because of ease of detection of the ABO blood group system, cross-matching, and scrutiny of the labels on the bags of blood before transfusion, isoimmune anemias can result from the sensitization to specific blood-group antigens after a blood transfusion. Depending on the extent of sensitization, the clinical features result from massive intravascular hemolysis and include chills, rigors, fever, jaundice, hypotension, and oliguria. Immediate or delayed reactions can occur. Laboratory findings include an elevated plasma Hb concentration, hemoglobinuria, reduced serum haptoglobin, and hyperbilirubinemia. Renal function may be reduced owing to haptoglobinemia. The timing of these studies is important to detect this, and they may need to be done serially. Elevated plasma Hb and hemoglobinuria are seen shortly after a transfusion reaction (within 1–2 hours) and, in severe cases, may not peak for 24 hours. Blood urea nitrogen and creatinine concentrations can also be abnormal within 24 hours but may take a week to become mildly elevated if hemolysis is mild and prolonged. A positive result with the direct antiglobulin (Coombs) test is common. In this test, antibody is detected on the surface of the patient's red cells using heterologous antisera prepared against human immunoglobulin.

The usual form of transfusion-induced hemolytic reactions involves IgG antibodies produced during an anamnestic response. Antibodies frequently are directed against the Rhesus (Rh), Kell, Kidd, and Duffy antigens. The antibodies coat the red cells, which are then sequestered by splenic macrophages or lysed in the intravascular space because of complement activation. The clinical and laboratory features of hemolysis are similar to those seen with IgM antibodies although they are less severe in nature. Fever and chills are common and can be delayed for several hours after completion of the transfusion. Laboratory results reflecting Hb catabolism can also be delayed, and hemolysis may be milder than that described in intravascular hemolysis associated with ABO incompatibility. Transfusion reactions due to alloimmunization represent a particular problem in patients with sickle cell anemia, as the donor pool of African-Americans is often limited for patients requiring red cell transfusion. By increasing the pool of African-American blood donors, transfusing with phenotypically marked blood, and carefully monitoring patients who received chronic transfusion therapy for alloantibodies or autoantibodies, this problem can be minimized.

Reactions due to IgM red cell abnormalities are less frequent, although they are dramatic and can be life-threatening; they usually begin after receipt of only small amounts of transfused blood. These antibodies cause rapid activation of complement on the cell membrane. This type of transfusion reaction is mainly associated with incompatibilities of the ABO blood group, and the degree of red cell destruction is proportionate to the amount of antibodies in the recipient's plasma, the quantity of A or B antigen on the transfused cells, and the volume of incompatible blood transfused. Red cells containing complement-activated antibodies on their surface are destroyed intravascularly or by the liver macrophages.

Hemolytic Anemia of the Newborn

Isoimmune hemolytic anemia in the newborn results from contamination of the maternal circulation with fetal red cells, and subsequent maternal sensitization and transplacental passage of maternal anti-fetal red cell antibody. This is most often the result of ABO or Rh incompatibility between the mother and the fetus but can also occur with minor blood group incompatibility because of Kell, Kidd, Duffy, and other rarer blood groups.

In hemolytic disease of the newborn (HDN), fetal red cells cross the placenta to the maternal circulation. If the mother lacks the antigen, IgG antibodies are produced and passively transfer back across the placenta to the fetal circulation. The fetal red cells become coated and hemolyze. In theory, any blood group that can produce IgG molecules and possesses sufficient antibody avidity potentially can cause the anemia.

ABO Incompatibility. In the case of anti-A and anti-B HDN, a mother with type O blood is specifically at risk for HDN. In most institutions, determining blood type and performing a Coombs test on umbilical cord blood are standard practice. Clinically, most cases go undetected. Frequently, the indirect Coombs test (which measures antibodies in plasma by incubating patient's plasma with a panel of red cells and subsequently with rabbit antihuman γ-globulin) yields a positive result, and the direct Coombs test result is negative or weakly positive. The findings within 24 hours after birth are hyperbilirubinemia and hemolysis. The peripheral smear shows moderate anisocytosis, microspherocytes, and a mild reticulocytosis. Except for the positive findings on the direct antibody test, these infants cannot be distinguished from children with hereditary spherocytosis. Disease caused by ABO antibodies differs from that caused by Rh incompatibility in that infants from the first pregnancy can be affected in ABO incompatibility.

Rh Disease. The antibody that binds to the newborn's red cells in this type of hemolytic anemia is produced by the mother's immune response to fetal red cells. It causes a more severe clinical hemolytic anemia than that seen in ABO disease. Rh disease does not usually affect the firstborn child unless the mother has been sensitized previously from transfusion or abortion and already possesses alloantibodies. Screening for these antibodies is performed on all Rh-negative pregnant women during their first trimester to identify pregnancies that require careful monitoring. Recently, methods have been reported to identify the Rh type of the fetus using molecular analysis of fetal amniocytes.

Hemolytic disease due to maternal-fetal Rh incompatibility is most commonly associated with anti-D, alone or in combination with anti-C or anti-E. Laboratory diagnosis depends on a strong positive result on Coombs testing of the infant's cord blood cells. The C, D, E phenotype can influence the variability of expression of the disease by affecting the potency of the D antigen. Therefore, knowledge of the maternal genotype may be predictive of disease severity. Serial titers of maternal antibody can be predictive of severe HDN. Rh sensitization and subsequent hemolytic disease of the newborn can be prevented or decreased in severity by careful monitoring of the Rh-negative mother. Rh immune globulin, when given in the second trimester, inhibits production of maternal Rh antibody. Detailed protocols for fetal monitoring during pregnancies affected by Rh sensitization are available and should be followed. Treatment of the affected newborn may require intrauterine transfusion or exchange transfusion at birth. Immune hemolysis can continue for several months after birth, requiring careful monitoring and occasional red cell transfusion.

Autoimmune Hemolytic Anemia

The term **autoimmune hemolytic anemia (AIHA)** is used to refer to a variety of warm antibody-mediated hemolytic anemias associated with various disorders, including postviral infection, systemic lupus erythematosus, lymphomas, and autoimmune disease. AIHA is associated with a wide variety of antibodies, the most common belonging to the Rh blood group. Red cell destruction is primarily due to macrophages in the spleen, which recognize the antibody and remove it, along with parts of the cell membrane, resulting in spherocytes. Extent of hemolysis is determined by the amount of IgG bound to the cell. When large amounts are found, complement (C3b) is also bound to the membrane, and red cells are thus sequestered in both the spleen and the liver.

Autoimmune hemolytic anemia can occur abruptly, usually after an acute viral infection. It often represents a pediatric emergency, as the decrease in Hb may be rapid and severe and immune-compatible blood is frequently impossible to obtain. When a milder, chronic picture is observed, it is important to rule out a defect in immune surveillance, which may be a consequence of primary immune deficiency diseases, a malignancy, or a collagen vascular disease.

The clinical features of AIHA include pallor, jaundice, and splenomegaly. The peripheral blood picture often shows a normal MCH and a variable MCV (depending on the reticulocyte count). Anisocytosis, polychromasia, and reticulocytosis are common, and spherocytes, schistocytes, and nucleated red cells can be present. In the acute form, children younger than 2–4 years are affected. Onset of hemolysis usually occurs after a viral infection. The child may present with severe anemia, jaundice, hemoglobinemia, and cardiorespiratory distress. The Hb concentration may be extremely low (< 2 g/dL). When red cells are needed to correct the severe anemia, blood is found to be incompatible, as evidenced by the strong positive Coombs test result. High and prolonged doses of corticosteroids are often required to treat this disease.

Products of Hb catabolism are present and include an elevated bilirubin, increased urinary urobilinogen, and increased serum lactic dehydrogenase. The direct Coombs test result is positive, and, in most cases, red cell coating with IgG molecules or complement binding can be demonstrated by using specific antisera. The component of complement most frequently involved is C3b.

Some antibodies react most efficiently with red cells at temperatures less than 37 °C and may optimally agglutinate at temperatures ranging from 4 to 25 °C. These antibodies are often IgM; they cause aggregation of red cells when blood is placed in the cold and therefore are called cold agglutinins. The antibodies are usually formed after viral infection (eg, *Mycoplasma* pneumonia) or infection with the Epstein-Barr virus; formation has been reported in cases of lymphomas and systemic lupus erythematosus. An association between the virus and the red cell agglutinin has been implicated in responsibility for the creation of a new antigenic site.

Clinical hemolysis can occur in patients with cold antibodies when the thermal range of the antibody is broad, and antibody binding can be demonstrated at temperatures up to 30 °C. The serologic findings show extremely high titers of a cold agglutinin often having anti-I (a red cell–associated antigen) specificity. The result of the direct Coombs test is positive, especially when an antiserum containing anticomplement components is used.

Another form of autoimmune hemolytic anemia in childhood is called **paroxysmal cold hemoglobinuria.** The IgG antibody responsible for this disease is the Donath-Landsteiner antibody. When this antibody is exposed to the cold, antigen-antibody complexes are formed; as the cells return to a normal temperature, these complexes bind complement, resulting in hemolysis. This uncommon disorder has been associated with syphilis, viral, and bacterial infections. The specificity of this antibody is against the P antigen. The laboratory features include a smear showing spherocytes, elevated reticulocyte count, and erythrophagocytosis. Hemoglobinuria is common. The direct result of the Coombs test is positive under cold conditions, 4–12 °C, and negative in warm conditions if antisera against IgG are. However, complement can be detected on the red cell surface. This type of antibody is not uncommon in children.

Drug-related mechanisms must be considered in the differential diagnosis of immune hemolytic anemia. Certain drugs can induce an immune hemolytic anemia by causing the formation of antibodies, either against the drug itself, which subsequently cross-reacts with the red cells, or against drug–red cell membrane complexes by possibly altering membrane antigenic structures (penicillin, cephalosporins, methadone). Other drugs (antihistamines, insulin, rifampin, quinidine, quinine, chlorinated hydrocarbons, insecticides, sulfonamides) cause immune-complex adsorption to red cells and activate complement. The result of the Coombs test may be positive for antibody or complement in these situations. If a patient found to have an immune hemolytic anemia is taking medication that could cause an immune response, the medication should be discontinued. When a causal relationship exists, hemolysis will subside.

MECHANICAL HEMOLYSIS & MICROANGIOPATHIC HEMOLYTIC ANEMIA

A hemolytic anemia can occur when red cells are fragmented by mechanical trauma, vascular inflammation, or thermal injury. A hemolytic anemia may develop in patients who have required heart-valve prostheses because of mechanical blood flow problems that cause red cell damage, a condition called the Waring Blender syndrome. In certain inflammatory states associated with infection or collagen vascular disease, fibrin deposition can occur across the microvascular bed; as a consequence, red cells are sheared as they pass through the fibrin meshwork. Notable findings on the peripheral smear include fragmented and distorted red cells (schistocytes), microspherocytes, and moderate thrombocytopenia due to platelet trapping in the fibrin strands. This type of hemolysis has been called microangiopathic hemolytic anemia. It can be found in the hemolytic uremic syndrome, thrombotic thrombocytopenic purpura, disseminated intravascular coagulation, systemic lupus erythematosus, acute glomerulonephritis, giant hemangiomas, and malignancies.

Acute hemolysis can also occur after thermal injury. The degree of hemolysis is often related to the severity of the burns and is believed to be caused by the irreversible denaturation of the red cell-membrane protein spectrin. Schistocytes and spherocytes are seen in the peripheral blood in these conditions, and spontaneous resolutions occur.

INADEQUATE RED CELL PRODUCTION

Processes that cause anemias as a result of inadequate cell production include nutritional deficiencies, dyserythropoiesis, chronic inflammatory diseases, and bone marrow atrophy or infiltration.

NUTRITIONAL DEFICIENCIES

Iron Deficiency Anemia

Iron deficiency is the most common form of anemia and exceeds all other causes in childhood by a factor of at least three. As the amount of iron in the newborn is approximately 75 mg/kg, a 3-kg infant will have approximately 225 mg total body iron at birth. If there is no iron in the diet, or if iron loss is greater than iron intake, by 6 months in full-term infants and as early as 3–4 months in premature infants, the iron stores present at birth will be depleted. The most common cause of iron deficiency is inadequate intake of iron during the rapidly growing childhood years. Excessive consumption of cow's milk associated with gastroenteritis and chronic blood loss and blood loss due to underlying diseases through the gastrointestinal tract, lungs, or kidney should be considered.

Iron reserves begin to decrease during the early stages of iron deficiency, resulting in a low serum ferritin concentration. Values less than 12 mg/mL have been considered diagnostic of iron deficiency. However, normal ferritin levels can exist in iron-deficient states when coexisting with a bacterial or parasitic infection, malignancy, or chronic inflammatory condition, as ferritin is an acute-phase reactant. As serum iron concentrations decrease, transferrin (total iron binding capacity [TIBC]) synthesis is stimulated, and the iron-transferrin ratio, called the transferrin saturation, decreases. A transferrin saturation less than 10% is consistent with iron deficiency.

The FEP concentration increases when the iron supply is low enough to impede Hb synthesis. The FEP is a simple, sensitive test for iron deficiency and can provide a guide to the adequacy of iron replacement therapy. Although the FEP was originally designed to detect lead poisoning, FEP levels in lead poisoning are usually very high. A careful environmental history should be taken to exclude lead poisoning as it can coexist with iron deficiency. Blood lead determination should be performed if there is any concern regarding lead poisoning.

With pronounced iron deficiency, the peripheral blood smear is remarkable for a microcytic, hypochromic anemia with severe anisocytosis and poikilocytosis. Basophilic stippling can occur, making such cases quite similar to thalassemia trait. Iron deficiency occurs over time; therefore, the red cell size is varied and the RDW is very high (> 14). This is in contrast to the thalassemia traits, in which the RDW is normal.

Physical findings associated with iron deficiency include pallor, lethargy, tachycardia, and tachypnea. Because iron deficiency develops over time, cardiorespiratory compensation is often quite remarkable, and some patients can tolerate Hb concentrations as low as 4 g/dL. In some cases of iron deficiency, growth retardation and neurodevelopmental delay can occur. In addition, protein-losing enteropathy can result as a consequence of iron depletion in the cells lining the gastrointestinal tract. Iron stores will be depleted before development of anemia, placing the infant at risk for the nonhematologic effects of iron deficiency.

Treatment of iron deficiency requires identification and correction of nutritional inadequacies, search for blood loss, and therapy with iron (2 mg elemental iron/kg twice daily). Iron therapy should be continued for several months after the red cell indices return to normal. Failure to respond to iron often reflects poor compliance. However, it may mean that the response is blunted by infection or that the diagnosis is incorrect. An adequate response to iron therapy is reflected by an increase of Hb concentration greater than 1 g/dL in 10 days. If measured, a reticulocytosis is usually evident within 3–5 days after starting oral iron supplementation. The FEP returns to normal when iron deficiency is corrected.

Megaloblastic Anemia

Vitamin B_{12} and folic acid deficiency are the most common causes of megaloblastic anemia. Rarely, megaloblastic anemia is due to inborn defects of pyridine (hereditary orotic aciduria) or purine metabolism (Lesch-Nyhan syndrome). Chemotherapeutic drugs such as methotrexate, cytosine arabinoside, and 5-fluorouracil commonly result in megaloblastic anemia.

The common biochemical abnormality in both folate and B_{12} deficiency is a defect in DNA synthesis, with lesser alterations in RNA and protein synthesis, leading to a state of unbalanced cell growth and impaired cell division. These cells, called **megaloblastic,** have greater quantities of DNA than do normal cells and are morphologically larger than normal. Nuclear maturation is dissociated from cytoplasmic maturation.

Megaloblastic anemia reflects only one component of the global cellular defect in DNA synthesis. Careful identification of the cause of megaloblastosis is required before initiation of therapy; these anemias can be confused with aplastic anemia or leukemia because they may lead to pancytopenia. Vitamin B_{12} deficiency causes severe neurologic disturbances in addition to its hematologic effects. Misdiagnosis and treatment of vitamin B_{12} deficiency as folate deficiency will result in hematologic improvement but will not correct the neurologic abnormality and can lead to permanent neurologic impairment.

Folic Acid Deficiency. Folic acid (pteroylmonoglutamate) is the commercially available parent compound for more than 100 compounds collectively referred to as **folates.** These are synthesized by microorganisms and by plants and are very thermolabile; thus, they are generally destroyed when food is boiled. A balanced Western diet can sustain folate balance because the daily requirement in children is approximately 0.3 mg/d. In the absence of dietary intake, folate stores can be depleted in weeks.

Food folates are hydrolyzed to an absorbable form by enzymes in the brush-border membranes of the small intestine; brush-border membrane folate-binding proteins facilitate active transport of folate into epithelial cells. Passive transport across the intestinal epithelium occurs with pharmacologic ingestion of folates. Ingested milk, which contains folate-binding proteins, can inhibit this process and decrease folate transport. Folate balance is maintained by both intestinal absorption and by an active enterohepatic circulation. Folate coenzymes are essential for the thymidylate cycle and for the methylation cycle, and defects in either of these cycles affect formation of methionine and inhibit DNA synthesis.

Folate receptors are present on all cells and are required for folate incorporation. These receptors can be upregulated or downregulated in various disease states. Congenital abnormalities in folate structure and function also exist. In the newborn, the concentrations of folate are maintained despite deficiencies in maternal folate. Once inside the red cell, folate is polyglutamated; this form associates with Hb. The level of intracellular folate is a more accurate predictor of folate status than serum folate concentration, and normal red cell folate levels can occur in conditions in which plasma levels are low.

Deficiencies of folate can occur in the following conditions: dietary intake is inadequate, demand is increased relative to intake (eg, during periods of active growth or in hemolytic anemias, there are increased requirements for hematopoiesis), drugs impair folate metabolism and inhibit absorption or use, gastrointestinal absorption of the vitamin is limited, and genetic abnormalities exist in the structure or activity of folate receptors or binding proteins.

Infant formulas and breast milk provide adequate folate for term and probably for low-birth-weight infants. Goat's milk is an extremely poor source of folate. In low-birth-weight infants who are given proprietary multivitamin supplements, folate must be administered separately because it is relatively unstable on storage. Infants require at least 10 times more folate for body weight than do adults. The recommended daily intake for infants is 20–50 µg/kg/d. Intestinal bacteria may augment folate supply, but prolonged use of antibiotics inhibits this source.

Folate deficiency occurs in chronic diarrheal states because of a secondary deficiency in intestinal conjugase, the enzyme required to convert dietary folate into an intestinally absorbable form, or interference with the enterohepatic circulation of folate. An extremely rare cause of congenital malabsorption of folate, manifested by 2–3 months of age, is the absence of cellular folate receptors. Folate analogues such as methotrexate and certain antibiotics such as trimethoprim (Septra, Bactrim) can cause folate deficiency by reacting with dihydrofolate reductase and interfering with the conversion of normal dihydrofolate substrates to the active tetrahydro forms. Oral contraceptives, phenytoin, and other anticonvulsants can interact with polyglutamates in the intestinal lumen and interfere with their digestion to the absorbable monoglutamate form. Understanding these mechanisms is important so that an appropriate form of folic acid is used to treat folate deficiency.

Folate deficiency should be considered in the evaluation of macrocytic anemia (see Figure 14–8). The reticulocyte count is normal or low, and neutropenia and thrombocytopenia may be found. The RDW is elevated, and red cell morphology is macrocytic and ovalocytic. The number of lobes within the granulocytes, called the **Arneth count,** is increased above the average of 3.4 nuclear lobes per cell if 100 cells are counted. Megaloblastic changes can be seen in all cell lines within the bone marrow, most notably in erythroid progenitors, in which nuclear maturation is markedly delayed compared with cytoplasmic maturation. A definitive diagnosis can be made by measuring the red cell folate content. Values less than 140 ng/mL are diagnostic. Although a serum folate content less than 3 ng/mL is also consistent with the diagnosis, serum levels are too sensitive to dietary fluctuations to be useful in many cases. If it is clear that megaloblastic anemia is secondary to folate deficiency and not vitamin B_{12} deficiency, folate can be given (0.5–1.0 mg/d). A response can be seen within several days. In cases in which it is not clear whether vitamin B_{12} deficiency has been excluded, the dose of folate should be reduced to 0.05–0.10 mg/d parenterally or 0.1 mg/d orally; this is adequate to produce a prompt reticulocyte response. A larger dose will cause a hematologic response in patients with B_{12} deficiency, although it will not affect the neurologic consequences of B_{12} deficiency.

Vitamin B_{12} Deficiency. This deficiency is uncommon in children; however, identifying and treating it is important because it can produce irreversible neurologic complications in addition to its hematologic effects. Humans receive their vitamin B_{12} exclusively from the diet, primarily from animal protein. Unlike folate, vitamin B_{12} is stable at high temperatures. The liver is the primary organ for B_{12} storage, and stores in children are capable of sustaining B_{12} needs for months. An efficient enterohepatic circulation preserves endogenous vitamin B_{12} and helps to prevent deficiencies when dietary inadequacy exists.

Once released by proteolysis from dietary protein, B_{12} is bound to a protein called R protein (so called because it migrates more rapidly in an electrophoretic field than does intrinsic factor [IF]) in the stomach. Pancreatic proteases digest R protein; as a consequence, B_{12} is released and rapidly combines with IF, which is resistant to digestion by pancreatic enzymes. IF is secreted in response to food in the stomach in a manner analogous to secretion of acid. In patients with pancreatic insufficiency, this process does not occur, and the B_{12} bound to protein is not absorbed. Specific receptors for IF exist in the ileum and account for the absorption of B_{12} by endocytosis. Within the enterocyte B_{12} is released from IF and is rapidly bound by transcobalamin II, which then transports B_{12} throughout the body. Vitamin B_{12} is incorporated into cells by a process of endocytosis.

The function of vitamin B_{12} within cells is to coordinate, with folate, the transfer of methyl groups required for DNA, RNA, and protein synthesis. Intracellular vitamin B_{12} is bound to methylmalonyl-CoA mutase and methionine synthetase and is required for their functions. This explains why patients with B_{12} deficiency have methylmalonic aciduria and why measurement of the concentration of this organic acid in the urine can be useful for the diagnosis of this vitamin deficiency. The polyglutamal form of tetrahydrofolate plays a central role in one-carbon metabolism required for these synthetic steps, and production of this important intermediate depends on both folate and vitamin B_{12}. Deficiencies of either vitamin result in similar defects in cell maturation and megaloblastic anemia; however, only vitamin B_{12} deficiency causes posterior lateral column disease and progressive neurologic impairment.

Vitamin B_{12} deficiency may be caused by nutritional inadequacy or by abnormal intragastric events. These include poor dissociation of food, deficient or defective IF, disordered mucous, or IF receptors, transenterocytic transport, and abnormal events in the small bowel (eg, inadequate pancreatic protease or usurping of luminal B_{12} by bacteria or intestinal worms).

If a child is fed a diet that completely lacks B_{12}, neonatal stores will be depleted by 6 months of age. Dietary inadequacy can be related to maternal deficiency, as seen in a breast-feeding mother who is a strict vegan and does not take B_{12}-containing supplements and whose child has megaloblastic anemia and neuropathy by 4 months of age.

The term **pernicious anemia** is applied to the anemia that results from a deficiency of IF. Juvenile pernicious anemia occurs in older children and is similar to pernicious anemia of adults. Gastric atrophy and decreased secretion of acid and pepsin are commonly associated with antibodies to intrinsic factor or to parietal cells. Selective immune deficiencies appear to contribute to the endocrinopathies associated with pernicious anemia and may be responsible for the entire clinical picture. Congenital pernicious anemia is usually manifest by 3 years of age. Although secretion of normally active IF is absent, other gastric functions and gastric morphology are normal. Furthermore, this disease has no immunologic component.

Because vitamin B_{12} is selectively absorbed by the distal half of the ileum, surgical removal of this portion of the small bowel for treatment of necrotizing enterocolitis, intussusception, regional enteritis, or congenital malformation results in a severe lifelong deficiency. Chronic regional enteritis can also cause B_{12} deficiency. Other rare causes of B_{12} deficiency are congenital absence or abnormal function of transcobalamin II and hereditary defects in enterocyte uptake of the B_{12}-IF complex.

The diagnosis of vitamin B_{12} deficiency is based on a high index of suspicion after a careful history and physical examination. Neurologic signs due to posterior and lateral column demyelinization in the spinal cord include parathesias, sensory deficits, loss of deep tendon reflexes, slowing of mental processes, confusion, and memory defects. Neurologic defects may precede anemia. Inappropriate administration of folate can result in a hematologic response in B_{12} deficiency but will have no effect on, or may aggravate, the neurologic effects.

Laboratory studies show macrocytic anemia and often pancytopenia. As with folate deficiency, the neutrophil lobe count is elevated. The serum B_{12} concentration is depressed to less than 100 pg/mL. The serum folate level is usually normal, but the red cell folate concentration may be decreased. Consequently, all three measurements—serum B_{12}, serum folate, and red cell folate—should be performed. When pernicious anemia is considered, a Schilling test should be performed, in which radiolabeled B_{12} is given with or without IF. IF can also be measured in gastric juice. Absence of gastric acid after histamine stimulation, and gastric mucosal morphology can distinguish forms of pernicious anemia.

The long-term treatment of vitamin B_{12} deficiency depends on its cause. In all cases, 25–100 µg/day vitamin B_{12} for several days may be used to initiate therapy followed by monthly injections of 50–100 µg. Hematologic improvement is prompt, and the extent of neurologic improvement depends on the extent of damage before onset of therapy.

CONGENITAL DYSERYTHROPOIETIC ANEMIAS

The congenital dyserythropoietic anemias are a rare group of hematologic disorders inherited in either an autosomal-recessive or an autosomal-dominant mode. They are characterized by anemia (usually hemolytic) and abnormal morphology in peripheral red cells and bone marrow erythroid progenitors. They affect all ethnic groups. Among the three major subtypes, there is marked clinical variability, ranging from mild to severe, life-threatening anemia. The central characteristic of the dyserythropoietic anemias is the failure to produce mature red cells in an orderly manner. Anemia with an inadequate reticulocyte response is often seen. Red cell destruction often occurs in the marrow. Type II, the most common form, is known by the acronym HEMPAS (hereditary erythroblastic multinuclearity with a positive acidified serum test), because multinucleated red cell precursors are seen in the marrow. The peripheral smear shows tear-drop cells and may demonstrate nucleated red cells. After incubation in an acid media, red cells are destroyed owing to their inability to prevent complement-mediated lysis. This laboratory picture is similar to that in patients with paroxysmal nocturnal hemoglobinemia.

ANEMIA SECONDARY TO INFLAMMATION

The anemia of chronic inflammation is due to impaired iron use, impaired production of erythropoietin, and hemolysis. Serum erythropoietin concentrations are often low, and serum iron is elevated because of a block in iron metabolism. Bone marrow iron stores are increased. The anemia is usually normochromic and normocytic with mild anisocytosis. The bone marrow shows mild normoblastic erythroid hyperplasia and elevated iron stores. In some cases, the diagnosis of anemia in chronic inflammatory conditions may be complex, as both iron deficiency and chronic inflammation may occur. For example, in cystic fibrosis, a combination of blood loss resulting in iron deficiency and chronic inflammation may be present.

Anemia that occurs during chronic inflammatory states develops within a few months of the primary disease. Red cell morphology is normochromic and normocytic, although hypochromia can develop over time. Anisocytosis is present, and FEP may be elevated. In contrast, the Hb concentration may be reduced 1–1.5 g/dL during acute inflammation. This anemia is normochromic and normocytic, and its cause is unknown. During acute inflammatory conditions, it is prudent to delay investigation of anemia, as the Hb concentration will increase to normal levels when the infection subsides. The anemia due to chronic inflammation will respond to treatment with erythropoietin. It will also resolve as the inflammatory condition resolves.

ANEMIA ASSOCIATED WITH DEFECTIVE BONE MARROW RESPONSE

Pancytopenia

The term **pancytopenia** refers to a reduction of erythrocytes, leukocytes, and thrombocytes. Pancytopenia may be due to bone marrow failure associated with the loss of stem cells; to inflammatory states that decrease stem cell production; to conditions that "crowd out" stem cells, such as malignancy, leukemia, or storage diseases; or to hypersplenism, which increases the number of peripheral blood cells residing in the spleen.

Acquired aplastic anemia refers to a situation of inadequate or complete cessation of hematopoietic activity within the marrow. It is often associated with bone marrow fibrosis. The cause is uncertain, but theories include acquired deficiencies of stem cells, deficiencies of environmental factors required for stem cell survival and function in the marrow, and immune-related disorders. Chemical and physical agents that have been associated with temporary or prolonged marrow suppression include cytotoxic drugs used for chemotherapy, benzene, sulfonamides, and chloramphenicol. Ionizing radiation also can cause injury to the bone marrow. Infections (eg, viral hepatitis and tuberculosis) can lead to marrow hypoplasia and aplastic anemia, and these must be excluded in a differential diagnosis. Most often, the cause of acquired aplastic anemia is idiopathic.

Quantitative abnormalities of all cell lines exist, as do qualitative abnormalities of maturation. The red cells exhibit anisocytosis, poikilocytosis, and macrocytosis, with an associated reticulocytopenia. The platelets appear small on a peripheral smear, if they are present at all. There is a concomitant increase in the bleeding time, and clot retraction is poor. Leukopenia is present; however, leukocyte morphologic abnormalities are not. Erythropoietin levels are markedly elevated, and the percentage of HbF may be increased. Serum iron concentrations are often high, as are the TIBC and transferrin saturation. The diagnosis is established on the appearance of the bone-marrow aspiration and biopsy specimens.

Treatment depends on the cause. In idiopathic cases, bone marrow transplantation is performed when compatible donors are available. Immunosuppressive agents are used if transplantation is not possible. Supportive care includes appropriate transfusions and aggressive treatment of infectious illness. Prognosis is poor if bone-marrow transplantation is not available.

Congenital aplastic anemia (Fanconi anemia) is a rare, autosomal-recessive hereditary disorder characterized by chromosome fragility and bone marrow hypoplasia. It is associated with a variety of congenital anomalies, including short stature, bony abnormalities associated with displacement of the thumb, abnormal skin pigmentation, and congenital abnormalities, such as single or horseshoe kidney. Affected individuals also have an increased predisposition to the development of leukemia. The bone marrow may be normocellular early in the disease, with a mild plasmacytosis, but ultimately becomes hypocellular. A normochromic and normocytic anemia is present at the outset, but macrocytosis can develop. There is an absolute reticulocytopenia. HbF concentrations usually are elevated, and nucleated red cells and immature leukocytes can be seen in the peripheral blood. The diagnosis of congenital aplastic anemia is usually not apparent until the end of the first decade, when thrombocytopenia is evident. However, if physical or radiographic findings are suggestive, specific cytogenetic abnormalities, such as chromosome breaks and abnormal cytogenetic changes after exposure to specific chemical agents, can be determined.

It is important to distinguish Fanconi anemia from idiopathic aplastic anemia, as Fanconi anemia has a better response to therapy with androgens and prednisone. In addition, the increased susceptibility to malignant transformation and associated clonal chromosomal abnormalities in Fanconi anemia must be recognized. Several recent reports of transplantation using cord blood, which is enriched in hematopoietic stem cells, obtained from siblings of patients with Fanconi anemia are encouraging. In all cases in which marrow transplantation might be indicated, this source of donor tissue should be considered.

Pure Red Cell Aplasia

Red cell aplasia is characterized by a selective decrease in red cell precursors in the presence of normal production of leukocytes and platelets. The two major groups of red cell aplasia in children are Diamond-Blackfan anemia and transient erythroblastopenia of childhood (TEC).

Diamond-Blackfan Anemia. This congenital form of red cell aplasia is characterized by a slowly progressive anemia usually beginning in infancy, like Fanconi anemia. Physical anomalies involving the skeletal and urogenital systems can be present in up to 25% of affected individuals. Children with this condition are often identified by 3–6 months of age, when anemia is detected and the reticulocyte count is very low. The presence of the low reticulocyte count is an important clue for suspecting the diagnosis. The anemia is eventually severe and is normochromic and normocytic. Macrocytosis may be seen, consistent with dyserythropoiesis. Other findings consistent with disordered erythropoiesis are elevated HbF level, elevated fetal "i" antigen, and a fetal pattern of red cell glycolytic and hexose-monophosphate shunt enzymes. Bone marrow examination reveals diminished or absent erythroid precursors and normal myeloid or erythroid precursors. The course is severe and prolonged, and patients are usually dependent on red cell transfusion, iron chelation, and steroids. Acute myelocytic leukemia has been reported in some patients. As immunologic mechanisms may be responsible for Diamond-Blackfan anemia, cyclosporin has been used with some success in patients not responsive to prednisone. Bone marrow transplantation is also an option if a suitable donor is available.

Transient Erythroblastopenia of Childhood. TEC, a relatively common, acquired form of pure red cell aplasia, usually presents in the 6-month to 4-year age group and is often preceded by a viral infection. Parvovirus B19 has been implicated in both normal children and in those affected by a hereditary hemolytic anemia. Patients with sickle cell anemia and HS may have aplastic episodes secondary to parvovirus infection. No physical stigmata are present, and spontaneous recovery occurs usually within weeks. Anemia is normochromic and normocytic. Neither macrocytosis nor elevated concentrations of HbF are noted, and fetal red cell antigens and enzymes are absent. Bone marrow aspirates show depressed or absent erythropoiesis but are otherwise normal. In patients with parvoviral infection, platelet counts may be elevated. Except for red cell transfusion, no therapy is required, and patients usually have complete remission within 4–6 weeks.

MORPHOLOGIC CLASSIFICATION

An approach to the diagnosis of anemia on the basis of red cell volume and Hb concentration is shown in Figure 14–8. As all patients have red cell indices performed during the evaluation for anemia, use of this information may facilitate the diagnostic evaluation.

MICROCYTIC ANEMIA

Microcytic hypochromic anemias encompass a subgroup of disorders involved with decreased Hb production, including iron deficiency, thalassemia, lead poisoning, sideroblastic anemia, and chronic blood loss. These anemias are characterized by an MCV less than 80 fL and MCHC less than 31%. The association of low cell volume

with decreased Hb concentration suggests a relationship between these two parameters.

The first step in the evaluation of a microcytic, hypochromic anemia is to take a careful history. A history of adequate dietary iron intake and a family history of refractory iron deficiency suggest thalassemia trait. Red cell indices and RDW will help to determine the subsequent workup. If the MCV is proportionately depressed for the degree of anemia and the RDW is elevated, iron deficiency should be considered. If the MCV is disproportionately depressed for the degree of anemia, (ie, Hb concentration, 8.5; MCV, 60) and the RDW is normal, consider α- or β-thalassemia trait. An elevated FEP level suggests iron deficiency or lead poisoning and is not consistent with α- or β-thalassemia trait. Blood lead levels will exclude lead poisoning. Elevated FEP levels can also be seen in children with heterozygote or mild forms of erythropoietic porphyria (Table 14–10).

NORMOCHROMIC NORMOCYTIC ANEMIA

Anemia associated with normal red cell indices can occur in diseases in which red cell production is decreased, or by increased red cell loss through hemorrhage or hemolysis. Included in this category are a wide range of primary or secondary bone marrow disorders, including hypoplastic anemias due to the bone marrow suppression from drugs, alcohol intoxication, infection, and bone marrow replacement (fibrosis, storage diseases, malignancies). Anemias associated with a normal bone-marrow response include acute blood loss, acute hemolysis, and hemoglobinopathies. Depression of erythropoietin production is usually secondary to renal disease or liver disease (impaired source of production), anemia of endocrine disorders (reduced stimulus), or anemia of chronic disease.

The reticulocyte count is the first decisive point in the investigation of normochromic, normocytic anemias. A corrected reticulocyte count should be calculated, as it is a prime indicator of bone marrow activity and, more specifically, of red cell production. Normal or reduced reticulocyte counts are present in situations with bone marrow suppression or replacement; consequently a bone marrow aspirate may help clarify the situation. Decreased reticulocyte counts with a normal marrow examination indicate a lack of marrow response in the presence of anemia.

MACROCYTIC ANEMIA

This subgroup includes the megaloblastic anemias that result from an asynchronous nuclear cytoplasmic maturation, such as vitamin B_{12} deficiency, folate deficiency, pernicious anemia, drug-induced states, and the congenital dyserythropoietic anemias. Macrocytic red cells develop in sickle cell patients treated with hydroxyurea. Bleeding

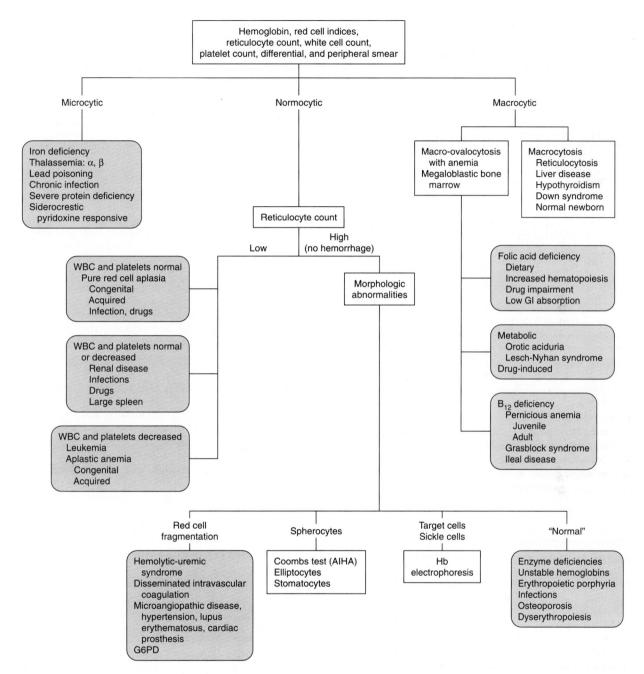

Figure 14–8. Algorithm diagramming the laboratory diagnosis of anemia. AIHA = autoimmune hemolytic anemia; GI = gastrointestinal; G6PD = glucose-6-phosphate dehydrogenase; Hb = hemoglobin; WBC = white blood cell count.

Table 14–10. Laboratory assessment of the common forms of microcytic anemia in children.[1]

	Iron Deficiency	α-Thalassemia Trait	β-Thalassemia Trait	Hemoglobin E Trait
Hemoglobin	Low/very low	Low	Low	Low
Mean cell volume	Low/very low	Very low	Very low	Very low
Red blood count	Low	High	High	Low
Relative distribution width	High	Normal	Normal	Normal
Free erythrocyte protoporphyrin	High	Normal	Normal	Normal
Hemoglobin electrophoresis	Normal	Normal	More A$_2$	Normal
Cord blood	Normal	Bart	Normal	F, A, E
Iron studies: ferritin	Low	Normal	Normal	Normal

[1]Relative scale: very low—low—normal—high.

disorders associated with reticulocytosis and liver disease may also show macrocytic characteristics. Newborns or individuals with elevated HbF values have macrocytic cells. Red cell macrocytosis is a common finding in individuals with Down syndrome, but it is usually not associated with anemia.

WHITE CELLS

Leukocytes include granulocytes, macrophages, and lymphocytes. Lymphocyte biology, function, and pathology are reviewed elsewhere in this text. Leukocytes originate from premature stem cells in the bone marrow, and their production and function are regulated by growth factors and cytokines. Leukocytes can be classified as **granulocytes,** the primary function of which is to ingest and kill bacteria, or as **mononuclear phagocytes,** which function as an important component in the reticuloendothelial system to remove abnormal cells or particles and participate in the immune response. Two pools of granulocytes exist in the circulation: One (which adheres to blood vessel walls) is called the **marginating pool,** and the other is the **circulating pool.** Fifty percent of white cells are usually found in each pool.

The phagocytes originate in the bone marrow from stem cells, circulate briefly in the blood stream, and exit to peripheral tissues. The neutrophils mature from myeloblast to mature polymorphonuclear neutrophils in 7 days and have an average half-life of 6–7 days in the peripheral circulation. Mononuclear phagocytes mature in 13 hours and have a circulating half-life of 8 hours. Survival in the tissues as macrophages may be as long as several months.

The macrophages reside principally in the spleen, liver, lymph nodes, lungs, and bone marrow; to a lesser extent, they are in the alimentary tract, central nervous system, mammary glands, and skin. In the spleen, the macrophages reside in close association with the lymphocytes in the germinal centers that make up the red pulp. The sluggish blood flow through the pulp allows sufficient time for the macrophages to perform a clearance function. Although the hepatic circulation is less sluggish than the splenic circulation, the contact time between the blood and the liver macrophages, the Kupffer cells, is still considerable. In the lymph nodes, macrophages are present throughout but are most abundant in the medullary zones, close to blood capillaries and efferent lymphatics. Here, macrophages play an important role in antigen presentation to T lymphocytes and, possibly, in the generation of specific immune response. Pulmonary macrophages reside in the alveolar sacs and within air spaces and clear inhaled microorganisms and inhaled matter. Macrophages reside abundantly in the bone marrow and may serve a clearance function in normal states or in pathologic states of ineffective erythropoiesis.

Granulocyte functions include phagocytosis and destruction of foreign particles. The process begins with stimulus recognition, then chemotaxis, adhesion, extravasation from the vascular space, activation of metabolic pathways to create microbicidal oxidative products, and phagocytosis of the smaller particles, with discharge of the lysosomal contents into the media. Defects in any of these processes can result in an impaired ability to fight infection.

QUANTITATIVE DISORDERS OF GRANULOCYTE FUNCTION

Little is known at the molecular level about the clinical conditions associated with abnormalities in the numbers of circulating granulocytes. Much, however, is known about the molecular basis of the pathophysiologic processes involved in ingestion and killing of bacteria.

NEUTROPENIA

Neutropenia is a condition in which inadequate numbers of granulocytes are produced. Normal neutrophil

Table 14–11. Normal leukocyte counts.[1,2]

Age	Total Leukocytes		Neutrophils[3]			Lymphocytes			Monocytes		Eosinophils	
	Mean	Range	Mean	Range	%	Mean	Range	%	Mean	%	Mean	%
Birth	—[4]	—	4.0	2.0–6.0	—	4.2	2.0–7.3	—	0.6	—	0.1	—
12 h	—	—	11.0	7.8–14.5	—	4.2	2.0–7.3	—	0.6	—	0.1	—
24 h	—	—	9.0	7.0–12.0	—	4.2	2.0–7.3	—	0.6	—	0.1	—
1–4 wk	—	—	3.6	1.8–5.4	—	5.6	2.9–9.1	—	0.7	—	0.2	—
6 mo	11.9	6.0–17.5	3.8	1.0–8.5	32	7.3	4.0–13.5	61	0.6	5	0.3	3
1 y	11.4	6.0–17.5	3.5	1.5–8.5	31	7.0	4.0–10.5	61	0.6	5	0.3	3
2 y	10.6	6.0–17.0	3.5	1.5–8.5	33	6.3	3.0–9.5	59	0.5	5	0.3	3
4 y	9.1	5.5–15.5	3.8	1.5–8.5	42	4.5	2.0–8.0	50	0.5	5	0.3	3
6 y	8.5	5.0–14.5	4.3	1.5–8.0	51	3.5	1.5–7.0	42	0.4	5	0.2	3
8 y	8.3	4.5–13.5	4.4	1.5–8.0	53	3.3	1.5–6.8	39	0.4	4	0.2	2
10 y	8.1	4.5–13.5	4.4	1.8–8.0	54	3.1	1.5–6.5	38	0.4	4	0.2	2
16 y	7.8	4.5–13.0	4.4	1.8–8.0	57	2.8	1.2–5.2	35	0.4	5	0.2	3
21 y	7.4	4.5–11.0	4.4	1.8–7.7	59	2.5	1.0–4.8	34	0.3	4	0.2	3

[1]Reproduced, with permission, from Dallman PR: Page 1222. In Rudolph AM et al (editors): *Rudolph's Pediatrics,* 20th ed. Appleton & Lange, 1996.
[2]Numbers of leukocytes are in × 10[9]/L or thousands per μL; ranges are estimates of 95% confidence limits, and percentages refer to differential counts.
[3]Neutrophils include band cells at all ages and a small number of metamyelocytes and myelocytes in the first few days of life.
[4]Insufficient data for a reliable estimate.

counts vary for age and race (Table 14–11). The absolute neutrophil count (ANC) is found by multiplying the white blood cell count by the total percentage of bands plus segmented (mature) neutrophils. **Mild neutropenia** is defined as an ANC of 1000–1500 cells/μL, **moderate neutropenia** as an ANC of 500–1000 cells/μL, and **severe neutropenia** as an ANC less than 500 cells/μL. This division into three categories is useful for determining the individual's risk for infection and the urgency of medical intervention. In severely neutropenic patients, endogenous bacteria are the most frequent pathogens, but neutropenic hosts often become colonized with a variety of nosocomial organisms.

Susceptibility to bacterial infection in neutropenic patients is quite variable and depends on the cause of the neutropenia and other associated problems. Many patients with chronic neutropenia have an elevated circulating monocyte count, which provides limited protection against pyogenic organisms. Patients who are neutropenic as a result of cytotoxic therapy (eg, chemotherapy or radiation) may be at an increased risk of infection because of the rate of decline of the neutrophil count, even before the ANC is reduced to less than 500 cells/μL. In addition, these patients can have altered phagocytic function related to their therapy and defects in cell-mediated, humoral, and macrophage-monocyte immunity. Malnutrition, splenectomy, and increased exposure to pathogens further weaken the host. All these factors must be considered when assessing the patient with neutropenia.

Neutropenia may be caused by defects in myelopoiesis, congenital or acquired, or may be secondary to factors extrinsic to the bone marrow. Intrinsic defects of myelopoiesis are rare but should still be included in the differential diagnosis of a newly identified patient with neutropenia, especially an infant.

Intrinsic Disorders of Myelopoiesis

Reticular dysgenesis is a rare disorder in which the early stem cells committed to myeloid and lymphoid lineages fail to differentiate. Infants with this disorder are vulnerable to fatal bacterial and viral infections and survive a few months at most. Although they lack neutrophils, T lymphocytes, B lymphocytes, and immunoglobulin formation, their erythroid and megakaryocytic lines are spared. Bone marrow transplantation has been successful in treating this inherited disorder.

Disorders of immunoglobulin formation, such as **X-linked agammaglobulinemia** and **dysgammaglobulinemia type I,** have been associated with neutropenia. Examination of the bone marrow reveals a maturation defect at the myelocyte stage. Clinical manifestations are variable and commonly include failure to thrive, frequent bacterial infections, and early death.

Severe congenital neutropenia, also known as **Kostmann syndrome,** is characterized by a lack of maturation of myeloid progenitors to the promyelocyte or myelocyte stage in the bone marrow. This is an autosomal-recessive disorder in which chronic neutropenia exists with an ANC usually less than 200 cells/μL. Patients with this disorder tend to have a monocytosis and moderate eosinophilia, yet frequent life-threatening infections develop starting from the first month of life. They have frequent febrile episodes, skin infections, stomatitis, and perineal abscesses and are susceptible to infection with the host's flora and opportunistic organisms. Since the introduction of granulocyte colony–stimulating factor (G-CSF) into the treatment of this disorder, quality and length of survival have dramatically improved. Studies have shown that these patients have normal levels of G-CSF, but the defect seems to reside at the level of the G-CSF receptor that can be overridden by pharmacologic doses of G-CSF. The therapy is well tolerated, and most patients maintain an ANC greater than 1000 cells/μL and do not have bacterial infections.

Cyclic neutropenia is a rare disorder characterized by regular periodic oscillations of the absolute neutrophil count every 19–21 days. Other blood cells, such as the platelets and reticulocytes, can also follow this oscillatory path. During the periods of neutropenia, the patient may have oral ulcers, lymphadenopathy, and, at times, serious infections including perineal ulcerations. The severity of the neutropenia determines the severity of the infection. During these episodes, bone marrow aspirates show maturation arrest at the myelocyte stage or myeloid hypoplasia. Between these episodes, patients usually are infection free and have normal neutrophil counts. The symptomatic periods tend to become fewer with age. There has been some evidence for a familial occurrence of this disorder, but most cases are sporadic. Animal studies support the hypothesis that cyclic neutropenia involves a regulatory defect in hematopoietic stem cells, although the exact nature of this defect has yet to be elucidated. Evaluation and management of these patients should start with determination of the individual's neutrophil cycle. A range of 14–36 days has been reported, with a median of 21 days. Infections during the neutropenic times should be treated aggressively, and appropriate precautions, especially good dental hygiene, should be taken to avoid infection. Preliminary studies using G-CSF to treat cyclic neutropenia appear promising.

Chronic Benign Neutropenia of Childhood

A particular group of children with chronic idiopathic neutropenia likely represents several poorly understood disorders. Many of these children have a benign course, hence the name **chronic benign neutropenia** of childhood. They often have mild to moderate neutropenia; the susceptibility to infection is roughly proportionate to the degree of neutropenia. The blood neutrophil count remains stable over years; however, in a subset of children the count becomes elevated in response to an infection. Spontaneous remissions at 2–4 years of age have been reported. Some cases appear to be familial. Affected individuals have normal life expectancies. Evaluation of the marrow shows decreased myelopoiesis (often with monocytosis), and there is considerable variability in the stage at which maturation is arrested. These patients are at low risk for development of serious infections, and no treatment is required except during infectious episodes. Some of these children resemble those with the lazy leukocyte syndrome, in which profound neutropenia is present with an apparently normal bone marrow and a characteristically poor response of the peripheral blood leukocytes to chemical or inflammatory stimuli. Some of the more symptomatic children may benefit from treatment with corticosteroids. Treatment with G-CSF is also being investigated.

ANCs are significantly lower in African-Americans than in whites. The explanation for these differences is unclear. Absolute neutrophil counts may be as low as 800/μL, yet they are not associated with infection, as an increase in absolute neutrophil count occurs in response to infection. Furthermore, bone marrow aspirate is normal with respect to myelopoiesis. Red cell and platelet counts are also normal. If the history for infections is unremarkable, neutropenia with counts greater than 500/μL in African-Americans requires no further investigation. If bacterial infections are present, these patients should have complete evaluation for neutropenia.

Extrinsic Causes of Neutropenia

Replacement of the bone marrow (as occurs with hematologic malignancies, glycogen storage diseases, granulomas associated with infection, and fibrosis related to chemical or radiation injury or osteoporosis) results in neutropenia. Frequently, the erythroid and megakaryocytic lines are also affected. Ineffective granulopoiesis can be seen in states of vitamin deficiency (vitamin B_{12} or folate), malnutrition (anorexia nervosa and marasmus), copper deficiency, and the Chédiak-Higashi syndrome (CHS).

The most common cause of transient neutropenia in childhood is viral infection. Viruses known to cause neutropenia include hepatitis A and B, influenza A and B, measles, rubella, varicella, and respiratory syncytial virus. Neutropenia corresponds to the period of acute viremia—the first 24–48 hours of the illness—lasting up to 1 week. Neutropenia occurring 1–2 weeks after viremia suggests an immune-mediated mechanism of neutrophil destruction or sequestration, and it should be determined whether titers of antineutrophil antibodies are elevated.

Bacterial sepsis is one of the more serious causes of neutropenia. Phagocytosis of microbes leads to release of toxic metabolites, which then activate the complement system, inducing neutrophil aggregation and adherence of leukocytes to the pulmonary capillary bed. Tumor necrosis factor and interleukin-1 (IL-1), released by the macrophages, likely accelerate this process. Activated granulocytes sequestered in the lungs may cause acute cardiopulmonary complications. Neonates have a limited granulocyte pool in their bone marrow, which can be exhausted rapidly during overwhelming bacterial sepsis. These infants may benefit from granulocyte transfusions or treatment with G-CSF.

Drug-induced neutropenia is a common and expected side effect of anticancer therapy. Many chemotherapeutic agents have a direct toxic effect on the early marrow stem cells. The severity and duration of the neutropenia depend on the particular medication, dosage, method of delivery, underlying disease, and state of nutrition and general health. These children should follow general supportive care guidelines for chronic neutropenia by taking prophylactic trimethoprim-sulfamethoxazole, to prevent *Pneumocystis carinii,* and antifungal medication; adhering to vigorous mouth care; avoiding exposure to crowds and sick individuals; and receiving prophylactic immunoglobulin for varicella exposures. Therapy with G-CSF or other granulocyte-mobilizing cytokines may shorten the period of severe neutropenia after chemotherapy.

Many other medications can induce neutropenia, including antibiotics (chloramphenicol, cephalosporins, penicillins, sulfonamides), anticonvulsants (phenytoin, valproic acid), anti-inflammatory agents, cardiovascular agents, tranquilizers, and hypoglycemic agents. The severity and duration of drug-induced neutropenia are variable. The underlying mechanism is not known, although studies with certain drugs have led to various hypotheses: immune-mediated, toxic effect of the drug or metabolites on the marrow stem cells, and toxic effects on the marrow microenvironment. After withdrawal of the drug, the marrow can repopulate with early myeloid forms in 3–4 days and appear morphologically normal by 1–2 weeks. The duration of neutropenia is likely related to the underlying mechanism; some chronic idiosyncratic drug reactions can last from months to years. Immune-mediated neutropenia usually resolves within 6–8 days of withdrawal of the offending agent.

Some cases of acquired neutropenia may represent an autoimmune disease with neutrophil specificity. Unlike in adults, immune neutropenia in children usually occurs in the absence of other diseases. These children have elevated titers of antineutrophil antibodies. The neutropenia is variable, ranging from mild to severe, and is often accompanied by monocytosis. Examination of the bone marrow usually shows myeloid hyperplasia, a response expected with increased peripheral destruction of the neutrophils. Treatment consists of aggressive management of infections with antimicrobials; in addition, steroid therapy is used for patients with severe neutropenia associated with recurrent infections. Splenectomy may be of only transient benefit and is not recommended. Use of high-dose intravenous immunoglobulin has been tried, but its efficacy remains unproved. Autoimmune neutropenia can also be a part of other autoimmune diseases such as Felty syndrome, a triad of rheumatoid arthritis, splenomegaly, and leukopenia. Immune neutropenia can also be associated with immune hemolytic anemia and thrombocytopenia (Evans syndrome).

Isoimmune neonatal neutropenia, analogous to Rh hemolytic anemia, can occur as a result of maternal sensitization to fetal neutrophil antigens during gestation. This results in the formation of IgG antibodies that cross the placenta and destroy the infant's neutrophils. The infants usually recover within 6–7 weeks, but fever and life-threatening infections can develop within the first few days after birth. Treatment of these infections may include use of antibiotics, plasma exchange, and infusion of maternal neutrophils known to lack the antigen to which the antibody is directed.

Organomegaly, in particular splenic enlargement from any cause, can cause sequestration of circulating neutrophils, resulting in neutropenia. Anemia and thrombocytopenia may also occur. Treatment of the underlying disease process often ameliorates the neutropenia.

Diagnostic Approach to the Child With Neutropenia

Evaluation of the child with neutropenia begins with a thorough history and physical examination. Included should be the child's family history, medication list, recent illnesses, age, and ethnicity. On examination, attention should be paid to any phenotypic abnormalities, adenopathy, splenomegaly, evidence of a chronic or underlying disease, and meticulous evaluation of the skin and mucous membranes (oral and perirectal). The laboratory evaluation helps establish the severity and duration (using periodic blood counts) of the neutropenia. Patients with chronic neutropenia should have blood counts checked twice a week for 6 weeks to evaluate for cyclic neutropenia. Additional studies include antineutrophil antibodies, assessment of cellular and serum immune status, and careful review of the peripheral smear for morphologic abnormalities of the white cells. Hematologic values, red cell indices, and platelet studies should also be done. A bone marrow aspirate and biopsy specimen may be necessary to identify granulocyte precursors and to search for defects in myeloid maturation. In addition, the bone marrow aspirate and biopsy specimen can be used to exclude hematologic malignancies, marrow infiltration, or fibrosis (Figure 14–9).

Management of the Child With Neutropenia

The management of neutropenia depends on many factors, including the nature of the neutropenia (acute or chronic), its severity, and the association with immune defects, underlying illnesses, or malignancies. Patients with acquired neutropenia arising from malignancy or chemotherapeutic drugs have a diminished inflammatory capability and are unusually susceptible to sepsis. Fever may be the earliest and only warning sign. Sepsis related to induced neutropenia remains a leading cause of mortality in these patients. Aggressive management of the febrile, neutropenic patient in the hospital has markedly reduced morbidity and mortality associated with infection.

In the neutropenic patient, the definition of fever is one episode of a temperature of 38.5 °C or higher or two temperatures of 38 °C or higher in a 24-hour period. The initial evaluation of the child with fever and neutropenia includes meticulous physical examination with particular attention to sites of occult infection (the oral cavity and perineum); peripheral and indwelling catheter blood cultures; urinalysis and urine culture; chest roentgenogram, if pulmonary symptoms are present; and cultures from sites of suspected infection, such as skin, throat, and stool. Blood cultures should be obtained every 24 hours in the persistently febrile patient. Broad-spectrum antibiotics must be started immediately and provide coverage for gram-negative and gram-positive organisms. A combination of an aminoglycoside and a β-lactam antibiotic provides initial broad coverage and is synergistic for *Pseudomonas* species. If the fever subsides, the cultures remain negative, and the clinical course improves, the antibiotics can be discontinued after 72 hours. Documented bacteremia should be treated with a full course of antibiotics. In the patient in whom infection of an indwelling

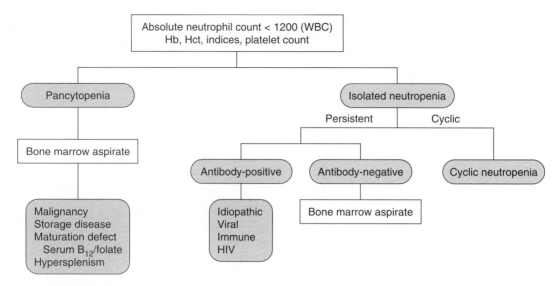

Figure 14–9. Algorithm diagramming the laboratory evaluation of the child with neutropenia. Hb = hemoglobin; Hct = hematocrit; WBC = white blood cell count.

catheter is a recurrent problem or the bacteremia persists beyond 48–72 hours, the catheter should be removed. In the persistently febrile, neutropenic patient, antifungal therapy with amphotericin should be begun by the fifth to seventh day and continued until the patient is no longer neutropenic and febrile. Many oncologists continue antibiotic therapy until the neutropenia resolves or there is some evidence of marrow recovery.

Evaluation of the Patient With Recurrent Infections

The differential diagnosis for a patient with recurrent infections is extensive. Although most of these patients will not have identifiable phagocytic disorders, defects of the host immune system should be considered. The algorithm in Figure 14–10 is presented to help organize this complicated workup.

NEUTROPHILIA

Neutrophilia refers to a circulating neutrophil count greater than 7500/μL in the child and 13,000/μL in infants. Neutrophilia may result from increased marrow production or changes between the circulating and marginating pools of neutrophils. Acute neutrophilia occurs after administration of epinephrine or corticosteroids, as well as after splenectomy. Chronic neutrophilia may be related to defective feedback mechanisms between circulating neutrophils and the marrow and may follow periods of prolonged administration of corticosteroids, infection, chronic inflammation, and chronic blood loss. A transient neutrophilia is seen after blood transfusions. Infections

such as tuberculosis, herpes simplex, and varicella may cause prolonged elevated neutrophil counts. Leukemoid reactions and leukocytosis resembling leukemia have been observed in neonates with Down syndrome and in association with sepsis. The benign neutrophilia of infancy resolves by the end of the first few weeks after birth.

QUALITATIVE DISORDERS OF GRANULOCYTE FUNCTION

Numerous rare inherited and acquired disorders have been described that are caused by abnormalities in one or more steps of phagocytic function, such as chemotaxis, adhesion, ingestion, degranulation, and oxidative metabolism. Affected individuals may have recurrent bacterial and fungal infections.

DISORDERS OF ADHESION

Leukocyte Adhesion Deficiency

Leukocyte adhesion deficiency (LAD) is a rare, autosomal-recessive disorder of impaired phagocyte adhesion, chemotaxis, and ingestion of complement (C3bi)-opsonized microbes. The molecular basis for this disease has been investigated, and mutations of the genes coding for specific neutrophil glycoprotein subunits have been found. Carriers can be identified, and prenatal diagnosis can be made if the genetic locations of the parental mutations are known.

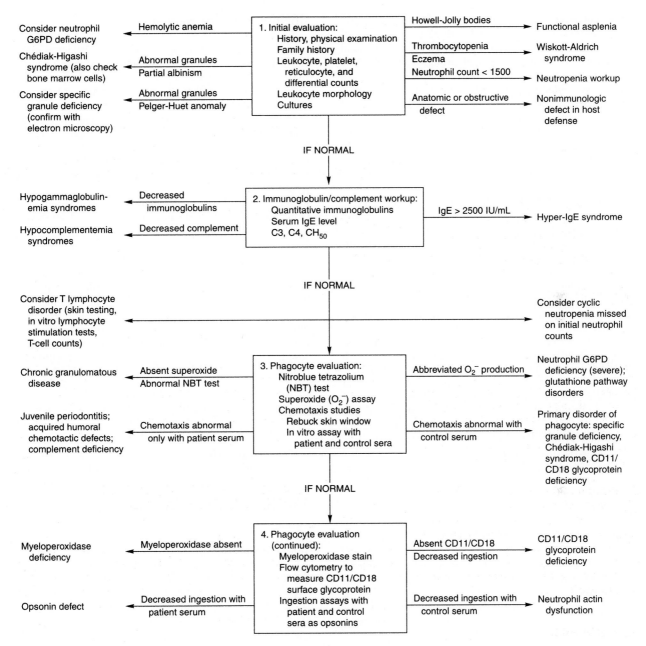

Figure 14–10. Algorithm diagramming laboratory evaluation of the patient with recurrent infections. G6PD = glucose-6-phosphate dehydrogenase. (Reproduced, with permission, from Lehrer RI: Neutrophils and host defense. Ann Intern Med 1988;109:127.)

To date, approximately 60 cases of LAD have been reported in the literature. Clinically, the disorder is characterized by repeated bacterial or opportunistic infections, severe gingivitis and periodontitis, frequent superficial bacterial infections with an invasive predisposition, and slow wound healing that is often first manifested as delayed umbilical cord separation. *Staphylococcus aureus* and gram-negative enteric bacteria are the most common

pathogens. Laboratory features include a persistent granulocytosis and failure of the neutrophils to accumulate at sites of infection.

The diagnosis of LAD should be suspected in any infant or newborn who presents with an unusually severe bacterial infection in the face of a striking granulocytosis (up to 100,000/μL). A leukemoid reaction may be mistakenly deemed the cause of the elevated white cell count.

Treatment depends on the clinical severity of the disorder, with phenotypes ranging from moderate to severe. In all patients, granulocytosis is the hallmark. Cutaneous and oral infections should be treated promptly. Prophylaxis with trimethoprim-sulfamethoxazole has been beneficial. Aggressive dental hygiene is advisable, with antimicrobial rinses such as chlorhexidine gluconate. Patients with LAD can have unusually severe infections, and the mortality rate is high, especially in patients younger than 2 years. Bone marrow transplantation has been used successfully to treat several cases and, at this time, may provide the only chance for survival.

Acquired Disorders of Adhesion

Exposure to a wide array of drugs can cause **decreased adhesiveness** of the neutrophils. Epinephrine and corticosteroids, the most common offenders, cause a dramatic increase in the total neutrophil count as the blood cells from the marginating pool within the vascular tree are released into the circulation. Epinephrine causes endothelial cells to release cyclic adenosine monophosphate (AMP), which impairs the neutrophil's ability to adhere. The mechanism by which corticosteroids alter adherence is unknown.

A variety of clinical situations can result in **increased neutrophil adherence** by complement activation. Such situations include thermal injuries, gram-negative bacterial sepsis, trauma, pancreatitis, and exposure to artificial membranes during hemodialysis and cardiopulmonary bypass. Neutrophils experience increased aggregation, and neutrophil clumps become trapped within small capillary beds, such as in the lung. These aggregated neutrophils generate toxic oxygen radicals and release proteases that damage structural proteins, such as collagen and elastin. These events can contribute to acute respiratory distress syndrome.

DISORDERS OF CHEMOTAXIS

Many mechanisms regulate the directed migration of phagocytes from the circulation to sites of infection and inflammation. Chemotactic factors must be generated in sufficient quantities to establish chemotactic gradients that promote granulocyte mobility. The phagocytes must have receptors for these agents as well as mechanisms for discerning the direction of the gradient. When these receptors are engaged, a series of intracellular metabolic events occurs that regulates the increased surface expression of adhesion-promoting molecules. Inflammatory mediators, such as IL-1, further direct the migration of phagocytes. Phagocyte-endothelial cell interactions play a central role in directing the tissue localization of neutrophils and monocytes during inflammation.

Many conditions may impair chemotaxis; this may be due to complement deficiency (C1, C2, C3, C4, C5), immunodeficiency syndromes (eg, Wiscott-Aldrich), or disorders of phagocyte function (leukocyte adhesion deficiency, CHS, and specific leukocyte granule deficiencies).

Chemotaxis in the Neonate

In the first few weeks after birth, infants are at an increased risk for the development of severe bacterial infections. The risk is even greater in preterm infants. Neonates may have defects in specific immunity and phagocyte-mediated immunity including splenic function. Defects in neutrophil adherence, chemotaxis, phagocytosis, and bacteriocidal activity have all been reported. The directed migration of neonatal neutrophils toward a variety of chemotactic agents (C5a, bacterial extracts) is reduced by 50% compared with adult neutrophils because of a defect in upregulation of cell-adhesion molecules. Neonatal neutrophils also display a diminished fusion of the specific granules within the plasma membrane after stimulation. Compounding these defects is a deficiency of antibodies directed against organisms that typically infect infants. Furthermore, with severe pyogenic infections, neonates can quickly exhaust their bone marrow granulocyte reserves. In addition to these granulocyte defects, the susceptibility of newborns to infections is further accentuated by defects in cellular and antibody-mediated immunity as well as in functional asplenia. Finally, as mentioned previously, the bone marrow reserve of granulocyte precursors is elevated in newborns, and neutropenia can occur with stress. All these abnormalities appear to correct within the first few months of life.

DISORDERS OF DEGRANULATION: CHÉDIAK-HIGASHI SYNDROME

Chédiak-Higashi syndrome is a rare, autosomal-recessive disease characterized by recurrent bacterial infections, partial oculocutaneous albinism, giant cytoplasmic inclusions in the granulocytes, and, in some patients, a mild bleeding diathesis. Peripheral and cranial neuropathies have also been described. A variety of tissues are affected. In melanocytes, the giant inclusions (**melanosomes**) prevent the even distribution of melanin, resulting in hypopigmentation of the hair, skin, iris, and ocular fundus. There are approximately 200 known cases of CHS; its rarity has made elucidation of the underlying molecular defect difficult. The lysosomal defect involves all blood cells. The neutrophils are most characteristic and contain giant coalesced azurophil-specific granules. The absolute neutrophil count ranges from 500 to 2000 cells/μL, reflecting intramedullary granulocyte destruction. Monocytes and lymphocytes are also affected, and the combined effects may contribute to abnormalities in specific immunity. Although the platelet count is normal, the platelets have a decreased number of dense granules and a storage pool deficiency of adenosine diphosphate (ADP) and serotonin. Platelet aggregation is often defective, and patients bruise easily and may have epistaxis and intestinal bleeding.

Individuals with CHS have recurrent infections involving the skin, respiratory tract, and mucous membranes, usually caused by both gram-positive (*S aureus*) and gram-negative bacteria, as well as fungi. Impaired bactericidal activity is a result of neutropenia and defective neutrophil function. Chemotaxis is markedly depressed. The large granules may impede the neutrophil's ability to travel through tight passages, such as between endothelial cells. Degranulation is delayed and incomplete, and there is a deficiency of antimicrobial protein production in the CHS neutrophils.

Affected individuals who survive beyond the first decade have a high risk of progressing to an accelerated phase of the disease, perhaps because of infection by Epstein-Barr virus. This phase is heralded by the onset of hepatosplenomegaly, lymphadenopathy, bone marrow infiltration by lymphohistiocytic cells, hemophagocytosis, and high fevers not attributable to infections. Thrombocytopenia develops and can worsen the bleeding disorder already present. The risk of overwhelming sepsis during this period is high, and many patients succumb.

The diagnosis of CHS is usually made by the history and physical examination and the finding of giant granules in the peripheral blood or bone marrow myeloid cells. In severely neutropenic patients, a bone marrow aspirate may be needed to confirm the diagnosis.

Management involves treatment of infections and supportive care measures as described for immune-compromised patients. The accelerated phase may respond to chemotherapeutic intervention but is frequently fatal. Bone marrow transplantation has been successfully performed on several patients during the chronic phase of the disease.

DISORDERS OF OXIDATIVE METABOLISM

Neutrophils contain a group of antimicrobial polypeptides that act as endogenous antibiotics. These are called **defensins.** Another class of microbicidal agents called **free radicals** is generated within the cell by the phagocyte respiratory burst pathway. In a series of reactions, molecular oxygen is converted initially to superoxide, and then to hydrogen peroxide (H_2O_2), hypochlorous acid (HOCl), and hydroxyl radical. The enzyme responsible for this burst of respiration is NADPH oxidase. Before this series of reactions, the neutrophil consumes little oxygen and relies primarily on anaerobic glycolysis for energy. Several clinically significant defects in the respiratory burst pathway have been identified and involve deficiencies of the regulatory enzymes: NADPH, G6PD, myeloperoxidase, glutathione reductase, and glutathione synthetase.

Chronic Granulomatous Disease

Chronic granulomatous disease (CGD) is a rare, genetically heterogeneous disorder, caused by a failure of respiratory burst activation in the phagocytes. At the molecular level, the defect has been localized to a defect in one of the NADPH subunits in the membrane or cytoplasm of the granulocyte. The symptoms of CGD appear

during the first year and are characterized by recurrent purulent bacterial and fungal infections. The most common pathogens are *S aureus, Aspergillus* species, and gram-negative bacilli, including *Serratia marcescens,* various *Salmonella* species, and *Pseudomonas cepaci.* Typical infections include pneumonia, complicated by empyema or lung abscess; suppurative lymphadenitis, usually involving the cervical nodes; cutaneous abscesses, paronychia, and perinasal impetigo; hepatic abscesses; osteomyelitis; and perirectal infections. In addition to pyogenic infections, a chronic inflammatory state is present with resultant formation of granulomas, one of the hallmarks of CGD. Hyperglobulinemia, short stature due to chronic illness, and anemia of chronic disease are evident in many affected individuals.

The unique susceptibility of CGD patients to specific infections is based on the inability of CGD phagocytes to produce hydrogen peroxide. Many bacteria, such as *S pneumoniae,* produce hydrogen peroxide and lack catalase, an enzyme that breaks down hydrogen peroxide. As a consequence, these organisms can be killed by CGD granulocytes.

The diagnosis of CGD is suspected from the history of infections, particular pathogens and sites of infection, and a family history of disease. A useful diagnostic test is the nitroblue tetrazolium (NBT) test. In dormant cells, NBT remains oxidized and is soluble and yellow. When normal neutrophils are stimulated to undergo a respiratory burst in the presence of NBT, which creates superoxide, this reduces the NBT and converts it to a deep purple color. Stimulated CGD neutrophils cannot reduce NBT dye, as they do not generate superoxide. Carrier states can also be identified using this method, with intermediate levels of NBT reduction seen in the phagocytes of autosomal-recessive carriers. However, NBT reduction may vary with the degree of X inactivation of the affected chromosome, and some carriers may be missed because of the selective advantage of the normal X chromosome. Molecular techniques can definitely establish a diagnosis and can be used for prenatal diagnosis as well.

The prognosis for patients with CGD is improving steadily. Many patients survive into their adult years with aggressive management of infectious episodes with antibiotics, antifungal agents, surgical drainage of abscesses, and prophylactic trimethoprim-sulfamethoxazole. Recently, the use of human recombinant interferon-γ has been shown to be useful in some patients and a well-tolerated treatment that reduces the frequency of serious infections. Allogenic bone marrow transplantation has been used successfully in several cases of CGD.

Glucose-6-Phosphate Dehydrogenase Deficiency

Leukocyte and erythrocyte G6PD are encoded by the same gene; however, clinically significant neutrophil G6PD deficiency is rare. This is explained in part by the neutrophil's high tolerance: Respiratory burst function is not adversely affected until the G6PD level is less than

5%. In addition, low levels of respiratory burst activity can be sufficient for host protection. In most types of G6PD deficiency, the neutrophil level is 20–75% of normal. Because of the neutrophil's short half-life, the effect of enzyme decay is not as significant as it is in the erythrocytes. This explains why leukocyte G6PD deficiency is not associated with clinical problems in African-Americans. The diagnosis of G6PD deficiency should be suspected in any patient with known erythrocyte G6PD deficiency, or in a patient with congenital nonspherocytic hemolytic anemia in association with recurrent infections. Treatment is aimed at prevention of infections with prophylaxis and with antimicrobials as indicated.

Myeloperoxidase Deficiency

This rare disorder is inherited in an autosomal-recessive mode. The deficiency of myeloperoxidase from the azurophilic granules of the neutrophils results in a pronounced delay in the killing of both catalase-positive and catalase-negative intracellular bacteria. Myeloperoxidase deficiency is the most common inherited disorder of phagocyte function, with a complete deficiency in 1:4000 individuals. Expression is variable and very mild. Neutrophils and monocytes are affected, but eosinophils show normal activity. The neutrophils have large residual stores of myeloperoxidase, and the respiratory burst seems to be augmented in these patients. In addition, the other oxidants produced by the respiratory burst, the various lysosomal antimicrobial proteins, and the activity of the normal eosinophils all contribute to provide sufficient host defense against most microorganisms. Usually, no treatment is required. Infections should be treated as in normal individuals, although these patients do have an increased susceptibility to candidal infections.

BASOPHILS & EOSINOPHILS

Eosinophils are leukocytes that are identified by their characteristic intracellular, refractile, eosinophilic staining granules. Eosinophils can be found in the bloodstream as well as in many body tissues. The epithelial lining of the intestine, especially the colon, is one of the most heavily populated areas. Eosinophils are capable of ingesting and killing bacteria and can enhance or suppress acute inflammatory reactions.

In normal children, the absolute circulating eosinophil count is 150–700/μL. Eosinopenia may occur as a result of adrenocortical hyperfunction or after the administration of pharmacologic doses of corticosteroids. Eosinophilia is most often due to allergy; asthma, hay fever, skin rashes, and allergic drug reactions are among the causes. Invasive parasitic infections, such as toxocariasis, trichinosis, echinococcal disease, ascaris, and, less commonly, intestinal parasites, can cause eosinophilia. Visceral larval migrans results in a large increase in the number of circulat-

ing eosinophils. Eosinophilia can be seen in premature infants and often occurs in infants who have chlamydial pneumonia. Gastrointestinal disorders, such as ulcerative colitis, Crohn disease, chronic hepatitis, and milk precipitin disease, may have an associated eosinophilia. Immunodeficiency syndromes, such as Wiscott-Aldrich syndrome, have associated eosinophilia. Cases of Hodgkin disease in which an eosinophilic factor is produced have moderate to severe eosinophilia. Eosinophilic leukemia is a rare form of leukemia and should be treated similarly to acute myelocytic leukemia. A rare group of hypereosinophilic syndromes of unknown etiology involves the cardiopulmonary system and includes disseminated eosinophilic collagen disease, Loeffler disease, endocarditis with endomyocardial fibrosis, and pulmonary infiltration with eosinophils.

Basophils are leukocytes that contain a few densely staining, basophilic granules. They account for less than 1% of the circulating leukocytes. Basophil granules are rich in histamine and heparin. Like eosinophils, basophils participate in allergic reactions. If basophilia is associated with leukocytosis and thrombocytosis, chronic myelogenous leukemia should be suspected. Basophilia can also occur with ulcerative colitis and myxedema.

PLATELETS

Megakaryocytes derive from the early stem cells, colony-forming unit stem cells (CFU-S); recently, a molecule called thrombopoietin (TPO) has been identified. TPO regulates the number of circulating platelets. Once the CFU-megakaryocyte becomes committed, the transitional megakaryocytes go through four stages of maturation. The megakaryoblasts are large and have globulated nuclei and basophilic cytoplasm containing granules and dense bodies. These cells then develop indented, horseshoe-shaped nuclei with more abundant and less basophilic cytoplasm with increased numbers of organelles. In the third stage of maturation, the megakaryocytes appear large with abundant granular eosinophilic cytoplasm. Finally, the megakaryocytes mature into cells with compact, dense nuclei and homogenous, intensely stained eosinophilic cytoplasm. The state of cytoplasmic maturation and its ploidy level determine the number of platelets contained by the megakaryocyte. Where and under what circumstances the platelets are released from the megakaryocytes has not yet been determined.

Mature platelets are small cells, approximately 1–4 μm in diameter. They are crucial in the initiation of hemostasis, forming the platelet plug. Excessive bleeding can occur if the platelets are dysfunctional or deficient in number. Bleeding secondary to platelet insufficiency typically involves the skin or mucous membranes and includes petechiae, ecchymoses, epistaxis, menorrhagia, hematuria, and gastrointestinal bleeding. Intracranial hemorrhages can occur but are rare. In response to marrow stress or thrombocytopenia, large platelets can be seen in the peripheral blood.

There are normally 150,000–400,000 platelets/µL in the peripheral circulation. Platelet mass is maintained at a constant rate under the control of TPO. Approximately one third of the platelets are sequestered in the spleen and serve as a reserve pool, released in times of hemostatic stress. The proportion of platelets sequestered is related directly to spleen size. Splenomegaly or asplenia must be considered when interpreting the circulating platelet concentration. Platelets survive 7–10 days once released from the marrow. Transfused platelets survive for a considerably shorter period, even if the patient's thrombocytopenia is due to decreased platelet production.

When the endothelial cell lining of the vessel wall is interrupted, platelets bind to the exposed adhesive proteins in the subendothelium. Primary hemostasis, or platelet plug formation, is initiated. During platelet adhesion, von Willebrand factor acts as a bridge between the platelet glycoprotein (GP) Ib/IX complex and the subendothelial matrix proteins. Platelets contract, extend pseudopods, and, during this activation process, release the contents of their granules (ADP, calcium, serotonin), thereby drawing other platelets to form a platelet aggregate. A network of platelet-platelet linkages via GP Ib/IIIa receptors results in formation of a platelet plug. Fibrinogen and von Willebrand factor are also important participants in this interaction. Arachidonic acid is released from the platelet membrane during the activation process, and its metabolic products initiate release of platelet granules. More platelets are recruited to the site of adherence, and the platelet framework facilitates the clotting cascade with the formation of a fibrin clot.

As with erythrocytes and leukocytes, disorders of platelet numbers can be secondary to increased destruction or storage in the spleen or decreased production. Qualitative platelet defects can also occur. Conversely, elevated platelet counts can be seen when the rate of production exceeds the rate of destruction or storage, as noted in acute inflammation, in postsplenectomy states (when the storage site for platelets is removed), or in acute hemorrhagic states.

QUANTITATIVE ABNORMALITIES OF THE PLATELETS

The initial evaluation of thrombocytopenia requires the confirmation of the platelet count on review of the peripheral smear, especially in the nonsymptomatic child. False values for platelet counts can result from aggregation of platelets in the syringe or collection tube; counting of small, nonplatelet particles (fragmented red or white cells) by automated cell counters; and pseudothrombocytopenia due to in vitro platelet agglutination by anticoagulant-dependent ethylenediamine tetra-acetic acid (EDTA) antibodies. In the latter case, review of the blood film may show clumps of agglutinated platelets at the periphery of the slide. The diagnoses of thrombocytopenia in children are shown in Table 14–12, and the approach to managing the child with thrombocytopenia is presented in Figure 14–11.

Table 14–12. Diagnoses of thrombocytopenia in pediatrics.

Destructive thrombocytopenias	
Immunologic	Idiopathic thrombocytopenic purpura
	Drug-induced
	Infection-induced
	Post-transfusion purpura
	Autoimmune disease
	Neonatal alloimmune
	Post-transplant
Nonimmunologic	Microangiopathic disease
	Hemolytic anemia and thrombocytopenia
	Hemolytic uremic syndrome
	Thrombotic thrombocytopenia purpura
	Cyanotic heart disease
Platelet consumption	Disseminated intravascular coagulation
	Giant hemangiomas
	Meconium aspiration
Neonatal problems	Pulmonary hypertension
	Polycythemia
	Respiratory distress syndrome
	Sepsis
	Prematurity
Impaired production	
Congenital and hereditary disorders	Thrombocytopenia–absent radius syndrome
	Fanconi anemia
	Bernard-Soulier
	Wiscott-Aldrich syndrome
	Glanzmann thrombasthenia
	May-Hegglin anomaly
	Amegakaryocytosis
Associated with chromosomal defects	Trisomy 13 or 18
Metabolic disorders and acquired processes	Marrow infiltration
	Malignancies
	Storage disease
	Myelofibrosis
	Aplastic anemia
	Drug-induced
Sequestration	
Hypersplenism	Hemolytic anemia, chronic
	Portal hypertension
	Glycogen storage disease

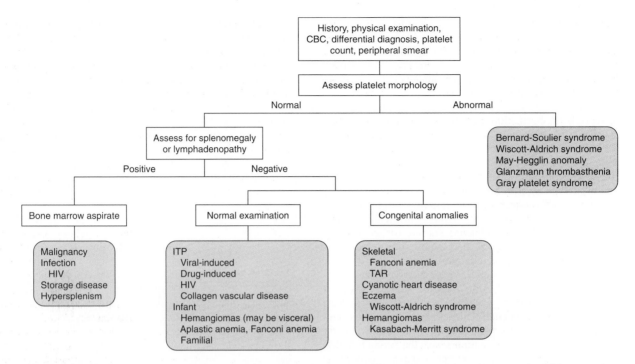

Figure 14–11. Algorithm diagramming the approach to the management of the child with isolated thrombocytopenia. CBC = complete blood count; ITP = idiopathic thrombocytopenic purpura; TAR = thrombocytopenia-absent radius syndrome.

DESTRUCTIVE THROMBOCYTOPENIA

Immune-Mediated Thrombocytopenia

The most common cause of destructive thrombocytopenia is immune-mediated platelet destruction. Shortened platelet survival can result from an IgG antibody directed against a platelet membrane antigen—either an autoantigen, or possibly neoantigen resulting from infection with a microorganism or drug exposure. IgM antibodies and complement activation are less frequently found but can also be seen in childhood immune idiopathic thrombocytopenia purpura (ITP).

Idiopathic Thrombocytopenia Purpura. ITP is an acute, self-limited disease of isolated thrombolytic thrombocytopenia that usually occurs in children aged 2–4 years; it usually resolves within 6 months. When ITP occurs in the child younger than 1 year or older than 10 years, the course is often chronic and associated with a generalized immune disorder. The otherwise healthy child presents with sudden onset of severe thrombocytopenia, manifest by petechiae, purpura, epistaxis, and, less frequently, hematuria and gastrointestinal hemorrhage. There may be a history of an antecedent viral illness within the past 1–3 weeks. Death from ITP is rare (< 1%) and usually due to intracranial hemorrhage.

Initial evaluation of the child with suspected ITP begins with a complete history and physical examination. Other than a possible antecedent illness and the acute onset of minor bleeding and bruising, the child is otherwise well. There is no hepatosplenomegaly or significant adenopathy (other than that seen with a mild viral illness). There should be no evidence of chronic disease, weight loss, fevers, or bone pain.

Review of the peripheral blood smear confirms a low platelet count, and the few remaining platelets are large. If platelet size is determined by an automated cell counter, it is elevated, consistent with young platelet age and rapid platelet destruction. The erythrocyte and leukocyte counts are normal, and there is no evidence of hemolysis or microangiopathic disease. Lymphocyte morphology may reflect the recent viral infection.

If any findings suggest another diagnosis, consideration should be given to performing bone marrow aspiration. The presence of immature megakaryocytes in normal or increased numbers in the marrow with normal erythroid and myeloid lineages confirms that the thrombocytopenia is due to increased peripheral destruction and supports the diagnosis of ITP. By convention, bone marrow aspiration is done on individuals with suspected ITP if steroids are to be part of the treatment plan, because of the small possibility that steroids may interfere with the diagnosis of leukemia.

A careful drug history should be obtained to identify agents that can cause thrombocytopenia, with particular attention to heparin, aspirin, aspirin-containing cold medications, and seizure medications. Agents that alter platelet function must be avoided. HIV infection should be considered when evaluating a patient with isolated thrombocytopenia, as this may be a first manifestation. One should screen for risk factors and test for HIV, if appropriate.

The physical examination should include particular attention to the presence of skeletal anomalies, as can be seen in thrombocytopenia-absent radius syndrome (TAR) and Fanconi anemia (short stature, radial limb dysplasia), diseases that can present with thrombocytopenia. Evidence of microangiopathic disease on the smear, fever, and central nervous system symptoms can be seen in thrombotic thrombocytopenia purpura and hemolytic uremic syndrome. Small platelets are seen in Wiscott-Aldrich syndrome, an X-linked disorder characterized by immunologic abnormalities, eczema, and recurrent infections. Patients with aplastic anemia may present initially with thrombocytopenia before progressing to pancytopenia.

A search for platelet antibodies should be conducted on all patients with acute thrombocytopenia. Assays for direct antibody measurement involve determining the antibodies coating the platelets, whereas indirect assays measure antiplatelet immunoglobulin in the plasma.

As the natural history of acute ITP is to resolve gradually and completely, the decision whether to treat the disorder becomes controversial. Many patients who have been observed carefully without pharmacologic intervention have done well. All patients and families should be counseled regarding rough play, contact sports, and the use of protective gear (helmets) and seat belts; intramuscular injections should be withheld until platelet counts increase.

For children with platelet counts below 20,000/μL, extensive oral or nasal mucosal hemorrhage, or retinal petechiae, the risk of central nervous system hemorrhage may be increased, and therapy with intravenous γ-globulin (IVIG) or corticosteroids is usually given. Treatment with IVIG, 1 g/kg over 4–6 hours, is often therapeutic. This treatment may need to be repeated 2–3 times for a total dose of 2–3 g/kg; doses should be given 24 hours apart. An increase in the platelet count is usually seen within 24–72 hours and peaks at approximately 9 days. γ-Globulin is thought to saturate the Fc receptors on the reticuloendothelial cells and therefore decrease the clearance of opsonized platelets. Side effects of IVIG are usually immediate and related to the rate of infusion and include nausea, lightheadedness, and headache. These symptoms can be alleviated with further doses by slowing the rate of infusion. Fever may also occur, and premedication with acetaminophen before the infusion is advisable.

Corticosteroids, rather than IVIG, have also been used in the medical management of ITP. Response is slightly slower than with IVIG. The usual steroid prescribed is prednisone, 1–2 mg/kg/d for 10–20 days, tapering the dosage over 2 weeks. Many patients respond to this treatment, but side effects may occur with repeated treatment or chronic use. An alternative to oral steroids has been pulse high-dose infusion of intravenous methylprednisolone. Some patients become thrombocytopenic after therapy and require retreatment. A relapse may be managed safely by observation and restriction of activity and medications, or with intermittent IVIG or pulse steroids.

If the patient has evidence of central nervous system hemorrhage and remains severely thrombocytopenic and unresponsive to IVIG and steroids, an emergency splenectomy should be considered. Continuous infusion of platelets is advised to control bleeding, and plasmapheresis should be considered, although the response is very limited.

Chronic ITP. In approximately 10–20% of children with acute ITP, chronic, persistent thrombocytopenia develops beyond 6 months. The child with chronic ITP may have an associated autoimmune disease or immunodeficiency state. Many patients with chronic ITP may not need treatment as the platelet count is often greater than 20,000/μL. Spontaneous remission can occur in these patients, and some remissions have been reported 2 years after the original diagnosis. Platelet count alone does not correlate with the risk of hemorrhage, as platelets are large and, consequently, have greater than normal procoagulant activity. In the rare patient with chronic, refractory ITP who has clinical hemorrhage or cannot tolerate the living restrictions imposed by the thrombocytopenia, splenectomy should be considered. Up to 85% of patients respond to splenectomy. Vinca alkaloids (vincristine and vinblastine), danazol, a nonvirilizing androgen, immunosuppressive agents (eg, azathioprine and cyclophosphamide), and infusion of RhoGAM, or anti-Rh (D) immunoglobulin, to individuals who are Rh-positive have been used with some success in selected patients requiring therapy. Ascorbic acid, cyclosporin, and interferon α-2β are other agents currently being investigated for use in chronic ITP.

Neonatal Alloimmune Thrombocytopenia. Neonatal alloimmune thrombocytopenia is a rare syndrome that occurs in approximately 1:5000 newborns. Immunization against platelet alloantigens can occur through either pregnancy or transfusion and can lead to severe thrombocytopenia in the fetal-newborn period, with a high risk of fatal hemorrhage. Several platelet antigens have been implicated, but the greatest number of cases can be related to PL^{A1} incompatibility. PL^{A1} is a platelet antigen that resides on the GP IIb/IIIa complex (the complex responsible for the fibrinogen receptor activity of platelets and important in aggregation and platelet-plug formation). Development of anti-PL^{A1} antibodies, therefore, not only can decrease platelet number, but can also interfere with normal platelet aggregation, resulting in a qualitative defect in the platelets in addition to thrombocytopenia. This likely explains the high incidence of serious bleeding in these infants after birth or in utero as compared with infants born to mothers with ITP who have antibodies that are not directed against PL^{A1}.

The typical presentation of the affected infant is an otherwise healthy newborn, without perinatal complications and with a normal maternal hematologic history, in whom petechiae, purpura, and extreme thrombocytopenia develop. For a mother with a previous low platelet count, the differential diagnosis includes maternal autoimmune or drug-dependent thrombocytopenia, infection, and preeclampsia. The infant who has birth asphyxia, infection, or congenital bone marrow hypoplasia, or who is premature, can also be thrombocytopenic. The presence of hepatosplenomegaly, intrauterine growth retardation, or intracranial calcifications with thrombocytopenia suggests a congenital viral infection. However, it is also important to exclude alloimmune thrombocytopenia by appropriate immunologic testing in these infants, as there is a potential recurrence of this complication in future pregnancies.

Most affected infants are first-born offspring, suggesting that antigenic exposure occurs early in pregnancy. The incidence of death and serious central nervous system disease is 10–15%, and many of these infants have had prenatal or perinatal intracranial hemorrhage. Evidence of intrauterine intracranial hemorrhage can be made by ultrasound. Even a platelet count less than 50,000/μL warrants concern, especially if the infant was born by vaginal delivery. Complications of early central nervous system hemorrhage include hydrocephalus, porencephaly, seizures, and fetal loss. Hyperbilirubinemia may occur owing to resolution of intracranial or intraorgan hemorrhage.

The thrombocytopenia is transient, lasting up to 4–6 weeks after delivery. An early platelet alloantigen evaluation of the newborn and parents is important, both to offer the affected infant treatment and to prevent such devastating complications with future pregnancies. Platelet typing should be done on the mother and father, looking for antigens responsible for alloimmunization in particular, as well as other platelet antigens frequently involved in alloimmune thrombocytopenia. The serum from the mother and infant should also be screened for antiplatelet antibodies. Studies should be done with maternal plasma and paternal or neonatal platelets to screen for antibodies.

Several treatment options are available for the infant with neonatal alloimmunization. Transfusion with antigen-negative platelets has been the mainstay of treatment. Because PL^A1 antigen-negative platelets are present in only 2% of the population, the most available source of platelets is from the mother. Random platelets may provide a transient increase, lasting 1–2 days, and should be used in cases of serious hemorrhage while antigen-negative platelets are being obtained and prepared. An alternative treatment is the administration of IVIG. The recommended dose is 1 g/kg/d for 1–3 days until the platelet count is 50,000–100,000/μL. Platelet transfusion may still be necessary with IVIG if immediate correction of the thrombocytopenia is needed.

A mother who has had one infant with neonatal alloimmune thrombocytopenia is at high risk for having subsequent infants with the same disease. The severity of antenatal and perinatal hemorrhage is also increased. Maternal antiplatelet antibody titers cannot be used to predict affected fetuses accurately. Fetal cord blood samples should be obtained periodically for determination of the platelet count starting at about 20 weeks of gestation, with ultrasound monitoring for hemorrhage. Studies done on mothers treated with IVIG 1 g/kg/w from midgestation until near term have shown increases in fetal platelet count in most cases; this approach should be considered. Delivery should be planned near term with an elective cesarean section or by planned induced vaginal delivery after documented increase in fetal platelet count after administration of maternal IVIG. Antigen-negative platelets should be obtained and prepared before delivery in the event of extreme thrombocytopenia or hemorrhage. The mother can undergo platelet phoresis before to delivery to obtain PL^A1-negative platelets. The infant's platelet count should be checked at birth and every 6–12 hours for 1–2 days, then daily, and be kept at or greater than 20,000/μL.

Drug-Induced Thrombocytopenia

In addition to immune-mediated mechanisms for thrombocytopenia induced by drugs, many bone marrow–suppressive agents used in chemotherapy cause thrombocytopenia, usually in the face of pancytopenia. Management is usually with platelet transfusion to prevent or treat bleeding. The bone marrow effects of these agents define their dose-limiting toxicities, and thrombocytopenia is a common and anticipated problem. These patients usually respond well to platelet transfusion, but their condition can become refractory because of the underlying illness, organomegaly and sequestration, sepsis, and other medications.

Non–Immune-Mediated Platelet Consumption

Several non–immune-mediated processes involve increased platelet consumption. Generalized platelet activation with trapping of microaggregates in the small vasculature contributes to the microangiopathic hemolytic anemia occurring in the hemolytic uremic syndrome and thrombotic thrombocytopenia purpura. Increased use of platelets may occur in active bleeding or infection. In disseminated intravascular coagulation (DIC), there is an imbalance between intravascular thrombosis and fibrinolysis, with increased platelet consumption, depletion of plasma clotting factors, and formation of fibrin. DIC can be activated by many etiologic events, including sepsis due to bacteria, viruses, or fungi; malignancy, particularly acute promyelocytic leukemia and neuroblastoma; hemolytic transfusion reactions; and trauma. Therapy is aimed at the underlying etiologic process; supportive care consists of platelet transfusion and plasma protein replenishment (cryoprecipitate, fresh-frozen plasma).

Thrombocytopenia can occur in the sick newborn for many reasons, most commonly infection, prematurity, asphyxia, respiratory distress syndrome, pulmonary hypertension, or meconium aspiration. These infants appear to have normal to increased platelet production but a decreased platelet life span for reasons that are unclear. Thrombocytopenia is a frequent occurrence in congenital cyanotic heart disease associated with compensatory polycythemia. Therapeutic phlebotomy may lessen the thrombocytopenia.

The association between thrombocytopenia and giant hemangiomas occurs in the infant with Kasabach-Merritt syndrome. The hemangiomas may be multiple and may involve only viscera. Therefore, in an infant with unexplained thrombocytopenia, imaging studies should be done to look for a vascular anomaly. Hemangiomas are proliferative lesions that grow rapidly for several months and then regress spontaneously. Platelet thrombi may develop in these lesions, and platelet life span may be decreased. These infants may also have a consumptive coagulopathy with low fibrinogen levels and elevated concentrations of fibrin degradation products. The lesions are prone to necrosis and infection. The size or location of a particular hemangioma cannot predict whether it will lead to platelet trapping and thrombocytopenia. These infants should be managed by close observation and hematologic monitoring, waiting for regression to occur. However, the lesions may become large enough to compromise the infant (impinge on the airway or vital organs, lead to compartment syndrome) resulting in serious illness or death. Corticosteroid treatment may be beneficial in a dose of 1–2 mg/kg/d until regression of the lesion and normalization of the platelet count occur, with subsequent tapering. Recently, interferon-α2 has been reported to be beneficial in correcting the platelet count and shrinking the lesion; it has been given in doses of 1–3 million U/m^2/d. This treatment, used alone or in combination with steroids, is under further investigation. Supportive transfusion therapy may be necessary when the infant is at risk of hemorrhage; platelet transfusions are given 1–2 times daily, as are plasma and cryoprecipitate if there is fibrinogen consumption. Antiplatelet medications (aspirin and dipyridamole) have been used to interfere with platelet trapping within the hemangioma, but they carry the risk of causing platelet destruction in addition to the thrombocytopenia.

THROMBOCYTOPENIA FROM DECREASED PLATELET PRODUCTION

Congenital amegakaryocytic thrombocytopenia, a rare cause of neonatal thrombocytopenia, may be caused by a congenital viral infection or an inherited disorder or may be idiopathic. Cytomegalovirus, rubella, and HIV all have been associated with hypoproductive thrombocytopenia. Neutropenia and anemia are often associated findings. The TAR syndrome is an autosomal-recessive disorder with variable thrombocytopenia despite normal erythroid and myeloid lineages. Many patients are transfusion dependent but may experience a spontaneous increase in megakaryocytopoiesis after 1 year of age. Fanconi anemia is another inherited disorder with both skeletal anomalies and hy-

poproductive thrombocytopenia, although other cell lines are affected. The cytopenia begins in early to late childhood and is associated with chromosomal instability. Infants with hypoproductive states without evidence of skeletal abnormalities may have other reasons for isolated thrombocytopenia, including Wiscott-Aldrich syndrome, viral infection, or an inherited giant platelet syndrome, such as the May-Hegglin anomaly or Bernard-Soulier syndrome. Evaluation of the peripheral smear and possibly a bone marrow aspirate may help confirm the diagnosis. Bone marrow transplantation, when a suitable HLA donor is available, should be considered for these disorders.

QUALITATIVE ABNORMALITIES OF THE PLATELETS

A number of molecular defects in platelet GP, receptors, and granules have been described and have furthered our understanding of platelet function. Some drugs and certain acquired metabolic conditions, such as renal failure, can affect platelet function.

The most useful screening test for qualitative platelet disorders in a patient with a normal platelet count is the bleeding time, which measures the length of time required for a platelet plug to form and cease bleeding from a small cut. This process requires normal platelet adhesion, activation, and aggregation in addition to normal vascular endothelium. In syndromes with defective blood vessels, such as Ehlers-Danlos and Marfan, the bleeding time may be prolonged despite normal platelet function. Also important is review of a peripheral blood smear with regard to platelet size and morphology. A number of congenital qualitative disorders are associated with either small or large platelets. Specific platelet aggregation studies can be done to measure the formation of platelet clumps in response to a variety of stimuli, which usually include ADP, epinephrine, collagen, arachidonic acid, and ristocetin. Normal agglutination requires that the platelet secretory granules (dense, α, lysosomes) respond appropriately to the stimulus. An intact platelet membrane and presence of normal GP and receptors are also necessary. These platelet reactions also initiate the coagulation cascade.

CONGENITAL DISORDERS OF PLATELET FUNCTION

Glanzmann Thrombasthenia

Glanzmann thrombasthenia is an autosomal-recessive disorder, with a normal platelet count and morphology, in which platelet deficient-type bleeding occurs (ie, epistaxis, petechiae, ecchymoses, menorrhagia, and gastrointestinal and mucous-membrane bleeding). The surface-membrane GP IIb and IIIa are decreased (partially or completely), leading to inadequate platelet-plug formation. On platelet aggregation studies, platelet aggregation is completely absent with all agonists. The diagnosis can be confirmed by documenting the absence of GP IIb/IIIa by sodium dodecyl sulfate polyacrylamide gel electrophoresis. The treatment of severe hemorrhage is platelet transfusion. Isoantibodies against the GP IIb/IIIa protein complex can develop in these patients after platelet transfusion, which limits the benefit of platelet transfusion.

Bernard-Soulier Syndrome

This syndrome is an autosomal-recessive disorder characterized by mild thrombocytopenia, very large platelets (5–6 μ), and a clinical syndrome of easy bruising and severe hemorrhage after trauma or surgery. These patients have deficiencies in the platelet GP Ib/IX and GP V. Challenge with ristocetin in platelet aggregation studies is abnormal, because the presence of von Willebrand factor and GP Ib is necessary for this stimulant. Treatment is the use of platelet transfusion at times of bleeding, but isoantibodies may develop against the glycoproteins missing from their own platelets and present on the transfused platelets.

Wiscott-Aldrich Syndrome

The Wiscott-Aldrich syndrome is a rare X-linked recessive disorder characterized by thrombocytopenia, very small platelets, severe eczema, and immunodeficiency. The clinical features, in particular the eczema and immune deficiency, may be mild at birth but become florid by 6–12 months of age. Management of these patients includes aggressive local therapy for the eczema, treatment of infections, and ultimately bone marrow transplantation.

PLATELET GRANULE DEFECTS

Platelets may be dysfunctional because of deficient granule content or lack of release of their contents on activation. Several families have been reported with severe forms of platelet-dense granule deficiency, also known as storage pool deficiency, reflecting an absence of ADP and ATP in the granules. Another rare defect involves absence of the contents of the α granules, resulting in a gray appearance of the platelet on Wright-stained smears. The gray platelet syndrome appears to be a result of a lack of packaging of the contents rather than lack of synthesis of the platelet-specific proteins. These patients can also have myelofibrosis caused by local effects of platelet-derived growth factor.

DRUG-INDUCED PLATELET DYSFUNCTION

A number of drugs impair platelet function, in particular aspirin and other nonsteroidal anti-inflammatory agents. Acetylsalicylic acid is a potent, irreversible inhibitor of the cyclooxygenase enzyme. When normal platelets are stimulated with an agonist (eg, ADP, epinephrine) arachidonic acid is released from the platelet membrane and then converted by cyclooxygenase to thromboxane A_2, a potent stimulant of platelet aggregation. Prostacyclin (PGI_2), an inhibitor of platelet aggregation, is released from the endothelial cells by the same mechanism. A balance exists between the platelet stimulatory effects of thromboxane production by platelets and the inhibitory effects of prostacyclin formation by the vascular endothelium. Aspirin interferes at both sites, and its effects on the platelets are permanent, for the duration of their life span (7–10 days). Aspirin in doses of 5–10 mg/kg causes a slightly prolonged bleeding time, without clinical sequelae. Individuals with mild intrinsic platelet defects may be particularly sensitive to an aspirin challenge, as measured by bleeding time before and after ingestion. Several nonsteroidal anti-inflammatory agents may also affect platelet function, although their inhibitory effects on platelet cyclooxygenase are reversed approximately 6 hours after removal of the drug. Anti-inflammatory agents that do not inhibit platelet function include choline salicylate and sodium salicylate.

SYSTEMIC DISEASES ASSOCIATED WITH PLATELET ABNORMALITIES

Uremia and chronic liver disease have been associated with severe hemorrhage and platelet dysfunction. Uremic patients have prolonged bleeding times and abnormal platelet aggregation, although the precise mechanism is unknown. The platelet receptor Ib may be defective, or there may be an inhibition of the platelet von Willebrand factor and GP Ib receptor interaction in uremic patients. These patients usually have normal or increased von Willebrand factor with normal activity. Nevertheless, administration of DDAVP (1-deamino-18-D-arginine vasopressin) increases levels of von Willebrand factor and transiently corrects the bleeding time. The bleeding time may also be corrected with cryoprecipitate infusion. Dialysis is a necessary part of the treatment of uremic patients; should they require surgery, they should undergo dialysis and receive DDAVP or cryoprecipitate to reduce the risk of hemorrhage.

Patients with liver disease have a multifactorial bleeding diathesis. Synthesis of all the plasma coagulation factors is markedly decreased. These patients may have associated portal hypertension with splenomegaly and shortened platelet survival. In addition, they may have an abnormality of platelet function, which may be transiently corrected with DDAVP or platelet transfusion.

HEMOSTASIS

Hemostasis requires the coordinate interaction between platelets, vascular endothelial cells, and plasma clotting factors. Hemostatic mechanisms can be classified into primary and secondary. In primary hemostasis, the platelets serve an important function in conjunction with the vascular endothelial cells. The clinical disorders that are associated with abnormalities of primary hemostasis are vascular abnormalities, qualitative abnormalities of the platelets, and VWD. An aberration in primary hemostasis is characterized by bleeding of the mucous membranes, epistaxis, and superficial ecchymoses. Typical manifestations are prolonged oozing from minor wounds or abrasions, or abnormal intraoperative bleeding. Abnormalities of secondary hemostasis are most frequently the result of coagulation factor deficiencies. Bleeding characteristically occurs from large vessels with subcutaneous, palpable hematomas, hemarthroses, or intramuscular hematomas. Patients with severe factor VIII or IX deficiency may bleed after trauma or surgery but may also have spontaneous bleeding.

History

Assessment of the child with a suspected or known bleeding diathesis begins with a complete history. A summary of important points in the history of the child with a bleeding disorder is presented in Table 14–13. The nature of the bleeding should be explored, with particular attention to location, duration, and frequency and the measures necessary to stop it. A previous history of bleeding associated with events such as trauma or surgery, dental extraction, circumcision, appendectomy, and tonsillectomy is also important. Inquiry should be made into a history of rash (petechial) or arthritis, with hemarthrosis, and of blood transfusion. The first episode of bleeding should be documented, and a careful history of bruising during the

Table 14–13. Obtaining a bleeding history.

Medical history
  Spontaneous bleeding
    Age of onset
    Bruising, petechiae (location)
    Joint bleeding, muscle bleeding
    Mucous membrane bleeding (epistaxis)
  Induced bleeding
    Injuries
      Duration of bleeding, nature of injuries
      Wound healing
      History of transfusions
    Surgical procedures
      Circumcision
      Tonsillectomy and adenoidectomy
      Dental work
      Appendectomy
  Menstrual history (duration and amount)
  Medications (over-the-counter, prescription, aspirin)
Family history
  Known bleeding diathesis
  Excessive hemorrhage after childbirth
  Gender of affected members
  Prepare family tree

toddler age is important. In girls, the duration and severity of menstrual bleeding should be documented.

A family history and pedigree are crucial, as many bleeding disorders are hereditary (see Chapter 5).

The history should also address the use of over-the-counter and prescription drugs that can induce bleeding. The most common offender is aspirin; it is important to ask the patient specifically about the use of medications for colds, sinus trouble, muscle aches, or headaches, as these drugs may contain aspirin. Some antibiotics, penicillin in particular, can affect platelet function or be associated with specific inhibitors of clotting. Anticonvulsants can cause thrombocytopenia, and procainamide has been associated with an acquired lupus anticoagulant.

Physical Examination

In addition to the routine examination, the skin should be scrutinized carefully for petechiae, purpura, and venous telangiectasias. The joints should be examined for swelling or chronic changes, such as contractures or distorted appearance with asymmetry related to repeated bleeding episodes. Mucosal surfaces, such as the gingiva and nares, should be examined for bleeding.

Laboratory Evaluation

An attempt should be made to classify the bleeding abnormality as being related to primary or secondary hemostasis. The following tests provide most of the information needed to make a laboratory diagnosis of a bleeding diathesis: examination of the peripheral smear, platelet count, bleeding time, prothrombin time (PT), partial thromboplastin time (PTT), and thrombin time (TT). Confirmatory tests include specific coagulation factor assays, fibrin degradation products, fragment F1.2, fibrinogen, inhibitor assays, and multimeric analysis of the factor VIII complex. The laboratory evaluation of the child with bleeding is presented in Figure 14–12.

The peripheral smear should be examined for morphology and number of platelets. It can also provide evidence of microangiopathic hemolytic anemia. The bleeding time is the single best test for evaluating primary hemostasis, as it requires a normal platelet count and normal platelet function in addition to normal vascular integrity. Patients with abnormal bleeding times may be thrombocytopenic, have qualitative platelet abnormalities (inherited or acquired), or have VWD. If bleeding time is abnormal, further studies include platelet aggregation studies and quantification of the components of the factor VIII complex (factor VIII:Ag, factor VIII:C, and factor VIII:RCoF). The bleeding time is not determined in a patient with a platelet count less than 50,000/µL, as it is expected to be abnormal.

Measurement of PT evaluates the extrinsic system of secondary hemostasis (factors VII, X, V, II, fibrinogen). Factor VII is unique to the extrinsic system, and PT is prolonged with a normal PTT in isolated factor VII deficiency. Factor VII is the first coagulation factor to be affected by oral anticoagulants, so PT is an excellent test for

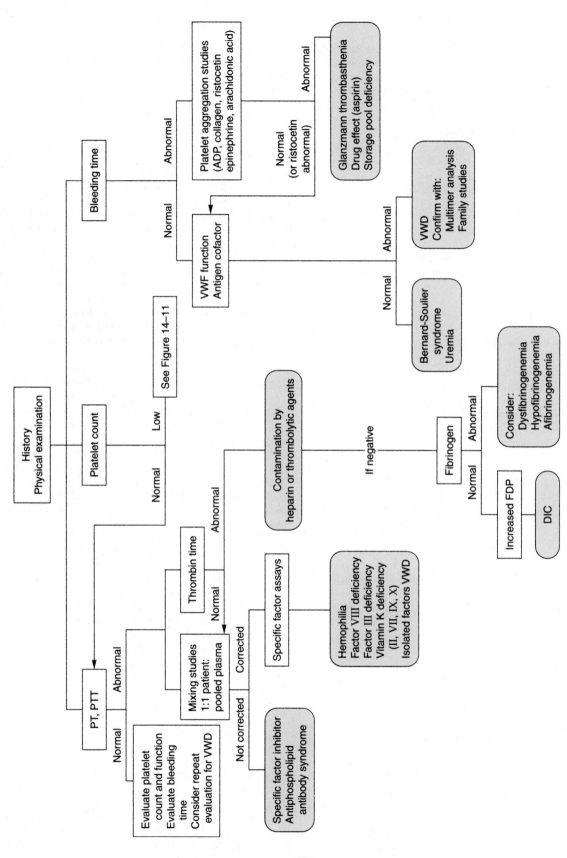

Figure 14–12. Algorithm diagramming the laboratory evaluation of the child with bleeding. ADP = adenosine diphosphate; DIC = disseminated intravascular coagulation; FDP = fibrin degradation products; PT = prothrombin time; PTT = partial prothrombin time; VWD = von Willebrand disease; VWF = von Willebrand factor.

monitoring oral anticoagulant therapy. Deficiencies in factors VII, X, V, II (prothrombin), or fibrinogen cause a prolongation of PT.

The partial thromboplastin time assesses the integrity of the intrinsic system of coagulation. For PTT to be normal, the coagulation factors involved need to be present with at least 30% activity. Patients with a normal PT but an abnormally elevated PTT typically have deficiencies of the factors unique to the intrinsic system (factors XII, XI, VIII, and IX, Fletcher factor, and Fitzgerald factor). Patients with the lupus anticoagulant can also have a normal PT but a prolonged PTT. PTT is widely used for monitoring heparin therapy, and a time 1.5–2.5 times longer than the upper limit of the normal range is desired for heparinization.

Thrombin time is abnormal when the plasma level of fibrinogen is decreased, when the fibrinogen is dysfunctional (hereditary or acquired), or when there are circulating anticoagulants (heparin) or fibrin degradation products. A modified thrombin test, because of its extreme sensitivity to heparin, is frequently used as a control for heparin contamination in assessing the coagulation status of the patient.

In the approach to the patient with a prolonged PTT, a circulating anticoagulant should be considered as the cause. To evaluate for an inhibitor, a 1:1 mixture of the patient's plasma and normal pooled plasma is prepared, and the PTT repeated. If the PTT is not corrected, the presence of an inhibitor can be assumed. If the PTT corrects, a deficiency of one or more coagulation factors probably exists, and specific factor assays should be performed. Some inhibitors are time dependent, such as factor VIII, and an incubation period before the PTT can assist in the diagnosis. The most frequent inhibitor encountered is heparin, and the second most frequent is the lupus anticoagulant. This inhibitor is present in 10% of patients with systemic lupus erythematosus, but lupus anticoagulant is common in patients with no evidence of underlying collagen vascular disease. Paradoxically, this anticoagulant is associated with clinical thrombosis rather than hemorrhage in up to 30% of patients. Therefore, an attempt to identify the nature of the anticoagulant is important. The anticardiolipin antibody test and lupus anticoagulant test can help with this distinction.

INHERITED BLEEDING DIATHESES

Von Willebrand Disease

Von Willebrand disease is a common, heterogeneous disorder of a thoroughly characterized GP called von Willebrand factor. This GP is responsible for the adherence of platelets to damaged endothelium and for the transport of factor VIII in the circulation. VWD is usually inherited in an autosomal codominant manner, but at least two variants of this disorder have been recognized: a rare autosomal-recessive form and an X-linked recessive type. The heterogeneity results from a variety of genetic defects, ranging from congenital absence of the von Willebrand protein to major dysproteinemias in which the molecular structure is abnormal. Von Willebrand factor is a large multimeric GP that is synthesized in megakaryocytes and endothelial cells. The activation of either endothelial cells or platelets at local sites results in a greatly increased local concentration of von Willebrand factor, thereby facilitating normal hemostasis. Desmopressin (DDAVP) can induce the release of von Willebrand factor from storage sites in the platelets and increase plasma levels in those whose levels were previously decreased. Once the von Willebrand factor causes the platelets to adhere via its GP Ib receptor, these platelets are activated, with subsequent recruitment of more platelets and platelet plug formation. Absence of von Willebrand factor leads to insufficient formation of both the platelet plug and fibrin clot. Von Willebrand factor also serves as a carrier protein for the plasma factor VIII molecule, and deficiency of this factor also results in a secondary deficiency of factor VIII. Infusion of plasma from patients deficient in factor VIII causes an increase in the factor VIII level in patients with VWD because hemophiliac plasma contains von Willebrand factor.

The clinical picture is variable, depending on whether the defect is a quantitative or qualitative deficiency of the von Willebrand factor. Males and females are similarly affected, and symptoms can be mild or as severe as hemophilia. There are several subtypes, categorized on the basis of factor VIII levels (antigen, Ristocetin cofactor, von Willebrand factor) and multimer structure. Those affected with VWD have mucocutaneous bleeding and posttraumatic and postsurgical bleeding. VWD should be suspected in the patient with platelet-type bleeding and a family history of a bleeding diathesis. The laboratory evaluation is summarized in Figure 14–12.

Treatment of VWD requires knowledge of the clinical subtype. Desmopressin is the treatment of choice in mild type I disease (the most common form) and may be of benefit with some of the other variants. However, desmopressin is contraindicated in certain variants (type IIB) as it may cause thrombocytopenia due to platelet activation and fail to generate a therapeutic response. A therapeutic trial of desmopressin is usually given with measurement of the bleeding time, PTT, and factor VIII levels before and after administration. A standard dose of 0.3 μg/kg is administered intravenously over 15–30 minutes, and follow-up studies are done 30–60 minutes after the infusion is completed. Patients who have severe VWD or the type IIB variant, or who are unresponsive to the desmopressin challenge, require replacement of von Willebrand factor from plasma-derived sources for bleeding episodes. Currently, no genetically engineered products are available. Humate P, a commonly used concentrate, has normal multimeric structure of von Willebrand factor and nearly normal levels of the protein. Treatment with factor concentrate is based on attaining a factor VIII level of 30–50%, with 1 IU/kg body weight of von Willebrand factor required to increase the plasma level by 2 IU/dL. If treatment is required for a prolonged period (eg, after trauma or surgery), treatment with desmopressin can result in tachyphylaxis and is therefore alternated with factor concentrate. Antifibrinolytics, such as epsilon amino caproic acid, are often used for oral bleeding and as an adjunct to therapy with dental surgery.

Hemophilia A, Factor VIII Deficiency

Classic hemophilia, or hemophilia A, is the most common hereditary clotting factor deficiency. The recessive gene is located on the X chromosome and linked closely to the genes for color blindness and G6PD. The disorder results from the deficiency of factor VIII antigen (factor VIII:Ag), a small subunit of the factor VIII molecule. Female carriers are usually unaffected, and the disease is seen almost exclusively in the male population.

Clinically, the first indication that a bleeding disorder is present may be from hemorrhage after circumcision or separation of the umbilical cord. However, a number of affected male infants have no difficulty during the neonatal period, and a negative history of bleeding after circumcision does not rule out the diagnosis of hemophilia. Mild hemophilia may go unsuspected for years until the patient experiences trauma or has a surgical procedure. Hemorrhage can occur spontaneously and be internal or external. Large hematomas can result in secondary conditions, such as hemarthrosis, disability, and joint degeneration. Significant blood loss can occur with muscular bleeds, and the leading cause of death is intracranial hemorrhage.

The diagnosis of factor VIII deficiency should be suspected in males with bleeding characteristic of factor deficiency, a family history of males with bleeding diatheses, and abnormal clotting studies (prolonged PTT). It can be confirmed by specific factor assays. The clinical severity range depends on the level of factor VIII present. A patient with mild hemophilia (factor VIII level, 10–30%) may experience bleeding only with surgery or trauma. Moderate hemophilia (factor VIII level, 2–10%) can be associated with severe hemorrhage after trauma, or occasionally with spontaneous hemorrhage. Spontaneous joint and soft tissue bleeding is characteristic of severe hemophilia (factor VIII level, 0–1%).

Treatment of patients with hemophilia and bleeding is by replacement of factor in a concentrated form. Many preparations are available, including recombinant products. Duration, frequency, and dosages of the treatments depend on the severity of the hemophilia and bleeding episode.

In all children with hemophilia, in addition to replacement of appropriate factor levels when bleeding has occurred and use of physical therapy programs to prevent or minimize chronic joint disease, comprehensive medical care must be given. Immunizations to prevent hepatitis B should be given as soon as possible after birth; appropriate consideration and screening procedures for HIV, prophylactic dental care, and aggressive management of hemarthrosis are required. Emotional support is essential to assist patients and families to cope with the emotional and social burden imposed by the disease. Prevention of chronic joint complications is crucial for the health and well-being of patients with hemophilia, and home care treatment should be used when possible.

Unfortunately, in approximately 10% of patients with severe hemophilia, antibody develops to administered concentrate containing the specific factor required for treatment. This prevents response to therapy and requires specific steps, such as consideration of immunosuppressive therapy, exchange transfusion, administration of prothrombin complex, and, in most cases, administration of sufficient factor product to block circulating antibody and still provide procoagulant activity.

Hemophilia B, Factor IX Deficiency

Factor IX deficiency is inherited as an X-linked recessive trait and is much less common than factor VIII deficiency, accounting for 12% of all patients with hemophilia. The clinical findings and initial evaluation are similar to factor VIII deficiency, although factor IX deficiency can be milder. Treatment of acute bleeding episodes is with specific factor concentrate. During the initial evaluation of a bleeding patient, if the identity of the specific coagulation factor deficiency has not been made, fresh-frozen plasma can be used to stop hemorrhage, as it contains all of the clotting factors.

Hemophilia C, Factor XI Deficiency

This coagulation defect is transmitted as an autosomal-recessive trait and occurs in both sexes, primarily in patients of Jewish ancestry. The homozygotes can have severe factor XI deficiency although the clinical manifestations are milder than those in patients with factor VIII or IX deficiency. Bleeding episodes can be managed by infusion of 10 mL/kg of fresh-frozen plasma.

Factor XIII Deficiency (Fibrin-Stabilizing Factor)

This coagulation abnormality is unique in that the patient presents with bleeding soon after birth similar to the types seen with classical hemophilia. However, standard laboratory assays such as PT, PTT, and TT are normal. A high index of suspicion is essential to establish the diagnosis, which can be accomplished by determining the solubility of the patient's clot in 5-M urea. Normal clots are insoluble because of the action of fibrin-stabilizing factor. Clots from patients with this deficiency are readily dissolved. The disorder can be treated with plasma infusions.

Other Rare Coagulation Abnormalities

α_2-Antiplasmin deficiency, factor XII deficiency, prekallikrein deficiency (Fletcher factor), high–molecular-weight kininogen (Fitzgerald factor) deficiency, hereditary afibrinogenemia or dysfibrinogenemia, and deficiencies of isolated prothrombin as well as factors V, VII, and X have all been identified using appropriate clotting measurements. Prekallikrein deficiency, high–molecular-weight kininogen deficiency, and factor XII deficiency all cause laboratory abnormalities but are not associated with clinical hemorrhage.

EVALUATION OF THE PATIENT WITH THROMBOSIS

Thrombotic disease and its complications are more prevalent in adults than in children. However, several inherited and acquired deficiencies of the physiologic inhibitors of coagulation can predispose the child to thrombosis; a search for these is required to initiate proper therapy. Quite possibly, the infrequency of reports of these disorders in children is because they are not usually considered in the differential diagnosis. Thromboses are occasionally seen with vascular stasis, malignancies, homocystinemia, renal disease, infection, and severe inflammatory disease and in patients with lupus anticoagulant.

The hemostatic system involves a balance between clot formation and clot lysis. Increase in the coagulation component without concomitant increase in clot lysis results in thrombosis. Alternatively, decrease in clot lysis without decrease in hemostasis results in thrombosis. Consideration of these physiologic events is necessary to identify defects resulting in thrombosis and to design appropriate interventions. In the child who does not have signs of systemic illness but presents with a thrombotic episode, a hereditary deficiency of a natural anticoagulant should be considered. The most common of these are the autosomal-dominant deficiencies of AT-III, heparin cofactor II, protein C, protein S, dysfibrinogenemia, and the autosomal-recessive defects of plasminogen (see Table 14–14).

Thrombosis can occur in certain heterozygotes. The premature infant, who has limited ability to synthesize many of these factors, may be at particular risk. Thrombosis is rare in the pediatric population but occurs most commonly in the second decade. The thrombosis may be spontaneous, induced by trauma, or associated with an indwelling catheter or mechanical valve. The diagnosis of a deep venous thrombosis is often suspected clinically but should be confirmed by Doppler ultrasound or computed tomographic imaging. If the venous thrombosis is thought to be recent (within 72 hours), thrombolytic therapy with urokinase should be started immediately and, if possible, be delivered in high dose in close proximity to the clot. Otherwise, systemic therapy can be administered. Anticoagulation may start with fibrinolytic therapy or afterward, depending on the size and location of the thrombus and the response to treatment. If the clot is thought to have been present 3–7 days or longer, treatment should proceed with anticoagulation with intravenous heparin. Conventional therapy is a 5 to 7-day course of intravenous heparin, followed by a warfarin-type oral anticoagulant. More recently, low–molecular-weight (LMW) heparin has been used successfully in adults and is being studied in pediatrics. It has been used safely and successfully in the neonatal and pediatric populations. LMW heparin is a promising alternative to oral anticoagulation with Coumadin, as it is safe and easy to administer (subcutaneous, daily or twice daily), has few side effects, and is easy to monitor (anti–factor Xa levels). Studies are in progress to determine optimal doses and clinical indications.

Early therapy of deep venous thrombosis is essential to prevent pulmonary embolus. If clinically suspected, however, appropriate studies should be obtained immediately (ventilation and perfusion scans, chest radiograph). Thrombolytic therapy and anticoagulation should start immediately. Duration of anticoagulant therapy is dependent on the underlying diagnosis, site of thrombus, and response to therapy but is usually at least 3–6 months.

Acquired disorders of coagulation can result in thrombotic disease. Conditions in which coagulation factor deficiencies are present, either because of lack of production or increased consumption, include vitamin K deficiency (newborn, liver disease, sepsis, chronic illness, malnutrition, prolonged antibiotic use), disseminated intravascular coagulation, cyanotic congenital heart disease with associated polycythemia, Kasabach-Merritt syndrome, and acquired inhibitors of hemostatic proteins (often related to infection or malignancy).

Therapy for these hereditary or acquired disorders can include replacement of the deficient or defective protein, fibrinolytic intervention to attempt to dissolve an existing clot, anticoagulant therapy with heparin or warfarin, and antiplatelet therapy. Decisions for specific therapy require a precise diagnosis and clinical assessment. Interventions in sick premature infants who have sepsis, or in children who exhibit postinfectious purpura fulminans, may require combinations of these approaches as well as coagulation factors to replace those that have been consumed. Acquired defects in clotting, such as the lupus anticoagulant (described above), may also require long-term anticoagulant therapy on the basis of the patient's clinical profile.

Table 14–14. Alterations of coagulation proteins associated with a prethrombotic state.

Deficiency	Screening Available
Antithrombin III deficiency	Functional assay of antithrombin III (heparin cofactor assay)
Protein C deficiency	Immunologic and functional assays of protein C
Protein S deficiency	Immunologic assays of total and free protein S
Dysfibrinogenemias	Screen for dysfibrinogenemias (immunologic and functional assays of fibrinogen, thrombin time)
Plasminogen deficiency	Fibrinolytic assays
Diminished plasminogen activator activity	Fibrinolytic assays
Lupus anticoagulant	Anticardiolipin antibody Lupus anticoagulant antibody

REFERENCES

Bain B (editor): *Blood Cells: A Practical Guide.* Lippincott, 1989.

Hoffman B et al (editors): *Hematology: Basic Principles and Practice,* 2nd ed. Churchill Livingstone, 1995.

Mentzer WC, Wagner GM (editors): *The Hereditary Hemolytic Anemias.* Churchill Livingstone, 1989.

Nathan DG, Oski FA (editors): *Hematology of Infancy and Childhood,* 4th ed. Saunders, 1993.

Reid CD et al (editors): *Management and Therapy of Sickle Cell Disease,* 3rd ed. National Institutes of Health, 1995.

15

Oncology

Carol A. Diamond, MD

Every year in the United States, cancer is diagnosed in about 6500 children aged younger than 15 years. Cancer is second to accidents as the most common cause of death in children; even so, more than 60% of children in whom cancer is diagnosed will survive. With more sophisticated approaches to the biologic analysis of malignancy and improved methods of disease evaluation and treatment, increased long-term survival with fewer side effects is expected. This chapter provides a basic introduction to our current understanding and practice of pediatric oncology.

LEUKEMIA

Acute leukemia is the most common malignancy in children, accounting for nearly 30% of all childhood cancer. Each year, about 2000 new cases are diagnosed in the United States. About 80% are of the lymphoblastic type; the remainder are nonlymphoblastic. Chronic leukemias are rare in children and are not discussed here.

ACUTE LYMPHOBLASTIC LEUKEMIA

The past 20 years have seen impressive progress in the successful treatment of children with acute lymphoblastic leukemia (ALL). This is due to better classification schemas, better understanding of the molecular biology of leukemia, and more aggressive treatment regimens.

Incidence & Epidemiology

The incidence of ALL is 4:100,000 children before age 15 years and peaks at age 4 years. ALL is more common in whites than in blacks and more common in boys than in girls.

Etiology

The exact etiology of ALL is unknown, but many predisposing genetic, environmental, viral, and immunologic factors have been suggested. For example, an increased risk of leukemia has been noted after ionizing radiation. In addition, siblings of affected children have an increased risk, as do children with abnormal chromosomes, such as trisomy 21, Fanconi, and Bloom syndromes. Oncogenes in association with chromosomal abnormalities are likely to be important in leukemogenesis.

Biologic Classification

Acute lymphoblastic leukemia is a heterogeneous disease, both clinically and biologically. Lymphoblast morphology, surface antigen populations, cytogenetic abnormalities, cytochemical staining characteristics, and clinical features are all considered in classifying children into specific risk groups. The French-American-British (FAB) cooperative working group established a universally accepted classification system on the basis of cellular morphologic characteristics. This system classifies cells into three groups—L1, L2, and L3 (Table 15–1). Patients with L1 cells have the best prognosis; the prognosis is worse among those with L2 and poorest among those with L3. Cell-surface antigens, determined by flow cytometry, have been useful not only in helping us understand the etiology of leukemia but also in prognosticating outcome.

Most cases of ALL arise from the monoclonal proliferation of B cell–committed progenitors. Those that are not derived from B cell–committed progenitors show various stages of intrathymic differentiation. Patients with T-cell ALL tend to be older boys with initial high white blood cell counts and more lymphomatous features, such as mediastinal masses, renal infiltrates, and pronounced adenopathy. The outcome for patients is best with early pre–B cell leukemia, intermediate for those with T-cell or pre–B cell leukemia, and worst for those with B-cell leukemia.

Cytogenetic abnormalities independently affect prognosis in ALL. Specific abnormalities, including abnormal

Table 15–1. French-American-British morphologic classification for acute lymphoblastic leukemia (ALL).

L1	Lymphoblasts with scanty cytoplasm and inconspicuous nucleoli (85% of patients with ALL).
L2	Lymphoblasts are usually larger but can be a variety of sizes; have more cytoplasm and more obvious nucleoli (14% of patients with ALL).
L3	Lymphoblasts are large, homogenous, deeply basophilic, abundant; vacuolated cytoplasm with prominent vesicular nucleoli; identical to Burkitt cells (1% of patients with ALL).

numbers of chromosomes, help identify children at particularly high risk of a poor outcome. About 60% of children with ALL have identifiable abnormalities in their leukemic cells. Hyperdiploidy and pseudodiploidy are the most common abnormalities detected. Children with hyperdiploid populations of cells do better than those without these cell populations.

Cytochemical and enzyme stains are becoming less important in characterizing lymphoblastic leukemic cells but are helpful in distinguishing lymphoid from nonlymphoid populations of cells. Terminal deoxynucleotidyl transferase (TdT) is the most common enzyme used to distinguish lymphoblastic from nonlymphoblastic leukemia. TdT is a DNA polymerase that catalyzes polymerization of deoxynucleotides in 70% of thymocytes and in fewer than 2% of bone marrow cells. Assays are positive for this enzyme in 90% of cases of ALL. Nonspecific esterases (NSE) are lysosomal enzymes used mostly for marking monocytic differentiation. Myeloperoxidase and Sudan black stains are also useful in distinguishing myeloid from lymphoid leukemias. However, now that flow cytometry and cytogenetics are easily accessible, these stains are less useful.

Clinical Presentation & Prognosis Factors

ALL is the uncontrolled proliferation of immature lymphoblasts with consequent suppression of normal hematopoiesis. These immature lymphoblasts can infiltrate the entire reticuloendothelial system, kidneys, brain, testicles, bone, and, uncommonly, skin. Symptoms at presentation thus are varied and include fever, pallor, bleeding, fatigue, weight loss, bone pain, headache, and gait disturbance. Lymphadenopathy and hepatosplenomegaly are common findings on physical examination. Infectious processes, autoimmune disorders, bone marrow failure syndromes, and other malignant neoplasms that infiltrate bone marrow must be distinguished from leukemia. Acute infection is commonly seen as part of the initial presentation of the child with ALL.

Several factors regarding clinical presentation carry prognostic significance. The two most important are the age of the patient and initial white blood cell count at diagnosis. Patients with very high white cell counts and children younger than 1 year or older than 10 years at diagnosis have the worst prognosis. With this clinical information, in combination with cytogenetic analysis of the leukemic cells and identification of cell-surface antigens, patients can be separated into good and poor risk groups for selection of appropriate treatment regimens. Specific therapy is designated for infants and for children with lymphomatous features and T-cell marker predominance and for children with specific cytogenetic abnormalities known to be associated with poor prognosis, such as t(9;22)(q34;q11), t(4;11)(q21;q23), or hypodiploidy. These groups of children are at particular risk for central nervous system (CNS) relapse with subsequent bone marrow relapse.

Treatment

Combination chemotherapy, either alone or with additional chemotherapeutic agents and radiation to the CNS and testicles (referred to as sanctuary sites), is the principal modality of therapy. Treatment regimens usually include an intensive initial induction phase, a consolidation phase aimed in particular at CNS prophylaxis, a reinduction period about 5 months into therapy, and a maintenance phase of 2–3 years. ALL regimens use some form of CNS prophylaxis to prevent involvement of the brain and meninges, which would otherwise occur in 60% of patients. Conventional induction treatment includes prednisone, L-asparaginase, and vincristine; in higher-risk patients, doxorubicin is added. With this therapy, 95% of patients go into remission within the first month of treatment. Methotrexate and 6-mercaptopurine with pulses of prednisone and vincristine (Oncovin) remain standard in maintenance protocols. The addition of combinations of cyclophosphamide, anthracyclines, 6-thioguanine, and cytosine arabinoside in a reinduction phase has improved the outcome markedly for many patients. Prophylactic therapy for the CNS is a crucial part of treatment for childhood ALL. Intrathecal administration of methotrexate with cranial radiation of 1800 cGy prevents CNS disease in more than 90% of children. In the small percentage of children who present with CNS disease, higher doses of radiation or triple intrathecal therapy with hydrocortisone, ara-C, and methotrexate is indicated. Experimental protocols, including bone marrow transplant for children in first remission with particularly high-risk ALL, are currently in progress.

Any reemergence of leukemic cells in a child receiving chemotherapy portends a poor outcome. The most common site of relapse is the bone marrow. After an isolated relapse in the bone marrow more than 6 months before completion of chemotherapy, intensive reinduction chemotherapy or allogeneic bone marrow transplant can prolong remissions in at least 30% of patients. Isolated relapse in extramedullary sites usually indicates a bone marrow relapse. The overall testicular relapse rate in boys with ALL is 30%; the patients at highest risk are those with T-cell type and lymphomatous features. CNS relapse while a child is receiving chemotherapy is often the precursor of a bone marrow relapse. It requires repeated induction therapy with intensive CNS therapy consisting of radiation and intrathecal medication.

Overall survival for patients with ALL in relapse is 40–50% at best, partly because of the cumulative toxicity from intensive therapy. Much work currently centers on better defining those patients who are at highest risk for early relapse and on detecting residual disease while a patient is receiving chemotherapy. In addition, a better understanding of drug resistance may improve the outlook for patients who experience relapse. Overall, continuous remission for 5 years in children with ALL is about 90%, but serious complications occur during and after therapy.

Complications of Therapy

Although the outlook for children with leukemia is brighter than in the past, progress has not come without a cost. The intensity of the treatment places a child at high risk for infection and bleeding and in need of attentive care by experienced personnel. The major complications of ALL treatment are directly related to the chemotherapeutic agents and their cytolytic effects. These include hyperleukocytosis with tumor lysis syndrome, infection associated with myelosuppression, and neurotoxicity.

Tumor lysis syndrome and hyperleukocytosis are often the first management problems the clinician faces in caring for the child with newly diagnosed ALL (Table 15–2). Patients with high initial white blood cell counts and bulky adenopathy in the mediastinum or renal involvement are at highest risk. These patients tend to be those with T-cell leukemia.

Tumor lysis syndrome is a metabolic derangement caused by rapid lysis of leukemic cells with release of intracellular phosphate, uric acid, and potassium at a rate that exceeds renal clearance. Uric acid, phosphate, and calcium can precipitate in the kidneys, causing obstruction, particularly at an acidic pH. Frequently one observes hyperkalemia, hyperphosphatemia, hypocalcemia, and hyperuricemia in serum electrolyte studies. The aim of treatment is to maximize urine output, alkalinize the urine to minimize precipitation of uric acid, and monitor cardiovascular status carefully and correct electrolyte abnormalities. Sometimes dialysis is necessary when renal failure is impending; in severe cases, the patient must frequently be managed in the intensive care unit.

Table 15–2. Guidelines for management of tumor lysis syndrome.

Hydrate 3000 mL/m²/d; strictly monitor intake and output.
Closely monitor cardiovascular status.
Administer allopurinol 300 mg/m²/d orally.
Begin alkalinization with sodium bicarbonate 150–200 meq/m²/d titrated to keep urine pH 7.0–7.5.
Give mannitol.
Give aluminum-phosphate binders as antacids orally.
Monitor calcium, phosphate, uric acid, electrolytes, magnesium every 6 hours and correct as needed until stable.
If hyperphosphatemia, hyperuricemia, and hyperkalemia persist in the face of decreased urine output, start renal dialysis.
Hold chemotherapy until stable.

Suppression of normal hematopoiesis is unavoidable in treating ALL. Most patients require support with packed red blood cells and platelets at some point during therapy, and myelosuppression puts the child at high risk for infection. Children with neutropenia should avoid crowds, individuals with known infectious disease, and individuals who have recently received live vaccines. Fever in a child with neutropenia must be considered to be due to an infection. Infections can rapidly be fatal if not treated promptly and correctly. In addition, they may be difficult to evaluate because of these patients' inability to mount a normal inflammatory response to an invasive pathogen. Staphylococci and gram-negative organisms are frequent causes, but the child should also be evaluated for fungal or viral processes. An empiric regimen of broad-spectrum antibiotics is recommended. Even if no organism is identified, antibiotics must be continued until the patient is no longer neutropenic. The use of granulocyte colony-stimulating factor (G-CSF) appears to be helpful in decreasing the degree and duration of neutropenia in patients treated with aggressive chemotherapy protocols.

The major long-term side effects in ALL are neurotoxic. These are mostly related to intrathecal methotrexate administration and radiation therapy. All children can expect a drop in IQ, and some children have severe neurotoxicity in the form of leukoencephalopathy with ataxia, seizures, and intellectual dysfunction; others have subtle learning problems or are asymptomatic and have white matter changes on neuroimaging.

ACUTE NONLYMPHOBLASTIC LEUKEMIA

Acute nonlymphoblastic leukemia (ANLL) is a heterogenous group of disorders in which immature malignant nonlymphoblastic precursors develop in the bone marrow and inhibit normal hematopoiesis. About 20–25% of all acute leukemias in childhood are nonlymphoblastic.

Incidence

Unlike ALL, which has a clear peak age of incidence, ANLL has a constant incidence from birth through adolescence and continues to be associated with a poorer long-term survival rate than ALL.

Etiology

The exact cause of ANLL is unknown, but the incidence is increased in children with trisomy 21, Fanconi, Bloom, Kostmann, and Diamond-Blackfan syndromes. A small percentage occurs in children who have previously been treated for Hodgkin disease and other malignant neoplasms. Another group of patients predisposed to ANLL includes those with myelodysplastic or myeloproliferative disorders.

Pathology

ANLL results from clonal proliferation of malignant

hemopoietic progenitors. Oncogenes, cytogenetic abnormalities, reactivity to monoclonal antibodies that recognize cell-surface antigens on normal nonlymphoblastic cells, cytochemical stains, and morphologic features have all been helpful in classifying the nonlymphoblastic leukemias.

ANLL is categorized by morphologic and cytochemical staining patterns. The subtypes are shown in Table 15–3. M0 is an undifferentiated leukemia, sometimes called a "stem cell leukemia." For practical purposes, the myeloid leukemias are FAB M1, M2, and M3; the mixed myeloid and monocytic leukemia is M4; pure monocytic leukemia is M5; erythroid leukemia is M6; and megakaryoblastic leukemia is M7. Myeloperoxidase is a useful stain for myeloid leukemias, whereas α-napthyl butyrate is detected in monocytic leukemia. There is no specific stain for erythroid leukemia, although erythroid leukemias do stain strongly with periodic acid-Schiff (PAS). Definitive diagnosis of M7 leukemia includes detection of platelet peroxidase activity by electron microscopy and reactivity with specific monoclonal antibodies directed against platelet surface antigens. M7 leukemia is the most common in children with Down syndrome.

Correlating FAB type with antigen expression has not been very successful. In general, the more differentiated leukemias tend to express early granulocyte antigens. Immunologic classification may be helpful prognostically; ie, My4, My7, and My8 are myeloid surface markers that are associated with a poorer prognosis. There is heterogenous antigen expression in ANLL.

Chromosome studies provide useful clinical data regarding certain groups of patients with ANLL. Almost all cases of ANLL have a demonstrable cytogenetic abnormality. The t(8;21)(22q, 11q) abnormality is the most frequent chromosome translocation and is more common in boys. Some abnormalities are frequently associated with specific types of ANLL; for example, the t(15;17) (22q, 11q) translocation is seen in progranulocytic leukemia, and inversion of chromosome 16 is associated with FAB M4. Monosomy 7 is associated with a myeloproliferative syndrome, pancytopenia, or ANLL; these children respond poorly to traditional chemotherapy and therefore should be considered for early bone marrow transplantation.

In nearly 20% of children with ANLL, the leukemia cells show characteristics of myeloid and lymphoid lineage. These cases are referred to as mixed lineage and are more common in patients with t(4;11) or t(9;11) cytogenetic abnormalities.

Clinical Features

Fever is the most common presenting symptom, occurring in up to 70% of children in whom ANLL is diagnosed. Anorexia, pallor, and bleeding are also common. Adenopathy is present in some, but not to the same degree as in ALL patients. In infants with ANLL, multiple skin nodules and subcutaneous extramedullary leukemia may occur. Baseline laboratory studies often reveal neutropenia with an elevated total white blood cell count, anemia, and thrombocytopenia. Abnormal coagulation tests may also be present. Disseminated intravascular coagulation (DIC) is most common in patients with profound leukocytosis and is most characteristic in those with acute progranulocytic leukemia. The DIC is presumably due to tissue thromboplastic activity from intracellular granules of the leukemic cells. Patients with extreme leukocytosis may present with lactic acidosis caused by sludging in small vessels, with resultant severe pulmonary, renal, or CNS compromise. The definitive diagnosis of ANLL is made when more than 30% of nonlymphoid blasts are seen in the bone marrow. Primary CNS disease is present at diagnosis in about 5% of patients; therefore, spinal fluid for cytologic examination must be obtained as well.

Prognosis

Prognostic factors in ANLL have not been defined as clearly as for ALL. Like ALL, however, high initial white blood cell counts appear predictive of decreased remission rates and increased relapses. Myelomonocytic or monocytic leukemia erythroid or megakaryoblastic subtypes are associated with poorer outcomes. Some cytogenetic subtypes and older age are associated with a somewhat more favorable outcome. As the overall outcome for children with ANLL improves, these factors become more important.

Treatment

The therapy necessary to induce remission for ANLL is more intensive and toxic than that used for ALL. As with ALL, the goal of induction therapy is to eliminate the malignant cell line and to reestablish normal hematopoiesis. Up to 80% of patients with ANLL achieve remission with induction therapy. Most relapse within 2 years, but patients who undergo a related allogeneic bone marrow transplantation in the first remission appear to have a 70% survival rate, versus 40–50% with conventional chemotherapy. The most effective induction regimens include daunomycin, cytosine arabinoside, dexamethasone, etoposide, vincristine, and G-thioguanine. Effective regimens used for induction lead to mucositis, liver toxicity, and severe bone marrow suppression and often require supplemental nutritional support. Coagulopathy is not uncommon. Support with blood products is virtually always necessary for the patient receiving induction therapy for ANLL. Perhaps the most life-threatening risk of induction

Table 15–3. French-American-British morphologic classification for acute nonlymphoblastic leukemia.

M0	Undifferentiated leukemia
M1	Acute myeloblastic leukemia without differentiation
M2	Acute myeloblastic leukemia with differentiation
M3	Acute promyeloblastic leukemia
M4	Acute myelomonoblastic leukemia
M5	Acute monocytic leukemia
M6	Erythroleukemia
M7	Acute megakaryoblastic leukemia

chemotherapy is infection from gram-negative organisms and fungus. Prolonged hospitalizations for antibiotic, nutritional, and blood product support are common.

CNS disease develops in approximately 5% of patients with ANLL; children particularly susceptible are those with M4 and M5 subtypes and any patient with a high white blood cell count at diagnosis. Although prophylactic therapy may decrease the incidence of CNS disease, it does not appear to affect overall outcome. A second remission in ANLL can be achieved in up to 50% of patients but is usually short-lived. Few long-term survivors have received chemotherapy alone after their leukemia recurred.

Allogeneic bone marrow transplantation is now considered the standard of care for patients with ANLL in first remission and has been more successful than chemotherapy alone for patients in second remission. Autologous purged bone marrow in first remission is also used but appears to be no more effective that conventional chemotherapy in first remission. This technique uses bone marrow that is collected after a patient is in remission; the marrow is purged of any residual leukemia cells by use of monoclonal antibody and chemotherapy. With continued improvement in supportive care and effective prevention and treatment of graft-versus-host disease, bone marrow transplantation in first remission has significantly improved disease-free survival.

Childhood ANLL comprises a small percentage of cases of acute leukemia in childhood but a considerable percentage of deaths. Improvement in supportive care, in conjunction with more aggressive induction chemotherapy, has improved our ability to achieve remission in ANLL patients over the past 15–20 years. It appears that related allogeneic bone marrow transplantation in the first remission is the best option for a patient. With expanded matched unrelated donor pools, it is likely that these will soon be considered in first remission as well. Continuing the quest for a better understanding of the biology of ANLL through cytogenetic analysis, oncogene manipulation to regulate leukemic clones, and more sensitive detection of residual disease will be helpful.

HODGKIN & NON-HODGKIN LYMPHOMA

HODGKIN LYMPHOMA

Hodgkin lymphoma constitutes a small portion of cases of childhood lymphoma but is associated with considerable satisfaction with regard to the development of a successful treatment program. More than 80% of pediatric cases of Hodgkin lymphoma are cured.

Incidence

Hodgkin and non-Hodgkin lymphoma together account for about 5% of pediatric malignancy, with an incidence of 6:1 million children younger than 15 years. In Hodgkin lymphoma, there is a bimodal age-specific incidence, with a peak in adolescence to young adulthood, and again later after age 50 years. The male-to-female ratio is 2:1, and before age 10 years, it is even more common in the male population than it is later in life. In early adolescence, girls are more commonly affected.

Genetics

Compared with the general population, Hodgkin lymphoma is more common in close relatives of affected patients, and multiple cases within families have been described. In most of these cases, the affected siblings share identical human leukocyte antigen (HLA) typing. There is no clear association with congenital syndromes, but it has been reported in ataxia-telangiectasia, inherited hypogammaglobulinemia, and AIDS.

Epidemiology & Etiology

In the United States, Hodgkin lymphoma appears less commonly in nonwhites and more commonly in higher socioeconomic groups, in which it occurs at a later age. Case clusters of Hodgkin lymphoma have been well described, suggesting a possible infectious etiology in some cases. Interest has centered on the Epstein-Barr virus, the virus responsible for endemic Burkitt lymphoma in Africa and associated with the formation of Reed-Sternberg cells in infectious mononucleosis. The etiology of Hodgkin lymphoma is unknown, but, as with other childhood malignancies, genetics, environmental factors, and relative immunocompetence probably lead to susceptibility.

Pathology & Biology

Although Hodgkin lymphoma is classified as a malignant lymphoma, the lymphocyte lineage of the abnormal cells remains unproved. Two groups of cells are seen in Hodgkin lymphoma, including stromal cells and the presumed malignant cells (the so-called Reed-Sternberg cells). These malignant cells usually account for less than 1% of the involved tissue. These cells probably originate in the monocyte-macrophage system rather than in lymphocyte.

Reed-Sternberg cells tend to occur singly or in clusters and are surrounded by stromal cells, which destroy the normal architecture of the lymph node. Depending on the degree of fibrosis and the predominant type of stromal cells present, four histologic appearances have been described: lymphocyte-predominant, mixed cellularity, lymphocyte-depleted, and nodular sclerosing. The prognosis of the first three types is usually proportionate to the ratio of abnormal cells to lymphocytes. The **lymphocyte-predominant type** is characterized by destruction of the lymph node architecture and significant infiltrates of normal lymphocytes surrounding a few Reed-Sternberg cells. Fibrosis is usually not seen. In **mixed-cellularity Hodgkin lymphoma,** Reed-

Sternberg cells are plentiful, there is some fibrosis, and the lymph node is usually completely effaced. Minimal necrosis may be present as well. In the **lymphocyte-depleted histology,** one sees primarily abnormal cells with a paucity of lymphocytes and significant fibrosis and necrosis. **Nodular sclerosing Hodgkin lymphoma** is morphologically distinct. Often the lacunar variant of Reed-Sternberg cells is seen with abundant pale cytoplasm. In most cases, a thickened capsule with proliferating bands of collagen divides the lymph node into distinct nodules. Mixed-cellularity or nodular sclerosing disease are the most common histologic appearances in children.

Hodgkin lymphoma is believed to arise in a single lymph node and spread first to adjacent nodes, then to other lymph node groups. Splenic involvement is almost always associated with the involvement of adjacent hilar nodes. As the disease spreads, the likelihood of dissemination to bone marrow, liver, lungs, and bone via the blood stream is greater. Early involvement of extranodal structures is usually associated with contiguous spread from adjacent lymph nodes.

Demonstrable cellular immunodeficiency is present in more than 50% of patients with Hodgkin lymphoma. It is suspected that the immune defect precedes the disease. The defect is manifest by decreased delayed hypersensitivity on skin testing and increased susceptibility to bacterial, fungal, and viral infections. This problem is further complicated by the treatment (which sometimes includes splenectomy), but some recovery of the immune deficiency can occur after treatment.

Clinical Presentation

More than 90% of children with Hodgkin lymphoma present with enlarged, painless lymph nodes or groups of lymph nodes in the cervical or supraclavicular area. The swelling usually is noted incidentally during examination for intercurrent illness. About 30% of children have systemic symptoms, including night sweats, fever, and loss of greater than 10% of body weight. The affected lymph node feels rubbery and is nontender. It can be single, matted with other nodes, or surrounded by normal reactive lymph nodes.

Diagnosis & Staging

The diagnosis of Hodgkin lymphoma is made by demonstrating typical histopathologic findings on a biopsy specimen. Fine-needle aspiration does not provide adequate material for diagnosis because the lymph node architecture must be assessed. Frozen sections of pathologic origin are notoriously inaccurate; therefore, it is important to wait for formal pathologic analysis. Baseline laboratory data should include a complete blood count, sedimentation rate, liver function tests, and chest radiograph. Sedimentation rate is useful as a marker of the success of treatment. A chest radiograph will demonstrate significant mediastinal adenopathy, which is not only useful for staging, but is also important if general anesthesia is to be used for the biopsy.

Once the diagnosis of Hodgkin lymphoma has been confirmed, clinical staging with computerized tomography (CT) of the chest, abdomen, and pelvis; bone marrow aspiration and biopsy; and gallium scan are recommended. Lymphangiography is recommended by some; however, it is not practical for many children and is contraindicated in patients with massive mediastinal adenopathy or in those with parenchymal lung disease. After identification of involved lymph node groups and the presence or absence of systemic symptoms, the clinical stage can be determined, as outlined in Table 15–4. This staging system acknowledges that extranodal disease caused by direct invasion from an affected node does not imply a worse prognosis than if only the single node was affected. The spleen is thus regarded as nodal tissue. Stage III has been further described with an "E" to denote extranodal disease and with an "S" to denote splenic disease. Patients without weight loss, fever, or night sweats are classified as "A" and have a better prognosis than those with systemic or "B" symptoms. As is true with other malignancies, higher stages carry a poorer prognosis.

Staging laparotomy is used for pathologic staging in some patients to assess intra-abdominal disease. It traditionally includes sampling of all node groups, biopsy of the liver, and splenectomy. In 30% of patients undergoing laparotomy, the clinical and pathologic staging differs. Both upgrading and downgrading of stage occur, with the difference most often being the unexpected involvement of the spleen. Whether to perform a laparotomy depends primarily on how the information gained from this procedure will affect treatment. Patients who may receive radiation therapy alone, such as those with stage I or II disease, probably should undergo lymphangiography if not laparotomy to rule out cryptic splenic involvement. However, if chemotherapy is planned, regardless of any new findings from the pathologic staging, a laparotomy is not needed. For example, a staging laparotomy is not indicated in patients with stage IV disease, as these patients all require radiation and chemotherapy. Although there is some operative risk to the patient undergoing laparotomy,

Table 15–4. Staging of Hodgkin lymphoma.[1]

Stage I	Involvement of a single lymph node region or a single extralymphatic site.
Stage II	Involvement of two or more lymph node regions on the same side of the diaphragm, or localized involvement of extralymphatic organ or site and of one or more lymph node regions on the same side of the diaphragm.
Stage III	Involvement of lymph node regions on both sides of the diaphragm, which may also be accompanied by localized involvement of extra lymphatic organ or site or by involvement of the spleen or both.
Stage IV	Disseminated involvement of one or more extralymphatic organs or tissues with or without lymph node enlargement.

[1]Patients with B symptoms (weight loss, fever, night sweats) have a worse prognosis.

the greatest risk probably is associated with splenectomy and the resulting decrease in immune function.

Treatment

Radiation therapy, which provided the first cures in Hodgkin lymphoma, is still the preferred treatment for some patients, particularly adults. However, the disadvantages for children include the need for laparotomy and splenectomy. In addition, the doses of radiation necessary for effective treatment often result in adverse musculoskeletal development. The advantage of radiation therapy is that it avoids the systemic toxicity and late complications of chemotherapy.

Standard chemotherapy for Hodgkin lymphoma is not established, but there has been considerable success with combinations of nitrogen mustard (mechlorethamine), vincristine, prednisone, procarbazine, doxorubicin (Adriamycin), bleomycin, vinblastine, and dacarbazine. The major disadvantages of chemotherapy alone are late relapses at the primary site and potential long-term side effects. The advantages of chemotherapy in early stages of the disease are that it obviates the need for a laparotomy and avoids the deforming effects of radiation therapy.

Combined modality therapy provides many potential benefits. As late relapses sometimes occur when chemotherapy alone is used, adding radiation to sterilize areas of local disease can be effective. In addition, when radiation is used with chemotherapy, lower doses of radiation can be used. The other major advantage is that a laparotomy need not be performed. Treatment usually lasts 6–8 months. After completion of treatment, the patient should be observed closely for evidence of relapse.

In more than two thirds of patients who experience relapse, the occurrence is within the first 2 years; few cases of relapse occur more than 4 years after diagnosis. If a patient has a relapse, different chemotherapy plus radiation or bone marrow transplantation can be offered.

Side Effects

The acute side effects of treatment for Hodgkin disease are similar to those for other tumors. However, because most patients with Hodgkin disease can expect to live full lives, the long-term side effects of radiation and chemotherapy take on greater meaning. Impaired growth and reproductive function are common, and the risk of second tumors and leukemias is significant. In addition, permanent end-organ damage can occur, resulting in significant morbidity for the patient. Organs particularly at risk for end-organ damage include the heart and lungs.

Several challenges remain in the understanding and treatment of Hodgkin disease. Continued effort to understand the etiology and biology of the disease is needed. In addition, better ways to stage the disease accurately and to provide adequate curative therapy with minimal toxicity and with decreased risk for second malignancy are needed.

NON-HODGKIN LYMPHOMA

Incidence & Epidemiology

Non-Hodgkin lymphoma (NHL) is about 1.5 times as common as Hodgkin lymphoma. Collectively, these tumors account for about 15% of childhood malignancies. The annual incidence is about 7:1 per million children, with a male predominance of 3:1. The peak age of incidence is 7–11 years, with a median age of 9 years. Occurrence before age 3 years is uncommon. A greater-than-usual risk of NHL occurs in children with congenital or acquired dysfunction of the immune system. In particular, several of the inherited disorders, such as ataxia-telangiectasia and Wiskott-Aldrich, Bloom, and Chédiak-Higashi syndromes, are associated with the development of NHL. Patients receiving chronic immunosuppressive therapy after organ transplant also have been shown to have an increased risk of NHL. The Epstein-Barr virus is implicated in the development of Burkitt lymphoma in African children. Chronic treatment with phenytoin has been associated with the development of Hodgkin lymphoma and NHL as well. Although the exact etiology of NHL is unknown, there are clear associations with other processes.

Pathology & Biology

Three major categories of NHL can be distinguished: large cell, lymphoblastic, and undifferentiated (Table 15–5). To some degree, these subgroups correlate with immunologic subtype and biologic behavior. Histopathologic classification schemes are based on cytomorphologic features and correlate with immunophenotype. Immunophenotypic studies on NHL cells show that about 40% of all cases are T cell–derived, and about the same percentage are B cell–derived. The remainder are non-T, non-B cell–derived neoplasms. Undifferentiated lymphomas (Burkitt and non-Burkitt type) are virtually all B-cell tumors, whereas lymphoblastic lymphomas are predominantly T-cell tumors. The large-cell lymphomas tend to be heterogenous immunologically; most are tumors of transformed B cells, some are T cell-derived, and a few appear to be derived from the macrophage-histiocytic lineage. The distinction between Burkitt and non-Burkitt subtypes is subjectively determined by the amount of cellular heterogeneity and has no clinical significance. All of these malignancies can invade the bone marrow and undergo leukemic transformation. Lymphoblastic NHL, the most common histologic type, is seen primarily in patients with disease above the diaphragm. Histiocytic undifferen-

Table 15–5. Histologic types of non-Hodgkin lymphoma.

Type	Percentage
Lymphoblastic	38
Burkitt	14
Non-Burkitt	20
Large cell	20
Other	8

tiated types are most common in patients with primary gastrointestinal disease.

Clinical Presentation

The wide variety of anatomic sites containing lymphoid tissue, including lymph nodes, Peyer patches, thymus, Waldeyer ring, and bone marrow, should create heterogeneity in clinical presentation (Table 15–6). Nevertheless, a few typical symptom complexes account for the majority of presentations. More than 30% of children affected with NHL present with gastrointestinal involvement, with right lower quadrant pain, nausea, vomiting, and abdominal distention. About 25% of children with NHL present with mediastinal involvement. These children frequently are preteen boys who have respiratory symptoms, cervical or supraclavicular adenopathy, or superior vena cava syndrome. **Superior vena cava syndrome** refers to a syndrome produced by extrinsic compression of the vena cava and its tributaries. Commonly, one sees plethora and edema of the face, neck, and upper chest, as well as visible, dilated collateral veins in these areas. Respiratory distress can be seen as a result of compression of the tracheobronchial tree. Less commonly, children present with regionally limited disease affecting the tonsils, nasopharynx, or Waldeyer ring. Systemic symptoms of erratic fever, night sweats, and weight loss are most common in advanced disease. The typical presentation of African Burkitt lymphoma is of massive tumor of the maxilla or mandible with or without orbital involvement. It is quite rare in the United States. Most children in the United States with Burkitt lymphoma present with abdominal disease, only occasionally involving CNS or bone marrow as well. Burkitt lymphoma grows very rapidly, with clinical signs and symptoms not lasting more than 6 weeks before presentation.

Diagnosis & Staging

In general, the role of surgery is limited to lymph node biopsy or, occasionally, excision of a mass. Laparotomy is necessary after an abdominal presentation of disease; in this setting, biopsy specimens of the liver, regional lymph nodes, para-aortic nodes, and any other suspicious nodes should be obtained. Radiographic imaging should focus on the area of the mass or its related symptoms. Initial evaluation should include chest radiograph; complete blood count, bone marrow aspirate, and biopsy; lumbar puncture; liver and renal function tests; serum uric acid, phosphorus,

calcium, and electrolyte concentrations; a gallium scan or technetium bone scan; and CT of chest, abdomen, and pelvis. Table 15–7 outlines staging classification for NHL.

Treatment

Tumor lysis syndrome should be expected during the treatment of any patient with lymphoma. This syndrome is most common in lymphoma patients with disseminated disease of the lymphoblastic type and is managed similarly to the tumor lysis syndrome seen in patients with leukemia. Dialysis must be instituted if hyperkalemia and hyperphosphatemia develop despite aggressive hydration, alkalinization, forced diuresis with mannitol, and use of phosphate binders.

Patients with localized lymphomas can expect a greater than 90% long-term survival. Patients with disseminated lymphoma do less well but continue to improve with aggressive chemotherapy protocols. Multidrug regimens, with many of the same agents used to treat leukemia, are effective. Surgery plays a role in resecting isolated abdominal lesions but must be combined with a course of chemotherapy. Radiation therapy is useful only for head and neck tumors. CNS prophylaxis consisting of radiation therapy and intrathecal chemotherapy probably is indicated only with parameningeal disease or advanced-stage disease. For patients with advanced disease, 1–2 years of intensive therapy is administered, with CNS prophylaxis.

Until the introduction of bone marrow transplantation, the outcome for patients who experienced relapse while receiving therapy was dismal. Up to 40% of children treated with allogeneic transplantation have shown prolonged survival. Allogeneic or autologous bone marrow transplantation is the treatment of choice for relapse of NHL off therapy as well.

NEUROBLASTOMA

Neuroblastoma is one of the most biologically fascinating of all childhood tumors. Spontaneous and induced

Table 15–6. Site distribution of primary non-Hodgkin lymphoma.

Site	Percentage
Mediastinum	26
Abdomen	35
Head and neck	3
Peripheral nodes	14
Other	22

Table 15–7. Staging of non-Hodgkin lymphoma (St. Jude's research scheme).

Stage I	A single node or extranodal site, except for abdomen or mediastinum
Stage II	A single extranodal tumor with regional nodal involvement
Stage III	Two or more extranodal sites on both sides of the diaphragm
	A primary thoracic tumor
	Extensive intra-abdominal disease
	All paraspinal or epidural tumors
Stage IV	Bone marrow or central nervous system involvement

maturation or regression may occur in some of these tumors. It is the most common solid tumor of childhood outside the CNS and accounts for about 50% of malignancies seen in infancy.

Incidence & Epidemiology

The incidence of neuroblastoma in the United States is about 8:1 million children. The median age of diagnosis is 2 years, and the tumor is slightly more common in boys. There may be a genetic predisposition for neuroblastoma, which has been reported in twins and siblings. Familial cases usually present at a slightly younger age and have a higher incidence of multiple primary tumors. The frequency of neuroblastoma is higher in children with Beckwith-Wiedemann syndrome, nesidioblastosis, and neurofibromatosis. It has also been described in the fetal hydantoin syndrome.

Genetics

Analysis of neuroblastoma cells has detected cytogenetic abnormalities in 80% of cases. The most consistent abnormality is a rearrangement or deletion in the short arm of chromosome 1. However, this is not specific to neuroblastoma and does occur in other malignant tumors. The second most common abnormality is seen in chromosome 17. The oncogenes n-*myc* and n-*ras* are amplified in neuroblastoma cells. The protooncogene n-*myc* is usually found as a single copy on the short arm of chromosome 2. Although n-*myc* is amplified, and multiple copies are found in 50% of patients with disseminated neuroblastoma, amplification of n-*myc* is unusual in localized tumors.

Pathology & Biology

Neuroblastoma is derived from the neural crest. Neural crest cells give rise to the adrenal medulla, sympathetic ganglia, thymus, Schwann cells, melanocytes, and membranous bone. Neural crest contains primitive stem cells that differentiate into sympathoblasts, the cells from which neuroblastomas are derived.

Neuroblastoma may develop anywhere along the sympathetic nervous system chain. The most common site of primary tumors within the abdomen is the adrenal gland, which accounts for 40% of tumors, and the paraspinal ganglion. Tumors are also found in the thorax, neck, and pelvis. Infants are more likely than older children to have thoracic tumors. About 50% of infants and 70% of older children show evidence of spread of tumor beyond the primary site. The most common metastatic sites are lymph nodes, bone marrow, bone, liver, and subcutaneous tissue.

Neuroblastoma consists of dense nests of cells separated by fibrillar bundles. Rosettes of cells surround a pink fibrillar center. Frequently, hemorrhage, necrosis, and calcifications are present. As maturation proceeds, cells differentiate toward ganglion cells, and increasing amounts of fibrillar material are present. Sometimes uniform maturation is interspersed with areas of undifferentiated cells. Completely differentiated cells result in a **gan-**glioneuroma, a tumor of well-differentiated ganglion cells, Schwann cells, and nerve bundles. Because the same tumors contain a spectrum of differentiated cells, multiple sections from all areas of a tumor mass must be sampled before a diagnosis of ganglioneuroma is made.

Urinary excretion of elevated amounts of catecholamine metabolites occurs in nearly 90% of patients with neuroblastoma. The metabolites measured most often are vanillylmandelic acid and homovanillic acid. Serum ferritin concentration is elevated in patients with higher-staged neuroblastoma and may be associated with a poorer prognosis. About 40–50% of patients with stage III and IV disease have high ferritin concentrations. In patients with normal ferritin values and stage II neuroblastoma, a slightly better prognosis can be expected.

It is sometimes difficult to differentiate neuroblastoma from lymphoma, Ewing sarcoma, rhabdomyosarcoma, and primitive neuroectodermal tumor by light microscopy. Electron microscopy of neuroblastoma reveals neurosecretory dense core granules in the peripheral cytoplasm and neural processes containing microtubules. With an antibody to neuron-specific enolase, neuroblastoma can be differentiated from other small round tumors of childhood except primitive neuroectodermal tumors. PAS staining produces a positive reaction in Ewing sarcoma and rhabdomyosarcoma but typically a negative reaction in neuroblastoma.

Clinical Presentation

The clinical presentation depends on the primary site and the degree of spread. Sometimes the presence of an abdominal mass is the first sign of disease. These masses usually are hard and irregular and often cross the midline. Thoracic masses are often detected in the posterior mediastinum when chest radiographs are obtained for other reasons. Cervical masses are sometimes misdiagnosed initially as infection, and cervical adenopathy representing neuroblastoma is more common on the left side than the right. The presence of a Horner syndrome or heterochromia iridis should suggest cervicothoracic neuroblastoma. Pelvic masses may present with bowel and bladder symptoms, resulting from direct compression by tumor or from compression of the spinal cord. The liver can be extremely large, which can lead to respiratory insufficiency, particularly in the infant. Large retroperitoneal masses often cause vascular compression resulting in edema of the lower extremities. Hypertension usually is due to compression of renal vasculature and rarely to elevated catecholamine concentrations. Paraspinal tumors at any site may extend through the foramina with subsequent spinal cord compression. Skin and subcutaneous nodules occur almost exclusively in infants. They are nontender, bluish, and mobile. Bone and bone marrow disease is often manifest by bone pain and limping. Sphenoid and retro-orbital bone involvement is common and results in orbital ecchymosis. Infiltration and replacement of the bone marrow by neuroblastoma results in pancytopenia with pallor, bleeding, and susceptibility to infection.

In older children, presenting symptoms are less specific and include intermittent fever, weight loss, and lethargy. One unusual presentation of neuroblastoma is the syndrome of opsoclonus, ataxia, and myoclonus. These patients have acute cerebellar and truncal ataxia with rapid eye movements. The pathophysiology of this disorder is not understood. It is often associated with a localized tumor, and symptoms improve after removal of the tumor. Even though these localized tumors are usually cured with surgery alone, 75% of patients are left with some permanent neurologic disability, including ataxia and mental retardation.

Diagnosis & Staging

Often the diagnosis of neuroblastoma is suspected from clinical features alone. Laboratory data, other than elevated catecholamine concentrations, are not specific for neuroblastoma. Pancytopenia may be present because of extensive bone marrow disease, or the hemoglobin concentration may be low because of bleeding within a large primary tumor. The platelet count is usually normal but may be decreased if DIC occurs, secondary either to metastatic disease or to tumor degradation after initiation of chemotherapy. Liver and renal function and coagulation studies usually are normal at time of diagnosis but are altered, at least intermittently, by chemotherapy.

Bone marrow aspiration and biopsy should be performed as well. Bone marrow studies can reveal infiltration with tumor, or an occasional cluster of cells can be found. Bone metastasis is rare without bone marrow disease, so if marrow appears not to be involved on initial evaluation when bone metastasis is present, multiple samples of bone marrow must be obtained. Spinal fluid needs to be studied only if the primary tumor is parameningeal or intracranial. These studies are needed for staging the tumor but are often diagnostic as well, obviating the need for a biopsy of the mass.

Imaging studies should include a CT scan of the chest, abdomen, and pelvis. The head and spine are better defined by magnetic resonance imaging (MRI). Radiographic findings depend on the primary site. Skeletal lesions are usually lytic and are found most commonly in proximal long bones, orbit, and skull. Technetium bone scan demonstrates these lesions and the primary tumor in 70% of cases. In abdominal primary tumors, calcifications are commonly seen within the tumor mass on CT. Frequently, hemorrhage is seen centrally in the tumor on MRI or CT. It is characteristic for neuroblastomas to displace and sometimes become adherent to adjacent kidney and liver but rarely to invade them. However, tumors can wrap around major structures causing obstruction and dysfunction.

The staging system for neuroblastoma is illustrated in Table 15–8. The distribution of patients by stage or extent of disease differs depending on the age at diagnosis, ie, infants are more likely to have localized or low-staged disease than are slightly older children.

Table 15–8. International staging for neuroblastoma.

Stage I	Localized tumor confined to area of origin; complete gross excision, with or without residual disease; identifiable ipsilateral and contralateral lymph nodes negative microscopically.
Stage 2A	Unilateral tumor with incomplete gross excision; identifiable ipsilateral and contralateral lymph nodes negative microscopically.
Stage 2B	Unilateral tumor with complete or incomplete gross excision; positive ipsilateral regional lymph nodes; identifiable contralateral lymph nodes negative microscopically.
Stage 3	Tumor infiltrating across the midline with or without regional lymph node involvement, or unilateral tumor with contralateral regional lymph node involvement, or midline tumor with bilateral regional lymph node involvement.
Stage 4	Disseminated tumor to distant lymph nodes, bone, bone marrow, liver, or other organs (except as defined in stage 4S).
Stage 4S	Localized primary tumor as defined for stage 1 or 2 with dissemination limited to liver, skin, or bone marrow.

Treatment

The primary modalities of therapy for neuroblastoma include surgery, chemotherapy, and radiation therapy. Because so many patients present with already disseminated disease, chemotherapy is necessary for cure except for those patients in stage 4S who are infants and have disease that is known to regress or differentiate spontaneously.

In most patients, surgical intervention is necessary at some point. Children with localized disease who have their tumor completely removed, or those who have microscopic residua, have a high likelihood of cure without the need for other therapy. In other cases, surgery mainly plays a diagnostic role or provides palliation when tumor is compressing vital organs. Many tumors are initially unresectable, and it is now common practice to establish the diagnosis first by biopsy of bone marrow or lymph nodes and then treat the tumor with intensive chemotherapy until it is more accessible for complete resection. This approach has several advantages: one can assess effectiveness of chemotherapy; definitive surgery may be safer, with greater salvage of normal tissue and greater opportunity for complete resection; and one need not delay treatment with chemotherapy until after postoperative recovery.

Radiation plays a limited role in treating neuroblastoma. Radiation therapy is indicated for control of tumors not responsive to chemotherapy, for tumors that cannot be totally resected, and for palliative treatment of unresectable lesions causing pain or organ dysfunction. It can also be useful to expedite regression of stage 4S tumors, for which fairly low doses are effective.

Chemotherapy is the mainstay of treatment for neuroblastoma. The chemotherapeutic agents used include cyclophosphamide, ifosfamide, platinum-based agents, doxorubicin, and epipophyllotoxin. Although improved survival of infants has been seen with these chemotherapeutic combinations, this is not the case for older children with advanced-stage disease. The trend now is to use these drugs in higher doses as continuous infusions.

Bone marrow transplant is a promising approach in patients with advanced disease who have achieved a complete or substantial partial remission with chemotherapy. These patients undergo conditioning with intensive regimens including chemotherapy and total body irradiation, followed by transplant with autologous bone marrow that has been purged of tumor cells or with allogeneic bone marrow.

Experimental therapies aimed at targeted delivery of therapy to tumor cells have been used in patients with neuroblastoma. These have included monoclonal antibodies that recognize epitopes on neuroblastoma cells and radioactively labeled drugs that are taken up preferentially by cells producing adrenergic neurotransmitters (I^{131} metaiodobenzylguanidine). In addition, drugs such as retinoic acid, which cause differentiation of neuroblastoma cells, are being investigated.

Prognosis

Many variables have been investigated as prognostic indicators in neuroblastoma, including ferritin, n-*myc* amplification, and histologic characteristics. However, probably the most important factors in long-term survival, other than the age of the patient and the stage and histopathology of the disease, are chemosensitivity and resectability of all disease not abolished by chemotherapy.

The most important factors in determining a patient's prognosis include clinical stage of disease, primary tumor site, and histologic characteristics of the tumor. The cure rate of infants with low stages of neuroblastoma is 85–90%. Older patients with more advanced disease have a progression-free survival rate of 15–38%. Patients with primary tumor in the adrenal gland or with less-differentiated histology tend to do more poorly than others, but this does not significantly contribute to the prognostic variables of age and stage.

With continuing clinical trials, further means of identifying patients at higher and lower risk will emerge, and therapy will be tailored more appropriately.

WILMS TUMOR

Incidence & Epidemiology

Wilms tumor, a tumor of the developing kidney, is the second most common malignant solid tumor in children outside the CNS. It accounts for 6–7% of all childhood cancer and is the most common renal tumor. The incidence is about 7:1 million children aged younger than 16 years, and the prevalence is about 1:10,000 children af-

fected. The incidence is similar throughout the world, with an equal distribution. Wilms tumor is rare in children younger than 6 months and older than 10 years. The peak age is 2–3 years.

Genetics

Wilms tumor has been associated with several congenital anomalies. The most common are hemihypertrophy, aniridia, and genitourinary anomalies, such as hypospadias, cryptorchidism, horseshoe kidney, fused kidney, ureteral duplication, and polycystic kidney. The incidence of a genitourinary anomaly with Wilms tumor is 5%.

Most patients with Wilms tumor have a normal karyotype; however, when there is an associated congenital aniridia, a deletion at 11p13 has been noted. Fifteen to 20% of patients inherit Wilms tumor, and 1% have one or more family members with Wilms tumor. Familial cases are more likely bilateral and occur at a younger age than do sporadic cases. A two-hit mutational model for Wilms tumor has been proposed in which the first mutation is in either the germ cell or somatic cell and the second mutation is postzygotic, such as a recombination or nondysjunction event. Recently, the candidate gene at 11p13 for Wilms tumor was cloned.

Pathology & Biology

Wilms tumor is pathologically diverse. It is characterized by metanephric blastema formations, and the prognosis is designated as favorable or unfavorable depending on the degree of cellular differentiation and nuclear atypia. Tumors can arise anywhere within the kidney and usually spread beyond a tumor pseudocapsule into the renal sinus or intrarenal lymphatics and blood vessels. Common sites of distant spread include lung, regional lymph nodes, and liver.

Clinical Presentation

Wilms tumor usually presents as an asymptomatic abdominal mass. The associated symptoms of abdominal pain, malaise, gross hematuria, and hypertension occur in about 30% of patients. Bleeding from the tumor can be enough to cause anemia, with resulting fatigue and pallor. Occlusion of the inferior vena cava by tumor thrombus can result in distended surface abdominal veins. In evaluating the child with suspected Wilms tumor, it is important to note hemihypertrophy, aniridia, and evidence of Beckwith-Wiedemann syndrome.

Diagnosis & Staging

The radiographic evaluation of a suspected Wilms tumor should begin with ultrasonography, not only to establish the organ of origin, but also to assess vena caval involvement and blood flow. A CT scan of the abdomen helps to define the extent of the tumor, and a CT scan of the chest will reveal the presence or absence of visible pulmonary metastasis. Initially, there is no need to evaluate bones or the brain unless there are suggestive symptoms, as metastasis to these areas is exceedingly uncommon.

The differential diagnosis in Wilms tumor is fairly limited; the major alternative with an abdominal mass being neuroblastoma. Other malignant diseases that can be confused with Wilms tumor are less common. Wilms tumors are intrarenal and cause intrinsic displacement of urinary collecting systems, whereas neuroblastomas, which usually arise from the adrenal gland or paravertebral sympathetic ganglia, displace rather than distort the kidney. Both tumors can have calcifications, but these are much more characteristic of neuroblastoma. Neuroblastoma occasionally arises in the kidney; therefore, biopsy is required before a diagnosis can be made. Staging of Wilms tumor is presented in Table 15–9.

Treatment

All patients with Wilms tumor require radical nephrectomy except for those with extensive bilateral disease or those with advanced-stage unilateral disease in which excessive risk is involved in performing a nephrectomy. For patients with massive abdominal disease, with or without renal vein and inferior vena cava involvement, preoperative chemotherapy and radiation therapy play a role in decreasing the risk of intraoperative rupture and decrease the amount of renal parenchyma that must be removed from patients with bilateral disease. It can also be helpful in downstaging disease.

Because advances in the treatment of childhood cancers occur quickly, assessing and defining optimal treatment at a given time is difficult. Currently, for patients with Wilms tumor and a favorable histologic diagnosis, radiation therapy is not required, and therapy with actinomycin and vincristine is adequate unless the tumor is in an advanced stage. Patients with an unfavorable histologic diagnosis should receive chemotherapy with vincristine, actinomycin, and doxorubicin with radiation therapy to the tumor bed unless it is a stage I tumor. The optimal length of therapy is not yet known.

Overall, more than 85% of cases of Wilms tumor are cured (Table 15–10). However, tumor recurs in about 20% of patients with a favorable histologic diagnosis and

Table 15–9. Clinicopathologic staging of Wilms tumor.

Stage I	Tumor limited to kidney and completely excised; no invasion through renal capsule, no kidney rupture, no distant spread.
Stage II	Tumor extends through capsule and into perirenal soft tissue and may infiltrate vessels outside the kidney, but is completely excised. There may be local spill of tumor into flank.
Stage III	Residual nonhematogenous dissemination of tumor confined to abdomen. Tumor may extend beyond surgical margin at resection and may involve lymph node tumor spill or peritoneal implants.
Stage IV	Hematogenous dissemination of tumor to lungs, liver, bone, brain, or distant lymph node dissemination.
Stage V	Bilateral renal involvement at diagnosis.

Table 15–10. Two-year relapse-free survival rate in Wilms tumor, based on national Wilms tumor study 3.

Stage	Survival Rate (%)
I	93
II	90
III	82
IV	65

stage II–IV disease and in about 50% of patients with unfavorable histologic diagnosis and stage II–IV disease. However, unlike other solid tumors that recur, many cases of recurrent Wilms tumor may be cured. Thus, early detection of recurrence is crucial, and close surveillance after completion of therapy is important.

A major goal of the current Wilms tumor study is to develop treatment plans that cause less acute and long-term toxicity. Radiation therapy of the trunk unfortunately is associated with scoliosis and trunk underdevelopment in some patients. Second cancers have been reported in long-term survivors of Wilms tumor, but most of these have occurred in irradiated areas and include thyroid cancers, breast cancers, and sarcomas.

SARCOMAS

Sarcomas are malignant solid tumors arising from primitive mesenchymal cells. Normally mesenchymal cells develop and differentiate into fibrous tissue, cartilage, muscle, and bone. When sarcomas develop, complete differentiation of mature structures does not occur, but sometimes a hint of maturation is seen, providing a clue to tissue specificity.

Rhabdomyosarcoma is the most common soft tissue sarcoma in children and arises from cells that normally would give rise to striated muscle. However, rhabdomyosarcoma can also arise in areas where striated muscle is not found normally. Undifferentiated sarcoma, another prominent sarcoma, appears to be derived from mesoderm, but the degree of maturity is so minimal that there is no indication of tissue specificity. Rhabdomyosarcoma and undifferentiated sarcoma constitute the main sarcomas of childhood.

Incidence & Epidemiology

Rhabdomyosarcoma accounts for 5–8% of all cases of childhood cancer and is the sixth most common childhood malignancy after acute leukemia, tumors of the CNS, lymphoma, neuroblastoma, and Wilms tumor. Like Ewing sarcoma, rhabdomyosarcoma is far more common in whites (8:1 million) than in blacks (3.9:1 million) and slightly more common in the male population. Sarcomas of the bladder and vagina occur primarily in infants and younger children, whereas tumors of the head and neck occur at all ages but are more common in children younger than 8 years.

Etiology

The etiology of rhabdomyosarcoma is unknown. A combination of genetic and environmental factors has been implicated. Preliminary evidence suggests that parents of children with rhabdomyosarcoma have had more exposure to chemicals than have case-control subjects.

Genetics

Associations have been established between rhabdomyosarcoma and neurofibromatosis, and an increased incidence in children of mothers who have had breast cancer, although no specific genetic factors have been identified. Tumors are now being studied for karyotypic abnormalities.

Pathology & Biology

Sarcomas of soft tissue can arise anywhere in the body and can spread to contiguous and distant areas. Regardless of the histologic subtype, all forms can infiltrate local structures and invade local lymphatic tissues or bloodstream. Because of this behavior, the site of origin, regional lymph nodes, bone marrow, lungs, and bones must be considered potential metastatic sites for rhabdomyosarcoma.

Establishing a diagnosis of rhabdomyosarcoma can be difficult. The feature most often sought in light microscopic evaluation is cross-striations imitating striated muscle. More specific and helpful studies include immunocytochemical stains and antibodies directed against specific components of skeletal muscle, including myosin, desmin, and actin. Electron microscopy is also useful, particularly in undifferentiated tumors. Once the diagnosis is established, it is useful to categorize the cell pattern, as this may affect prognostic and treatment considerations. Most tumors can be classified as embryonal or alveolar in pattern. Embryonal rhabdomyosarcoma has spindle-shaped cells that appear to float in an abundant myxoid matrix. The alveolar pattern has a picture similar to lung alveoli but is lined by densely packed, high-grade, non–spindle-shaped tumor cells.

Clinical Presentation

Sarcoma has two major presentations in childhood: appearance of a mass lesion with or without pain and obstruction or pain of an involved or adjacent organ, which on investigation reveals a mass lesion. Signs and symptoms leading to a diagnosis of rhabdomyosarcoma are specific to the primary tumor site.

Approximately 25% of head and neck rhabdomyosarcomas are in the orbit, and 50% arise in other parameningeal sites of the head and neck. The sex ratio is equal, and the average age at diagnosis is 6 years. Orbital tumors present with proptosis and sometimes ophthalmoplegia. Tumors

in this location tend to be diagnosed before dissemination. Nonorbital parameningeal sarcomas arise most often in the nasopharynx, middle ear, mastoid region, pterygoid infratemporal fossa, and paranasal sinuses. These tumors usually present with nasal, aural, or sinus obstruction, with or without mucopurulent or sanguineous discharge. The presence of cranial nerve palsy may suggest involvement of adjacent meninges. Headache, vomiting, and systemic hypertension may result from intracranial extension. Craniocervical sarcomas arising in areas other than the orbit and parameningeal sites often present simply as a painless mass.

The genitourinary tract is another major site for rhabdomyosarcoma. Most of these sarcomas arise in the prostate and bladder. Bladder tumors tend to grow intraluminally, usually in or near the trigone. Hematuria, urinary obstruction, and occasionally extrusion of mucosanguineous tissue can occur. Children most commonly affected tend to be younger than 4 years. A prostate tumor usually presents as a large pelvic mass with or without accompanying urethral obstruction and constipation. As opposed to bladder tumors, prostate tumors tend not to remain localized and may present with spinal cord compression. Paratesticular tumors usually present as painless unilateral masses in the inguinal or scrotal region in prepubertal and postpubertal males. Up to 40% of patients have involved regional lymph nodes at the time of diagnosis. Embryonal histology tends to predominate in sarcomas of the genitourinary tract and in the head and neck.

Tumors of the trunk and extremities present with painless swelling in the affected body part. About 50% of these tumors have the alveolar histology, and regional lymph node involvement is rare unless the histology is of the alveolar type. Intrathoracic and retroperitoneal tumors tend to become quite large, with local invasion of adjacent tissues and lymph nodes before they are diagnosed. Often these tumors are not amenable to complete resection. These patients tend to do poorly, with recurrence likely despite aggressive multimodal therapy. Perineal tumors are uncommon and tend to be of alveolar histology. They frequently present with regional lymph node involvement. Biliary tract, brain, and liver sarcomas are rare.

Diagnosis & Staging

As opposed to masses or obstructive processes due to infection, sarcomas usually are nontender and impart no unusual hue to overlying skin. In this setting, a biopsy should be performed after radiographic imaging. MRI or CT scans are good for characterizing and determining the extent of the mass. MRI is probably superior for imaging the brain, spine, and pelvis. To evaluate for the presence of metastatic disease, a CT scan of the chest, a technetium bone scan, and a bone marrow biopsy are indicated. When parameningeal sites are involved, spinal fluid should be obtained for cytologic analysis. Baseline laboratory work includes a complete blood count; liver and renal function studies; and measurements of serum electrolyte, calcium, phosphorus, and uric acid concentrations in anticipation of chemotherapy. Assessing extent of disease at the onset is crucial for treatment planning. Table 15–11 outlines staging and grouping of sarcomas currently defined.

Prognosis

Several prognostic variables have been defined for rhabdomyosarcoma. Patients who present with localized disease fare much better than do those with metastatic disease at time of diagnosis. The histologic type also carries prognostic significance, as those with alveolar histology do more poorly than do those with embryonal rhabdomyosarcoma. The primary tumor site is also important prognostically. Patients with extremity or retroperitoneal tumors do very poorly. Sites less accessible to the surgeon make total resection less likely, and certain sites are more likely than others to be associated with lymphatic spread. In addition, the radiotolerance of some sites and their adjacent structures is greater than others and thus affects treatment.

Treatment

Treatment of sarcomas involves surgical resection if possible, radiation therapy for control of residual tumor, and systemic chemotherapy. Primary surgery is the fastest way to ablate disease and should be used when subsequent function or appearance will not be significantly impaired. When microscopic residua are found after an initial excision, or when the initial excision was performed without knowledge of the neoplasm, reexcision of the area should precede nonsurgical management. Sometimes debulking procedures are purposefully performed to decrease the field of radiation therapy when complete excision is not feasible. When local relapse occurs, therapy should include radical surgery when feasible, followed by radiation therapy when possible, with further intensive chemotherapy.

Radiation as a local control plays a major role in the treatment of children with rhabdomyosarcoma and undifferentiated sarcoma. It is particularly important in killing residual tumor cells from sites where surgery alone cannot ablate the tumor mass. Without radiation therapy, 75% of tumors will recur locally.

Chemotherapeutic agents useful in rhabdomyosarcoma include vincristine, cyclophosphamide, and actinomycin D. Ifosfamide and adriamycin have been associated with clinical responses as well. Timing of the radiation and chemotherapy depends on the clinical group of the tumor. Overall, chemotherapy is continued for about 1 year, with close surveillance after completion of therapy.

BONE TUMORS

Primary bone tumors are rare in childhood, and successful treatment remains a major challenge. Bone tumors are the seventh most common group of malignancies in children; however, in adolescents they are the third most common group of malignancies, exceeded only by leukemia and lymphoma. In the United States, the incidence of primary bone tumors is about 5:1 million children. This section presents only the two most common malignant bone tumors in young patients—osteosarcoma and Ewing sarcoma.

OSTEOSARCOMA

Epidemiology & Etiology

Osteosarcoma accounts for 60% of malignant bone tumors in the first two decades of life, with a peak incidence in late adolescence. It is equally common in boys and girls.

Although the etiology is unknown, certain associations have been established. As osteosarcoma frequently occurs in the long bones of children older than 13 years, it appears to be associated with a period of rapid bone growth in children. It is also more common in children who are taller than average. About 4% of cases are associated with previous radiation therapy. An association with retinoblastoma is well recognized, and it can occur in previously radiated areas or in distant bones. Retroviruses have been shown to induce bone sarcomas in animals, and it has been speculated that viruses play a role in human disease. Although a history of trauma often brings the child to medical attention, there is no evidence to suggest that trauma is an etiologic factor in osteosarcoma.

Pathology & Biology

Osteosarcoma usually originates in the osteon of medullary bone. The connective tissue stroma in osteosarcoma typically appears as a mixture of atypical, large, highly malignant spindle cells interspersed with osteoid production and calcium. Several histologic types are clas-

Table 15–11. Surgical-pathologic grouping system for rhabdomyosarcoma.

Group I	Localized disease, completely resected
	A. Confined to organ or muscle of origin
	B. Infiltration outside organ or muscle of origin; regional nodes not involved
Group II	Total gross resection with evidence of regional spread
	A. Grossly resected tumors with microscopic residual disease
	B. Regional disease with involved nodes, completely resected with no microscopic residual disease
	C. Regional disease with involved nodes, grossly resected, but with evidence of microscopic residual disease and/or histologic involvement of the most distal regional node (from the primary site) in the dissection
Group III	Incomplete resection or biopsy specimen with presence of gross residual disease
Group IV	Distant metastasis present at onset

sified by the relative preponderance and character of the matrix within the tumor. The four major types are osteoblastic, chondroblastic, fibroblastic, and telangiectatic. Another biologic variant of osteosarcoma without particular histologic specificity is multifocal osteosarcoma. This form has a particularly poor prognosis. Osteosarcoma develops most commonly in the distal femur, proximal tibia, and proximal humerus. These three sites account for 60% of tumors. Ninety percent of osteosarcomas develop in the metaphysis, and 10% develop in the diaphysis.

Clinical Presentation

Most patients seek medical care after about a 4-month history of pain in the affected area. A history of trauma is usual and can play a role in delaying diagnosis. Lower extremity tumors can present with a limp, and pain is severe, often causing awakening at night. On physical examination, a mass can be palpated in 60% of patients, often associated with local warmth. In advanced tumors, increased vascular markings can be seen over the mass. Range of motion usually is decreased secondary to pain.

Systemic symptoms other than intermittent fever are rare unless disease is metastatic at the time of presentation. At diagnosis, 20% of patients have radiographically visible metastatic disease in the lungs. Other, less common sites of metastasis include bone, pleura, lymph node, kidney, and brain. At diagnosis, about 80% of patients have elevated serum alkaline phosphatase concentration. This finding is associated with an increased likelihood of disease progressing to pulmonary metastasis.

Diagnosis & Staging

The initial evaluation usually includes a plain radiograph, which is sometimes diagnostic. Extension of tumor through the periosteum may result in a sunburst-like appearance in 60% of cases. Periosteal reaction with new bone formation can produce an "onion peel" sign as well, but this is less common. MRI is useful in determining the extent of cortical bone involvement, the presence of intramedullary spread, the presence of noncontiguous lesions, and invasion into adjacent soft tissue. Nonetheless, a biopsy is required for diagnosis even though MRI imaging is very suggestive. A staging workup after diagnosis should include a technetium bone scan to identify other possible bone lesions and a CT scan of the chest to rule out metastatic disease in the lung, the most common site for metastatic disease. In preparation for chemotherapy, a complete blood count and tests for hepatic and renal function should be obtained.

The differential diagnosis of osteosarcoma includes a variety of benign and malignant conditions that present with pain, swelling, and an abnormal radiograph. Of the malignant disorders, fibrosarcoma, rhabdomyosarcoma, Ewing sarcoma, and metastatic disease from other malignancies are major considerations. Benign neoplastic processes to consider in the differential diagnosis include giant cell tumor, aneurysmal bone cyst, unicameral bone cyst, osteoblastoma, osteochondroma, and chondroblas-

toma. Non-neoplastic processes that must be differentiated from osteosarcoma include a stress fracture, osteomyelitis, and a subperiosteal hematoma.

Treatment

Before the use of chemotherapy for osteosarcoma, even with amputation, more than 80% of patients died. Currently, standard treatment includes neoadjuvant chemotherapy with some combination of high-dose methotrexate, cisplatin, doxorubicin, and ifosfamide for 8–10 weeks, followed by a surgical procedure, either amputation or limb salvage, which is then followed by more chemotherapy to complete a treatment course of approximately 1 year. Chemotherapy before surgery not only presumably destroys micrometastasis and prevents delay in postoperative recovery secondary to chemotherapy, but also allows one to determine effectiveness of therapy. Response to preoperative chemotherapy can be assessed by clinical radiographic and pathologic parameters. In addition, killing the primary tumor enhances the chance that tumor cells will be absent around the margins at surgery and can decrease the likelihood of hematogenous seeding at that time.

Over the past 20 years, limb salvage procedures have become an integral part of therapy for specific candidates with osteosarcoma. The decision to perform amputation versus a limb salvage procedure depends on the size and location of the tumor and patient preference.

Prognosis

With chemotherapy and complete resection of tumor, approximately 70% of patients experience disease-free survival. Metastases develop most commonly within the first 2 years after diagnosis; the sooner patients have metastatic disease, the poorer their overall outcome. Long-term survival after the development of metastasis is rare but can be achieved with surgical resection of pulmonary disease. The effectiveness of further chemotherapy and radiation therapy has not been demonstrated.

Several prognostic features may be important. Historically, patients younger than 10 years have a poorer prognosis. Tumors of the extremities are associated with a slightly better outlook than are those of the axial skeleton. Probably the most significant prognostic factor in osteosarcoma is the effectiveness of chemotherapy against the tumor, combined with an effective surgical procedure. Future work is focused on finding more effective chemotherapy, continued improvement in detecting residual disease, and developing better surgical approaches. Currently, the effectiveness of an immune-regulated agent in preventing the development of metastatic disease is being studied in a clinical trial.

EWING SARCOMA

Until about 20 years ago, fewer than 20% of patients with Ewing sarcoma survived regardless of the extent of disease at diagnosis. Today, with better understanding of the biologic behavior of this disease, better chemotherapy, and better radiation therapy, a more optimistic outlook has emerged.

Incidence & Epidemiology

Ewing sarcoma accounts for about 1% of all childhood cancer and about 30% of malignant childhood bone tumors. The annual incidence is about 2.69:1 million cases in whites and 0.28:1 million cases in blacks. There is a distinct male predominance of approximately 70%, and, like osteosarcoma, Ewing sarcoma is more common in taller individuals. Although several cases of familial occurrences of Ewing sarcoma have been reported, the evidence has not been substantial enough to suggest an inherited genetic susceptibility.

Etiology

There is no known etiology. Unlike osteosarcoma, there is no association between Ewing sarcoma and ionizing radiation. A translocation between chromosome 11 and 22 has been identified in many tumor specimens. This is not specific for Ewing sarcoma, as it can be seen with tumors of neuroepithelial origin as well and appears to result in a disrupted transcription factor.

Pathology & Biology

The small, round, blue cell tumors of childhood (neuroblastoma, Ewing sarcoma, rhabdomyosarcoma, lymphoma) provide a diagnostic dilemma for the pathologist. Many pathologists base their diagnosis on a corroborative history, physical examination, radiographic findings, and a positive PAS stain. Under light microscopy, a fairly uniform population of homogenous small cells with hyperchromic nuclei is noted. The typical Ewing sarcoma is undifferentiated, with scant cytoskeletal formations, absence of membrane or cytoplasmic products, and no appreciable extracellular matrix. It is speculated that Ewing sarcoma is derived either from a stem cell that resides in the mesenchymal component of the medullary canal of bone and in extra-axial soft tissue or from primitive neuroepithelial origins. Flow cytometry is useful in the diagnosis of Ewing sarcoma, in that Ewing sarcoma cells stain positively for the c-*myc* tumor marker. However, lymphoblastic lymphoma may produce a positive stain as well. Other markers must be used to differentiate these malignancies.

Clinical Presentation

It is difficult to distinguish Ewing sarcoma from other malignant bone processes on the basis of clinical findings alone. There are no pathognomonic radiologic lesions, and diagnosis can be verified only with open biopsy. Apart from osteosarcoma, the two conditions most often mistaken for this tumor are osteomyelitis and histiocytosis. The time from onset of symptoms to diagnosis varies but is usually 1–5 months. Patients manifest pain and sometimes a palpable mass. Systemic symptoms, including fever and anemia, are more common in Ewing sar-

coma than in osteosarcoma. Like osteosarcoma, Ewing sarcoma is a disease of older children and adolescents; the median age at diagnosis is 13 years, a slightly younger age of diagnosis than that found with osteosarcoma.

The femur is the bone most commonly involved, but virtually any bone can be affected. Most osteolytic lesions are in the metaphysis. Medullary expansion and thickening of cortical bone and major soft tissue component are common. As with osteosarcoma, Ewing sarcoma originates from the medullary cavity. It can metastasize virtually anywhere, but lungs and lymph nodes are the usual initial sites, and late recurrences tend to metastasize to the brain.

Diagnosis & Staging

The radiographic appearance of Ewing sarcoma is variable; a diffuse lytic lesion in the metaphysis of a long bone is the most common finding. When tumor occurs in flat bones, a sclerotic reaction is not infrequent. This so-called onion skinning represents periosteal new bone formation. After a plain film radiograph, an MRI is the imaging study of choice to evaluate the primary lesion. Metastatic disease is present at diagnosis in 15–35% of patients. A bone scan is useful to rule out multiple bony sites, and a CT scan of the chest is important to detect visible lung metastasis. A bone marrow biopsy and aspirate should be performed as well, because Ewing sarcoma does metastasize to bone marrow. One need not evaluate the brain or spinal column unless the primary site is adjacent to these areas or there are suggestive symptoms and signs. Baseline studies before chemotherapy should include a complete blood count and hepatic and renal function tests. No biochemical serum studies are of use in Ewing sarcoma. As with osteogenic sarcoma, an open biopsy is the diagnostic procedure of choice in establishing histologic diagnosis.

Prognosis

Like osteosarcoma, the more distal from the axial skeleton, the better the likelihood of long-term survival. In addition, patients with widely metastatic disease have a much poorer outcome than do those with an isolated lesion. Girls have been suggested to have a slightly better long-term survival than boys. Again, as with osteosarcoma, probably the most important factors are responsiveness of the primary tumor to chemotherapy and the ability to have excellent local control with complete resection or high-dose radiation, or some combination of the two.

Treatment

Chemotherapy, radiation, and surgery historically have played important roles in the treatment of Ewing sarcoma. The decision to radiate or locally excise the tumor depends primarily on the location of the tumor. Unfortunately, pathologic fractures are too common in radiated bones. The later development of osteosarcoma in the radiated bone can occur in up to 5% of patients. Standard therapy consists of chemotherapy with doxorubicin, cyclophosphamide, and vincristine for 1 year with surgery or radiation to the primary tumor at about week 10 of therapy. Newer treatments are being explored, including other chemotherapeutics, hyperfractionated delivery of radiation therapy, and autologous bone marrow transplant for widely metastatic disease. For pelvic tumors, presurgical chemotherapy and radiation therapy help to shrink the tumor, allowing complete surgical resection in some.

Even with intensive radiation therapy and chemotherapy, 10–20% of patients experience a local recurrence. The 3-year survival rate is 60–70%. Patients with metastatic disease still have a very poor prognosis, and salvage with late relapse is also poor. The risk of relapse decreases for patients who are free of disease for 3 years; however, relapses as late as 8 years have been reported.

HISTIOCYTOSIS

Biology

The histiocytoses are characterized by infiltration and accumulation of cells of the monocyte-macrophage type. Recently, the histiocytoses have been classified pathologically. This schema is based on how these lesions relate to normal histiocytic and reticulocyte subsets. This system provides a conceptual framework for diagnosis and treatment of these lesions.

Class I. This group includes disorders in which the central cell has histiopathic features of the Langerhans cell. The Langerhans cell is a normal skin cell that processes antigens. **Langerhans cell histiocytosis (LCH),** formerly known as **histiocytosis X,** is not a true neoplasm but a proliferative lesion, possibly secondary to a defect in immunoregulation. The characteristic "tennis racket" appearance of Birbeck granules seen on electron microscopy is found in normal histiocytes as well. The significance of the presence of Birbeck granules is not known. Langerhans cells stain positively for S100 and CD_{1a}. Grossly, the class I histiocytoses are granulomatous lesions and are either pure histiocytic infiltrates or mixed with eosinophils. Recent evidence suggests that LCH is a clonal disorder, but this is not yet proved.

Class II. This group of histiocytoses, representing the largest group of those disorders, includes the nonmalignant histiocytoses in which the accumulating mononuclear cell is of the phagocytic antigen-processing cell. This is different from class I cells, which are also reactive histiocytes but of the antigen-presenting or dendritic cell type. In class II histiocytoses, the normal monocyte-macrophage is the predominant cell type, frequently in a mixed lymphohistiocytic infiltrate. There is no cytologic atypia in this type, which includes familial erythrophagolymphohistiocytosis (FEL) and infection-associated histiophago-

cytic syndrome. Most affected sites include red pulp of the spleen, hepatic sinusoids, bone marrow, and lymph node sinuses. Prominent phagocytosis of platelets, red cells, and leukocytes is common.

Class III. This group comprises true malignant disorders of mononuclear phagocytes, including histiocytic sarcoma, acute monoblastic leukemia, and malignant histiocytosis. Acute monoblastic leukemia occurs when bone marrow–derived monoblasts proliferate. Malignant histiocytosis occurs when malignant clones of mononuclear phagocytes are intermediately differentiated between monocytes and monoblasts and fixed-tissue histiocytes. This malignancy is a systemic process involving the whole reticuloendothelial system. Erythrophagocytosis may be present but is not a prominent feature. Histiocytic lymphoma is rare; it is a malignancy of the mononuclear phagocyte system at the stage of the fixed-tissue histiocyte. The lesions are localized and discrete. Without specialized diagnostic tests, this tumor would be in the category of large-cell immunoblastic lymphoma.

Clinical Presentation

Presentation in the **class I** histiocytoses is variable and includes chronic draining otitis media, chronic rash, fever, adenopathy, bone pain, diabetes insipidus, weight loss, hemolytic anemia, and hepatosplenomegaly. The differential diagnosis rests on identifying Birbeck granules. The clinical hallmark of LCH is the presence of lytic bone lesions. In infants, LCH can present with wasting, hepatosplenomegaly, generalized lymphadenopathy, anemia, and sometimes pancytopenia. Milder forms are seen in older children. All tissues can be involved, but the most common include bone, skin, liver, spleen, lymph nodes, and bone marrow. Only 25% or less involve lungs, eyes, orodental tissues, ear, CNS, or gastrointestinal tract.

The outcome of class I histiocytoses is variable. In most cases, the disease resolves itself. The two most important prognostic factors appear to be age at diagnosis and degree of organ involvement. Children younger than 2 years at the time of diagnosis have a higher mortality rate than do older children. This probably represents a more aggressive form of disease seen in the younger children rather than any other factor. In addition, the presence of organ dysfunction has been a poor prognostic sign; the involvement of multiple organs has an additional negative effect on survival. Approaches to treatment have varied. Because treatment does not appear to affect prognosis, less intensive therapy is the current trend. Therapies usually include either low-dose radiation therapy, prednisone, vinblastine, or some combination. All treatment is directed against developing irreversible damage to tissues.

Class II histiocytic processes presumably are secondary to a primary underlying disease process; with effective treatment of the disease, the histiocytic process should resolve. FEL is characterized by hemophagocytosis and a positive family history. It is rare and almost always rapidly fatal. Currently, bone marrow transplant is the treatment of choice. Affected children, usually younger than 4 years at the time of diagnosis, manifest fever of unknown origin and weight loss. Erythrophagocytosis is marked. The diagnosis rests on identifying lymphohistiocytic infiltrates with conspicuous erythrophagocytosis. Infection-associated hemophagocytosis is associated with a variety of viral, fungal, bacterial, and parasitic infections. Usually it occurs in the setting of an acquired immunodeficiency or in T-cell lymphoid malignancy. Clinical features include coagulopathy, fever, liver disease, and anemia. The diagnosis is usually made by bone marrow aspirate, which demonstrates frequent, benign-appearing histiocytes containing platelets and red cells.

Class III histiocytoses are the most uncommon form. Fever, wasting, hepatosplenomegaly, and lymphadenopathy are seen. The diagnosis is best made by lymph node biopsy. Treatment is based on an accurate diagnosis and involves chemotherapy and bone marrow transplantation.

CHEMOTHERAPY BASICS

Chemotherapy has provided more benefit to children with cancer than to affected adults, and many principles of modern chemotherapy are based on the experience in children.

Most chemotherapeutic agents are cytotoxic and produce cytotoxic effects by interfering with the synthesis or function of DNA (Table 15–12). Only actively proliferating cells are susceptible to the effects of these agents; therefore, anticancer drugs are most effective in cancers with a high growth fraction. Because growth fraction decreases as tumor size increases, most chemotherapy is more effective against microscopic disease than bulk disease.

Using chemotherapy in a rational manner in children has been difficult, as many of the quantitative actions have not been defined and pharmacokinetic studies in children have not been performed. Thus, drug dosage and schedule have for the most part been empiric. Antitumor drugs are fairly nonselective and have the lowest therapeutic index of any group of drugs. Toxicities are common and frequently must be tolerated to achieve therapeutic effect.

The selection of the drugs used to treat a child with cancer is made mostly by tumor histology and stage. Active drugs are usually used in combination to ensure the greatest chance of achieving a good response. This provides a broader range of coverage against naturally occurring drug resistance and decreases the chances of acquired resistance. Some combination regimens include drugs with known activity as single agents, whereas other combinations exploit biochemical interactions between the drugs.

Table 15–12. Classes of chemotherapies and their mode of action.

Class	Mode of Action
Alkylating agent Nitrogen mustard Cyclophosphamide Ifosfamide, Cisplatin Nitrosurea, DTIC	Covalently binds alkyl group, damaging intrastrand DNA links, DNA-protein cross-links.
Antimetabolites 6-Mercaptopurine 6-Thioguanine Cytosine arabinoside 5-Fluorouracil	Structurally analogous to important intermediates in biosynthetic pathways; either inhibits synthesis of macromolecules or incorporated to make a faulty molecule.
Antitumor antibiotics Anthracyclines Bleomycin Dactinomycin	Most naturally occurring of these drugs—derived from *Streptomyces* bacteria.
Plant alkyloids Vincristine, Vinblastine Epipodophyllotoxins VP-16, VP-26	Inhibit mitotic spindle formation or cause breaks in DNA strand.
Corticosteroids Prednisone Dexamethasone	Lympholytic? Mediated through glucocorticoid receptors.
L-asparaginase	Catalyzes the conversion of amino acid L-asparagine to aspartic acid and depletes circulating pool of L-asparagine.

DTIC = decarbazine.

Ideally, each drug is given in optimal dosage with the shortest possible interval between courses of therapy. If possible, drug combinations with overlapping and additive toxicity are avoided.

Acute toxicities of chemotherapy include myelosuppression, nausea and vomiting, alopecia, mucositis, allergic or cutaneous reactions, and local tissue burn from subcutaneous extravasation of drug. Some drugs have unique toxicities, such as anthracycline with cardiotoxicity and vincristine with neuropathy. With the increasing use of colony-stimulating factors after chemotherapy courses, shorter durations of neutropenia are seen, and fewer episodes of fever with neutropenia are experienced by the patient. Transfusions with platelets and packed red blood cells are necessary for many patients during their course of treatment. Nausea and vomiting are well controlled with antiemetics in most patients.

Long-term side effects of chemotherapy are a growing concern as more children enjoy long-term survival. The major adverse side effects include impaired growth and development, impaired reproductive function, and the possibility of permanent cardiac, pulmonary, or renal damage. In addition, patients treated with chemotherapy for one malignancy are at a greater risk than the general population for the development of a second malignancy. The long-term toxicities of radiation are a particular concern for children as well. Not only are there increased risks for second malignancies but also for impaired growth, especially to the musculoskeletal system, and for impaired organ function. With new approaches to the delivery of radiation and effective combinations of chemotherapy and lower-dose radiation, we hope to see fewer long-term side effects from radiation.

Drug resistance has long been encountered but recently has been better understood. Drug resistance most likely develops from genetic alterations, resulting in changes in gene products or in cellular metabolism. A great deal of research is in progress aimed at finding avenues to bypass drug resistance.

Although chemotherapy is not without risk for the child with cancer, its use has greatly improved survival for this group of patients. Research continues toward the development of more specific, more effective, and safer agents.

APPROACH TO THE CHILD WITH LYMPHADENOPATHY

The differential diagnosis of lymphadenopathy in children is large; however, the overwhelming majority is due to infectious processes (see Chapter 9). **Lymphadenopathy** is defined as a nontender lymph node larger than 10 mm at all anatomic sites, except in the epitrochlear area, where nodes larger than 5 mm are considered abnormal, and in the inguinal area, where a node must be larger than 15 mm to be considered abnormal. Lymphadenopathy, especially when it persists longer than 6 weeks, often raises the concern of an ongoing malignant process.

It is sometimes difficult for the clinician to differentiate infectious from malignant lymphadenopathy. Several clues should raise one's suspicion of a malignancy. Although many of the systemic symptoms of infection are similar to those of a malignancy, in general, weight loss, fever, malaise, bone pain, and bleeding should suggest a malignancy rather than a simple infectious process. On physical examination, matted nodes, particularly in the low cervical or supraclavicular regions, likewise raise the suspicion of a malignancy. The lymphadenopathy associated with metastatic neuroblastoma, or sarcoma, is characteristically hard and frequently immobile. However, in lymphoma and leukemia, the nodes can be rubbery and mobile. Lymphadenopathy associated with a malignant process is rarely associated with tenderness, erythema, or warmth unless a secondary infection is ongoing.

Most lymphadenopathy associated with a viral process resolves spontaneously in approximately 2–6 weeks. The lymphadenopathy of cat scratch fever is frequently seen by the pediatric oncologist. Bacterial processes can cause significant adenopathy which may require antibiotics to improve. If the lymphadenopathy persists, nonspecific studies should be undertaken, including a complete blood count and the specific tests for various infectious causes of lymphadenopathy. Other screening tests often considered useful include a purified protein derivative, chest radiograph, and erythrocyte sedimentation rate. If still no etiology is found, a fine needle aspirate with cultures should be considered. However, if one is particularly suspicious of a malignant process, a lymph node biopsy should be performed so that the lymph node architecture can be assessed; adequate tissue will be available for further studies. Probably the most important rule to avoid missing adenopathy associated with malignancy is to take a very careful history and to follow the patient's status closely with repeated physical examinations.

APPROACH TO THE CHILD & FAMILY WITH CANCER

The diagnosis of cancer in a child is an incomprehensible tragedy for a family. Approaching the family with sensitivity and care is crucial to establishing a long-term working relationship. Determining the family structure and resources and identifying the primary caretakers are important first steps in directing information and initiating future discussions.

Because disbelief, terror, and shock characterize the typical initial response to the suspected diagnosis of cancer in a child, one should keep early discussions brief, frequent, and concrete in nature. Thorough and thoughtful explanations of the diagnostic evaluation and procedures are crucial for preparing the child and family and play an instrumental part in building trust.

Once the diagnostic evaluation is complete and the diagnosis is confirmed, a family conference should be held. This conference should include members of the family, key caretakers, and the health care team, comprising the oncology nurse specialist, social worker, pediatric oncologist, and primary care physician. Encouraging the family to bring a tape recorder to the session provides the opportunity for them to review the discussion. It is also wise to provide the family with educational materials before the conference so that they may prepare questions in advance.

The family conference should cover the cause of the disease, the outcome without treatment, treatment options, study protocols, and the team's specific recommendations for treatment. Information should be given on how chemotherapy works, acute and chronic effects of chemotherapy, and side effects of the specific chemotherapy to be used. In addition, the psychological impact of the experience on the patient and the family should be discussed. This is also the time when consent is obtained to proceed with treatment. Perhaps the most important function of the meeting, besides conveying information about the disease and treatment, is to emphasize that treating a child with cancer is a team effort in which the family plays a crucial role. The family should be told that, besides curing cancer, the goal of treatment is to promote and maintain as normal a childhood as possible for patients and their siblings. Emphasizing the importance of the family as educated advocates for the child not only ensures knowledge of the treatment and expected side effects, but also allows the family to experience some sense of control and usefulness.

Frequently, the family and child manifest myriad behaviors and emotions in response to the cancer. Acknowledging these and guiding the family to productive coping strategies aids in the child's overall well-being. Particular attention to the special needs and responses of siblings is important. It is not uncommon to see school problems, acting out, and depression in the siblings of children in whom cancer is diagnosed. The combined insights of the medical team members should be shared in regular discussions with the family to ward off predictable and anticipated problems throughout the course of treatment. Involving the family in a support group may be helpful and should be recommended to all families.

In summary, responding to both the child and the family with respect, patience, and honesty is crucial to success in the complicated, often lengthy process of treating cancer in a child.

REFERENCES

LEUKEMIA

Pui CH, Crist WM: Biology and treatment of acute lymphoblastic leukemia. J Pediatr 1994;124:491.

Smith M et al: Uniform approach to risk classification and treatment assignment for children with acute lymphoblastic leukemia. J Clin Oncol 1996;14:18.

Wells RJ et al: Treatment of newly diagnosed children and adolescents with acute myeloid leukemia: A Childrens Cancer Group study. J Clin Oncol 1994;12:2367.

HODGKIN & NON-HODGKIN LYMPHOMA

Reiter A et al: Non-Hodgkin's lymphomas of childhood and adolescence: Results of a treatment stratified for biologic subtypes and stage—a report of the Berlin-Frankfurt-Munster Group. J Clin Oncol 1995;13:359.

NEUROBLASTOMA

Matthay KK et al: Allogeneic versus autologous purged bone marrow transplantation for neuroblastoma: A report from the Childrens Cancer Group. J Clin Oncol 1994;12:2382.

WILMS TUMOR

Tournade MF et al: Results of the Sixth International Society of Pediatric Oncology Wilms' Tumor Trial and Study: A risk-adapted therapeutic approach in Wilms' tumor. J Clin Oncol 1993;11:1014.

SARCOMAS

Pappo AS et al: Biology and therapy of pediatric rhabdomyosarcoma. J Clin Oncol 1995;13:2123.

BONE TUMORS

Link MP et al: The effect of adjuvant chemotherapy on relapse-free survival in patients with osteosarcoma of the extremity. N Engl J Med 1986;314:1600.

16

Kidneys & Electrolytes

Anthony A. Portale, MD, Robert S. Mathias, MD, Diana C. Tanney, MD, & Donald E. Potter, MD

EVALUATION OF RENAL FUNCTION

In healthy individuals, the kidneys excrete water, solutes, and metabolic wastes in amounts that permit the maintenance of a relatively constant internal milieu despite the consumption of a widely varied diet. Cellular integrity depends on the maintenance of a narrowly regulated extracellular fluid (ECF) osmolality. In response to information from osmoreceptors and volume receptors, the brain and kidneys produce hormones and vasoactive substances that allow rapid and precise regulation of salt and water excretion by the kidney.

The kidneys produce urine via glomerular ultrafiltration of plasma and selective tubular reabsorption of water and solutes; tubular secretion of solutes also plays an important but lesser role. The kidneys receive approximately 20% of the cardiac output via the renal arteries. In an individual with a cardiac output of 5 L/min, renal blood flow is 1 L/min and renal plasma flow is 550 mL/min, assuming a hematocrit of 45%. As a consequence of the Starling forces, which favor filtration, and a highly permeable glomerular capillary membrane of large surface area, approximately one fifth of the plasma flowing through the glomerular capillaries is filtered into the Bowman space. The rate of formation of ultrafiltrate is termed the **glomerular filtration rate (GFR).** In a 70-kg adult man, the GFR is approximately 125 mL/min, or 180 L/d. Because the GFR is determined in part by cardiac output and renal plasma flow, both of which are a function of body size and sex, the GFR in children is lower than that in adults. Rather than establishing normative values for children of various ages and sizes, it is customary for the measured GFR to be normalized to a body surface area of 1.73 m_2 using the following formula:

$$\text{GFR (mL/min/1.73 m}^2\text{)} = \frac{\text{GFR (mL/min)} \times 1.73 \text{ m}^2}{\text{SA (m}^2\text{)}}$$

where SA equals the surface area of the patient.

Within each nephron, the ultrafiltrate of plasma passes from Bowman's space into the renal tubule, where its composition is changed by reabsorptive and secretory transport processes. More than 99% of the filtered water, sodium, chloride, and bicarbonate is reabsorbed by the renal tubule and returned to the blood. The daily filtered load of sodium is approximately 25,000 meq; the tubules reabsorb this amount minus an amount equal to the daily dietary intake of sodium, 100–250 meq/d, which is excreted. Failure to reabsorb nearly all the sodium filtered would quickly result in life-threatening sodium and volume depletion. The kidneys also excrete the daily load of endogenous acid produced because of diet and metabolism and remove metabolic wastes, such as urea nitrogen, creatinine, phosphorus, and uric acid.

GLOMERULAR FILTRATION RATE

The need to assess renal function in children arises when they have symptoms or signs suggestive of renal disease, such as abnormal urinary findings, peripheral edema, or hypertension. The GFR is an important measure of renal function, as it reflects the overall excretory function of the kidney and, therefore, the number of functioning nephrons. GFR is not measured directly, but can be estimated experimentally by measuring the clearance from plasma of a marker substance such as inulin. Inulin, a low-molecular-weight sugar, is an ideal marker for estimating GFR because it is not bound to plasma proteins and is freely filtered by the glomerulus, without being reabsorbed, secreted, or metabolized by the renal tubules. **Renal clearance** of any substance is defined as the volume of plasma completely cleared of that substance per unit time. When inulin is infused intravenously at a constant rate to achieve a steady-state plasma inulin level, all the inulin filtered by the glomerulus is excreted in the urine, thus completely clearing the volume of plasma filtered.

The clearance of inulin (C_{inulin}) is calculated according to the following equation:

$$\text{GFR} \cong C_{inulin} \text{ (mL/min)} = \frac{U_{inulin} \times V \text{ (mL/min)}}{P_{inulin}}$$

where U_{inulin} equals urinary inulin concentration, V equals the volume of urine passed during a given time, and P_{inulin} equals the plasma inulin concentration. Normative values for GFR (corrected to 1.73 m^2), measured by inulin clearance in children, are listed in Table 16–1.

The clearance of creatinine (C_{creat}), the metabolic end-product of normal muscle metabolism, is commonly used to estimate GFR in the clinical setting. At steady state, the rate of creatinine produced from muscle metabolism remains relatively constant from day to day and is matched by an equal rate of creatinine excretion. In normally proportioned individuals, the rate of creatinine excretion is approximately 15 mg/kg/d in children to 20 mg/kg/d in adults; this difference reflects the proportionate increase in muscle mass that occurs with growth. The C_{creat} is usually measured from a urine specimen collected over a 24-hour period; the plasma creatinine value is determined at the end of the urine collection period. The C_{creat} is calculated according to the following equation:

$$C_{creat} \text{ (mL/min)} = \frac{U_{Cr} \text{ (mg/dL)} \times V \text{ (mL/min)}}{P_{Cr} \text{ (mg/dL)}}$$

The C_{creat} tends to overestimate the GFR because, in addition to being filtered across the glomerulus, creatinine is also secreted into the renal tubular lumen. When renal function is normal, C_{creat} overestimates the GFR by approximately 10–20%; the degree of overestimation increases substantially, however, as renal function worsens, because a greater percentage of the creatinine excreted comes from tubular secretion. Despite these limitations, C_{creat} determination remains a useful and readily obtainable estimate of the GFR. Repeated measurements made over time provide useful information about the rate of disease progression or regression.

Radionuclide imaging studies also can be used to esti-mate the GFR. The low-molecular-weight filtration markers, diethylenetriaminepenta-acetic acid (DTPA) and iothalamate, can be conjugated to radioisotopes and then injected intravenously into the patient. Their rate of appearance in and disappearance from the kidneys is monitored by external radiation counters. Estimates of GFR obtained with this technique are comparable to those obtained by inulin clearance measurements. Performance of a radionuclide study requires less time than does a C_{creat} determination and does not necessitate blood or urine collection; its disadvantages are a relatively high cost, the need for intravenous access, and the radiation exposure, albeit low.

In clinical practice, the plasma creatinine concentration is the most commonly used index of kidney function. It can be seen from Equation 3 that the C_{creat}, which estimates the GFR, varies inversely with the plasma creatinine (P_{Cr}) concentration:

$$C_{creat} = \frac{\text{Constant}}{P_{Cr}}$$

where Constant equals the daily amount of creatinine excreted in urine. To see how C_{creat} and P_{Cr} are inversely related, consider a patient with a GFR of 120 mL/min and serum creatinine concentration of 1.0 mg/dL. A decrease in GFR to 60 mL/min (a 50% decrease) will be accompanied by an increase in serum creatinine concentration to 2.0 mg/dL. An important hazard of using P_{Cr} to monitor renal function is that the largest actual reduction in GFR is accompanied by the smallest numerical increase in the serum creatinine concentration. For example, in a healthy 4-year-old child in whom the serum creatinine concentration normally is 0.4 mg/dL, a 50% decrease in GFR (from 120 mL/min to 60 mL/min) will result in a doubling of the serum creatinine concentration to 0.8 mg/dL, an increase of only 0.4 mg/dL. A further limitation of the serum creatinine concentration is that a mild to moderate decrease in GFR is accompanied by an increase in the rate of tubular secretion of creatinine. The increased tubular secretion of creatinine limits the increase in serum creatinine concentration that would be expected from the decrease in GFR. When creatinine secretory activity is maximally increased, further decreases in the GFR are more directly associated with increases in serum creatinine concentration.

An easily obtainable estimate of GFR is often needed when evaluating patients with renal disease or determining the correct drug dosage for medications that undergo renal metabolism or excretion. Various formulas have been developed that allow estimation of the C_{creat} from the serum creatinine concentration and some parameter of body size. The following formula (Schwartz formula), which was derived from measurements of height, serum creatinine concentration, and C_{creat} values, can be used in children:

$$C_{creat} \text{ (mL/min/1.73 m}^2\text{)} = \frac{K \times \text{Height (cm)}}{P_{Cr} \text{ (mg/dL)}}$$

Table 16–1. Glomerular filtration rate (GFR) measured by inulin clearance at different ages.

Age	GFR (Inulin Clearance) Mean and Range ($\pm$ 2 SD) (mL/min/1.73 m^2)
Premature	47 (29–65)
2–8 d	38 (26–60)
4–28 d	48 (28–68)
35–95 d	58 (30–86)
1–6 mo	77 (41–103)
6–12 mo	103 (49–157)
12–19 mo	127 (63–191)
2–12 y	127 (89–165)
Adult men	131 (88–174)
Adult women	117 (87–147)

where K is a coefficient that accounts for differences in body size and thus in muscle mass in children of different ages and sexes. The appropriate values of K to be used in this equation are listed in Table 16–2.

URINALYSIS

A complete urinalysis includes both chemical and microscopic examination of a urine specimen; the specific determinations are listed in Table 16–3. The general appearance of urine can provide useful information, as frothy or foamy urine may indicate proteinuria; pink, red, or tea-colored urine usually indicates hematuria.

The urine **specific gravity** is a measurement of the density of urine compared with that of water. Under most circumstances, the urine specific gravity reflects the osmolality of the urine, which in turn reflects the action of antidiuretic hormone (ADH; arginine vasopressin) on the renal tubule. The normal range of urine specific gravity is 1.001–1.030, corresponding to a urine osmolality of 40–1200 mOsm/kg. In patients with diabetes insipidus, the urine specific gravity is very low, usually 1.000–1.005, whereas in those with the syndrome of inappropriate antidiuretic hormone (SIADH) secretion, urine specific gravity is high, 1.015–1.030. Osmolality is the preferred measurement of renal concentrating capacity, as the presence of glucose, protein, or contrast media can give rise to an increase in the measured specific gravity without a change in urine osmolality.

Chemical tests can be performed on urine specimens using reagent-impregnated dipsticks that yield semiquantitative results. Urinary **pH,** measured with the dipstick, or less commonly with a pH electrode, ranges from approximately 4.5 to 8.0 throughout the course of the day; first morning specimens typically are acidic (ie, < 6.0). Measurement of urinary pH during acid or bicarbonate loading of a patient with suspected renal tubular acidosis can help to delineate the precise location of the renal tubular defect.

The dipstick detects urinary **protein concentration.** A positive result by dipstick can reflect either an increased quantity of urinary protein or a normal quantity of protein in a concentrated specimen. Collection of a timed urine specimen is necessary to quantitate urinary protein excretion precisely (see this chapter, Proteinuria).

The presence of **glucose** in the urine, in the absence of

Table 16–3. Components of a urinalysis.

General appearance	
Color	Odor
Turbidity	Foam
Specific gravity	
Chemical tests (dipstick)	
pH	Bilirubin
Protein	Urobilinogen
Glucose	Nitrite
Ketones	Leukocyte esterase
Blood	
Microscopic examination	
WBC, WBC casts	Hyaline, granular casts
RBC, RBC casts	Bacteria
Epithelial cells	Crystals

RBC = red blood cell; WBC = white blood cell.

hyperglycemia, suggests an impairment in the tubular handling of glucose, as occurs in the Fanconi syndrome, a disorder in which proximal tubular reabsorption of phosphate, amino acids, and bicarbonate also is impaired.

Urine dipsticks test positive for blood when either hemoglobin or myoglobin is present in the urine. Hemoglobin is detected when either erythrocytes or free hemoglobin are present; the latter can occur in patients with intravascular hemolysis. Myoglobinuria occurs during rhabdomyolysis. On microscopic examination of urine, the finding of erythrocytes confirms the presence of hematuria, and the finding of red blood cell casts confirms that the kidney is the source of the hematuria. The presence of white blood cells (WBCs) suggests an infection of the urinary tract; WBC casts accompanied by a positive urine culture are diagnostic of pyelonephritis. Other types of casts, such as hyaline or granular casts, can be found in normal individuals and are therefore nondiagnostic.

Crystals can form in the urine in a pH- and temperature-dependent manner. In acid urine, calcium oxalate and uric acid crystals are most commonly seen; both may be present in the urine of normal individuals. Cystine crystals are always abnormal and indicate that the patient has either cystinosis or cystinuria. In alkaline urine from healthy individuals, calcium carbonate, calcium phosphate, and triple phosphate crystals can be seen. Triple phosphate crystals are also seen in patients with urinary tract infections (UTIs) caused by urease-producing bacteria.

Table 16–2. K values for children of various ages for use in Schwartz formula.

Age	K Value
Low-birth-weight infants < 1 y	0.33
Full-term infants < 1 y	0.45
Children 2–12 y	0.55
Girls 13–21 y	0.55
Boys 13–21 y	0.70

EVALUATION OF HEMATURIA

Hematuria is defined as the excretion of an excessive number of erythrocytes in the urine. Normal individuals may excrete as many as 1 million red blood cells (RBCs)

per day, which gives rise to 1–2 RBCs per high-power field (HPF) on microscopic examination of centrifuged urine. Hematuria in children is defined as the finding of more than 5 RBCs/HPF. In large study populations of healthy, school-aged children, the incidence of hematuria, when only a single urinalysis is performed, is 4–5%. When documented on at least 2 of 3 consecutive urinalyses, the incidence is significantly lower, 0.5–1%, indicating that hematuria is frequently transient. Most children with hematuria have benign conditions that require no intervention and have an excellent prognosis. Thus, time-consuming and expensive diagnostic studies should be reserved for patients who, by history, physical examination, and initial laboratory screening tests, are deemed to be at high risk for serious renal or extrarenal disease. Fortunately, a determination of risk can be readily made during the initial evaluation.

Hematuria may be readily apparent as a bright red or brownish discoloration of the urine, in which case it is termed **macroscopic** or **gross hematuria.** Visible hematuria is usually alarming to patients and families and prompts medical evaluation. On the other hand, microscopic hematuria usually is found in asymptomatic children undergoing routine dipstick screening of urine. Commercially available dipsticks are impregnated with reagents that change color in the presence of hemoglobin, yielding a positive result for blood. Using this methodology, the presence of as few as 5 RBCs/HPF will yield a positive test for blood. A positive dipstick test for blood indicates the presence of RBCs, hemoglobin, or myoglobin but cannot distinguish among them. For this reason, a positive dipstick must be followed by microscopic examination of a properly centrifuged, freshly obtained urine specimen (15 mL of urine spun at 2000 RPM for 5 minutes) to confirm the presence of RBCs before the diagnosis of hematuria is made.

Once the diagnosis of hematuria is confirmed, an attempt should be made to determine the site of blood loss. Macroscopic hematuria of renal origin is classically brownish, tea-colored, or Coca-Cola–colored, is not associated with pain or blood clots, and is strongly suggested by the additional findings of proteinuria, hypertension, edema, or azotemia. Conversely, macroscopic hematuria of extrarenal origin is bright red and frequently associated with pain and blood clots.

On microscopic examination, the morphologic appearance of urinary erythrocytes has been shown to reflect their site of origin, ie, glomerular versus nonglomerular. Presumably because of their deforming journey through small disruptions in the glomerular capillary wall, RBCs of glomerular origin become dysmorphic. They are smaller than their isomorphic counterparts and have distorted, irregular contours. Phase contrast microscopy is the traditional method for examining RBC morphology in urine specimens. With the use of the supravital stains, Eosin-Y and Sternheimer-Malbin, regular light microscopy can also be used reliably to detect dysmorphic erythrocytes. Red blood cells of nonglomerular origin dis-

play a normal morphologic appearance. The finding of urinary RBC casts is diagnostic of glomerular or tubular origin for the hematuria and is not seen with extrarenal bleeding. A mild degree of proteinuria due to the release of hemoglobin from RBCs may be found in cases of macroscopic hematuria. The most common causes of hematuria in children are listed in Table 16–4.

PATIENT EVALUATION

History

Evaluation of a child with confirmed hematuria begins with a thorough history. Important historical features and physical findings and the most likely corresponding diseases are listed in Table 16–5.

Physical Examination

The physical examination begins with the accurate recording of blood pressure in all children regardless of age, using an appropriately sized cuff. Height and weight measurements should be plotted on standardized growth charts. The patient's skin should be assessed for rash, petechiae, purpura, pallor, and edema. The abdominal examination should evaluate for palpable masses (hydronephrosis, polycystic kidney disease, Wilms tumor) and areas of

Table 16–4. Causes of hematuria in children.

Renal diseases—glomerular
Acute glomerulonephritis (poststreptococcal)
IgA nephropathy
Alport syndrome
Benign familial hematuria (thin basement membrane disease)
Chronic glomerulonephritis (focal segmental glomerulosclerosis, membranoproliferative glomerulonephritis, membranous glomerulopathy)
Systemic vasculitis (Henoch-Schönlein purpura, systemic lupus erythematosus)
Hemolytic uremic syndrome

Renal diseases—extraglomerular
Pyelonephritis
Interstitial nephritis
Polycystic kidney disease
Acute tubular necrosis
Renal venous or arterial thrombosis
Sickle cell nephropathy
Wilms tumor
Hydronephrosis
Papillary necrosis

Nonrenal diseases
Cystitis, urethritis
Urethral or vaginal foreign body or trauma
Vigorous exercise
Vesicoureteral reflux
Hypercalciuria
Nephrolithiasis
Hemorrhagic cystitis (cyclophosphamide, ticarcillin)
Tumors (sarcoma botryoides, rhabdomyosarcoma)
Coagulopathy
Vascular malformations

Table 16–5. Evaluation of the child with hematuria.

Historical Features	Relevance
Recurrent gross hematuria	IgA nephropathy (most likely) Benign familial hematuria Alport syndrome
Dysuria, urinary frequency suprapubic or flank pain	Urinary tract infection Nephrolithiasis
Recent upper respiratory tract infection or sore throat, impetigo	Poststreptococcal glomeru-lonephritis
Recent therapy with penicil-lins, nonsteroidal anti-inflammatory drugs	Allergic interstitial nephritis
Trauma	Renal contusion, hydronephro-sis
Family history	
Hearing deficit	Alport syndrome
Microscopic hematuria	IgA nephropathy Benign familial hematuria Alport syndrome Hypercalciuria
Renal insufficiency or failure	Alport syndrome Polycystic kidney disease
Nephrolithiasis	Hypercalciuria
Sickle cell disease/trait	Sickle cell nephropathy
Physical findings	
Edema	Minimal change nephropathy Focal segmental glomeruloscle-rosis Membranoproliferative glomerulonephritis Membranous glomerulopathy Other forms of glomeru-lonephritis
Petechiae, purpura, rash	Henoch-Schönlein purpura Systemic lupus erythematosus
Pallor	Hemolytic uremic syndrome
Abdominal mass	Tumor Hydronephrosis

pain or tenderness (UTI). The external genitalia should be inspected for signs of inflammation or trauma, or the presence of a foreign body.

Laboratory Evaluation

A complete urinalysis should be obtained for each patient with hematuria. Of particular importance are the findings of leukocytes (infection, interstitial nephritis), WBC casts (pyelonephritis), RBC casts (acute glomerulonephritis, other glomerular diseases), proteinuria (quantity, nephrotic versus non-nephrotic amount), and dysmorphic RBCs (renal versus nonrenal origin).

ETIOLOGY OF HEMATURIA

The more commonly encountered diseases causing hematuria in children are discussed below in detail. With the information obtained from the history, physical examination, and urinalysis, a differential diagnosis can be

made for the individual patient on the basis of a knowledge of the likely etiologies and their characteristic features. Figure 16–1 provides an algorithm for the evaluation of children with persistent hematuria.

Glomerulonephritis

Acute poststreptococcal glomerulonephritis (APSGN) and IgA nephropathy are discussed later in this chapter (see Glomerulonephritis).

Urinary Tract Infection

Both cystitis and pyelonephritis are common causes of hematuria, either microscopic or macroscopic. Symptoms of cystitis include dysuria, frequency, urgency, and suprapubic abdominal pain. Pyelonephritis in infants is distinguished by fever, vomiting, and irritability and in older children by the additional findings of costovertebral angle tenderness, flank pain, and dysuria. The presence of urinary RBCs, if due to infection, should be accompanied by leukocytes. Newer urine dipsticks that test for nitrite and leukocyte esterase suggest the presence of infection if positive. A urine culture should be performed in all patients with hematuria to rule out bacterial infection, even in the absence of dysuria.

Diagnosis of UTI depends on the isolation of more than 100,000 bacterial colonies per milliliter from the culture of a clean-catch urine specimen. Colony counts of less than 100,000 organisms per milliliter are considered to be positive if the urine has been obtained by either suprapubic aspiration or urethral catheterization. Cultures obtained from U-bag specimens are unreliable unless meticulous skin preparation is ensured and the specimen is delivered promptly to the laboratory for processing. With antibiotic therapy and resolution of the infection, urinary tract discomfort and hematuria resolve. Viral cystitis also may cause gross hematuria, dysuria, and suprapubic pain. In this case, the urine culture is negative for bacteriologic pathogens, and the hematuria usually resolves within 1 week without specific therapy.

Alport Syndrome

Alport syndrome, also known as **progressive heredi-tary nephritis,** is characterized by glomerulonephritis, sensorineural deafness, and ocular abnormalities, including anterior lenticonus and perimacular pigmentary changes. Symptoms of the disease include hematuria, proteinuria, and progressive renal insufficiency. The hearing deficit, which is usually in the high-frequency range, may not appear until the teenage years and may require formal audiologic testing for detection.

Since the first description of Alport syndrome in the early 1900s, many kindreds have been identified. Pedigree analysis indicates the presence of autosomal-dominant, autosomal-recessive, and X-linked dominant patterns of inheritance in different families. Males are more severely affected than females, even within the same family. In most females with Alport syndrome, persistent microscopic hematuria is the only manifestation of the disease,

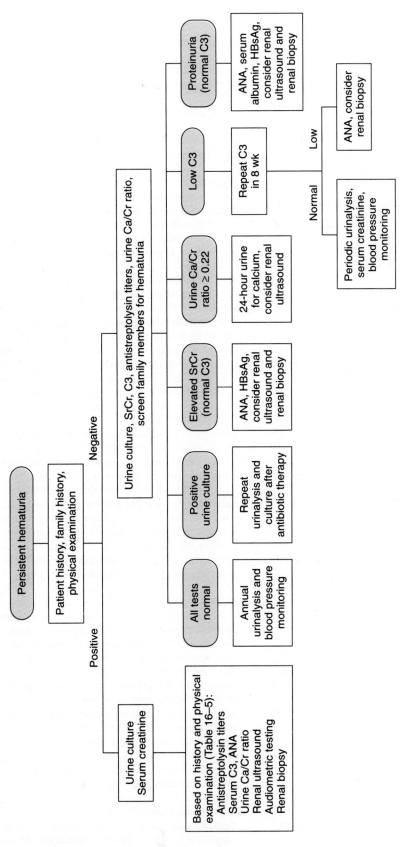

Figure 16–1. Algorithm for the diagnostic evaluation of children with persistent hematuria. ANA = antinuclear antibody; HBsAg = hepatitis B surface antigen; Ca/Cr = calcium, creatinine; SrCr = serum creatinine.

and progression to end-stage renal failure is rare. In affected males, on the other hand, persistent microscopic or recurrent macroscopic hematuria typically is observed in early childhood, and progression to end-stage renal failure occurs by 20–30 years of age.

No specific laboratory findings aid in the diagnosis. Alport syndrome should be strongly considered in a child with microscopic hematuria in whom a positive family history is obtained for either Alport syndrome or sensorineural deafness with progressive renal insufficiency. Such children should undergo audiologic evaluation. The definitive diagnosis requires a renal biopsy. The diagnostic findings of Alport syndrome are seen by electron microscopy (EM) rather than by light microscopy. On EM, the lamina densa of the glomerular basement membrane appears thickened and split and is sometimes referred to as having a "basket weave" appearance.

The management of patients with Alport syndrome includes close attention to fluid, electrolyte, and acid-base status and treatment of hypertension, as with other forms of progressive glomerulonephritis (see section on Chronic Renal Failure). To date, there is no specific therapy to alter the progressive course of Alport nephritis. Dialysis and renal transplantation are appropriate for patients whose disease progresses to end-stage renal failure. Alport nephritis does not recur in the transplanted kidney; however, a small percentage of patients with Alport syndrome who undergo transplantation have antiglomerular basement membrane nephritis, which can result in loss of the transplanted kidney.

Benign Familial Hematuria (Thin Basement Membrane Disease)

This condition manifests in children and young adults as persistent microscopic hematuria with or without proteinuria. If proteinuria occurs, it is usually mild and rarely results in the nephrotic syndrome. Although this disease is known to cluster in families, no particular mode of inheritance has been elucidated. Benign familial hematuria differs from Alport syndrome in several important ways: (1) deafness and ocular abnormalities are not seen, (2) deterioration of renal function is rare, and (3) thickening and splitting of the glomerular basement membrane are not seen in renal biopsy specimens examined by EM.

The diagnosis of benign familial hematuria should be strongly considered in a patient with persistent microscopic hematuria in whom dipstick screening of family members reveals microscopic hematuria or in whom the family history reveals the presence of hematuria without deafness or progressive renal insufficiency. Definitive diagnosis requires EM examination of renal tissue obtained by biopsy. The distinctive finding is decreased thickness (265 nm or less) of the peripheral glomerular capillary basement membranes. The light microscopic appearance of the glomerulus is normal. Despite the persistence of microscopic hematuria for many years, this condition is benign and nonprogressive in virtually all patients and thus requires no therapy.

Idiopathic Hypercalciuria

Ionized and complexed calcium are freely filtered by the renal glomerulus, and 98–99% of the filtered calcium load is reabsorbed by the tubules. In healthy children, urinary calcium excretion is less than 4 mg/kg/d. **Hypercalciuria,** defined as urinary calcium excretion in excess of this amount, is present in approximately 3% of healthy children. Increased dietary intake of calcium-containing foods does not cause hypercalciuria because the normal gastrointestinal tract limits its absorption. Idiopathic hypercalciuria is the result of either excessive gastrointestinal absorption of dietary calcium or a renal leak of calcium due to decreased tubular reabsorption. With increased gastrointestinal absorption of calcium, the resultant increase in the filtered load of calcium results in hypercalciuria, which appropriately returns the serum calcium level to normal.

As many as 25% of children with isolated hematuria have idiopathic hypercalciuria as a cause. The hematuria is painless and can be either microscopic or macroscopic; the bleeding is thought to result from mechanical trauma to tubular and uroepithelial cells caused by calcium crystals. Invariably, RBC casts and proteinuria are absent. Although hematuria does not occur in all children with hypercalciuria, they are all at increased risk for the development of calcium-containing stones and frequently have a positive family history of nephrolithiasis. The inheritance pattern of hypercalciuria resembles that of an autosomal-dominant trait.

An easily performed screening test for hypercalciuria is the calculation of the ratio of urine calcium to creatinine concentration, determined in a randomly obtained urine sample. A ratio greater than 0.22 in a fasting morning specimen suggests excessive urinary calcium excretion, although infants may have higher ratios. If the result of the screening test is positive, a confirmatory 24-hour urine collection should be obtained to determine the calcium excretion rate quantitatively. All children with isolated hematuria of unknown etiology should be screened for hypercalciuria.

For children with hypercalciuria without a history of renal stones, conservative therapy is appropriate. This includes dietary salt restriction, which decreases urinary sodium excretion. In children whose dietary intake of calcium greatly exceeds the Recommended Dietary Allowance (RDA), limitation of calcium intake to the RDA level may decrease calcium excretion. Restriction of calcium intake below the RDA is inadvisable in growing children. High fluid intake is advisable, as this will dilute urinary calcium and avoid supersaturation, a condition necessary for stone formation. Hypercalciuric children with a history of renal stones may require thiazide diuretics, if limitation of the intake of salt and calcium (to the RDA) do not result in resolution of the hypercalciuria. Thiazide diuretics reduce calcium excretion by increasing calcium reabsorption in the distal tubule.

Miscellaneous

Isolated hematuria also may be due to strenuous exercise, blunt trauma, a bleeding disorder, or sickle-cell trait or disease. The first three of these should be apparent from a careful history. Although blunt trauma to an otherwise normal kidney can cause hematuria, the occurrence of macroscopic hematuria after minimal trauma should raise the possibility of a hydronephrotic or cystic kidney. Any patient at risk for carriage of the sickle-cell trait, particularly African-Americans, should be tested for the presence of hemoglobin S. Heterozygotes as well as homozygotes for hemoglobin S can have hematuria secondary to medullary ischemia, which is caused by the sickling of RBCs within the renal medulla.

Hematuria also is seen in allergic interstitial nephritis, a condition usually caused by exposure to certain medications and characterized by hematuria, proteinuria, and a decreased GFR. The medications most often responsible for this condition are nonsteroidal anti-inflammatory agents, penicillin, methicillin, cephalosporins, phenytoin, cimetidine, furosemide, and thiazide diuretics. A history of recent or current use of one of these medications in a patient with hematuria should raise the possibility of this diagnosis. A positive Wright stain demonstrating urinary eosinophils lends further support for this diagnosis. Therapy for allergic interstitial nephritis is withdrawal of the offending medication. In most patients, urinary abnormalities resolve and the GFR returns to normal after the medication has been discontinued.

GLOMERULONEPHRITIS

Glomerulonephritis is defined histologically as inflammation of the glomeruli. There is proliferation of one or more of the glomerular cell types—mesangial cells, endothelial cells, and epithelial cells—and exudation of leukocytes. Other glomerular diseases, which are not characterized by inflammation, are often included under the term glomerulonephritis but are more properly known as glomerulopathies, eg, minimal change disease and membranous glomerulopathy. Hematuria and proteinuria are nonspecific clinical expressions of all glomerular diseases and cannot reliably distinguish between proliferative and nonproliferative types. Nevertheless, hematuria tends to predominate in the true glomerulonephritides, and proteinuria in the glomerulopathies. In this section, glomerulonephritis is used as a generic term for both types of disease. Only those glomerulonephritides that occur with some frequency in children are considered.

Glomerulonephritis can be acute, subacute, or chronic. Clinical features of acute glomerulonephritis are both gross and microscopic hematuria, including the presence of RBC casts, proteinuria, pyuria, edema, oliguria, hypertension, flank pain, and increased serum concentrations of both urea nitrogen and creatinine (azotemia) (Table 16–6).

Table 16–6. Clinical and laboratory features of acute glomerulonephritis.

Clinical Features	Laboratory Findings
Gross hematuria	Microscopic hematuria
Edema	Red blood cell casts
Hypertension	Proteinuria
Flank pain	Pyuria
Oliguria	Elevated antistreptolysin O, anti-hyaluronidase, and anti DNAse-B titers
Fever (uncommon)	Decreased CH_{50} and C3 levels
	Elevated erythrocyte sedimentation rate
	Leukocytosis

Although the classic form of glomerulonephritis, acute poststreptococcal glomerulonephritis (APSGN), often presents as a serious illness with many of these features, glomerulonephritis also may be detected incidentally by the findings of microscopic hematuria or proteinuria on a routine urinalysis.

Glomerulonephritis occurs in many forms, which have been classified histologically, by characteristic patterns observed by light, electron, and immunofluorescence microscopy. These types can exist as primary renal diseases or as renal manifestations of systemic diseases. For example, diffuse proliferative glomerulonephritis can be a primary renal disease, most frequently ASPGN, or it can be the renal manifestation of a systemic disease, such as systemic lupus erythematosus. In addition, systemic diseases such as systemic lupus erythematosus can be associated with glomerulonephritis of different histologic types, eg, focal glomerulonephritis, membranous glomerulopathy, or diffuse proliferative glomerulonephritis, either in different patients or in the same patient at different times. Because of this variability, hybrid classifications of the glomerulonephritides, on the basis of both clinical and histologic descriptions, are commonly used (Table 16–7).

The causes of most forms of glomerulonephritis, whether intrinsic to the kidney or part of a systemic disease, are unknown, but their pathogenesis often involves

Table 16–7. Classification of glomerulonephritis.

Intrinsic Renal Diseases	Systemic Diseases
Diffuse proliferative glomerulonephritis	Systemic lupus erythematosus
Poststreptococcal glomerulonephritis	Henoch-Schönlein purpura
Mesangial proliferative glomerulonephritis	Hepatitis B virus infection
IgA nephropathy	Chronic infection: infective endocarditis, ventriculo-atrial shunts
Focal segmental glomerulosclerosis	HIV type 1 infection
Membranoproliferative glomerulonephritis	Polyarteritis nodosa
Membranous glomerulopathy	Goodpasture syndrome
Rapidly progressive glomerulonephritis	Wegener granulomatosis
	Diabetes mellitus
	Sickle cell disease

immune mechanisms, such as the deposition of antigen-antibody complexes in the glomeruli. Anti-inflammatory and immunosuppressive drugs, such as corticosteroids and cytotoxic agents, are frequently used to treat these diseases. However, for most of the diseases, controlled studies have not been performed to test the efficacy of these drugs. The prognosis of most of the glomerulonephritides is better in children than in adults; nevertheless, chronic glomerulonephritis is one of the most common causes of end-stage renal disease in older children and adolescents. The two most common forms of glomerulonephritis in children, APSGN and IgA nephropathy, are discussed.

ACUTE POSTSTREPTOCOCCAL GLOMERULONEPHRITIS

The occurrence of glomerulonephritis after streptococcal infections has been recognized for more than 150 years. After pharyngeal or skin infections with certain strains of group A streptococci, glomerulonephritis may develop after a latent period of 1–3 weeks. A number of nephritogenic strains of streptococci have been identified, but the occurrence rate of nephritis after infection with any one of these strains is variable. APSGN is primarily a disease of children, with a peak incidence at age 7 years; it is rare in infants. Boys are affected twice as often as girls. The incidence of the disease in North America decreased after 1940, related to a decreased incidence and severity of streptococcal infections in general, but there has been an apparent resurgence in recent years. The disease can present in both sporadic and epidemic forms.

Pathogenesis & Pathology

The pathogenesis is incompletely understood but appears to involve the deposition of a streptococcal antigen, streptokinase, in the glomeruli with subsequent activation of plasminogen and complement leading to an inflammatory reaction. APSGN is a diffuse proliferative glomerulonephritis and is the classic example of this pathologic form, although the same pathology also can be observed in glomerulonephritis that follows pneumococcal, staphylococcal, and viral infections, including mumps and varicella. There is proliferation of all three types of glomerular cells—mesangial, endothelial, and epithelial—as well as accumulation and exudation of polymorphonuclear leukocytes in the glomerulus. In severe cases, glomerular capillary lumens can be obliterated by proliferating cells, or the glomerular tuft can be compressed by epithelial cell crescents. EM demonstrates the presence of electron-dense humps, which are thought to be immune complexes, on the epithelial side of the glomerular basement membrane. Immunofluorescence microscopy reveals a granular pattern of staining of immune globulins, primarily IgG and complement, outlining the capillary loops.

Clinical Features

There is marked variability in the clinical presentation and course of the disease. Patients usually seek medical attention because of the onset of periorbital edema or gross hematuria, which is often described as tea-colored or brown urine. Hypertension, oliguria, urinary RBC casts, and proteinuria are also common, and the child may complain of headache, malaise, flank pain, and fever. Renal failure severe enough to necessitate the use of dialysis occurs in a small percentage of patients, as does the nephrotic syndrome. On the other hand, many cases are so mild as to go unnoticed, as evidenced by the fact that urinalyses performed on apparently healthy siblings of index cases often show microscopic hematuria and proteinuria. Therefore, in patients with microscopic hematuria who report a recent pharyngeal or skin infection, serologic evidence of streptococcal infection should be sought.

Laboratory findings include leukocytosis, mild anemia, an elevated erythrocyte sedimentation rate, increased serum levels of creatinine and urea nitrogen, decreased serum levels of total hemolytic complement (CH_{50}) and C3, and increased serum levels of antibodies against streptococcal antigens. The most sensitive tests of the latter are the anti-hyaluronidase and anti-DNAse B titers for skin infections, and the antistreptolysin O (ASO) titer for pharyngitis.

The overt signs and symptoms of nephritis usually subside within 1–2 weeks, although microscopic hematuria and, especially, low-grade proteinuria may persist for months or even years. Complete recovery occurs in more than 95% of children but in only 70–85% of adults.

Diagnosis

The diagnosis of APSGN depends on the demonstration of elevated serum titers of antibodies against streptococcal antigens and decreased serum complement levels in a child with glomerulonephritis. Antibody titers to streptococcal antigens remain elevated for 4–6 months, whereas serum complement levels return to normal within 10 days to 8 weeks after the onset of nephritis. In virtually all cases, serum complement levels return to normal within 8 weeks of onset. The finding of persistently decreased complement levels suggests the glomerulonephritis of systemic lupus erythematosus or membranoproliferative glomerulonephritis.

Treatment

Most patients can be managed at home. Indications for admission to the hospital are hypertension, which usually is caused by oliguria with fluid retention, and acute renal failure. The treatment is symptomatic and includes salt and fluid restriction and the use of diuretics, such as furosemide, and antihypertensive drugs, such as hydralazine and nifedipine. Antibiotics are indicated if a streptococcal infection is still present, but they do not shorten the duration of the nephritis.

IgA NEPHROPATHY

IgA nephropathy, or Berger disease, was first described in 1968 and has subsequently been recognized as the most common form of glomerulonephritis in both children and adults. Because the diagnosis of IgA nephropathy is dependent on a renal biopsy specimen, its incidence is unknown, but it has been found in approximately 20% of children undergoing biopsy for evaluation of hematuria. IgA nephropathy is primarily a disease of children and young adults and is rare in infants. Males are involved twice as frequently as females. The etiology and pathogenesis are unknown. The finding of identical patterns of deposition of IgA both in glomeruli and in subdermal capillaries in patients with IgA nephropathy and Henoch-Schönlein purpura suggests that these two entities may be different expressions of the same disease.

Pathology

Immunofluorescence microscopy reveals the characteristic feature, which is the presence of IgA deposited throughout the mesangial areas of the glomerulus. The deposits usually contain IgG, IgM, C3, and properdin as well, but in lesser amounts. By light microscopy, the glomeruli may appear normal but, more frequently, exhibit focal or diffuse mesangial cell proliferation and increased mesangial matrix, sometimes accompanied by focal necrotizing lesions, segmental glomerulosclerosis, capsular adhesions, or epithelial crescents. Patchy areas of tubular atrophy and interstitial mononuclear cell infiltration often accompany glomerular disease.

Clinical Features

The most common presenting feature is the occurrence of intermittent and recurrent episodes of gross hematuria, or the finding of microscopic hematuria with or without proteinuria on routine urinalysis. Gross hematuria characteristically occurs during or shortly after an upper respiratory tract infection and resolves spontaneously after several days. This is in contrast to the hematuria of patients with poststreptococcal glomerulonephritis, in whom pharyngitis precedes the onset of hematuria by 1–2 weeks. Loin pain may be present. Between episodes, the urine may be clear or contain small numbers of red cells and, occasionally, protein. In most children with IgA nephropathy, blood pressure and renal function are normal at the time of diagnosis.

The natural history is incompletely characterized. In the largest pediatric experience, 15 years after the onset of disease 11% of the children had chronic renal failure whereas 71% were in complete remission. Features of the disease predicting a poor prognosis include heavy proteinuria and pathologic findings of diffuse mesangial proliferation and a high percentage of glomeruli with sclerosis or crescents. Although there is a high recurrence rate of IgA nephropathy in patients who receive renal transplants, the disease in the transplanted kidney is invariably mild and nonprogressive.

Diagnosis

Although definitive diagnosis depends on histologic findings, the pattern of gross hematuria occurring in association with upper respiratory infection is so characteristic of IgA nephropathy that a presumptive diagnosis can be made without a renal biopsy. This pattern also occurs in children with hereditary nephritis (Alport syndrome) and benign familial hematuria, but these entities usually can be excluded on the basis of a negative family history and the fact that many children with Alport syndrome have sensorineural hearing loss. The renal histologic findings in IgA nephropathy are indistinguishable from those in patients with nephritis due to Henoch-Schönlein purpura, a systemic vasculitis characterized by a purpuric rash, abdominal pain, joint swelling or pain, and glomerulonephritis.

Treatment

Since IgA nephropathy usually is a benign disease in children, treatment usually is reserved for patients with poor prognostic features. Treatments that have been used with varying degrees of success include fish oils, corticosteroids, and intravenous immune globulin (IVIG).

EVALUATION OF PROTEINURIA

In healthy individuals, protein is excreted in the urine in very small amounts; the amount varies with age (Table 16–8). The composition of urinary proteins is complex and consists of albumin (40%), immunoproteins (15%), Tamm-Horsfall proteins (40%), and various peptides (5%). Important immunoproteins that appear in the urine are IgA, IgG, and β_2-microglobulin. Tamm-Horsfall proteins are mucoproteins derived from tubular epithelium of the distal nephron. Peptides or hormones that are present in the urine include parathyroid hormone, vasopressin, insulin, vitamins, and various binding proteins.

MECHANISMS OF RENAL HANDLING OF PROTEIN

The composition and quantity of urinary protein are determined by a number of renal and extrarenal factors. The GFR influences the filtration of protein macromolecules by affecting both the glomerular capillary plasma flow rate and transcapillary hydraulic pressure gradient. The glomerular capillary wall permits free passage of water and

Table 16–8. Urinary protein excretion in healthy infants, children, and adolescents.

Age	Mean (Range) (mg/m²/d)
5–30 d	182 (88–377)
7–30 d	145 (68–309)
2 mo–4 y	100 (37–244)
5–10 y	85 (21–234)
11–16 y	63 (22–181)

small solutes but restricts the passage of plasma proteins depending on their size, charge, and overall configuration. The clearance of proteins is inversely related to their molecular size. Moreover, negatively charged proteins, such as albumin, are repulsed by the negatively charged glomerular capillary wall, thus preventing their filtration and excretion. The proximal tubule not only reabsorbs most filtered amino acids, but also reabsorbs and degrades albumin and low-molecular-weight proteins that have traversed the glomerular barrier. Most of these proteins are absorbed from the tubular lumen by either endocytic or pinocytic processes, then transferred to lysosomal compartments where they are catabolized by proteolytic enzymes.

DETECTION & QUANTIFICATION OF PROTEINURIA

The dipstick method is the most commonly used screening test for detection of proteinuria. With this method, protein in the urine induces a color change of the indicator dye tetrabromphenol; the change is proportionate to the concentration of the protein. The results are graded from negative (yellow) to 2+ (green, 100 mg/dL) to 4+ (dark green, > 2000 mg/dL). The lower limit of detection for urinary protein by the dipstick method is 10–20 mg/dL. A false-negative result can occur when the urine is very dilute (specific gravity < 1.018) or contains a non–albumin-like protein, and a false-positive result can occur when the urine is strongly alkaline (pH > 7.0) because the indicator dye is buffered to maintain a pH of 3.0. Because of the variability of daily urine flow rates and the limit of detection of urinary protein, the dipstick method is not useful as a quantitative test for urinary protein.

Urinary protein can also be detected by the turbidimetric method in which reagents such as sulfosalicylic acid, trichloroacetic acid, or heat cause a denaturation of urinary proteins, resulting in their precipitation. The degree of turbidity of the urine sample is compared against a set of standards, thus permitting semi-quantification of the urinary protein concentration. For precise measurements, a third method using spectrophotometry can be used (Biuret, Coomassie blue, or Lowry methods).

ETIOLOGY OF PROTEINURIA

In healthy children aged 3 weeks to 18 years, the prevalence of asymptomatic proteinuria varies from 1.8 to 11.6% on a single random urine test and is 0.6% when two or more consecutive urine specimens are analyzed. The prevalence is highest in adolescence and appears to be greater in girls than in boys. The causes of proteinuria in children are listed in Table 16–9.

Transient Proteinuria

Transient proteinuria can be associated with many conditions, such as stress, heavy exercise, extreme cold, heart

Table 16–9. Causes of proteinuria in children.

Transient	
Fever	Extreme cold
Orthostatic	Epinephrine
Exercise	Seizures
Stress	Congestive heart failure

Persistent
Orthostatic
Benign (sporadic or familial)
Increased plasma concentration of protein
   Multiple myeloma, primary amyloidosis, lymphoma, chronic lymphocytic leukemia
Decreased tubular reabsorption of protein
   Hereditary: Fanconi syndrome associated with Wilson disease, cystinosis, Lowe syndrome
   Acquired: drugs (aminoglycosides, phenacetin, lithium), acute tubular necrosis, interstitial nephritis, radiation nephritis
Glomerular
   Primary: Minimal change disease, focal segmental glomerulosclerosis, membranous nephropathy, membranoproliferative glomerulonephritis, IgA nephropathy
   Secondary:
      Infectious: poststreptococcal glomerulonephritis, endocarditis, hepatitis
      Immune/multisystem: systemic lupus erythematosus, Goodpasture syndrome, rheumatoid arthritis, Henoch-Schönlein purpura, ulcerative colitis, polyarteritis
      Metabolic: diabetes mellitus
      Hereditary: Alport syndrome, Fabry disease
      Drugs: nonsteroidal anti-inflammatory agents
Structural abnormalities of the urinary tract, congenital or acquired
Polycystic kidney disease: autosomal recessive or dominant
Hydronephrosis: posterior urethral valves, ureterovesical or ureteropelvic obstruction
Hypoplastic-dysplastic disease
Reflux nephropathy

failure, fever, seizures, and epinephrine administration. Under these conditions, the proteinuria is postulated to result from hemodynamic changes that produce a decrease in renal plasma flow out of proportion to GFR. These hemodynamic changes result in an increase in the protein concentration in glomerular capillaries, which enhances its concentration gradient and thus its movement into the urinary space. With resolution of these conditions, the proteinuria disappears.

Orthostatic Proteinuria

Orthostatic proteinuria is a condition in which protein excretion is considerably greater in the standing than in the recumbent position. Although this phenomenon occurs in most healthy individuals, the amount of protein excreted in the standing position is below the detection limit of the dipstick method. In patients with orthostatic proteinuria, the amount of proteinuria ranges from 0.5 to 1.5 g/24 h. Orthostatic proteinuria is found most commonly in the adolescent population. Renal biopsy specimens of affected individuals have revealed either normal glomeruli or mild glomerular changes; the long-term clinical course is benign. Although the mechanism is not completely understood, orthostatic proteinuria is believed to result from increased transglomerular passage of albumin. This condition may be transient or long-standing.

Persistent Proteinuria

Persistent proteinuria typically is a sign of glomerular disease, although it can also be caused by conditions associated with renal tubular disease or an increased filtered load of protein. Both the site and degree of injury are important determinants of the magnitude of proteinuria. With tubular injury, the amount of proteinuria is usually less than 2 g/24 h. Proteinuria can occur in patients with proximal tubular dysfunction, such as the Fanconi syndrome, or in patients receiving aminoglycoside antibiotics, which are known to be toxic to the proximal tubule. Removal of the toxin usually restores tubular function to normal, and the proteinuria resolves. In adult patients with multiple myeloma, in which the proteinuria is due to an increased filtered load of low-molecular-weight proteins (immunoglobulin light chains), measurement of serum proteins and the urinary immuno-electrophoresis pattern are useful for diagnosis.

Persistent proteinuria can be caused by glomerular disease that is either primary (disorders in which the glomeruli are the sole or predominant tissue involved) or secondary to a systemic disease (see Table 16–9). Depending on the severity of the glomerular injury, urinary protein excretion can range from less than 1 g to more than 20 g per day. The clinical course, response to therapy, and prognosis of patients with proteinuria vary greatly depending on the underlying cause. In patients with benign persistent proteinuria, the outcome is excellent and no therapy is warranted; in postinfectious glomerulonephritis, the outcome usually is favorable, and only supportive therapy is necessary for the acute complications. By contrast, in certain primary glomerular diseases, moderate or severe proteinuria associated with the nephrotic syndrome (protein excretion > 50 mg/kg/d, hypoalbuminemia, edema, and hyperlipidemia) can be persistent and unresponsive to therapy, and progression to renal insufficiency can occur, requiring dialysis and subsequent transplantation. Congenital disease with or without associated structural anomalies of the urinary tract can also cause persistent proteinuria. Diagnosis of these conditions usually is made on the basis of their clinical, radiologic, or, rarely, histologic features.

EVALUATION OF ISOLATED PROTEINURIA

The finding of isolated proteinuria (Figure 16–2) in a child should be confirmed on at least two subsequent urinalyses. Urine for analysis is preferably obtained in the morning when it is concentrated (specific gravity > 1.018) and acidic (pH < 6.0). If neither of the repeated urinalyses is positive for protein, transient proteinuria is likely and further evaluation is not warranted. However, if proteinuria is confirmed, a detailed medical history and physical examination are required. A history of recent infections, signs and symptoms of other renal or systemic disease, previous abnormal urinalysis results, exposure to potential renal-toxic medications (eg, aminoglycosides, ifosfamide), and a family history of renal disease or deafness are important pieces of information that assist in differentiating among the various glomerular diseases. The physical examination should focus on the detection of growth retardation and hypertension, as these can be the first signs of renal dysfunction. Generalized edema and signs of respiratory difficulty may occur when proteinuria is severe.

If the urine dipstick reveals proteinuria of 1+ or less and the findings of both the physical examination and the remainder of the urinalysis are normal, the child should be observed, with a physical examination and complete urinalysis performed annually. However, if the urine dipstick reveals proteinuria of 2+ or greater, one should evaluate the patient (older children and adolescents) for orthostatic proteinuria. This is performed by collecting the first urine specimen (specimen 1) when the patient has arisen in the morning and the second specimen after the patient has ambulated for 2–4 hours (specimen 2). Both specimens are checked for protein by the dipstick method. If specimen 1 is free of protein and specimen 2 contains protein, the test result is positive for orthostatic proteinuria. A confirmatory test should be performed in all patients. If orthostatic proteinuria is confirmed and renal function is normal, the patient can be observed with an annual physical examination and urinalysis. However, if both specimens are positive for protein, orthostatic proteinuria is probably not the cause. Blood urea nitrogen and serum creatinine concentrations should be determined in all patients.

If proteinuria is persistent and not orthostatic, further evaluation is warranted. The proteinuria should be quantitated, and the 24-hour urine collection permits the most precise determination of total protein excretion. Proteinuria is considered abnormal when it exceeds the upper limit of normal for age (see Table 16–8). In the same collection, a C_{creat} should be determined not only to estimate the GFR but also to verify the adequacy of the collection. In addition to obtaining a serum creatinine specimen for C_{creat} measurement, a serum albumin and total protein concentration should be determined. One can estimate the magnitude of proteinuria on a random, untimed urine sample by computing the ratio of the urinary total protein concentration to the urinary creatinine concentration. As a guide, values less than 0.1 are considered normal, 0.1–1 mild, greater than 1.0–5.0 moderate, and greater than 5.0 severe proteinuria; the last category correlates with nephrotic range proteinuria.

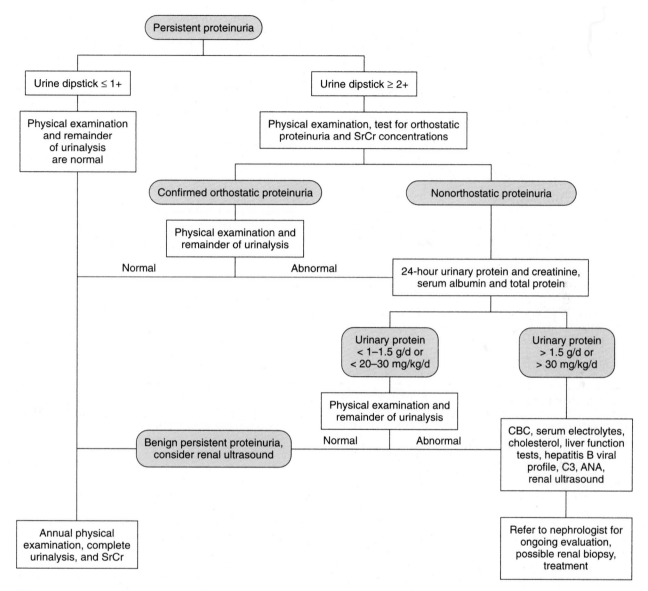

Figure 16–2. Algorithm for the diagnostic evaluation of children with persistent proteinuria. ANA = antinuclear antibody; CBC = complete blood count; SrCr = serum creatinine.

If urinary protein is less than 1.0–1.5 g or less than 20–30 mg/kg/d, and if the findings from serum chemistries, remainder of urinalysis, and physical examination are normal, the patient can be observed with an annual physical examination, urinalysis, and serum creatinine determination. Patients with more significant proteinuria, with or without edema, require further diagnostic tests, which include serum electrolytes, cholesterol, complete blood count, liver function tests, hepatitis B virus profile,

C3 level, and an antinuclear antibody (ANA) test (see section below, Nephrotic Syndrome). A renal ultrasound study should be performed to determine whether cystic disease or structural abnormalities are present (eg, polycystic, dysplastic, or reflux nephropathy), although nephrotic range proteinuria is rare in these patients. The decision whether to intervene with therapy or to perform a renal biopsy is determined by the clinical presentation and the initial evaluation.

NEPHROTIC SYNDROME

The nephrotic syndrome is defined by a constellation of clinical and laboratory findings that includes severe proteinuria, hypoalbuminemia, edema, and hyperlipidemia. The severe proteinuria usually is a result of glomerular injury that leads to increased glomerular capillary wall permeability to serum proteins. In contrast, the hypoalbuminemia, edema, and hyperlipidemia are a consequence of the heavy urinary protein loss. Over the years, it has become clear that nephrotic syndrome has diverse etiologies with distinct glomerular histopathology and clinical courses. This discussion focuses on the causes of primary or idiopathic nephrotic syndrome in children (Table 16–10). Nephrotic syndrome associated with multisystemic disease or with metabolic, hereditary, infectious, malignancy-associated, or drug-induced glomerular diseases is not discussed in detail; these secondary causes are listed in Table 16–11.

EPIDEMIOLOGY

In patients younger than 16 years, the nephrotic syndrome is the most frequent presentation of persistent glomerular disease; the incidence is 2–7 new cases per 100,000 persons per year. The prevalence is approximately 16 cases per 100,000 children. In early childhood, cases in boys predominate with a ratio of 2:1; however, in adolescence and adulthood, the distribution between genders is equal.

CLINICAL & LABORATORY FEATURES

Most children with nephrotic syndrome come to medical attention because of the onset of edema, expressed as swelling of the eyes in the morning and of dependent areas, such as the genitals, legs, and feet, at the end of the

Table 16–11. Secondary causes of nephrotic syndrome in children.

Multisystemic disease: systemic lupus erythematosus, Goodpasture syndrome, Henoch-Schönlein purpura (IgA nephropathy), amyloidosis, Wegener granulomatosis
Malignancy: Hodgkin disease, leukemia, multiple myeloma
Drugs: mercurial compounds, gold, penicillamine, captopril, nonsteroidal anti-inflammatory agents
Toxins: bee sting, diphtheria, pertussis, tetanus toxoid
Infectious:
  Bacterial: poststreptococcal glomerulonephritis, infective endocarditis, tuberculosis
  Viral: hepatitis B, cytomegalovirus, HIV type 1, Epstein-Barr virus
Metabolic disease: Diabetes mellitus
Familial:
  Infancy: Congenital nephrotic syndrome (Finnish-type, diffuse mesangial sclerosis)
  Beyond infancy: Alport syndrome, sickle cell disease
Miscellaneous (rare): massive obesity, reflux nephropathy, chronic renal graft rejection

day. In most cases, the swelling is preceded by a nonspecific prodromal illness. A few children present with a history of allergies and previous treatment with antihistamines; on rare occasions, there is a history of edematous periods followed by spontaneous remissions. On physical examination, the peripheral edema is characteristically soft and pitting. With an increase in the severity of the edema, ascites and pleural effusions can occur.

The "gold standard" laboratory test for determining the degree of proteinuria is the timed 24-hour urine collection, although less precise estimates can be made from a single untimed urine specimen (see this chapter, Proteinuria). **Nephrotic-range proteinuria** is defined as a urinary protein excretion rate in children of greater than 40 mg/m^2/h or greater than 50 mg/kg/d, or in adults, greater than 3.5 g/24 h. When the rate of urinary protein loss exceeds the capacity of the liver to synthesize new protein, hypoalbuminemia occurs.

One of the principal functions of albumin is to generate oncotic pressure within the intravascular compartment. When the plasma albumin concentration decreases significantly, a decrease in plasma oncotic pressure promotes the movement of fluid from the intravascular to the interstitial space, which results in the development of edema. The intravascular depletion leads to activation of the renin-angiotensin system, retention of sodium and water, and worsening of the edema. Clinically apparent edema usually does not occur until the plasma albumin concentration decreases to less than approximately 2 g/dL. In some patients with nephrotic syndrome, there is primary renal retention of sodium and water, which results in expansion of the plasma volume and suppression of the renin-angiotensin system. The expanded plasma volume increases capillary hydrostatic pressure, which further promotes loss of fluid into the interstitial space and the development of edema (Figure 16–3).

Table 16–10. Histologic classification of primary idiopathic nephrotic syndrome in children.

	Percent (n = 464)
Minimal change disease	78
Glomerular sclerosis	9
Segmental	(7)
Global	(2)
Mesangial proliferation	2
Membranoproliferative glomerulonephritis	7
Membranous glomerulopathy	1
Other	3

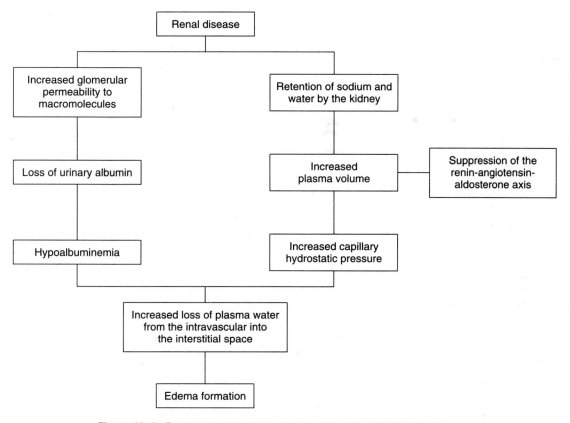

Figure 16–3. Proposed mechanisms of edema formation in nephrotic syndrome.

EXTRARENAL COMPLICATIONS

In most patients with nephrotic syndrome, serum concentrations of total cholesterol and triglycerides are elevated. Recent data suggest that either the hypoalbuminemia and consequent reduction in plasma oncotic pressure or the enhanced urinary loss of an unknown regulatory factor, or both, results in enhanced hepatic production of very-low-density lipoproteins (VLDL) and reduced peripheral use and catabolism of lipoproteins.

In nephrotic syndrome, plasma proteins, in addition to albumin, are lost in the urine. Decreased concentrations of IgG and factor B, important components of the alternate pathway of complement activation, may play a role in the unusual susceptibility to infection by encapsulated bacteria observed in patients with massive proteinuria.

In patients with nephrotic syndrome, there is an increased risk of thrombosis of the renal vein, pulmonary artery or vein, or peripheral arteries or veins, and of pulmonary emboli. The mechanisms responsible for the hypercoagulable state of these patients are not well understood. Antithrombin III levels may be severely depressed because of urinary losses and may play an important role. Plasma protein C and protein S levels may be normal or

elevated, but their functional activity may be reduced. Factors IX and XII concentrations are reduced in nephrotic syndrome, whereas factors V, VII, VIII (von Willebrand factor), and X are elevated. In addition to these disturbances in the coagulation system, increased platelet aggregation or enhanced erythrocyte aggregation may play a role. Another contributing factor is volume depletion with its associated stasis, hyperviscosity, and hyperlipidemia.

The most common site of thrombosis is the renal vein, and affected patients may present with flank pain, hematuria, and an acute decline in GFR. Acute pain or other symptoms at other sites, such as the leg or chest, may suggest the development of thrombosis. Useful diagnostic studies include renal ultrasound, peripheral venous Doppler, arteriogram, pulmonary ventilation-perfusion ($\dot{V}/\dot{Q}$) scan, or magnetic resonance imaging.

Another group of proteins that may be lost in the urine is the important metal and hormone-binding proteins. For example, zinc deficiency may contribute to poor wound healing and impaired cell-mediated immunity. Deficiency of thyroxine-binding globulin may lead to a hypothyroid state. Urinary losses of vitamin D–binding globulin may cause a vitamin D deficiency state.

PRIMARY IDIOPATHIC NEPHROTIC SYNDROME

In the next section, the clinical spectrum, histopathology, natural history, and response to therapy of the more common disease entities classified as primary idiopathic nephrotic syndrome are discussed (see Table 16–10). The frequency of the various diseases varies according to the age at the time of presentation. For example, minimal change disease is found in 80–85% of children with nephrotic syndrome, whereas membranous glomerulonephritis is the most common cause in patients older than 60 years. The classification of renal diseases is based on the histologic appearance of renal tissue obtained by biopsy. However, although the histologic appearance of renal tissue may be classified as a distinct entity, it may in fact arise from one of several different disorders, each with a different pathogenesis, which culminates in a similar histologic picture.

Minimal Change Disease

Minimal change disease, also known as **lipoid nephrosis,** is the most common cause of primary idiopathic nephrotic syndrome in children, with a peak occurrence between the ages of 2 and 6 years. In many cases, a viral upper respiratory illness precedes the onset of the proteinuria, and, occasionally, there is a history of allergies or previous immunizations. Although the pathogenesis of minimal change disease is unknown, considerable evidence suggests that a disorder of the immune system is involved (Table 16–12).

The initial clinical manifestation of nephrotic syndrome typically is the appearance of edema. The edema usually is dependent and demonstrated by swollen eyes in the morning and swelling of the feet at the end of the day. With progression of the disease, more severe edema, marked weight gain, abdominal distention with ascites, and respiratory distress with pleural effusion are commonly seen. Both blood pressure and renal function are normal in most patients; however, a subset of patients may have mild hypertension and azotemia. In addition to heavy proteinuria, approximately 10% of patients present with microscopic hematuria; gross hematuria or the presence of RBC casts are not consistent with the diagnosis of minimal change disease. Serum C3 levels are normal. Thus, the diagnosis of minimal change disease should be strongly considered in children younger than 6 years with nephrotic syndrome in whom hematuria, hypertension, azotemia, and hypocomplementemia are absent.

On pathologic examination, the characteristic feature on light microscopy is the absence of glomerular alterations; occasionally, an increase in mesangial cellularity is seen. Immunofluorescence studies fail to demonstrate IgG or complement; however, occasional mesangial deposits of IgM are seen. EM reveals effacement of the foot-processes of the glomerular capillary epithelial cells. As the proteinuria resolves, the epithelial cells resume their normal ultrastructural appearance.

Therapy

Most children with a diagnosis of minimal change disease can receive treatment on an outpatient basis. Indications for hospitalization include severe anasarca requiring aggressive diuretic therapy, inability to take oral medications, infections such as peritonitis, or the need for a renal biopsy. The management of edema includes dietary restriction and the judicious use of diuretics. Salt restriction is accomplished by eliminating foods with a high salt content and by not adding salt during preparation or serving of food. A high protein intake offers no advantage in compensating for the severe urinary protein loss. The most commonly used diuretics are loop diuretics, such as furosemide. One should be familiar with the known side effects of prolonged use of loop diuretics, such as hypokalemia, hyperchloremic metabolic acidosis, and, rarely, interstitial nephritis; their occurrence necessitates frequent monitoring of these patients.

The striking feature of minimal change disease is its characteristic response to steroid therapy; specifically, an accelerated diuresis and the elimination of proteinuria. The International Study of Kidney Diseases in Children revealed that 93% of 363 patients with minimal change disease responded to 8 weeks of therapy, defined as 3 or more days of "protein-free" urine (< 1+ by Albustix). A suggested protocol for the treatment of minimal change disease with prednisone is shown in Table 16–13; other similar protocols have been used. In patients with minimal

Table 16–12. Evidence for a disorder of immune function in the pathogenesis of minimal change nephrotic syndrome.

Remission associated with measles infection
Remission induced by corticosteroids and cytotoxic drugs
Occurrence in Hodgkin disease
Sera from nephrotic patients inhibits lymphocyte proliferation in response to mitogens; no inhibition during remission
Increased incidence of allergic disease
Decreased immunoglobulin levels

Table 16–13. Treatment of nephrotic syndrome with corticosteroids.

Initial treatment	Prednisone, 2 mg/kg daily orally bid or tid until urine is free of protein for 1 wk
	2 mg/kg every other morning for 2 wk
	Taper over 4–5 wk
	Total duration of treatment is 8–10 wk
Treatment of relapses	Same as above
Treatment of frequent relapses	Same as above
	Tapering schedule should be extended over 8–16 wks, depending on clinical response

change nephrotic syndrome who receive an initial 8-week course of prednisone therapy, approximately 93% respond with resolution of the proteinuria (Figure 16–4). Several patterns of responsiveness to subsequent courses of prednisone in children with minimal change nephrotic syndrome have been observed, including (1) nonrelapsers—complete remission without relapses; (2) relapsers—complete remission, with relapses of proteinuria occurring when prednisone has been discontinued for at least 2 weeks; (3) steroid dependence—complete remission with relapse of proteinuria occurring when prednisone is tapered; and (4) steroid resistance—failure to induce complete remission of proteinuria. In patients with frequent relapses (> 3 per year), a prolonged course of alternate-day low-dose steroids may be beneficial in preventing further relapses.

In patients with frequent relapses or steroid dependency, untoward effects of long-term steroid therapy can occur, such as growth suppression, obesity, striae, gastritis, or bleeding, and, less commonly, hypertension, diabetes mellitus, osteoporosis, or cataracts. When these occur, most pediatric nephrologists recommend that a renal biopsy be performed (Table 16–14) and that cytotoxic drug therapy with either cyclophosphamide or chlorambucil be initiated. In addition to determining the renal histology, the biopsy specimen assists in providing information regarding the response to therapy and long-term prognosis. Cyclophosphamide is the most frequently used cytotoxic agent. Several studies have shown that treatment with 2–3 mg/kg/day for 8–12 weeks is effective in inducing a sustained remission of proteinuria. Cyclophosphamide toxicity includes both acute effects, such

Table 16–14. Relative indications for renal biopsy in nephrotic syndrome.

Secondary causes of nephrotic syndrome
Age > 10–12 y
Significant hematuria, hypertension, or azotemia
Low C3 for more than 8 wk
Initial nonresponse to corticosteroids
Before using cytotoxic agents
Steroid toxicity

as bone marrow suppression, gastritis, alopecia, and hemorrhagic cystitis, and the potential long-term effects of cancer and gonadal dysfunction. The latter complications appear to be minimized when the total cumulative dose administered is less than 168 mg/kg.

The long-term follow-up of children with biopsy-proved minimal change nephrotic syndrome is highly favorable. The estimated 10-year survival rate of steroid-responsive patients with minimal change disease is greater than 95%. Progression to renal failure does not occur, and major reasons for increased morbidity and mortality are associated with the side effects associated with therapy, such as infection.

FOCAL SEGMENTAL GLOMERULAR SCLEROSIS

Most patients with focal segmental glomerular sclerosis (FSGS) present in a fashion similar to those with minimal

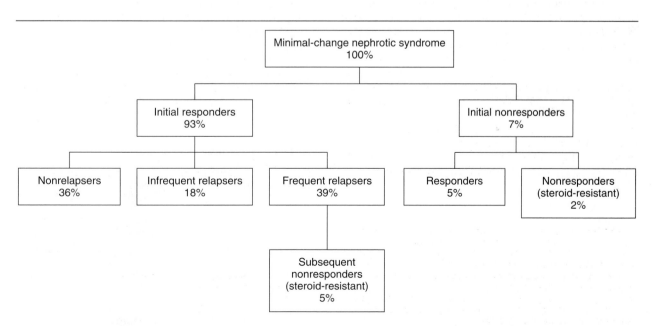

Figure 16–4. Response to prednisone therapy in children with minimal change nephrotic syndrome.

change nephrotic syndrome. However, a subset of patients may present with asymptomatic proteinuria noted on routine urinalysis. FSGS is found in about 7–15% of children with nephrotic syndrome and is the second most common lesion seen in children. Typically, the diagnosis is made when a renal biopsy is performed in a child with presumed minimal change nephrotic syndrome who is unresponsive to a course of steroids or in a patient with a history of frequent relapses or steroid dependency.

The pathogenesis of FSGS is unknown. It may be idiopathic or associated with other glomerular or systemic diseases. On light microscopy, the lesion is characterized by focal and segmental sclerosis of the glomerular tuft associated with increased mesangial matrix and basement membrane. Lesions preferentially affect the juxtaglomerular glomeruli. IgM and C3 can often be seen in the affected segments, but IgG and IgA are less common. EM reveals effacement and diffuse or segmental alterations of the foot processes.

Most patients with FSGS (50–70%) demonstrate persistent proteinuria, progressive decline in GFR, and hypertension that are unresponsive to therapy. However, spontaneous remission without progressive renal failure can occur in approximately 20–35%, and exacerbation of proteinuria and nephrotic syndrome with a late onset of renal failure can occur in 10–15%. Treatment with cytotoxic agents, cyclosporine, or nonsteroidal anti-inflammatory agents has been ineffective in altering the course of this disease. However, two recent uncontrolled studies, one in which prolonged high-dose intravenous steroids combined with cytotoxic therapy was used and the other in which high-dose oral cyclosporine A was used, have demonstrated some effectiveness in inducing and maintaining remission in patients previously resistant to conventional steroid therapy. For patients who progress to renal failure, dialysis and transplantation are therapeutic options. Unfortunately, the risk of recurrence of FSGS in the transplanted kidney is reported to be as high as 40%.

MEMBRANOPROLIFERATIVE GLOMERULONEPHRITIS

Although rare (7%) in childhood, more than 50% of patients with membranoproliferative glomerulonephritis (MPGN) show evidence of edema associated with the nephrotic syndrome. Many of these patients have hematuria, hypertension, and mild azotemia. A persistently reduced serum C3 level is a characteristic finding in MPGN, in contrast to the transient reduction observed in patients with poststreptococcal glomerulonephritis.

The clinical course of MPGN in children is variable. In patients with serum creatinine concentrations of 2 mg/dL or greater, most have end-stage renal failure within 3 years. Other patients may have prolonged periods of hematuria and proteinuria followed by the development of edema, subsequent azotemia, and end-stage renal failure. Only a small percentage of patients go into complete remission.

Pathologically, two major variants of MPGN have been described (although some groups have reported a third variant). Both variants demonstrate increased mesangial cellularity and matrix and C3 deposition in both the glomerular capillary wall and mesangium. In type I MPGN, the glomerular capillary wall is thickened, with a "tram-track" appearance, and EM reveals electron-dense deposits in subendothelial areas. In type II MPGN, EM reveals widened glomerular basement membranes associated with the presence of dense deposits. The pathogenesis of type I MPGN is thought to involve chronic glomerular deposition of immune complexes; the pathogenesis of type II is unknown.

Poor prognostic indicators in MPGN are hypertension, reduced GFR, and the nephrotic syndrome. Various therapeutic regimens have been used in an attempt to slow the progression of disease. There is some evidence to suggest that low-dose, long-term, alternate-day steroid therapy with close observation may be beneficial.

MEMBRANOUS GLOMERULOPATHY

The histologic lesion of membranous glomerulopathy (MGN) is rare in the pediatric age group. MGN appears to be more common in older children and adolescents, although it can occur at any age. Most patients are asymptomatic and are often referred to the pediatric nephrologist because of significant proteinuria on routine urinalysis or nephrotic syndrome unresponsive to steroid therapy. Other patients may present with edema and hematuria, either microscopic or macroscopic. The pathogenesis of MGN is unknown; however, there is evidence that immune complex–mediated mechanisms are involved. MGN has been associated with various infections, the most frequent being the hepatitis B virus.

The clinical course of patients with MGN is highly variable. Most patients have persistent proteinuria; however, isolated hematuria has been reported. Edema and the nephrotic syndrome may or may not be present throughout the course of the disease. In most patients, serum complements concentrations are normal.

The histologic lesion is characterized by diffuse and uniform thickening of the glomerular capillary wall without significant mesangial proliferation. Immunofluorescence microscopy characteristically reveals diffuse granular staining along the capillary loops with IgG and C3. EM reveals immune complexes as dense deposits in the subepithelial space.

Even though the clinical course is variable in children, the overall prognosis is excellent, with spontaneous remission of proteinuria occurring is 50–60%. Renal failure has been reported to occur in 13–30% of patients with MGN. Children with nephrotic syndrome are at greatest risk of long-term complications; alternate-day steroid therapy may improve their prognosis.

In summary, the course, natural history, and ultimate outcome of primary idiopathic nephrotic syndrome in children are determined primarily by the underlying histologic lesion. As discussed, one often cannot determine the underlying histologic lesion on the basis of the presenting symptoms alone. After consultation with a pediatric nephrologist, a reasonable therapeutic approach to children with nephrotic syndrome who have no risk factors for serious underlying diseases that may require renal biopsy (see Table 16–12) would be a short course of treatment with prednisone. In patients in whom the nephrotic syndrome resolves with prednisone therapy, the most likely lesion is minimal change disease. Unfortunately, such patients can later have unresponsiveness to steroids and, when a renal biopsy is performed, can be shown to have FSGS.

ACUTE RENAL FAILURE

Acute renal failure (ARF) is a clinical syndrome characterized by a sudden decrease in renal function sufficient to cause retention of metabolic wastes. It is reflected by an increase in the serum concentrations of urea nitrogen and creatinine. When ARF is due to hypovolemia or shock, oliguria usually occurs; when it is due to toxic or inflammatory injury to the kidney, urine output may be decreased or may be normal (nonoliguric ARF). ARF that is caused by ischemic or toxic injury to the nephron is often referred to as **acute tubular necrosis (ATN).**

Common causes of ARF in children are listed in Table 16–15. ARF can occur when there is inadequate perfusion of the kidneys, as with severe dehydration, hemorrhage, or shock (prerenal causes). If the circulating blood volume is promptly restored in such cases, oliguria and azotemia often can be reversed. However, if renal hypoperfusion is prolonged, established renal failure may result. Intrinsic renal causes of ARF are nephrotoxic, inflammatory, or renovascular disorders, and the postrenal causes are obstructive lesions of the urinary tract. In newborn infants, acute onset of renal failure can be due to ischemic or toxic injury to the kidney but can also be due to congenital renal abnormalities, such as multicystic dysplasia of the kidneys; bilateral renal agenesis, polycystic kidney disease; or obstructive lesions, such as posterior urethral valves.

HISTORY

The history provides clues as to the underlying cause of ARF. A prerenal cause is suggested by a history of severe vomiting and diarrhea, hemorrhage, shock due to cardiac arrest, sepsis, or anaphylaxis. It also is suggested by hypovolemia due to severe nephrotic syndrome, diabetic ketoacidosis, or burns. Patients with renal concentrating defects, such as those with preexisting chronic renal insufficiency, polycystic kidney disease, or diabetes insipidus, are more susceptible to prerenal ARF.

An intrinsic renal cause of ARF is suggested by a history of exposure to nephrotoxins, such as aminoglycoside antibiotics, amphotericin B, radiocontrast agents, or drugs that can cause tubulointerstitial nephritis, such as the penicillins or nonsteroidal anti-inflammatory agents (indomethacin). The last group of drugs also can reduce renal blood flow in patients with cardiac dysfunction. A history of gross hematuria suggests acute glomerulonephritis; a history of bloody diarrhea, oliguria; and pallor, hemolytic

Table 16–15. Causes of acute renal failure in children.

Prerenal	Intrinsic Renal	Postrenal
Hypovolemia	Nephrotoxins	Ureteral obstruction
Severe dehydration	Aminoglycosides, cephalosporins, amphotericin B	Calculi, clot, tumor
Hemorrhage	Radiocontrast agents	Ureteropelvic junction
Burns	Heavy metals	Ureterovesical junction
Diabetic ketoacidosis	Organic solvents, pesticides	Urethral obstruction
Hypotension/hypoperfusion	Myoglobin (crush syndrome)	Posterior urethral
Shock (cardiogenic, septic, anaphylactic)	Parenchymal disorders	valves
Cardiac surgery	Acute glomerulonephritis	Diverticulum, stricture
Severe nephrotic syndrome, hepatic cirrhosis	Hemolytic uremic syndrome	Ureterocele
Hepatorenal syndrome	Systemic vasculitis	Hydrocolpos
	(Henoch-Schönlein purpura, systemic lupus erythematosus, polyarteritis, Wegener granulomatosis)	Tumor
	Acute interstitial nephritis (bacterial, allergic)	
	Tubular obstruction (tumor lysis syndrome, uric acid, oxalic acid)	
	Acute tubular necrosis (prolonged ischemia)	
	Vascular disorders	
	Renal artery thrombosis or embolism	
	Renal vein thrombosis	
	Indomethacin ($\downarrow$ renal blood flow)	

uremic syndrome (HUS), which is discussed in detail below.

Obstructive disorders are suggested by a history of abdominal or flank pain, dysuria or UTI, poor urinary stream, passage of renal stones, prior administration of cancer chemotherapeutic agents, renal tubular acidosis, or instrumentation of the urinary tract.

PHYSICAL EXAMINATION

The physical examination may reflect the underlying cause of ARF and should focus initially on assessing the patient's state of hydration. Hypovolemia is revealed by sunken eyes, decreased skin turgor, tachycardia, and orthostatic hypotension; intravascular volume overload is revealed by periorbital or pedal edema, hypertension, or congestive heart failure. A palpable flank mass or enlarged kidneys suggest hydronephrosis, polycystic kidney disease, or renal vein thrombosis; a palpable bladder suggests urethral obstruction.

LABORATORY FINDINGS

The following measurements are essential for evaluation of the patient with ARF: complete blood count and determination of serum concentrations of sodium, potassium, chloride, total carbon dioxide, urea nitrogen, creatinine, calcium, phosphorus, total protein, and albumin. Urine should be obtained for urinalysis and culture; evaluation of the urinary sediment can be particularly helpful (Table 16–16). The urine osmolality and concentrations of sodium and creatinine should also be measured; it is important that this be done before a diuretic agent is administered. In patients in whom acute glomerulonephritis is suspected, one should measure the ASO and anti-DNAse B titers, as well as serum complement and ANA levels (see this chapter, Glomerulonephritis).

Oliguria is defined as a urine volume of less than 0.8

Table 16–16. Urinary sediment in acute renal failure.

No or scant abnormalities
    Prerenal or postrenal azotemia
    Hepatorenal syndrome
Red blood cells and casts
    Acute glomerulonephritis
    Hemolytic uremic syndrome
    Systemic vasculitis
White blood cells
    Pyelonephritis
    Interstitial nephritis (eosinophils)
Tubular epithelial cells casts, coarse granular casts, mild proteinuria, few red blood cells and white blood cells
    Acute tubular necrosis
Crystalluria
    Uric acid—tumor lysis syndrome
    Calcium oxalate—nephrolithiasis

mL/100 kcal/h in children, less than 1.0 mL/kg/h in infants, and less than 400 mL/d in adolescents and adults. In patients with oliguria, the chemical composition of the urine is a valuable aid in distinguishing established intrinsic renal failure from prerenal azotemia (Table 16–17); the latter is potentially reversible if the patient's intravascular volume is restored promptly. In virtually all patients with unexplained ARF, one should perform a renal ultrasound study to rule out urinary tract obstruction. A chest radiograph and electrocardiogram (ECG) should be performed when volume overload and hyperkalemia, respectively, are present.

TREATMENT

The objectives of the initial management of the patient with ARF are the assessment of intravascular volume status, treatment of life-threatening complications, and diagnosis of acute urinary tract obstruction. Diagnostic evaluation of the underlying cause of ARF should be initiated after initial stabilization of the patient.

Initial Measures

For patients with oliguria and signs of intravascular volume depletion, isotonic fluid (0.9% sodium chloride, Ringer lactate, or colloid) should be given intravenously, 10–20 mL/kg over 15–30 minutes, or blood, 10 mL/kg, should be given until skin turgor, pulse, blood pressure, and central venous pressure (if available) are normal. If the urine output increases, a prerenal cause of ARF is likely. If oliguria persists, furosemide, 1–2 mg/kg intravenously, or mannitol, 0.5–1 g/kg intravenously over 15–30 minutes, should be administered. If oliguria still persists, then ARF due to intrinsic renal disease is established, and the patient's fluid intake should be restricted to insensible water loss, estimated at 35 mL/100 kcal/d, plus other losses. If urine output increases with administration of diuretics (a positive response is urine output of 5–10 mL/kg over 1–3 h), ARF may be nonoliguric, and efforts to maintain a diuresis should be continued. Patients with ARF due to intrarenal obstruction by uric acid crystals (tumor lysis syndrome) may benefit from a sustained diuresis induced by mannitol, achieved by infusing a solution of 3% mannitol in 0.25% saline at a rate equal to that of urine output.

Specific Treatments

Acute life-threatening complications of ARF that require immediate treatment are severe intravascular volume overload, with congestive heart failure and pulmonary edema, severe hypertension, and severe hyperkalemia. Patients with severe ECF volume overload require urgent dialysis. The treatment of severe hypertension is discussed below (see Evaluation of Hypertension). Treatment of ARF includes the following:

Energy & Protein Intake. To minimize protein catabolism and progressive azotemia, energy intake of 70–100

Table 16–17. Laboratory findings in acute renal failure.

Test	Prerenal	Intrinsic Renal	Postrenal
Ultrasound	Normal	Normal/increased size or echogenicity	Dilated pelvis, ureter, bladder
Urine osmolality (mOsm/kg)	> 500	< 350	Urinary indices not helpful
Urine/plasma creatinine	> 14:1	< 14:1	
Urine sodium (meq/L)	< 20	> 30	
Fractional excretion of sodium (%)[1]	< 1	> 2	
	> 2.5 in neonates	> 2.5 in neonates	
Urinary sediment	Minimal findings	Trace to 2 + protein	Unremarkable; white blood cells with infection
	Few granular casts	Few white blood cells, red blood cells	
		Brown granular casts	
		Tubular epithelial cells	

[1]Fractional excretion of sodium (%) = $\dfrac{U_{Na}(meq/L)}{U_{creat}(meq/L)} \times \dfrac{S_{creat}(mg/dL)}{S_{Na}(mg/dL)} \times 100$

kcal/kg/d combined with protein intake of 0.7–1 g/kg/d should be provided, either orally or with central intravenous alimentation.

Electrolytes. Sodium and potassium should be restricted in patients with oliguria. In nonoliguric patients, urinary electrolyte and water losses should be replaced as necessary to maintain normal intravascular volume and electrolyte concentrations. Hyponatremia occurring during the oliguric phase of ARF is due to excessive administration of water; thus, water intake should be reduced further, rather than giving sodium.

Hyperkalemia. Hyperkalemia is common and is due to release of potassium from cells as a result of catabolism, hemolysis, acidosis, and transfusion of blood products. If the serum potassium level is greater than 6.0 meq/L and the ECG pattern is normal or reveals peaked T waves, sodium polystyrene sulfonate (Kayexalate) (Table 16–18) should be given to reduce the potassium level over a period of several hours and repeated as necessary. If more severe ECG changes are present or the potassium

level is greater than 7.5 meq/L, urgent additional therapy is required, as outlined in Table 16–18. If hyperkalemia persists or worsens despite these measures, then acute dialysis is indicated.

Hypocalcemia. Treatment is indicated when tetany, either overt or latent, is present. Latent tetany may be demonstrated by eliciting the Chvostek sign (twitching of the muscles at the margin of the lips when the facial nerve is stimulated by tapping over the zygoma) or the Trousseau sign (carpal spasm induced when a blood pressure cuff is inflated to 20 mm Hg above systolic pressure for 3 minutes). Intravenous calcium should be given as a 10 mg/kg dose of elemental calcium over 5–10 minutes, as 10% calcium gluconate (94 mg elemental calcium per 10-mL ampoule), 1 mL/kg per dose, or as 10% calcium chloride (270 mg elemental calcium per 10-mL ampule), 0.3–0.5 mL/kg/dose.

Hyperphosphatemia. Phosphorus-containing foods should be restricted. If the serum phosphorus level is greater than approximately 6 mg/dL, the phosphate-bind-

Table 16–18. Treatment of hyperkalemia.

Drug	Effect	Onset of Action	Duration of Action	Dose	Comments, Complications
Calcium	Stabilizes myocardium	Immediate	Minutes	10% calcium gluconate, 0.5 mL/kg intravenously over 2–4 min	Bradycardia, hypercalcemia. Requires ECG monitoring
NaHCO$_3$	Shifts K$^+$ into cells with increased blood pH	30–60 min	Hours	2–3 meq/kg over 30–60 min	Hypernatremia, hypervolemia, alkalosis, hypocalcemia
Glucose and insulin	Shifts K$^+$ into cells	30 min	Hours	Glucose 0.5 g/kg with insulin 0.3 U/g glucose over 30 min	Hyperglycemia or hypoglycemia
Sodium polystyrene sulfonate	Exchanges Na$^+$ for K$^+$ in gut and thus removes K$^+$ from patient	1 h	Hours	1 g/kg orally or 1.5 g/kg rectally, with 3 mL 70% sorbitol per gram resin. Repeat at 4 to 6-hr intervals	Fecal impaction; hypernatremia with repeated doses

ECG = electrocardiogram.

ing agent calcium carbonate, 2–3 g with each meal, or 3 times per day in patients without oral food intake, should be administered.

Acidosis. Severe metabolic acidosis (pH < 7.1; plasma sodium bicarbonate, 12–15 meq/L) should be treated with intravenous sodium bicarbonate, 2–3 meq/kg per dose administered over 30–60 minutes. Care should be taken when administering alkali to patients who are both acidotic and hypocalcemic; there is an increased risk of inducing tetany when systemic pH is rapidly increased because of increased binding of ionized calcium to albumin. In severely hypocalcemic patients, calcium should be given intravenously before giving alkali. Milder degrees of acidosis should be treated with sodium bicarbonate, 1–3 meq/kg/d, either orally or intravenously.

Dialysis. Urgent dialysis, either peritoneal dialysis or hemodialysis, is required for children who do not respond to initial treatment of the above complications. Less urgent indications for dialysis are severe acidosis, hyponatremia, azotemia complicated by central nervous system depression or bleeding, and a serum urea nitrogen level greater than 125–150 mg/dL.

OUTCOME

Children with ARF should be hospitalized. After initial stabilization, they require full evaluation to determine the cause of the ARF and treatment in consultation with a pediatric nephrologist. Frequent monitoring of blood pressure, cardiovascular status, and urine output, and meticulous fluid and electrolyte management are essential components of care. Children with ECF volume overload, hypertension, or electrolyte abnormalities should be admitted to a pediatric critical care unit; less ill patients may be managed on a pediatric ward.

HEMOLYTIC UREMIC SYNDROME

HUS is characterized by the classic triad of ARF, microangiopathic hemolytic anemia, and thrombocytopenia. In children, HUS is the most common cause of ARF requiring acute dialysis. It is primarily a disease of childhood, but any age can be affected. Seasonal variation has been observed, with most cases occurring in late spring, summer, and early fall.

Two groups of patients may be distinguished on the basis of their presentation, either epidemic (typical, classic) or sporadic (atypical). In the former group, most patients present with a gastrointestinal prodrome, characterized by abdominal pain, vomiting, and diarrhea with or without blood. In the latter group, patients have no prodrome at all. Familial and recurrent forms of the atypical variant have been described, with both types having high morbidity and mortality rates. HUS also has been associated with ingestion of drugs (cyclosporin, mitomycin, and oral contraceptives), the postpartum period, collagen vascular disease, malignant disease, and bone-marrow and solid organ transplantation. Such secondary cases of HUS are seen more commonly in adult patients than in children (Table 16–19).

HISTOPATHOLOGY

→ *thrombosis within small blood vessels*

The histopathologic lesion of HUS is characterized as thrombotic microangiopathy, with the major sites of involvement being the kidney, brain, skin, pancreas, heart, spleen, and adrenal. The picture of thrombotic microangiopathy is described as comprising (1) agglutinated platelets in arterioles and capillaries out of proportion to fibrin deposition, (2) endothelial swelling, and (3) minimal inflammatory infiltrate; these abnormalities of the microvasculature can be focal. Activation of platelets and the coagulation cascade probably occurs with deposition of platelets and fibrin-like material within the lumen of the glomeruli and, occasionally, the arterioles. In the glomeruli of the kidney, there is endothelial injury with detachment of the basement membrane and interposition of fluffy-appearing material similar to that in the capillary lumen. Three categories of renal histopathologic lesions have been defined: cortical necrosis, predominance of glomerular injury, and predominance of arteriolar injury. Although there is no correlation between the various lesions with the typical or atypical forms of HUS, there is some suggestion that predominantly glomerular lesions are seen in typical cases and predominantly arteriolar lesions in atypical cases.

PATHOPHYSIOLOGY

The initial pathogenic event is thought to be injury to the endothelial cells of the renal microvasculature caused by bacterial toxins, with subsequent activation and aggregation of platelets. In many patients with classic HUS, gastrointestinal disease has been associated with *Escherichia coli* infection. For example, in an epidemic of

Table 16–19. Etiologic classification of hemolytic uremic syndrome.

Idiopathic (atypical)
Infectious (typical): *Escherichia coli*, *Shigella dysenteriae* type 1, *Streptococcus pneumoniae*
Hereditary: autosomal recessive, autosomal dominant
Recurrent: sporadic (atypical), post-transplantation
Associated with:
  Drugs: cyclosporine, oral contraceptives, mitomycin
  Pregnancy
  Radiation
  Transplantation: bone marrow, kidney
  Malignancy

HUS that occurred in a nursing home, infection with E coli O157:H7 was found in 12 of 55 affected residents. This strain of *E coli* has been shown to produce a specific toxin, known as verotoxin, which is directly toxic to endothelial cells in vitro. HUS has been associated with both gastrointestinal and respiratory infection due to other organisms, including *Shigella dysenteriae* type I, *Campylobacter jejuni, Salmonella typhi,* and *Streptococcus pneumoniae.*

Additional mechanisms that promote platelet activation and aggregation may play a role in the pathogenesis of HUS. In some patients with HUS, a deficiency of prostacyclin or of circulating von Willebrand factor multimers, both known to inhibit platelet aggregation, has been seen. However, whether these disturbances in platelet aggregation are primary or secondary to the endothelial injury is not clear.

CLINICAL FEATURES & LABORATORY FINDINGS

After the typical gastrointestinal prodrome, most patients have hematuria and proteinuria with mild renal insufficiency, anemia, and thrombocytopenia. However, a number of patients have ARF with oliguria or anuria and severe azotemia. The anuria may last from a few days to several weeks. In a significant minority of patients, hypertension, due to either intrinsic renal disease or fluid overload, or both, develops.

The microangiopathic hemolytic anemia results primarily from physical destruction of RBCs in the microcirculation and their subsequent removal from the circulation by the spleen. The degree of hemolysis varies from mild to severe and usually parallels the course of renal involvement. Evidence of hemolysis is demonstrated on the peripheral blood smear by the presence of schistocytes, as well as Burr and target cells. This hemolytic process is associated with reticulocytosis, hemoglobinemia, reduced serum haptoglobin levels, and a negative Coombs test result. Jaundice may develop as a result of the hemolysis and indirect hyperbilirubinemia. The thrombocytopenia is caused by intravascular clumping and removal of damaged platelets by the reticuloendothelial system and varies in severity and duration. Occasionally, petechiae or purpura are noted on the skin. Leukocytosis is present, and evidence of a coagulopathy is typically absent.

Extrarenal and extrahematologic manifestations also can be seen in patients with HUS. Involvement of the central nervous system occurs in approximately one third of patients and ranges in severity from mild to severe. Irritability, personality changes, drowsiness, seizures, transient cortical blindness, hemiparesis, and coma are observed. Seizures may be caused by hypertension, electrolyte disturbances, or brain microthrombi. Cardiac involvement is rare in childhood and may be manifested by a cardiomyopathy, aneurysm, or myocarditis. A subset of patients can have severe disease of the gastrointestinal tract, which is due to injury of the gastrointestinal microvasculature, characterized by severe abdominal pain, and sometimes associated with intussusception, perforation, frank necrosis, or stricture. Insulin-dependent diabetes mellitus may develop as a result of pancreatic dysfunction and can be transient or permanent. Other organ systems that may be involved during the course of HUS are the liver, with a transient elevation of enzymes, the skeletal muscle, and the eye.

TREATMENT

Therapy usually is guided by the degree of organ involvement and the severity of clinical manifestations. Because children with typical HUS have an excellent prognosis, they can be managed conservatively with judicious transfusion of blood products for anemia and thrombocytopenia, treatment of hypertension, seizure control, and careful control of electrolyte and water disturbances. Either peritoneal dialysis or hemodialysis should be performed in patients with prolonged anuria who have severe azotemia, hyperkalemia, acidosis, or signs of severe intravascular volume overload such as pulmonary edema and hypertension. Such a comprehensive regimen of supportive therapy is primarily responsible for the decline in the mortality rates from 40–50% in the 1950s to the current rate of 5–10%.

Over the years, multiple therapeutic modalities have been used in an attempt to improve the clinical course. These include immunosuppressive agents, steroids, antiplatelet agents, anticoagulants, prostacyclin and plasma infusions, and plasmapheresis. Unfortunately, none of these therapies have been convincingly demonstrated to improve the outcome of this disorder. Therefore, it is recommended that patients with HUS be managed conservatively with supportive therapy.

OUTCOME

Important determinants of morbidity and mortality in children with HUS are the type of presentation, the severity and duration of renal involvement, and the severity of neurologic disease. Patients with a typical diarrheal prodrome have a good prognosis, whereas those with atypical presentations generally have a worse prognosis. The anuria associated with severe renal disease ranges in length from a few days to several weeks. Although in some studies prolonged anuria has been associated with a worse prognosis, most such patients eventually have complete resolution of disease and normalization of renal function. Nevertheless, a few patients have either irreversible renal failure during the acute episode or progressive renal insufficiency and end-stage renal failure months to years later. Such patients require chronic dialysis treatment and renal transplantation. In patients with seizures, hemiparesis, or coma during the acute illness, persistent neurologic involvement is rare.

CALCIUM & PHOSPHOROUS METABOLISM

Calcium and phosphorous are essential for normal growth and mineralization of bone and for other important metabolic processes. The plasma concentrations of calcium and phosphorus are maintained by the interaction between the three major organ systems—bone, intestine, and kidney—and are regulated within a narrow physiologic range by the actions of three hormones—1,25-dihydroxyvitamin D (1,25-$(OH)_2$D), parathyroid hormone (PTH), and calcitonin (CT). Abnormalities of calcium and phosphorus metabolism are often seen in the context of disordered renal function and therefore are discussed in this chapter.

Calcium in plasma exists in three fractions: protein-bound calcium (40%), which is not filtered by the renal glomerulus, and ionized calcium (48%) and complexed calcium (12%), which are filtered. Albumin accounts for 90% of the protein-bound calcium in plasma, and conditions that affect the serum albumin concentration, such as nephrotic syndrome or hepatic cirrhosis, will affect the measurement of total calcium concentration. Ionized calcium is the fraction of plasma calcium that is important for a variety of physiologic processes. Phosphorus exists in plasma in two forms, an organic form (57%) and an inorganic form (43%); in clinical settings, only the inorganic form is routinely measured. Most inorganic phosphorus (85%) is freely filterable by the kidneys.

VITAMIN D

The major source of vitamin D in humans is the cutaneous conversion of 7-dehydrocholesterol to vitamin D_3 **(cholecalciferol),** which occurs on exposure of the skin to ultraviolet light. Little vitamin D is present naturally in foods, and fortification of certain foods, such as milk, with vitamin D_2 **(ergocalciferol),** or administration of supplemental vitamin D_2 often is necessary to prevent the occurrence of vitamin D deficiency in infants and adolescents and in those with limited exposure to sunlight. Vitamin D is subsequently hydroxylated in the liver to 25-hydroxyvitamin (25-OHD), the major circulating form of vitamin D. Both vitamin D and 25-OHD represent storage, not active, forms, of this hormone. Conversion of 25-OHD to its physiologically active form, 1,25-$(OH)_2$D, occurs in the proximal tubules of the kidney. The principal factors that stimulate renal synthesis of 1,25-$(OH)_2$D are

hypocalcemia, increased serum concentrations of PTH, and hypophosphatemia. The active hormone 1,25-$(OH)_2$D acts primarily on the intestine to increase its absorption of calcium and phosphorus, on the skeleton to increase calcification of osteoid and mobilization of skeletal mineral, and on the parathyroid gland to decrease synthesis and secretion of PTH.

PARATHYROID HORMONE

PTH is an 84–amino acid polypeptide that is synthesized and secreted by the four parathyroid glands, which are derived from the third and fourth pairs of branchial pouches, usually located just posterior to the thyroid gland. In healthy adults, the total weight of the four glands is less than 200 mg. The plasma ionized calcium concentration is the principal regulator of PTH secretion. A decrease in ionized calcium induces a rapid increase in synthesis and secretion of PTH, whereas an increase in ionized calcium induces a decrease in PTH secretion. Severe hypomagnesemia can impair PTH secretion in response to hypocalcemia. PTH secretion also is inhibited by increased concentrations of 1,25-$(OH)_2$D.

Parathyroid Hormone Testing

Whereas intact active PTH has a half-life of only minutes, inactive PTH metabolites remain in the serum for hours. These inactive fragments of PTH are excreted by the kidneys and thus are retained in the circulation in patients with renal insufficiency. With the recent development of PTH assays that measure the "intact," biologically active hormone, clinical determination of serum PTH concentrations is readily performed. Given that PTH release is regulated by plasma calcium concentration, rational interpretation of measured PTH concentrations requires knowledge of the simultaneously measured calcium concentration (Figure 16–5).

CALCITONIN

CT is a 32–amino acid peptide synthesized and secreted by the parafollicular or C cells of the thyroid gland. Secretion of CT is stimulated by hypercalcemia and inhibited by hypocalcemia. CT acts primarily on bone to decrease bone resorption, and the principal physiologic effect of the hormone is to decrease the serum calcium concentration.

EXTRACELLULAR CALCIUM HOMEOSTASIS

A decrease in the plasma calcium concentration induces a rapid increase in secretion of PTH from the parathyroid gland. PTH acts on the kidney to decrease excretion of calcium, increase excretion of phosphorus, and stimulate

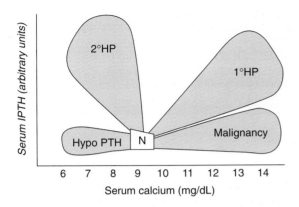

Figure 16–5. Interpretation of measured parathyroid hormone (PTH) concentrations and simultaneous calcium concentration. 1°HP = primary hyperparathyroidism; 2°HP = secondary hyperparathyroidism; IPTH = inactive parathyroid hormone; N = normal; Hypo PTH = hypoparathyroidism. (Reproduced, with permission, from Andreoli TE et al: Page 521 in: *Cecil Essentials of Medicine,* 2nd ed. Saunders, 1990.)

Table 16–20. Differential diagnosis of rickets.

Abnormalities of vitamin D metabolism
  Deficient dietary vitamin D and lack of sunlight exposure
  Fat malabsorption with reduced vitamin D absorption
  Increased metabolic clearance secondary to anticonvulsant therapy
  Liver disease (impaired 25-hydroxylation of vitamin D)
  Renal insufficiency (impaired 1-hydroxylation of 25-hydroxy-vitamin D)
  1α-hydroxylase deficiency (vitamin D–dependent rickets type 1)
  Vitamin D receptor/postreceptor defect (vitamin D–dependent rickets type 2)

Dietary calcium deficiency (rare)

Dietary phosphorus deficiency (rare after infancy)

Impaired renal reabsorption of phosphorus
  X-linked hypophosphatemic rickets
  Hereditary hypophosphatemic rickets with hypercalciuria
  Fanconi syndrome (renal proximal tubular dysfunction)
  Renal tubular acidosis
  Post-renal transplantation hypophosphatemia
  Tumor-induced hyperphosphaturia (oncogenic osteomalacia)

production of 1,25-$(OH)_2$D. PTH, together with 1,25-$(OH)_2$D, acts on bone to stimulate release of calcium and phosphorus. 1,25-$(OH)_2$D acts on the intestine to promote absorption of calcium and phosphorus. These actions of PTH and 1,25-$(OH)_2$D on their target issues result in an increase in plasma calcium concentration to normal values. Because of the phosphaturic effect of PTH, phosphorus released from bone is excreted in the urine; thus, there is little change in serum phosphorus concentration. Conversely, with an increase in plasma calcium concentration, release of PTH and production of 1,25-$(OH)_2$D are decreased, and release of CT is stimulated. The combined effects of these hormonal changes on bone, kidney, and intestine are opposite to those occurring with hypocalcemia; the result is a decrease in calcium concentration to normal values.

DISORDERS OF CALCIUM HOMEOSTASIS

Rickets

In growing children, rickets can occur when the availability of calcium and phosphorus are not sufficient to permit normal mineralization of newly formed bone osteoid. In the most common form of rickets, calcium and phosphorus deficiency are secondary to deficiency of vitamin D, which results from inadequate dietary intake of vitamin D combined with limited exposure to sunlight. Congenital or acquired disorders of vitamin D metabolism (Table 16–20) also can give rise to deficiency of the hormone. Vitamin D deficiency results in impaired intestinal absorption of calcium and phosphorus, hypocalcemia, secondary hyperparathyroidism, increased bone resorption, hyperphosphaturia, hypophosphatemia, and impaired bone

mineralization. In industrialized countries, the incidence of vitamin D–deficient rickets has been greatly reduced because of the routine fortification of foods such as milk and supplementation of breast-fed infants with vitamin D. Nevertheless, vitamin D–deficient rickets remains a major public health problem in many countries.

The clinical and radiographic signs of rickets vary greatly with age of onset, duration, and severity of vitamin D deficiency. The signs predominate in those areas in which bone growth is rapid, namely the epiphyses of long bones and the costochondral junctions. Palpable enlargement at the wrists and ankles and at the costochondral junctions ("rachitic rosary") are characteristic clinical signs of florid rickets. With weight bearing in older infants and children, bowing of the femur and tibia can be seen. Radiographs reveal characteristic abnormalities of the epiphyseal regions of the long bones. There is widening of the radiolucent space between the metaphyseal lines and the epiphysis that reflects the accumulation of uncalcified cartilage. The metaphyseal lines often are irregular, frayed, and hollowed ("cupping"). The shafts of the long bones usually reveal thinning of the cortices. The biochemical findings in patients with rickets, noted above, vary greatly depending on the etiology, duration, and severity of the disease.

Hyperparathyroidism

Disorders of increased PTH production are uncommon in children. The clinical manifestations of these disorders are varied and are summarized in Table 16–21. There are many causes of hypercalcemia (Table 16–22). Primary hyperparathyroidism may result from an adenoma, hyperplasia, or carcinoma; can occur in either familial or nonfamilial patterns; and may be isolated or occur in association with multiple endocrine adenomatoses syndromes I

Table 16–21. Signs and symptoms of hyperparathyroidism.

General	Renal
Weakness	Polyuria/polydipsia
Fatigability	Stones
Weight loss	
Gastrointestinal	Bones
Peptic ulcer	Pain
Chronic pancreatitis	Osteopenia
Nausea/vomiting	
Pain	
Central nervous system	
Headache	
Depression	
Delusion/confusion	
Lethargy/coma	

Table 16–23. Clinical signs of hypocalcemia.

Tetany
Convulsions
Muscle cramps
Carpopedal spasm—Trousseau sign
Facial twitching—Chvostek sign
Laryngeal stridor
Paresthesias

and II. Treatment of primary hyperparathyroidism usually involves surgical removal of adenomatous, hyperplastic, or carcinomatous parathyroid glands. Secondary hyperparathyroidism typically occurs in patients with chronic renal insufficiency or nutritional deficiency of vitamin D, and treatment involves administration of vitamin D or its active metabolites.

Hypoparathyroidism

Most patients with inadequate secretion of PTH present with symptoms associated with hypocalcemia and hyperphosphatemia (Table 16–23). These include tetany, convulsions, muscle cramps, laryngeal stridor, and paresthesias. Because the ability to secrete PTH can be limited even in normal infants, feeding of a high-phosphorus–containing formula, such as cow's milk, can give rise to hypocalcemia. A number of disorders are associated with decreased secretion of PTH (Table 16–24). DiGeorge syndrome results from the abnormal embryologic development of the third and fourth pharyngeal pouches. Most infants (60%) with DiGeorge syndrome present within 48 hours after birth with cardiovascular defects, most often an interrupted aortic arch or truncus arteriosus, and have hypocalcemia secondary to PTH deficiency at a medial age of 8 days after birth. Other associated findings include hypertelorism, antimongoloid slant of the eyes, cleft palate, carp-shaped mouth, and micrognathia. Some affected infants have thymic dysplasia with a variable degree of cellular immune deficiency. The prognosis of such infants depends on the extent and ability to correct their immunodeficiency and cardiac anomalies.

Pseudohypoparathyroidism

Pseudohypoparathyroidism (PHP) results from a failure of end-organ responsiveness to PTH. In patients with PHP, serum concentrations of PTH are increased, but hypocalcemia and hyperphosphatemia occur, similar to that seen in patients with hypoparathyroidism. Three types of PHP have been described. PHP type Ia is associated with variable dysmorphic features, including short stature, round face, and short metacarpal bones; many patients are mentally retarded. This type of PHP, which is often familial, is associated with deficient activity of the G_S protein, which couples the PTH receptor to adenylate cyclase, resulting in defective stimulation of cyclic adenosine monophosphate (cAMP) in response to PTH. Patients with PHP Ib have normal G_S activity and are often normal in appearance. Patients with PHP type II appear to have a defect in PTH signaling distal to the formation of cAMP.

CHRONIC RENAL FAILURE

In patients with chronic renal failure, a slow deterioration of renal function is caused by a variety of renal and urologic diseases and results in a symptom complex involving multiple abnormalities of body composition and metabolism, hormonal regulation, and organ system functioning.

Table 16–22. Causes of hypercalcemia.

Hyperparathyroidism	Adrenal insufficiency
Excessive vitamin D intake	Sarcoidosis
Hypervitaminosis A	Milk-alkali syndrome
Hypercalcemia of malignancy	Thiazide diureticis
Immobilization	Williams syndrome (idiopathic
Familial hypocalciuric hyper-	hypercalcemia of infancy)
calcemia	Subcutaneous fat necrosis
Hyperthyroidism	

Table 16–24. Conditions associated with hypoparathyroidism.

Parathyroid destruction
  Surgery
  Autoimmune
    Polyglandular autoimmune syndromes—type 1
Magnesium deficiency
DiGeorge syndrome
Transient
Familial

ETIOLOGY & PATHOGENESIS

The more common causes of chronic renal failure in children are listed in Table 16–25. In infants and young children, congenital abnormalities of the kidneys and urinary tract and inherited diseases predominate, whereas in older children, various forms of glomerulonephritis are more common. In many of the conditions listed, renal failure is caused by the gradual destruction of renal parenchyma by an ongoing inflammatory, immunologic, or metabolic disease. In other conditions, however, after an initial insult to the kidneys, further gradual deterioration occurs despite the absence of an ongoing disease process. These conditions include such diverse entities as renal hypoplasia and dysplasia, surgically corrected renal reflux, and the slowly progressive renal failure that follows an episode of HUS. The common denominator in these conditions is a reduction in the number of nephrons, which is known to result in compensatory hypertrophy of the remaining nephrons. Studies in experimental animals have demonstrated that this hypertrophy response is mediated by an increase in intraglomerular plasma flow, hydrostatic pressure, and filtration rate and that this process eventually leads to glomerular scarring and obsolescence. The pathogenesis of this so-called hyperfiltration injury, and its significance in the progression of renal failure in humans, is incompletely defined and is the subject of continuing studies.

PATHOPHYSIOLOGY

As a consequence of nephron destruction in chronic renal failure and subsequent hypertrophy of the remaining nephrons, patients with mildly to moderately reduced GFR can maintain normal body fluid homeostasis. Although the amount of glomerular filtrate formed each day in these patients is greatly diminished, the tubules of surviving nephrons are sufficiently able to increase the fractional excretion of salt and water so that intake and output of these substances are balanced. This adaptive process, however, has limits. The ability of damaged kidneys to increase salt and water excretion in response to acute volume loads and to conserve salt and water in response to acute dehydration becomes progressively compromised as the GFR decreases.

CLINICAL FINDINGS

With kidney failure, there is retention in the body of a variety of substances that are normally excreted by the kidneys. These include urea nitrogen, creatinine, uric acid, potassium, phosphorus, hydrogen ions, sodium chloride, and water. The retention of these substances and a number of other, less–well-defined "uremic toxins" causes a variety of pathologic processes in the body, which include metabolic and hormonal abnormalities, decreased immune responsiveness, and organ-system dysfunction. In addition, blood concentrations of hormones normally synthesized and secreted by the kidneys, such as erythropoietin and $1,25\text{-}(OH)_2D$, are decreased, and the level of the renal hormone renin may be increased.

Some of the clinical and biochemical manifestations of the uremic state are listed in Table 16–26. The pathogenesis of many of these abnormalities is poorly defined but is thought to involve the action of as-yet unidentified uremic toxins. Some of the described abnormalities, such as decreased immune responsiveness, are of limited clinical significance, whereas others, such as peripheral neuropathy, occur only in patients with long-standing severe renal failure and are rarely seen in those who receive appropriate medical care, including the timely initiation of dialysis.

Table 16–25. Causes of chronic renal failure in children.

	Percentage of Total
Glomerulonephritis	25
Urinary tract malformations	25
Reflux nephropathy and obstructive uropathy	
Renal hypoplasia/dysplasia	16
Cystic diseases	10
Medullary cystic disease and autosomal-recessive polycystic disease	
Cystinosis	4
Hemolytic uremic syndrome	3
Alport syndrome	3
Henoch-Schönlein syndrome	2
Other	12

Table 16–26. Clinical manifestations of chronic renal failure.

Cardiovascular
    Hypertension, pulmonary edema, pericarditis, cardiomyopathy
Nervous system
    Drowsiness, obtundation, seizures, peripheral neuropathy
Gastrointestinal
    Anorexia, nausea and vomiting, gastritis, colitis, malnutrition
Musculoskeletal
    Rickets, osteomalacia, osteitis fibrosa, metastatic calcification, myopathy
Hematopoietic
    Anemia, coagulation disorders
Metabolic
    Acidosis with increased anion gap, glucose intolerance, hypertriglyceridemia
Hormonal
    Increased parathyroid hormone, increased renin-angiotensin, increased prolactin and luteinizing hormone, decreased 1,25-dihydroxyvitamin D, decreased erythropoietin
Immunologic
    Decreased cellular immunity

DIAGNOSIS

Although renal failure is readily diagnosed by a constellation of findings, including increased serum concentrations of creatinine and urea nitrogen, anemia, and acidosis, the cause of the renal failure and its duration are not always apparent. Findings that suggest chronicity are small kidney size, growth retardation, and renal osteodystrophy, although these are not invariably present in chronic disease. The definitive test, both to diagnose the underlying kidney disease and to determine its acuity or chronicity, is a renal biopsy.

TREATMENT

When there is no specific therapy for the underlying cause of renal failure, the management of chronic renal failure consists of instituting nonspecific measures that may retard the progression of renal failure and prevent or treat the complications of renal failure. The progression of renal failure may be retarded by aggressive treatment of hypertension and by dietary restriction of protein and, perhaps, phosphorus. Although hypertension can be a consequence of renal disease and renal failure in many patients, hypertension also can cause kidney damage, and effective control of blood pressure has been shown to retard the progression of renal failure in patients with a variety of renal diseases.

Restriction of dietary protein can decrease glomerular hydrostatic pressure and GFR and, in animals with reduced renal mass, has been shown to prevent compensatory hypertrophy and to slow the progression of renal failure. Although studies of the effects of protein restriction on the progression of renal failure in humans have been difficult to perform and have yielded uncertain results, most nephrologists prescribe protein restriction early in the course of renal failure. Malnutrition and, in children, growth retardation are possible complications of protein restriction.

The most important clinical manifestations of renal failure in children, which require prevention or treatment, are metabolic acidosis, disorders of calcium and phosphorus metabolism, renal osteodystrophy, hypertension, anemia, and nutritional and growth disturbances.

Metabolic Acidosis

The acidosis of renal failure is caused by the inability of the kidneys to excrete the 1–3 meq/kg of hydrogen ion that children generate daily. Acidosis can be a cause of the poor growth that is characteristic of children with renal failure. It is treated with sodium bicarbonate or sodium citrate, 1–3 meq/kg/d.

Renal Osteodystrophy

In severe renal failure, renal excretion of phosphorus is reduced, which results in hyperphosphatemia. Renal production of $1,25\text{-}(OH)_2D$ also is reduced, which results in decreased calcium absorption by the intestine. As a consequence, hypocalcemia and secondary hyperparathyroidism occur, which leads to excessive resorption of bone (**osteitis fibrosa**). Other forms of bone disease have been described and characterized by impaired bone mineralization (**osteomalacia**), a combination of osteitis fibrosa and osteomalacia (**mixed**), and one caused by accumulation of aluminum in bone (**aplastic**). When the product of the calcium times phosphorus concentration in serum exceeds 70, calcium phosphate may be deposited in soft tissues, such as blood vessels, viscera, and skin; the latter is manifested by pruritus.

These abnormalities are treated by restriction of dietary phosphorus, the use of drugs that bind phosphorus in the gut, such as calcium carbonate or calcium acetate, and the administration of 1,25-dihydroxyvitamin D_3 (calcitriol).

Hypertension

Hypertension can be caused by salt and water retention and plasma volume expansion, by increased secretion of renin by the kidneys, and by less–well-understood mechanisms, such as overactivity of the sympathetic nervous system and decreased renal production of vasodilator prostaglandins and kinins. In advanced renal failure, salt and water retention is the most common mechanism. The diagnosis of volume-dependent hypertension is made when other signs of increased plasma volume are present, such as edema and cardiomegaly, whereas the diagnosis of renin-dependent hypertension depends on the finding of increased plasma renin activity.

Volume-dependent hypertension is best managed by dietary salt restriction and treatment with a thiazide diuretic or furosemide. Renin-dependent hypertension can be treated with a β-blocker or, preferably, with more potent drugs affecting the renin-angiotensin system, specifically the angiotensin-converting enzyme inhibitors. Drugs commonly used to treat chronic hypertension in patients with renal failure are presented in the section, Evaluation of Hypertension.

Anemia

The anemia of chronic renal failure is caused primarily by decreased renal production of erythropoietin, although RBC survival is shortened in uremic patients, presumably owing to the effect of a uremic toxin. The anemia is readily corrected by the parenteral administration of erythropoietin, initially given in a dose of 100 U/kg, three times a week. Coexisting iron deficiency must be treated before erythropoietin can be effective.

Nutrition & Growth

Growth retardation is common in children with chronic renal failure, especially in those with congenital renal diseases. Causes of growth retardation include poor calorie intake, acidosis, renal osteodystrophy, and, possibly, resistance to the effects of growth hormone and decreased efficiency of calorie utilization by the body. The most important of these is poor calorie intake, which is the result of anorexia, probably related to high serum concentrations of urea nitrogen or some other product of protein metabolism. The treatment involves protein restriction when the blood urea nitrogen concentration exceeds 80 mg/dL, although this value is arbitrary, and protein restriction may be appropriately initiated at an earlier stage of renal failure to prevent hyperfiltration injury. Protein should not be restricted to less than the RDA for the child. In the infant and young child, protein restriction is best accomplished by substituting a low-protein formula, such as Similac PM60/40 (Ross Laboratories), which also has decreased concentrations of sodium, potassium, and phosphorus, for cow's milk.

Despite protein restriction and the maintenance of low blood urea nitrogen concentrations, calorie intake may be insufficient for growth. Added calories, in the form of carbohydrate or fat suspension, can be prescribed. If children are unable or unwilling to take these orally, nasogastric or gastrostomy tube feeding is sometimes undertaken. In some children, growth remains poor despite the provision of adequate calories and the correction of acidosis and renal osteodystrophy. In recent years, the use of human recombinant growth hormone, 0.05 mg/kg/d, has significantly improved the growth of such children.

EVALUATION OF HYPERTENSION

Hypertension is uncommon in children. Mild hypertension may be secondary to obesity or have no demonstrable cause, but severe hypertension, especially in prepubertal children, is almost always secondary to some medical condition. When defining and evaluating hypertension in children, special attention must be paid to techniques of blood pressure measurement and to recognizing that blood pressure levels normally increase with age throughout childhood. The goal of the evaluation of a child with hypertension is primarily to discover the cause of the hypertension and, secondarily, to determine whether the hypertension has resulted in damage to other organs.

MEASUREMENT OF BLOOD PRESSURE

The size of the blood pressure cuff must be appropriate to the size of the child. The bladder of the cuff should encircle, or nearly encircle, the upper arm, and the width of the cuff should be at least two-thirds the length of the upper arm. A smaller cuff results in spuriously high blood pressure measurements.

The child must be quiet when blood pressure is measured. The measurement of blood pressure in infants and toddlers is often difficult. In this age group, as well as in older children, it may be easier to obtain accurate measurements of blood pressure by machines that use oscillometric or Doppler techniques than by traditional auscultatory techniques. The blood pressure should be taken three times, and the last measurement, or the mean of the last two measurements, should be recorded.

DEFINITION OF HYPERTENSION

Hypertension is defined as a systolic or diastolic blood pressure, or both, determined on three separate occasions, equal to or greater than the 95th percentile of the blood pressure of normal children of the same age and sex (Table 16–27). In adolescents, a blood pressure of 140/90 mm Hg or greater is also considered to represent hypertension, although it may be less than the 95th percentile for normal children.

ETIOLOGY OF HYPERTENSION

Hypertension in children can be primary (essential) or secondary. Studies of blood pressure in large school populations have identified small numbers of mildly to moderately hypertensive children; in many of these children, no cause for the hypertension could be found. In contrast, in studies of children admitted to tertiary care hospitals because of severe hypertension, a cause has almost always been discovered. Primary hypertension is rare in young children but becomes more common in adolescents, especially in black males and in children with a strong family history of hypertension.

Secondary hypertension can be associated with a variety of acute illnesses but is more often a consequence of obesity or of chronic diseases, congenital malformations, or tumors of organs known to affect the regulation of blood pressure (Table 16–28). Hypertension can also result from the ingestion of drugs and toxins and can occur in children with Turner syndrome and Williams syn-

Table 16–27. Classification of significant hypertension by age group.

Age Group	Blood Pressure (mm Hg)	
	Systolic	Diastolic
Newborn		
7 d	≥ 96	—
8–30 d	≥ 104	—
Infant < 2 y	≥ 112	≥ 74
Children		
3–5 y	≥ 116	≥ 76
6–9 y	≥ 122	≥ 78
10–12 y	≥ 126	≥ 82
Adolescents		
13–15 y	≥ 136	≥ 86
16–18 y	≥ 142	≥ 92

Table 16–28. Causes of hypertension in children.

Persistent Causes by Organ System	Acute and Miscellaneous Causes
Obesity	Ingestions
Renal	Contraceptives, steroids, cocaine, amphetamines, phencyclidine
Chronic glomerulonephritis, pyelonephritis, renal failure	
Malformations (cystic, etc)	Lead intoxication
Obstructive uropathy	Turner syndrome
Renal artery stenosis or thrombosis	William syndrome
Endocrine	Bronchopulmonary dysplasia
Cushing syndrome	Acute renal disease
Congenital adrenal hyperplasia	Burns
Primary hyperaldosteronism	Orthopedic traction
Dexamethasone-suppressible hyperaldosteronism	Poliomyelitis
Apparent mineralocorticoid excess	Guillian-Barré syndrome
	Cyclic vomiting
Hyperthyroidism (systolic)	Hypercalcemia
Cardiovascular	Genitourinary surgery
Coarctation of the aorta	
Takayasu arteritis	
Central nervous system	
Increased intracranial pressure	
Dysautonomia	
Tumors	
Pheochromocytoma	
Neuroblastoma	
Wilms tumor	

Table 16–29. History and physical examination of the hypertensive child.

Historical Features	Relevance
Family history of hypertension	Essential hypertension Dexamethasone-suppressible hypertension
Ingestion of contraceptive pills, steroids, amphetamines, cocaine, phencyclidine, lead	Drug or toxin-induced hypertension
Heat intolerance, restlessness	Hyperthyroidism
Headaches, sweating, pallor, palpitations	Pheochromocytoma
Previous urinary tract infections	Chronic pyelonephritis

Physical Findings	Relevance
Obesity	Obesity-related hypertension
Signs of increased intracranial pressure	
Moonface, buffalo hump, striae	Cushing syndrome
Webbed neck, low hairline, widely spaced nipples	Turner syndrome
Elfin facies, mental retardation	Williams syndrome
Café-au-lait spots	Renal artery stenosis Pheochromocytoma
Warm skin, hyperactive reflexes, large thyroid	Hyperthyroidism
Decreased blood pressure and pulses in legs	Coarctation of the aorta
Abdominal masses	Wilms tumor, neuroblastoma, cystic or obstructed kidney
Abdominal bruits	Renal artery stenosis
Virilization, hypogonadism, pseudohermaphroditism	Congenital adrenal hyperplasia
Retinal arteriolar changes	Severity, chronicity of hypertension

drome; in the latter conditions, the hypertension usually is related to renal or vascular anomalies. The most common causes of severe persistent hypertension are chronic pyelonephritis and glomerulonephritis, renal anomalies, coarctation of the aorta, and renal artery stenosis. Endocrine causes of hypertension are much less common.

EVALUATION OF THE HYPERTENSIVE CHILD

A careful history and physical examination and a few laboratory tests usually are sufficient to diagnose the common causes of hypertension or to indicate the need for further evaluation of a suspected cause. Many of the causes of acute hypertension listed in Table 16–28 are identified by the clinical setting. If the cause is not apparent after the initial evaluation, further tests for less common causes can be performed. The need for extensive or invasive testing is determined by the severity of the hypertension. Items in the history and physical examination that are important in establishing the cause of hypertension are listed in Table 16–29, and useful laboratory and imaging tests are listed in Table 16–30.

History

It is important to elicit a family history of hypertension. The presence of a strong family history of essential hypertension in an adolescent with mild to moderate hypertension suggests that the adolescent's hypertension is pri-

mary and decreases the need for evaluation of secondary causes. A rare form of hypertension, dexamethasone-suppressible hypertension, is an autosomal-dominant condition that is suggested by the early onset of hypertension in family members. In adolescent girls, the use of contraceptive pills should be ascertained, because this is the most common cause of hypertension in this population.

Physical Examination

Determination of blood pressures and pulses in the arms and legs is important to exclude coarctation of the aorta. Hyperthyroidism, Cushing syndrome, and adrenogenital syndrome should be suggested by the characteristic physical signs of these disorders, and the presence of an abdominal mass suggests Wilms tumor, neuroblastoma, or a hydronephrotic or cystic kidney. Café-au-lait spots suggest neurofibromatosis, which is associated with an increased incidence of renal artery stenosis and, less commonly, of pheochromocytoma.

Initial Laboratory Evaluation

Laboratory tests used to diagnose the causes of hypertension are divided into two categories in Table 16–30: Initial Evaluation and Extended Evaluation. The basic tests are those used to detect structural abnormalities or chronic diseases of the kidneys, which are the most common causes of severe hypertension in children and which

Table 16–30. Laboratory and imaging evaluation of the hypertensive child.

Test	Relevance
Initial Evaluation	
Urinalysis	Chronic pyelonephritis, glomerulonephritis, renal anomalies
Urine culture (girls)	Chronic pyelonephritis
Serum blood urea nitrogen, creatinine	Renal insufficiency
Serum electrolytes	Hypokalemia and alkalosis (hyperaldosteronism)
Renal ultrasound	Renal anomalies, hydronephrosis, renal scars, Wilms tumor, neuroblastoma
Extended Evaluation	
Plasma renin concentrations	Increased: renal artery stenosis
	Decreased: primary hyperaldosteronism, dexamethasone-suppressible hypertension
Plasma aldosterone concentrations	Increased: renal artery stenosis, primary hyperaldosteronism, dexamethasone-suppressible hypertension
Plasma deoxycorticosterone	Increased: congenital adrenal hyperplasia
Urinary steroids	Apparent mineralocorticoid excess
	Congenital adrenal hyperplasia
Urinary catecholamines, metanephrines, VMA	Pheochromocytoma, neuroblastoma
DMSA scan	Chronic pyelonephritis
Renal Doppler ultrasound	Renal artery stenosis
Captopril renal scan	Renal artery stenosis
Renal arteriography	Renal artery stenosis

DMSA = dimercaptosuccinic acid; VMA = vanillylmandelic acid.

are often occult. These tests usually are not helpful in the diagnosis of renal artery stenosis, although the finding of a decreased serum potassium level and an increased serum carbon dioxide level suggests hyperaldosteronism. In the absence of other evidence of renal disease, it is not necessary to perform a renal ultrasound study when evaluating an adolescent patient with mild or moderate hypertension and a family history of essential hypertension.

Extended Evaluation

If the history, physical examination, and basic laboratory evaluation have not revealed the cause of the hypertension and the hypertension is mild, no further testing is indicated, but the child's blood pressure should be checked periodically. If the hypertension is severe or if there is evidence of damage to the heart, as determined by echocardiography, or to the eyes, as determined by examination of the ocular fundi, extended testing should be performed to detect occult renal disease, renal artery stenosis, disorders of adrenal steroidogenesis, or catecholamine-secreting tumors. Chronic pyelonephritis without a history of UTIs is diagnosed by dimercaptosuccinic acid (DMSA) renal scan. The definitive test for renal artery stenosis, which is much more common than either hyperaldosteronism or pheochromocytoma, is renal arteriography. Less invasive screening tests for renal artery stenosis are available, such as plasma renin activity, Doppler imaging of the renal arteries, and the captopril renal scan, but their sensitivity is less than 90% and they cannot reliably exclude the diagnosis of this condition. Primary hyperaldosteronism, which is rare in childhood and may be associated with familial dexamethasone-suppressible hypertension, is diagnosed by elevated plasma aldosterone levels and decreased plasma renin activity. Pheochromocytoma, which is also rare, is diagnosed by elevated levels of catecholamines in a 24-hour urine specimen. The interpretation of tests in the extended evaluation can be difficult and often requires consultation with an endocrinologist or a nephrologist.

Treatment

In children with mild hypertension, nonpharmacologic intervention is indicated; this includes restriction of dietary salt intake, weight reduction, and an increase in physical exercise. In adult patients with essential hypertension, approximately 50% appear to respond to salt restriction with a lowering of blood pressure. Data also suggest that weight loss is effective in lowering blood pressure in obese patients. In the adolescent population, however, both motivation and compliance with dietary restrictions are poor. Therefore, patient education along with a dietary regimen of moderate sodium allowance, in contrast to strict salt restriction, increase the likelihood of compliance.

In children with moderate or severe hypertension, pharmacologic therapy is indicated, especially in patients with evidence of damage to other organs (left ventricular hypertrophy, change in optic fundi, proteinuria). For acute and long-term treatment of hypertension, agents used in children are shown in Tables 16–31 and 16–32, respectively. Once optimal lowering of blood pressure has been achieved (diastolic blood pressure < 90th percentile) with a minimum of side effects, it is recommended that antihypertensive medication be continued for 6–12 months. At that time, a trial reduction in the amount of medication can be attempted with close monitoring of the blood pressure.

RENAL TUBULAR ACIDOSIS

NORMAL RENAL ACIDIFICATION

In healthy individuals, the kidneys participate in regulating the acid-base composition of ECF by regulating the

Table 16–31. Pharmacologic treatment of acute hypertension.

Agent	Mechanism of Action	Dose/Route	Onset of Action	Comments/ Side Effects
Nifedipine	Calcium channel blocker	0.25–0.5 mg/kg po or sl; may repeat q 10–20 min ×1	10 min	Flushing, headache, nausea, tachycardia, edema
Labetalol	α- and β-adrenergic blocker	0.25–2 mg/kg/h IV	3–5 min	Dizziness, tiredness, nausea
Diazoxide	Direct arteriolar vasodilator	2 mg/kg IV push, may repeat q 5–10 min ×2	3–5 min	Nausea, vomiting, flushing, hyperglycemia
Hydralazine	Direct arteriolar vasodilator	0.2–0.4 mg/kg IV; repeat q 4 h	5–10 min	Tachycardia, palpitations, flushing, headache
Sodium nitroprusside	Arteriolar and venous vasodilator	0.5–8 µg/kg/min by continuous IV infusion	Instantaneous	Monitor serum thiocyanate concentrations in intensive care unit setting

IV = intravenous; sl = sublingual; po = oral.

plasma concentration of bicarbonate at normal levels. To do this, the kidneys must reabsorb nearly all the bicarbonate filtered at the glomerulus and must excrete acid as titratable acid ($H_2PO_4^-$) and ammonium (NH_4^+). In the proximal tubule, secretion of hydrogen ion (H^+) results in reabsorption of approximately 80–90% of the filtered load of bicarbonate at normal plasma bicarbonate concentrations. In the distal nephron, principally the cortical and medullary collecting tubules, secretion of H^+ results in reabsorption of the remaining 10–15% of filtered bicarbonate, thereby decreasing the pH of tubular fluid to less than approximately 6.4. As the pH of tubular fluid decreases further to 4.5–5.5, the secreted H^+ titrates further the major urine buffers, HPO_4^{2-} and ammonia (NH_3), to form $H_2PO_4^-$ and NH_4^+. The amount of H^+ excreted as titratable acid and ammonium is referred to as **net acid excretion.** Excretion of net acid results in the generation of new bicarbonate in an amount equal to that lost in buffering the endogenous load of noncarbonic acid generated from diet and metabolism; this amount averages approximately 1 meq/kg/d in normal adults ingesting typical North American diets and approximately 1–3 meq/kg/d in healthy infants and young children.

RENAL TUBULAR ACIDOSIS

Renal tubular acidosis (RTA) is a clinical syndrome in which the kidneys fail to maintain a normal plasma concentration of bicarbonate in the setting of a normal rate of acid production from diet and metabolism. The syndrome is characterized by metabolic acidosis with hyperchlore-

Table 16–32. Pharmacologic treatment of chronic hypertension in children.

Class of Drug	Examples	Dosage	Interval	Comments/ Side Effects
Calcium channel blockers	Nifedipine	0.25 mg/kg	q 4–6 h	Flushing, nausea, headache, tachycardia, edema
	Nifedipine extended release	30–60 mg	q 12–24 h	
β-Adrenergic blockers	Propranolol	0.5–2 mg/kg	q 12 h	Avoid in asthma
	Atenolol	25–50 mg	q 24 h	
Central α-adrenergic stimulators	Clonidine	0.05–0.3 mg	q 8–12 h	Rebound hypertension on withdrawal
	Clonidine skin patch	Nos. 1–3 (delivers 0.1–0.3 mg/d)	One every 7 d	
Vasodilators	Hydralazine	0.5–1 mg/kg	q 6–8 h	Tachycardia, palpitations, flushing, headache
	Minoxidil	0.2–0.5 mg/kg	q 24 h q 8 h	
Angiotensin converting enzyme inhibitors	Captopril	0.15–2 mg/kg	q 12–24 h	Hyperkalemia, can lower GFR
	Enalapril	2.5–20 mg		
Combined α- and β-adrenegic blocker	Labetalol	1–1.5 mg/kg	q 12 h	Dizziness, tiredness, nausea
Diuretics	Chlorothiazide	5–10 mg/kg	q 12–24 h	Hypokalemia, hyperuricemia, hyperglycemia (thiazides)
	Hydrochlorothiazide	0.5–1 mg/kg	q 12–24 h	
	Furosemide	0.5–2 mg/kg	q 8–12 h	Hypokalemia, hypercalciuria, ototoxicity (furosemide)

GFR = glomerular filtration rate.

mia and often an inappropriately high urine pH. When the acidification disorder results in reduced reclamation of filtered bicarbonate by the proximal nephron, the disorder is called **proximal RTA** or **type 2 RTA.** When the disorder results in reduced excretion of $H_2PO_4^-$ and NH_4^+ (net acid) by the distal nephron, it is called **distal RTA** or **type 1 RTA;** when the reduction in net acid excretion is accompanied by hyperkalemia, the disorder is called **hyperkalemic RTA** or **type 4 RTA.** The disorder of renal acidification can occur with little or no reduction of renal mass, which distinguishes RTA from the acidosis that accompanies chronic renal insufficiency.

Proximal (Type 2) Renal Tubular Acidosis

In patients with proximal RTA, the capacity of the proximal tubule to reabsorb bicarbonate is reduced. Thus, at normal plasma bicarbonate concentrations, substantial bicarbonaturia occurs, net acid excretion ceases, and metabolic acidosis ensues. As the plasma bicarbonate concentration decreases, the amount of bicarbonate that escapes reabsorption by the impaired proximal tubule becomes sufficiently small that it can be completely reabsorbed by the otherwise normal distal nephron. Bicarbonaturia then ceases, urine pH decreases to less than 5.5, and net acid excretion becomes equivalent to acid production from diet and metabolism. The excessive urinary loss of bicarbonate enhances secretion of potassium by the distal nephron and results in hypokalemia; the hypokalemia worsens when sodium bicarbonate is given.

Proximal RTA occurs in a variety of diseases, usually as part of the Fanconi syndrome, a generalized dysfunction of the proximal tubule characterized by impaired reabsorption of bicarbonate, amino acids, phosphate, glucose, low-molecular-weight proteins, and, sometimes, uric acid. The causes of the proximal RTA are listed in Table 16–33. The cellular mechanisms by which bicarbonate reabsorption is impaired in proximal RTA have not been defined.

Children with proximal RTA associated with the Fanconi syndrome typically have hypophosphatemia and sometimes mild hypocalcemia and hypomagnesemia; bone age may be retarded, rickets or osteomalacia often occur, and nephrocalcinosis and nephrolithiasis typically are not observed.

Classic Distal (Type 1) Renal Tubular Acidosis

In patients with classic distal (type 1) RTA, the collecting tubule is unable to lower urine pH appropriately to less than approximately 6.0, which results in incomplete reabsorption of bicarbonate and a reduction in urinary excretion of $H_2 PO_4^-$ and NH_4^+; metabolic acidosis thus ensues. The urine anion gap, which is thought to reflect urine NH_4^+ concentration (see below), is zero or positive. Renal reabsorption of glucose, amino acids, and phosphate by the proximal tubule is not impaired. In children with distal RTA, the amount of bicarbonate excreted in the urine can be as much as 15% of the filtered bicarbonate load; such severe "renal bicarbonate wasting" is more common in infants and young children, particularly in the weeks to months after initiation of alkali therapy when growth velocity has greatly increased. In older children and adult patients with distal RTA, the magnitude of bicarbonaturia is less, approximately 1–3 meq/kg/d.

The characteristics of type 1 RTA are a consequence of a reduced **net** rate of H^+ secretion by the collecting tubule. Such a reduction might result from either a reduced unidirectional rate of active H^+ secretion from cell to lumen or from increased permeability of the cell membrane that permits passive backleak of secreted H^+ from lumen to cell, or of HCO_3^- from cell to lumen.

Renal wasting of sodium and potassium are characteristic of untreated type 1 RTA; these abnormalities are corrected by alkali therapy in most but not all patients. The urinary excretion of calcium and renal clearance of phosphorus are increased, and urinary excretion of citrate is reduced in patients with type 1 RTA; these abnormalities are thought to result in the occurrence of medullary nephrocalcinosis and recurrent nephrolithiasis in these patients. The sustained correction of acidosis tends to reverse these abnormalities, and although nephrocalcinosis and nephrolithiasis persist, stones may be passed less frequently.

Type 1 RTA may occur either alone or in association with a number of acquired or genetically transmitted systemic diseases (Table 16–34). In children, type 1 RTA most commonly occurs alone as either a sporadic or familial disorder. Autosomal-dominant and autosomal-recessive modes of transmission have been recognized; the latter has been associated with sensorineural hearing loss and nephrocalcinosis.

Table 16–33. Causes of proximal (type 2) renal tubular acidosis with Fanconi syndrome.

Primary—sporadic or familial
Familial systemic diseases—cystinosis, Lowe syndrome, hereditary fructose intolerance, galactosemia, Wilson disease
Vitamin D deficiency with low Ca, PO_4, and high parathyroid hormone—malabsorption syndromes
Drugs or toxins—acetazolamide, lead, cadmium
Other—medullary cystic disease, renal transplantation

Table 16–34. Causes of distal (type 1) renal tubular acidosis.

Primary—sporadic or familial
Systemic diseases—sickle cell anemia, osteopetrosis
Autoimmune—Sjögren syndrome, chronic active hepatitis
Disorders causing nephrocalcinosis—hypercalciuria, primary hyperparathyroidism, vitamin D intoxication
Drugs or toxins—amphotericin B, lithium, analgesics
Other—pyelonephritis, obstructive uropathy, renal transplantation

Hyperkalemia (Type 4) Renal Tubular Acidosis

In patients with hyperkalemic (type 4) RTA, most commonly those with chronic tubulointerstitial renal disease and moderate reduction in GFR, metabolic acidosis is associated with hyperkalemia and decreased renal clearance of potassium, and the severity of the acidosis and hyperkalemia is disproportionately great for the degree of renal insufficiency. Urine pH can decrease to less than 5.5 during acidosis, yet urinary excretion of NH_4^+ and hence of net acid are low. This reflects a suppression of renal ammonia production by the hyperkalemia in these patients. Proximal tubule function is not impaired.

The physiologic characteristics of type 4 RTA are those predicted to occur as a consequence of aldosterone deficiency or impairment in its renal effect. In the normal mammalian distal nephron, aldosterone is a major determinant of the secretion of both hydrogen ion and potassium; the resulting maintenance of a normal plasma potassium concentration enhances ammonia production and thus net acid excretion.

Clinical Variants. Type 4 RTA occurs in a wide variety of clinical disorders, either with or without associated renal parenchymal disease (Table 16–35). The most common cause is tubulointerstitial renal disease, in which deficiency of aldosterone is caused by a deficiency of renin, so-called hyporeninemic hypoaldosteronism. Type 4 RTA and aldosterone deficiency also can occur in clinical conditions in which renal parenchymal injury is absent, as in infants with the salt-wasting form of congenital adrenal hyperplasia, 21-hydroxylase deficiency, or in patients with bilateral adrenal insufficiency. In some patients with type 4 RTA, there is evidence for end-organ resistance to the renal action of aldosterone. In infants with congenital pseudohypoaldosteronism, failure to thrive, dehydration, hyponatremia, hyperkalemia, and hyperchloremic acidosis occur, plasma renin activity and urine and plasma aldosterone levels are greatly increased, and glucocorticoid hormone levels are normal.

DIAGNOSIS OF RENAL TUBULAR ACIDOSIS

Clinical Features

The child with RTA who has not received treatment has nonspecific symptoms, such as failure to thrive, polydipsia and polyuria, constipation, anorexia, vomiting, and listlessness. The presence of certain signs and symptoms suggest a particular type of RTA. Rickets and osteomalacia may be a prominent presenting feature in patients with the Fanconi syndrome, often in association with hypophosphatemia and mild hypocalcemia. Nephrocalcinosis is common in patients with type 1 RTA, but not in those with types 2 or 4 RTA. Muscle weakness may be a prominent feature in patients with untreated hypokalemia who have either type 1 RTA or the Fanconi syndrome.

Laboratory Evaluation

The metabolic acidosis of patients with RTA is associated with hyperchloremia and thus with a normal plasma anion gap, calculated as serum concentrations of $[Na - (Cl + HCO_3^-)]$ (normal range, 8–16 meq/L). Other disorders that can cause metabolic acidosis with a normal anion gap are listed in Table 16–36. When metabolic acidosis is associated with the retention in plasma of the anions of endogenously produced or exogenously administered (non–chloride-containing) acids, the plasma anion gap is increased (see Table 16–36).

To evaluate acid-base status, one should obtain an arterial or arterialized venous blood sample for measurement of blood pH, partial pressure of carbon dioxide (Pco_2), and total carbon dioxide concentration and, nearly simultaneously, a urine sample for measurement of pH and urine anion gap (see below). In healthy infants and young children, the normal values for blood Pco_2 and plasma bicarbonate and total carbon dioxide concentrations are lower than those in healthy adults; the values increase with age. For measurement of urine pH, the sample should be taken up in a syringe promptly to prevent loss of carbon dioxide, which can increase the pH; pH should be measured using a pH meter.

Table 16–35. Clinical spectrum of hyperkalemic (type 4) renal tubular acidosis.

Aldosterone deficiency
  Primary–Congenital adrenal hyperplasia, Addison disease
  Secondary–Tubulointerstitial renal disease with hyporeninemia, diabetes mellitus, obstructive uropathy, analgesic nephropathy
Aldosterone resistance
  Pseudohypoaldosteronism
  Tubulointerstitial renal disease
  Drugs—Spironolactone, amiloride
Uncertain pathogenesis
  Chronic pyelonephritis, lupus nephritis, renal transplantation

Table 16–36. Differential diagnosis of metabolic acidosis.

Normal Anion Gap	Increased Anion Gap
Gastrointestinal loss of HCO_3	Ketoacidosis
Diarrhea	Lactic acidosis
Small bowel or pancreatic drainage	Uremic acidosis
Ureterosigmoidostomy	Toxins
Renal loss of HCO_3	Salicylate
Renal tubular acidosis	Ethylene glycol
Diamox	Methanol
Dilutional acidosis	Paraldehyde
Administration of NH_4Cl, arginine HCl	Inborn errors of metabolism
Postrespiratory alkalosis	

Assessment of Urine Acidification

Because the urine pH reflects only the concentration of free H+ in urine, which accounts for less than 1% of the total amount of H+ excreted, urine pH by itself may not adequately reflect urine net acid excretion during acidosis. In normal individuals, the kidneys respond to chronic acidosis by substantially increasing the urinary excretion of ammonium. Because urinary NH_4^+ is not measured routinely in hospital laboratories, it has been proposed that the urinary NH_4^+ concentration can be indirectly estimated by the urine anion gap, calculated as urine concentrations of $[Na^+]$ + $[K^+]$ − $[Cl^-]$. In nonacidotic healthy individuals, the urine anion gap is positive, approximately 30–35 meq/L, and becomes progressively negative as the rate of NH_4^+ excretion increases during acidosis. In acidotic patients with type 1 or type 4 RTA, the anion gap remains inappropriately positive, consistent with their very low NH_4^+ excretion. In patients with proximal RTA, the urine anion gap would be predicted to be zero or positive, although negative values have been observed in children with proximal RTA. Thus, the diagnosis of RTA should be strongly considered in a patient with persisting hyperchloremic metabolic acidosis in whom extrarenal causes of the acidosis have been excluded and in whom the urine anion gap is zero or positive; the urine pH typically is inappropriately high (> 5.5–6). When the urine anion gap is negative, it can be inferred that the kidney is responding appropriately to the acidosis; thus, a nonrenal cause for the acidosis is likely.

In a patient with probable RTA and moderate metabolic acidosis (plasma total carbon dioxide concentration of approximately 18 meq/L), and in whom urine pH is approximately 6.0 or greater, it is recommended that oral ammonium chloride be given to increase the severity of the acidosis in order to distinguish classic distal RTA from proximal or type 4 RTA. Before doing so, one should correct any existing ECF volume contraction or hypokalemia. If urine pH decreases to less than 5.5, the diagnosis of distal (type 1) RTA can be ruled out; if it does not, the diagnosis of type 1 RTA is likely. In patients with proximal RTA associated with the Fanconi syndrome, the fractional renal clearance of phosphate, amino acids, glucose, and potassium is increased, and hypophosphatemia and hypokalemia typically occur.

The finding of hyperchloremic acidosis and hyperkalemia suggests type 4 RTA; urine pH may or may not be appropriately acidic (ie, < 5.5) during acidosis, either spontaneously or after ammonium chloride. The GFR may be mildly to moderately reduced. Evaluation of the status of renin-aldosterone activity helps to distinguish aldosterone deficiency from aldosterone-resistant states.

Treatment & Prognosis

Distal (Type 1) RTA. In some acidotic patients with type 1 RTA, hypokalemia severe enough to cause respiratory depression can occur; if so, it should be corrected with intravenously administered potassium before acidosis is corrected. In infants and children, sustained correction of acidosis can be achieved by oral administration of sodium bicarbonate or sodium citrate, 3–14 meq/kg/d in 4 divided doses, until the plasma bicarbonate concentration becomes normal. In adult patients, 1–2 meq/kg/d of alkali is usually sufficient. In some patients, potassium supplements may also be required to sustain normokalemia; if so, 20–50% of the alkali requirement can be given as potassium bicarbonate or potassium citrate. Sustained correction of acidosis in infants is associated with an increase in growth velocity; within 3–6 months, normal stature can be attained and maintained. Older children may require several years to attain normal height. With correction of acidosis, urinary calcium and phosphorus excretion decreases, and citrate excretion increases; nephrocalcinosis can be prevented by alkali therapy.

Proximal (Type 2) RTA. Correction of acidosis in patients with type 2 RTA requires administration of alkali in amounts ranging from 3 to 20 meq/kg/d; alkali requirements must be determined empirically for each patient. In the rare patient with isolated type 2 RTA, acidosis can be corrected by giving sodium bicarbonate alone. In patients with type 2 RTA and Fanconi syndrome, correction of hypokalemia should be achieved by giving a substantial fraction, often 50% or more, of the alkali requirement as potassium bicarbonate or potassium citrate. Supplemental oral phosphorus and sometimes magnesium and vitamin D may be required. When type 2 RTA is associated with Fanconi syndrome, treatment is directed where possible toward removal of those substances crucial to its causation, as in the case of hereditary fructose intolerance, galactosemia, Wilson disease, and tyrosinemia.

Hyperkalemic (Type 4) RTA. In patients with type 4 RTA who have tubulointerstitial renal disease and reduced GFR, administration of mineralocorticoid in either physiologic replacement doses (fludrocortisone, 0.10–0.15 mg/d) or superphysiologic amounts can increase net acid excretion and substantially ameliorate metabolic acidosis and hyperkalemia. However, mineralocorticoid should be used cautiously as it may exacerbate hypertension or increase the ECF volume in some patients. Restriction of dietary potassium, administration of furosemide, or administration of sodium bicarbonate, 1–2 meq/kg/d, has also been shown to ameliorate acidosis and hyperkalemia. When type 4 RTA is due to deficiency of aldosterone, physiologic doses of mineralocorticoid should be administered; in patients with pseudohypoaldosteronism, administration of supplemental sodium chloride often suffices.

CONGENITAL ANOMALIES OF THE URINARY TRACT

The overall incidence of structural genitourinary anomalies in the general population is approximately 4%, on the basis of autopsy studies. Many urinary tract anomalies are not symptomatic and remain undetected or are discovered accidentally. Most children with clinically significant urinary tract anomalies come to medical attention in one of the following ways: (1) an abnormal finding on a prenatal ultrasound, (2) detection of an abdominal or flank mass in the newborn period, (3) appearance of Potter syndrome at birth, (4) diagnosis of UTI, (5) detection of hypertension, or (6) development of renal insufficiency or failure. The most common, clinically significant anomalies of the urinary tract are listed in Table 16–37.

CLINICAL PRESENTATIONS OF URINARY TRACT ANOMALIES

This section discusses the clinical presentation of common urinary tract anomalies and the appropriate diagnostic evaluation and differential diagnoses for each.

Abnormal Prenatal Ultrasound

Fetal ultrasonography has become a routine part of prenatal care and can identify urinary tract anomalies as early as 15 weeks postconception. The incidence of congenital urologic anomalies as detected by prenatal ultrasound ranges between 0.2% and 1.5%, depending on the study. Ultrasound examination of the fetal kidneys can determine their number, location, and size. The renal pelvis and calyces become discernible when they are dilated, and renal cysts are detectable as echolucent areas within the renal parenchyma.

Hydronephrosis, or dilatation of the renal pelvis and calyces, is the most common urinary tract abnormality found on prenatal ultrasound examination; it may be unilateral or bilateral. Of the causes of hydronephrosis listed in Table 16–38, the most common is obstruction of the ureteropelvic junction (UPJ). The obstruction usually is unilateral and incomplete; therefore, fetal urine output is adequate and oligohydramnios does not occur. Severe UPJ obstruction may lead to cystic changes within the affected kidney(s), which are detectable on prenatal ultrasound. Postnatally, confirmation of the diagnosis of UPJ obstruction is made by a diuretic-augmented renal scan and/or an intravenous pyelogram.

Table 16–37. Significant congenital anomalies of the urinary tract.

Renal	Bladder
Agenesis	Vesicoureteral reflux
Hypoplasia	Ectopic ureterocele
Dysplasia	
Polycystic kidney disease	Urethral
	Posterior urethral valves
Ureteral	
Ureteropelvic junction obstruction	
Prune-belly syndrome	

Table 16–38. Abnormal fetal renal ultrasound findings and their causes.

Hydronephrosis
  Ureteropelvic junction obstruction
  Posterior urethral valves
  Duplex ureter with ureterocele
  Transient, idiopathic
Renal cysts
  Multicystic dysplasia
  Dysplasia with cysts
  Polycystic kidney disease

Renal cysts detected prenatally, as with hydronephrosis, may be associated with many diseases, the most common of which are listed in Table 16–38. When cysts are large, they may be difficult to distinguish from severe hydronephrosis on prenatal ultrasound examination, whereas postnatal ultrasound examination, with its improved resolution, and radionuclide renal scans usually can distinguish between these two entities.

Oligohydramnios, a decrease in the volume of amniotic fluid, is a worrisome prenatal ultrasound finding. Because urine is the primary component of amniotic fluid, oligohydramnios is often the result of either renal dysfunction with decreased urine production or urinary tract obstruction. Renal dysfunction may be due to bilateral renal agenesis, bilateral multicystic dysplasia, or polycystic kidney disease. Obstructive causes of oligohydramnios are posterior urethral valves and bilateral obstruction of the ureteropelvic or ureterovesical junctions. In the past few years, attempts have been made to bypass the obstruction surgically in utero in an effort to relieve back-pressure on the developing kidneys and improve amniotic fluid volume, with varying success. However, most patients with urinary tract anomalies detected by prenatal ultrasound do not have oligohydramnios. Such patients usually are asymptomatic at birth and can safely undergo further diagnostic evaluation later in the newborn period.

Potter Syndrome

At birth, children with nonfunctioning or severely obstructed kidneys often present with the classic signs and symptoms of Potter syndrome. Oligohydramnios, resulting from decreased urine output, causes compression of the fetus by the uterine walls and results in limb deformities and abnormal facial features termed **Potter facies** (epicanthal folds, low-set ears, flattened nose, and receding chin). Because amniotic fluid volume plays an important role in normal lung development, oligohydramnios also is associated with hypoplasia of the lungs. Pulmonary hypoplasia/respiratory failure is responsible for most of the deaths in newborns with renal failure and oligohydramnios.

The leading causes of Potter syndrome are bilateral renal agenesis, bilateral cystic, malformed kidneys (multicystic dysplasia), and bilateral obstructed kidneys. In evaluating a newborn infant with this syndrome, one should first perform a renal ultrasound study. Important features to note on the renal ultrasound are the kidney sizes and the presence of renal cysts, hydronephrosis, hydroureter, the size of the bladder, and the thickness of the bladder wall. With this information, the level of the obstruction, if present, usually can be localized. Evidence of obstruction necessitates urgent urologic consultation, and if urethral obstruction is present, a bladder catheter should be placed. Renal function should be assessed immediately and repeatedly over time.

Abdominal Mass

More than 50% of palpable abdominal masses in newborn infants are renal in origin. The vast majority of these are hydronephrotic or multicystic dysplastic kidneys. Noncongenital causes, such as renal vein thrombosis and tumors, account for fewer than 7% of renal masses.

The infant with a palpable abdominal mass should undergo renal ultrasound as soon as possible. When hydronephrosis is severe, the renal pelvis and calyces may be massively dilated and surrounded by only a thin rim of renal parenchyma. Patients with multicystic dysplasia have detectable cysts within the renal parenchyma; the cysts may be so large as to be indistinguishable from the dilated renal pelvis of a hydronephrotic kidney. A renal scan (DMSA) can be used to distinguish between these two entities. In multicystic dysplasia, the kidney is nonfunctional and will demonstrate no uptake of radioactive tracer, whereas in hydronephrosis, uptake of tracer will be visible in the rim of renal parenchyma surrounding the dilated pelvis.

The diagnosis of hydronephrosis, either unilateral or bilateral, should prompt a search for an obstructive malformation. The site of obstruction usually can be determined from the ultrasound study on the basis of the location of the dilatation and the size and appearance of the bladder. Obstruction of the UPJ most commonly causes unilateral hydronephrosis without dilatation of the ipsilateral ureter. Obstruction of the ureterovesical junction, either unilateral or bilateral, causes hydroureteronephrosis of the affected side(s). Bladder outlet obstruction, as in male infants with posterior urethral valves, usually results in bilateral hydronephrosis with dilatation of both ureters and a thickened bladder wall.

Urinary Tract Infection

Both during and after the newborn period, infants with significant urinary tract anomalies often present with a UTI. The flow of urine is abnormal within cysts; dilated, obstructed collecting systems; or refluxing, incompletely emptying systems, predisposing the patient to infection. Children with a documented UTI should undergo a renal ultrasound study and a voiding cystourethrogram (VCUG) to determine whether anomalies, obstruction, or reflux are present. Boys should be evaluated after their first UTI, regardless of age, because UTIs in boys are highly associated with urinary tract anomalies. UTIs are more common in girls, particularly those aged 7–10 years, and less fre-

quently associated with anomalies. Thus, it is recommended that girls older than 8 years with uncomplicated cystitis be evaluated radiographically after their second UTI, and girls younger than 8 years after their first infection. All children, regardless of age, with pyelonephritis or with cystitis caused by an unusual organism should undergo prompt evaluation with renal ultrasound; ideally, the VCUG should be performed 3–4 weeks after the infection has resolved. Prophylactic antibiotics should be administered after completion of the therapeutic course until it is determined that vesicoureteral reflux (VUR) is not present.

Hypertension

Although acquired renal disease accounts for most cases of hypertension in children (see this chapter, Hypertension), congenital urinary tract anomalies and their complications are responsible for a significant number. The most common congenital anomalies that cause hypertension are unilateral renal agenesis, VUR with kidney scarring, polycystic kidney disease, and multicystic dysplasia. The evaluation of renal causes of hypertension is discussed elsewhere.

Chronic Renal Insufficiency

Unfortunately for many children, congenital anomalies may remain undetected until renal insufficiency becomes severe and symptoms of uremia develop. Congenital anomalies that can progress to end-stage renal failure include hypoplasia, dysplasia, polycystic kidney disease, VUR complicated by infection, and obstructive uropathies.

SPECIFIC CONGENITAL URINARY TRACT ANOMALIES

This section discusses in more detail the various congenital anomalies listed in Table 16–37. Normal development of the kidney requires the presence and interaction of two embryologic structures—the ureteric bud and the metanephrogenic blastema. Each structure exerts a developmental influence on the other. The ureteric bud ultimately becomes the trigone of the bladder, the ureter, the renal calyces and pelvis, and the collecting ducts, whereas the metanephros gives rise to the epithelial cells of the glomeruli, the proximal and distal tubules, and the loops of Henle. Absence of either of these embryologic structures or their failure to achieve the necessary contact with one another results in malformations of the kidney and/or the urinary tract.

Renal Anomalies

Agenesis is defined as the failure of formation of the kidney; it may be unilateral or bilateral. Bilateral agenesis is incompatible with long-term extrauterine life, whereas unilateral agenesis is asymptomatic if the contralateral kidney is normal. This malformation arises when the ureteric bud, because of either its absence or malposition, fails to induce the metanephros.

The term **hypoplastic** designates a small kidney owing to a reduced number of otherwise normal nephrons; the remainder of the urinary tract is normal. When the ureteric bud has an abnormal origin, it contacts only a portion of the metanephros, and thus fewer nephrons develop; those present then become hypertrophied. Hypoplasia is clinically significant when both kidneys are affected. Patients with bilateral hypoplasia have polydipsia and polyuria during infancy, and inevitable progression to end-stage renal failure occurs by late childhood.

Dysplastic kidneys lack normally developed nephron structures. Strong evidence suggests that the abnormal development results from urinary tract obstruction in utero. More than 90% of dysplastic kidneys are associated with obstruction of the lower urinary tract, most commonly at the UPJ obstruction, the posterior urethra, or the distal ureter from an obstructing ureterocele. Dysplastic kidneys are characterized histologically by the presence of primitive ducts, metaplastic cartilage, and immature glomeruli. The extent of renal functional impairment reflects the degree of morphologic abnormalities and depends largely on the severity of the obstruction. The gross appearance of these kidneys is potentially quite varied and may be solid, cystic, small, large, reniform, or misshapen.

The most severe form of dysplasia, which results from atresia of the ipsilateral ureter, is termed **multicystic dysplasia.** These kidneys are large, contain macroscopic cysts, and usually are detected by prenatal ultrasound or as abdominal masses in the early newborn period. Approximately 30% of children with unilateral multicystic dysplastic kidneys have structural abnormalities of the contralateral kidney.

Polycystic kidney disease occurs as either an autosomal-recessive (ARPKD) or an autosomal-dominant (ADPKD) disease. The autosomal-recessive form has previously been called **infantile polycystic kidney disease** because it commonly presents in the first year after birth. Babies presenting with ARPKD have extremely large kidneys with innumerable small (1–8 mm diameter) cysts of the collecting ducts. Many such infants tend to be critically ill owing to pulmonary hypoplasia, and most die within a few days of birth. Those with fewer cysts and therefore more functioning renal parenchyma present at a later age and have a better prognosis for survival, although many eventually progress to end-stage renal failure and require dialysis and transplantation. The outcome of patients with ARPKD is complicated by the associated liver disease characterized by periportal fibrosis and biliary duct dilatation. By contrast, ADPKD usually remains asymptomatic until the fifth or sixth decade of life.

Ureteral Anomalies

Obstruction of the UPJ is the most common site of urinary tract obstruction in children. The obstruction may be caused by a segment of the ureter that lacks peristaltic activity, by muscular bands, or by aberrant vessels that cause external compression of the UPJ; unilateral cases predominate (75% of total). Complete UPJ obstruction is associated with severe renal dysplasia. Lesser degrees of obstruction result in hydronephrosis with a consequent increased risk of UTI and its sequelae. Treatment requires surgical removal of the obstructed segment and reanastomosis of the normal ends (pyeloplasty). The amount of function of the involved kidney should be determined by a renal radionucleotide scan before surgery, as an obstructed kidney with little or no function should probably be removed rather than repaired.

The **prune-belly syndrome** (Eagle-Barrett syndrome) consists of the triad of absent abdominal wall musculature, urinary tract anomalies, and cryptorchidism. The urologic anomalies range from mild, asymptomatic dilatation of the urinary tract to severe hydroureteronephrosis with renal dysplasia and renal failure; the dilatation almost always exists in the absence of obstruction. The diagnosis usually can be made at birth on the basis of the appearance of the abdominal wall. Evaluation of these children should include imaging of the urinary tract and assessment of renal function.

During normal micturition, contraction of the bladder wall musculature compresses the distal ends of the ureters, thereby preventing the passage of urine from the bladder into the ureters. Congenital VUR results from inadequate tunneling of the distal ureter through the bladder wall, due to either malposition or maldevelopment of the ureteric bud. Reflux can also develop in patients with obstruction of the bladder outlet in whom high intravesical pressures are generated by contraction of the bladder wall, as occurs with a neurogenic bladder and posterior urethral valves. VUR may range from mild to severe, as judged by the extent of reflux seen on a routine VCUG; the severity is routinely graded from 1 to 5 according to the system of the International Reflux Study Committee (Figure 16–6).

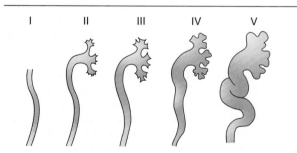

Figure 16–6. Grades of vesicoureteral reflux (International Classification): *I:* involving the ureter only; *II:* involving the ureter, pelvis, and calyces without dilatation; *III:* same level as II but with mild to moderate dilatation of ureter and pelvis; *IV:* same as III but with blunting of calyceal fornices and increased dilatation; *V:* increased dilatation and tortuosity of ureter and papillary impressions in calyces lost.

Reflux results in incomplete emptying of the bladder during voiding, predisposing the patient to infection. Furthermore, with more severe grades of reflux, urine may enter the renal collecting tubules under high pressure. Reflux of infected urine into the kidney is known to cause renal scarring; the evidence is compelling but still inconclusive as to whether reflux of sterile urine causes renal injury. In children with mild forms of reflux (grades 1–3) who have normal renal function and little or no renal scarring, it is recommended that prophylactic antibiotics be administered to prevent renal injury from occurring or progressing. The milder degrees of VUR tend to resolve as children age. Breakthrough infections due to noncompliance or the development of resistant organisms are common. In children with severe reflux (grades 4 and 5) or those with lesser grades of reflux but decreased renal function, surgical correction of reflux is often necessary because the likelihood of spontaneous resolution of VUR is low. Surgical correction of reflux has not been shown to be superior to medical therapy in preventing progressive renal injury.

Complete **duplication** of the ureter occurs when two separate ureters each drain a different pole of a single kidney, and each ureter empties into the bladder. The ureter draining the lower pole frequently is malpositioned and consequently refluxes; the ureter draining the upper pole also is malpositioned and may be obstructed by a ureterocele, a cystic dilation of the distal end of the ureter, leading to hydronephrosis or dysplasia of the upper pole. Evaluation of a duplex system requires a renal ultrasound or intravenous pyelogram and a VCUG. The obstruction caused by a ureterocele is treated surgically.

Urethral Anomalies

Posterior urethral valves, when present in boys, obstruct the outflow of urine from the bladder. The obstructing tissue appears as a diaphragm with a slitlike orifice that is obliquely placed within the prostatic or posterior urethra; the embryologic defect responsible for urethral valves is unknown. Severe obstruction causes dysplastic development of both kidneys in utero, and the diagnosis is made in such severely affected children either prenatally or shortly after birth. Children with milder obstruction present when it is noticed that they strain to urinate or have a weak urinary stream or when they have a UTI.

The diagnosis of posterior urethral valves is made with a VCUG, which demonstrates that the posterior urethra is elongated and dilated from the bladder neck to the level of the valves, or by direct visualization under urethroscopy. The bladder wall is invariably thickened secondary to muscular hypertrophy. Half these bladders have trabeculations or diverticula, and approximately 60% of patients with urethral valves have secondary VUR.

Achievement of adequate urine drainage, either through a bladder catheter or vesicostomy, should be the immediate goal. Definitive therapy requires surgical ablation of the valves, which can be performed transurethrally with an endoscope, and reimplantation of the ureters.

PARENTERAL FLUID THERAPY

BODY COMPOSITION

Water is the major constituent of the body; total body water (TBW) accounts for approximately 70–75% of body weight in the term newborn infant. TBW decreases to approximately 65% of body weight in infants and children and to approximately 60% of body weight in the adult man. Because the water content of fat is low, TBW represents a smaller fraction of body weight both in obese individuals and in women (55%), in whom body content of fat is higher than in men. Body water has two components: intracellular fluid (ICF), which constitutes 35–40% of body weight, and extracellular fluid (ECF), which constitutes 25% of body weight in children and about 20% in the adult. The ECF is composed of intravascular (plasma) fluid (5%), interstitial fluid (15%), and transcellular fluid (1–3%), the last of which consists of gastrointestinal secretions and pleural, peritoneal, and synovial fluids.

The amount of water in the body is precisely regulated to maintain the plasma osmolality constant at 285–295 mOsm/kg water, despite daily fluctuations in water and solute intake. This regulation occurs via a close feedback interaction between the hypothalamic osmoreceptors and volume receptors in the aortic arch and cardiac atrium, the posterior pituitary, and the collecting ducts of the kidney. When a decrease in water intake or an increase in solute intake induces an increase in plasma osmolality of 1–2%, thirst is stimulated, which leads to an increase in water intake and release of ADH, which increases water retention by the renal collecting ducts. Both thirst and release of ADH are also stimulated by a decrease in ECF volume of approximately 8% or more, as can occur with hemorrhage or dehydration. Conversely, a decrease in plasma osmolality of approximately 1–2% results in suppression of ADH release. These homeostatic responses result in a return of plasma osmolality to normal values. In certain circumstances, the stimulatory effect of reduced intravascular volume on ADH release can override the suppressive effect of an increased plasma osmolality.

MAINTENANCE PARENTERAL FLUID THERAPY

It is convenient to separate parenteral fluid therapy in children into two phases or categories: **maintenance therapy,** which is intended to replace ongoing normal and abnormal losses of fluid and electrolytes, and **deficit therapy,** which is intended to replace fluid and electrolytes previously lost because of illness, such as dehydration, with the goal being to return ECF volume and body composition to normal.

The goal of maintenance intravenous fluid therapy is to provide water and electrolytes in amounts that equal daily physiologic losses of these substances from the body. The daily requirements for water and electrolytes depend not on body size, but on the rate of metabolism and thus the caloric expenditure of the patient. For example, an increase in the rate of metabolism results in an increase both in heat production, which increases evaporative water loss from the skin, and in endogenous generation of solutes requiring renal excretion, which increases urine water loss at any given urine osmolality.

The energy expenditure of the average hospitalized patient can be estimated from the body weight (Table 16–39). These estimates, which include basal metabolic expenditure plus an average increment for activity in bed, are higher per kilogram body weight in younger patients than in older ones. The initial estimate must be modified in patients whose metabolic rate is affected by a specific circumstance; for example, with fever, the caloric expenditure is increased by 12% per degree Celsius increase in body temperature above normal and, with hypermetabolic states (hyperthyroidism, salicylate intoxication), the caloric expenditure is increased by 25–75%. Conversely, caloric expenditure is reduced in patients with hypothermia or hypometabolic states.

Water

Water is lost from the skin owing to evaporation and from the lungs owing to normal respiration; these losses are referred to as **insensible water loss (IWL).** Daily insensible water loss is approximately 45–50 mL for each 100 kcal of energy expended; of this, approximately one third is lost through the lungs and the remaining two thirds through the skin. **Daily urine water loss** can vary widely and depends on the amount of solute requiring excretion and on renal concentrating ability. When the urinary solute load is average and the urine osmolality is approximately equal to that of plasma, ie, there is neither significant concentration nor dilution of urine, urine water loss is approximately 65 mL/100 kcal/d. These insensible and urinary water losses are offset in part by water that is generated endogenously during metabolism, an amount estimated at 12–15 mL/100 kcal/d. Losses of water from sweat or in formed stools usually are negligible. Thus, the daily provision of 100 mL water per 100 kcal energy expended meets physiologic water losses in most patients (Table 16–40). In the presence of sweating, an additional 10–25 mL/100 kcal/d should be added.

Table 16–40. Maintenance water requirements.

	mL/100 kcal/d
Insensible water loss	45–50
Lungs	30
Skin	15
Urine water loss[1]	60–80
Hidden intake (water of oxidation)	12–15
Usual requirements	100

[1]Urine water loss depends on renal solute load and renal concentrating ability.

Electrolytes

Electrolytes (sodium, potassium, and chloride) are provided in amounts that meet their daily losses in the urine, without requiring either maximal renal conservation or maximal excretion of these substances. It is customary to provide 3 meq of sodium and 2 meq of potassium per 100 kcal per day as the chloride salts, ie, as sodium and potassium chloride.

Energy

In patients with only short-term illness and without preexisting malnutrition, full replacement of calories is not necessary. Rather, provision of approximately 20% of the estimated caloric expenditure as glucose will prevent ketosis and minimize endogenous breakdown of protein. This is accomplished by administering 5% dextrose in water.

For example, the daily maintenance requirements in a healthy 9-year-old girl who weighs 30 kg are as follows: energy expenditure, 1700 kcal; water, 1700 mL; sodium, 54 meq; potassium, 34 meq; chloride, 88 meq; and glucose, 85 g. These would be provided by administering 5% dextrose in water containing 30 meq/L of sodium chloride and 20 meq/L of potassium chloride, at a rate of 70 mL/h for 24 hours. These guidelines are appropriate for use in children of all ages except newborn infants, in whom insensible and renal losses vary depending on gestational and postnatal age.

Abnormal Losses

In certain circumstances or disease states, ongoing insensible and renal losses of water and electrolytes differ from those estimated, and their replacement during maintenance therapy must be adjusted accordingly. Examples of states of abnormal loss and the appropriate modifications to maintenance therapy are given in Table 16–41.

APPROACH TO THE PATIENT WITH DEHYDRATION

Clinical Features

The normal rate of turnover of water, electrolytes, and foodstuffs in infants and children is about three times that in the adult; as a consequence, infants and children are more susceptible to the adverse effects of disorders of

Table 16–39. Calculation of energy expenditure in children.

Body Weight (kg)	Energy Expenditure (kcal/kg/d)
3–10	100
10–20	1000 + 50 kcal/kg
> 20	1500 + 20 kcal/kg

Table 16–41. States of abnormal loss and modifications in maintenance therapy.

Fever	Increase caloric estimate by 12% per 1 °C increase in body temperature.

Hypermetabolism
  Salicylism
  Hyperthyroidism
	Increase caloric estimate by 25–75%.

Sweating	Increase water allowance by 10–25 mL/100 kcal; increase Na and Cl allowance by 0.5–1 meq/100 kcal.

Obligatory oliguria
  Renal insufficiency
  Congestive heart failure
  Edematous states
  Syndrome of inappropriate
    ADH secretion
	Decrease water allowance by 20–50%.

Obligatory polyuria
  Diabetes insipidus
  Renal tubular disease
  High solute load
	Increase water allowance.

Gastrointestinal loss
  Nasogastric suction
  Small bowel drainage
  Diarrhea
	Replace with equal volume of solution with equivalent electrolyte composition.

Third space loss
  Postoperative, burns,
    trauma
	Replace with isotonic solution.

ADH = antidiuretic hormone.

fluid balance. Deficits of water, sodium, and potassium can occur in a wide variety of clinical disorders that affect children; the most common of these is acute gastroenteritis, in which diarrhea and vomiting lead to dehydration. In children with acute gastroenteritis, water and electrolytes are lost from the gastrointestinal tract in considerable excess of their intake, which leads to contraction of the ECF volume and the appearance of clinical signs of dehydration.

The patient's state of hydration is evaluated by the physical examination, although historical information, such as the frequency of urination or the patient's prior body weight, can be helpful. On the basis of the physical findings (Table 16–42), the magnitude of dehydration is judged to be mild, moderate, or severe, which corresponds to a relatively acute (3–5 days) loss of body weight in the infant of 5%, 10%, or 15%, respectively, or in older children and adults, of 3%, 6%, or 9%, respectively. The physical findings described and the corresponding estimates of the degree of dehydration apply to patients in whom dehydration develops over 3–5 days and in whom the serum sodium concentration is relatively normal (130–150 meq/L), so-called isotonic dehydration. In such patients, approximately 60% of body fluid is lost from the extracellular space and approximately 40% from the intracellular space. With hypertonic dehydration (serum sodium concentration > 150 meq/L), the ECF volume is better maintained owing to greater movement of water from the intracellular to the extracellular space. As a consequence, the clinical signs of dehydration are less severe for a given loss of body weight. Conversely, with hypotonic dehydration (serum sodium < 130 meq/L), the ECF volume is less well maintained; thus, the clinical signs of dehydration are more severe for a given loss of body weight.

Laboratory Findings

Patients hospitalized with dehydration should have the following laboratory tests performed: complete blood count; serum electrolyte, total carbon dioxide, urea nitrogen, and creatinine concentrations; venous blood gas determination; and urinalysis. On the basis of the serum sodium concentration, dehydration is judged to be isotonic, hypertonic, or hypotonic; this information assists in the clinical assessment of the patient, as noted previously, and in therapy. Patients with diarrheal dehydration frequently have metabolic acidosis, which can have several causes, including loss of bicarbonate to the gastrointestinal tract, reduced urinary excretion of acid due to oliguria, and poor peripheral perfusion with accumulation of lactic acid. The urinalysis should be consistent with the diagnosis of dehydration, ie, the urine should be concentrated with an osmolality usually greater than 500 or specific gravity greater than 1.020. A dilute urine (specific gravity < 1.010, osmolality < 300 mOsm/kg) in a dehydrated patient with frequent urination suggests that a defect in the urine-concentrating mechanism is present.

Table 16–42. Clinical assessment of hydration.

	Magnitude of Dehydration		
	Mild	**Moderate**	**Severe**
Body weight loss (< 2 y of age)	5%	10%	15%
(> 2 y of age)	3%	6%	9%
Skin turgor	nl, sl ↓	↓↓	↓↓↓
Mucous membranes	nl, sl dry	very dry	parched
Skin color	pale	gray	mottled
Urine output	sl ↓	oliguria	marked oliguria and azotemia
Blood pressure	normal	± normal	reduced
Pulse rate	↑	↑↑	↑↑↑, weak

nl = normal; sl = slight.

Treatment

The objectives of treatment are to provide water, electrolytes, calories, and other nutrients in amounts that will replace the existing deficits of these substances and meet their ongoing losses, both normal and abnormal. These objectives should be accomplished safely and over a relatively brief period of time. Rehydration therapy can be administered either orally or intravenously; oral therapy is appropriate for patients with mild to moderate dehydration. For patients with severe dehydration and shock, isotonic fluid should be administered intravenously until intravascular volume is restored; oral therapy can be considered when the child is more stable.

The treatment of the infant or child with dehydration is traditionally viewed as occurring in three phases:

1. Phase 1: In this phase the goal is rapid expansion of the intravascular volume to treat or prevent shock, to improve peripheral perfusion, and to restore normal renal functioning. This phase lasts one to several hours, depending on the severity of dehydration.
2. Phase 2: The remaining deficits of water and sodium are largely replaced, the deficits of potassium are partially replaced, acid-base status is normalized, and water and electrolytes are administered in amounts that meet ongoing abnormal losses plus maintenance requirements. This phase lasts approximately 24 hours.

Table 16–43. Intravenous treatment of dehydration.

I. Restore circulating blood volume:
  A. Administer *isotonic* fluid, 20–40 mL/kg over 20–40 min: lactated Ringer 0.9% saline, plasma.
  B. Monitor perfusion, blood pressure, urine output; give additional isotonic fluid until these normalize.
II. Calculate and replace deficits of water and electrolytes:
  A. With isotonic or hypotonic dehydration, replace deficits over 12–24 h. For severe hyponatremia, serum Na < 115 meq/L, or seizures, infuse 3% NaCl to increase serum Na to 120 meq/L (3% NaCl contains 0.5 meq/mL Na). With hypernatremic dehydration, replace deficits over 48–72 h (rate of serum sodium correction is < 5 meq/L per 12 h).
  B. Replace ongoing abnormal losses with appropriate fluid.
  C. Provide normal maintenance requirements.
III. Restore K^+ deficit over 2–4 d and nutritional deficit over days to weeks.

3. Phase 3: The remaining body deficits of potassium are replaced, and nutritional deficits are restored. This phase lasts several days to weeks.

Patients should be monitored closely during the first two phases of therapy. Parenteral therapy of dehydration is outlined in Table 16–43.

REFERENCES

EVALUATION OF RENAL FUNCTION

Geyer SJ: Urinalysis and urinary sediment in patients with renal disease. Clin Lab Med 1993;13:13.

Rose BD: *Clinical Physiology of Acid-Base and Electrolyte Disorders,* 4th ed. McGraw-Hill, 1994.

Schwartz GJ et al: The use of plasma creatinine concentration for estimating glomerular filtration rate in infants, children, and adolescents. Pediatr Clin North Am 1987;34:571.

EVALUATION OF HEMATURIA

Bodziak KA et al: Inherited diseases of the glomerular basement membrane. Am J Kidney Dis 1994;23:605.

Stapleton FB: Hematuria associated with hypercalciuria and hyperuricosuria: A practical approach. Pediatr Nephrol 1994;8:756.

Yadin O: Hematuria in children. Pediatr Ann 1994;23:474.

GLOMERULONEPHRITIS

Cole BR, Salinas Madrigal L: Acute proliferative glomerulonephritis and crescentic glomerulonephritis. In: Holliday MA et al (editors): *Pediatric Nephrology,* 3rd ed. Williams & Wilkins, 1994.

Donadio JV et al: A controlled trial of fish oil in IGA nephropathy. N Engl J Med 1994;331:1194.

Wyatt RJ et al: IGA nephropathy: Long-term prognosis of pediatric patients. J Pediatr 1995;127:913.

EVALUATION OF PROTEINURIA

Dodge WF et al: Proteinuria and hematuria in schoolchildren: Epidemiology and early natural history. J Pediatr 1976;88: 327.

Feld LG et al: Evaluation of the child with asymptomatic proteinuria. Pediatr Rev 1984;5:248.

Vehaskari VM: Orthostatic proteinuria. Arch Dis Child 1982;57:729.

West CD: Asymptomatic hematuria and proteinuria in children: Causes and appropriate diagnostic studies. J Pediatr 1976;89:173.

NEPHROTIC SYNDROME

Grupe WE: Primary nephrotic syndrome in childhood. Adv Pediatr 1979;26:163.

International Study of Kidney Disease in Children: Nephrotic syndrome in children: Prediction of histopathology from clinical and laboratory characteristics at time of diagnosis. Kidney Int 1978;13:159.

Lewis MA et al: Nephrotic syndrome: From toddlers to twenties. Lancet 1989;1:255.

Trompeter RS: Immunosuppressive therapy in the nephrotic syndrome in children. Pediatr Nephrol 1989;3:194.

ACUTE RENAL FAILURE

Brady H et al: Acute renal failure. Page 1200 in: Brenner BM (editor): *Brenner and Rector's The Kidney*, 5th ed. Saunders, 1996.

HEMOLYTIC UREMIC SYNDROME

Fong JSC et al: Hemolytic-uremic syndrome. Current concepts and management. Pediatr Clin North Am 1982;29:835.

Kaplan BS et al: Recent advances in understanding the pathogenesis of the hemolytic uremic syndromes. Pediatr Nephrol 1990;4:276.

Siegler RL: Management of hemolytic-uremic syndrome. J Pediatr 1988;112:1014.

Siegler RL et al: Long-term outcome and prognostic indicators in the hemolytic-uremic syndrome. J Pediatr 1991;118:195.

Upadhyaya K et al: The importance of nonrenal involvement in hemolytic-uremic syndrome. Pediatrics 1980;65:115.

CHRONIC RENAL FAILURE

Brenner BM et al: Dietary protein intake and the progressive nature of kidney disease: The role of hemodynamically mediated glomerular injury in the pathogenesis of progressive glomerular sclerosis in aging, renal ablation, and intrinsic renal disease. N Engl J Med 1982;307:652.

Fine RN et al for the Genentech Cooperative Study Group: Growth after recombinant human growth hormone treatment in children with chronic renal failure: Report of a multicenter randomized double-blind placebo-controlled study. J Pediatr 1994;124:374.

Wassner SJ: Conservative management of chronic renal insufficiency. In: Holliday MA et al (editors): *Pediatric Nephrology,* 3rd ed. Williams & Wilkins, 1994.

EVALUATION OF HYPERTENSION

Loggie JMH (editor): *Pediatric and Adolescent Hypertension.* Blackwell, 1992.

National High Blood Pressure Education Program Working on Hypertension Control in Children and Adolescents: Update on the 1987 Task Force on High Blood Pressure in Children and Adolescents. A Working Group Report from the National High Blood Pressure Education Program.

RENAL TUBULAR ACIDOSIS

Portale AA: Renal tubular acidosis. In: Holliday MA et al (editors): *Pediatric Nephrology,* 3rd ed. Williams & Wilkins, 1994.

CONGENITAL ANOMALIES OF THE URINARY TRACT

Belman AB: A perspective on vesicoureteral reflux. Urol Clin North Am 1995;22:139.

Tripp BM, Homsy YL: Neonatal hydronephrosis: The controversy and the management. Pediatr Nephrol 1995;9:503.

PARENTERAL FLUID THERAPY

Avery ME, Snyder JD: Oral therapy for acute diarrhea: The underused simple solution. Curr Concepts 1990;323:891.

Hellerstein S: Fluid and electrolytes: Clinical Aspects. Pediatr Rev 1993;14:103.

17

Circulation

Michael M. Brook, MD, Phillip Moore, MD, & George F. Van Hare, MD

CARDIAC PHYSIOLOGY

The purpose of the circulation is to deliver oxygen to the tissues of the body to support their metabolic activities. To achieve this, the heart pumps blood, initiated by intrinsic electrical activity, through vessels to the lungs and body.

OXYGEN DELIVERY

Oxygen tissue delivery is determined by two main factors: the amount of oxygen carried by blood and the volume of blood the heart pumps to the body with each beat (stroke volume). Oxygen is carried by blood predominately bound to hemoglobin in red blood cells, although a small amount is dissolved. This means that the amount of oxygen in blood depends predominately on the patient's hemoglobin concentration and the oxygen saturation. Cyanosis and anemia decrease oxygen delivery.

CARDIAC FUNCTION

The pump function of the heart is best determined by the cardiac output, which is the volume of blood (in liters) the heart pumps to the body per minute. Because of the variable size among the pediatric population, cardiac output typically is divided by the child's body surface area and reported as cardiac index (L/min/m^2). Cardiac output equals stroke volume (L/beat) times heart rate (beats/min). Three factors determine stroke volume: preload, afterload, and contractility. Therefore, heart rate, preload, afterload, and contractility are the major determinants of cardiac function (Table 17–1).

Heart Rate

Although it would seem that an increase in heart rate should increase cardiac output, this usually is not the case because of adjustments in diastolic filling. Very fast or slow rates affect stroke volume through changes in preload and contractility. Because the duration of systole is relatively constant as heart rate changes, increases in heart rate diminish the time available for diastolic filling of the ventricle. At very fast heart rates, as seen during an episode of paroxysmal ventricular tachycardia, cardiac output may be reduced dramatically because of poor diastolic filling, resulting in decreased preload. Mild bradycardia allows for increased diastolic filling, which improves stroke volume. The heart maintains a normal cardiac output, because the increase in stroke volume compensates for the decreased rate. As bradycardia becomes more severe, however, cardiac output is reduced as the decrease in rate overwhelms the limited increase in preload. Increasing heart rate has a direct effect on improving contractility acutely; however, chronic fast rates, such as occur in various forms of supraventricular tachycardia (SVT), can cause decreased contractile function leading to tachycardic cardiomyopathy.

In addition to rate, cardiac rhythm plays a role in cardiac function. With atrioventricular dissociation, such as in second or third degree heart block, the normal atrial contribution to active filling of the ventricle is lost, adversely affecting preload and diminishing cardiac output. Bundle-branch block, ventricular pacing, and ventricular tachycardia all cause poorly organized ventricular contraction leading to decreased cardiac output.

Preload

In isolated strips of myocardium, preload refers to the amount of stretch applied to the muscle before contraction. Increased stretch results in increased force of contraction to a maximum; contraction then declines as stretch becomes more extreme. This relationship is known as the Starling mechanism.

Precontraction myocardial stretch in the beating heart is best represented by the end diastolic volume of the ventri-

Table 17–1. Determinants of left ventricular output.

Determinant	Clinical Measurement (In Order of Decreasing Reliability)
Heart rate	Pulse
	Ventricular rate on ECG
Preload	End diastolic volume
	End diastolic pressure
	Mean left atrial pressure
	Mean pulmonary capillary wedge pressure
Afterload	Left ventricular end systolic wall stress
	Systemic vascular resistance
	Mean aortic pressure
	Diastolic aortic pressure
Contractility	Slope of end systolic pressure-volume relation
	Slope of velocity of shortening — end systolic wall stress
	Left ventricular ejection fraction
	Left ventricular % fractional shortening

ECG = electrocardiogram.

cle. Increased end diastolic ventricular volume results in increased stretch on the ventricular myocytes, causing an increase in stroke volume. Unfortunately, there is no easy and accurate way to measure end diastolic volume short of placing special catheters into the beating ventricle. There is, however, a nonlinear relationship between diastolic pressure and volume in the ventricle. This allows us to estimate ventricular diastolic volume, and therefore preload, from measurements of ventricular end diastolic pressure, such as the mean central venous pressure (for the right ventricle) and the mean left atrial or pulmonary arterial wedge pressure (for the left ventricle). All these pressures are easily and routinely monitored in critically ill children, particularly those recovering from cardiac surgery. Caution must be exercised in the interpretation of these pressures because of the nonlinearity of the ventricular end diastolic pressure-volume relationship. Compliance in the ventricle decreases with increasing stretch so that at higher end diastolic pressures, large increases in pressure may be seen with very little change in ventricular volume and therefore very little change in actual preload. A rough indication of ventricular preload may be obtained by assessing organs or vessels "upstream" from the ventricle in question. Distended neck veins and an enlarged liver suggest elevated right ventricular preload, whereas pulmonary rales suggest pulmonary edema and elevated left ventricular preload.

If poor cardiac output is primarily due to inadequate preload resulting from reduced blood volume, such as with active bleeding or severe dehydration, dramatic increases in cardiac output are easily obtained by increasing preload, ie, the infusion of blood, colloid, or crystalloid. If cardiac output is low for another reason, such as high afterload, low heart rate, or poor contractility, the preload usually is normal and often may be increased to compensate. Further increases in preload may result in limited and temporary increases in cardiac output, but optimal man-

agement should be directed to treatment of the primary problem, eg, afterload reduction, pacing, or infusion of inotropic agents. In fact, when preload is high as a compensatory mechanism, it often is the cause of many symptoms. For example, the compensatory increase in left atrial pressure that occurs with left ventricular failure may lead to pulmonary edema because of high pulmonary venous pressures, resulting in respiratory distress.

Afterload

Afterload refers to the resistance that isolated muscle works against during contraction, ie, the force resisting shortening of the muscle. Although this force can be easily and accurately measured in isolated muscle, it is impossible to measure it directly in the beating heart. In the beating heart, the analogous concept is the resistance against which the ventricle contracts. For a given preload and intrinsic myocardial contractility, the cardiac output will decrease as the resistance or afterload increases. This resistance is provided by the semilunar valves, arteries, and capillary beds downstream and is influenced by the shape and thickness of the ventricle itself. The most accurate technique for estimating afterload is the measurement of systolic wall stress, which considers chamber size, thickness, and intraventricular pressure. This is impractical, however, as it requires simultaneous, continuous measurement of ventricular or arterial pressure with echocardiographic images of ventricular chamber size and thickness.

The practical clinical approach to evaluating afterload is to measure arterial blood pressure (P) and blood flow (Q) and calculate mean vascular resistance (R = ΔP/Q). This is an extreme oversimplification and limited estimate of afterload. Because mean vascular resistance is directly related to mean pressure and inversely related to mean flow, it assumes that the heart generates continuous, rather than pulsatile, flow. Even more problematic, mean vascular resistance reflects mainly the contribution of the peripheral vascular bed to afterload and ignores central vessel compliance, semilunar valve resistance, and ventricular size and shape. Despite these significant limitations, mean vascular resistance is a reasonable estimate of afterload in most patients. Exceptions include those patients with abnormalities of their proximal arterial tree (eg, coarctation of the aorta, pulmonary artery banding, nondistensible conduit placement, and dilated aortic or pulmonary roots), semilunar valve stenosis, or significant ventricular dilation and/or hypertrophy (eg, dilated cardiomyopathy, idiopathic hypertrophic subaortic stenosis [IHSS], and subaortic stenosis).

Increased afterload may result in significant impairment of cardiac function in children. Common examples include infants who are in shock and have severe aortic stenosis (AS) or coarctation or patients who have long-standing malignant hypertension. Often, even though increased afterload is not the primary cause of low cardiac output, it is a contributing factor. Compensatory mechanisms, such as endogenous catecholamine release, may increase systemic vascular resistance markedly. This elevation in afterload may be poorly tolerated by a ventricle with poor contractile function or mitral regurgitation. Careful use of afterload-reducing agents, such as nitroprusside, captopril, or prazosin, may improve cardiac output dramatically in these circumstances.

Contractility

Contractility refers to the inotropic state of the heart, or the intrinsic contractile characteristics of the myocardium not related to preload or afterload. Within a myocyte, this is determined by the activity of the contractile proteins actin and myosin. Contraction begins when an action potential depolarizes the myocyte by sequential influx of sodium and calcium. This results in intracellular calcium release from the sarcoplasmic reticulum, which binds to troponin causing a conformational change that interferes with the binding of troponin to actin. This allows the formation of cross-bridges between actin and the myosin head. The chemical energy of adenosine triphosphate (ATP) rotates the myosin head, which displaces actin to the center of the sarcomere resulting in shortening of the myocyte. The amount of force developed by the contracting myocyte is, in part, dependent on the number of cross-bridges formed. The contractile state of the heart therefore depends on many factors, including the size and number of healthy myocytes, the availability of intra- and extracellular calcium, and the amount of circulating catecholamines.

For the beating heart, contractility is the potential for cardiac muscle to do work, ie, eject blood. An increase in contractility results in greater shortening of the myocardium at a constant preload and afterload. The Starling curve is shifted up and leftward, so that for a given preload and afterload the ventricular output is increased (Figure 17–1). Unfortunately, neither in the laboratory nor at the bedside is an independent measure of myocardial contractility readily available. The best independent index of contractility is the end systolic pressure-volume relationship. If one measures both pressure and volume in an ejecting ventricle during the entire cardiac cycle, determines the point at which end systole occurs, and then varies the loading conditions, the slope of the line formed by these end systolic pressure-volume points is a good measure of contractility. When contractility is increased, the degree of shortening is increased for any end systolic pressure, and the attained end systolic pressure is higher for any end systolic volume. In effect, the end systolic pressure volume relation is shifted to the left (Figure 17–2). These curves can be obtained invasively during cardiac catheterization, with the use of special catheters placed directly in the left ventricle. A less invasive estimate of contractility is the relationship between the velocity of shortening of the myocardium with the end systolic wall stress. This relationship can be determined by simultaneous continuous measurement of arterial pressure with echocardiographic images of ventricular contraction.

Clinically, there is no reliable way to measure cardiac

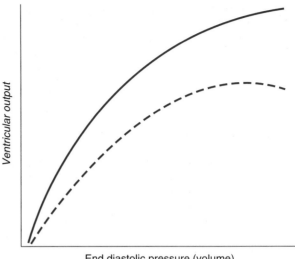

Figure 17–1. An increase in end diastolic volume (preload) results in an increase in ventricular output. When contractility is increased *(solid line)*, the output is lower at the same preload.

contractile state. The cardiac output should be assessed by physical examination and invasive techniques, such as cardiac output measurements by thermodilution technique or evaluation of the systemic arterial-venous O_2 saturation differential. Noninvasive measurement of left ventricular ejection fraction (the percentage of the left ventricular di-

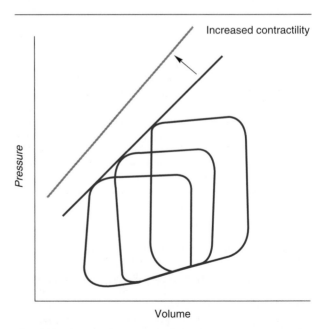

Figure 17–2. An increase in contractility (ie, catecholamine infusion) increases and shifts the end systolic pressure-volume relation to the left with a higher slope.

astolic volume that is ejected) and subjective assessment of myocardial wall motion by echocardiography should be obtained. However, preload and afterload also must be evaluated. If the cardiac output is low and the ejection fraction is dramatically reduced, there is no evidence of increased afterload, and preload is adequate, then contractile function is decreased. On the other hand, if reduced cardiac output and ejection fraction occurs in the setting of severe AS or coarctation (fixed increased afterload), it is impossible to separate the effects of the increased afterload on the left ventricle from those of contractility.

The specific treatment of decreased cardiac contractility involves the use of inotropic agents. Digoxin is the most commonly prescribed digitalis preparation and the only liquid oral preparation available in the United States. For the acute management of contractile dysfunction, intravenous (IV) digoxin may be used; however, more potent catecholamine agents, such as dopamine, dobutamine, isoproterenol, and epinephrine, are used more commonly. In addition, the phosphodiesterase inhibitors, such as amrinone and milrinone, can be used. All these agents have additional affects on the circulation, specifically with respect to heart rate and venous and/or arterial vessel tone. The most appropriate agent is chosen on the basis of the state of the child's preload, afterload, and heart rate (Table 17–2). In addition to inotropic support, patients with decreased contractility may benefit from direct alterations in preload, afterload, and heart rate.

CIRCULATION

To understand congenital heart disease fully, one must recognize fetal blood flow patterns in the central circulation and the changes in these flow patterns with birth. With very few exceptions, serious structural cardiac disease diagnosed in the newborn period is completely compatible with a relatively normal intrauterine existence. It is the transition to extrauterine life that makes the cardiac lesion hemodynamically significant. The best example of this principle is the infant with pulmonary atresia. While

Table 17–2. Properties of inotropic agents for the acute management of decreased cardiac contractility.

Agent	Contractility	Afterload	Heart Rate
Amrinone/milrinone	↑	↓↓	(↑)
Isoproterenol	↑	↓↓	↑↑↑
Dobutamine	↑↑	(↓)[1]	(↑)[1]
Dopamine	↑↑	↑↑[1]	↑↑[1]
Epinephrine	↑↑	↑↑	↑↑

[1]Severity of effect very dose dependent.

the infant is in utero, very little blood flow needs to be delivered to the lungs because oxygenation is provided by the placenta. With closure of the ductus arteriosus after birth, however, pulmonary blood flow may be inadequate to oxygenate the infant, leading to a rapidly fatal condition if no intervention is undertaken.

FETAL CIRCULATION

In the normal fetus, as in the normal newborn, there are two atria, two ventricles, and two great vessels. The fetus, however, has additional structures: a patent foramen ovale, a patent ductus arteriosus (PDA), and a patent ductus venosus, as well as the placenta (Figure 17–3). The placenta serves as the site of gas exchange. Because pulmonary arteriolar vasoconstriction maintains high resistance in the pulmonary circuit, most right ventricular blood traverses the ductus arteriosus, rather than the branch pulmonary arteries and lungs. The right ventricle, therefore, provides blood to the descending aorta and the placenta via the ductus. The left ventricle supplies the ascending aorta and the upper body, including the brain, and sends a small amount down the descending aorta to mix with right ventricular output. Therefore, there is a functional, but not absolute, separation in the systemic circulation in the fetus, with the right ventricle supplying the lower body and placenta and the left ventricle supplying the upper body.

Oxygenation occurs in the placenta, and blood of higher oxygen content passes from the placenta into the umbilical vein. Umbilical venous blood is distributed to both lobes of the liver, and about half bypasses the liver through the ductus venosus directly into the inferior vena cava. Portal venous blood is distributed almost completely to the right liver lobe.

Blood in the ascending aorta has a higher oxygen content than that in the descending aorta, and so the brain receives blood with a higher oxygen content than does the placenta. This separation in oxygen content is caused by the patterns of streaming in the right atrium. Blood from the superior vena cava, low in oxygen content, preferentially crosses the tricuspid valve and is sent by the right ventricle via the ductus to the descending aorta and placenta for reoxygenation. Blood from the inferior vena cava, higher in oxygen content because of the contribution from the placenta, preferentially crosses the foramen ovale to fill the left atrium and left ventricle and is sent predominantly to the upper body, brain, and coronary circulation.

TRANSITION TO EXTRAUTERINE CIRCULATION

A number of complex events occur with birth (Figure 17–4). Occlusion of the umbilical cord removes the low-resistance capillary bed from the systemic circulation.

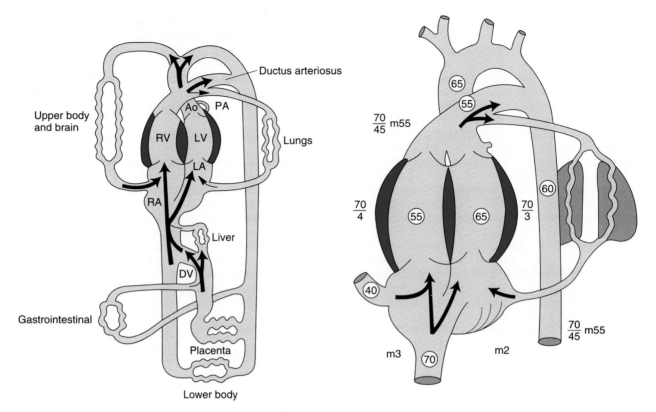

Figure 17–3. Diagrams of the fetal circulation. **Left:** Blood is oxygenated in the placenta and returns to the fetus through the umbilical vein. About half the umbilical venous blood passes through the liver, and the remainder bypasses the liver through the ductus venosus (DV) directly into the inferior vena cava. Inferior vena caval blood is distributed partly through the foramen ovale to the left atrium (LA) and partly through the tricuspid valve to the right ventricle (RV) **(left and right panels).** Superior vena caval blood passes almost exclusively into the right ventricle. Blood ejected from the right ventricle passes mainly through the ductus arteriosus to the descending aorta, and only a small amount enters the lungs. **Right:** Numbers in circles show oxygen saturations in cardiac chambers and great vessels. Numbers alongside are pressures (mm Hg). Ao = ascending aorta; LV = left ventricle; PA = pulmonary artery; RA = right atrium.

Breathing results in a marked decrease in pulmonary resistance. Two distinct mechanisms are responsible for this effect on the pulmonary vessels. Rhythmic physical expansion of the lungs releases a prostaglandin, probably prostacyclin (PGI_2). An increase in alveolar oxygen level stimulates production of nitric oxide, a powerful pulmonary vasodilator. The increased pulmonary blood flow returns to fill the left atrium, and this increased left atrial filling closes the foramen ovale, limiting and eventually eliminating flow from the inferior vena cava into the left atrium. Because blood that returns from the lungs is much more completely oxygenated than that which was provided by the placenta, arterial oxygen saturation increases. This increase in arterial oxygen saturation and, in particular, the loss of endogenous prostaglandins produced by the placenta eventually brings about closure of the ductus arteriosus and ductus venosus. Finally, the foramen ovale becomes nonpatent. Most of the transition from fetal to neonatal circulation takes place in the first several minutes after birth owing to changes in vascular resistance. Func-

tional closure of the ductus arteriosus takes place within 10–15 hours after birth, but anatomic closure occurs only after several days to 2 weeks. The foramen ovale typically remains patent with no flow through it for weeks or months and, in fact, may remain patent into adulthood in some individuals.

PULMONARY VASCULAR BED

Whereas the first breath is accompanied by a sudden and dramatic decrease in pulmonary vascular resistance, a further decrease in resistance occurs over the first several days of life, as pulmonary arterioles relax and subsequently lose much of the smooth muscle in the media. In normal infants, the pulmonary vascular bed resembles the adult pattern both in resistance and in histologic appearance by several weeks of age. In some individuals, however, this maturation of the pulmonary vascular bed may not occur or may occur over a longer time course. Two

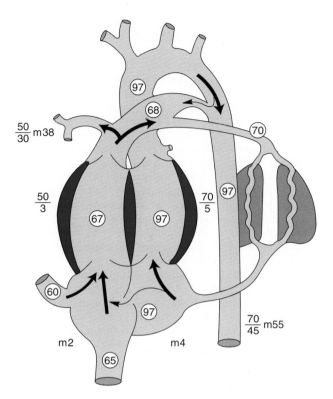

Figure 17–4. Neonatal circulation. Placenta has been removed. The foramen ovale has closed, and the ductus arteriosus has almost closed. Pulmonary arterial pressure has fallen from fetal levels but is still higher than adult levels. Numbers in circles show oxygen saturations in cardiac chambers and great vessels. Pressures (mm Hg) are shown alongside.

factors may be responsible. First, alveolar hypoxemia maintains pulmonary vasoconstriction after birth, as in babies born at high altitude or with lung disease. Second, pulmonary hypertension may be responsible. An example is the infant with a large ventricular septal defect (VSD). In such an infant, the presence of the defect allows transmission of systemic left ventricular systolic pressure to the right ventricle and in turn to the pulmonary artery and peripheral vascular bed. This pulmonary hypertension interferes with the normal decrease in pulmonary vascular resistance described previously. In such a patient, resistance may remain high until 1–2 months of age and does not decrease to normal levels while pulmonary arterial pressure remains elevated.

In any infant with a congenital heart lesion comprising a large communication between the ventricles or aorta and pulmonary artery, pulmonary arterial pressure remains elevated. The normal disappearance of smooth muscle in the media does not occur, and this contributes to the maintenance of an increased pulmonary vascular resistance. If the cardiac defect is corrected, the pulmonary vessels lose the medial muscle layer and assume normal adult charac-

teristics. If the pulmonary hypertension persists, secondary changes in the arterioles develop. Intimal proliferation, with migration of smooth muscle cells into the intima and then fibrosis, results in a progressive increase in pulmonary vascular resistance. These changes are permanent, and correction of the defect at this stage does not improve the pulmonary vascular resistance. For this reason, cardiac defects are repaired early. The intimal proliferative and fibrotic changes usually do not begin to develop before age 6 months, but they increase progressively, becoming severe as early as 9–12 months or as late as adolescence. The progressive increase in pulmonary vascular resistance results in a decrease of left-to-right shunt and subsequently in the development of a right-to-left shunt, with clinical cyanosis. Patients with high pulmonary blood flow but normal or only slightly elevated pressure, such as with a large atrial septal defect (ASD), undergo the normal decline in pulmonary vascular resistance after birth, but the intimal proliferative and fibrotic changes may occur, usually after adolescence.

CARDIAC ELECTRICAL ACTIVITY

Cardiac impulses are formed by cardiac cells that exhibit **pacemaker activity,** or **spontaneous automaticity.** In adults, such cells are found primarily in the sinus and atrioventricular nodes and, to a lesser extent, in atrial muscle and the His-Purkinje (distal conducting) system. The sinus node develops quite early in gestation as a well-demarcated structure at the junction of the right atrium and superior vena cava.

Cardiac muscle cells have the ability to transmit electrical impulses to adjacent cells via **gap junctions,** specialized structures that make the cytosol of adjacent cardiac cells electrically continuous. An action potential that spreads down one cardiac cell will be transmitted easily to adjacent cardiac cells, leading to propagation throughout the heart. Instead of homogenous conduction in all directions, propagation is known to be more rapid along the long axis of cardiac cells than along the transverse axis. The velocity of impulse propagation in cardiac muscle depends on a number of factors, including fiber orientation; passive properties of cardiac muscle, such as membrane excitability threshold, resistance, and capacitance; and active properties related to the action potential. The most important of these factors is the rate of increase of phase 0 of the action potential, also known as dV/dT or maximum velocity (V_{max}). Conduction velocity is directly related to the magnitude of V_{max}, and factors that affect V_{max} also affect conduction velocity.

Phase 0 of the action potential occurs when the membrane potential is increased from its resting negative value to its excitability threshold (Figure 17–5). In cardiac muscle cells, or fast-response cells, this results in the opening of voltage-sensitive sodium channels, the rapid entry of positively charged sodium ions, and the further increase in the membrane potential toward 0 potential. The sodium channel is time dependent and inactivates, allowing other ionic mechanisms eventually to return the membrane potential to its resting potential. Antiarrhythmic agents, such as procainamide and quinidine, are thought to exert their effects by blocking fast sodium channels, thereby slowing the rate of increase of phase 0 and consequently decreasing conduction velocity.

In pacemaker, or slow-response, cells like those found in the sinus and atrioventricular node, the upstroke of the action potential, and therefore the velocity of conduction, is much slower than in fast-response cells found elsewhere (Figure 17–5). Phase 0 of the action potential is not mediated by the opening of fast sodium channels, but instead by the slow inward calcium current.

In normal sinus rhythm, the spread of cardiac excitation proceeds from the sinus node through the atrial muscle to excite both right and left atria. Excitation reaches the atrioventricular node by way of cell-to-cell intra-atrial conduction. The atrioventricular node gives rise to a bundle (**bundle of His**) that penetrates the central fibrous body and then divides to form the left and right bundle branches, made up of Purkinje cells. The atrioventricular node is made up of slow-response cells that are histologically similar to those found in the sinus node. The slower upstroke of the action potential in the atrioventricular node is associated with a lower conduction velocity than elsewhere in the heart, and the atrioventricular node is responsible for introducing a significant delay between atrial and ventricular contraction.

Nodal conduction time is age related. Little is known about conduction time in the node during fetal life. However, atrioventricular nodal conduction is normally quite short at birth (20–40 msec) but increases progressively with age to as long as 200 msec in adulthood. Conduction in the distal conducting system (His bundle and bundle branches), normally 20 msec at birth, increases to 40–50 msec in adulthood.

In addition to introducing a delay, the atrioventricular node also limits the number of atrial impulses that may conduct to the ventricles. This function is adaptive; arrhythmias, such as atrial flutter or fibrillation, occur with atrial rates as high as 500–600 beats/min. Refractoriness in the atrioventricular node limits the resulting ventricular rate. Refractoriness is also age dependent. In late fetal life and in the newborn period, the atrioventricular node may conduct atrial rates as high as 300 beats/min without block; however, with increasing age, atrioventricular block occurs at progressively slower atrial rates. Atrioventricular node refractoriness is also quite sensitive to autonomic influences.

The adult heart is well invested with nerve fibers, and both the sympathetic and parasympathetic nervous systems influence cardiac automaticity and conduction. Sympathetic fibers reach the sinus node, atrioventricular node, bundle branches, and atrial and ventricular myocardium, whereas vagal fibers are more limited in distribution, affecting mainly the atrial myocardium and the sinus and atrioventricular nodes. Innervation of the ventricles by the vagus nerve is limited, but vagal stimulation can lead to mild decreases in ventricular contractility.

Sympathetic stimulation leads to increased automaticity

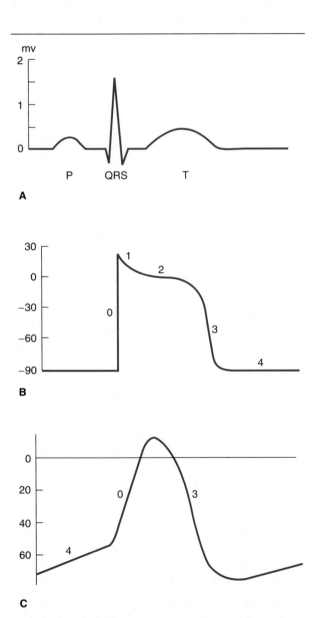

Figure 17–5. *A:* Typical electrocardiogram, lead II. *B:* Transmembrane potential of cardiac muscle cell. *C:* Transmembrane potential of pacemaker cell. (Reproduced, with permission, from Stanger P, Van Hare GF: Arrhythmias. Page 1441 in Rudolph AM [editor]: *Rudolph's Pediatrics,* 20th ed. Appleton & Lange, 1996.)

of both the sinus and atrioventricular nodes, shortening of refractory periods and conduction times through the atrioventricular node, and shortening of refractory periods in both atrial and ventricular myocardium. In short, sympathetic stimulation increases heart rate by increasing both the firing rate of the sinus node and the conduction rate of electricity through the heart. Sympathetic stimulation, of course, may have a host of other effects on the circulation, including increased contractility, changes in blood pressure, and effects on the coronary circulation. Vagal stimulation produces effects that, in general, are the opposite of those produced by sympathetic stimulation. Therefore, decreases in sinus and atrioventricular node automaticity and increases in atrioventricular node conduction time are demonstrable. Sympathetic and parasympathetic effects on the heart are age related and change during fetal and postnatal development. The two opposing influences may develop at different rates during fetal life. Heart rate is thought to be primarily under vagal control at the time of birth. In humans, sympathetic development is not complete at birth but is completed later.

DIAGNOSTIC TECHNIQUES

The evaluation of the child with suspected heart disease involves the interpretation of many diagnostic modalities, at each step forming and refining a list of possible diagnoses on the basis of the information available. In most patients, particularly infants, a probable diagnosis can be obtained before, or even without, obtaining a diagnostic study such as an echocardiogram. It is more important to determine the physiologic process accounting for the symptomatology and to begin treatment of the symptoms while a definitive diagnosis is being established.

CLINICAL ASSESSMENT

History

As in all children, a complete birth history is important. With respect to cardiac disease, prematurity and maternal rubella infection increase the risk of PDA and pulmonary artery stenosis. Medications used during pregnancy may act as teratogens; for example, lithium increases the risk of Ebstein anomaly in the fetus. In the family history, siblings or other family members with congenital heart disease should be noted. If an immediate family member is affected, the risk of congenital heart disease increases from 0.8 to 2–3%. A history of sudden death, seizures, or arrhythmias may be important in diagnosing the long-QT syndromes. The history of the present illness should include inquiry into all possible cardiac symptoms, including failure to thrive, feeding difficulty, cyanosis, squatting, respiratory distress, sweating, pallor, chest pain, palpitations, dizziness, and syncope. Specific questions regarding feeding are often helpful, eg, the volume of formula an infant consumes per feeding, how long the feeding takes, and causes for slow feeding. Comparing the child's activity level to that of siblings and playmates is a good indicator of early fatigability.

Physical Examination

The approach to physical diagnosis of the cardiovascular system in children must, of course, be tailored to the age of the child as well as to the suspected cardiac problem. Percussion is rarely performed as part of the cardiac examination, particularly in children. Inspection, palpation, and auscultation are discussed below. Of these, careful auscultation is the most important, and often the most difficult, in children.

Various strategies for auscultation may be used, depending on the age of the child. Although adolescents and older school-aged children usually are quite cooperative, younger children may not be. Infants several months of age or younger may be quieted with a pacifier or bottle or by nursing. In older infants, simple eye contact may quiet a child for long enough to obtain at least an initial examination. Bright objects brought into the field of view may also help distract the infant. Once a child is old enough to recognize strangers, careful auscultation may become difficult or impossible. Some may be quieted by partially redressing the child, and others may become quiet when carried down the hall just out of view of their parents.

General Examination. Most important, an assessment of whether the child appears healthy or sick should be made, as this will modify the subsequent examination greatly. Children who appear acutely or chronically ill, of course, are approached with a much higher degree of suspicion. Identification of cyanosis is of great importance. Whereas peripheral cyanosis may be due to a cold room (especially in infants), central cyanosis suggests arterial deoxygenation, in turn suggesting cardiac or pulmonary disease, or both. The earliest signs of central cyanosis are in the perioral area. When one is in doubt about the presence of central cyanosis, pulse oximetry, which is becoming increasingly available, has the advantages of being noninvasive and confirmatory (see below). However, estimation of oxygen saturation based on the intensity of cyanosis can be quite inaccurate. The intensity of cyanosis is determined by the concentration of desaturated hemoglobin, rather than by the actual oxygen saturation. Therefore, babies who are markedly polycythemic may appear quite cyanotic, despite relatively minor arterial desaturation, because of the high absolute concentration of desaturated hemoglobin. On the other hand, infants with significant anemia appear relatively pink despite significant arterial desaturation. The latter situation is most common at 1–2 months of age, when normal physiologic anemia may occur. Infants who are somewhat cold, especially in the delivery room, may manifest impressive peripheral cyanosis that does not reflect central arterial desaturation. Arterial desaturation may be a sign of (1) right-to-left shunting of blood, as is seen in a variety of congenital heart lesions and in persistent fetal circulation; (2) transposition of the great vessels, with delivery of systemic venous blood directly to the aorta; (3) pulmonary venous desaturation due to alveolar hypoxia, as with pulmonary edema, pneumonia, or atelectasis with perfusion of unventilated alveoli; or (4) a combination of these factors.

The degree of **respiratory distress** should be noted, as this can provide a clue to the cause of the problem. Respiratory distress should be distinguished from tachypnea. Distress implies increased work of breathing. This is manifested by increased accessory muscle use, resulting in retractions and nasal flaring, and attempts to increase intrathoracic pressure, causing grunting or sighing. In general, cardiac lesions with reduction in pulmonary blood flow present without significant respiratory distress, unless cyanosis is profound. Lesions with poor systemic output and acidosis, as well as those with increased pulmonary blood flow, present with respiratory distress. Finally, infants with primarily pulmonary disease, as well as those with superimposed pulmonary disease, have respiratory distress.

Careful assessment of the **pulses** and **peripheral perfusion** is crucial in the infant with suspected heart disease. The femoral pulses are compared with an upper extremity pulse, usually the radial or brachial pulse, in assessing the possibility of aortic coarctation. Most experienced clinicians believe that such a careful comparison by palpation is more reliable than the determination of four-limb blood pressures (see below). Conditions that cause a decreased pulse in all sites include any condition with decreased systemic blood flow, especially those lesions that depend on the patency of the ductus arteriosus for systemic flow, such as hypoplastic left ventricle.

Palpation. The precordium is palpated, noting location of the impulse, as well as the degree of precordial activity and the location of any thrills. An impulse from the left ventricle is normally palpated at the apex. An impulse along the left sternal border is due to the right ventricle and usually is not present normally. A right ventricular or increased left ventricular impulse reflects increased volume or pressure load in the particular ventricle. In addition to being present precordially, a thrill may be felt at the suprasternal notch, where it usually indicates aortic or, occasionally, pulmonic valvar stenosis. The presence of a thrill is never normal, with the possible exception of the occasionally felt supraclavicular thrill associated with a loud venous hum.

The spleen tip may be palpable normally in infants but is otherwise not normally felt. The liver edge is palpated in most infants; it is sharp and normally felt as much as 2 cm below the right costal margin. An enlarged liver is a sign of congestive heart failure (CHF), and the liver edge may often be felt to extend to the left upper quadrant and to below the umbilicus. One should remember that pulmonary hyperinflation, as is seen in asthma and bronchi-

olitis, may push the liver down and make it appear enlarged when it is not. In this case, the edge is sharp and not felt to the left of the xiphoid process. Also, one should remember that in children with abnormal cardiac and abdominal situs, the liver may be entirely to the left or mainly at the midline.

Auscultation. A complete cardiac auscultatory examination includes use of both the bell and diaphragm of the stethoscope in each of the precordial areas. These areas typically are referred to as the aortic, pulmonic, tricuspid, and mitral areas; however, in children it is best to describe them by chest landmarks, because in many types of congenital heart disease, the cardiac structures may not be positioned normally. Therefore, one listens at the upper right and left sternal borders (second intercostal space), along the lower left sternal border (third and fourth intercostal space), and at the apex and describes the position where the murmur or cardiac sound is maximal. One also listens for radiation of pulmonic murmurs to both clavicles, axillae, and lung fields and of aortic murmurs to the carotid arteries.

In children, although the sounds are louder than in adults, the heart rate is significantly faster, making accurate auscultation challenging. At each location, one should pay attention to each sound separately before moving to the next sound. For example, one should concentrate on the first heart sound, ignoring all other sounds, then concentrate on the second heart sound, and so on. In this way, one may avoid missing more subtle findings in patients with prominent murmurs.

First Heart Sound. The first heart sound is normally heard maximally at the apex, is of low frequency, and is normally single. Splitting of the first heart sound may often be noted normally. It may be differentiated from early systolic clicks by the low frequency of the sound, as opposed to clicks, which have a higher frequency. Variability of intensity of the first heart sound may be caused by atrioventricular dissociation caused by complete atrioventricular block.

Second Heart Sound. The importance of accurately assessing the second heart sound cannot be overemphasized. Normally, in children and infants beyond several weeks of age, the second heart sound is split with inspiration and narrow or single with expiration, and the aortic and pulmonic components are of about equal intensity and frequency. It is best heard at the base, and splitting is best evaluated at the upper left sternal border. Pulmonary hypertension causes earlier closure and accentuation of P_2, and so one may hear a loud and single second heart sound. Such a finding is of crucial importance, particularly in patients with correctable congenital heart defects, such as atrioventricular canal defect, as it involves the risk of progression to irreversible pulmonary vascular disease. In infants and children who have a normal arterial oxygen saturation, the loudness of the second heart sound often is more helpful than splitting, which can be masked by the fast heart rate. Pulmonic stenosis may cause delay and softening of P_2. Transposition of the great vessels may be associated with a single second heart sound at the upper left sternal border because of malposition of the semilunar valve. Splitting often is appreciated in such patients at the third intercostal space at the left sternal border, with a soft P_2 due to the posterior position of the pulmonic valve in transposition.

Third & Fourth Heart Sounds. In children, when listening in a quiet room with the bell, third heart sounds often are heard normally at the apex. Fourth heart sounds are not normally heard, and a loud third or a fourth heart sound suggests the presence of poor ventricular compliance, as might be present in dilated cardiomyopathy or CHF. Soft mid-diastolic murmurs often are mistaken for third or fourth heart sounds and are caused by increased flow across a normal tricuspid or mitral valve, as might occur in atrial or VSDs with a left-to-right shunt.

Clicks. Ejection and nonejection clicks may be appreciated. Ejection clicks occur early in systole, just after the first heart sound, and are thought to be caused by sudden tensing of the walls of the great vessel during ventricular ejection, rather than by actual valve movement. Aortic ejection clicks are heard best at the third left intercostal space, are slightly higher frequency than first heart sounds, and do not vary with respiration. They are caused by valvar AS or by idiopathic aortic root dilatation. Pulmonic ejection clicks are heard best at the upper left sternal border, are quite high frequency, and become softer with inspiration. They are due to valvar pulmonic stenosis or to pulmonary root dilation. Nonejection clicks, also known as midsystolic clicks, occur well after the first heart sound, are heard best in the upright or standing patient, are of medium frequency, and typically do not vary with respiration. They usually are due to mitral valve prolapse.

Murmurs. The evaluation and description of murmurs involve assessment of several factors. The loudness of the murmur is described from grades 1 to 6: Grade 1 murmurs are clearly softer than the heart sounds, grade 2 murmurs are approximately as loud as the heart sounds, grade 3 murmurs are clearly louder than the heart sounds, thrills are present with grade 4 murmurs, grade 5 murmurs can be heard with the edge of the stethoscope, and grade 6 with the stethoscope off the chest or with the naked ear. Grade 5 and 6 murmurs are very rare. The **frequency** of each murmur should be assessed. This may also be referred to as the "pitch" of the murmur. In general, the frequency will be determined by the difference in pressure between the two chambers creating the murmur. Therefore, in patients with small VSDs, a high-pitched murmur will be heard because of the difference between systemic pressure in the left ventricle and normal low pressure in the right ventricle. In addition, **form or shape** of the murmur (diamond-shaped or crescendo-decrescendo murmurs are termed ejection murmurs), the relation to the first heart sound (beginning with the first heart sound, obscuring the first heart sound, or well separated from the first heart sound), and the cardiac phase (systolic, diastolic, continuous) should be described. In general, ejection murmurs are due to semilunar valve or vessel stenosis. Murmurs that start with the first heart sound but do not obscure it and are not of ejection quality are termed **long systolic, or decrescendo,** murmurs and are caused by atrioventricular valve insufficiency. Murmurs that obscure the first heart sound at the point when they are maximal are termed **holosystolic** murmurs, even if they end slightly before the second heart sound, and are usually caused by some form of VSD.

Finally, the **position and radiation** of the murmur, defined as the origin of the murmur, should be noted. They usually are determined by the area in which the murmur is loudest. Some murmurs, however, are heard throughout the chest. In these cases, the area in which the frequency or pitch of the murmur is highest defines the origin, because high frequencies transmit less well than low ones. Certain murmurs have classic patterns of radiation, such as valvar pulmonary stenosis (PS) or pulmonary artery stenosis; these murmurs often are easily heard in the axillae, as well as in the left upper sternal border.

An example of a complete description of a murmur would be a "grade 2/6 medium-frequency, short systolic murmur at the lower left sternal border without radiation." This description is consistent with a small muscular VSD.

Early diastolic decrescendo murmurs that start with A_2 or P_2 are caused by semilunar valve regurgitation. Mid-diastolic murmurs may be caused by atrioventricular valve stenosis or by increased flow across a nonstenotic atrioventricular valve, as might be heard in patients with left-to-right shunts.

Continuous murmurs, which continue through systole and diastole, are most commonly caused by a PDA or by some other condition in which shunting continues throughout the cardiac cycle, such as with a surgical aortopulmonary (AP) shunt or a pulmonary arteriovenous (AV) fistula. Continuous murmurs should be differentiated from the coexistence of separate systolic and diastolic murmurs.

Blood Pressures. Blood pressure measurement is more helpful for following changes in hemodynamic condition than for diagnosing particular defects. This is true both for standard cuff pressures and for those obtained automatically by machine, because the act of inflating a cuff in a conscious infant often is associated with agitation and straining on the part of the infant. Because nonsimultaneous measurements reflect from somewhat different hemodynamic states, comparisons of upper and lower extremity pressures are unreliable. One approach to increase the reliability of such comparisons is to use two automatic machines simultaneously on the upper and lower extremities and then to switch the machines and repeat the procedure. The difference between the two readings is averaged to correct for intermachine variation.

Beyond the newborn period, however, blood pressure should be routinely measured in all children, even when heart disease is not suspected. Children with mild to moderate coarctation of the aorta often are asymptomatic until they present with hypertension in the arm during puberty.

Radiography

The chest radiograph may provide subtle information concerning possible types of heart disease, but the most common use is for assessment of heart size and determination of pulmonary blood flow. To determine heart size, the width of the cardiothymic silhouette is measured and compared with the width of the chest at its largest dimension. The ratio should be 0.65 or less. As true posteroanterior projections are unusual in infants, the measurement is made using an anteroposterior chest film. The most reliable measurements are from films on which a good inspiration was obtained, with the diaphragms seen at the ninth or tenth posterior rib margin. The heart may falsely appear enlarged if the film is taken on expiration. One should remember that the heart, thymus, and pericardial fluid may be seen as part of the cardiothymic silhouette. The degree of pulmonary vascularity should be noted as normal, increased, or decreased. In addition, the presence or absence of interstitial fluid, which is seen in pulmonary edema, should be noted.

The position of the cardiac apex on the cardiac silhouette should be evaluated; right ventricular enlargement causes an upturned apex, whereas left ventricular enlargement pushes the apex to the diaphragm. The size and distribution of pulmonary vasculature, particularly in cyanotic infants, can give clues to etiology. For example, patients with obstruction to pulmonary blood flow, as seen in tetralogy of Fallot (TOF) and related lesions, often have a hypoplastic pulmonary vasculature, termed "black lung fields." Patients with transposition complexes, however, have large pulmonary arteries, resulting in a picture of hypervascularity and whiter lung fields. The presence or absence of the pulmonary artery knob at the upper left heart border provides information regarding the position or size of the main pulmonary artery. Finally, the width of the mediastinum can provide information regarding great artery position and size. A narrow mediastinum, for example, often is seen in transposition of the great arteries because the great vessels are superimposed in the anterior/posterior projection.

Electrocardiography

The interpretation of pediatric electrocardiograms (ECGs) is a large and complicated topic that is covered only superficially here. When interpreting an ECG, it is important to develop a stepwise, systematic approach. This ensures that all pertinent findings will be seen and allows better integration of the various features. First, the rate should be determined as normal, fast, or slow. Second, the rhythm should be determined as regular or irregular: If the rhythm is irregular, does it display a repeating pattern or is it inconsistent? The association of P and QRS waves should be determined: Are they at the same rate? Is there a 1:1 relationship, a 2, 3, or 4:1 relationship, or no relationship? Next, the P waves should be evaluated. In normal sinus rhythm, the P wave is upright in leads I, II, and III. Tall P waves in lead II indicate right atrial enlargement, whereas prolonged and biphasic P waves sug-

gest left atrial enlargement. The P-R interval should be measured and compared with normal values for age. The duration of the QRS and the QT interval also should be measured, and the QT corrected for heart rate. Machine interpretation of the QT interval never should be trusted. The QRS axis should be determined (Figure 17–6). The presence of normal septal Q waves in leads II, III, aVF, V_5, and V_6 should be sought. The precordial R and S wave amplitudes should be compared against normal values. Finally, the ST segments and T wave pattern should be determined, particularly in the right precordial leads.

The utility of the ECG in the diagnosis of congenital heart disease is largely in the diagnosis of ventricular hypertrophy. Normal newborns have relative predominance of the right ventricle over the left ventricle. This predominance shifts to left ventricular predominance in the first year of life because of the decrease in pulmonary arterial pressure and consequent decrease in right ventricular systolic pressure. All ECG interpretations in children must be made relative to the normal right or left ventricular predominance that exists at that particular age. Therefore, one never interprets a normal newborn ECG as showing "right ventricular hypertrophy, normal for age." Right ventricular hypertrophy at that age would require larger-than-normal right ventricular forces for a newborn. A rough idea of ventricular predominance may be determined by remembering that the right ventricle is oriented to the right, superior, and anterior, whereas the left ventricle is oriented to the left, inferior, and posterior. One chooses leads for examination that represent these orthogonal directions fairly well. Lead V_5 is a good right-left lead, aV_F is a good superior-inferior lead, and V_2 is a good anterior-posterior lead. One may then compare the forces present in these leads with normal standards for age to arrive at a judgment of relative ventricular predominance (Table 17–3). One may also examine the T wave axis as an aid in diagnosing right ventricular hypertrophy, again remembering the normal shift that occurs with development. Normally, the T wave is upright in leads V_1, V_{3R}, and V_{4R} for the first week after birth but inverts by 8 days and remains inverted until about 8 years of age. If it is upright between 8 days and 8 years, right ventricular hypertrophy is likely. Finally, the axis may be an aid to diagnosis in newborns (Figure 17–6).

Unfortunately, with the exception of its use in the diagnosis of arrhythmias, the ECG rarely is diagnostic in the evaluation of the newborn with cardiac disease. Several points deserve emphasis, however. Although one might suppose that a lesion obstructing the left ventricle (eg, aortic coarctation) would produce left ventricular hypertrophy, in the newborn such lesions are seen more often with right ventricular hypertrophy. This is most likely because in the intrauterine circulation, the right ventricle is responsible for a larger amount of the combined ventricular output when the left ventricle is obstructed. The same often is true of lesions obstructing the right ventricle, which may be associated with left ventricular hypertrophy. The ECG picture varies a great deal within each of

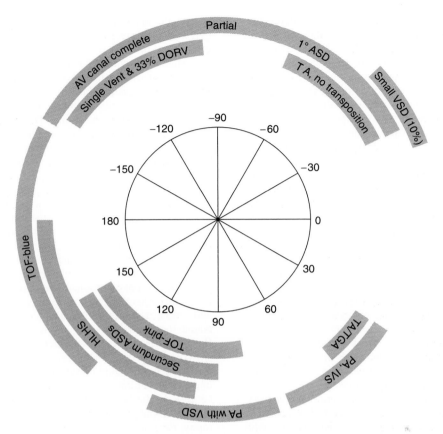

Figure 17–6. Typical frontal plane electrocardiogram axis in children presenting with various congenital heart defects in the newborn period. 1° = primum; ASD = atrial septal defect; AV = atrioventricular; DORV = double-outlet right ventricle; HLHS = hypoplastic left heart syndrome; IVS = intact ventricular septum; PA = pulmonic atresia; TA = tricuspid atresia; TGA = transposition of the great arteries; TOF = tetralogy of Fallot; Vent = ventricle; VSD = ventricular septal defect.

Table 17–3. Normal electrocardiographic voltages by age (95th percentile).

Age	V₅		A_{VF}		V₂	
	R	S	R	S	R	S
0–24 h	18.0	24.0	*	*	28.1	33.8
1–7 d	19.3	16.2	10.5	3.1	31.1	34.1
8–30 d	27.0	12.3	12.4	3.8	29.0	25.7
1–3 mo	20.7	12.7	13.8	3.1	27.4	34.1
3–6 mo	25.5	15.4	18.5	3.4	28.6	26.5
6–12 mo	24.7	8.0	16.4	3.7	24.4	30.1
1–3 y	27.7	7.0	16.6	3.8	22.5	32.1
3–5 y	30.0	5.8	16.7	3.0	22.8	28.8
5–8 y	31.2	6.6	14.8	3.4	22.0	35.3
8–12 y	30.0	4.4	17.8	3.7	16.9	35.6
12–16 y	26.7	5.0	19.7	3.8	18.4	41.0

Reproduced, with permission, from Liebman J et al (editors): Page 61 in: *Pediatric Electrocardiography.* Williams & Wilkins, 1982.

the diagnostic groups, and the ECG pattern may be completely normal in infants with serious disease, such as transposition. In practice, the clinician uses the ECG as a confirmatory test to establish that heart disease is present and that the ECG fits the suspected diagnosis. An example is the pattern seen in infants with complete atrioventricular canal defects, who have an abnormally superior axis in the frontal plane (northwest axis). Consider a child presenting with signs of a VSD, with a loud holosystolic murmur, signs of CHF, and little or no cyanosis at 1 month of age. If the ECG shows the typical abnormally superior axis, the diagnosis is probably atrioventricular canal defect rather than simple VSD.

Pulse Oximetry

Pulse oximetry provides an excellent method for assessing arterial oxygen saturation noninvasively by using a probe attached to the palm or foot in the infant. Even though the measurement of arterial blood gas tension is always useful, pulse oximetry avoids a painful needle stick, which can cause agitation, struggling, and breath-holding, making such direct measurements somewhat unreliable. Measurements should always be made from the right hand and from a foot to provide information about ductus arteriosus flow patterns. For example, patients with severe aortic coarctation or interruption and a PDA providing flow from the pulmonary artery to the descending aorta have a much lower saturation in the feet than in the hands. On the other hand, patients with transposition may have a much higher saturation in the feet than the hands, because pulmonary arterial blood is highly saturated and passes from the pulmonary artery into the ductus and descending aorta. To avoid problems created by intermachine variability, it is helpful to use two machines simultaneously and then switch the leads. The final reading is the average difference between the upper and lower extremity readings.

Hyperoxic Test

The hyperoxic test is a method to help differentiate blood oxygen desaturation due to cardiac disease from that due to pulmonary disease. It does not distinguish this difference alone, however, and always should be interpreted in the context of all other data. Right-arm and lower-body measurements always should be made simultaneously to evaluate the pattern of ductus arteriosus shunting. Pulse oximetry is sufficient if the saturation measures less than 92–93%; otherwise, an arterial blood gas should be obtained. Measurements are made at baseline conditions, ideally room air, and then after breathing 100% oxygen for approximately 5 minutes. Patients with pulmonary disease alone usually have an increase in partial pressure of oxygen (Po_2) greater than 20–30 mm Hg or an increase in oxygen saturation greater than 10%. Those with a fixed right-to-left shunt may have a small increase in oxygenation, but it usually is less than these amounts. The term **fixed right-to-left shunt** refers to lesions in which no increase is possible in either pulmonary blood flow or in mixing of systemic and pulmonary venous return. In such patients, therefore, pulmonary venous blood is already nearly completely oxygenated, and little additional oxygenation is possible. A good example is TOF, in which there is a high resistance to pulmonary flow because of PS and a right-to-left shunt through a VSD. Patients with large left-to-right shunts and systemic hypoxemia may have large increases in oxygenation because added inspired oxygen normalizes pulmonary venous saturation, which may be low because of pulmonary edema and the accompanying oxygen diffusion gradient. Patients with mixing of pulmonary and systemic venous return and no obstruction to pulmonary flow may also have a large increase in oxygen saturation because additional inspired oxygen may cause a large increase in pulmonary venous Po_2. In addition, oxygen may cause pulmonary vasodilation and a further increase in pulmonary blood flow. The best example of this phenomenon is total anomalous pulmonary venous return (TAPVR) without obstruction, in which there is a large amount of pulmonary flow, but cyanosis is present because of mixing

that occurs in the right atrium. Supplemental inspired oxygen may increase arterial saturation somewhat. The same effect may be seen with the use of pulmonary vasodilators, such as prostaglandin E_1 (PGE_1).

A variant of this test involves repeating the measurements while making the child cry. This is particularly helpful at increasing differential saturation caused by right-to-left shunting through a PDA. If either the upper or lower body is predominantly supplied by ductal flow, the saturation usually will decrease, whereas the other saturation (that supplied by pulmonary venous blood) will remain stable.

Echocardiography

Cardiac ultrasonography is the definitive diagnostic method for the evaluation of infants with suspected cardiac disease. It is noninvasive and safe, can be done at the bedside of sick newborn infants, and can be used successfully in premature infants of all sizes. The resolution is sufficient to make complete anatomic diagnoses in even the smallest hearts. The use of Doppler echocardiography and, more recently, color Doppler flow mapping has added the ability to study intracardiac and extracardiac flow patterns for the assessment of valve function and sites of obstruction. The quality of the diagnostic information is such that many infants who previously would have undergone cardiac catheterization now undergo cardiac surgery on the basis of the echocardiogram alone. There are two important issues to note concerning echocardiography. First, it is expensive; therefore, it cannot be used in every infant with the slightest suspicion of cardiac disease. Patients must be recommended for echocardiography on the basis of a cardiac evaluation, including physical examination, oxygen saturation measurement, and other modalities. Second, echocardiography must be guided by a knowledge of the infant's presenting signs and the results of the evaluation to date. Knowing the patient's clinical status allows the experienced echocardiographer to have an appropriate differential diagnosis and ensure a complete and accurate examination. Otherwise, important and often subtle findings may be missed.

Echocardiography is now also used to guide both interventional catheterization and surgical procedures. Many institutions now routinely perform balloon septostomy for D-transposition or other lesions under echocardiographic guidance rather than catheterization. In addition, the advent of transesophageal echocardiography allows evaluation of detailed anatomy in the operative suite and has decreased the incidence of postoperative residual defects substantially by allowing immediate assessment of the surgical repair.

Catheterization

The need for cardiac catheterization to diagnose cardiac defects has decreased dramatically, as the accuracy of ultrasound technology has allowed for more complete noninvasive initial evaluation. Certain features, however, remain beyond the scope of echocardiography, such as measurement of vascular pressures and accurate shunt flows. In addition, the peripheral pulmonary vasculature is best viewed by angiography. Finally, postoperative evaluation often includes catheterization because scarring can impair ultrasound examination. Recently, therapeutic catheterization has become very successful at correcting or palliating several conditions previously amenable only to surgical therapy. Valvar aortic and pulmonary stenosis are best treated initially with balloon valvuloplasty performed in the catheterization laboratory. Closure of PDA in nonpremature infants is accomplished easily, with minimal expense and hospital stay, by using implantable coils. Closure of intracardiac defects with devices delivered percutaneously remains experimental.

Catheterization can be performed safely at any age. In newborn infants, the umbilical vessels provide ready access to both the venous and arterial circulation. When this route is unavailable, arterial access in infants is associated with increased risk of pulse loss. Currently, few patients require intubation and mechanical ventilation for catheterization.

COMMON PROBLEMS

INFANT WITH CYANOSIS

Cyanosis is a bluish discoloration of the skin and mucous membranes caused by deoxygenated or reduced hemoglobin (for a detailed discussion, see Chapter 4). It is crucial to determine the cause of cyanosis in a newborn rapidly, as it often can be life-threatening. Initial assessment should include evaluation of the extent and location of cyanosis (central versus peripheral), heart rate, presence and intensity of pulses, blood pressure, respiratory rate, and presence of respiratory distress. This evaluation, together with a few laboratory studies, can pinpoint the cause of the cyanosis (Figure 17–7).

Peripheral cyanosis refers to the skin, particularly the extremities, whereas **central cyanosis** refers to involve-

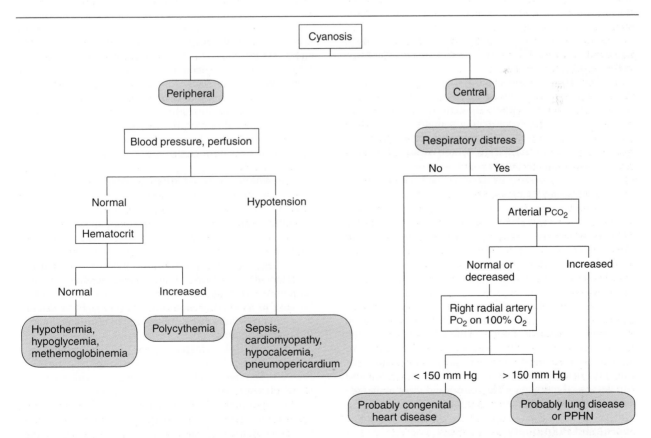

Figure 17–7. Algorithm showing evaluation of infants with cyanosis. Pco_2 = partial pressure of carbon dioxide; PPHN = persistent pulmonary hypertension of the newborn; Po_2 = partial pressure of oxygen.

ment of the mucous membranes of the mouth and tongue. Skin color in newborns is very sensitive to changes in temperature and arterial or venous vasoconstriction. Isolated peripheral cyanosis is not associated with structural heart disease but can be caused by low cardiac output with decreased peripheral perfusion, as with sepsis, cardiomyopathy, hypocalcemia, or pneumopericardium. It can be caused by decreased peripheral perfusion with normal cardiac output, eg, with hypoglycemia or hypothermia. In addition, abnormally high amounts of deoxygenated hemoglobin in the blood, eg, with polycythemia or methemoglobinemia, may cause profound peripheral cyanosis.

Central cyanosis suggests hypoxia due to lung disease or structural heart disease resulting in some degree of right-to-left shunting. Differentiating between these two can be difficult. Any infant with significant central cyanosis and no respiratory distress has structural heart disease until proved otherwise. Severe polycythemia or methemoglobinemia can present this way, although it would be unusual. If the infant has respiratory distress and tachypnea, with or without retractions, a blood gas should be obtained from either the right radial or temporal artery. Significant elevation in partial pressure of arterial carbon dioxide ($Paco_2$) suggests lung disease, but if the $Paco_2$ is normal or only mildly elevated, a hyperoxia test should be performed. The infant should be placed in 100% oxygen, and simultaneous blood gases drawn from both the right radial and pedal (or umbilical) arteries. If the Pao_2 is greater than 150 mm Hg in the right radial (or temporal) arterial blood, structural heart disease is extremely unlikely.

If the initial evaluation suggests that central cyanosis is due to structural heart disease, treatment with IV fluids (80 mL/kg/d) and PGE_1 (0.05 µg/kg/min) should be initiated, as should consultation with a pediatric cardiologist. PGE_1 is a potent vasodilator, and infants often need an IV fluid bolus of 10–20 mL/kg crystalloid at its initiation to maintain an adequate intravascular volume. In addition, because PGE_1 may cause apnea, intubation with mechanical ventilation may be necessary. Oxygen should be given in nontoxic doses ($\leq$ 60% Fio_2) to minimize any associated lung disease; one should remember, however, oxygen will have little effect on cyanosis because of right-to-left shunting from structural heart disease. Metabolic acidosis should be corrected first with adequate fluid administration; if there is no response, IV sodium bicarbonate should be given.

Once treatment has been initiated, a more definitive diagnosis of the type of congenital heart disease can be made with further evaluation, including a chest radiograph and ECG (Figure 17–8). In general, infants who have cyanosis as their most prominent presenting feature for congenital heart disease fall into one of two groups: those with decreased pulmonary blood flow and those with normal or increased pulmonary blood flow.

Decreased Pulmonary Blood Flow

Pulmonary blood flow may be reduced in lesions associated with obstruction on the right side of the heart, such as atresia, hypoplasia, or stenosis of either the pulmonary arteries, pulmonary valve, right ventricle, or tricuspid valve. These patients all have in common decreased pulmonary blood flow on chest radiograph and obligatory right-to-left shunting across either the atrial or ventricular septum causing cyanosis. These lesions include pulmonary atresia with an intact ventricular septum (PA/IVS) or with a VSD (PA/VSD), critical valvar PS, single ventricle with associated subvalvar or valvar PS (SV with PS), TOF, tricuspid atresia (TA), and the Ebstein anomaly (dysplastic tricuspid valve resulting in insufficiency, and subvalvar PS).

ECG findings can differentiate this group further. Infants with TOF, PS, or PA/VSD have findings of right ventricular hypertrophy and right axis deviation (> 120 degrees).

Tetralogy of Fallot. TOF consists of four main features: PS, a large VSD, right ventricular hypertrophy, and dextroposition of the aorta so that it overrides the septal defect. The PS causes a systolic murmur that is easily audible over the left upper sternal border. Because of the large, unrestrictive VSD and the overriding aorta, there is significant right-to-left shunting through the ventricular septum, causing cyanosis. Patients may present late with hypercyanotic episodes, known as "tetralogy spells," in which vigorous crying results in increasing cyanosis because of reduced pulmonary blood flow. Hypercyanotic spells are treated acutely with administration of oxygen, morphine for sedation, and phenylephrine to increase systemic vascular resistance. PA with VSD is similar to TOF except that all pulmonary flow comes from either the ductus arteriosus or from aorta to pulmonary artery collateral vessels. Therefore, instead of a systolic PS murmur at the left upper sternal border, there may be a continuous murmur under the left clavicle or over the back because of continuous flow through the ductus arteriosus or collateral arterial circulation.

Pulmonary Valve Stenosis & Atresia. Infants with critical pulmonary valve stenosis have a systolic murmur over the left upper sternal border and may be profoundly cyanotic because of right-to-left shunting at the atrial level as the ductus arteriosus closes. Severe right ventricular hypertension, much greater than systemic levels, may result in tricuspid regurgitation. The treatment of choice is catheter balloon dilation of the stenotic valve. Infants may remain mildly cyanotic for several weeks after treatment because of slow regression of the severe right ventricular hypertrophy, which causes persistent right-to-left shunting through the foramen ovale.

An axis of 0–120 degrees on the ECG with evidence of left ventricular hypertrophy suggests the diagnosis of PA/IVS. The right ventricle is hypoplastic with no egress, so the pressure commonly is suprasystemic, leading to tricuspid regurgitation, which may produce a high-pitched systolic murmur at the left lower sternal border. Cyanosis is due to right-to-left shunting through the atrial septum, and pulmonary blood flow is supplied by a PDA. Sinusoidal vessels may connect the right ventricle with the

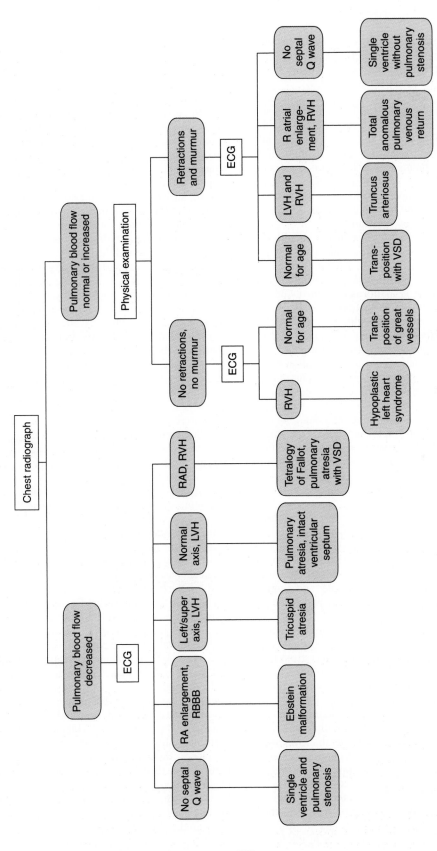

Figure 17–8. Algorithm of approach to specific diagnosis in infants with cyanotic congenital heart diseases. ECG = electrocardiogram; LVH = left ventricular hypertrophy; RAD = right axis deviation; RBBB = right bundle-branch block; RVH = right ventricular hypertrophy; VSD = ventricular septal defect.

coronary arteries; this may limit the surgical options and ultimate prognosis. The initial treatment is to increase pulmonary blood flow with PGE$_1$; then, a surgical shunt from the systemic to pulmonary artery is performed.

Tricuspid Atresia. The ECG in infants with TA shows a leftward superior axis (0 to −90) and left ventricular hypertrophy. Because these infants have no communication between their right atrium and right ventricle, all systemic venous blood crosses the atrial septum and mixes with pulmonary venous blood. TA often is associated with PS or a restrictive VSD, so pulmonary flow is obstructed. The initial treatment is to increase pulmonary blood flow with prostaglandin infusion; then, an AP communication should be achieved surgically.

Ebstein Anomaly. The Ebstein anomaly should be suspected if the ECG shows right bundle-branch block with right atrial enlargement. Up to 30% of patients will have delta waves suggestive of Wolff-Parkinson-White syndrome. The tricuspid valve is malformed, with displacement of the septal and posterior leaflets into the right ventricle. This results in tricuspid regurgitation, particularly in the newborn infant with high pulmonary artery pressures. As pulmonary pressures decrease during the first week after birth, cyanosis and tricuspid regurgitation may resolve. Almost the entire right ventricle may be part of the right atrium ("atrialized"), resulting in severe tricuspid regurgitation. The displaced leaflet may obstruct the right ventricular outflow tract, further limiting pulmonary blood flow and increasing the right-to-left shunt across the atrial septum. These patients require a surgical systemic-to-pulmonary shunt to maintain adequate pulmonary blood flow.

Normal or Increased Pulmonary Blood Flow

The second group of infants with cyanotic congenital heart disease comprises those with normal to increased pulmonary blood flow. Pulmonary and systemic venous blood mixes within the heart chambers. These conditions include transposition of the great arteries, truncus arteriosus, TAPVR, hypoplastic left heart syndrome, and single ventricle. They can be differentiated easily by physical examination and ECG findings (Figure 17–8).

Transposition of the Great Arteries. Infants with transposition of the great arteries, in which the aorta arises from the right ventricle and the pulmonary artery from the left ventricle, have a normal ECG for age and often no audible murmur. Because the desaturated systemic venous blood is delivered directly to the aorta, these infants can be profoundly cyanotic unless they have mixing of their saturated pulmonary venous blood through either an atrial or VSD or a PDA. If there is considerable mixing, cyanosis may not be marked; if mixing is minimal, severe cyanosis occurs. In the immediate newborn period, PGE$_1$ may relieve cyanosis by opening the ductus. Emergency management of a profoundly cyanotic infant with transposition of the great arteries involves tearing a hole in the atrial septum by performing a balloon atrial septostomy. The cardiologist may do this procedure either at the bed-

side with the use of ultrasound guidance or in the catheterization laboratory. Definitive treatment is a surgical switch of the pulmonary artery and aorta so that they arise from the correct ventricles.

Truncus Arteriosus Communis. In truncus arteriosus, there is no pulmonary valve. The pulmonary artery arises directly from the aorta (trunk) just above the aortic (truncal) valve, which straddles a large VSD. Complete mixing occurs in the proximal ascending aorta, causing cyanosis. The ECG typically shows biventricular hypertrophy, and there may be a loud systolic click on examination because of the large anterior abnormal aortic (truncal) valve. Definitive treatment for these patients is surgical correction, consisting of closure of the VSD and placement of an artificial pulmonary artery and valve between the right ventricle and the branch pulmonary arteries.

Total Anomalous Pulmonary Venous Return. Infants with TAPVR typically have right atrial enlargement and right ventricular hypertrophy on ECG. The chest radiograph characteristically shows a normal heart size with pulmonary edema, which is often severe. The pulmonary veins, instead of entering the left atrium normally, form a confluence behind the left atrium and drain to the right atrium. This may be via a vertical vein to the left innominate vein; to the superior vena cava, coronary sinus, or right atrium directly; or via a common pulmonary vein, which descends below the diaphragm and joins with the inferior vena cava via a portal vein and the ductus venosus. Complete mixing takes place in the right atrium with right-to-left shunting through the foramen ovale to fill the left ventricle and maintain an adequate cardiac output. If there is obstruction to the pulmonary venous return, as is almost always present with veins draining below the diaphragm, cyanosis is very prominent because of both complete mixing and respiratory distress associated with pulmonary edema. If the hole in the atrial septum is restrictive, the left ventricle cannot fill and cardiac output will be compromised. Definitive treatment of TAPVR is surgical anastomosis of the pulmonary vein confluence directly to the left atrium.

Hypoplastic Left Heart Syndrome. Hypoplastic left heart syndrome can also present with cyanosis if the ductus arteriosus remains open. Because there is obstruction at the mitral valve/hypoplastic left ventricle, all pulmonary venous blood shunts through the atrial septum to mix in the right atrium. Total systemic blood flow is derived through the ductus arteriosus from the pulmonary artery. If the ductus arteriosus is open, the patient will have normal pulses and a normal examination except for cyanosis. The ECG shows right ventricular hypertrophy with markedly decreased left-sided voltages. As the ductus closes, these infants present with shock because systemic blood flow is reduced. Oxygen administration may result in ductus arteriosus constriction and therefore must be used with caution in these infants. Treatment options include a series of two or three palliative surgeries to create a single ventricle physiology or heart transplantation.

Single Ventricle. Infants with a single ventricle typically have an associated ASD as well as atrioventricular valve abnormalities; therefore, mixing occurs both at the atrial and ventricular levels. ECG findings vary but always show an absence of the normal Q wave in the lateral chest leads (V_6 and V_7), indicating the absence of a ventricular septum. Infants may have associated valvar or subvalvar PS, causing reduced pulmonary flow, or no associated stenosis with markedly increased pulmonary flow. Initial treatment is determined by the amount of pulmonary blood flow. For infants with too much pulmonary blood flow, pulmonary artery band surgery is performed to reduce flow. For those with too little pulmonary blood flow, a shunt is placed from the aorta to the pulmonary artery to augment flow.

INFANT WITH SHOCK

Shock is defined as the inability to generate sufficient cardiac output to meet tissue metabolic needs. In the face of inadequate output, the peripheral vasculature constricts to shunt blood to the crucial central organs. This results in a profound decrease in peripheral circulation. As cells convert to anaerobic metabolism, lactate is generated, resulting in acidemia. Profound acidemia can compromise cardiac output further, initiating a dangerous cycle that results in severe organ failure and, eventually, death.

When presented with an infant in shock, the clinician should consider sepsis first and treat the infant accordingly until another cause becomes evident. Initial management should be directed toward the "ABCs," (*A*irway, *B*reathing, *C*irculation), including 100% oxygen administration, aggressive fluid management, and correction of acidosis (see Chapter 10). Cardiac involvement should be considered if appropriate fluid resuscitation does not result in improvement (Figure 17–9). **Hepatomegaly** suggests poor cardiac function associated with either primary cardiac disease or impaired cardiac function secondary to metabolic derangement. The liver in infants is an excellent general indicator of volume status and cardiac output. In general, shock in an infant with sepsis is associated with profound intravascular volume depletion, caused by a combination of dehydration and vasodilatation, requiring large amounts of volume resuscitation. The cardiac output in these infants initially is normal or increased. As a result, the liver usually is not palpable. An enlarged liver suggests volume overload or impaired cardiac function, often both. In this situation, a cardiac etiology of shock should be considered. As described above, severe acidemia can impair cardiac function. Therefore, hepatomegaly can develop in infants with profound acidemia associated with sepsis because of poor cardiac function. Even in these patients, however, hepatomegaly is an indication for inotropic support of cardiac function, as opposed to further volume resuscitation. **Cardiomegaly** also suggests cardiogenic shock, particularly in patients with myocarditis or cardiomyopathy, who often have a heart that appears to fill the entire chest.

Left Heart Obstruction. The most common cardiac cause of shock is **left heart obstruction** (see Figure 17–9). An infant with obstruction to left ventricular inflow or outflow can decompensate rapidly if systemic output is dependent on the right ventricle via the ductus arteriosus. As the ductus arteriosus closes, systemic blood flow is compromised, and shock develops. The major clinical findings in these infants are **decreased or absent peripheral pulses,** either globally or in the lower extremities, and hepatomegaly. **Differential cyanosis** may be present, suggesting that the ductus arteriosus is partially patent and supporting the systemic output from the right ventricle via the pulmonary artery. Murmurs may be audible, which can be suggestive either of outflow obstruction (systolic murmur at the left sternal border) or of inflow obstruction (diastolic murmur at the apex). The ECG usually shows right ventricular hypertrophy with decreased left-sided forces because of the persistence of fetal right ventricular dominance. ST and T wave changes may occur in the left precordial leads.

Children with shock due to left heart obstruction represent a spectrum, from hypoplastic left heart syndrome to simple coarctation of the aorta. All present with shock when the ductus arteriosus closes. After initiation of PGE_1, evaluation, including chest radiograph and ECG, can further delineate the specific diagnosis.

Hypoplastic Left Heart Syndrome. In this condition, there is severe stenosis of both the mitral and aortic valves, often with atresia of both valves and a very small left ventricle. The left ventricle has no effective output; therefore, all left atrial blood must cross the atrial septum and mix with systemic venous return, resulting in oxygen desaturation. The entire output, both systemic and pulmonary, is supplied by the right ventricle. If the ductus arteriosus is open, these patients have normal pulses and examination except for arterial O_2 desaturation. Physical examination is often unremarkable, but a third heart sound may be heard because of the high flow through the tricuspid valve. There is no differential in pulses or O_2 saturation between upper and lower extremities. The chest radiograph often is unremarkable but can show a relatively small heart with increased pulmonary vascularity. The ECG shows right ventricular hypertrophy with markedly decreased left-sided voltages. When the ductus arteriosus closes, systemic blood flow cannot be maintained, and weak pulses with pallor develop; because of inadequate blood flow and oxygen to the tissues, metabolic acidosis results. Treatment options include a series of two or three palliative surgeries to create a single ventricle physiology or heart transplantation.

Aortic Stenosis. In AS, there is a variable degree of obstruction to left ventricular outflow. When the obstruction is moderate to severe, the ventricle is unable to provide adequate cardiac output through the dysplastic, usually monocuspid, valve. Physical examination often shows differential O_2 saturation, associated with ductal supply to the lower body, but may not show pulse differential because there is no aortic obstruction. Auscultation shows a

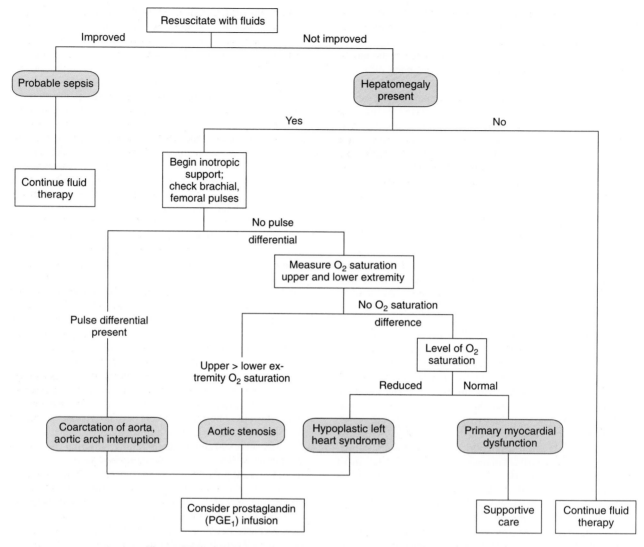

Figure 17–9. Algorithm of assessment and approach to infants with shock.

systolic ejection murmur at the left sternal border, which can radiate to the neck, and there may be a thrill in the suprasternal notch. Chest radiograph may show cardiomegaly. The ECG usually shows right ventricular hypertrophy. Definitive treatment usually involves balloon valvuloplasty performed at cardiac catheterization. If this cannot be achieved, surgical relief of the obstruction is indicated.

Aortic Arch Interruption. This results when the normal left fourth fetal aortic arch abnormally regresses. Right-arm and head blood flows are provided by the left ventricle, whereas left-arm and lower-body flows depend entirely on the ductus arteriosus. Physical examination often reveals a systolic murmur at the left sternal border. Upper/lower body O_2 saturation differences usually are present, and pressure differences develop when the ductus arteriosus constricts. Chest radiograph may show a narrow upper mediastinum because the thymus often is absent. Aortic arch interruption frequently is associated with the DiGeorge syndrome of absent thymus and parathyroid glands. Hypocalcemia and immune deficiency may be important features. ECG findings often are indistinguishable from those with other left heart obstructions but can show normal or increased left forces, particularly after the immediate newborn period. Surgical correction of the interruption is required.

Coarctation of the Aorta. This is the most common obstructive lesion of the left side of the heart. A ledge or ring of tissue is present just distal to the left subclavian artery opposite the ductus arteriosus. Patients may be asymptomatic, except for a higher upper body blood pressure when the obstruction is mild. Newborn infants are asymptomatic until the ductus closes but can have decreased lower body O_2 saturation, particularly when crying. As the ductus closes, the lower-extremity pulses are decreased or absent. Auscultation often shows a systolic murmur at the upper right sternal border, because 40–60% of patients also have a bicuspid aortic valve. The chest radiograph of infants usually is normal until the ductus closes; however, if left ventricular failure develops, cardiomegaly occurs. The ECG usually shows right ventricular hypertrophy during infancy but may show biventricular hypertrophy. The standard treatment has been surgical resection of the narrowing, but balloon arterioplasty is equally effective beyond the early newborn period.

Myocardial Lesions. Patients with myocarditis, cardiomyopathy, or coronary anomalies may present with shock because of very poor cardiac function, but more commonly present with CHF after the first months postnatally (see below, Child With Respiratory Distress/Congestive Heart Failure). Initial treatment is supportive and includes inotropic support and mechanical left ventricular assist if necessary.

Myocardial Dysfunction. This is the second major cardiac cause of shock. Myocardial dysfunction has many causes; severe anemia and acidemia are two of the more common causes. Viral myocarditis and cardiomyopathy represent the major causes of cardiogenic shock in infants. These infants present with shock, poor peripheral pulses and perfusion, acidemia, pulmonary edema, severe cardiomegaly, and hepatomegaly. The presenting features are not substantially different from those of left heart obstruction. The ECG may show a lack of ventricular hypertrophy and classically shows low voltages in the setting of myocarditis or severe biventricular hypertrophy in patients with hypertrophic cardiomyopathy (HCM).

When cardiogenic shock is considered in an infant, initial management should be directed toward supporting the cardiac output, correcting any metabolic defects, and opening the ductus arteriosus. An IV infusion of dopamine or dobutamine (5–10 µg/kg/min) or epinephrine (0.05–0.10 µg/kg/min) should be initiated, and the dose titrated to achieve an adequate cardiac output and blood pressure. Calcium should also be considered to increase the strength of cardiac contraction; this is of particular importance in preterm infants in whom hypocalcemia may occur. Sodium bicarbonate should be administered to correct any acidosis; anemia, if present, should be treated with packed red blood cells. PGE_1 should be administered (0.05 µg/kg/min) to maintain ductus arteriosus patency if left-sided obstruction is suspected. A pediatric cardiologist should be consulted.

INFANT WITH RESPIRATORY DISTRESS

Two major cardiac pathophysiologies should be considered in an infant who presents with respiratory distress.

Increased pulmonary arterial flow causes transudation of fluid into the interstitium, thereby decreasing lung compliance and increasing the work of breathing. As a result, the infant becomes tachypneic and dyspneic. As the course progresses, alveolar fluid may accumulate, further increasing the work of breathing and resulting in retractions. The main cardiac cause of increased pulmonary arterial flow in an infant is a left-to-right shunt, either intracardiac or at the level of the great artery. **Pulmonary venous congestion,** an increase in pulmonary venous and capillary pressure, results in interstitial fluid accumulation and respiratory distress. Pulmonary venous congestion is due mainly to elevated left atrial pressure, either from poor cardiac function or from obstruction to left ventricular inflow (see Shock, above).

In an infant with respiratory distress, it can be difficult to distinguish cardiac disease from pulmonary disease. In both instances, tachypnea and retractions are usually present. The child with cardiac disease usually has a hyperactive, often visible, precordial impulse, indicating an increased volume load on the heart. The chest radiograph will not show focal infiltrates or atelectasis but usually shows cardiomegaly, with increased pulmonary arterial markings. The ECG is helpful, in that most patients with respiratory distress have right ventricular hypertrophy. The causes of respiratory distress generally fall into three categories: arterial runoff into either the pulmonary or venous system, complete intracardiac mixing with no restriction to pulmonary blood flow, and obligate left-to-right shunting. An obligate shunt is defined as one that is not dependent on a decrease in pulmonary resistance, eg, a communication between the left ventricle and right atrium, or between a systemic artery and vein.

Initial treatment of respiratory distress is always supportive. The ABCs of initial resuscitation should always be followed (see Chapter 10). Oxygen should be administered, although it may not improve the pulmonary venous desaturation if pulmonary edema is marked. Diuretics will decrease interstitial pulmonary fluid, thus decreasing the work of breathing. When the distress is severe, mechanical ventilation should be considered. In addition to removing the work of breathing from the patient, positive pressure ventilation will also help to decrease alveolar edema. Inotropic agents, such as digoxin, may not be necessary in the acute setting but may improve symptoms if severe. In premature infants, the use of indomethacin to close a PDA should be considered. In severely symptomatic infants, IV inotropic agents, such as dopamine or dobutamine, may be indicated.

When cardiac disease is considered, initial evaluation of the arterial pulses can begin to distinguish various defects. Bounding pulses and a wide pulse pressure indicate a runoff from the arterial system, either into the pulmonary arteries, as occurs in truncus arteriosus, AP window, or large PDA, or into the venous system from an AV malformation (Figure 17–10). In atrioventricular canal defect, "single ventricle" defects, and TAPVR, there is no arterial runoff; therefore, the pulses are normal or decreased.

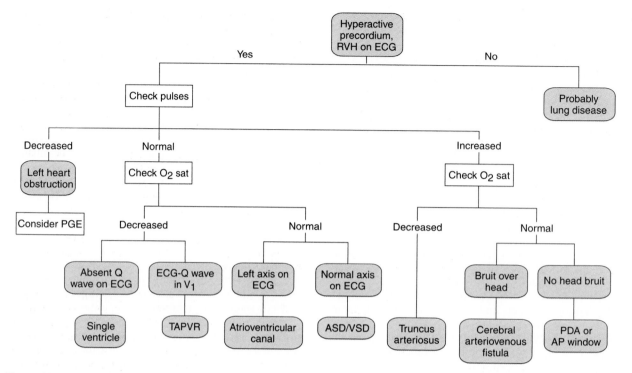

Figure 17–10. Algorithm showing approach in evaluating infants with respiratory distress. AP = aortopulmonary; ASD = atrial septal defect; ECG = electrocardiogram; PDA = patent ductus arteriosus; PGE = prostaglandin E; RVH = right ventricular hypertrophy; TAPVR = total anomalous pulmonary venous return.

The arterial saturation distinguishes lesions that include a right-to-left, as well as left-to-right shunt, from those with a pure left-to-right shunt. A patient with bounding pulses and arterial desaturation most likely has truncus arteriosus. Infants with AP window, PDA, and AV malformation usually have normal arterial saturation. In the patient with AV malformation, a bruit often is heard over the area of the malformation. Patients with total pulmonary venous return, complex heart disease, and "single ventricle" physiology have normal pulses and O_2 desaturation, whereas infants with atrioventricular canal or large atrial and ventricular defects usually are fully saturated.

Although the ECG usually shows right ventricular hypertrophy, it can be helpful in the differential diagnosis. A left or indeterminate axis is seen in AV canal defects, common in infants with Down syndrome but not in atrial and ventricular defects. Children with TAPVR often have a Q wave in the right chest leads indicative of severe right ventricular hypertrophy, whereas those with single ventricle often have an absence of Q waves throughout the precordium because of an absent or very abnormally placed ventricular septum.

Total Anomalous Pulmonary Venous Return. In TAPVR, the pulmonary veins do not enter the left atrium normally; rather, they form a confluence behind the left atrium and drain to the right atrium. The infant with TAPVR and obstruction to pulmonary venous return presents with severe cyanosis (see Cyanosis, above). Without obstruction, the presentation is respiratory distress with mild desaturation. There is a large increase in pulmonary blood flow, resulting in respiratory distress, and complete mixing, producing desaturation. The physical examination shows a hyperactive precordium with a widely split S_2. The chest radiograph shows cardiomegaly and can show a "snowman" appearance. This characteristic picture is seen in TAPVR via a vertical vein and is caused by enlargement of the vertical vein and superior vena cava above the heart. ECG typically shows right atrial enlargement and right ventricular hypertrophy. Definitive treatment is surgical anastomosis of the pulmonary vein confluence directly to the left atrium.

Atrioventricular Canal Defect. This is a common cardiac defect, particularly in Down syndrome, being present in approximately 20% of these children. Atrioventricular canal defect forms as a result of failure of fusion of the endocardial cushions, structures normally responsible for separation of the common atrioventricular valve into tricuspid and mitral valves and for septation of the lower portion of the atria and upper posterior portion of the ventricles. As a result, children with this defect have a large common defect involving both the atria and ventricles. In addition, a single atrioventricular valve with five leaflets often is present. The combination of large atrial and ventricular defects results in a large left-to-right shunt and also can result in almost complete mixing of pulmonary and systemic venous blood. Physical examination shows a loud S_1 caused by closure of the valve and can show a holosystolic murmur of atrioventricular valve insufficiency, commonly present in this lesion. Pulmonary hypertension often results, and the S_2 also is increased. Chest radiograph shows cardiomegaly, often out of proportion to the degree of vascular markings. The ECG is often characteristic, with a "northwest" axis (180–270 degrees). Biventricular hypertrophy often is present. Surgical correction usually is required and is performed at 3–6 months of age.

Truncus Arteriosus. In this defect, there is no pulmonary valve. The pulmonary artery arises directly from the aorta (trunk) just above the aortic (truncal) valve, which straddles a large VSD. Complete mixing occurs in the proximal ascending aorta causing cyanosis. Because pulmonary resistance is lower than systemic, pulmonary flow is increased, causing respiratory distress. Children most commonly present in the first weeks postnatally. Physical examination shows a loud, single S_2, often with an ejection click, and a continuous murmur due to flow through the pulmonary arteries. Systolic and diastolic murmur caused by stenosis and insufficiency of the common valve also may be heard. The pulses usually are bounding because of the large aortic runoff. The ECG typically shows biventricular hypertrophy. Definitive treatment for these patients is surgical correction consisting of closure of the VSD and placement of an artificial pulmonary artery and valve between the right ventricle and the branch pulmonary arteries.

Aortopulmonary Window & Arteriovenous Malformation. Other types of arterial communications, such as AP window and AV malformation, are uncommon. AP window is a large communication between the ascending aorta and main pulmonary artery, just above the valve level. It usually occurs as an isolated defect. AV malformations are abnormal vessels that bypass the capillary bed, providing a very–low-resistance communication between the arterial and venous systems. They occur most commonly in the brain, liver, and skin. In both these lesions, there is an increased pulmonary blood flow but no mixing; therefore, arterial O_2 saturation is normal. Physical examination shows bounding pulses from arterial runoff. In AV malformation, a bruit may be heard over the anterior fontanelle or the liver. Patients with AP window have a loud systolic murmur, which can be mistaken for a VSD. In patients with AV malformation in the brain, chest radiograph may show enlargement of the superior vena cava, whereas in AP window findings usually are not specific. The ECG will show right ventricular hypertrophy. Treatment of both lesions is surgical: AP windows can be corrected by closing the defect, whereas AV malformations require embolization of the abnormal vessels, which are often multiple.

Single Ventricle. Patients with many different complex congenital defects can be grouped into what is termed **single ventricle physiology.** This includes lesions such as double-inlet left ventricle, in which both atrioventricular valves feed into the left ventricle, and double-outlet right ventricle, in which both the aorta and pulmonary artery arise from the right ventricle. In all these complex lesions, the physiology is that of a single atrium and ventricle, which results in complete mixing of pulmonary and systemic venous return. Systemic and pulmonary blood flows are determined by the relative resistances in these circulations. When there is no right-sided obstruction, the pulmonary flow is increased, often two to three times normal. These children present as early as the first week after birth with respiratory distress. Oxygen saturation is decreased because of complete mixing, often to 88–93% in room air. Physical examination can be deceptively normal. Some patients have dextrocardia, a clue to the severity of their disease. Likewise, the chest radiograph is not diagnostic but shows cardiomegaly. ECG may show an ectopic atrial rhythm, or various degrees of atrioventricular block. There often is right ventricular or combined ventricular hypertrophy. For infants with increased pulmonary blood flow, a pulmonary arterial banding procedure is performed. For those with too little pulmonary blood flow, a shunt is placed from the aorta to the pulmonary artery to augment flow.

Large intracardiac shunts, such as a combination of a larger ASD and moderate or large VSD, can present with distress very early, within the first weeks. The systolic shunt of the VSD increases the diastolic shunt of the ASD to produce a rapid increase in pulmonary arterial flow. Finally, milder forms of left heart obstruction can present with respiratory distress as a primary symptom. More commonly, poor perfusion is present (see above). Mild coarctation of the aorta and AS can result in elevated left atrial pressure and, thus, pulmonary venous pressure, resulting in pulmonary edema and distress.

ASYMPTOMATIC MURMUR

Innocent Murmurs

Asymptomatic murmurs in children are extremely common. The challenge for the pediatrician is to determine whether the murmur signifies cardiac disease and, if so, which evaluation and treatment are necessary. Innocent or "normal" murmurs occur in approximately 30–50% of children. They are heard most often in young school-aged children but are not infrequent in infants or adolescents. A heart murmur noted in the first 24 hours after birth carries a 1:12 risk of congenital heart disease; one heard first at 6 months, a 1:7 risk; and one heard first at 12 months, only a 1:50 risk. However, if a murmur detected at birth persists for 12 months, the risk of congenital heart disease is 3:5. Innocent murmurs usually can be recognized with the use of skilled auscultation and bedside maneuvers without the need for extensive and expensive diagnostic testing.

Innocent murmurs have several general characteristics that set them apart from murmurs associated with cardiac disease (Table 17–4). With the exception of the venous hum, which is continuous, innocent murmurs occur only in systole and tend to be short, peaking in the first half of systole. They usually are soft, rarely greater than a grade 2 (on a scale of 1 to 6) in intensity and tend to be well localized. Again with the exception of the venous hum, there are no innocent thrills. The most common innocent heart murmurs are described below.

Still Murmur. This vibratory, musical, medium-frequency, grade 1–2, systolic ejection murmur is localized midway between the left lower sternal border and the apex. It decreases in intensity with inspiration and upright position and increases with exercise, excitement, or fever. It is most commonly heard in children aged 2–7 years. It appears to originate in the left ventricle and may be related to vibrations of false chordae tendineae, although this remains controversial.

Innocent Pulmonary Ejection Murmur. This high-frequency, grade 1–2, crescendo-decrescendo systolic ejection murmur is well localized to the second left intercostal space along the sternal border. It is louder when the patient is supine and is accentuated by exercise, excitement, and fever. The murmur usually disappears immediately with the Valsalva maneuver. This murmur is identical in quality with the murmur of an ASD, except that it is associated with a normal second heart sound. It is caused by relatively high velocity flow in the pulmonary artery and proximity of the pulmonary artery to the chest wall.

Cervical Venous Hum. This low-frequency, grade 1–2, continuous murmur is heard loudest at either the upper left or the right sternal border just above or below the clavicle. Because of its location and continuous nature, it often is mistaken for a PDA. It is loudest when the patient is sitting and diminishes or disappears when the patient is supine. The murmur usually can be accentuated by turning the patient's head away from the side of the murmur and obliterated by pressing lightly over the jugular vein. It is caused by turbulent flow in the jugular veins.

Supraclavicular Arterial Bruit. This grade 1–3, crescendo-decrescendo systolic murmur is heard best above the clavicles with radiation to the neck. The intensity is increased with exercise but not affected by posture or respiration. Compression of the subclavian artery against the first rib or hyperextension of the shoulders will diminish or abolish the murmur and can be used to differentiate it from the murmur of AS. It is thought to be caused by turbulent flow at the origin of the brachiocephalic vessels from the aorta.

Peripheral Pulmonic Stenosis. This is characterized by a grade 1–2, systolic ejection murmur heard best in the axilla or back and more softly over the left upper sternal border. It often is heard in the newborn infant and disappears by several months of age. It is not caused by structural cardiac disease but by the normal reduction in diameter of the proximal branch pulmonary arteries arising from the pulmonary trunk during early infancy, resulting in turbulence of blood flow. Once identified, reexamination of the infant at age 4 months is necessary to document resolution and ensure that the murmur is not due to pathologic pulmonary artery stenosis.

Pathologic Systolic Murmurs

In general, pathologic systolic murmurs tend to be louder, longer, and harsher than innocent murmurs and do not vary with respiration. Pathologic systolic murmurs are due to either a hole in the heart, such as a VSD or ASD; stenosis of the aortic or pulmonic valves or outflow tracts; stenosis of the pulmonary artery or aorta; or regurgitation of the mitral or tricuspid valves. Each abnormality has distinct features of the cardiac examination that distinguish it from the others (Table 17–5).

Ventricular Septal Defect. A VSD is a hole in the septum between the right and left ventricles; this results in a left-to-right shunt causing increased pulmonary blood flow, which can lead to CHF. VSD is the most common congenital heart defect, occurring in 3/1000 live births and comprising 16% of all children with heart disease. Only 15% of VSDs are of a size sufficient to require diagnostic

Table 17–4. Innocent murmurs.

Murmur	Location	Intensity	Quality	Other
Cervical venous hum	Right or left upper sternal border below clavicle	Grade 1–2 continuous	Low frequency	Diminishes with jugular vein compression
Peripheral pulmonic stenosis	Left upper sternal border with louder radiation to back or axilla	Grade 1–2 systolic ejection	Crescendo-decrescendo, low frequency	Newborn to age 4 mo
Pulmonary ejection	Left upper sternal border	Grade 1–3 systolic ejection	Crescendo-decrescendo, medium frequency	Decreases with Valsalva maneuver
Still	Midway between left lower sternal border and apex	Grade 1–2 systolic ejection	Vibratory, musical, low frequency	Decreases intensity with inspiration
Supraclavicular arterial bruit	Above right or left clavicle with radiation to neck	Grade 1–3 holosystolic	Crescendo-decrescendo, medium to high frequency	Decreases with shoulder hyperextension

Table 17–5. Diagnostic features of the common causes of pathologic murmurs in children.

Diagnosis	Chest Radiograph	Pulses	Electrocardiogram	Auscultation
Shunt lesions				
Ventricular septal defect	Increased pulmonary vascularity	Normal	LVH ± RVH, LAE	≥ Grade 3 holosystolic murmur LLSB, P2 normal to increased
Atrioventricular canal defect	Increased pulmonary vascularity	Normal	RVH ± LVH, superior axis	≥ Grade 3 holosystolic murmur LLSB, P2 normal to increased
Patent ductus arteriosus	Increased pulmonary vascularity	Increased	LVH ± RVH, LAE	≥ Grade 2 continuous murmur ULSB, P2 normal to increased
Intrinsic				
Myocarditis	Pulmonary edema	Decreased	ST & T abnormal, low voltage ± LVH	Sounds soft, S3 may be heard
Cardiomyopathy	Pulmonary edema	Decreased	ST & T abnormal, inferior axis, low voltage ± LVH	Soft sounds, S3 may be heard
Ischemia	Pulmonary edema	Decreased	ST & T abnormal, deep Q waves	Soft sounds, S3 may be heard
Obstruction				
Aortic stenosis	Pulmonary edema	Decreased	LVH ± ST abnormalities	≥ Grade 3 systolic ejection murmur URSB, ejection click
Coarctation of aorta	Pulmonary edema	Upper extremity > lower extremity	LVH	Grade 2–3 systolic murmur, possibly also in diastole paraspinally

LLSB = left lower sternal border; LVH = left ventricular hypertrophy; RVH = right ventricular hypertrophy; LAE = left atrial enlargement; RAE = right atrial enlargement; ULSB = upper left sternal border; URSB = upper right sternal border.

or therapeutic intervention; the remainder either close spontaneously or are so small that they have no hemodynamic effect. The murmur, due to turbulent blood flow through the defect, is medium- to high-frequency, is grade 2–4, occupies the whole of systole, and is loudest at the fourth intercostal space to the apex. Treatment for small VSDs is limited to antibiotic prophylaxis to minimize the small risk (0.7%/y) of bacterial endocarditis. Large VSDs should be closed surgically to prevent the development of pulmonary vascular disease.

Atrial Septal Defect. An ASD is a hole in the septum between the right and left atrium. It results in a left-to-right shunt, causing right ventricular volume overload and increased pulmonary blood flow; this can lead to CHF and pulmonary hypertension but usually not until the second or third decade of life. Approximately 3–5% of children with significant heart disease have an ASD, making it the third most common congenital heart defect. Most children are asymptomatic and present with a murmur at age 2–5 years. Small ASDs may close spontaneously, but this rarely occurs after the age of 2 years. Physical examination is remarkable for a medium- to high-frequency systolic ejection murmur heard loudest at the left upper sternal border because of the increased blood flow across the normal pulmonary valve. In addition, because of the increased pulmonary flow, the pulmonary valve takes longer to close, resulting in a widely split second heart sound. The widely split second heart sound differentiates an ASD from an innocent pulmonary ejection murmur. Small ASDs less than a few millimeters in diameter require no treatment and do not require antibiotic prophy-

laxis. Larger ASDs require surgical closure, but new catheter-directed closure techniques are being developed.

Aortic Stenosis. AS, a congenital abnormality of the aortic valve, consists of thickening and fusion of one or more of the valve leaflets, resulting in limited opening of the valve during systolic ejection. Neonates with severe, or "critical," AS present in shock (see Shock, above). Infants and children usually present asymptomatically with a systolic murmur, most often at age 5–15 years. By the third decade, AS is the second most common congenital heart defect, after VSD. Physical examination reveals a harsh, medium-frequency systolic ejection murmur at the second right intercostal space associated with an ejection click over the lower left sternal border; in addition, a thrill often is palpable in the suprasternal notch. The natural history of AS is to worsen over time; most children require treatment at some time during childhood or young adulthood. Treatment consists of either catheter balloon dilation or surgical repair. Antibiotic prophylaxis is needed both before and after treatment because, despite a good physiologic result from treatment, the valve remains abnormal and therefore at risk for endocarditis.

Pulmonary Stenosis. PS is a congenital abnormality of the pulmonic valve consisting of thickening of the valve leaflets, resulting in limited opening of the valve during systolic ejection. It occurs in about 8% of children with congenital heart disease, making it the second most common lesion during childhood. Neonates with severe ("critical") PS present with cyanosis, but most patients present asymptomatically as infants or preschool-aged children with a systolic murmur. Physical examination is significant for a harsh, medium-frequency systolic ejection murmur at the second left intercostal space associated with an ejection click along the left sternal border. In contrast to AS, there is no suprasternal notch thrill, although in severe cases a thrill may be palpable over the left upper sternal border. Mild PS may not require treatment other than antibiotic prophylaxis. However, the degree of stenosis may progress, so careful routine follow-up is required. Moderate or marked degrees of PS result in right ventricular hypertrophy on the ECG. The treatment of choice for moderate to severe PS is catheter balloon dilation.

Valvar Regurgitation. Isolated regurgitation of either the mitral or tricuspid valves is a rare cause of asymptomatic murmurs in children. The exception is tricuspid regurgitation in the newborn. The elevated pulmonary pressures can persist 24–48 hours after birth and often cause tricuspid regurgitation despite a normal tricuspid valve. This murmur may be difficult to distinguish from a VSD murmur, as it is a medium-frequency holosystolic murmur heard loudest at the left lower sternal border. This murmur disappears during the first week after birth as pulmonary arterial pressure decreases.

Pathologic Continuous & Diastolic Murmurs

With the exception of a venous hum, which can be made to disappear with maneuvers (see above), a continuous or diastolic murmur always should be considered pathologic until proved otherwise. A continuous murmur usually is due to a PDA, although continuous flow lesions, such as a fistulae (cerebral, hepatic, pulmonary, or coronary), AP window, or AP collateral circulation, may cause continuous murmurs. Diastolic murmurs are due either to aortic or pulmonic regurgitation or to mitral stenosis. Fortunately, these last three lesions are rare and usually associated with other cardiac defects.

Patent Ductus Arteriosus. PDA is a common lesion in children younger than 1 year (making it the sixth most common lesion in congenital heart disease). PDAs are common in preterm infants; the more premature the infant, the greater the likelihood that ductus patency will persist after birth. If it is not necessary to close the ductus pharmacologically with indomethacin or surgically because of symptoms, it usually closes spontaneously within several weeks after birth. Ductus patency is the abnormal persistence of a normal fetal vessel that connects the main pulmonary artery with the descending aorta. After birth, it results in left-to-right shunting to the pulmonary arteries, which can cause CHF, with enlargement of the left atrium and ventricle and pulmonary hypertension. In addition, a PDA carries a substantial risk of developing endocarditis. Symptoms are dependent on the size of the PDA, which determines the amount of the left-to-right shunt. Most children have small- to moderate-sized PDAs and present asymptomatically with a murmur. Cardiac examination is significant for increased pulse volume and a continuous medium- to low-frequency murmur heard loudest just inferior to the left clavicle. Treatment is closure, either by surgical ligation or a new catheter coil closure technique.

CHILD WITH RESPIRATORY DISTRESS/CONGESTIVE HEART FAILURE

CHF may be defined as inadequate contractile heart function for the specific hemodynamic needs. There may be normal requirements for flow but poor myocardial contractility (eg, cardiomyopathy), or flow requirements may be dramatically increased in the face of normal or even increased myocardial contractility (eg, VSD with large left-to-right shunt and increased pulmonary blood flow). The inadequacy of contractile function may be manifested as inadequate systemic output for metabolic needs, as in a child with CHF caused by a large left-to-right shunt who does not grow and gain weight. Alternatively, it may be associated with adequate systemic output, but compensatory mechanisms may result in other clinical problems, such as a large left-to-right shunt in a child who has an enlarged liver.

In practical terms, the signs and symptoms of CHF in children include respiratory distress (tachypnea and/or retractions), increased cardiac activity (tachycardia and/or a hyperdynamic precordium), and cardiac enlargement (detected either by chest radiograph or echocardiogram). Two physiologic mechanisms can result in heart failure in children. The most common is a large left-to-right shunt, as with a large ASD, VSD, atrioventricular canal defect, or PDA, causing markedly increased pulmonary blood flow and interstitial fluid accumulation. The large left-to-right shunt is a volume load for the atria and ventricles. To maintain an adequate cardiac output, the heart compensates by enlarging and by beating faster and with greater force, which leads to the cardiac enlargement and increased precordial activity. The second physiologic mechanism occurs when there is intrinsic myocardial dysfunction, as with myocarditis. Because of the dysfunction, cardiac output decreases and ventricular filling pressures increase, resulting in elevated left atrial and pulmonary vein pressures. This causes pulmonary edema, leading to respiratory distress. Because of the low cardiac output, the kidneys retain free water, which increases intravascular volume, causing cardiac dilation. The heart tries to maintain output by increasing heart rate.

The differential diagnosis of CHF in children includes a large left-to-right shunt (ASD, VSD, PDA, atrioventricular canal, or AV fistula), left-sided obstruction leading to myocardial dysfunction (severe coarctation or AS), or intrinsic myocardial dysfunction (myocarditis, cardiomyopathy, or infarct due to anomalous coronary artery). The evaluation should include a thorough physical examination, measurement of pulse oximetry, chest radiograph, and ECG. If the respiratory distress is marked, treatment must be initiated immediately. An echocardiogram should be performed to define the lesions.

Large shunt lesions can be differentiated from obstructive lesions or intrinsic myocardial dysfunction on the appearance of the chest radiograph. Shunt lesions will have increased pulmonary artery size but minimal pulmonary edema, whereas obstructive or intrinsic dysfunction lesions will have predominately pulmonary edema. The specific physical and ECG findings of left-to-right shunt lesions and left-sided obstructive lesions in children are similar to those for infants (see above). Cardiac examination in a child with intrinsic myocardial dysfunction is characterized by tachypnea, rales, tachycardia, a hyperdynamic precordium, a gallop rhythm heard loudest over the left lower sternal border or apex, and often a systolic murmur at the apex due to mitral regurgitation. In myocarditis, the ECG findings are nonspecific with diminished voltages throughout the chest leads and nonspecific ST-T wave abnormalities. ECG findings in patients with cardiomyopathy often include left atrial enlargement and left ventricular hypertrophy. Ischemic myocardial dysfunction due to an anomalous coronary artery may show ECG findings of ST-T wave elevation consistent with myocardial ischemia or Q waves suggestive of previous myocardial infarction.

Infants with a single ventricle typically have an associated ASD as well as atrioventricular valve abnormalities; therefore, mixing occurs both at the atrial and ventricular levels. ECG findings vary but always show an absence of the normal Q wave in the lateral chest leads (V_6 and V_7), indicating the absence of a ventricular septum. Infants may have associated valvar or subvalvar PS, causing reduced pulmonary flow, or no associated stenosis with markedly increased pulmonary flow. Initial treatment is determined by the amount of pulmonary blood flow. For infants with too much pulmonary blood flow, pulmonary artery band surgery is performed. For those with too little pulmonary blood flow, a shunt is placed from the aorta to the pulmonary artery to augment flow.

CHILD WITH STRIDOR— VASCULAR RINGS

Stridor is a common symptom of upper airway disease, including croup and bronchomalacia (see Chapter 18). It also can be a symptom of heart disease, specifically vascular rings. A **vascular ring** is an aortic arch anomaly in which the esophagus and trachea are completely surrounded by vascular structures. Although this condition is rare compared with airway abnormalities, it nonetheless represents an important cause of stridor and feeding difficulties in infants. When vascular rings are diagnosed and treated, appropriately complete correction usually is possible.

In infants, the history associated with vascular rings is very similar to that with tracheomalacia: "noisy breathing" since birth, which worsens during an upper respiratory infection or when the child is agitated. Children can have difficulty feeding or have reflex apnea with feeding.

In older children, a history of choking on food or difficulty in swallowing solids is common. A careful history reveals that these children often had respiratory symptoms early in life that were attributed to "bronchitis." In children with other heart disease and respiratory symptoms, these difficulties may be attributed to their heart disease. Rings that cause little compression can be asymptomatic and found incidentally when an imaging study is obtained for another reason.

Diagnosis

If a vascular ring is considered, a barium swallow is the initial diagnostic procedure of choice. A posterior pulsatile indentation of the esophagus is the classic feature. Endoscopy shows similar features. Bronchoscopy shows an anterior pulsatile mass, representing the ascending aortic portion of the ring. Magnetic resonance imaging (MRI) provides a definitive diagnosis in most cases by clearly showing the anatomy of the head and neck vessels. Echocardiography can show the features of a vascular ring, particularly when a right aortic arch is present, but is not completely reliable. Angiography usually is not necessary, except in complex vascular anomalies. Barium swallow, followed by MRI, usually provides a definitive diagnosis for surgical correction. However, in patients with a ligamentum arteriosum (remnant of a ductus arteriosus), it may be difficult to demonstrate the lesion by any technique; the condition should be suspected in a patient with symptoms of a vascular ring and the presence of an anomalous subclavian artery.

Treatment

In nearly all cases, surgery successfully eliminates the vascular ring. In double aortic arch, the smaller of the two arches is divided, opening the ring. With pulmonary slings and aberrant right subclavian arteries, reimplantation is possible. With the right aortic arch, aberrant left subclavian artery, and left ligamentum arteriosum complex, simply dividing the ligamentum is all that is necessary.

Although surgery may successfully eliminate the ring, these patients often have severe bronchomalacia or tracheomalacia, which may be responsible for their continued respiratory symptoms. In some, these symptoms gradually improve with time and with growth of the trachea; in others, they remain a problem.

Types of Vascular Rings

Vascular rings can be classified as complete (those that form a complete circle) and incomplete (those that form a "C" around the trachea and esophagus but still cause compression). Incomplete rings are more common but also more variable in the symptoms they produce.

The most frequent form of incomplete ring is the aberrant right subclavian artery. In this condition, the right subclavian artery does not arise as a branch of the first vessel from the arch (the innominate artery); instead, it arises as a branch from the normal aorta as it descends on the left. To reach the right arm, it must pass from the left descending aorta and behind the esophagus, occasionally causing some compression.

Pulmonary artery slings are very rare but more frequently symptomatic. In this condition, the left pulmonary artery does not arise normally; instead, it arises from the right pulmonary artery and then passes to the left lung between the esophagus and trachea. The most frequent symptoms are those of expiratory obstruction, with wheezing, because the site of obstruction is well below the thoracic inlet. Because compression is more severe to the right mainstem bronchus, asymmetric air trapping may occur. This may be a clue to the diagnosis. Pulmonary artery sling should be considered in the differential diagnosis of wheezing, particularly when it does not seem responsive to bronchodilators and especially when it is associated with persistent hyperinflation of the right lung.

The most common form of complete vascular ring is the double aortic arch (Figure 17–11). In this condition, the ascending aorta branches into an anterior (left) and posterior (right) branch. The posterior limb passes behind the trachea and esophagus. The two limbs join to re-form the descending aorta, to complete the ring. The carotid and subclavian arteries usually arise from both anterior and posterior limbs as four discrete vessels. Often, one of the two arches is dominant, and the other is substantially smaller.

The other common form of complete ring is the association of a right aortic arch with an aberrant retroesophageal left subclavian artery and a left-sided ductus or ligamentum arteriosum. This condition is similar to aberrant right subclavian artery.

A right aortic arch is common and often is associated with congenital heart disease, especially truncus arteriosus and TOF. Typically, the first vessel to arise is a left innominate artery; a right-sided ductus arteriosus originates from the base of the right subclavian artery. When the left subclavian artery arises aberrantly from the descending aorta and passes retroesophageally to the left arm, and when it gives rise to a left-sided ductus arteriosus, a complete vascular ring exists. This is because the trachea and esophagus are encircled by the ascending aorta to the right, the retroesophageal left subclavian artery behind, and the ligamentum arteriosum to the left, which passes to the pulmonary artery in front.

CHILD WITH PALPITATIONS/ ARRHYTHMIAS

Complaints of abnormalities of rhythm are very common. They are often described as irregular beats, extra beats, "strange" or skipped beats, fast or "racing heart," or "jumping in the chest." Fortunately, most of these symptoms do not represent serious arrhythmias; however, potentially serious arrhythmias can present with mild symptoms initially. Determining the underlying diagnosis, as well as which children may need more thorough investigation, often is difficult because of the periodic nature of the symptoms and the lack of other associated findings.

The history often is nonspecific, but particular attention should be paid to a past history of syncope (see below) or lightheadedness and chest pain. A complete family history of structural heart disease or of sudden death should be elicited. The association of the sensation with exercise, position, or food intake, particularly caffeine-containing substances, should be determined. In general, the findings of the physical examination are unremarkable, except for the arrhythmia. Diagnosis and treatment therefore become dependent on documentation of the rhythm.

Documenting an abnormal rhythm can be difficult, particularly when the symptoms are periodic and infrequent. An ECG should always be obtained. A sinus arrhythmia is a common, normal finding in children, as are occasional premature atrial contractions. Pre-excitation, when present, suggests reentrant tachycardia. More serious abnormalities, such as atrioventricular block or a prolonged QT interval, warrant immediate referral to a pediatric cardiologist. The ECG, however, often is normal. If the suspected arrhythmia is frequent, such as every day or every few days, a 24-hour Holter monitor recording is indicated. However, the episodes often occur weekly or even less frequently, and the Holter monitor record is likely to be normal. In these instances, an event recorder is helpful. The patient carries an event recorder, which is placed on the chest when the arrhythmia is experienced, recording the rhythm. This allows capture of even infrequent events. Alternatively, patients occasionally are asked to come to

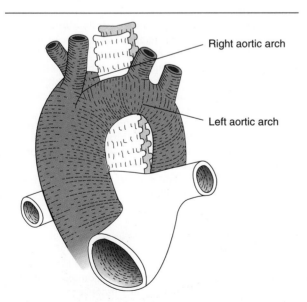

Figure 17–11. Double aortic arch. Arch bifurcates into left (anterior) and right (posterior) branches to encircle the trachea and esophagus. The two branches rejoin behind the esophagus to form a single descending aorta. (Reproduced, with permission, from Shuford WH, Sybers RG [editors]: *The Aortic Arch and Its Malformations.* Thomas, 1974.)

Right aortic arch

Left aortic arch

the emergency department or clinic as soon as they experience symptoms, but this is reserved for those in whom diagnosis is very difficult. Treadmill testing can be performed when symptoms are associated with exercise or to determine the severity of the arrhythmia for recommendations regarding athletic participation.

Premature Beats

The new onset of frequent premature beats often is the clue to underlying conditions, such as digoxin toxicity, other drug ingestions, myocarditis, hypoxia, hypokalemia, hypercarbia, or acidosis.

Causes

Supraventricular Premature Contractions. These are recognizable as narrow-QRS beats that occur early. They may also have wide-QRS complexes caused by bundle branch aberration. Those that originate in the atrium may be recognizable by finding a premature P wave superimposed on the previous T wave, deforming it. This sign may be very subtle, however, and may require examination of multiple leads.

Ventricular Premature Complexes. These are recognizable as wide, often bizarre, early beats, usually without preceding P waves. The differentiation between ventricular contractions and aberrantly conducted supraventricular contractions is sometimes difficult or impossible from the surface ECG. Although traditionally premature ventricular beats may be differentiated from supraventricular beats by the presence of a full compensatory pause, this sign is somewhat unreliable. The identification of fusion beats, in which a sinus beat occurs simultaneous with a premature beat, thus creating an intermediate morphology, is very helpful and establishes the premature beat as ventricular in origin.

Treatment. In the absence of tachycardia, patients only rarely need to be treated for premature beats of any kind. Supraventricular premature contractions virtually never require treatment. Ventricular premature contractions may require treatment in a few situations:

1. when they are multiform
2. when they occur in couplets or short runs of ventricular tachycardia
3. when they are seen in association with a recently converted ventricular tachycardia
4. when they exhibit the "R on T" phenomenon; ie, they fall repeatedly on the early part of the T wave of the preceding beat.

Abnormal Tachycardia

Tachycardia in children is much more common than bradycardia. Tachycardia is classified by the duration of the QRS. A narrow-QRS tachycardia is one in which the QRS duration is similar to that during normal sinus rhythm, or in the normal range for age if a baseline ECG is not available. A wide-QRS tachycardia is one in which the QRS duration is substantially longer than the duration in normal sinus rhythm, or longer than the 95th percentile

for age. Nearly all narrow-QRS tachycardias in children are supraventricular in origin, and nearly all wide-QRS tachycardias are ventricular in origin. Any form of narrow-QRS tachycardia may manifest aberration, defined as widening of the QRS complex. Aberration usually is due to rate-dependent bundle-branch block. The onset of aberration may be progressive; once established, aberration may persist until termination of the tachycardia. Because the QRS complex widening results from rate-dependent bundle-branch block, it usually resembles a right or left bundle-branch block pattern. Aberration with SVT often occurs at the onset of the tachycardia in the absence of preexisting bundle-branch block, but sustained bundle-branch aberration with SVT is rare in children.

Narrow QRS tachycardia is by far the most common major arrhythmia encountered in childhood. Most patients do not have underlying structural heart disease. Presentation can occur at any age. The arrhythmia can be an incidental finding or can present with nonspecific symptoms, including irritability, sleep or feeding difficulty, lethargy, or even cardiovascular collapse. The rate of the tachycardia depends on both the age at presentation and the underlying etiology. The differential of narrow QRS tachycardia includes **atrioventricular reentrant tachycardia (AVRT),** more commonly known as the standard SVT, atrial ectopic tachycardia, atrial fibrillation, atrial flutter, and junctional tachycardia. Of these, reentrant tachycardia is most common. The term "reentrant" refers to the circular movement of impulses between the atria and ventricles

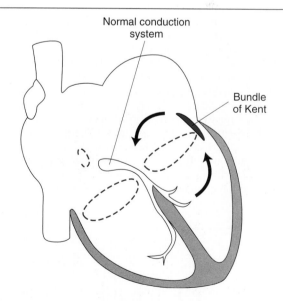

Figure 17–12. Diagram of reentrant circuit in Wolff-Parkinson-White syndrome. Impulses proceed down the normal conduction system to the ventricle and then retrograde up the bundle of Kent (accessory pathway) back to the atrium where they may then reenter the normal conduction system.

(Figure 17–12). During normal rhythm, the ECG can be normal or can show pre-excitation caused by antegrade conduction via the bundle of Kent. A premature atrial contraction can block in the bundle, then conduct via the atrioventricular node. The impulse travels via the ventricle to the bundle and is conducted retrograde, setting up the circular transmission. Therefore, during tachycardia, the QRS is often normal. P waves may be seen after the QRS but are often buried in the T wave. The tachycardia rate can be as high as 280–300/min in infants (Figure 17–13) and 220–250/min in older children. The rhythm is extremely regular, such that a bedside monitor will read exactly the same rate consistently over several minutes.

Atrial ectopic tachycardia is due to increased automaticity of atrial tissue outside the sinus node. It appears similar to AVRT but often shows occasional atrioventricular block, or variability of rate, which confirms the diagnosis. Atrial flutter is a reentrant tachycardia in which the entire reentrant circuit is located within the atrium. It can present with rates as fast as 360/min in young infants but also can present with fractions of that rate because of variable atrioventricular block. When atrioventricular block is present, a characteristic "sawtooth" pattern of atrial activity can be seen. **Atrial fibrillation** is very unusual in the absence of underlying congenital heart disease and shows an "irregularly irregular" rhythm. Often, no two R-R intervals are of the same length. **Junctional tachycardia** is extremely rare outside the immediate postoperative period.

Immediate Therapy for Narrow-QRS Tachycardia. For critically ill patients with any form of narrow-QRS tachycardia, synchronized DC cardioversion is indicated. The correct initial dose for cardioversion or defibrillation is 0.5–2 J/kg. Narrow-QRS tachycardias should always be converted in synchronous mode, in which the shock is timed to fall on the next QRS complex, to avoid delivery on the T wave. Ventricular fibrillation should always be defibrillated in asynchronous mode. In general, with wide-QRS tachycardias, an initial attempt using synchronous mode should be made. However, some forms of ventricular tachycardia appear almost sinusoidal, and the cardioverter-defibrillator may not sense R waves well. In these cases, the use of asynchronous mode may be necessary. For seriously ill patients in whom there may be signs of CHF but who have a measurable blood pressure and are conscious, the clinician must make a judgment about the stability of the patient's hemodynamic status. If the patient's condition is judged unstable, the patient should undergo electrical cardioversion after placement of an IV line. Patients whose condition is more stable are managed with the use of vagal maneuvers, followed by pharmacologic therapy; electrical cardioversion is an option if these measures should fail.

In a child with narrow complex tachycardia whose condition is stable, it is important to document both the rhythm and the attempts at conversion, because in many patients it may not recur, and the rhythm during conversion or attempted conversion often is diagnostic. If the patient is well, general vagal maneuvers can be attempted. Carotid massage and orbital pressure should not be performed in children. The carotid sinus region is not easily located in infants. Orbital pressure may be dangerous because eye injury could occur. In infants, rectal stimulation (by taking the rectal temperature) frequently is effective. Gagging with a nasogastric tube occasionally is effective. The diving reflex may be elicited by placing a bag filled with ice over the face (and covering the ears) for 15 seconds. Older children may be coached to perform a standard Valsalva maneuver. These maneuvers should be performed with an IV line in place and should not be continued longer than 5 minutes in seriously ill patients before one proceeds to other modalities. Although helpful, vagal maneuvers often are unsuccessful, and pharmacologic conversion is indicated.

Adenosine is valuable in the acute diagnosis and management of SVTs that involve the atrioventricular node as part of the reentrant circuit. This agent, when given rapidly by IV injection, induces a brief episode of complete atrioventricular block, thereby interrupting the reentrant circuit. The onset of effect is less than 1 minute, the half-life in blood is less than 10 seconds, and the resulting atrioventricular blockade is therefore brief and self-limited. The successful conversion of AVRT with adenosine is evidence against other forms of tachycardia, such as atrial tachycardia, that do not involve the atrioventricular node as part of the reentrant circuit.

Although adenosine usually converts only AVRT, it can be extremely useful in the diagnosis of other types of narrow complex tachycardia. By inducing complete atrioventricular block, it slows the ventricular rate, allowing better determination of atrial rate. In atrial ectopic tachycardia, atrial flutter, and atrial fibrillation, adenosine in-

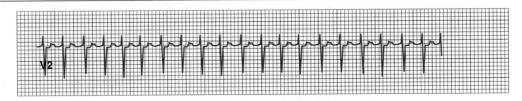

Figure 17–13. Narrow QRS tachycardia in an infant, aged 1 week, with atrioventricular reentrant tachycardia (AVRT). Notice the rapid rate (285 beats/min), extreme regularity of the rhythm, and lack of obvious P waves.

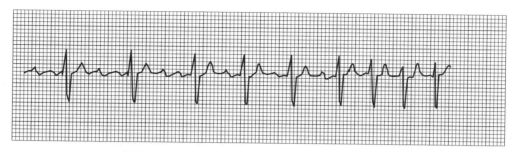

Figure 17–14. Diagnosis of atrial flutter by administration of adenosine. Adenosine-induced atrioventricular block slows the ventricular rate, allowing visualization of the characteristic "sawtooth" pattern of atrial flutter. After metabolism of the adenosine and rapid ventricular response, the flutter is much less apparent.

duces ventricular slowing, but the atrial activation is unaffected (Figure 17–14), and the diagnosis may be made easily. Adenosine is given as a rapid IV bolus, beginning at 50–100 µg/kg and gradually increasing until the desired effect, atrioventricular block, is achieved. Further increases in dosage are not indicated, nor is repeated administration to convert the rhythm transiently without other pharmacologic treatment.

Verapamil has been used for conversion in the past but is rarely indicated today because of the severe hypotension that it may cause, especially in infants. In addition, asystolic cardiac arrests have been reported in infants younger than 6 months.

Digoxin is an effective agent for the treatment of most pediatric narrow-QRS tachycardias. A disadvantage is the relatively long period necessary to digitalize a patient safely. One approach to IV digitalization is to give 10 µg/kg as a first IV dose, followed by a second dose 2 hours later and a third dose at 6–12 hours. It should not be given if hypokalemia is present or if there is a suspicion of digoxin toxicity.

Immediate Therapy for Wide-QRS Tachycardia. Because most children presenting with wide-QRS tachycardia have ventricular tachycardia (Figure 17–15) rather than SVT with aberration, and because it is often nearly impossible to differentiate these possibilities firmly in children by using only a surface ECG, patients with wide-QRS tachycardia are managed as if they had ventricular tachycardia. In practice, this means that electrical cardioversion is indicated in nearly all cases. In patients who are neither seriously nor critically ill, one may defer cardioversion while pharmacologic agents are administered. In this situation, procainamide would be a good choice because it is effective both for ventricular and supraventricular arrhythmias. Lidocaine may be used if there is certainty that the diagnosis is ventricular tachycardia. *Verapamil, however, should never be given to patients with wide-QRS tachycardia;* if the diagnosis is actually ventricular tachycardia, and verapamil fails to convert the rhythm to sinus rhythm, the resulting hypotension in the face of continued tachycardia may be life-threatening.

Abnormal Bradycardia
Causes
Sinus Bradycardia. Sinus bradycardia is recognized as a regular slow atrial rate with normal P waves and 1:1 conduction. Causes include hypoxia, acidosis, increased intracranial pressure, abdominal distension, and hypo-

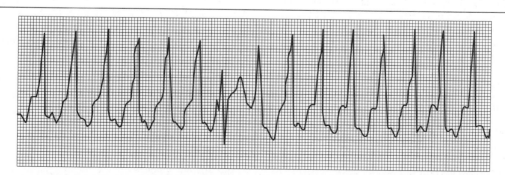

Figure 17–15. Ventricular tachycardia: Very wide QRS complexes are seen. A single capture beat is seen and occurs with a narrow QRS complex, proving the presence of ventricular tachycardia. (Reproduced, with permission, from Van Hare GF: Dysrhythmias. In Grossman M, Dieckmann RA [editors]: *Pediatric Emergency Medicine. A Clinician's Reference.* Lippincott, 1991.)

glycemia. Drugs such as digoxin and propranolol may also cause significant sinus bradycardia. Mild slowing may be due to increased vagal tone or cardiac conditioning.

Atrioventricular Block. **Complete atrioventricular block** may be congenital or surgically induced or may occur suddenly because of myocarditis. It is recognized as atrioventricular dissociation, with regular RR intervals, regular PP intervals, an atrial rate greater than ventricular rate, and an absence of capture beats.

Second-degree atrioventricular block should be classified as Mobitz type 1 (Wenckebach) or Mobitz type 2. Wenckebach conduction is characterized by progressive PR interval prolongation followed by a blocked beat, followed by recovery of conduction. Type 2 block lacks this characteristic PR prolongation with shortening after the blocked beat. Type 1 generally has a better prognosis than type 2 and responds to medication readily.

Other causes of bradycardia are sinus exit block, in which sinus P waves intermittently disappear owing to blockage of impulses leaving the region of the node, and frequent premature atrial contractions, which occur too early to be conducted to the ventricles and therefore slow the resulting ventricular rate.

Treatment. The hemodynamic effect of a slow heart rate depends on how different it is from the patient's usual heart rate. Sudden decreases in rate may be poorly compensated by increases in stroke volume, particularly in those with preexisting poor cardiac function. Moderate bradycardia in normal children rarely requires treatment. Exceptions include the sudden occurrence of complete atrioventricular block or pacemaker failure. The urgency of treatment is dictated by the hemodynamic status. Underlying causes, such as hypoxia, should be corrected.

If treatment is indicated, initial treatment with atropine, followed by continuous isoproterenol infusion, will increase sinus rates, improve atrioventricular conduction, and may increase the rate of subsidiary pacemakers. After initial stabilization with medications, temporary transvenous pacing should be instituted, particularly in patients with very low ventricular rates (< 30/min) or in those with hemodynamic compromise. Subsequently, implantation of a permanent pacemaker may be necessary if bradycardia does not improve.

CHILD WITH SYNCOPE

Syncope is a sudden, brief loss of consciousness caused by diffuse transient impairment of cerebral function. The sudden loss of consciousness often is associated with loss of postural tone and falling, with a quick recovery of consciousness once in the supine position. The fall may cause physical trauma. If the child cannot fall to the supine position, as when trapped upright in a school desk, recovery to consciousness may be delayed, and a tonic-clonic seizure may develop. Syncope is a common presenting symptom in older children and adolescents. Often patients present with presyncope symptoms, including lightheadedness, dizziness, weakness, pallor, cold sweat, or blurred vision. Although it most often is benign, syncope can be the presenting symptom for significant cardiac, neurologic, or metabolic disease and even the harbinger of sudden death (Table 17–6). Therefore, a careful evaluation to elucidate the cause is mandatory.

Evaluation of a child with syncope begins with a careful and detailed history and physical examination. The history should detail events leading up to the episode, and describe the episode. This description should include the duration; observations during the episode, such as incontinence, vomiting, associated injuries, and tonic-clonic movements; and duration of the neurologic state during the recovery. If the history and physical examination findings suggest a neurologic cause, an electroencephalogram or a computed tomographic (CT) or MRI scan of the brain might be indicated. If a metabolic cause is implicated, laboratory studies, including serum glucose and electrolyte levels and blood count, should be obtained. An ECG, 24-hour Holter monitor, echocardiogram, tilt-table test, and electrophysiology study might be necessary if the initial evaluation suggests a cardiac cause.

The most common cause of syncope in children is neurally mediated syncope. The classic example is the cadet who passes out while standing at attention for hours in the hot sun. This is benign except for the risk associated with falling during the episode. The mechanism is a sudden decrease in systemic venous return that results in less filling of the left ventricle and a decreased left ventricular end diastolic volume. In response, increased contractility and stimulation of cardiac vagal fibers lead to reflex bradycardia, vasodilation, and hypotension, which in turn lead to transient hypoperfusion of the brain, causing syncope. Once the supine position is attained, perfusion to the brain is restored, as is normal systemic venous return, abolishing the transient reflex. There are three clinical types of neurally mediated syncope, identified on the basis of the predominate features: the first, vasodepressor, starts with and is dominated by hypotension; the second, cardioin-

Table 17–6. Causes of syncope.

Cardiac	Neurologic	Metabolic
Neurally mediated syncope	Seizures	Hypoglycemia
Bradyarrhythmia	Breath-holding	Electrolyte abnormalities
Sick sinus syndrome	Hyperventilation	malities
Atrioventricular block		Severe anemia
Tachyarrhythmia		
Supraventricular		
Ventricular tachycardia		
Prolonged QT interval		
Hypertrophic cardiomyopathy		
Aortic stenosis		
Pulmonary hypertension		

hibitory, starts with and is dominated by marked bradycardia; and the third, mixed response, is a mixture of both. Neurally mediated syncope is exacerbated by anything that predisposes to decreased systemic venous return (eg, physical exhaustion, prolonged recumbency) or to peripheral vasodilation (eg, exercise, hot weather, and emotional stress).

The diagnosis often can be made from a typical history, normal physical examination findings, and lack of evidence for a neurologic, cardiac, or metabolic cause. If necessary, the definitive diagnosis is made with a positive tilt-test result. The patient lies supine on a table for 10 minutes while baseline heart rate and blood pressure are measured. The patient is then rapidly tilted to an upright position with continuous monitoring of the blood pressure and heart rate. If the symptoms develop and are associated with hypotension and/or bradycardia, the diagnosis is clear. Treatment for a single episode should be conservative. For recurrent episodes, expansion of intravascular volume by increasing salt intake or treating with fluorocortisone (Florinef, 0.1–0.3 mg) may be adequate. Treatment with β-adrenergic blockers, such as propranolol, can be effective. In the cardioinhibitory type, if symptoms are severe, cardiac pacemaker placement has been effective.

Other cardiac causes of syncope include arrhythmias and lesions that impair cardiac output. Either severe bradycardia, sick sinus syndrome or atrioventricular block, or supraventricular or ventricular tachycardia may cause syncope. All except SVT are extremely rare in children without congenital heart disease. Syncope may occur with SVT, although most children complain of chest discomfort, fatigue, weakness, or dizziness. Prolonged QT syndrome must be considered, as it is associated with serious ventricular tachycardia (torsades de points) and ventricular fibrillation, which often result in syncope or even sudden death. QT prolongation may be associated with congenital deafness and autosomal-recessive inheritance (Jervell-Lange-Nielson) or autosomal-dominant inheritance with deafness (Romano-Ward syndrome). Electrolyte abnormalities and some anti-arrhythmic drugs (eg, quinidine, procainamide, and amiodarone) can prolong the QT interval. Evaluation should include a 12-lead ECG with careful measurement of the corrected QT interval. In addition, a 24-hour Holter monitor or event recorder may be necessary to record the abnormal rhythm. Treatment is directed at the specific type of arrhythmia and may include anti-arrhythmic medications, a cardiac pacemaker, or an implantable defibrillator.

Transient decreased cardiac output due to left ventricular outflow tract obstruction may result in syncope, especially during or immediately after exercise. The inability to increase cardiac output leads to increased parasympathetic tone and systemic vasodilation by stimulating left ventricular baroreceptors. The lesion most frequently associated with syncope is HCM (see above). Severe fixed obstruction, such as severe AS, also may be responsible. Patients with severe pulmonary hypertension may present with syncope associated with low output during a pulmonary hypertensive crisis. Rarely, a child with dilated cardiomyopathy, anomalous left coronary artery, or a cardiac tumor presents with syncope. The cardiac examination will have an abnormality, which should be confirmed and defined with an echocardiogram. Treatment is directed at the specific cardiac abnormality.

Noncardiac causes of syncope are extensive, and a detailed discussion is beyond the scope of this chapter (see Table 17–6). Seizure disorder is the most common. Psychogenic causes, such as breath-holding in toddlers and hyperventilation in teenagers, also occur frequently. Metabolic abnormalities, including hypoglycemia, electrolyte imbalance, and severe anemia, may cause syncope.

CHILD WITH CHEST PAIN

Chest pain is a common complaint, particularly in the school-aged child. Viral illness and emotional and physical stress, as well as trauma and cardiac disease, can all produce what is described as "chest pain." When evaluating a child with pain, one should determine the degree of acute illness. Chest pain can be grouped by the initial presentation: acute onset versus chronic and recurring.

Acute Onset

Children with acute-onset chest pain usually seek urgent relief from their pain. In these children, the etiology of their pain should be determined quickly, and treatment initiated. Acute-onset chest pain is by nature more severe than chronic and recurring pain and is more likely to be caused by a serious medical illness. A focused history should be obtained, with specific attention to a history of trauma, viral illnesses, drug or toxin ingestions, and palpitations. The severity, location, and radiation of the pain; factors that exacerbate or relieve symptoms; and other symptoms should be determined. The position in which the child prefers to lie should be noticed. Physical examination should focus on the degree of acute illness, skin color, respiratory effort, and peripheral pulses and perfusion. Auscultation should focus on the breath and heart sounds, with specific attention to unequal breath sounds or muffled heart sounds. Laboratory examination is directed by the results of examination.

Pericarditis. This represents an inflammation of the pericardial sac, with resultant fluid production and tension in the perinatal pericardium. It can be caused by viral or bacterial illness and is associated with many autoimmune diseases. In children with pericarditis, pain is acute, substernal, and squeezing, and they are often quite ill. The description is very similar to anginal pain. There often is a history of viral illness. The child prefers to lie very still, leaning forward, which relaxes the pericardium and decreases pain. Pressure on the chest, breathing, and movement exacerbate the pain. Examination can show thready peripheral pulses and a paradoxical pulse, indicating impending cardiac tamponade. Auscultation reveals tachycardia and distant heart sounds and sometimes a friction rub; this may not be heard with a large effusion. Echocardiography confirms the presence of an effusion. Initial treatment when signs of tamponade are present is emergent drainage. Other treatment is directed toward the underlying cause.

Chest Trauma. Chest trauma, particularly blunt trauma, can result in hemopericardium. The presentation and characteristics of this pain are very similar to those of acute pericarditis, except that, in addition, chest wall tenderness usually is present at the site of trauma. These children should be quickly evaluated for signs of tamponade, undergo an echocardiogram for confirmation, and receive emergent pericardial drainage. They also should be evaluated for other mediastinal bleeding by CT scan after initial stabilization.

Myocardial Ischemia or Infarction. Fortunately, these are rare causes of pain in children. Most children at risk for myocardial ischemia have known underlying heart disease and are under the care of a pediatric cardiologist. Ischemic pain in children has two main causes: severe ventricular hypertrophy and coronary artery disease. Ischemia can develop in patients with **severe ventricular hypertrophy,** particularly of the left ventricle. With marked hypertrophy, the subendocardium is poorly perfused when the oxygen supply cannot meet demand, as during exercise. The history is typical for ischemia, except in very small children. Physical examination confirms the presence of the lesion. Initial treatment is directed at the underlying cause of hypertrophy or is directed at relieving symptoms when the cause is not apparent.

Coronary Artery Disease. Coronary artery disease is rare in children. Congenital anomalies of the coronary arteries, such as pulmonary origin of the left coronary artery (POLCA), more commonly present with CHF in the first year of life. Acquired coronary artery disease, such as the aneurysms seen in Kawasaki disease, can present with chest pain. In general, however, the diagnosis is known and treatment initiated before the development of disease. Ischemia may occur after recovery if thrombosis develops in an aneurysm, obstructing coronary flow.

Arrhythmias. Children with arrhythmias can present with acute chest pain. This pain usually is not severe, and the child usually appears well. The pain is less localized and is associated with lightheadedness and the sensation of palpitations or fast heart rate. Physical examination findings usually are unremarkable, except for the rhythm abnormality. ECG confirms the diagnosis (see Child With Palpitations/Arrhythmias, above).

Pulmonary Disease. Pulmonary disease, such as pneumothorax, pneumonia, or pleural effusions, can present with chest pain. The pain often is unilateral, but smaller children cannot localize this. There usually is dyspnea, and blood oxygen desaturation often is present. Examination reveals decreased or absent breath sounds on the side involved. Chest radiograph confirms the diagnosis (see Chapter 18).

Esophageal Disease. Esophageal disease, such as acute esophagitis, gastroesophageal reflux, or foreign body ingestion, can mimic the pain of pericarditis or ischemia. It is substernal but has a more burning quality, is associated with dysphagia, and often is relieved by antacids. Physical examination findings often are nonspecific. The diagnosis is suspected from the history. Direct esophageal examination or imaging confirms the underlying etiology.

Chronic & Recurrent Pain

Chronic, recurring chest pain is much more common than acute-onset pain. It usually is milder, and care is not sought until the pain has persisted for some time. The diagnosis can be difficult to establish because the child usually is seen when not experiencing pain. A thorough history, including potential emotional stressors, should be obtained. Major anxiety regarding severe underlying cardiac disease often is present. History should focus on trauma, viral illnesses, and the relationship between the pain and movement, breathing, and daily activities, such as school or play. The periodicity, locality, radiation, if any, and severity of the pain should be determined. Physical examination should focus on signs of trauma, which can be subtle; symptoms of a viral, particularly upper respiratory, illness; and general state of the patient. One should always attempt to reproduce the pain by thoroughly and firmly palpating the chest or by placing the child in the position that reportedly produces the pain. Auscultation is directed primarily toward the intensity of the heart sounds and the presence of abnormal heart sounds or murmurs.

The most common cause of recurrent pain is not associated with any organic pathology. The terms **idiopathic, psychogenic,** and **growing pains** are used, although the term psychogenic should be avoided because of the negative connotation this gives to the family. The history often reveals an association between the pain and major stressful activities, such as school work. It usually is not associated with either exercise or enjoyable activities. The pain is very vague and localized as an oval over the entire chest. When challenged, the child cannot localize the pain. Most patients believe that the heart is the cause of their pain. Physical examination usually is normal but should be complete, even repeating some portions to reassure the patient and family that the heart is normal. Explanation of all the normal portions of the examination is helpful. Laboratory examination usually is not necessary. The situation should be explained thoroughly to the patient and family, without giving the impression that it is "all in their head."

Chest wall pain due to costochondritis is the next most common cause of recurrent pain. There often is a history of a preceding viral illness. The pain is sharp, very short in duration, easily localized by the patient with a single finger, and associated with movement or exercise. In general, the child is well. The pain often can be reproduced by careful, firm palpation of the area in question. Laboratory examination is rarely indicated. Symptomatic pain treatment with anti-inflammatory medication usually is sufficient.

INFECTIONS OF THE HEART

PERICARDITIS

Infections of the pericardium are discussed under The Child with Chest Pain, above.

MYOCARDITIS & CARDIOMYOPATHY

In this section, disorders of the myocardium are discussed, including acute inflammatory conditions, termed **myocarditis,** and those without specific evidence of inflammation, termed **cardiomyopathy.**

Myocarditis

Myocarditis is an active inflammation of the myocardium. This inflammation may result from many causes (Table 17–7). Tissue injury results from cytotoxic cell destruction and antibody complement–mediated destruction of myofibrils by the virus.

Many conditions causing myocarditis also may involve the pericardium and produce effusions and pericarditis. Inflammation and necrosis of cardiac muscle most frequently causes poor contractile function; this leads to cardiac dilation with an increase in left ventricular volume and mitral regurgitation. Left ventricular end diastolic pressure increase is transmitted to the left atrium and pul-

Table 17–7. Most frequent causes of myocarditis.

Infectious	
Coxsackievirus B and A	Diphtheria
Influenza virus A and B	Typhoid fever
Echovirus	Lyme disease
Mumps virus	Rocky Mountain spotted fever
Rubella	Chagas disease (trypanosomiasis)
Rubeola	Trichinosis
HIV	Toxoplasmosis
Infectious mononucleosis	
Varicella/zoster	
Inflammatory	
Systemic lupus	Ulcerative colitis
erythematosus	Polymyositis
Scleroderma	Sarcoidosis
Acute rheumatic fever	
Kawasaki disease	
Toxic	
Doxorubicin (Adriamycin)	Acetazolamide
Sulfonamides	Amphotericin B
Cyclophosphamide	Scorpion bites
Neuromuscular	
Muscular dystrophies	Friedreich ataxia
Metabolic	
Beriberi	Hypothyroidism

monary veins, resulting in pulmonary edema. Clinical findings include a soft third or fourth heart sound with displacement of the left ventricular impulse laterally, both indicating cardiomegaly. A systolic murmur of mitral regurgitation often is heard at the apex. A patient may complain of exercise intolerance or shortness of breath. If they occur in a patient with current or recent evidence of an infectious or inflammatory process, myocarditis should be suspected. Less frequently, myocarditis may present primarily with arrhythmia, and the new onset of palpitations in a patient with such evidence of infection or inflammation should also suggest myocarditis. A chest radiograph shows cardiomegaly with pulmonary edema. An ECG shows ST and T wave changes, often with low QRS voltages.

The most frequent cause of myocarditis is viral, and coxsackievirus A and B groups are most important. Myocarditis may follow a nonspecific prodrome that sometimes includes fever and an erythematous rash. Infants in the first year of life may be affected; in these patients, the disease may be fatal. Other viruses implicated in myocarditis include echovirus, influenza, and rubella. In many patients, however, a viral etiology of myocarditis is suspected, but no specific agent is isolated.

Other infectious etiologies, more rarely seen in North America, include typhoid fever, diphtheria, toxoplasmosis, and trichinosis. Of increasing importance is the myocarditis that sometimes occurs with Rocky Mountain spotted fever and with Lyme disease. Specific therapy often is available for myocarditis caused by these agents.

The clinical course depends on the degree to which the myocardium is damaged. Some patients experience slow resolution of symptoms and cardiomegaly, which gradually improves over several months or even years. In others, chronic CHF develops. Infants may experience a rapidly progressive course, including severe CHF, cardiogenic shock, and death. There is no effective treatment for viral myocarditis; intensive support must be provided until the disease has run its course. Support includes positive pressure ventilation, diuretics, and inotropic agents. The use of IV immunoglobulins has been suggested but is controversial. Mechanical myocardial support with a ventricular assist device and extracorporeal membrane oxygenation (ECMO) has been helpful in severe cases.

Myocarditis is rarely seen as the only manifestation of a more generalized inflammatory disease; more often, the disease may be diagnosed by the other inflammatory manifestations, including pericarditis. During acute rheumatic fever, acute cardiac decompensation may occur. In some patients, this is due to severe valvular dysfunction; in others, it is due to myocarditis with severe contractile dysfunction. The collagen vascular diseases may rarely be seen with major myocardial involvement, although pericardial involvement is more common. Examples include systemic lupus erythematosus and rheumatoid arthritis. Of great importance is the cardiac involvement in Kawasaki disease (see Chapter 8).

As in the viral forms, specific therapy is not available

for myocarditis that occurs in association with systemic inflammatory disease. Although anti-inflammatory agents often are used, there is little or no evidence that they are effective in preventing or reversing myocarditis. This includes myocarditis in association with rheumatic fever. There is evidence that the administration of IV immunoglobulin early in the course of Kawasaki disease improves myocardial function and decreases the subsequent incidence of coronary arterial aneurysms.

Cardiomyopathy denotes damage to cardiac muscle in which no inflammatory process can be defined. It is associated with many storage diseases and has many causes (Table 17–8).

Patients with **dilated cardiomyopathy** present with signs of ventricular systolic (contractile) dysfunction and are found to have cardiac dilatation on chest radiography, which usually is mainly caused by left ventricular chamber enlargement. This enlargement occurs as a compensatory mechanism for poor cardiac contractile function. These patients may have signs of CHF, or they may be well compensated with little more than signs of cardiac enlargement. They may also manifest symptoms suggestive of arrhythmia, such as syncope or palpitations.

In most cases of dilated cardiomyopathy, no cause can be found; therefore, these are termed **idiopathic dilated cardiomyopathy.** In some cases, there may be a familial pattern. Rarely, there may be a familial carnitine deficiency or other abnormality of mitochondrial function. Infiltrative diseases, such as sarcoidosis and amyloidosis, which involve the myocardium in adults, are very unusual in children with dilated cardiomyopathy. In children receiving doxorubicin (Adriamycin) for cancer chemotherapy, the occurrence of dilated cardiomyopathy is related to the dose. Approximately 5% of patients have symptomatic cardiotoxicity after a cumulative dose of 500 mg/m^2; with higher doses, however, the incidence reaches 50%. The incidence of an identifiable cause of cardiomyopathy is extremely low, despite the use of techniques such as endomyocardial biopsy. Furthermore, even if a cause is found on the biopsy specimen, definitive treatment is unlikely to be available. Endomyocardial biopsies are performed to identify those rare cases for which treatment might be available, as well as to provide the patient and family with a prognosis.

The clinical course of dilated cardiomyopathy is variable. Spontaneous resolution is not uncommon in younger children; in both older children and adults, however, progression is more common. Progressive development of CHF requires gradual intensification of medical management, including the use of afterload-reducing agents. Eventually, many such patients become candidates for cardiac transplantation. A particularly disturbing development in a patient with dilated cardiomyopathy is the occurrence of syncope or documented ventricular arrhythmias. Repeated syncope in a patient with dilated cardiomyopathy is an ominous sign and may signal the possibility of sudden death. Such patients are considered for cardiac transplantation even if their hemodynamic status is otherwise compensated. Finally, such patients may have mural thrombi that subsequently may embolize and cause strokes or other problems. This is a particular problem in patients with dilated cardiomyopathy in whom chronic atrial fibrillation has developed. Antiplatelet agents, such as aspirin or dipyridamole, should be used to prevent the development of mural thrombi. Anticoagulants, such as warfarin, should be used in patients in whom thrombi have already developed.

Restrictive cardiomyopathy differs from the dilated form in that there is no ventricular dilatation. Instead, the ventricle may be contracted and small, whereas the atria may be dilated because of the high ventricular diastolic pressures. Clinically, this often appears as cardiomegaly on the chest radiograph, despite the normal or small ventricular chamber sizes. There also may be evidence of passive congestion with pulmonary edema.

The main problem in restrictive cardiomyopathy is a dramatically reduced ventricular compliance, with an abnormally high pressure at normal ventricular volumes and therefore reduced ventricular diastolic filling. Although there may also be systolic dysfunction with reduced ejection fraction, the clinical picture is mainly that of diastolic dysfunction with pulmonary and hepatic congestion and atrial enlargement. Chronic atrial dilatation may lead to severe atrial arrhythmias, such as atrial flutter, which may be very poorly tolerated in such patients. Patients may have atrial thrombi and subsequent systemic embolization, as do patients with dilated cardiomyopathy.

In children, the principal course of restrictive cardiomyopathy is endocardial fibroelastosis, a disease featuring deposition of dense fibrous tissue over the ventricular endocardium, particularly over the ventricular apex and mi-

Table 17–8. Forms of cardiomyopathy.

Form (Etiology)	Distinguishing Features
Dilated 　Idiopathic 　Doxorubicin toxicity 　Carnitine deficiency 　Sarcoidosis 　Amyloidosis	Enlarged left ventricular chamber size, poor systolic function; ventricular arrhythmias common with severe cardiomyopathy
Restrictive 　Subendocardial 　　fibroelastosis 　Gaucher disease	Small left ventricular chamber size, diastolic dysfunction, pulmonary edema, atrial dilation and atrial arrhythmias common
Hypertrophic	Obstructive and nonobstructive forms; obstruction increases with exercise; may present with exercise-related chest pain or exercise intolerance; atrial or ventricular arrhythmias may be fatal, not related to degree of obstruction
Arrhythmogenic right 　ventricular dysplasia	Right ventricle dilated on echocardiogram; fatty infiltration on magnetic resonance imaging; ventricular arrhythmias are most prominent feature

tral valve apparatus. A rare cause of restrictive cardiomyopathy in children is Gaucher disease, a deficiency of the enzyme glucocerebroside-β-glucosidase, which primarily affects the nervous system.

In the diagnosis of restrictive cardiomyopathy, it is important to rule out constrictive pericarditis, as this condition may also cause high venous pressures with atrial dilation and small ventricles. Patients with restrictive cardiomyopathy should not have significant pulsus paradoxicus, whereas most patients with constrictive pericarditis do. Echocardiographic indices of ventricular filling may also separate the two conditions. At cardiac catheterization, patients with constrictive pericarditis have similar elevations in right and left ventricular end diastolic pressures, whereas patients with restrictive cardiomyopathy who have predominant involvement of the left ventricle usually have much higher left than right ventricular end diastolic pressures.

The prognosis is poor for patients with extensive restrictive cardiomyopathy. No specific therapy is available, although there are reports of symptomatic improvement with the administration of calcium channel–blocking agents, such as verapamil. Patients with this condition eventually may require referral for cardiac transplantation.

Hypertrophic cardiomyopathy refers to the condition of severe hypertrophy of the left ventricle, which is not secondary to a hemodynamic cause, such as hypertension or AS. In such patients, there may be concentric and symmetric hypertrophy of the ventricles or asymmetric septal hypertrophy, with the interventricular septum being thicker than the left ventricular free wall. HCM is known by several other names, including idiopathic hypertrophic subaortic stenosis (IHSS). The cause of HCM most often is idiopathic. In some patients, a familial relationship has been noted, indicating genetic associations. When symmetric hypertrophy is present, metabolic diseases must be considered, such as glycogen storage disease type II (Pompe disease), carnitine deficiency, and pyruvate metabolism disorders. Extensive hypertrophy leads to a ventricle that is hypercontractile, with an abnormally high ejection fraction. This may cause dynamic subaortic obstruction, particularly if asymmetric septal hypertrophy is present. There may be evidence of diastolic dysfunction with atrial dilatation and higher than normal venous pressures. There usually is a family history of HCM or sudden death. Histologically, the hypertrophied ventricular muscle is abnormal, with myocyte degeneration and myofibrillar disarray. In patients with Pompe disease, glycogen deposition is apparent in myocytes on light or electron microscopy.

Patients with HCM may present with dyspnea on exertion, chest pain, dizziness, palpitations, or syncope. They may also present with sudden death as the first manifestation, although it is rare for a previously asymptomatic patient with HCM to die suddenly. Clinically, one may divide the condition into cases with left ventricular outflow obstruction and those without obstruction. When obstruction occurs, it is dynamic and related to the asymmetric septal hypertrophy, with dramatic narrowing of the left ventricular outflow tract during systole. Such narrowing is worsened with exercise, increased inotropic state, and dehydration. Dyspnea on exertion, chest pain, and exercise intolerance are most prominent in patients who have the obstructive form of HCM, as these symptoms are thought to be due to dynamic left ventricular obstruction. In either group, arrhythmias that are unrelated to the degree of left ventricular obstruction may occur. These arrhythmias may be atrial or ventricular and are thought to be responsible for syncope and sudden death in these patients.

Clinically, one suspects HCM in patients with the above symptoms who also have a positive family history, particularly if the family history includes sudden death. Although the cardiac examination may suggest a problem, increased left ventricular impulse, loud ejection murmur, and paradoxical splitting of the second heart sound make the condition difficult to diagnose on the basis of examination. The ECG usually shows evidence of left ventricular hypertrophy, often with additional left septal hypertrophy. There also is an increased incidence of the Wolff-Parkinson-White syndrome in this condition. The echocardiogram remains the best modality for establishing the diagnosis of HCM, as it demonstrates the ventricular and/or septal hypertrophy, atrial dilation, and the lack of another cause for hypertrophy.

In treating this condition, one must differentiate between the symptoms of obstruction and those of arrhythmia, as these two manifestations are, for the most part, unrelated to one another. Agents that increase the inotropic state, such as digoxin, are not usually necessary, as there is little or no systolic dysfunction. Furthermore, these agents may be contraindicated, as they may increase the outflow obstruction, which is dynamic and related to contraction. Diuretic agents, which decrease filling pressures, also may worsen obstruction. The two agents used effectively for patients with symptoms are propranolol, a β-adrenergic blocker, and verapamil, a calcium channel blocker. Of the two, propranolol probably is used more often in children. Cardiac contractility may be reduced by both agents, thereby decreasing dynamic obstruction. Evidence indicates that these agents are effective in improving symptoms of HCM; unfortunately, however, they have not influenced the incidence of sudden death, which may be as high as 3–7% per year. Patients with syncope or dizziness are probably at higher risk of sudden death, and consideration in such patients should be given to the use of high-dose β-blocking agents or amiodarone; in preliminary investigations, both have appeared to decrease the risk of death. Any patient with HCM must be restricted from vigorous exercise.

Arrhythmogenic right ventricular dysplasia is a rare cardiomyopathy occurring primarily in adults and, infrequently, in adolescents. It is characterized by fatty replacement of ventricular myocardium, limited to the right ventricular free wall. Although extensive fatty replacement may adversely affect cardiac function leading to hemodynamic derangements, the primary mode of presentation is of ventricular arrhythmias. Typically, these occur with exercise and may be responsible for sudden death. Management of such patients is directed at controlling the ventricular arrhythmia. In severe cases, surgical resection of the involved myocardium has been performed.

INFECTIVE ENDOCARDITIS

Definition

The term **infective endocarditis** denotes a condition in which a bacterial or fungal infection involves the endocardial surface of the heart, most commonly the cardiac valves, or the endothelial surfaces of central vessels. Such infection may lead to destruction of the valves with resulting CHF, or it may lead to disseminated sepsis. In the preantibiotic era, this condition was almost uniformly fatal. Currently, despite the availability of antimicrobial agents effective against nearly all pathogens responsible for endocarditis, the disease carries a mortality rate of 15–20%. Therefore, the importance of prevention, as well as early diagnosis and institution of treatment, cannot be overstated.

Pathophysiology

Whereas bacterial and fungal pathogens may cause endocarditis in any person, the patients at greatest risk are those with preexisting cardiac structural abnormalities. Because rheumatic heart disease has become rare in children, this group consists of children with congenital heart disease. All forms of congenital heart disease are associated with an increased risk of endocarditis; however, this increased risk is smallest in patients with ASDs and highest in those with defects such as TOF and VSDs. Within these groups, those patients who have undergone palliative cardiac surgery, and particularly those who have had placement of artificial tissue grafts, are at the highest risk.

The pathophysiology of the disease begins with the introduction of pathogens into the bloodstream. Although certain high-risk events, such as dental extractions and IV drug abuse, produce bacteremia, nearly all persons are thought to experience bacteremia occasionally, eg, after tooth brushing and other activities. Once introduced into the bloodstream, the pathogen adheres to the endocardium. In general, these sites are determined by the hemodynamic environment, and areas of greatest turbulence are most often infected. For example, in patients with surgical shunts placed between the aorta and the pulmonary artery, infection develops in the pulmonary artery opposite the aortic jet. Such "jet lesions" are thought to be created by turbulent flow and to encourage the development of endocarditis. However, endocarditis has often been reported to involve nonturbulent areas of the endocardium, and invasive organisms can cause endocarditis even in patients whose hearts apparently are completely normal. The adherence of the pathogen to the endocardium leads to the deposition of platelets and thrombin, which form the vegetation. The growth of this vegetation may be associated with progressive valve destruction, damage to the blood vessels, or the occurrence of embolization as pieces of the vegetation break off and travel to distant sites. The chronic presence of bacteria or fungi may lead to the development of immune complexes, which may in turn cause a serum sickness–like reaction.

A great many pathogens have been found to cause endocarditis (Table 17–9). The viridans streptococci, which are normal mouth flora, have been the most common. However, recent reports have shown that *Staphyloccocus aureus* has been increasing in frequency and now accounts for nearly as many cases in children. Other pathogens include the enterococcus, the gram-negative enteric organisms, the pneumococcus, *Staphyloccocus epidermidis,* and *Candida albicans.* In immune-compromised patients, more indolent, slow-growing pathogens may be involved.

Diagnosis

In the past, infective endocarditis has been classified as either "acute" or "subacute" bacterial endocarditis. Although the classification is useful for remembering the different possible modes of presentation of the illness, few patients present with either classic picture. More often, features of both presentations are present (Table 17–10).

Patients with an acute presentation have a short duration of illness, high fever, and signs of progressive CHF because of valve destruction. They may also manifest signs of serious embolization, which may include pulmonary embolus, stroke, hematuria, or peripheral emboli. Valve destruction may be so rapid that signs of cardiac failure are present. Patients with a subacute presentation have a long (often more than 2 weeks) duration of illness, low-grade or even absent fever, and signs of immune complex disease, such as glomerulonephritis, arthritis, and skin rash. Findings such as the presence of petechiae, Osler nodes (small digital nodules), Janeway lesions (hemorrhagic or purpuric skin lesions), and Roth spots (retinal hemorrhagic lesions) are helpful in making the diagnosis but are rarely seen in children. A new or changed cardiac murmur may be appreciated, but one must be careful: The presence of fever often amplifies trivial cardiac murmurs in children. Signs of CHF usually are not part of the subacute presentation.

The diagnosis of infective endocarditis rests on clinical findings as well as on the results of blood cultures. Infec-

Table 17–9. Organisms most frequently isolated in endocarditis.

Viridans streptococci
Staphylococcus aureus
Enterococci
Streptococcus pneumoniae
Enteric gram-negative organisms (*Escherichia coli, Klebsiella species,* etc)
Candida albicans
Staphylococcus epidermidis

Table 17–10. Acute and subacute presentation of endocarditis.

Acute Presentation	Subacute Presentation
New murmur	New murmur
Cardiac decompensation	Little or no decompensation
Short duration of illness (< 2 wk)	Longer duration of illness (> 2 wk)
Major emboli	
	Splenomegaly
	Petechiae
	Osler nodes
	Janeway lesions
	Roth spots
	Splinter hemorrhages

tive endocarditis produces a constant low-grade bacteremia, rather than episodic high-grade bacteremia. Therefore, multiple blood cultures are very helpful. One normally obtains four to six blood cultures, if possible, before the institution of therapy. When at least five of six cultures are positive for the same organism, endocarditis is likely, whereas simple bacterial sepsis is less likely.

Echocardiography may be quite helpful in establishing the diagnosis in patients who have endocarditis but is not useful for ruling out the disease in patients who do not have it. This is because the prominent echocardiographic findings often are not present in patients who do have the disease. Diagnostic echocardiographic findings can include vegetations, dilatation of the aorta or pulmonary artery in patients with invasion of these vessels, and the presence of previously absent valvular regurgitation indicating valve destruction.

Treatment

The decisions that must be made in the treatment of endocarditis are complicated by two somewhat conflicting needs: the need to establish a microbiologic diagnosis and the need to institute therapy as quickly as possible to minimize valve destruction. The institution of broad-spectrum therapy before adequate blood cultures have been obtained may lead to uncertainty in the diagnosis and the possibility of prolonged unnecessary therapy with multi-

ple toxic agents. On the other hand, excessive delay in the institution of therapy to obtain cultures may lead to rapid valve destruction and progressive CHF or septic shock. In practice, one must consider both competing issues. In patients with a more "subacute" presentation, rapid valve destruction and sepsis are less likely, and 12–24 hours for obtaining adequate cultures is reasonable. In patients with a more "acute" presentation, therapy should be delayed for no more that 2 hours, and six cultures should be rapidly obtained in that time.

Initial therapy should include coverage for the viridans streptococci as well as for *S aureus* and enterococcus. This is true both for patients with community-acquired infections as well as for those who have undergone cardiac surgery. In the latter group, coverage for multiple drug–resistant organisms (such as *S epidermidis*) should be included, as well as coverage for whatever locally prominent nosocomial pathogens are present in the hospital. Once the pathogen has been identified, more specific therapy may be substituted on the basis of the antibiotic sensitivities of the pathogen.

All patients being treated for infective endocarditis should receive daily repeated blood cultures, beginning 12–24 hours after institution of therapy. Persistent positive cultures despite theoretically adequate antibiotics represent the potential for therapeutic failure. Therefore, higher doses of the antibiotic or additional agents will be necessary. Continued surveillance is vital for signs of emboli, for ECG changes that might indicate invasion of the cardiac conduction system, and for progression of cardiac valvular dysfunction.

Early surgical consultation should be sought because surgery for débridement or for valve replacement may become necessary. The generally accepted indications for surgery include progressive CHF despite medical therapy, persistent infection despite theoretically adequate antimicrobial treatment, serious systemic embolization, infection involving a prosthetic cardiac valve, and, perhaps, the presence of fungal endocarditis. Timing of surgery will be dictated by the hemodynamic condition.

It is well established that relapse after successful treat-

Table 17–11. Antibiotic regimen for prophylaxis of bacterial endocarditis in children.[1]

Procedure	Standard Regimen	For Penicillin-Allergic Individuals
Dental, oral, respiratory tract, or esophageal	Amoxicillin 50 mg/kg (max, 3.0 g) 1 h before procedure	Clindamycin 20 mg/kg or cephalexin or cefadroxit 50 mg/kg or azithromycin or clarithromycin 15 mg/kg 1 h before procedure
	Unable to Take Oral Medications	**For Penicillin-Allergic Individuals**
	Ampicillin 50 mg/kg IV or IM (max. 2.0 g) within 30 min before procedure	Clindamycin 20 mg/kg IV or cefazolin 25 mg/kg IV or IM within 30 min before procedure
Gastrointestinal, genitourinary (excluding esophageal) procedures or high-risk patients	Ampicillin 50 mg/kg plus gentamicin 1.5 mg/kg IV or IM 30 min before; amoxicillin 25 mg/kg orally or ampicillin 25 mg/kg IV or IM 6 h later	Vancomycin 20 mg/kg IV over 1–2 h plus gentamicin 1.5 mg/kg IV or IM, complete infusion/injection within 30 min of starting procedure

[1]Based on recommendations of the American Heart Association. JAMA 1997;277:1794.

ment occurs, and, in the past, occurred more often after short courses of antibiotic therapy. Therefore, most patients should receive a prolonged course (commonly 4–6 weeks) of IV antimicrobial therapy.

Prevention

Most cases of infective endocarditis do not follow an identifiable invasive procedure or event. Therefore, the disease is by no means completely preventable. However, certain high-risk procedures have been identified, and one may perhaps lower the risk of the development of endo-

carditis if antibiotic prophylaxis is given in association with these events. Such procedures include dental work; surgery on the gastrointestinal, respiratory, or genitourinary tracts; and childbirth. Nearly all patients with congenital heart disease should receive antibiotic prophylaxis during these procedures. The exceptions include patients who have had successful repairs of PDA, ASD, and simple VSD. Antibiotic regimens for prevention of bacterial endocarditis for these procedures have been proposed by the American Heart Association (Table 17–11).

REFERENCES

Committee on Rheumatic Fever, Endocarditis, and Kawasaki Disease: Prevention of bacterial endocarditis: Recommendations by the American Heart Association. JAMA 1990;264: 2919.

Fyler DC et al: Report of the New England Regional Cardiac Program. Pediatrics 1980;65(Suppl):375.

Gillette PC, Garson A Jr (editors): *Pediatric Arrhythmias, Electrophysiology, and Pacing.* Saunders, 1990.

Kaplan EL: Infective endocarditis in children: The changing profile. J Cardiac Surg 1989;4:310.

Klaus MH, Fanaroff AA (editors): *Care of the High-Risk Neonate.* Ardmore Medical Books, 1986.

Liebman J et al (editors): *Pediatric Electrocardiography.* Williams & Wilkins, 1982.

Richards MR et al: Frequency and significance of systolic cardiac murmurs in the first year of life. Pediatrics 1955;15:169.

Roberts NK, Gelband H (editors): *Cardiac Arrhythmias in the Neonate, Infant and Child.* Appleton-Century-Crofts, 1983.

Rudolph AM: *Congenital Diseases of the Heart.* Year Book, 1974.

Shuford WH, Sybers RG (editors): *The Aortic Arch and Its Malformations.* Thomas, 1974.

Special Writing Group of the Committee on Rheumatic Fever, Endocarditis, and Kawasaki Disease of the Council on Cardiovascular Disease in the Young of the American Heart Association: Guidelines for the diagnosis of rheumatic fever. Jones Criteria, 1992 update. JAMA 1992;268:2069.

18

Respiratory Diseases

Robert W. Wilmott, MD, & Mark E. Dato, MD, PhD

The lungs represent a unique gas-exchanging interface between the host and the environment. The airways are a series of dichotomously branching tubes that connect to the alveolar space; the alveolar space is a gas-exchanging interface with an area the size of a tennis court. The normal 5-year-old child respires at least 5000 L of air per day, and, because of the exposure to inhaled microorganisms and inhaled antigens, the lungs have developed sophisticated host defense mechanisms, both specific and nonspecific. These exposures make the lungs susceptible to a wide variety of diseases.

HISTORY

A systematic medical history should be obtained in a comfortable environment free of distractions and interruptions. The chief complaint should be identified. The history of the presenting complaint should be documented in detail with regard to time of onset and duration. In addition, relieving or precipitating factors should be identified. Treatments that have been attempted should be noted, and those that were most effective should be evaluated. The environment and the circumstances under which the presenting complaint developed may be important. Symptoms should be evaluated in terms of their quality, severity, and timing.

Respiratory diseases are often affected by environmental factors, such as changes in temperature, and exposure to noxious agents, such as exhaled cigarette smoke or a stove used for domestic heating. The physician should obtain a detailed description of the child's home, including type of heating, condition of the home, proximity to urban or rural sources of potential allergens, and history of household pets, such as dogs, cats, and birds (budgerigars, parrots, or pigeons). The type of bedding used and the presence of soft furnishings or soft toys in the child's bedroom should be noted. The presence or absence of animal or vegetable fibers in feather pillows, eiderdowns, or soft furnishings, as well as the systems in use for air purification, air filtration, air conditioning, or humidification, should be recorded.

Pulmonary symptoms are often precipitated by trigger factors. Exercise is an important trigger factor for coughing and wheezing. In children with asthma, excitement, change in climate, exercise, or exposure to cold, dry air may produce symptoms. Often laughter will produce coughing or wheezing in these children. Eating may bring on symptoms of respiratory disease if food is aspirated on swallowing or if the child has gastroesophageal reflux.

The composition of the household may provide clues; for example, the presence of young siblings may be important in terms of exposure to viral infections. If unusual infections are in the differential diagnosis, ask about recent travel to unusual areas, exposure to exotic animals, and potential drug abuse or high-risk behavior by the patient or parents.

Typical symptoms of respiratory disease are coughing, wheezing, chest tightness, sputum production, noisy breathing, fever, shortness of breath, cyanosis, and chest pain. The past medical history should be obtained. An important aspect is the birth history; specifically, whether the pregnancy was normal and whether the child was premature should be determined. The feeding history also may be important, particularly in younger children. A history of current medications, as well as a history of any drug allergies, should be obtained.

The family history also should be obtained. Some diseases of the respiratory tract in children have a genetic basis; for example, cystic fibrosis (CF) and antitrypsin deficiency are autosomal-recessive diseases. Other diseases, such as the immune deficiency disorder chronic granulomatous disease, are X-linked recessive conditions that may have serious pulmonary complications.

Important aspects of the social history are the child's schooling and how the child is performing at school. The structure of the family, the occupations of the parents, the coping strategies of the family, and the type of social support that the family has are important details.

The final part of the history is a review of organ systems, which is best performed systematically. In the interest of time, as well as relevance, this is often performed during the physical examination.

PHYSICAL EXAMINATION

One of the most important aspects of the physical examination, which is sometimes neglected in the enthusiasm to evaluate the organ systems, is the general examination. The patient should be examined for general health and the presence or absence of cyanosis, anemia, and tachypnea. The more serious pulmonary diseases, such as CF, are associated with failure to thrive, which may be evident on general appearance. However, it is important to measure the child's height and weight, to obtain previous height and weight measurements if possible, and to plot these measurements on a percentile chart. Failure to thrive will then be evident as a crossing of the percentile chart in a downward direction (see Chapter 1).

A very important physical sign to be elicited on physical examination is the presence or absence of digital clubbing. Digital clubbing is an abnormal sign in which the ends of the fingers are swollen with an increased amount of connective tissue under the base of the fingernail. This can be determined by visual inspection or palpation or by looking for the absence of the normal diamond formed between the nail bases when two identical fingers are opposed; in North America, this is known as the Scamroth sign (Figure 18–1). The causes of digital clubbing are shown in Table 18–1.

Table 18–1. Causes of digital clubbing.

Pulmonary
    Bronchiectasis
    Cystic fibrosis
    Immotile cilia syndrome
    Bronchiolitis obliterans
    Pulmonary abscess
    Empyema
    Malignant tumors (primary or secondary)
    Interstitial fibrosis
Cardiac
    Cyanotic congenital heart disease
    Subacute bacterial endocarditis
    Chronic congestive heart failure
Hepatic
    Biliary cirrhosis
    Biliary atresia
Gastrointestinal
    Crohn disease
    Ulcerative colitis
    Chronic infective diarrhea
    Polypolis coil
Other
    Thyrotoxicosis

Much can be learned by simple observation, especially in a young child who may become uncooperative as the examination continues. The physician should observe the child for respiratory rate, rhythm, and effort. Use of accessory muscles of respiration indicates respiratory distress that may be associated with increased airway resistance due to asthma or decreased lung compliance due to interstitial fibrosis. Very high breathing rates are seen in children with decreased compliance of the respiratory system, fever, anemia, exertion, and metabolic acidosis. Anxiety can also cause hyperventilation. A slow respiratory rate can occur in children with central nervous system depression or metabolic alkalosis. Normal values for respiratory rate according to age are shown in Figure 18–2.

Abnormalities of the rhythm of breathing can be a normal finding in infants younger than 3 months, who often have respiratory pauses for up to 10 seconds. Children also may have cycles of increasing and decreasing tidal volume separated by apnea, so-called Cheyne-Stokes breathing, with congestive heart failure or increased intracranial pressure.

Increased respiratory effort is an important physical finding, and the signs include subcostal retractions, intercostal retractions, supraclavicular retractions, movement of the trachea (a tracheal tug), use of the sternocleidomastoid muscles for respiration, and movements of the alae nasi. Movement of the chest wall should be evaluated visually. Normally, the chest wall and abdomen move outwardly during inspiration. Inward movement of the chest during inspiration characterizes paradoxical breathing. This occurs when the chest wall loses its stability, as seen in children with paralysis of intercostal muscles from a spinal cord lesion. This abnormality can be normal in young infants, who have a very flexible rib cage. Paradoxical

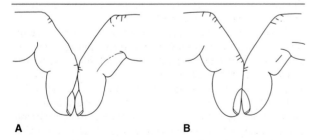

A   **B**

Figure 18–1. **A:** A normal child has a diamond-shaped window present between the nail bases when the fingers are opposed. **B:** The appearance of digital clubbing where the diamond-shaped window has been obliterated by the increased amount of soft tissue under the base of the nail. (Reproduced, with permission, from: Pulmonology. Page 502 in: Polin RA, Ditmar MF [editors]: *Pediatric Secrets,* 2nd ed. Hanley & Belfus, 1997.)

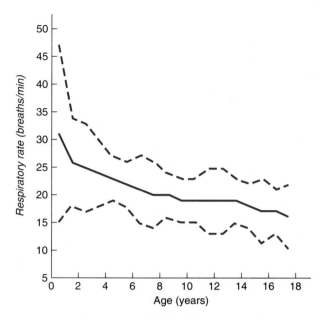

Figure 18–2. Mean values *(solid line)* ± 2 SD *(dashed lines)* of the normal respiratory rate at rest. There is no significant difference between the sexes, and the regression line represents data from both boys and girls. The respiratory rate decreases with age and shows the greatest normal variation during the first 2 years of life. (Data from Iliff A, Lee VA: Child Dev 1952;23:237; reproduced, with permission, from Pasterkamp H: The history and physical examination. In: Chernick V, Kendig EL [editors]: *Disorders of the Respiratory Tract in Children.* Saunders, 1990.)

breathing also may occur in patients with upper airway obstruction. Children with difficulty in breathing often have inspiratory in-drawing of the lower lateral chest, which eventually produces a depression called a Harrison groove. This is sometimes seen in children with severe asthma.

Inspection of the respiratory system should then focus on the upper airway. The nose should always be examined, and nasal patency should be evaluated. The turbinates are best examined with the use of an otoscope. Nasal polyps are commonly found in children with CF, and the turbinates may appear boggy and violet in children with allergies. The oropharynx should be inspected for the presence of cobblestoning from chronic sinusitis and for malformations, such as cleft palate. Examination of the oropharynx may reveal enlarged tonsils. The frontal and maxillary paranasal sinuses should be palpated for tenderness; transillumination of the sinuses in a darkened room may be attempted, but this approach is insensitive for the detection of reduced pneumatization.

PALPATION

Palpation usually commences with the cervical lymph nodes, followed by the trachea. A slight deviation of the trachea to the right is normal because of the presence of the descending aorta on the left side. Marked deviation to one side may signify atelectasis on one side or overexpansion of the other side, as seen with pneumothorax.

PERCUSSION

Percussion of the chest is best performed by tapping lightly with the middle finger (the plexor) of the dominant hand on the middle phalanx of the other hand's middle finger (the pleximeter). The pleximeter should be placed firmly (of course, the hand should be warm!), and percussion should be gentle, with quick perpendicular movements. The anterior, lateral, and posterior surfaces of the chest should be examined by comparing symmetric sites between the right and left sides. Reduced resonance will be noted in the presence of consolidation or pleural effusion. Increased resonance will be present if there is replacement of lung by more air than normal, as seen with emphysema or pneumothorax.

AUSCULTATION

Auscultation of the chest is performed by using the diaphragm of the stethoscope. The breath sounds should be evaluated; they should be equal and have a normal vesicular quality. Because of the smallness of the chest in young children, it is possible to hear tubular breath sounds in the periphery originating from the large airways; this is a normal finding. The quality and symmetry of the breath sounds also should be evaluated. Adventitial respiratory sounds are best considered in two categories: crackles and wheezes. Crackles are nonmusical, interrupted lung sounds that can be classified as fine or coarse, depending on the duration and frequency of the sounds. Fine crackles that occur during late inspiration are common in interstitial pulmonary fibrosis and in the early stages of pulmonary edema. Coarse crackles may be heard in early inspiration and during expiration; they are often heard at the mouth. Coarse crackles are caused by increased airway secretions or pneumonic consolidation.

Wheezes are musical, continuous sounds that originate from narrowed airways. Widespread narrowing of the airways in asthma leads to multiple sources for these sounds and various pitches, or "polyphonic" wheezes. A fixed obstruction in a large airway, for example, an inhaled foreign body, produces a "monophonic" wheeze in a constant location that may be present on inhalation and exhalation. The intensity of expiratory wheezing is related to respiratory effort, and the patient may need to cooperate with deep, forced inhalations and exhalations for wheezes to become evident. In younger children, it often helps to squeeze the upper part of the chest manually during exhalation to elicit a wheeze while holding the diaphragm of the stethoscope below the clavicle. This technique is called the way to "squeeze a wheeze."

DIAGNOSTIC PROCEDURES

RADIOLOGY

Anteroposterior and lateral chest radiographs are valuable tools in evaluating children with suspected lung disease. Right and left lateral decubitus films are used to demonstrate the presence of an inhaled foreign body or to evaluate pleural effusions. Inspiratory and expiratory x-ray films to locate a foreign body are helpful in older patients who can cooperate, but they are not useful in younger children. Fluoroscopy of the diaphragm can be used to assess diaphragmatic motion and phrenic nerve function, although this technique is now being replaced by ultrasound.

COMPUTED TOMOGRAPHIC SCAN

High-resolution computed tomography (CT) is useful to evaluate the pulmonary interstitium for diseases such as idiopathic pulmonary fibrosis. CT scans are also useful to evaluate anatomic structures in the parenchyma, such as cysts and solid lesions, and mediastinal structures, such as vascular malformations, airway compression, and enlarged lymph nodes. Contrast enhancement may be helpful in diagnosing sequestrations and pulmonary arteriovenous fistulae.

BRONCHOSCOPY

Fiberoptic bronchoscopy has revolutionized pulmonary medicine. Although this technique was developed for use in adults, it is possible to examine young children if pediatric flexible bronchoscopes are used together with sedation and topical anesthesia. Direct visualization of the airways allows the diagnosis of congenital airway anomalies and airway obstruction by foreign bodies or mucous plugs. Mucous plugs can be treated very effectively with lavage by using the suction channel of the instrument; foreign bodies are more easily removed with a rigid bronchoscope. Bronchoalveolar lavage is used to obtain bronchial secretions for microscopy and culture. Protected sterile brushes can be used to obtain reliable cultures; this technique avoids contamination of the specimen with normal bacterial flora from the upper airways. Transbronchial biopsy and transbronchial needle aspiration are more useful in adults than in children. The flexible fiberoptic bronchoscope is also very useful for selective bronchography and difficult endotracheal intubations.

THORACENTESIS

Children who have pleural effusions may have pneumonia, malignancy, tuberculosis, hypoproteinemia, or abnormal lymphatic drainage of the thorax. Fluid may be aspirated from the pleural space for diagnostic purposes or for relief of respiratory distress. The fluid is then examined by Gram stain, aerobic and anaerobic cultures, and measurement of glucose and protein levels, white and red cell counts, pH, and lactate dehydrogenase levels. These measurements allow the fluid to be classified as a transudate or an exudate (Table 18–2). Cytologic analysis should be performed on the pleural fluid if there is the possibility of a malignancy.

PULMONARY FUNCTION TESTS

Pulmonary disease may be evaluated noninvasively with the use of pulmonary function tests. These allow quantification of the extent of pathology, evaluation of responses to therapy, and objective follow-up of chronic diseases, such as asthma and CF. Exercise-induced asthma can be diagnosed by evaluating pulmonary function before and after a standardized exercise provocation test.

The two main types of pulmonary function abnormality are restrictive defects and obstructive diseases. In restrictive defects, lung volumes are reduced by fibrosis or by chest wall deformity. Obstructive diseases are characterized by airflow obstruction from asthma, CF, or bronchopulmonary dysplasia.

The simplest device for evaluating pulmonary function is the peak flow meter. This device measures the maximal velocity of gas in the mouth when the patient exhales forcefully; this measurement is reduced in obstructive disease. Measurement of peak flow rate is very useful in the evaluation of asthma; it can be used in the daily monitoring and adjustment of the dose of inhaled medications. Peak flow rate usually can be measured in children by 5 years of age and sometimes in younger children. It has the disadvantage of being very effort dependent.

BLOOD GAS & OXYGEN SATURATION MEASUREMENTS

Arterial blood is used to assess acid-base balance, oxygenation, and carbon dioxide excretion. Carbon dioxide is

Table 18–2. Laboratory tests to distinguish pleural exudates from pleural transudates.

	Exudate	Transudate
Protein	> 2.6 g/dL	< 2.6 g/dL
Pleural–plasma protein ratio	> 50%	< 50%
Lactic dehydrogenase	> 200 IU	< 200 IU
pH	< 7.20	> 7.20

retained and oxygenation is reduced in children with respiratory failure. Acid-base disturbances can be classified into respiratory or metabolic causes of acidosis or alkalosis. The drawing of arterial blood gases has the disadvantage of being quite uncomfortable, which is a particular problem with children. An approximation of acid-base balance and carbon dioxide excretion can be obtained by drawing a venous blood gas. The arterial hemoglobin oxygen saturation can be measured by pulse oximetry with the use of a probe that measures the differential absorption by the capillary blood of two wavelengths of red light. The combination of a venous blood gas and oxygen saturation measurement is often sufficient to make clinical decisions.

SWEAT TEST

The sweat test is used to diagnose CF with the finding of increased concentrations of chloride and sodium in the sweat. The test must be performed by an experienced laboratory using pilocarpine iontophoresis as described by Gibson and Cooke. The sweat is collected on a weighed filter paper or gauze for 30 minutes and then analyzed for chloride concentration. A value greater than 60 meq/L in a sample weighing at least 75 mg is diagnostic of CF, although the test should be repeated for confirmation. A value in the range 40–60 meq/L is in the "grey zone," and the test should be repeated. Although the test is accurate, there are many recognized causes of false-positive and false-negative sweat test results (Table 18–3).

Table 18–3. Causes of false-positive and false-negative sweat test results.[1]

False-Positive Results	False-Negative Results
Laboratory error	Laboratory error
Malnutrition	Administration of the anti-
Renal diabetes insipidus	biotic cloxacillin
Untreated adrenal insufficiency	Peripheral edema
Untreated hypothyroidism	
Anorexia nervosa	
Familial cholestasis	
Celiac disease	
Fucosidosis	
Ectodermal dysplasia	
Hypogammaglobulinemia	
Hypoparathyroidism	
Type I glycogen storage disease	
Klinefelter syndrome	
Atopic dermatitis	
Mucopolysaccharidosis	
Pupillotonia-areflexia and seg-	
mental hypohidrosis	

[1]Adapted, with permission, from Ruddy RM, Scanlin TF: Abnormal sweat electrolytes in a case of celiac disease and a case of psychosocial failure to thrive. Clin Pediatr 1987;26:83.

COMMON CLINICAL PROBLEMS

PERSISTENT COUGH

Children often present with chronic or persistent coughing. The cough may be infrequent, or it may be debilitating and disruptive to both the patient and the family. The cough mechanism serves the dual purpose of protecting the tracheobronchial tree from the penetration of foreign substances and removal of endogenous materials with subsequent expectoration.

Chronic cough is defined as one that persists for 3–6 weeks; recurrent cough shows periods of intermittent resolution. The cough mechanism is dependent on the coordination of inspiratory and expiratory muscles, normal laryngeal function, intact irritant receptor reflex, and a functional diaphragm. Cough may be voluntary or involuntary. The cough center is located in the pons, and voluntary input is supplied from the cerebral cortex.

Persistent cough in infants should always be regarded as abnormal. Aggressive workup for anatomic abnormalities, functional abnormalities (such as gastroesophageal reflux), congestive heart failure, or infectious diseases should be pursued. Involuntary coughing is the end result of stimulation of irritant receptors located in the upper and lower airways, including the sinuses, external ear, pleura, diaphragm, and pericardium; the highest concentrations are found at points of airway bifurcation, such as the carina. Stimulation may occur with allergies, infections, or the inhalation of noxious agents or foreign bodies in the aerodigestive tract. Ineffective coughing may also result in a persistent cough because of the inability of the cough to clear endogenous materials and persistent stimulation of irritant cough receptors. Voluntary coughing may become persistent in individuals with psychological problems.

Causes of Chronic or Recurrent Cough

There are many causes of chronic cough in children (Table 18–4), but most cases are associated with only a few causes. An algorithm for the evaluation of cough is provided in Figure 18–3. In cases of acute onset, the physician must be aggressive in the workup and diagnosis to provide alleviation of possible life-threatening events. The child with acute onset of coughing may be at high risk for progressive airway obstruction and respiratory distress.

Trauma. Ingestion and inhalation of foreign bodies is common in children aged 1–3 years. Impaction of the foreign body in the airway results in persistent coughing, and a localized, unilateral wheeze is highly suspicious. A chest radiograph with asymmetric hyperinflation, secondary to a ball-valve effect, warrants immediate action. The radiograph may be confirmatory if the object is ra-

Table 18–4. Causes of chronic cough.

Infection	Inflammatory
Sinusitis	Asthma
Pneumonia	Allergic rhinitis
Pharyngitis	Cystic fibrosis
Laryngitis	Recurrent aspiration
Tracheobronchitis	Chemical
Pertussis	Smoke
Parapertussis	Strong fumes
Influenza	Hydrocarbon ingestion
Bronchiolitis	Congenital
Tuberculosis	Laryngotracheomalacia
Immune deficiency	Tracheoesophageal fis-
Neoplastic	tula
Lymphoma	Vascular ring
Mediastinal tumors	Lobar sequestration
Trauma	Miscellaneous
Aspirated foreign body	Gastroesophageal reflux
Foreign body in external	Psychogenic
auditory canal	Congestive heart failure

diopaque. In the United States, the most common inhaled foreign body is the peanut. Children who have inhaled foreign bodies can be asymptomatic until secondary infection ensues. A foreign body in the external auditory canal can also stimulate irritant receptors and cause a reflex cough.

Gastroesophageal Reflux. Gastroesophageal reflux, with or without aspiration, causes a chronic cough by stimulation of esophageal receptors resulting in bronchoconstriction, as well as irritation of cough receptors in the hypopharynx or larynx. If the chest radiograph shows chronic parenchymal changes in the child with chronic cough, recurrent aspiration should be considered.

Cystic Fibrosis. Any child with unexplained chronic cough, with or without evidence of gastrointestinal malabsorption, should undergo a sweat chloride analysis.

Sinusitis & Postnasal Drip. Irritation of receptors in the posterior pharynx by drainage of nasal secretions from chronic sinusitis is a common cause of a chronic cough. Sinusitis may also aggravate underlying reactive airways disease with resultant bronchoconstriction and exacerbation of cough. Parents often report an increase in coughing at night when their child is in the supine position. Overt nasal discharge may not be present. Careful examination of the posterior pharynx often will show tenacious mucus on the posterior pharyngeal wall and a cobblestone appearance of the mucosa.

Asthma. Airway hyperreactivity with inflammation of the airways is an extremely common cause of chronic coughing. Cough-variant asthma, which is not associated with wheezing, is a well-recognized entity in children; aggressive treatment often relieves the problem.

Infection. In early childhood, viral infections, such as parainfluenza, adenovirus, and influenza, are common respiratory infections. Acute infection, resulting in pharyngitis, laryngitis, laryngotracheal bronchitis (croup), and acute epiglottitis, is a common cause of acute cough. Per-

tussis or parapertussis should be considered in the child with a paroxysmal cough. Diagnosis of pertussis may be made by fluorescent antibody testing of a nasopharyngeal swab; confirmation must be obtained by culture. Viral pneumonias, causing low-grade airway inflammation, are common infections of early childhood; the common agents are respiratory syncytial virus (RSV), influenza, and parainfluenza. *Mycoplasma pneumoniae* can cause a persistent cough in school-aged children that may last 8–10 weeks.

Environmental Toxins. Inhalation of cigarette smoke has been shown to cause an increase in otitis media in children, as well as an increased number and duration of upper respiratory infections. Chronic exposures to inhaled irritants should be sought in the history. Other environmental agents that may cause direct irritation of the airways are insecticides and industrial emissions.

Congenital Anomalies. Congenital malformations of the airway, including tracheoesophageal fistula, laryngotracheal clefts, and other anomalies that increase the risk of aspiration, can cause a persistent cough. Congenital anomalies of the lung parenchyma, including sequestration and cystic adenomatoid malformation, should be considered in the differential diagnosis. Vascular malformations and congenital heart disease can contribute to chronic cough through pulmonary edema or compressive effects on the airway.

Evaluation of the Patient With a Chronic Cough

Careful history taking is very important when examining a child with a chronic cough. Precipitating factors, including association with feedings and position in the young infant, should be sought. The age at onset of symptoms is valuable in considering congenital anomalies. The quality of the cough, as well as possible mucous production, should be ascertained. The quality of the cough can suggest the diagnosis. A dry, barking cough is classically seen in croup and epiglottitis. Paroxysmal coughing suggests the presence of an infectious disease, such as pertussis or *Chlamydia*.

Alleviating or exacerbating factors should be considered. Coughing after strenuous exercises is suggestive of exercise-induced bronchospasm. A cough that stops during sleep is suggestive of psychogenic causes. Coughing associated with seasonal variation may indicate allergic rhinitis. A child who is unaffected at school but has persistent cough at home may have environmental allergies. Any treatments that seem to improve the child's cough are valuable diagnostically; these may include bronchodilator or antibiotic therapy.

Physical Examination. The general state of health and nutrition is important. Children with immunodeficient states, CF, or chronic gastrointestinal disease typically have a chronically ill appearance. Careful examination of the oropharynx, external auditory canals, and nasal passages is also important. Examination of the chest for evidence of retractions or increased anteroposterior diameter

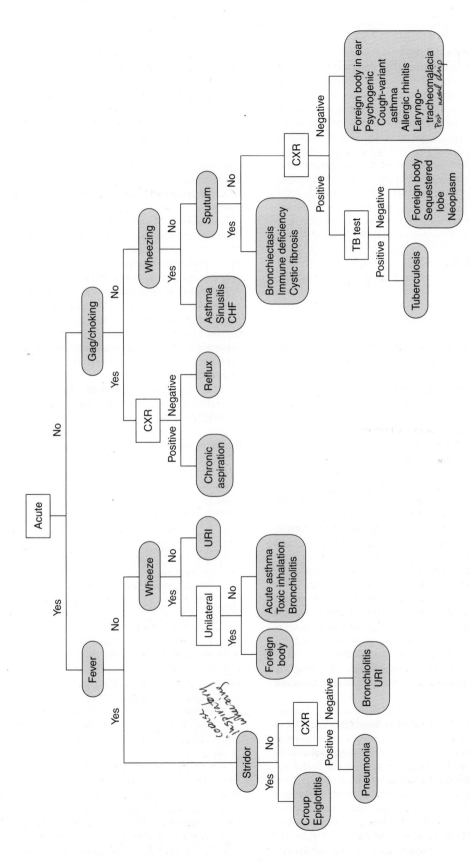

Figure 18–3. An algorithm for the evaluation of chronic and acute cough. CHF = congestive heart failure; CXR = chest radiograph; TB = tuberculosis; URI = upper respiratory infection.

→obstr. of bronchioles c̄ fibrous granulation tissue 2° mucosal irritation/ulceration (irritant gases, pneumonia)

may suggest obstructive diseases, such as asthma or bronchiolitis obliterans. Auscultation may demonstrate a localized wheeze, as heard in foreign-body aspiration. Diffuse, polyphonic, musical wheezes are consistent with asthma or bronchiolitis. Coarse crackles are the result of mucopurulent plugging of small airways and can be associated with CF, bronchiectasis, or pneumonia. Fine end-inspiratory crackles suggest interstitial lung disease with pulmonary fibrosis or pulmonary edema. Careful palpation of the abdomen for hepatosplenomegaly is warranted; subdiaphragmatic abscess with resultant diaphragmatic irritation can cause a persistent cough. Examination of the extremities for digital clubbing should not be overlooked. Evidence of recurrent infections of the skin can be seen in immunodeficiency syndromes with neutrophil dysfunction. All children with chronic or persistent cough warrant a chest radiograph. Evidence of gas trapping, peribronchial thickening, alveolar infiltrates, or cardiomegaly should be noted. Symmetry of the left and right hemithorax should be checked. Pulmonary function tests can be valuable in children able to participate, generally those older than 5 years. Pre- and post-bronchodilator studies may demonstrate reversible obstruction, as seen in asthma. Airway obstruction, either intrathoracic or extrathoracic, may be diagnosed; the former might suggest airway compression from adenopathy or lymphoma.

RECURRENT OR PERSISTENT PNEUMONIA

↗ 2x in 1 year or 3x total *↗ lasting > 1 month.*

Examination of the child with recurrent or persistent pneumonia requires a systematic approach to obtain the time course of both symptoms and radiographic changes. Pneumonia is an illness manifested clinically by fever, coughing, upper or lower respiratory symptoms, and dyspnea or tachypnea. Associated physical findings include dullness to percussion, fine crackles, and decreased breath sounds; wheezing may or may not be present. This constellation of signs and symptoms, in conjunction with a chest radiograph showing an alveolar infiltrate, constitutes clinical evidence of pneumonia. A period of at least 1 month, and possibly a minimum of 3 months, has been proposed as the definition of persistence. Recurrent pneumonia is defined as two episodes of pneumonia during the same year or three episodes of pneumonia during any time period.

The first step in examining a child with recurrent pneumonia is to review the history and radiographs carefully to determine whether they meet the criteria for recurrent pneumonia or whether they represent repeated evaluations of improperly treated or resolving pneumonia. Careful serial review of all available radiographs with a pediatric radiologist is very helpful. A careful history should be taken to ascertain whether the child has had symptom-free periods between the suspected bouts of pneumonia and to establish the general baseline health of the child. Because recurrent pneumonias in children may be the manifesta-

tion of a more protean disease state, a careful review of systems, including the general nutritional status of the child and any other recurrent infections, is important. Daytime and nighttime symptomatology of the child should be elicited, together with the history of attendance at day care and exposure to cigarette smoke. The child's medication history should be obtained, especially the chronic or recurrent use of antibiotics. In developing a differential diagnosis, it should be realized that pulmonary infections generally come from two possible sources: direct inoculation from the airways and hematogenous spread.

Because the physician relies on the chest radiograph to diagnose pneumonia, it is important to have an appreciation for the time scale of normal resolution of pneumonia in the pediatric patient without complications. A community-acquired pneumonia, such as *Streptococcus pneumoniae,* usually shows radiographic resolution in 6–7 weeks. Severe RSV or adenoviral pneumonia may take as long as 12–15 months, depending on the severity of the initial infection. Therefore, careful longitudinal follow-up of these patients is necessary to make the diagnosis of recurrent or persistent pneumonia, as well as to appreciate improving symptoms or radiographs.

After recurrent or persistent pneumonia is diagnosed, a logical stepwise approach to understanding its etiology is necessary (Table 18–5). It is helpful to approach recurrent or persistent pneumonia by determining whether the pneumonia is unilobar or multilobar, as seen on the chest ra-

Table 18–5. Differential diagnosis of persistent or recurrent pneumonia.

	Unilobar	Multilobar
Aspiration syndromes		
Central nervous system abnormalities	+	+
Gastroesophageal reflux	+	+
Myopathies	+	+
Anatomic causes of aspiration		
Tracheoesophageal fistula	+	+
Laryngotracheal cleft	+	+
Cleft palate	+	+
Congenital anomalies		
Sequestration	+	
Bronchogenic cyst	+	
Cystic adenomatoid malformation	+	
Pulmonary hypoplasia	+	
Tracheal bronchus	+	
Heart disease		+
Mucociliary dysfunction		
Cystic fibrosis		+
Chronic bronchitis		+
Primary ciliary dyskinesia		+
Luminal obstruction		
Foreign body	+	
Bronchial stenosis	+	
Tracheobronchomalacia		+
Hilar adenopathy	+	
Vascular compression	+	
Immunodeficiency syndromes		+

diograph; the age of the child should also be considered. Recurrent pneumonias are usually caused by aspiration syndromes, abnormal airway clearance from obstruction or dysfunctional cilia, or congenital abnormalities of the cardiopulmonary system. Immunologic deficiencies also cause recurrent pulmonary infections. In the latter case, the history will reveal other evidence of immunologic dysfunction, including recurrent sinus disease, middle ear infection, failure to thrive, or recurrent skin infections.

In the child with asthma or airway hyperreactivity, a recurrent pneumonia is often diagnosed on the basis of radiographic evidence of an increased density in the right middle lobe. The child's asthma is exacerbated by intercurrent upper respiratory infections and mucous plugging, leading to fever, wheezing, crackles, and diminished breath sounds. Intraluminal obstruction due to inspissated mucus in the airway causes inflammation and obstruction. Aggressive treatment of the underlying reactive airways disease includes techniques to improve clearance of the airway. Chest physiotherapy is often all that is needed in these patients. It is important to demonstrate normalization of the radiograph.

Unilobar Pneumonia

Single-lobe disease is indicative of three possible processes. The most common is a congenital structural abnormality, such as bronchogenic cysts, a sequestered lobe, or congenital cystic adenomatoid malformation of the lung. Another type of abnormality contributing to unilobar recurrent pneumonia is intraluminal or extraluminal obstruction. A history of acute choking or a witnessed episode of aspiration of a foreign body is most relevant. Extremely rare causes of intraluminal obstruction in childhood include bronchial adenomas and bronchial hamartomas. Any pathology causing extrinsic compression of the airway (extraluminal) can lead to recurrent pneumonia distal to the compression. These anomalies include vascular rings, congenital heart disease with enlargement of the atria or pulmonary arteries, and prior surgical repairs of congenital heart defects. Other extraluminal causes of obstruction include tumors of the mediastinum, such as lymphomas and neuroblastomas. Parahilar adenopathy from tuberculosis, histoplasmosis, coccidioidomycosis, or other infectious diseases is a common cause of extraluminal bronchial obstruction. Treatment of the underlying disease process usually results in resolution. Aspiration syndromes are generally thought to be multilobar processes; however, unilobar disease has been described in some children. A history of choking or feeding intolerance with increased respiratory distress after meals is helpful in discerning this problem.

Multilobar Pneumonia

Multilobar pneumonia is common with reflux and aspiration in young infants who are often in the supine position. When bilateral upper lobe infiltrates are noted on the chest radiograph of an infant, a complete workup for aspiration should ensue. A thorough neurologic examination

of such children is essential. Myopathies or neuromuscular disorders and their associated esophageal dysmotility carry a high risk for aspiration. Congenital anomalies, such as laryngotracheal clefts, tracheoesophageal fistulas (whether undiagnosed or previously repaired), and esophageal webs or strictures, all lead to a higher incidence of aspiration. Signs and symptoms of gastroesophageal reflux should not be overlooked, as this condition is amenable to medical or surgical treatment.

Dynamic anomalies of the airway may also lead to recurrent pneumonia, probably by poor clearance of the airway secretions and mucus. Laryngomalacia, tracheomalacia, and bronchomalacia may cause noisy breathing and recurrent pneumonia. Diseases such as CF are associated with abnormal mucociliary function, and any child with recurrent pneumonia should undergo a sweat chloride test.

Bronchiectasis may develop in children with recurrent pneumonia; therefore, a chest CT scan should be considered in a child with recurrent pneumonia and signs of chronic pulmonary disease. Flexible bronchoscopy is also indicated to diagnose infectious disease. Environmental irritants often cause ciliary dysfunction with resultant mucous plugging. These irritants include second-hand cigarette smoke, strong fumes from solvents, recurrent viral infections from day care, and antigen exposure from cats or birds. Primary ciliary dyskinesia also results in poor airway clearance associated with recurrent sinus disease, bronchiectasis, and airway inflammation due to chronic infection. Functional studies of the cilia or electron microscopic examination of ciliary biopsy material can confirm this diagnosis. Aspiration syndromes can be diagnosed with the use of various tests, including modified barium swallows, gastric-emptying scans, and pH probes. Direct visualization of the glottis by fiberoptic endoscopy is helpful in the child with a swallowing incoordination who may have intermittent aspiration according to food thickness. Congenital abnormalities of the upper airway, including laryngotracheal clefts, laryngomalacia, esophageal strictures, and webs, can be seen best by rigid laryngoscopy and esophagoscopy. Malacia of the trachea or the distal or mainstem bronchi is best visualized by flexible bronchoscopy with the patient sedated and breathing spontaneously. Allergic pneumonitis, such as a hypersensitivity pneumonitis, is suspected when the patient's symptoms seem to resolve when removed from the potential antigen exposure.

ASTHMA

Asthma, the most common chronic lung disease in children, affects 4–8% of children younger than 17 years. Approximately 11 million school days are missed each year because of asthma-related illness. It also accounts for approximately 13 million physician visits and more than 200,000 hospitalizations per year. In 1990, approximately $1.8 billion was spent in the treatment and prevention of asthma. Approximately 80–90% of children who are affected by asthma have their first episode by 5–6 years of age. The prevalence of asthma has increased over the past 10 years, and African-Americans are disproportionately affected. Socioeconomic factors show that the poor are affected more than the affluent, and boys tend to be affected more than girls up to the age of 10 years.

Pathophysiology

Asthma, or **reactive airways disease (RAD),** is caused by reversible airway obstruction. Airway hyperresponsiveness leads to exaggerated constriction of the bronchi when an individual is exposed to airway irritants, chemicals, and pharmacologic agents. Children with asthma have symptoms of coughing, wheezing, and shortness of breath after exposure to "triggers" such as viral infections, allergens, strong fumes, cold air, and exercise.

Airway hyperresponsiveness is an invariable part of asthma, and the severity of disease correlates with the degree of hyperresponsiveness. Hyperresponsiveness can be measured in the laboratory with a pharmacologic challenge, such as methacholine or histamine, or with a physiologic challenge involving exercise. Possible mechanisms causing airway hyperreactivity include airway inflammation, abnormal autonomic regulation of airway caliber, changes in bronchial smooth muscle function, and loss of bronchial epithelial integrity. The most important of these is airway inflammation. Pathologic studies have demonstrated the presence of inflammatory cells in the airways of patients with either mild or severe asthma. Patients with asthma have altered cellular immunity and increased levels of inflammatory mediators, particularly in the airway. This has led to the use of anti-inflammatory drugs, such as systemic steroids, inhaled steroids, disodium cromoglycate, and nedocromil sodium; these drugs can reduce the symptoms associated with a reduction in airway hyperresponsiveness.

The mechanism of airflow obstruction has three components: bronchospasm, mucosal edema, and mucous plugging of the lumen. Bronchodilators effectively relieve bronchospasm, whereas anti-inflammatory drugs affect all three components.

Allergy is an important trigger factor in many children with asthma. There is a correlation between serum IgE level and the risk of sensitization to environmental allergens. School-aged children with asthma commonly have positive skin test results to inhaled allergens, such as house dust mite, cockroach, molds, cat dander, and grass and tree pollen. Allergies are a less important factor in preschool children, in whom viral infections are common triggers. In the child with allergies, asthma may be associated with allergic rhinitis, conjunctivitis, or eczema.

Clinical Features

Clinical manifestations of asthma are the result of diffuse airway obstruction and include wheezing, dyspnea, recurrent coughing, and accessory muscle use. Airway narrowing is due to bronchospasm and mucosal edema with subsequent mucus plugging by thick, tenacious mucus. Air trapping occurs during the expiratory phase of respiration and results in a hyperinflated barrel chest.

Numerous triggers stimulate the hyperreactive airways of asthma. Well-recognized triggers include viral infections, sinus infections, tobacco smoke, strong fumes, and allergens such as dust mites, animal hairs or fur, and cold air. Exercise-induced bronchospasm is seen in some children. In addition, asthma symptoms can be seen with emotional disturbances.

Classically, asthma has been divided into intrinsic and extrinsic types. Extrinsic asthma is IgE-mediated (allergic), whereas intrinsic asthma does not have an allergic etiology. This division is academically interesting; however, in the treatment of either type, the basic physiology of chronic inflammation and increased mucous production leading to airway hyperreactivity is the same. A key point in the clinical history is the history of recurrent exacerbations provoked by known triggers. The episodic nature of asthma should allow the patient to have periods of normal breathing between attacks; a history of persistent noisy breathing should lead the physician to suspect other causes. Symptoms can also occur predominantly at night and may be indicative of gastroesophageal reflux or exposure to allergens, such as house dust mites in the child's bedroom. Eczematous skin rashes and seasonal rhinitis are common in children with asthma (the "atopic triad"). A family history of asthma is common. If one parent has reactive airways disease, the child has a 25% likelihood of having it as well. This risk doubles if both biologic parents have asthma.

The physical examination is important in the diagnosis of asthma or reactive airways disease. Polyphonic musical wheezing throughout the chest and evidence of atopy are key to the diagnosis, although wheezing has many other causes (Table 18–6).

Diagnosis

The diagnosis of asthma is supported by objective demonstration of reversible airflow obstruction. Spirometry showing a decrease in the forced expiratory flow rate in 1 second (FEV_1) with a normal or decreased expiratory flow volume curve (FVC) is consistent with airflow obstruction. Scooping on the expiratory flow volume loop further supports this diagnosis (Figure 18–4). Demonstra-

Table 18–6. Causes of wheezing by age.

Infants and Children	Adolescents and Adults
Asthma	Asthma
Bronchiolitis	Chronic bronchitis (smoking,
Cystic fibrosis	substance abuse)
Foreign body	Infections
Gastroesophageal reflux	Cystic fibrosis
Aspiration pneumonitis	Angiotensin-converting
Congenital heart disease	enzyme inhibitors
Bronchopulmonary dysplasia	β-Adrenergic blockers
Ciliary dyskinesia	

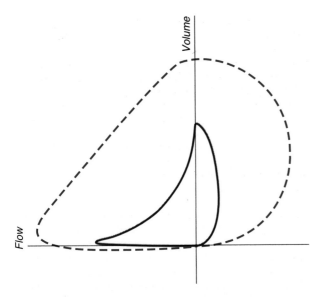

Figure 18–4. Flow-volume loop in a patient with intrathoracic airway obstruction because of small airway disease **(solid line).** A normal flow-volume loop **(dashed lines)** is shown for comparison. The loop sags because of progressively increasing small airway obstruction at lower lung volumes. (Reproduced, with permission, from: Evaluation of the airway. In: Myer CM et al [editors]: *The Pediatric Airway: An Interdisciplinary Approach.* Lippincott, 1995.)

tion of the reversibility of the airflow obstruction by bronchodilators strongly supports the diagnosis of asthma.

Bronchial hyperresponsiveness may be demonstrated by pharmacologic challenge with histamine or methacholine or by exercise provocation. The methacholine bronchial provocation test has the greatest sensitivity and specificity but is time-consuming; this test probably is not required in most children with asthma, in whom a clinical diagnosis can be made confidently.

Clinical Management

Peak expiratory flow (PEF) rates, measured by hand-held meters, are extremely helpful in managing asthma on an outpatient basis. These objective measurements can be communicated to the physician during periods of illness. A step-care plan based on the patient's expected and personal best flow rates is helpful in establishing a clear plan. Other diagnostic tests are not necessary unless clinical suspicion warrants them (eg, a history suggestive of foreign-body aspiration). Allergy testing may help to define suspected triggers (see Chapter 19). Clinical severity may be divided into mild, moderate, or severe asthma (Table 18–7).

The management of patients with reactive airways disease is threefold:

1. Education
2. Self-recognition of clinical deterioration
3. Pharmacology.

Education & Self-recognition. Asthma education gives the patient an understanding of the logical approach to medications used in asthma. In addition, it allows clear communication of symptoms to the physician on an outpatient basis. Asthma is episodic, and recognition of changing clinical status by the patient is helpful. The use of PEF meters gives the patient the ability to monitor baseline flow rates and to detect any deterioration. It also allows objective changes to be communicated to the physician by telephone.

Pharmacologic Approach. Pharmacologic reversal of chronic airway inflammation, airway obstruction, and airway hyperresponsiveness is the cornerstone of treatment (Table 18–8; Figures 18–5 to 18–8). The first-line drugs in the treatment of mild asthma are the β_2-adrenergic agonists, which have the ability to relax airway smooth muscle and have rapid onset of action. These drugs provide the patient with immediate relief of symptoms; however, their limited duration of action may require repeated dosing. In addition, the β_2 agonists are associated with side effects, including dysrhythmias, tachycardias, hypokalemia, and systemic hypertension. They are administered by metered-dose inhaler, nebulizer, or mouth. Long-acting β_2 agonists are now available, but these agents should not be used on an acute basis, as their onset of action is delayed and repeated dosing may lead to toxicity with cardiac dysrhythmias. The anticholinergic bronchodilators, such as ipratropium bromide,

Atrovent

Table 18–7. Severity classification of asthma.

Mild	Moderate	Severe
Cough/wheeze < 3 times/wk	Cough/wheeze > 2 times/wk	Daily wheezing with frequent exacerbations
Nocturnal symptoms < 3 times/mo	Nocturnal symptoms 2–3 times/wk; emergent care < 3 times/y	Nightly symptoms
PEFR > 80% predicted; ≤ 20% variability	PEFR 60–80% predicted; 20–30% variability	PEFR < 60% predicted; > 30% variability
Good exercise tolerance	Wheezing between exacerbations	Poor exercise tolerance
Few symptoms between exacerbations	Signs of airway obstruction	Hospitalizations > 2 times/y
> 15% bronchodilator response	> 15% bronchodilator response	Substantial obstruction; incomplete reversibility

PEFR = peak expiratory flow rate.

Table 18–8. Dosages for therapy in childhood asthma.[1]

β_1-Adrenergic agonists	
Inhaled (albuterol, metaproterenol, bitolterol, terbutaline, pirbuteral)	
Metered-dose inhaler	2 puffs q 4–6 h
Dry powder inhaler	1 capsule q 4–6 h
Nebulizer solution[2]	
Albuterol	5 mg/mL; 0.10–0.15 mg/kg in 2 mL of saline q 4–6 h, maximum 5 mg
Metaproterenol	50 mg/mL; 0.25–0.50 mg/kg in 2 mL of saline q 4–6 h, maximum 15 mg
Oral	
Liquids:	
Albuterol	0.10–0.15 mg/kg q 4–6 h
Metaproterenol	0.3–0.5 mg/kg q 4–6 h
Tablets	
Albuterol	2- or 4-mg tablet q 4–6 h
	4-mg sustained-release tablet q 12 h
Metaproterenol	10- or 20-mg tablet q 4–6 h
Terbutaline	2.5- or 5.0-mg tablet q 4–6 h
Cromolyn sodium → *stabilize mast cell membranes*	
Metered-dose inhaler 1 mg/puff; 2 puffs bid–qid	
Dry powder inhaler 20 mg/capsule; 1 capsule bid–qid	
Nebulizer solution 20 mg/2 mL ampule; 1 ampule bid–qid	
Theophylline → *bronchodilators, unknown mech.* *may inhibit PDE sterase*	
Liquid	
Tablets, capsules	
Sustained-release tablets, capsules	
Dosage to achieve serum concentration of 5–15 µg/mL	
Corticosteroids	
Inhaled[3]	
Beclomethasone	42 µg/puff 2–4 puffs bid–qid
Triamcinolone	100 µg/puff 2–4 puffs bid–qid
Flunisolide	250 µg/puff 2–4 puffs bid
Oral[4]	
Liquids:	
Prednisone	5 mg/5 mL
Prednisolone	5 mg/5 mL
Tablets:	
Prednisone	1, 2.5, 5, 10, 20, 25, 50 mg
Prednisolone	5 mg
Methylprednisolone	2, 4, 8, 16, 24, 32 mg

[1]Reproduced, with permission, from National Asthma Education Program: *Guidelines for the Diagnosis and Management of Asthma.* Expert Panel Report. US Department of Health and Human Services, Public Health Service, National Institutes of Health, August, 1991.
[2]Premixed solutions are available. It is suggested that the dosage per kilogram recommendations be followed.
[3]Consider use of spacer devices to minimize local adverse effects.
[4]For acute exacerbations, doses of 1–2 mg/kg in single or divided doses are used initially and are then modified. Reassess in 3 days, as only a short burst may be needed. There is no need to taper a short (3- to 5-day) course of therapy. If therapy extends beyond this period, it may be appropriate to taper the dosage. For chronic dosage, the lowest possible alternate-day dosage should be established.

act by blocking vagal pathways and have minimal systemic absorption or side effects. Some evidence suggests that they effectively relieve bronchospasm from gastroesophageal reflux. Methylxanthines, specifically theophylline, have mild to moderate bronchodilator activity and some anti-inflammatory activity and may augment respiratory muscle function. The intravenous administration of these drugs for acute exacerbations of asthma has become less common because of toxicity (affecting the cardiovascular system, central nervous system, and gastrointestinal tract) and questionable efficacy. In patients with moderate to severe asthma, the chronic use of slow-release preparations of theophylline may allow the physician to reduce the use of systemic steroids.

Because asthma is a state of chronic airway inflammation, the use of both steroidal and nonsteroidal anti-inflammatory agents has been emphasized since the publication of guidelines by the National Heart, Lung & Blood Institute (see Table 18–8; Figures 18–5 to 18–8). Cromolyn sodium and nedocromil sodium are the best examples of nonsteroidal anti-inflammatory agents. The mechanism of action of these drugs is poorly understood but is thought to involve stabilization of mast cell membranes. The drugs are used prophylactically and inhibit both early- and late-phase allergic reactions. Four to six weeks of treatment are needed to determine the efficacy of these medications before treatment failure can be evaluated. Some patients experience coughing when given these agents, particularly the dry powder formulations.

Corticosteroids are the most effective anti-inflammatory drugs. They inhibit inflammatory cell migration and cytokine production; they also increase the response to β_2 agonists. Early use of these agents in asthma prevents progression of airway obstruction. In children with moderate to severe asthma, corticosteroids are essential to control airway inflammation. Systemic corticosteroids have many adverse effects, including increased appetite, truncal obesity, glucose intolerance, mood alteration, hypertension, fluid retention, and cataract formation. The formulation of inhaled steroids, using metered-dose inhalers, has enabled us to use steroids without systemic side effects.

Inhaled steroids have been shown to be extremely effective in moderate and severe asthma. They should be the first-line medication in someone who has coughing or wheezing more than twice per week or has nocturnal symptoms more than two to three times per week. In general, they do not have systemic effects at doses up to 800 µg per day. Oral thrush is a major side effect of metered-dose inhaled steroids. In young children, there appears to be no linear growth inhibition with conventional doses. The use of inhaled steroids has enabled previously systemic steroid–dependent children to be weaned from their treatment.

The overall management of the child with asthma is based on the understanding of the disease process by the family and physician, the ability to measure deterioration in the child's status subjectively and objectively, and the appropriate use of medications to provide bronchodilation and quell the ongoing chronic inflammation of the airways. It is also important to recognize asthma triggers and to avoid them as much as possible. A step-care plan often enables children to control their asthma independently and allows a method of communication between the physician and family during times of deterioration. Good communication between the physician and family typically leads to a better outcome, as well as a decrease in the frustration that this disease can present to families.

Clinical characteristics	Assessment of lung function (FEV₁ or PEFR)	Therapy[1]	Outcome

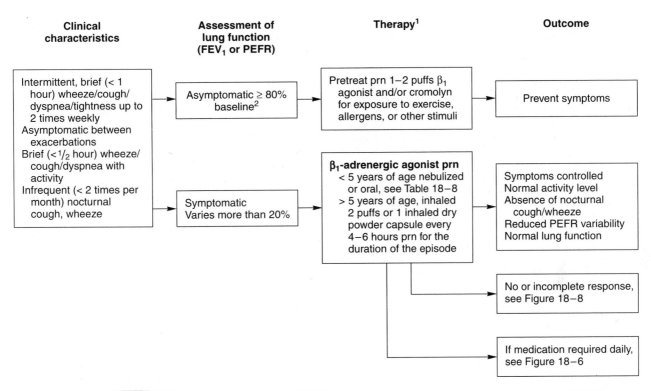

Figure 18–5. An algorithm for the management of asthma in children (chronic mild asthma). [1]All therapy must include patient education about prevention (including environmental control where appropriate) as well as control of symptoms. [2]Percentage of peak expiratory flow rate (PEFR%) baseline refers to the norm for the individual, established by the clinician; this may be the percentage predicted of standardized norms or percentage of patient's personal best. FEV_1 = forced expiratory volume in 1 second. (Reproduced, with permission, from the National Asthma Education Program: *Guidelines for the Diagnosis and Management of Asthma.* Expert Panel Report. US Department of Health and Human Services, Public Health Service, National Institutes of Health, 1991.)

Prognosis

Asthma is a chronic disease, and most children have persistent symptoms and persistent pulmonary function test abnormalities, even though the disease may become milder as they become older. In general, pulmonary function tracks throughout life according to earlier patterns; thus, patients who were mildly affected in the past will tend to have mildly affected pulmonary function test results in the future. Lung volumes and flow rates increase through childhood until early adolescence, when they stabilize until the beginning of the aging process. This is the most probable explanation for the improvement seen in many children with asthma; however, even if their symptoms are minimal and the pulmonary function test results are mildly affected, such children still have an increased risk for the development of chronic obstructive pulmonary disease in adult life and for the recurrence of symptoms. Approximately half of all children with asthma have a remission of their symptoms by early adulthood. The probability of resolution is less in children with severe asthma; only 5% of these patients have prolonged remissions. Children with asthma that begins before 2 years of age and has an allergic basis have a worse prognosis in terms of severity and persistence of symptoms than do children with asthma that begins later. Children with severe asthma that starts early in life also have a worse prognosis than do those with mild asthma. Many children who have symptoms in early childhood associated with viral respiratory tract infections become symptom free in later childhood. Asthma tends to be more severe if the child has other associated allergic diseases, such as eczema, or has a positive family history. Fortunately, death from asthma is unusual, although there has been concern in recent years about the increased numbers of sudden death associated with asthma. The reasons for this increase are unclear but are likely to be undertreatment, late presentation for medical care, and, possibly, overuse of β_2 bronchodilators.

CYSTIC FIBROSIS

CF is the most common lethal autosomal-recessive disease that affects the white population, with an incidence of approximately 1:3300. The incidence among African-

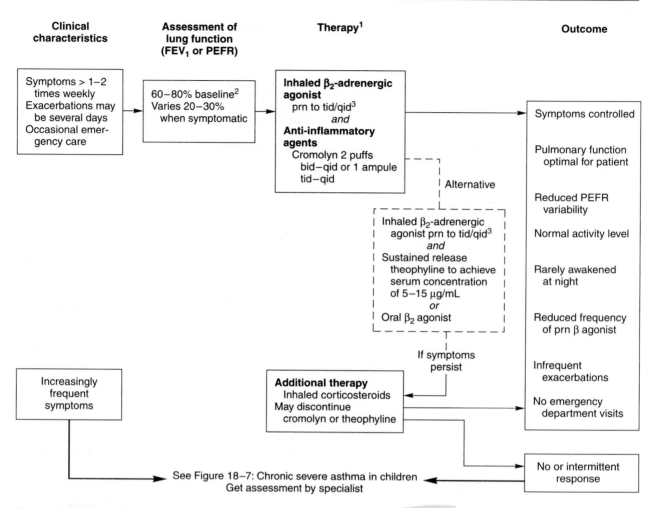

Figure 18–6. An algorithm for the management of asthma in children (chronic moderate asthma). [1]All therapy must include patient education about prevention (including environmental control where appropriate) as well as control of symptoms. [2]Percentage of peak expiratory flow rate (PEFR%) baseline refers to the norm for the individual, established by the clinician; this may be the percentage predicted of standardized norms or percentage of patient's personal best. [3]If exceed three to four doses a day, consider additional therapy other than inhaled β_2-adrenergic agonist. FEV_1 = forced expiratory volume in 1 second. (Reproduced, with permission, from the National Asthma Education Program: *Guidelines for the Diagnosis and Management of Asthma.* Expert Panel Report. US Department of Health and Human Services, Public Health Service, National Institutes of Health, 1991.)

Americans is approximately 1:15,000, and among Native Americans, approximately 1:32,000. The disease affects three main organ systems: the lungs, with recurrent lower respiratory tract infections and progressive obstructive pulmonary disease; the gastrointestinal tract, with pancreatic exocrine insufficiency; and the sweat glands, with production of hypertonic sweat rich in sodium and chloride. Abnormal hyperviscous secretions characterize the disease and are probably responsible for the clinical manifestations.

Pathophysiology

The basic defect of CF is a mutation in a gene that is 250,000 base pairs long and resides on chromosome 7.

This gene produces the CF transmembrane conductance regulator (CFTR) protein. Mutation of the CFTR protein causes an abnormality of cyclic adenosine monophosphate–regulated chloride conductance in epithelial cells. In 1989, the *CF* gene was identified and cloned, leading to a period of rapid and exciting advances in understanding the basic mechanisms underlying CF. In North America, approximately 75% of affected individuals with CF have a point mutation that results in deletion of the amino acid phenylalanine at the 508 position of CFTR, thus designated ΔF508. Currently, there are more than 500 known mutations of the *CF* gene. Defective chloride transport due to mutant CFTR can be seen in epithelial cells of the respiratory, gastrointestinal, hepatobiliary, pancreatic, and

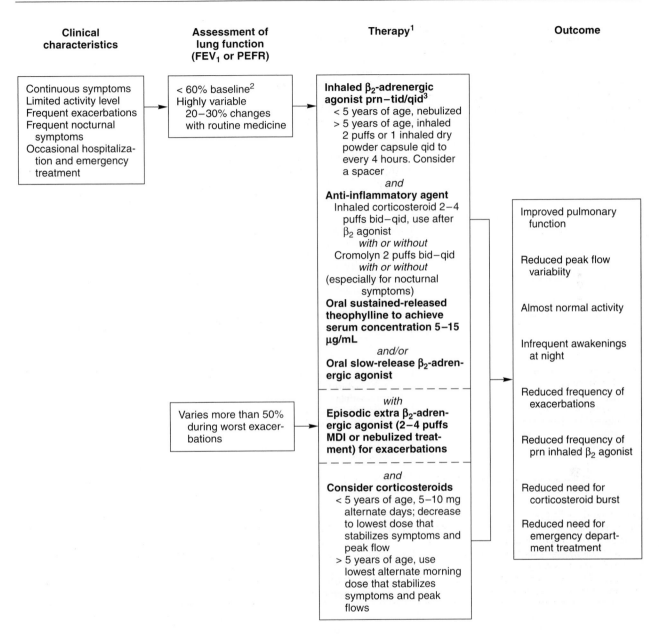

| Clinical characteristics | Assessment of lung function (FEV₁ or PEFR) | Therapy[1] | Outcome |

Figure 18–7. An algorithm for the management of asthma in children (chronic severe asthma). Note: Individuals with severe asthma should be evaluated by an asthma specialist. [1]All therapy must include patient education about prevention (including environmental control where appropriate) as well as control of symptoms. [2]Percentage of peak expiratory flow rate (PEFR%) baseline refers to the norm for the individual, established by the clinician; this may be the percentage predicted of standardized norms or percentage of patient's personal best. [3]If exceed three to four doses a day, consider additional therapy other than inhaled β_2-adrenergic agonist. MDI = metered-dose inhaler; FEV₁ = forced expiratory volume in 1 second. (Reproduced, with permission, from the National Asthma Education Program: *Guidelines for the Diagnosis and Management of Asthma.* Expert Panel Report. US Department of Health and Human Services, Public Health Service, National Institutes of Health, 1991.)

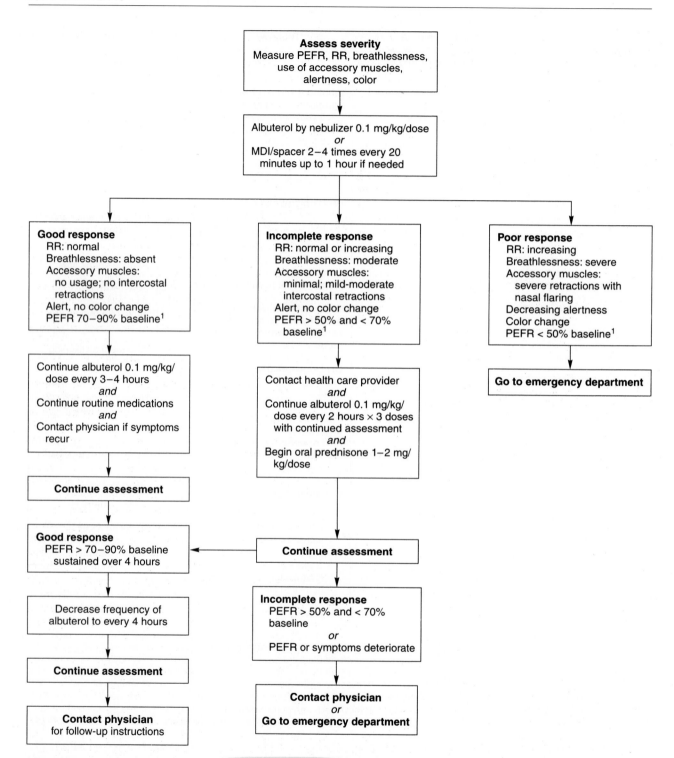

Figure 18–8. An algorithm for home management of acute exacerbations of asthma in children. [1]Percentage of peak expiratory flow rate (PEFR%) baseline refers to the norm for the individual, established by the clinician; this may be the percentage predicted of standardized norms or percentage of patient's personal best. MDI = metered-dose inhaler; RR = respiratory rate. (Reproduced, with permission, from the National Asthma Education Program: *Guidelines for the Diagnosis and Management of Asthma.* Expert Panel Report. US Department of Health and Human Services, Public Health Service, National Institutes of Health, 1991.)

reproductive tracts. CFTR has regulatory effects on other chloride channels as well and controls sodium reabsorption by epithelial cells. The net result of failure of CFTR function in the epithelial surfaces of tissues is dehydrated, viscous secretions with reduced mucociliary clearance.

Clinical Features

The primary organ systems affected by CF are the pulmonary, gastrointestinal, and reproductive systems. Inspissated mucus in the airways of patients leads to recurrent infections of the lower respiratory tract with bacteria such as *Pseudomonas aeruginosa* and *Staphylococcus aureus*. This leads to a chronic endobronchial inflammation with airflow obstruction. The airflow obstruction progresses, becoming worse with each intercurrent pulmonary infection, although usually it responds to treatment with antibiotics. Over a period of years, there is progressive loss of lung function, eventually leading to severe airflow obstruction, ventilation perfusion mismatching, and hypoxemia. The hypoxemia, in turn, leads to an increased pulmonary vascular resistance and pulmonary hypertension, so that most CF patients eventually die of respiratory failure complicated by right ventricular failure. Common pulmonary complications are bronchiectasis due to repeated bacterial infections of the airway causing permanent weakening of the airway wall; atelectasis, particularly in young children with smaller airways; and hemoptysis, which may be minor or, on occasion, massive. The latter problem occurs when an ulcerating airway lesion erodes a hypertrophied bronchial artery.

Gastrointestinal manifestations are caused by exocrine pancreatic insufficiency, which is thought to be due to thick pancreatic secretions. The result is destruction of the exocrine portion of the pancreas, leading to malabsorption of fat, carbohydrates, and proteins. This leads to the clinical symptoms of steatorrhea, diarrhea, and failure to thrive in infancy. Approximately 18% of infants affected by CF are born with an obstruction in the small intestine caused by thick inspissated meconium, so-called meconium ileus. Men affected by CF usually are infertile because of obstruction of the vas deferens. Most probably, chronic inspissation of secretions in utero leads to abnormal cannulation of the vas deferens and obstructive azoospermia. In young women with CF, fertility rates are decreased to approximately 50% of normal; delayed menarche occurs in approximately 20% of patients.

Hypochloremic, hypernatremic dehydration with alkalosis occurs in very young infants with CF because of excessive loss of salt from sweat glands. It tends to occur in hot weather, particularly if oral intake of salt and water is decreased.

The **distal intestinal obstructive syndrome (DIOS)**, formerly known as meconium ileus equivalent, can develop in patients with CF. This functional intestinal obstruction probably results from abnormal CFTR function in the mucous-secreting glands of the intestine. Patients presenting with either abdominal distention or constipation must be examined. Early intervention with mucolytic or osmotic agents is often successful and may obviate surgical intervention.

In approximately 15–20% of adolescents with CF, hepatobiliary disease, typically focal biliary cirrhosis, develops. This leads to intralobular cirrhosis with resultant portal hypertension, varices, and increased risk for gastrointestinal bleeding. Repeated and continued scarring of the pancreas, as well as a relative insulin resistance, results in diabetes mellitus in approximately 20% of adults with CF.

Diagnosis

The diagnosis of CF is based on the following criteria: the occurrence of at least one typical clinical symptom of CF or a positive family history, combined with a positive sweat test result on two occasions; the finding of two CF mutations on analysis of the CF locus; or the finding of abnormal nasal potential difference measurements on two occasions. Nasal potential difference refers to the measurement of bioelectrical potentials in the nose using a perfusion method. The transepithelial potential difference is increased in CF because of the abnormal secretion of chloride. See Table 18–3 for causes of false-positive and false-negative sweat test results.

In approximately 60% of patients with CF, the diagnosis is determined during the first 12 months after birth; in 85% of patients, the diagnosis is determined by the age of 5 years, and in 90–94%, by 10 years. Delayed diagnosis may be due to wide variations in the clinical manifestations of CF, resulting in mild disease or misdiagnosis of the clinical presentation. Approximately 18% of affected newborns present with meconium ileus or rectal prolapse; any infant with these signs should undergo sweat testing when clinically stable. The diagnosis of CF should also be considered in a newborn with prolonged neonatal jaundice, failure to thrive, or any pulmonary manifestation, such as wheezing, coughing, or tachypnea and retractions, that cannot be explained clinically. Segmental or lobar atelectasis may be the presenting manifestation of pulmonary disease in an affected infant. In the slightly older child, the diagnosis is often considered if there is recurrent wheezing, recurrent pneumonia, chronic cough, bronchiectasis, staphylococcal pneumonia, chronic recurrent pansinusitis, or nasal polyps. Nasal polyps occur in approximately 10–24% of children and more than 50% of adolescents with CF. The presence of nasal polyps at any age requires investigation by sweat chloride analysis. Digital clubbing is almost always associated with cardiopulmonary or hepatic disease, and CF is an important cause of clubbing in children (see Table 18–1). Any patient with *P aeruginosa* recovered from sinuses, sputum, or epiglottic culture should be assumed to have CF until the diagnosis is disproved. Gastrointestinal symptoms include steatorrhea and malabsorption syndrome. Infants and children with failure to thrive or episodes of partial obstruction of the small or large intestine must also undergo a sweat test.

Clinical Management

The treatment of CF is threefold:

1. Treatment of recurrent, chronic endobronchial infections
2. Augmentation of hyperviscous secretions from the airway
3. Pancreatic enzyme replacement with the subsequent alleviation of malabsorption

Augmentation of caloric intake by nutritional supplementation has also shown to be a benefit to patients with CF.

Pulmonary Management. Early pulmonary disease is manifested by endobronchial infection initially caused by *S aureus*, *Haemophilus influenzae*, and gram-negative bacilli, such as *Escherichia coli*. By 8–10 years of age, virtually all patients with CF have become colonized with *P aeruginosa*, and this is the predominant organism in their sputum. Patients with CF have intermittent pulmonary exacerbations requiring the use of either oral or intravenous antibiotics on the basis of symptomatology and culture results. At these times, they often report an increased frequency of coughing with an increase in sputum quantity and tenacity. They often have increased shortness of breath, decreased exercise tolerance, and decreased appetite. On physical examination, they may demonstrate an increased work of breathing with increased use of accessory muscles of respiration. Usually, they have weight loss and abnormal pulmonary function test results. Auscultation demonstrates coarse crackles either locally or globally; the crackles represent mucous plugging of small airways associated with chronic inflammation and increased production of hyperviscous mucus.

In the younger child, antibiotic coverage should include *H influenzae*, as well as *S aureus*; oral antibiotics, such as cephalexin, amoxicillin-clavulanate, cefprozil, and clarithromycin, are commonly prescribed. In the child with known *Pseudomonas* colonization, anti-pseudomonal combinations of a β-lactam with an aminoglycoside are appropriate. Common choices are ceftazidime and tobramycin, or ticarcillin and tobramycin. Most of these combinations require intravenous therapy. Newer, orally absorbed drugs in the quinolone class (such as ciprofloxacin) can be prescribed; however, data about their safety in children are limited, and *Pseudomonas* can become resistant to their actions. Increasing emergence of multidrug-resistant, gram-negative organisms, such as *Burkholderia cepacia*, *Xanthomonas maltophilia*, and multidrug-resistant *P aeruginosa* is a problem. This most likely reflects the increasing use of antibiotics, as well as the increased survival of patients.

Gastrointestinal Management. Nutritional management is important in CF, as it seems to improve the overall prognosis and the resistance to pulmonary infections. The basic treatment is replacement of the missing exocrine pancreatic function by taking oral pancreatic supplements with food. This comes in the form of purified pancreatic enzymes (pancrelipase) prepared in microsphere or microtablet form and packaged in capsules. Children with CF will take several capsules with each meal and one or two capsules with each snack, so that the enzymes are ingested just before food. A minority of patients with CF have sufficient pancreatic function and therefore do not require these enzyme supplements. Even with enzyme therapy, there may be ongoing mild steatorrhea, which tends to deplete the patient of fat-soluble vitamins. Therefore, the standard practice is to supplement vitamin intake with a multivitamin that includes A, D, E, and K. Children with CF have increased calorie requirements and may need as many as 30% more calories per kilogram. These increased requirements are met with calorie supplements. Children with mild disease can increase their caloric intake by consuming more snacks and larger meals. Children with more severe symptoms may require supplementation with special food or even overnight enteral feeding through a nasogastric, gastrostomy, or jejunal tube. Increased salt losses should be addressed in hot weather, particularly if the patient is going to exercise in high environmental temperatures. Usually, it is sufficient to allow them free access to table salt. They may enjoy salty snacks, such as saltine crackers and pretzels. Some patients who have high sodium requirements require treatment with sodium chloride tablets.

Prognosis

Even with optimal medical management, complications result from progression of the underlying disease (Table 18–9). Currently, the median age of survival in patients with CF is more than 29 years, and patients born with CF today are expected to have life expectancies greater than 40 years. The current average life expectancy represents a doubling in the past 20 years. This is believed to be due to increased understanding of the pathophysiologic mechanisms associated with CF, use of anti-pseudomonal antibiotics, aggressive treatment of malabsorption, and improved methods for airway clearance.

The clinical expression of disease in CF is wide ranging. Many patients can lead relatively normal lives, and

Table 18–9. Complications in patients with cystic fibrosis.

Pulmonary	Gastrointestinal
Atelectasis	Pancreatic insufficiency
Pneumothorax	Rectal prolapse
Hemoptysis	Intestinal obstruction
Respiratory acidosis	Failure to thrive
Pulmonary hypertension	Cholecystitis
Respiratory failure	Focal biliary cirrhosis
Nose and throat	Portal hypertension
Nasal polyps	Pancreatitis
Chronic sinusitis	Endocrine
Cardiac	Diabetes mellitus
Cor pulmonale	Reproductive
Orthopedic	Azoospermia
Hypertrophic pulmonary osteoarthropathy	Decreased fertility in women

many women with mild disease have successfully borne children. General pediatricians and other physicians are going to become increasingly involved in the care and management of patients with CF, as this disease is common and the life expectancy is improving.

BRONCHOPULMONARY DYSPLASIA

Bronchopulmonary dysplasia (BPD), one of the chronic lung diseases of infancy, is a relatively new disease. It has been recognized only in the past 20–30 years as a consequence of our ability to keep alive infants of extreme prematurity with very low birth weights, as well as nonpremature infants who have had severe respiratory distress.

Most, but not all, infants with BPD are premature. BPD appears to be the result of the lungs' response to initial injury and the lungs' ability to repair and recover from that injury. The initial injury, in the case of low-birth-weight infants, is pulmonary immaturity and injury resulting from necessary support measures, such as increased fraction of inspired oxygen (FiO_2), barotrauma from mechanical ventilation, resultant inflammation, and infections. BPD is also seen in children with chronic respiratory distress from meconium aspiration, congestive heart failure, severe neonatal pneumonia, diaphragmatic hernia with associated pulmonary hypoplasia, and pulmonary hemorrhage. The diagnosis of BPD depends on the clinical, radiographic, and histologic features (when available). More than 75% of cases involve premature infants with a birth weight of less than 1000 g; in addition, approximately 20% of ventilated newborns are affected with BPD. This represents approximately 3000–7000 affected infants in the United States each year. BPD is more common in boys than in girls. It is also more common in white infants than in African-American infants. The incidence of BPD varies between medical centers, which is probably a reflection of variations in patient population demographics, as well as variations in treatment.

The classic definition of BPD is chronic respiratory distress with tachypnea, increased work of breathing, air trapping, a persistent oxygen requirement after 28 postnatal days, and consistent chest radiograph findings. The disease has been altered in recent years by changes in ventilator pressures and therapeutic modalities, use of exogenous surfactant, nutritional support, recognition of hyperoxia in lung injury, improved ability to regulate and restrict fluids to the very low birth weight infant, and medical and surgical approaches to patent ductus arteriosus. Because of prematurity, normal lung growth and development are disrupted by exposure to adverse environmental stimuli. The immature lung is most susceptible to oxidant and pressure-related injury. Antioxidant levels are greatly reduced in premature infants compared with full-term infants. The premature lung also appears to have immature repair mechanisms, the cellular regulation of which may be dysfunctional during the repair phase of lung injury.

Pathophysiology

Most infants with BPD are premature. Soon after birth, the infant manifests respiratory distress with tachypnea, chest wall retractions, and nasal flaring often associated with cyanosis and grunting. Overall, there is greatly increased work of breathing. These infants require a high FiO_2 (often greater than 60%) and often require ventilatory support. Hyperoxia causes injury to the epithelial and endothelial barriers, which leads to an increase in permeability of the alveolar capillary membrane. There is direct injury to type II pneumocytes, demonstrated by microscopic swelling. The combination of decreased surfactant production with protein leak into the alveolus leads to a decrease in lung compliance and worsening atelectasis. Often, at the end of the first week, there is a slight improvement, which usually heralds the proliferative or repair phase of BPD. Bronchoalveolar lavage studies of infants with BPD show an increase in number of inflammatory cells. Various mediators, including leukotrienes, thromboxane, platelet-activating factor, and cytokines (eg, interleukin-1), have been found in the lavage samples, which supports the notion that inflammation of the airway and alveolar units causes the disease. With the institution of positive-pressure ventilation, damage to the lungs occurs by barotrauma. Compliance of the tracheobronchial tree is greater than that of the alveolar unit, leading to overdistention of the airways, distal gas trapping, and regional hyperinflation. Classic chest radiograph findings show areas of atelectasis mixed with areas of hyperinflation.

Features of BPD are summarized in Table 18–10. One functional abnormality of the airway is increased airway resistance. Older children with BPD show increased airway hyperreactivity to methacholine challenge, as well as cold air challenge. Children with BPD have periods of clinical improvement and deterioration, usually with chronic hypercapnia and persistent oxygen requirements. Any cardiovascular lesion that leads to increased left-to-right shunting must be identified. Such lesions include patent ductus arteriosus, ventricular septal defects, and atrial septal defects. Other sources of lung injury need to be minimized, especially aspiration syndromes and gastroesophageal reflux.

Long-term abnormalities in BPD include pulmonary

Table 18–10. Pathophysiologic abnormalities in bronchopulmonary dysplasia.

Pulmonary	Cardiovascular
Increased airway resistance	Pulmonary hypertension
Increased mucous production	Systemic hypertension
Increased airway hyperreactivity	Ventricular hypertrophy
Decreased compliance	Right heart failure
Decreased mucociliary clearance	Gastrointestinal
Pulmonary edema	Increased gastroesophageal reflux
Increased incidence of tracheobronchomalacia	Oral-motor hypersensitivity

hypertension, right ventricular hypertrophy, and left ventricular hypertrophy, even in the absence of pulmonary or systemic hypertension. Large systemic-to-pulmonary collateral arteries, which increase the pulmonary blood flow, are often seen on autopsy. Long-term intubation of the airway can lead to subglottic stenosis, inability to establish oral feedings, and increased incidence of pneumonia. Gastroesophageal reflux and electrolyte abnormalities secondary to diuretic therapy are common complications.

Clinical Management

The goals of clinical management are to treat hypoxemia, optimize ventilation with subsequent reduction in hypercarbia, minimize inflammation of the airways, and optimize somatic growth. Oxygen therapy is prescribed to keep arterial blood oxygen saturations between 92 and 95% while the infant is awake, asleep, and feeding. This has been shown to decrease the pulmonary vascular resistance and to optimize the growth of the child.

Chronic drug therapy for patients with BPD is aimed at bronchodilatation, control of inflammation, and minimization of fluid retention. Bronchodilators used include the β_2-adrenergic agonists and the anticholinergic bronchodilators, such as ipratropium bromide. These have been shown to improve lung compliance and airway resistance.

Steroidal and nonsteroidal anti-inflammatory agents are often used for more severe cases of BPD. Systemic steroids are the mainstay of treatment on both an acute and a chronic basis. The clinician has to measure carefully the risk and benefit of steroid use. Inhaled steroids have few systemic toxicities and could be a useful treatment for these children; there are few data on their efficacy in BPD.

Diuretic therapy is extremely effective in BPD. In the acute phase, loop diuretics are needed to minimize fluid retention. This may lead to hypokalemia and hyponatremia, resulting in a hypochloremic metabolic alkalosis. Hypercalcuria can lead to nephrocalcinosis and decreased bone density.

The caloric requirements of the infant with BPD are increased compared with the needs of children without chronic lung disease. The etiology of the increased caloric requirement is not fully understood; however, the increased work of breathing accounts for some of this increase. Meeting the caloric requirement of children with BPD and providing true weight gain and growth are essential to the long-term prognosis. Oral-motor dysfunction from delayed introduction of oral feedings often necessitates long-term placement of feeding tubes. The ability of the infant to feed orally should be promoted by using a team approach involving speech pathology and occupational therapy.

Prognosis

School-aged children with a history of BPD still have evidence of airflow obstruction and air trapping on pulmonary function tests. They also have a higher incidence of airway hyperreactivity on methacholine challenge. Infants with chronic lung disease of infancy have an increased incidence of viral respiratory infections, as well as recurrent pneumonia in the first 2 years. Their pulmonary reserve is less, and their clinical deterioration with infections is usually more acute. The ability to promote the growth of the infant with optimal nutrition provides the best long-term outcome for these children.

NOISY BREATHING

Noisy breathing in infants and children is a common presenting complaint to the pediatrician. This may represent a benign problem, or it may be indicative of life-threatening airway obstruction. The physician therefore must have a logical and organized approach in the evaluation.

Noise during breathing is due to turbulent airflow caused by airway obstruction. The key to evaluation is to discern the level and severity of the obstruction. The obstruction may exist anywhere between the nares and the distal tracheobronchial tree (Table 18–11).

Examination of the Patient

History and physical examination are important in the workup of noisy breathing for the physician to generate a precise differential diagnosis and to initiate treatment. Newborns and very young infants may present at birth with noisy breathing or stridor. Changes in the quality of the cry or hoarseness, persistent coughing, and any periods of apnea or cyanosis should be noted. Alleviation of symptoms by positional change is also important information. Worsening of symptoms related to feedings is indicative of aspiration syndromes, which may be caused by laryngotracheal clefts or tracheoesophageal fistulae. It is also important to note whether the abnormal sounds are persistent, or

Table 18–11. Causes of noisy breathing.

Anatomic	Infectious
Choanal atresia	Croup
Subglottic stenosis	Epiglottitis
Laryngeal web	Retropharyngeal abscess
Vascular rings/compression	Bronchiolitis
Tracheoesophageal fistula	Mononucleosis
Craniofacial anomalies	Upper respiratory infection
Micrognathia	Functional
Macroglossia	Laryngomalacia
Functional	Tracheomalacia
Foreign body	Gastroesophageal reflux
Congenital heart disease	Obstructive sleep apnea
Metabolic	Neurologic
Cystic fibrosis	Encephalocele
Connective tissue disease	Cerebral palsy
Storage diseases	Vocal cord paralysis
Neoplasm	Hypotonia/hyporeflexia
Laryngeal neoplasms	Hemangioma
Papilloma	Neurofibromas
	Mediastinal tumors
	Hygroma
	Angiofibroma

whether there are periods of alleviation. The quality of breath sounds during sleep, when the child's spontaneous tidal volume is lower, should be noted. A history of snoring while sleeping is suggestive of obstructive sleep apnea, commonly due to adenoidal or tonsillar hypertrophy. Functional abnormalities, such as laryngotracheomalacia, improve during periods of calm or quiet breathing. Any associated abnormalities of swallowing should also be ascertained. A history of foreign body ingestion should be explored in all children of toddler age. In the school-aged child and adolescent, dyspnea or chest pain may be indicative of neoplastic growth in the mediastinum. Symptoms of gastroesophageal reflux should be sought, and any associated cough and its quality should be noted.

Physical Examination

The general appearance of the child should be noted, and height, weight, and head circumference should be plotted on standard growth curves. The general appearance of the child should be noted for evidence of dysmorphic features consistent with congenital syndromes. The examination of the head should include palpation of the cervical region for masses and inspection for evidence of midline dimples or tracts consistent with structural remnants. Inspection of the nasal passages is important for signs of obstruction. In all children, thorough examination of the oropharynx with notation of the mandibular structure, tongue size, palate integrity, and posterior pharynx contour is important. Elicitation of a gag reflex must also be carried out. Inspection of the chest for evidence of retractions, as well as quality of chest excursion, is important. Auscultation can be most revealing when the phase of the respiratory cycle is correlated with the aberrant breathing sounds. Stridor is indicative of upper airway obstruction and occurs during the inspiratory phase. Large airway noises commonly associated with tracheomalacia are heard in the expiratory phase; however, with severe obstruction, biphasic sounds are heard. Auscultation over the mouth and the lateral neck should be performed to differentiate upper airway noises from lower airway noises, which may be transmitted in the small child. In a calm child, the examiner may purposely agitate the patient to elicit abnormal breathing sounds and to check for augmentation of existing sounds with increased tidal volume. In infants, the breathing sounds should be evaluated in both a supine and a prone position, as supralaryngeal obstruction is usually worse when supine. Palpation of the liver and spleen during the abdominal examination is useful for possible evidence of storage diseases, which may contribute to abnormal breathing sounds, secondary to infiltration of laryngeal structures. The presence of clubbing or cyanosis of the nail beds should be noted. A careful neurologic examination is important, and evidence of hypotonia or dysreflexia should be sought.

Diagnostic Evaluation

Anteroposterior and lateral chest radiographs should be obtained in all children with noisy breathing. Silhouettes of the heart and great vessels should be examined for proper size and orientation. Lung parenchymal disease may be secondary to aspiration, infection, or associated cardiac disease. Careful examination is necessary to detect tumors of the thorax, as compression of airway structures from tumors often results in noisy breathing.

High kilovolt airway films in both the anteroposterior and lateral views are useful for evaluation of upper airway obstruction. These may be helpful in acute settings, such as croup or epiglottitis; however, normal airway films do not rule out all underlying pathologies.

Direct visualization of the respiratory tract is the most revealing investigation for noisy breathing. The flexible bronchoscope allows one to evaluate the nasal passages, laryngeal structures, and tracheobronchial tree. Dynamic compression is best seen with a flexible bronchoscope, because the patient is lightly sedated and spontaneously breathing. Structures of the posterior larynx often require rigid bronchoscopy for complete evaluation.

CT scan may be indicated in patients when tumors of the head, neck, or mediastinum are being considered. Choanal stenosis and atresia is best visualized by this [*opening into the nasopharynx of the nasal cavity*] technique. Vascular anomalies that may be causing external compression of the airway, such as aortic arch anomalies, innominate artery compressions, and compressions of the left or right mainstem bronchus by the pulmonary arteries, are well visualized by magnetic resonance imaging (MRI). MRI scans should be obtained only after evidence of external compression has been demonstrated by bronchoscopy. Either MRI or CT may be used to evaluate the head of a neurologically abnormal child. Testing for metabolic diseases should be pursued when clinically indicated.

The use of a pediatric sleep laboratory is helpful in the child with noisy breathing. Neurologic, cardiac, and respiratory data are gathered and are used to measure the clinical severity of any obstruction and to help understand its etiology.

The child with noisy breathing presents a diagnostic challenge to the clinician. With a complete history and careful clinical examination, the physician can narrow the diagnostic possibilities considerably. Carefully chosen diagnostic tests are used systematically to ascertain the etiology of the noisy breathing. Referral of these patients to a pediatric subspecialist is often necessary for treatment of the airway anomalies.

REFLUX & ASPIRATION

Gastroesophageal reflux is defined as the movement of gastric contents into the esophagus due to a dysfunction of the lower esophageal sphincter, and aspiration is the introduction of foreign material into the tracheobronchial tree. Aspiration of foreign material may be clinically inapparent and occurs in normal individuals, but aspiration of a foreign body or large volumes of foreign material may be life-threatening. Aspiration is often a chronic, repetitive event resulting in repeated lung injury, chronic inflammation, and irritation of the airways and lung parenchyma.

Three mechanisms are responsible for the proper movement of contents down the esophagus into the stomach. The first is the complex process of mastication, food bolus formation, and presentation to the esophagus. Second, peristaltic waves propel the contents toward the stomach. Coordination of this peristaltic wave depends on an intact neuromuscular system and an esophagus that is patent and free of strictures. The third is entrance into the stomach through the lower esophageal sphincter (LES), a 2- to 3-cm region of increased tone at the distal end of the esophagus. Dysfunction of the LES is the most common cause of clinically apparent gastroesophageal reflux. The acute angle formed between the distal esophagus and stomach enhances sphincter competence by creating a flap valve. Vagally mediated signals cause relaxation of the normally tonic LES during swallowing and allow passage of food into the stomach.

Reflux of gastric acid causes inflammation in the esophageal mucosa. Moderate to severe esophagitis results in a dysfunctional clearance of acid contents, perpetuating the esophagitis and dysfunctional clearing. Gastric contents can reach the upper esophagus and larynx, causing irritation of the vocal cords with laryngospasm and subsequent stridor. Penetration of the glottic opening by the refluxed material results in aspiration. Vagally mediated neuroreceptors that line the esophagus and upper aerodigestive tract can cause reflex bronchospasm when subjected to low pH material. Reflux with or without aspiration can cause respiratory dysfunction by one of three mechanisms: (1) direct mechanical obstruction, that is, foreign body or large volume aspiration; (2) chronic aspiration pneumonitis; and (3) bronchospasm. Pulmonary complications due to gastroesophageal reflux and aspiration are significant (Table 18–12).

Various disorders leave the patient at high risk for aspiration (Table 18–13). Increased incidence of gastroesophageal reflux is seen in obstructive lung diseases, including asthma, BPD, and CF. Pharmacologic agents used to treat various pulmonary diseases, such as methylxanthines and β-adrenergic drugs, cause a decrease in LES pressure and increased reflux. Coughing and autogenic drainage techniques used by patients with chronic lung disease also increase the likelihood of gastroesophageal reflux.

Diagnosis

The physician must remain vigilant for signs of gastroesophageal reflux and aspiration (Table 18–14). Careful

Table 18–13. Causes of aspiration.

Anatomic	Neuromuscular	Functional
Micrognathia	Immature swallow reflex	Gastroesophageal reflux
Tracheoesophageal fistula	Seizure disorder	Dysphagia
Laryngotracheal cleft	Vocal cord dysfunction or paralysis	Achalasia
Cleft palate	Myopathies	
Esophageal stricture	Hydrocephalus	
Vascular ring		

↠ *small jaw, esp. mandible*

observation by the parents or caretaker is helpful because the signs and symptoms are intermittent and can be quite subtle. Objective documentation of reflux, with or without aspiration, also may be difficult because of the intermittent nature of the disease. The physician must correlate historical data with the results of physical examination and objective testing to make the diagnosis.

Diagnostic Tests

Once the clinical suspicion of reflux and aspiration has been raised, the clinician must determine a testing approach on the basis of the suspected cause of aspiration. No single test is diagnostic, and all modes of testing have limitations (Table 18–15). Direct observation of the child during and after feeding in the examination room can help determine the underlying etiology.

Bronchoscopy is valuable for direct visualization of the supraglottic, glottic, and subglottic areas. Anatomic abnormalities, such as laryngotracheal clefts, vocal cord paralysis, and possibly tracheoesophageal fistulas, can be ruled out, and lipid-laden macrophages obtained by bronchoalveolar lavage lend supporting evidence for aspiration.

Therapy

Therapy is based on the underlying mechanism of disease (Table 18–16). Anatomic abnormalities causing aspiration are surgically corrected if possible. Medical management of reflux may prove successful and cost-effective. Pharmacologic management is typically twofold:

1. Neutralize or reduce gastric acids
2. Decrease gastric transit time with the use of prokinetic agents.

Table 18–12. Complications of untreated gastroesophageal reflux.

Recurrent wheezing	Bronchiectasis
Recurrent pneumonia	Interstitial fibrosis
Obstructive lung disease	Restrictive lung disease

Table 18–14. Signs and symptoms of gastroesophageal reflux and aspiration.

Emesis	Congested breathing
Apnea or bradycardia	Laryngospasm and stridor
Coughing or choking with feedings	Hoarseness
Chronic recurrent wheezing	Failure to thrive
Feeding refusal	

Table 18–15. Diagnostic tests for gastroesophageal reflux and aspiration.

Test	Advantages	Disadvantages
Chest radiograph	Demonstrates lobar infiltrates; evaluates hyper-inflation; may show bronchiectasis	Pathophysiology not elucidated
Upper gastrointestinal radiograph	Anatomic configuration of upper gastrointestinal tract; evaluates patency of esophagus; can demonstrate aspiration	Approximately 60% sensitive for gastroesophageal reflux; large amount of liquid used
Modified barium swallow	Examines swallow mechanism by fluoroscopy; small amount of liquid/paste used; patient in upright position	Increased radiation exposure; highly dependent on expertise of radiologist
Gastric emptying scan	Rate of gastric emptying evaluated; 75% sensitive for gastroesophageal reflux; delayed lung scan may detect aspiration	Specialized equipment needed; images dependent on prolonged patient immobilization; no anatomic information generated
pH probe	Considered "gold standard" for reflux; prolonged recording period with the patient in various positions; can establish association between clinical symptoms and pH data	Does not demonstrate aspiration; results dependent on scoring system of raw data
Video endoscopic swallow study (VESS)	Evaluation of upper airway structures; direct observation of swallow mechanism; direct visualization of laryngeal penetration by various food types; no radiation	Does not evaluate reflux; success dependent on speech pathologist and the availability of an experienced endoscopist
Bronchoscopy with lavage for lipid-laden macrophages	Lipid-laden index very sensitive for aspiration; lavage cultures revealing oral flora may be helpful	Invasive; highly dependent on pathologist for accurate assessment of specimen; low specificity

When medical management of gastroesophageal reflux fails, surgical intervention is necessary to protect lungs from recurrent soiling. Fundal plication, with or without placement of a gastrostomy tube, may be indicated.

The clinician must be aggressive in treating gastroesophageal reflux and aspiration to minimize irreversible structural and functional damage to the lungs.

PNEUMOTHORAX

Intrapleural accumulation of air is termed pneumothorax. The introduction of intrapleural air occurs from either the direct penetration of the parietal pleura or penetration of the visceral pleura, secondary to alveolar rupture. Severe penetrating trauma may result in disruption of both the parietal and visceral pleura.

Pneumothoraces may be categorized as spontaneous or traumatic. Certain disease processes are associated with an increased risk of spontaneous pneumothorax (Table 18–17). Pneumothorax can also be divided into static and progressive. Progressive pneumothoraces result in tension pneumothorax. Tension pneumothoraces may be life-threatening, secondary to compression of mediastinal structures, causing decreased cardiac output.

Pathophysiology

Blunt trauma to the chest wall may cause pneumothorax, secondary to rib fracture with parenchymal penetration. Shear forces may cause disruption of peripheral small airways and peripheral alveolar units with subsequent escape of gas. Common iatrogenic causes of traumatic pneumothoraces include thoracentesis, thoracotomy, central line placement, and tracheostomy. In general, disease processes that cause spontaneous pneumothoraces are associated with obstruction of segmental or distal airways, resulting in a ball-valve effect with subse-

Table 18–16. Therapy for gastroesophageal reflux.

Nonpharmacologic
  Thicken feedings
  Upright position during and after feedings
  Increase frequency and decrease quantity of feedings
Pharmacologic
  Antacid
  Ranitidine *Zantac* 2–6 mg/kg/d divided bid (maximum 300 mg/d)
  Omeprazole *Prilosec* 0.7–3.3 mg/kg/d divided bid
  Prokinetic
    Metoclopramide 0.4–0.8 mg/kg/d divided qid
    Cisapride 0.2 mg/kg/dose tid–qid
  Surgical
    Fundoplication
    Relief of gastric outlet obstruction if present

Table 18–17. Diseases associated with spontaneous pneumothorax.

Congenital bullae	Histiocytosis X
Congenital lobar emphysema	Malignancy
Cystic fibrosis	Pertussis
Marfan syndrome	Pulmonary abscess
Asthma	

quent hyperinflation of the distal air space unit. Resultant forces on the overlying parenchyma are responsible for disrupting the pleura, leading to pneumothorax. Direct disruption of the visceral pleura can be seen in disorders such as histiocytosis X and metastatic disease. Congenital anomalies, such as congenital lobar emphysema, may result in spontaneous pneumothorax from both overexpansion of the airway unit and disruption of abnormal structural integrity.

Physical Findings

The onset of pneumothorax is acute with sudden onset of chest pain, progressive shortness of breath, tachypnea, and often shoulder pain on the ipsilateral side. Rapid hemodynamic deterioration in a patient with suspected pneumothorax suggests a rapidly expanding pneumothorax or "tension pneumothorax" and requires immediate intervention. Any patient with rapid onset of respiratory distress, tachypnea, hypotension, and hypoxemia, in conjunction with absent or diminished breath sounds, requires the introduction of a large bore needle or chest tube for immediate evacuation of air.

Physical findings in static or nonprogressive pneumothorax may include chest asymmetry, splinting of the thorax on the affected side, pleuritic pain on deep inspiration, shoulder pain, and decreased or absent breath sounds on the affected side. Palpation of the trachea for deviation and the neck for subcutaneous air may be helpful in the diagnosis.

The upright anteroposterior chest radiograph is extremely sensitive for the diagnosis of pneumothorax. It allows the amount of intrapleural air and degree of mediastinal shift to be evaluated.

Treatment

Treatment is based on the clinical status of the patient and underlying etiology. Surgical intervention may be necessary for penetrating chest trauma or persistent air leak, secondary to blunt trauma. Small pneumothoraces in asymptomatic or mildly symptomatic patients usually resolve without treatment; these patients may benefit from the use of high FiO_2 to augment the reabsorption of intrapleural air. Larger collections of intrapleural air (> 25% of the volume on the affected side) usually need evacuation by needle or chest tube placement. Chest tube placement with continuous suction augments the reexpansion of the affected lung. Persistent air leak into the pleural space due to bronchopulmonary fistula formation is possible and necessitates medical or surgical pleurodesis. The end result of these procedures is adhesion of the parietal and visceral pleuras to seal the persistent air leak.

PLEURAL EFFUSIONS

Pleural effusions, which are abnormal collections of fluid in the pleural cavity, are common. The pleural space is formed by the approximation of the parietal and visceral pleuras, which join at the hila of the lungs.

The pleura is composed histologically of a single layer of mesothelial cells. The space between the visceral and parietal layers is 10–20 μm in width. Liter quantities of fluid may collect in this space, resulting in respiratory distress. Lesser quantities of fluid may exist in the pleural space and be clinically inapparent. In normal, healthy individuals, 0.1–0.2 mL/kg of pleural fluid exists between the parietal and visceral pleuras. The pleuras are supplied by systemic vessels and lymphatics. Hydrostatic and oncotic pressures maintain an equilibrium that is responsible for the normal circulation of pleural fluid. Disease states may alter these forces (Table 18–18).

Pleural effusions can be divided into transudates and exudates on the basis of chemical properties. Transudates are ultrafiltrates of serum, as they have low levels of protein and markers such as lactate dehydrogenase (LDH). Conversely, exudates have high levels of protein and LDH. See Table 18–2 for the chemical composition distinguishing transudates and exudates.

Exudates are produced by disease states that cause inflammation of the pleura with subsequent disruption of its barrier filtration properties. Transudates are the result of changes in hydrostatic or oncotic pressures that cause accumulation of ultrafiltrate in the pleural space. In general, transudates are the result of systemic disease, whereas exudates are the result of inflammatory disease processes in the chest or adjacent organs of the upper abdomen. When either transudates or exudates contain inflammatory cells and infectious agents, such as bacteria, an empyema results. Various causes of pulmonary effusions, both transudative and exudative, are shown in Table 18–19.

Diagnosis

The medical history may contain symptoms that are highly suggestive of pleural effusion. In the previously healthy child, complaints of chest pain, shortness of breath, exercise intolerance, or a persistent irritating cough can be found. The patient may also find a position of comfort that relieves some or all of the symptoms. Fever may or may not be present, depending on the etiology of the effusion. Exudative effusions, secondary to bacterial pneumonia, often will have increased coughing and sputum production. Pulmonary causes must be considered in the patient with gastrointestinal complaints, especially with upper-quadrant abdominal pain. A history of trauma to the thoracic cage may result in pulmonary contusion or disruption of the thoracic duct with secondary

Table 18–18. Pathophysiologic mechanisms of pleural effusion.

Increased hydrostatic pressure (systemic or venous hypertension)
Decreased oncotic pressure (hypoalbuminemia)
Decreased pleural space pressure (asthma, choking)
Increased microvascular permeability (infection)
Decreased lymphatic drainage (lymphangiectasia) → dilation of lymphatic vessels
Movement of fluid from peritoneal space

Table 18–19. Causes of pulmonary effusions.

Exudative	Transudative
Infectious	Congestive heart failure
Bacterial	Neoplastic syndrome
Viral	Cirrhosis
Fungal	Hypoalbuminemia
Mycobacterial	Nephrotic syndrome
Gastrointestinal	Protein-losing
Subdiaphragmatic abscess	enteropathy
Pancreatitis	Chylothorax
Splenic infarct	Collagen vascular diseases
Neoplastic	Miscellaneous
Leukemia	Uremia
Lymphoma	Drug induced
Neuroblastoma	Radiation
Metastatic	Pulmonary embolism
Trauma	Pulmonary contusion
Hemothorax	

chylothorax. Unexplained joint pain or skin rashes may suggest autoimmune or collagen vascular disease.

Physical Examination

The general appearance of the patient and overall nutritional status are important. The posture of the patient can be indicative of pleural irritation, as the patient will splint the chest on the affected side. With larger effusions, percussion of the chest will be dull in areas of fluid collection, and auscultation will reveal decreased breath sounds. Differentiation of pleural effusion from parenchymal consolidation, which will also result in dullness to percussion and decreased breath sounds, can be ascertained by attempting to elicit tactile vocal fremitus and egophony. Palpation of the trachea and cardiac impulse may show displacement toward the contralateral side.

Chest Radiograph

The minimum amount of fluid that can be visualized by a standard chest radiograph depends on the size of the child's thorax when upright. Blunting of the costophrenic angles, obliteration of the hemidiaphragms, and fluid tracking up the lateral margin of the chest should be identified. The position of the trachea and mediastinal structures should be noted. By placing the patient in the lateral decubitus position, with the affected hemithorax down, as little as 50 mL of free-flowing effusion can be detected. The decubitus position may also demonstrate a subpulmonic or subdiaphragmatic collection.

Thoracentesis

Thoracentesis, the withdrawal of fluid from the pleural space, is done for diagnostic or therapeutic indications, or both. Occasionally, ultrasound guidance is necessary to sample a loculated effusion. With massive effusions, tube thoracostomy is necessary.

Fluid analysis should include its gross appearance and its cytologic makeup. The fluid should also be submitted for biochemical analysis, including protein content, LDH

level, and pH. Microbiologic analysis should consist of culture for bacterial, fungal, and mycobacterial organisms. Other tests may be warranted depending on the suspected cause; for example, triglyceride analysis may be needed if chylothorax is suspected.

Treatment

Treatment is dependent on the accurate diagnosis of the cause of the effusion. Underlying infectious diseases should be appropriately treated. Repair of structures injured by trauma or previous surgery may require surgical intervention. Systemic diseases often require aggressive systemic management. Repeated or continued drainage of pleural effusions may be indicated when oxygenation and ventilation become compromised, whereas mild effusions may be easily managed on an outpatient basis in the mildly symptomatic or asymptomatic individual.

LESS COMMON CLINICAL PROBLEMS

IMMOTILE CILIA SYNDROME

The immotile cilia syndrome is an inherited genetic disease with abnormalities of the ultrastructure of the respiratory cilia. The disease affects the ciliated epithelium in the paranasal sinuses, middle ear, and the airway. Because the ultrastructural defect is also present in spermatozoa, males affected by this disease have abnormal sperm mobility. Fifty percent of individuals with this disease have situs inversus.

The characteristic feature of this disease is discoordinate beating of the respiratory cilia, resulting in reduced mucociliary clearance. Three well-recognized structural defects are usually inherited in an autosomal-recessive manner: (1) absent dynein arms, (2) radial spoke defect, and (3) deletion of the central pair with translocation of a peripheral doublet (Figure 18–9).

Clinical Features

The clinical features result from abnormal clearance of the mucous blanket from the respiratory tract. Characteristically, children with immotile cilia syndrome have recurrent otitis media and sinusitis with recurrent coughing and wheezing. They may have situs inversus, although this is not a diagnostic criterion. Infertility occurs in men, whereas fertility is usually normal in affected women.

Symptoms often start in infancy and are relatively mild compared with children who have CF. Most children with the immotile cilia syndrome have productive coughing with recurrent sinusitis and otitis media. Thirty percent have bronchiectasis, 20% have nasal polyps, and 20%

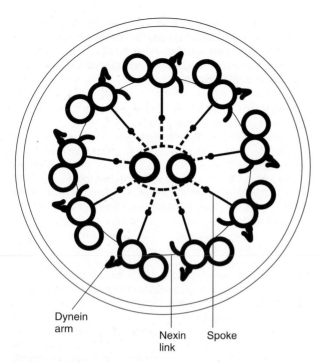

Figure 18–9. Diagram of the cross-section of a cilium. (Reproduced, with permission, from Eliasson R et al: The immotile cilia syndrome. A congenital ciliary abnormality as an etiologic factor in chronic airway infections and male sterility. N Engl J Med 1977;297:1.)

have digital clubbing. Sputum cultures are positive for a variety of bacteria, including *H influenzae, S aureus,* and *Streptococcus viridans.*

The diagnosis is based on the clinical association of bronchiectasis, situs inversus, sinusitis, otitis media, and male infertility (Kartagener syndrome). The diagnosis is confirmed by electron microscopic examination on ciliated epithelium obtained from the respiratory tract. This can be obtained in the outpatient setting by brushing the nasal epithelium with a cytology brush, after administration of a local anesthetic. Optimally, the cilia should be examined at two sites; therefore, a bronchial mucosal biopsy specimen is often obtained by bronchoscopy.

Treatment is symptomatic and involves controlling the recurrent infections with antibiotics, treating airways obstruction with bronchodilators, and improving mucociliary clearance with chest physical therapy. Surgical treatments are sometimes necessary for sinusitis, middle ear infections, and nasal polyps. Pulmonary resections may be indicated if there are isolated segments of bronchiectasis causing persistent symptoms. In general, the prognosis is good.

CONGENITAL MALFORMATIONS OF THE LUNG

Congenital Lobar Emphysema

Congenital lobar emphysema is the congenital overinflation of a pulmonary lobe; this most commonly affects the upper lobes, particularly the left upper lobe. Overinflation is usually caused by gas trapping by a ball-valve anomaly affecting the airway, so that the lobe may inflate but not deflate. The most commonly identified airway anomaly is segmental bronchomalacia, although folds of bronchial mucosa or polyps can produce similar lesions. In 50% of cases, no precise cause is found.

This is a relatively uncommon pulmonary malformation. It occurs more often in boys than in girls, and 14–20% of cases are associated with congenital heart disease. The most common cardiac lesions are patent ductus arteriosus and ventricular septal defects. Some cases are associated with renal malformations or rib cage anomalies. One third of cases of congenital lobar emphysema present at birth, and half have presented by 4 weeks of age. The presentation is usually with moderate respiratory distress that worsens as the lobe inflates. Cyanosis is usually present. Some cases are asymptomatic.

Physical examination shows hyperinflation of the affected hemithorax with reduced breath sounds over the affected lobe. The chest radiograph shows a large, hyperlucent lobe with indistinct lung and vessel markings. There is mediastinal shift away from the affected lobe and atelectasis of the normal ipsilateral lung. The diagnosis can be confirmed by CT scan. Treatment usually involves lobectomy. In some patients, however, who are asymptomatic or have mild symptoms, treatment has involved only observation; this approach is controversial.

Pulmonary Sequestration

Pulmonary sequestration refers to a segment of nonfunctioning, isolated pulmonary tissue with a systemic blood supply. There is neither pulmonary arterial blood supply nor communication with the tracheobronchial tree. The arterial blood supply usually arises from the thoracic or abdominal aorta. There are two types of sequestration: (1) extralobar and (2) intrapulmonary. Extralobar sequestrations are surrounded by their own pleural investment, whereas intrapulmonary sequestrations are located within a lobe, without a discrete separation. They have similar histologic structures. Intrapulmonary sequestration is much more common than extralobar sequestration; both types occur predominantly in the left lower lobe in the posterior basal segment.

Many cases of intrapulmonary sequestration are asymptomatic or they present in late adolescence, when detected on routine chest radiographs. Sometimes these lesions become infected and present as pneumonia or a pulmonary abscess. Extralobar sequestrations are usually detected in the first year of life because, in up to 50% of cases, they are associated with other congenital malformations, including diaphragmatic defects, pulmonary vascular lesions, esophageal communications, and duplication of the colon. The diagnosis of sequestration is made by chest CT scan. If the diagnosis is unclear, a definitive diagnosis can be made by angiography to delineate the feeding vessel and the venous system. MRI studies can also display the vessels clearly. An upper gastrointestinal series should be considered to rule out possible communication with the gastrointestinal tract.

Treatment involves surgical resection. Even if the patient is asymptomatic, surgery should be recommended because of the risk of infection.

Cystic Adenomatoid Malformations

Cystic adenomatoid malformation occurs when there is an overgrowth of the terminal bronchioles, causing an adenomatous appearance on histology. This malformation occurs early in fetal development, probably around 35 days' gestation. The lesions have intracystic communications and are connected to the tracheobronchial tree. The cysts receive their blood supply from the bronchial circulation.

Cystic adenomatoid malformations affect all lobes equally, although usually only one lobe is involved. The most common presentation is with acute respiratory distress because of the cyst expanding and compressing surrounding structures. Cystic adenomatoid malformation can be detected on routine chest radiographs or may present as recurrent pneumonia.

Chest radiographic findings are variable and depend on the type of cyst. There are commonly multiple air-filled cysts with depression of the ipsilateral diaphragm and mediastinal shift away from the lesion.

Cystic adenomatoid malformations can easily be confused with diaphragmatic hernias, because the air in a multiloculated cyst can mimic bowel in the thoracic cavity. Placement of a nasogastric tube in the stomach and instillation of contrast medium will help distinguish the diaphragmatic hernia. A chest CT scan can help delineate the size and nature of the lesion, although this is not essential. Treatment involves surgical removal of the affected lobe.

Bronchogenic Cysts

Bronchogenic cysts represent islands of bronchial tissue left behind during the branching of the airways in early fetal development. If the bronchial tissue is separated from the airways early in gestation, the cyst tends to be placed in the mediastinum; if it occurs later in gestation, the cyst develops in the pulmonary parenchyma. The separation occurs before complete formation of the conducting airways by 16 weeks' gestation. Bronchogenic cysts are thin walled and have a ciliated columnar epithelial lining. The wall contains the histologic components of airways: smooth muscle, bronchial glands, cartilage, and nervous tissue. Cysts commonly contain serous or mucoid fluid.

Bronchogenic cysts are usually single, unilocular, and round; they average 2–10 cm in diameter. Most commonly, they are mediastinal and located close to the carina; many are located between the trachea and esophagus. The cysts are often asymptomatic. Moderate to severe respiratory distress can occur with airway compression, and this is a common presentation in infancy. Pulmonary bronchogenic cysts occur later in gestation and are usually found in the lower lobes. These cysts often become infected and may present in this way.

Bronchogenic cysts can be diagnosed by chest radiograph and confirmed by CT scan. Treatment usually involves surgical removal. Arguably, the status of these lesions could be followed by chest radiograph or CT scan. However, there is a small risk of malignant change in the lesions, and the best approach is removal and histologic examination.

Pulmonary Cysts

Congenital pulmonary cysts develop early in fetal life, at a time when the terminal airways have formed and alveolarization is occurring. No specific cause has been determined. These are characteristically thin-walled cysts lined by columnar epithelium.

Pulmonary cysts are usually singular and multilocular. They are usually greater than 1 cm in diameter and affect just one lobe. They are peripherally located and usually communicate with the airways, so they are air filled. Pulmonary cysts may present with respiratory distress because the ventilation is poor, and gas trapping can occur with inflation of the cyst and compression of the surrounding structures. Later in life, presentation with infection is more common.

The chest radiograph reveals a thin-walled, rounded, cystic lesion containing faint strands of lung tissue. If the cyst is large enough, there will be mediastinal shift and flattening of the ipsilateral diaphragm. Large pulmonary cysts and congenital lobar emphysema can be difficult to distinguish but are readily differentiated by CT scan. Treatment involves surgical resection of the cyst.

Pulmonary Agenesis, Aplasia, & Hypoplasia

Pulmonary agenesis, aplasia, and hypoplasia represent a spectrum of lung malformations characterized by underdevelopment of the lung. In pulmonary agenesis, there is no development of the bronchial tree, pulmonary tissue, or pulmonary vasculature; in pulmonary aplasia, there is a rudimentary bronchial pouch. In pulmonary hypoplasia, which is the most common, there is a decrease in the number and size of the airways, alveoli, and pulmonary vasculature. These malformations are commonly associated with other congenital malformations. Pulmonary hypoplasia can occur as a complication of diaphragmatic hernia, oligohydramnios, or pleural effusion in utero.

Patients may remain asymptomatic or present with respiratory distress, according to the severity of hypoplasia. Common symptoms are tachypnea and cyanosis, and laboratory studies may show hypoxia, hypercarbia, and acidosis.

The radiologic findings are small, underdeveloped lungs, unilaterally or bilaterally. The diaphragms may be elevated. In the case of congenital chest wall lesions, such as asphyxiating thoracic dystrophy, the thoracic cage may be bell shaped. In pulmonary agenesis or aplasia, there is a homogenous density on the affected side with absence of a normally aerated lung. Often, there is herniation of the normal lung from the other side that is best visualized on a lateral film, where it appears in the anterior mediastinum.

Chest CT will confirm the herniation of the normal lung from the opposite side and will show the absence of pulmonary parenchyma and tracheobronchial tree. Bronchoscopy reveals the absence of the mainstem bronchus in the case of agenesis, or of one or more mainstem bronchi in the case of hypoplasia or aplasia. Angiography can be used to investigate the pulmonary vasculature to the affected side.

The treatment of pulmonary agenesis or hypoplasia is supportive. These patients appear to be at increased risk of infection, and broad-spectrum antibiotics should be used when they have respiratory infections. Chest physical therapy may help maintain clearance of respiratory secretions, and supplemental oxygen is necessary if a patient has low oxygen saturation.

The prognosis of these abnormalities depends on the severity of the lesion and the associated anomalies.

RESTRICTIVE LUNG DISEASES

Chest Wall

Diseases of the chest wall can cause an excessively stiff or small thoracic cage (reduced compliance) or one that is unstable and unable to generate sufficient inspiratory force (increased compliance or decreased respiratory muscle strength). The abnormalities that can cause restrictive lung disease by affecting the chest wall include neuromuscular diseases, spinal deformities, chest wall deformities, trauma, obesity, and diaphragmatic deformities.

Neuromuscular Diseases

Neuromuscular diseases weaken the muscles of respiration and may decrease chest wall compliance. They include muscular dystrophy, Guillain-Barré syndrome, poliomyelitis, and spinal cord injury. The earliest mani-

festations are easy development of respiratory fatigue; with increasing weakness, patients have hypoventilation that tends to be particularly severe during sleep. This in turn leads to increased pulmonary vascular resistance, pulmonary hypertension, right ventricular hypertrophy, and the development of cor pulmonale. Many diseases characterized by respiratory muscle weakness are associated with kyphoscoliosis, which may compromise even further the respiratory muscle weakness. Sometimes there is difficulty swallowing secretions, which may predispose to aspiration pneumonia. The major symptoms of respiratory muscle weakness are dyspnea, tachypnea, and headaches. Patients feel anxious and may prefer to sit up; they complain of being unable to sleep lying down. Physical signs include tachypnea, reduced thoracic excursions, paradoxical respiration, weight loss, and easy fatigability.

Assessment of respiratory muscle weakness includes pulmonary function tests, maximal inspiratory and expiratory pressures, maximal voluntary ventilation, and measurement of arterial blood gases. General supportive therapy includes physical therapy, optimal nutrition, and a pulmonary rehabilitation program based on exercise.

If respiratory failure, either acute or chronic, develops, ventilatory support should be considered. Whether this is appropriate will depend on the underlying condition and prognosis; consideration of the family's wishes and feelings is very important. Acute deterioration can be precipitated by infection, general anesthesia, or a sudden deterioration in the underlying condition. If the precipitating cause is reversible, intubation and mechanical ventilation should be considered. Long-term ventilation will require a tracheotomy. We have had some success with negative pressure ventilation using either a cuirass or a poncho-style "raincoat" ventilator for this problem. Nasal mask ventilation or face mask ventilation may be sufficient to support children in the early stages of respiratory failure from neuromuscular diseases. Details concerning the pathophysiology, diagnosis, and treatment of the neuromuscular diseases that cause respiratory failure are described in Chapter 21. A list of neuromuscular diseases that cause respiratory failure is presented in Table 18–20.

Severe abnormalities of the chest wall, such as depression of the sternum (pectus excavatum), can cause restrictive lung disease. Most cases of pectus excavatum do not lead to significant physiologic limitation of either respira-

Table 18–20. Neuromuscular diseases that cause respiratory failure.

Rapid	Moderately Fast	Slow
Spinal cord injury (C3–5)	Werdnig-Hoffman disease	Juvenile spinal muscular atrophy
Poliomyelitis	Pompe disease	Duchenne muscular dystrophy
Guillain-Barré syndrome	Myasthenia gravis	Becker muscular dystrophy
Drug toxicities	Congenital myotonic	Congenital muscular dystrophy
Tick paralysis	dystrophy	Chronic inflammatory
Botulism	Congenital muscular	demyelinating polyneuropathy
Myasthenia gravis crisis	dystrophy	(chronic Guillain-Barré
Acute polymyositis	Nemaline myopathy	syndrome)
Dermatomyositis	Fukuyama disease	Mitochondrial myopathy

tory or cardiac function. The most severe forms may become more pronounced with increasing age and lead to restrictive pulmonary disease. This defect is sometimes associated with mitral valve prolapse, Wolff-Parkinson-White conduction defects, or Marfan syndrome. The severe forms of pectus excavatum are unattractive, and surgical correction for cosmetic appearance is often appropriate. Surgical correction does not usually improve pulmonary function.

Kyphoscoliosis

The abnormal curvature of the spine due to kyphoscoliosis may be idiopathic. It can also be a secondary abnormality from myelomeningocele, von Recklinghausen disease, congenital vertebral anomalies, or neuromuscular diseases. Severe kyphoscoliosis causes a restrictive defect on pulmonary function testing. The results of pulmonary function tests are usually normal unless the scoliosis exceeds 60 degrees, and respiratory symptoms usually do not develop unless the angle exceeds 90 degrees. Severe kyphoscoliosis is associated with recurrent airway infections, atelectasis, and respiratory failure.

Treatment consists of prevention of the progression of the angle by bracing, spinal fusion, or insertion of paravertebral rods. Severe cases require mechanical ventilation for respiratory support.

Interstitial Diseases

Interstitial pulmonary diseases represent a class of uncommon pulmonary diseases characterized by restrictive defects on pulmonary function testing and a reticulonodular pattern of shadowing on the chest radiograph. The underlying pathologic feature of these diseases is inflammation of the alveolar septal tissue with fibrosis and an increasing number of inflammatory cells, both in the septa and in the alveoli. This group of diseases in children has been reviewed extensively. Interstitial lung disease in children has a large number of known causes (Table 18–21).

Characteristically, children with interstitial lung disease have progressive dyspnea associated with coughing, tachypnea, poor weight gain, and exercise intolerance. Examination reveals digital clubbing and fine end-inspiratory crackles; wheezing may be present if airways disease is a feature. When pulmonary hypertension develops in severe cases, there is an accentuated pulmonary second sound. These diseases are often progressive, depending on the underlying etiology.

The diagnosis is initially suspected from chest radiograph and confirmed by chest CT scan. A high-resolution CT scan is most informative; it is more sensitive than regular CT scans for detecting the early stages of interstitial diseases. However, high-resolution CT has limitations in younger children because of motion artifact introduced by rapid respiratory movements. Sedation or general anesthesia may be necessary to obtain good images.

Pulmonary function tests show restricted pulmonary defects with a reduced carbon monoxide diffusion rate. Hy-

Table 18–21. Causes of interstitial lung disease in children.[1]

Infectious or postinfectious	Environmental inhalants, toxic
Viral	substances, foreign mater-
Cytomegalic virus	ials, or antigenic dusts
HIV	Inorganic dusts
Respiratory syncytial virus	Silica
Adenovirus	Asbestos
Influenza virus	Talcum powder
Parainfluenza viruses	Zinc stearate
Mycoplasma	Organic dusts
Measles	Hypersensitivity
Mycobacterial	pneumonitis
Fungal	Bird-fancier's lung
Pneumocystis carinii[2]	Farmer's lung
Aspergillus species	Fumes
Bacterial	Sulfuric acid
Mycobacteria	Hydrochloric acid
Legionella pneumophila	Gases
Bordetella pertussis	Chlorine
	Ammonia
Drug-induced disorders	Nitrogen dioxide
Antineoplastic drugs	Lymphoproliferative disorders
Cyclophosphamide	Familial erythrophagocytic
Nitrosoureas (carmustine,	lymphohistiocytosis
lomustine)	Angioimmunoblastic
Azathioprine	lymphadenopathy
Cytosine arabinoside	Lymphoid interstitial
6-Mercaptopurine	pneumonitis
Vinblastine	Pseudolymphomas of the
Bleomycin	lung
Methotrexate	Metabolic
Miscellaneous drugs	Storage disorders
Nitrofurantoin	Hermansky-Pudlak
Penicillamine	syndrome
Gold salts	Pulmonary lipidosis
Neoplastic diseases	Gaucher disease
Leukemia	Niemann-Pick disease
Hodgkin disease	Disorders of ion transport
Non-Hodgkin lymphoma	Cystic fibrosis
Histiocytosis X	Other
Letterer-Siwe disease	Cardiac failure
Hand-Schüller-Christian	Renal disease
disease	Degenerative disorders
Eosinophilic granuloma	Idiopathic pulmonary alveo-
Neurocutaneous syndromes	lar microlithiasis
with interstitial lung disease	
Tuberous sclerosis	
Neurofibromatosis	
Ataxia-telangiectasia	

[1]Adapted, with permission, from Hilman BC: Interstitial lung disease in children. Page 362 in: Hilman BC (editor): *Pediatric Respiratory Disease: Diagnosis and Treatment.* Saunders, 1993.
[2]*P carinii*, previously considered a protozoan, is now classified as a fungus.

poxemia is characteristically present, especially with exercise. Lung biopsy is often necessary to confirm the diagnosis of interstitial lung disease.

Therapy of the idiopathic interstitial lung diseases is directed toward reducing the inflammatory processes in the pulmonary interstitium to prevent the progression to fibrosis. Immunosuppressive therapy may include corticosteroids and cytotoxic or immunosuppressive drugs, such as azathioprine, cyclophosphamide, and methotrexate. Supportive therapy includes supplemental oxygen and nutritional support. Patients in whom supportive therapy has failed and who are progressing to end-stage disease should be considered for lung transplantation.

THORACIC TUMORS

Thoracic tumors are very uncommon in children, who may present with weight loss, chest pain, or hemoptysis. The more common pulmonary malignancies are presented in Table 18–22.

Diagnosis of pulmonary malignant disease is determined by CT scan followed by lung biopsy. Treatment involves resection of operable lesions and chemotherapy or radiation therapy for inoperable lesions.

Mediastinal Tumors

Mediastinal tumors may cause coughing, wheezing, difficulty in swallowing, shortness of breath, fever, weight loss, lower respiratory tract infections, or recurrent atelectasis. The most common cause of a mediastinal tumor is enlarged lymph nodes from malignancy, infection, or inflammatory disease. A list of tumors that may develop in the anterior, middle, or posterior mediastinum is presented in Table 18–23.

The diagnosis of a mediastinal mass is determined by CT scan and biopsy. Other possible tests include a tuberculin test, bone marrow aspiration, or barium swallow, depending on the probable cause. Treatment will depend on the cause.

ABNORMALITIES IN RESPIRATORY CONTROL

Central Hypoventilation Syndrome

Central hypoventilation syndrome (CHS) may be present at birth or soon afterward and results in severe hypoventilation or even apnea. This disease is associated with a congenital defect in respiratory drive. In some cases, there is a history of injury to the central nervous system, and there may be a genetic component. The dis-

Table 18–22. Pulmonary neoplasms in childhood.

Malignant
  Bronchogenic carcinoma
  Leiomyosarcoma (often arising from airway smooth muscle)
  Fibrosarcoma
Metastatic tumors
  Wilms tumors
  Lymphoma
  Osteogenic sarcoma
  Sarcomas
Benign
  Hamartoma
  Bronchial adenoma
  Papilloma of the trachea or bronchi

Table 18–23. Mediastinal masses in children.[1]

	Common	Rare

Anterior mediastinum	Thymic lesion
	  Hyperplastic cyst
	Angiomatous tumor
	  Hemangioma
	  Lymphangioma
	Teratoma
	Lymphoma
	  Hodgkin disease
	  Non-Hodgkin
	    disease
		Substernal thyroid
		Thymic tumor

Middle mediastinum	Lymphoma Lymphadenopathy Bronchogenic cyst Granuloma	Pericardial cyst
Posterior mediastinum	Neurogenic tumor Duplication cyst	Pheochromocytoma Anterior menin- gocele Hemangioma

[1]Modified, with permission, from Brecher ML: Pediatric mediastinal masses: Your role in management. J Respir Dis 1986;7:73.

ease is rare. There is no abnormality of the heart, lungs, or chest wall that would account for hypoventilation. Ventilation is often normal while awake but depressed when asleep; it can be abnormal even when awake during periods of infection or with exercise. Less severe forms of CHS are associated with a partial pressure of carbon dioxide (Pco_2) of 45–50 mm Hg when awake; with hypoventilation during sleep, the partial pressure of arterial carbon dioxide ($Paco_2$) may increase to 80–90 mm Hg.

The cause of CHS is not well defined. There appears to be a defect of the central chemoreceptors located in the medulla of the brain, so that there is apnea during non–rapid eye movement sleep when these chemoreceptors have an important role in maintaining respiratory drive. The diagnosis of CHS is often made clinically in an infant who retains carbon dioxide and requires mechanical ventilation in the absence of cardiac, pulmonary, or neuromuscular disease. Tests of ventilatory responses to hypoxia and hypercapnia can be used to demonstrate a blunted response. Other evaluations include polysomnographic sleep studies and a CT or MRI scan of the brain.

Treatment in the first year relies on positive-pressure ventilation. This can be achieved with nasal or face-mask ventilation, but most infants require a tracheotomy and nighttime mechanical ventilation. After 1 year of age, children with CHS can be managed with phrenic nerve pacing in combination with nighttime mechanical ventilation. This will allow for increased mobility and normal activities during the day. For pacing, bilateral phrenic nerve electrodes must be implanted. A tracheotomy is maintained because children with CHS often have difficulty maintaining a patent upper airway. Around-the-clock pacing is not recommended because of the risk of producing damage to the phrenic nerves. Respiratory stimulants, such as theophylline and doxapram, are not usually effective.

Table 18–24. Differentiation of hemoptysis from hematemesis.[1]

	Hemoptysis	Hematemesis
Color	Bright red and frothy	Dark red or brown
pH	Alkaline	Acid
Consistency	May be mixed with sputum	May contain food particles
Symptoms	Preceded by gurgling noise; accompanied by coughing	Preceded by nausea; accompanied by retching

[1]Reproduced, with permission, from Rosenstein BJ: Hemoptysis. Page 533 in: Hilman BC (editor): *Pediatric Respiratory Disease.* Saunders, 1993.

PULMONARY HEMORRHAGE

Pulmonary hemorrhage is usually suggested by a combination of hemoptysis with anemia and diffuse alveolar infiltrates on the chest radiograph. Sometimes it is difficult to distinguish hemoptysis from hematemesis. Clinical points of differentiation are listed in Table 18–24. The possible causes of pulmonary hemorrhage in children, listed in Table 18–25, should be kept in mind when obtaining the history and performing the physical examination. It is particularly important to ask about the possibility of foreign body inhalation and to elicit symptoms that might suggest an underlying infection, such as a chronic cough, sputum production, or fever. Substance abuse or exposure to toxins may be relevant, and it is important to ask about overseas travel that might involve exposure to parasitic infections and tuberculosis. Many individuals have recently immigrated to the United States from Southeast Asia, where paragonimiasis is endemic; this is an important cause of pulmonary hypertension and hemoptysis that is otherwise asymptomatic. The nose and oropharynx should be examined carefully to ensure that the bleeding is from the lower respiratory tract. Sometimes nasopharyngoscopy or laryngoscopy is helpful.

The next phase of evaluation is a chest radiograph. It may show diffuse alveolar infiltrates from diffuse pulmonary hemorrhage, atelectasis, or interstitial infiltrates. Localized air trapping would suggest airway obstruction, for example, by an inhaled foreign body.

Laboratory Evaluation

Laboratory evaluation may include coagulation studies,

Table 18–25. Causes of pulmonary hemorrhage.

Retained foreign body	Lung tumors
Infection	Benign
Bacterial	Hamartoma
Pneumonia	Malignant
Lung abscess	Carcinoma of the bronchus
Bronchiectasis	Bronchial adenoma
Tuberculosis	Pulmonary infarct
Fungal	Pulmonary embolism
Actinomycosis	Vaso-occlusive crisis
Aspergillosis	Cardiovascular
Histoplasmosis	Vascular
Coccidioidomycosis	Arteriovenous malformation
Parasitic	Familial telangiectasia
Hydatid disease	Pulmonary hemangioma
Strongyloides	Cardiac
Paragonimiasis	Mitral stenosis
Autoimmune	Trauma
Goodpasture syndrome	Crush injury
Pulmonary	Penetrating injury
hemosiderosis	Thoracic surgery
Wegener granulomatosis	
Collagen vascular	
disease	

hemoglobin measurement, arterial blood gases, tuberculin test, sputum cultures, sputum cytology, examination of gastric aspirates for acid-fast bacilli or hemosiderin-laden macrophages, and an examination of stool for ova and parasites. In patients with renal involvement and hemoptysis, renal function should assessed by measuring blood urea nitrogen and creatinine concentrations; the presence or absence of antiglomerular basement membrane antibodies should be determined as well. Renal biopsy may be needed to make this diagnosis.

A CT scan of the chest is the best method to define the anatomy of any abnormal structures. Angiography is used to define congenital malformations of pulmonary vessels, such as arteriovenous malformations or pulmonary telangiectasia. MRI is useful to examine mediastinal structures, such as the great vessels.

Endoscopy is useful to identify the source of bleeding, to obtain samples for culture and acid-fast stains, and to obtain specimens for cytology. Bronchoscopy is also used for treatment in the case of inhaled foreign bodies or endobronchial lesions such as polyps.

Treatment of pulmonary hemorrhage will vary according to the specific etiology.

REFERENCES

Abman SH, Groothius JR: Pathophysiology and treatment of bronchopulmonary dysplasia. Current issues. Pediatr Clin North Am 1994;41:277.

Chernick V (editor): *Kendig's Disorders of the Respiratory Tract in Children,* 5th ed. Saunders, 1990.

Gibson LE, Cooke RE: A test for concentration of electrolytes in sweat in cystic fibrosis of the pancreas utilizing pilocarpine by iontophoresis. Pediatrics 1959;23:545.

Hardie W et al: Pneumococcal pleural empyemas in children. Clin Inf Dis 1996;22:1057.

Hilman BC (editor): *Pediatric Respiratory Disease: Diagnosis and Treatment.* Saunders, 1993.

Hulka GF et al: Evaluation of the airway. Page 25 in: Meyer CM III et al (editors): *The Pediatric Airway: An Interdisciplinary Approach.* Lippincott, 1995.

National Asthma Education Program: *Guidelines for the Diagnosis and Management of Asthma. Expert Panel Report.* US Department of Health and Human Services, Public Health Service, National Institutes of Health, 1991.

Orenstein SR, Orenstein DM: Gastroesophageal reflux and respiratory disease in children. J Pediatr 1988;112:847.

Ramsey BW: Management of pulmonary disease in patients with cystic fibrosis. N Engl J Med 1996;335:179.

Richardson MA, Cotton RT: Anatomic abnormalities of the pediatric airway. Pediatr Clin North Am 1984;31:821.

Rudolph CD: Gastroesophageal reflux and airway disorders. Page 327 in: Meyer CM III et al (editors): *The Pediatric Airway: An Interdisciplinary Approach.* Lippincott, 1995.

Sahn, SA: The pleura. Am Rev Respir Dis 1988;138:184.

Schidlow DV: Cough in children. J Asthma 1996;33:81.

Wald E: Recurrent and non-resolving pneumonia in children. Semin Respir Infect 1993;8:46.

Wilmott RW: Cough. Page 164 in: Schwartz MW (editor): *Principles and Practices of Clinical Pediatrics.* Year Book Medical Publishers, 1987.

Wilmott RW, Fiedler MA: Recent advances in the treatment of cystic fibrosis. Pediatr Clin North Am 1994;41:431.

Allergy: Mechanisms & Disease Processes

Richard S. Shames, MD

Allergy defines an immunopathologic process in which specific IgE antibodies mediate a hyperactive immune response against normally harmless environmental agents (type I immediate hypersensitivity; see below). The terms allergy and **atopy** are often used interchangeably, although atopy more specifically refers to the inherited tendency to have a persistent IgE response to common, naturally occurring inhalant and ingested agents, known as **allergens.** Allergens possess **immunogenicity,** that is, the ability to stimulate the production of antibody responses, and **reactivity,** that is, the ability to react with preformed antibody. Atopy may be subclinical. Several allergic diseases often coexist in the same patient. The triad of allergic rhinitis, atopic dermatitis, and asthma represents common conditions in pediatric practice. Other primarily allergic conditions include urticaria, angioedema and anaphylaxis, food hypersensitivity, and drug allergy. Asthma and atopic dermatitis are discussed in detail in Chapters 18 and 12, respectively.

SIGNIFICANCE OF ALLERGIC DISEASE

Allergic disease affects 12–20% of the population worldwide. It is estimated that 40 million Americans have asthma or other allergic diseases. Allergic rhinitis, the most common allergy, has a prevalence of 10–12%, with a peak incidence in childhood and adolescence. Asthma affects 5–10% of children, and allergy is the predominant etiology in 80–90%. Complications of allergic rhinitis include sinus disease and eustachian tube dysfunction, causing morbidity into the adult years. Allergic disease accounts for significant use of medical services; 9% of patient visits to a physician's office involve allergic diseases.

HYPERSENSITIVITY IMMUNE RESPONSES

Gel and Coombs devised a classification scheme to divide the mechanisms of immune responses to antigen into four distinct types of reactions to allow for clearer understanding of the immunopathogenesis of the disease. Allergy is classically defined as type I hypersensitivity.

Type I. Anaphylactic or immediate hypersensitivity reactions occur after the binding of antigen to preformed IgE antibodies attached to the surface of the mast cell or basophil. These reactions result in the release of inflammatory mediators (see below, Pathophysiology of the Allergic Response) that produce the clinical manifestations. Examples of type I–mediated reactions include anaphylactic shock, allergic rhinitis, allergic asthma, and acute drug allergic reactions.

Type II. Cytotoxic reactions involve the binding of either IgG or IgM antibody to antigens covalently bound to cell-membrane structures. Antigen-antibody binding activates the complement cascade and results in the destruction of the cell to which the antigen is bound. Examples of tissue injury by this mechanism include immune hemolytic anemia and Rh hemolytic disease in the newborn. Another example of type II–mediated disease process is autoimmune hyperthyroidism, a disorder in which thyroid-stimulating antibodies simulate the thyroid tissue, or thyroid-stimulating hormone (TSH)–binding inhibitory antibodies inhibit the binding of TSH to its receptor. Similarly, in myasthenia gravis, antibodies are directed to the acetylcholine receptor, blocking this neuromediator from interacting with its receptor. In these latter diseases, cytolysis is not a component of these reactions.

Type III. Immune complex–mediated reactions occur when immune complexes are formed by the binding of antigens to antibodies. Complexes usually are cleared from the circulation by the phagocytic system. However, deposition of these complexes in tissues or in vascular endothelium can produce immune complex–mediated tissue injury by leading to complement activation, anaphylatoxin generation, chemotaxis of polymorphonuclear leukocytes, phagocytosis, and tissue injury. Serum sickness, certain types of nephritis, and certain features of bacterial endocarditis are clinical examples of type III–mediated diseases.

Type IV. Delayed hypersensitivity reactions are not mediated by antibody, but rather are mediated primarily by T lymphocytes (cell-mediated immunity). Classic examples are the tuberculin skin test reactions and contact dermatitis.

ETIOLOGIC FACTORS

The development of allergy results from an interaction of genetic and environmental factors. Individuals who are genetically predisposed to the development of specific IgE responsiveness require repeated exposure to the offending allergen as well as other modifying factors for the expression of clinical disease.

GENETICS OF IMMUNE RESPONSE

A family history of allergic disease is by far the most important predisposing factor in the development of allergy. Family and twin studies indicate that total serum IgE concentration has a heritability of greater than 50%. Specific human leukocyte antigen (HLA) types are possibly associated with sensitivity to specific allergens. Heritable factors may influence the regulation of IgE biosynthesis, control of specific immune responses (including IgE antibody expression) by immune response genes, control of the release of endogenous mediators of inflammation, and regulation of overall immune responsiveness. Recent sibling pair studies suggest that five markers in chromosome 5q31.1 are linked with a gene modulating total serum IgE concentration. Evidence was found for the linkage of 5q31.1 and the interleukin-4 (*IL-4*) gene (see below), suggesting that *IL-4* or a nearby gene in this chromosome locale regulates overall IgE production.

AGE, SEX, & RACE

The onset of allergic disease peaks in childhood, although it may develop at any age. Most patients with a positive family history of allergy manifest signs before 10 years of age, suggesting a possible crucial exposure period.

Allergic rhinitis usually has its onset later than asthma. Atopic dermatitis usually begins in childhood. In infancy, gastrointestinal symptoms may herald the onset of allergy.

Before the age of 10 years, allergy occurs twice as often in males, whereas females appear to catch up during the teens and twenties. Racial patterns of allergic disease are difficult to separate from environmental influences and immigration patterns. Changes in allergic expression in immigrants who have moved to a new location suggest a significant influence of environmental and dietary factors.

ENVIRONMENTAL FACTORS

Although genetic tendencies predispose individuals to the development of allergic disease, exposure to environmental factors is necessary to trigger the onset of clinical symptoms. Both allergens and nonallergic factors, such as infectious agents and pollutants, appear to influence the development of allergic disease.

Allergens

Allergens consist of protein, glycoprotein, and carbohydrate materials of animal or vegetable origin. Airborne substances, including house dust mite, animal danders, fungal spores, and plant pollens, have a direct impact on respiratory mucosa and elicit the development of respiratory allergy in predisposed individuals. Injected allergens, such as stinging insect (Hymenoptera) venom, drugs, and less, well-characterized ingested allergens in food substances elicit respiratory, skin, gastrointestinal, or cardiovascular symptoms in certain individuals.

Improved immunochemical methods have led to the isolation of highly purified allergens, permitting structural characterization of these agents. Allergens usually have a molecular weight of 5000–60,000, but specific properties that account for the allergenicity of certain molecules are not known. Acarine mites primarily of the *Dermatophagoides* species constitute the primary allergen in house dust. Its major antigenic determinant (Der p 1) is found in the proteinaceous membranes of mite fecal particles. The mite allergens become readily airborne and settle primarily on mattress surfaces, fabric-upholstered furniture, and floor carpeting. New radioimmunoassay techniques allow measurement of mite allergen content in house dust samples. The most important cat allergen (Fel d 1) exists in cat saliva, in extracts of cat hair, dander, and pelt, and in certain sebaceous glands of the skin. Dog allergens have been found in hair, dander, pelt, saliva, and serum proteins. Among pollen allergens, weed and grass species are important sources of seasonal respiratory allergy. Tree pollens are less important allergenic agents because of their relatively short pollination season.

Allergens derived from natural rubber latex are an increasingly important public health concern because of the growing prevalence of hypersensitivity in certain individuals. There appear to be at least 20 recognized allergens found in many common dipped or molded latex products, such as surgical gloves, balloons, catheters, and rubber toys. Latex proteins may induce hypersensitivity by mucocutaneous, intracutaneous, or aerosolized exposure. Certain individuals with frequent exposure to latex (eg, children with spina bifida or congenital urogenital anomalies, health care workers, and latex factory workers) are at increased risk of latex hypersensitivity.

Infection

Viral agents in particular may influence the development and exacerbation of allergy. These appear to induce damage to epithelial cells and subsequent inflammation, thus exposing nerve endings that control airway reactivity to increased stimulation and antigen absorption. Certain viruses, such as respiratory syncytial virus (RSV), may further induce the development of viral-specific IgE. Products of respiratory agents may also stimulate mast cells and inflammatory cells directly, thus inducing an allergic response.

Air Pollutants

Although both indoor and outdoor air pollutants may increase the activity of existing allergic disease, they have not been clearly established as triggers for the onset of allergy. Increased incidence of allergic disease in urban populations may indicate a causal role for air pollutants, although a recent epidemiologic study found increasing morbidity and mortality from asthma in a large urban population despite declining levels of air pollutants. Sulfur dioxide, emitted from the combustion of sulfur-containing fuels, can alter bronchial mucociliary clearance and has been found to impair expiratory flow rates and vital capacity in adolescents with asthma. Cigarette smoke, the primary indoor pollutant, has been considered a potential factor in the development of allergic disease and otitis media. Studies suggest greater development of asthma in smokers compared with nonsmokers. Tobacco polyphenols induce IgE responsiveness in animals, a finding that may underscore the in utero effects of smoke exposure in humans. Exposure to passive smoking increases the incidence of lower respiratory infection in infants and possibly triggers the onset of asthma. Furthermore, environmental exposure to tobacco smoke has been found to be a significant risk factor in the development of reactive airways disease in infants and young children.

MECHANISMS OF ALLERGY

ANTIBODY STRUCTURE & FUNCTION

Immunoglobulins (antibodies) are proteins that combine specifically with antigens to initiate the humoral (antibody-mediated) immune response. Circulating immunoglobulins have unique specificity for one particular antigenic structure, as well as the diversity to encounter a broad range of antigenic materials. This diversity arises from complex DNA rearrangements and RNA processing within antibody-producing B cells. All immunoglobulin molecules share a four-chain polypeptide structure consisting of two heavy and two light chains (Figure 19–1). Each chain includes an amino-terminal portion containing the variable (V) region and a carboxy-terminal portion containing four or five constant (C) regions. V regions are highly variable structures that form the antigen-binding site, whereas the C domains are relatively invariant and mediate effector functions of the molecules. The five classes, or **isotypes,** of immunoglobulins are termed **IgG, IgA, IgM, IgD,** and **IgE** and are defined on the basis of differences in the C region of the heavy chains. Digestion of an immunoglobulin molecule by the enzyme papain produces two Fab (antigen-binding) fragments and one Fc fragment. Pepsin digestion of the immunoglobulin mole-

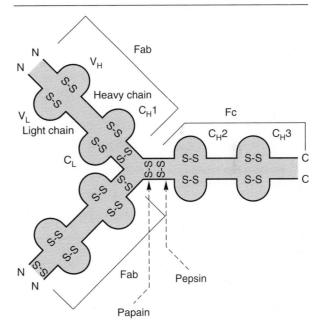

Figure 19–1. Immunoglobulins are four-chain structures consisting of two heavy chains and two light chains. The amino-terminal ends (V region) function as the antigen-combining site, while carboxy-terminal domains (C regions) define the isotype. Interchain and intrachain disulfide bonds (S-S) are essential to the three-dimensional structure of the molecule. Sites of enzyme cleavage by pepsin and papain are shown. C_L = constant region of light chain; Fab = antigen-binding fragment; Fc = crystallizable fragment; V_H = variable region of heavy chain; V_L = variable region of light chain. (Reproduced and modified, with permission, from Page 74 in: Middleton E et al: *Allergy: Principles and Practice,* 4th ed. Mosby, 1988.)

cule results in two Fab-like fragments joined by a disulfide bond. Immunoglobulins serve a variety of secondary biologic roles, including complement fixation, transplacental passage, and facilitation of phagocytosis, all of which participate in host defense against disease. The IgE molecule is a monomeric structure with a molecular weight of 190,000. It constitutes only 0.004% of the total serum immunoglobulins but binds with high affinity to mast cells and basophils via a site in the Fc region. IgE mediates specifically the release of chemical mediators from mast cells and basophils in allergic hypersensitivity diseases as well as in host defense against parasites.

IgE SYNTHESIS & REGULATION

The inappropriate production of IgE in response to allergen defines allergic hypersensitivity. Induction of B cells to synthesize IgE is primarily a function of the interaction of three cytokines, IL-4, IL-13, and γ-interferon (IFNγ) (Figure 19–2). IL-4 is a crucial factor for isotype-switching to IgE and is sufficient to initiate germ-line transcription of IgE. IL-13 has about 30% structural homology to IL-4 and shares many of the same activities on mononuclear cells and B lymphocytes. Compared with IL-13, IL-4 tends to be an earlier and more transient signal. Additional B-cell activation factors triggered through the B-cell–membrane receptor CD40 are required for the expression of mature messenger RNA (mRNA) and subsequent IgE synthesis. In humans, a variety of secondary signals synergize with IL-4. Multiple cytokines can modulate IL-4–dependent IgE synthesis; IL-5 and IL-6 may upregulate the synthesis of IgE, whereas INFγ is inhibitory. Therefore, an imbalance favoring IL-4 over INFγ may induce IgE formation. In one study, reduced IFNγ at birth was associated with clinical atopy at 12 months of age. A defect in IFNγ secretion may be due to a post-transcriptional defect in secretion.

T cells play a central role in the induction of allergic and inflammatory responses, both as a source of IL-4 and in delivery of secondary signals after interaction with B cells. Antigens, processed by antigen-presenting cells such as macrophages or by B cells directly, elicit the activation of CD4+ T-helper lymphocytes. The activated T cells elaborate cytokines to direct B cells or to recruit and activate other cells, such as eosinophils, neutrophils, and macrophages (Figure 19–3). Two subsets of CD4+ cells have been recognized on the basis of a characteristic pattern of cytokine release. TH$_1$ cells elaborate IFNγ and tumor necrosis factor β (TNFβ) but not IL-4 and IL-5 and have been found to participate in delayed hypersensitivity reactions (type IV). TH$_2$ cells secrete IL-4, IL-5, and IL-9 but not IFNγ and TNFβ and have been implicated in allergic and inflammatory responses. As discussed, IL-4 is crucial to isotype switch to IgE. IL-5 promotes maturation, activation, and chemotaxis of eosinophils, and IL-9 is a mast-cell and T-cell growth factor. Activated T cells and their characteristic cytokines have been demonstrated at sites of allergic inflammation in both skin and airway disease. The demonstration of in vitro allergen-specific T-cell lines, which proliferate and secrete large amounts of IL-4 when exposed to relevant antigen, further supports the existence of specific TH$_2$-like clones. What drives undifferentiated CD4 T lymphocytes to become either TH$_1$ or TH$_2$ cells is not known, although the specific cytokine milieu in which the TH-cell differentiation occurs appears to be important in determining the direction of differentiation. The major determinant of TH$_2$ differentiation is the cytokine IL-4, whereas the cytokine IL-12 appears to drive the differentiation to TH$_1$ cells.

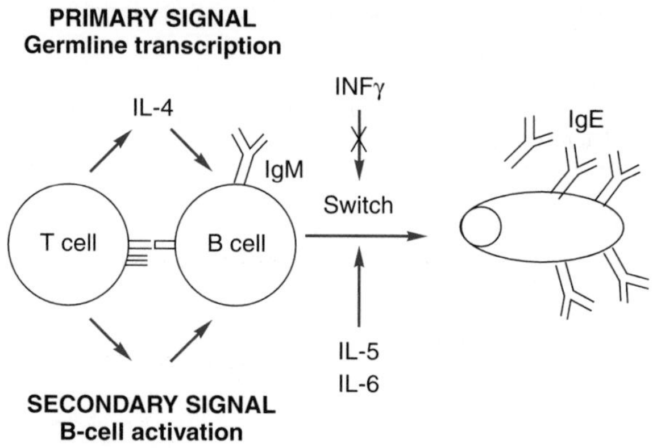

PATHOPHYSIOLOGY OF THE ALLERGIC RESPONSE

Allergic responsiveness consists of an IgE-mediated activation of previously sensitized tissue mast cells and basophils. **Sensitization** from early antigen exposure defines the subclinical induction of an allergic immune response. Reexposure of the individual to the offending allergen induces the clinical basis of the allergic response.

Allergic Sensitization. Allergen-specific IgE binds to high-affinity Fc receptors on tissue mast cells and basophils as well as to low-affinity receptors on macrophages, eosinophils, and platelets, thus sensitizing these cells for future allergen encounters. Sensitization is indicated by in vivo skin test reactivity or an in vitro radioallergosorbent test (RAST), even if clinical expression of disease is not apparent.

PRIMARY SIGNAL
Germline transcription

SECONDARY SIGNAL
B-cell activation

Figure 19–2. Induction of IgE synthesis by B cells requires two signals. Activated T cells elaborate interleukin (IL)-4, the primary signal that influences isotype switching to IgE at the transcriptional level. Secondary B-cell activation factors are required for mature expression of IgE. IL-4–dependent IgE synthesis is inhibited by interferon-γ (INFγ) and stimulated by IL-5 and IL-6. (Modified, with permission, from Vercelli D, Geha RS: Regulation of IgE synthesis in humans: A tale of two signals. J Allergy Clin Immunol 1991;88:285.)

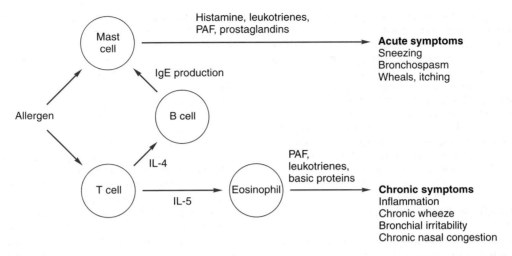

Figure 19–3. T lymphocytes play an important role in the induction of allergic and inflammatory responses. Processed antigen presented to T-helper lymphocytes (CD4+) elicits the release of cytokines, including interleukin (IL)-4 and IL-5, which in turn induce IgE production by B lymphocytes and activation of eosinophils, respectively. IgE-directed mast cell activation elicits the acute allergic response, whereas activated eosinophils in part mediate the chronic inflammatory state. PAF = platelet activating factor. (Reproduced, with permission, from Kay AB: "Helper" [CD+] T cells and eosinophils in allergy and asthma. Am Rev Respir Dis 1992;145[Suppl]:S22.)

Allergen Stimulation of Mediator Release. On re-exposure to allergen, the sensitized individual can mount an accelerated hypersensitivity response. Mast cells, armed with antigen-specific IgE on their surfaces, can bind and cross-link allergen. Bridging of cell-bound IgE requires that two IgE molecules be linked by multivalent antigen; a single Fab monomer is unable to induce the subsequent reaction. Binding and cross-linking of specific antigen initiates a physical approximation of surface IgE receptors, triggering a sequence of biochemical events that results in the degranulation of mast cells and basophils.

Mediators of Inflammation. Activation of mast cells and basophils triggers both release of preformed mediators (histamine, chemotactic factors, and enzymes) and synthesis and release of membrane-derived mediators (prostaglandins [PG], leukotrienes, and platelet-activating factor) (Table 19–1). Histamine and the newly generated mediators interact with surface receptors on blood vessels, smooth muscle, and glands, inducing vascular leakiness, smooth muscle constriction, and mucus secretion. Preformed chemotactic mediators, leukotrienes, and platelet-activating factor elicit the accumulation of inflammatory cells, including eosinophils, neutrophils, and mononuclear cells. Enzymes, including neutral proteases and acid hydrolases, participate in the chemical modification of intermediate compounds and in the formation of toxic oxygen metabolites. Mast cells, basophils, lymphocytes, and granulocytes also have the ability to synthesize and release proinflammatory cytokines, growth factors, and regulatory factors, which interact in complex networks. Mediator and cytokine release can thus precipitate a sustained inflammatory response, resulting in localized edema, mucus secretion, epithelial disruption, and influx of eosinophils, neutrophils, and mononuclear cells. Studies of atopic individuals challenged intranasally with pollen al-

Table 19–1. Mast cell and basophil mediators classified in terms of vasoactive and smooth muscle–constricting, chemotactic, and enzymatic functions.[1]

Vasoactive and smooth muscle–constricting mediators
Preformed
Histamine
Generated
Arachidonic acid metabolites (PGD_2, LTC_4)
Platelet-activating factor (PAF)
Adenosine
Chemotactic mediators
Eosinophil-directed
Eosinophil chemotactic factor of anaphylaxis (ECF-A)
ECF oligopeptides
PAF
Neutrophil-directed
High-molecular-weight neutrophil chemotactic factor
Leukotriene B_4
PAF
Enzymatic mediators
Neutral proteases
Tryptase
Chymase
Lysosomal hydrolases
Other enzymes
Superoxide dismutase
Peroxidase

[1]Modified, with permission, from Stites DP, Terr AI: In: *Basic and Clinical Immunology,* 7th ed. Appleton & Lange, 1991.
PGD_2 = prostaglandin D_2; LTC_4 = leukotriene C_4.

lergen or with cold, dry air provide evidence of a clear biphasic pattern of mediator release, characterized by an initial early response at 15–30 minutes and a late delayed response at 6 hours, the latter of which does not require reexposure to allergen.

Early & Late Phase Responses. The **early phase response (EPR),** or "classic" allergic reaction, occurs in a sensitized individual within minutes of an antigen exposure and is marked by the release of vasoactive and bronchoconstrictor mediators including histamine, TAME esterase, leukotrienes, PGD_2, kinins, and kininogens. The **late phase response (LPR),** which may either follow the EPR (dual response) or occur as an isolated event (Figure 19–4), begins 2–4 hours after initial antigen exposure, reaches maximal activity at 6–12 hours, and resolves within 12–24 hours. The LPR, marked predominantly by an influx of eosinophils and mononuclear cells with recruitment of both monocytes and T cells, is thought to most closely mimic

clinical disease. Mediators (except PGD_2) of the EPR reappear during the LPR in the absence of antigen rechallenge. Absence of PGD_2, an exclusive product of mast cell release, suggests that basophils are a potentially important source of mediators in the LPR. From such inflammatory cells, elaboration of cytokines and histamine-releasing factors may perpetuate the LPR, leading to a sustained hyperresponsiveness of the target tissue, eg, bronchi, skin, or nasal mucosa. Products of activated eosinophils, such as major basic protein, may be destructive to bronchial epithelial tissue and predispose to persistent airway reactivity. Epithelial damage is a feature of both atopic dermatitis and asthma. Pathophysiologic events of the LPR thus characterize a persistent inflammatory state.

Late phase reactivity has been described in allergic rhinitis and conjunctivitis, asthma, food-sensitive atopic dermatitis, and anaphylaxis. Inflammatory changes in the airways are recognized as crucial attributes of chronic

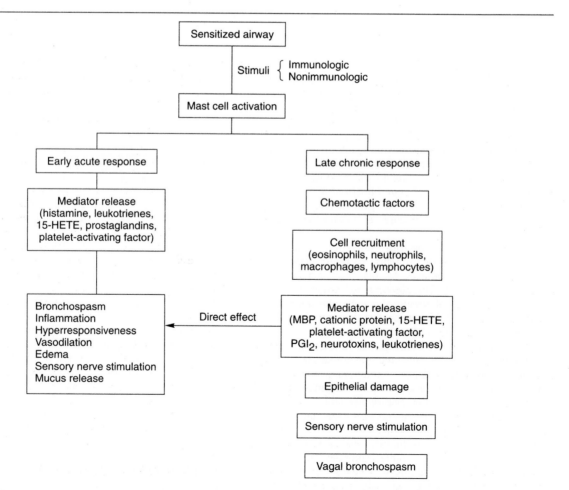

Figure 19–4. Progression of early (acute) and late (chronic) asthma responses, indicating major chemical mediators and cells involved in progression to clinical asthma. HETE = hydroxyeicosatetraenoic; MBP = major basic protein; PGI_2 = prostaglandin I_2 (prostacyclin).

asthma and other allergic diseases. Therefore, therapeutic interventions that prevent or reverse inflammatory processes that characterize the LPR are most effective in the control of chronic and severe disease (see below).

APPROACH TO THE PATIENT WITH SUSPECTED ALLERGY

Fundamental to the evaluation of the patient with suspected allergic disease is a thorough history and physical examination. Specific laboratory tests confirm the diagnosis of allergy.

HISTORY

Symptoms. Allergic rhinitis is characterized by paroxysmal sneezing; itching of the nose, eyes, palate, or oropharynx; nasal stuffiness; and rhinorrhea with or without postnasal drip. **Pruritus** results from the actions of histamine secreted by mast cells and basophils during the EPR and is the hallmark symptom of allergy. Sinusitis, serous otitis media, or eustachian tube dysfunction are frequent complications of underlying allergic disease. Asthma is indicated by intermittent and recurrent cough, wheeze, dyspnea, and chest tightness, although cough may be the sole presentation in 5% of children with asthma. Atopic dermatitis is suggested by a recurring pruritic skin rash in a symmetric distribution with predilection for certain sites. Loss of well-being and irritability may accompany symptoms of allergic disease, although primary behavioral disorders are not likely allergic in nature. Skin and airway disease often coexist in atopic patients.

Patterns of Disease. Allergic disease commonly begins in childhood. Neonatal onset of symptoms suggests other etiologies (eg, chronic lung disease and tracheoesophageal fistula), although infants may be sensitized in utero. Although allergic symptoms may be chronic and continuous, they are frequently episodic and may vary with seasonal exposure, location, and time of day. Symptoms commonly occur immediately after allergen exposure (eg, housework, animal exposure, and foods), irritant exposure (perfumes, odors, smoke), viral illness, ambient temperature change, or exercise.

Environmental History. Exposure to indoor pets; dust mite from stuffed toys, bedding, and bedroom carpeting; and mold may trigger allergic reactivity. Infants and young children attending day care and preschool have frequent exposures to viral illnesses, which are common nonallergic causes of upper and lower respiratory disease. Similarly, parental smoking can act as a nonallergic trigger for respiratory symptoms.

Previous and Current Therapy. Previous therapeutic response to allergy avoidance measures, elimination diets, and pharmacotherapy can suggest a diagnosis of allergy. Discontinuing topical nasal vasoconstrictors after prolonged use may result in rebound congestion, known as rhinitis medicamentosa.

Family History. Atopy in one or both parents or in siblings presents significant risk for development of allergic disease.

PHYSICAL EXAMINATION

A complete, detailed examination, emphasizing the skin as well as upper and lower respiratory systems, should be performed. Growth parameters in allergic disease are usually normal but may be impaired in chronic severe asthma. Impaired growth in the setting of chronic nasal and airway disease should prompt an evaluation for immune deficiency, cystic fibrosis (CF), or metabolic disease.

Characteristic signs of allergic disease include a horizontal nasal crease from frequent nose rubbing and allergic "shiners" representing bilateral infraorbital edema. Chronic nasal obstruction and mouth-breathing from allergic rhinitis may result in long facies, narrow maxilla, flattened malar eminences, overbite, and a high-arched palate ("adenoid facies"), which can lead to orthodontic problems.

Examination of the nose may reveal deformities from previous trauma, polyps, or septal deviation, suggesting structural etiologies of rhinitis. An examination by nasal speculum should *always* be performed. Pale, bluish, edematous turbinates are characteristic but seen in only 50% of cases. Nasal polyps are infrequent in allergic rhinitis in children and may indicate aspirin-sensitive asthma or CF. Clear and watery nasal secretions suggest allergy, whereas chronic or recurrent mucopurulent secretions may indicate rhinosinusitis, ciliary defects, or immune deficiency.

Tearing, scleral or conjunctival injection, and periorbital swelling suggest allergic involvement. Evidence of persistent middle ear fluid and hearing impairment may indicate chronic rhinitis and eustachian-tube dysfunction.

Acute or chronic patchy skin lesions involving the face and extensor surfaces of the extremities suggest atopic dermatitis (**eczema**) in infants and children. Later, the lesions show a flexural pattern of distribution, with predilection for the antecubital and popliteal areas and the neck. Superinfected lesions may be observed.

Wheezing may be noted in acute asthma. A prolonged expiratory phase or audible wheezing on exhalation indicates acute or chronic airway obstruction.

LABORATORY PROCEDURES

Specific diagnostic tests may support a history and examination suggestive of clinical allergy.

Antigen-Specific IgE

In vivo skin testing and in vitro RAST provide evidence for antigen-specific IgE. Identification of specific environmental allergens is essential for directing specific avoidance measures and for consideration of immunotherapy.

Skin testing represents the primary tool for the evaluation of antigen-specific IgE sensitivity. Improved characterization of allergen immunochemistry and standardization of testing devices have rendered testing increasingly sensitive. Major advantages to skin testing include simplicity, rapidity of performance, and low cost. This test measures sensitization but does not imply clinical disease; correlation with history and examination is essential.

Percutaneous or intradermal administration of dilute concentrations of specific antigens elicits an immediate wheal and flare response in a sensitized individual. The response usually peaks within 10–15 minutes and occasionally up to 30 minutes. Although reactions usually indicate clinical allergy when the diameter of the wheal exceeds 3 mm, comparison with a positive control (histamine) is essential. Skin testing cannot be performed on patients currently taking antihistamine drugs, which suppress skin test reactivity. It also may be difficult in patients with extensive eczema.

Positive skin test reactions to inhalant allergens, combined with a history and examination suggestive of allergy, strongly incriminate the allergen as a cause of the symptoms. Negative skin tests with an unconvincing allergy history favors a nonallergic etiology. Skin testing for food allergens is less reliable than for inhalant allergens because only 40–50% of positive skin test reactions for food allergens correlate with controlled food challenge. Negative skin test reactions for food allergens is helpful in excluding suspected hypersensitivity to specific foods. Skin testing with insect venoms is an obligate confirmation of clinical evidence of allergic reactivity.

RAST provides quantitative in vitro assays of allergen-specific IgE (Figure 19–5). The patient's serum is reacted initially with antigen bound to a solid phase material and then labeled with a radioactive or enzyme-linked anti-IgE antibody. RAST shows a 70–80% correlation with skin testing to pollens, dust mites, and danders. This test is useful in patients receiving chronic antihistamine therapy and in patients with extensive dermatitis.

Total Serum IgE Level

Elevated IgE levels may occur with atopic diseases, but diagnostic usefulness is limited by considerable overlap of levels with normal individuals. IgE levels greater than 200 IU/mL suggest allergy, whereas values less than 20 IU/mL make allergy unlikely. Serum IgE levels vary with age (see Chapter 7) and are usually not useful in the diagnosis of allergic rhinitis. In children with asthma highly associated with atopy, an elevated serum IgE concentration is common and suggests an allergic etiology. Serum IgE levels are considerably increased in more than 90% of patients with atopic dermatitis. The presence of IgE in

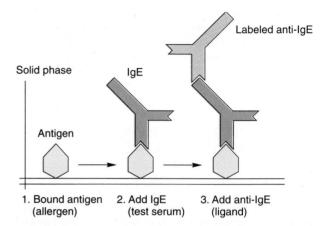

Figure 19–5. Radioallergosorbent testing (RAST) provides a quantitative in vitro measure of antigen-specific IgE. Patient serum is reacted with solid-phase bound antigen and labeled with a radioactive or enzyme-linked anti-IgE.

cord serum has been demonstrated to be a predictor of subsequent atopy. Nonatopic conditions, including immunodeficiency syndromes, neoplasm, and parasitic disease, are associated with marked elevations of IgE concentration.

Total Eosinophil Count

Although eosinophils play an important role in the inflammatory response of allergic disease, the eosinophil is primarily a tissue-dwelling cell. It is present 100-fold more frequently in the marrow and tissues than in peripheral blood. Circulating cells reflect only trafficking between sites of production and function. Peripheral eosinophilia is therefore of limited value in the diagnosis of allergic disease.

Nasal Cytology

Examination of nasal secretions for eosinophils is useful in the diagnosis of allergic rhinitis. Atopic specimens usually show high numbers of eosinophils, basophils, and neutrophils, whereas nonatopic secretions demonstrate an absence of basophils and eosinophils, with few neutrophils and bacteria. The degree of nasal eosinophilia is related to the extent of allergic exposure and symptomatology. Specimens may be obtained from blown secretions or by nasal scraping with a plastic curette from the medial third of the inferior turbinate. Specimens may be stained with Wright or Hansel stain. Both techniques have 70% sensitivity and 94% specificity.

Lung Function Testing

Spirometric testing and bronchoprovocation are discussed in Chapter 18. Bronchial obstruction is assessed by spirometry and airway hyperreactivity by pharmacologic or nonpharmacologic bronchoprovocation; these methods represent important tools for the evaluation of suspected asthma. Although pharmacologic bronchoprovocation with histamine or methacholine is highly sensitive in the diagnosis of asthma, positive test results indicating airway hyperreactivity may be found in patients with allergic rhinitis during pollen season, in individuals after a viral respiratory infection, and in some relatives of patients with asthma.

Sinus Evaluation

Acute and chronic sinusitis are common complications of allergic airway disease. In some patients with chronic asthma and sinusitis, asthma relief occurs only after treatment of the sinus disease. Assessment of sinus involvement may be made by radiograph, computed tomography (CT) scan, or direct visualization. Radiographic or CT evidence of air-fluid levels, opacification, and thickening of sinus membrane tissue (> 6 mm thickness) are associated with sinus infection. Plain films of the sinuses have less sensitivity than CT scan for the diagnosis of chronic sinusitis, although a single Waters view can provide a helpful screening for maxillary and frontal sinus disease. Flexible nasopharyngoscopy (**rhinoscopy**) permits direct visualization of the upper airway and may be useful in the evaluation of persistent nasal obstruction, epistaxis, and laryngeal symptoms.

Other Tests

A number of other diagnostic modalities are important in the differential diagnosis of suspected allergy. Gastrointestinal studies, including stool pH, ova, and parasite studies; esophageal pH monitoring; and endoscopy may help to exclude diagnoses that mimic gastrointestinal allergy. Recurrent sinopulmonary infection with chronic rhinitis and otitis media warrant evaluation for immunodeficiency, ciliary dyskinesia syndrome, and CF. Quantitative immunoglobulins with functional testing of antibody responses to protein and polysaccharide antigens are indicated to rule out immunodeficiency. Persistent nasal obstruction should prompt consideration of tonsillar or adenoidal hypertrophy or polyps. The presence of a foreign body in the nasal passage can cause chronic unilateral purulent drainage.

BASIC APPROACHES TO THERAPY

Therapy of clinical allergy includes patient education, avoidance of incriminated allergens, pharmacologic management, and immunotherapy.

PATIENT EDUCATION

Providing information about basic elements of allergic disease, the role of environmental allergens, and the mechanisms and appropriate use of drug therapy represents an important aspect of patient management. Thoughtful and specific educational strategies permit patients to acquire the skills and confidence essential for successful management of their disease. Education should be continuous from the point of initial diagnosis.

ENVIRONMENTAL CONTROL

Identification of relevant allergens by history and skin testing provide the basis for environmental control measures. Avoidance of indoor allergens such as dust mite, cockroach, animal danders, and molds and avoidance of pollens to the extent possible can reduce the allergen load for an individual, thus reducing symptoms and medication requirements. Beneficial effects of dust mite control are apparent from controlled studies in which rigorous dust control in hospitalized settings resulted in significant clinical improvement in mite-sensitive asthma patients. Because mites thrive in high humidity and allergen loads are greatest in bedding and floor carpeting, mite control measures stress the use of covers for mattresses, box springs, and pillows, removal of bedroom carpet, and maintenance of low humidity. Additional measures include frequent washing of sheets and bedding in hot water, removal of upholstered furniture and stuffed toys from bedrooms, and the use of chemicals that kill mites.

Animal exposures, particularly to household cats, represent potent allergenic sources. Although removal of the family pet often is emotionally difficult, such a measure can produce dramatic improvement. Some studies suggest that weekly bathing of a cat in water may remove considerable amounts of allergen and result in clinical improvement. Although pollen avoidance may be difficult, air-conditioned environments and reducing outdoor activity on high–pollen-count days, may prove helpful.

Avoidance of environmental irritants, such as exposure to cigarette smoke, strong odors, and perfumes, may reduce threshold reactivity to allergenic loads.

PHARMACOLOGIC THERAPY

Symptomatic Treatments

Antihistamines are effective for the treatment of nasal itching, sneezing, and rhinorrhea, although less effective for the control of nasal congestion. They are most effective in the treatment of seasonal or episodic allergic rhinitis. These agents act primarily through competitive inhibition at histamine H_1 receptor sites. The major side effect is sedation, although this effect becomes less problematic after initial usage and may be limited by nighttime dosing.

Seldane   Hismanal   Claritin

Newer antihistamines (terfenadine, astemizole, and lorata-dine) are nonsedating but are not yet available in liquid formulation. Cetirizine is a potent low-sedating antihista-mine recently approved in the United States. None of the newer antihistamines is approved for use in children younger than 12 years. *Zyrtec*

α-Adrenergic agents constitute a class of sympatho-mimetics that induce vasoconstriction by stimulation of α-adrenergic receptors. Oral agents may be effective in temporarily reducing nasal congestion and mucosal edema and are often used in conjunction with antihistamines in the treatment of acute allergic rhinitis. Topical vasocon-strictors have limited usefulness in patients with chronic allergic rhinitis because overuse can result in rhinitis medicamentosa.

Prophylactic & Anti-inflammatory Agents

Intal

Topical cromolyn preparations, such as cromolyn sodium, have proved effective in the prophylactic treat-ment of allergic rhinitis, conjunctivitis, and asthma. Cro-molyn can block early and late phase reactivity in aller-gen-challenged patients. It is an exceptionally safe drug but cannot reverse or terminate an allergic response once it has started.

As the most effective anti-inflammatory agents avail-able, **corticosteroids** have become indispensable therapy in the management of chronic allergic disease. Topical preparations for dermatologic, nasal, and pulmonary dis-ease in the form of skin creams and aerosols are highly potent, locally active, and rapidly metabolized drugs with no significant systemic effects. Oral corticosteroids are re-served for short-term use in patients with extremely se-vere and intolerable allergic airway disease. Long-term use of oral corticosteroids is rarely indicated in the treat-ment of nasal or dermatologic allergy.

Corticosteroids interfere with arachidonic acid meta-bolism and therefore limit the generation of inflam-matory mediators and prevent directed migration and activation of inflammatory cells. These agents also upreg-ulate β-receptors, rendering β-stimulatory agents more ef-fective. Corticosteroids block late phase, but not early phase, reactivity in allergen-challenged sensitized individ-uals.

1) beclomethasone
• Vanceril
• Beclovent
2) flunisolide
• AeroBid
3) fluticasone
• Flovent
4) triamcinolone
acetonide
• Azmacort

Aqueous nasal steroid sprays are highly effective in maintenance treatment of moderate to severe seasonal or perennial allergic rhinitis. No adverse long-term effects have been demonstrated, although the potential for mu-cosal atrophy and septal perforation exists with prolonged improper use of the nasal inhaler.

Immunotherapy

Immunotherapy (desensitization or hyposensitization) involves the subcutaneous administration of increasing quantities of allergen extract in sensitized individuals to reduce the threshold for the development of clinical symp-toms. Although this form of therapy has been used for more than 80 years, controlled studies to document its ef-fectiveness have been available for only 20–30 years. Proper use of immunotherapy requires an accurate assess-ment of individual sensitivity by skin testing and correla-tion with symptom patterns. Effective treatment of anti-gen-specific allergies requires long-term administration of high doses of allergen (6–12 μg of allergen per injection). Optimally, these extracts should be standardized using the most modern techniques. Use of low-dose immunotherapy or administration by sublingual or oral route is of no proven value.

Immunotherapy represents an adjunct to the pharmaco-logic and environmental management of patients with allergic rhinitis and selected individuals with allergic asthma. Treatment is generally reserved for patients who cannot avoid relevant allergens and have had a suboptimal response to, or poor tolerance of, pharmacotherapy. Im-munotherapy represents the primary treatment for insect sting (Hymenoptera) anaphylaxis. Treatment is not indi-cated for management of atopic dermatitis or food-related disorders.

Hymenoptera venom immunotherapy has demonstrated considerable effectiveness in preventing subsequent sting anaphylaxis. Treatment of allergic rhinitis with various antigens, including dust mite, cat, ragweed, grass, and tree pollens, has also been proved effective. Although data supporting effectiveness of immunotherapy in asthma are less clear, treatment appears to be most effective in pa-tients with relevant and unavoidable allergic triggers, in-cluding cat, house dust mite, grass, and tree pollen. Stud-ies have been difficult to assess in part because of differing methodologies and confounding nonallergic trig-gers in asthma.

The mechanism of action of immunotherapy has not been precisely defined. Many immunologic changes have been demonstrated, but their significance is unclear. Levels of antigen-specific IgE increase initially but then diminish; subsequent seasonal increase in pollen-spe-cific IgE is blunted. Increased levels of antigen-specific IgG (blocking antibodies) are thought to preclude IgE-me-diated responses but do not correlate with clinical im-provement. Additional immunologic changes include increased antigen-specific suppressor cells, decreased lymphokine production, and reduced LPR to antigen chal-lenge.

Although immunotherapy is generally safe, administra-tion should be undertaken only by specially trained physi-cians. Local reactions, primarily erythema and swelling at the injection site, are normally insignificant and transient and help to safely gauge dosing. Infrequently, patients may manifest systemic reactions, including generalized hives, angioedema, bronchospasm, and anaphylaxis. Early recognition and aggressive treatment of generalized reac-tions are essential. No adverse long-term effects from im-munotherapy have been observed. Patients who become pregnant during the course of immunotherapy may con-tinue receiving injections if they are receiving mainte-nance therapy.

DISEASES OF IMMEDIATE HYPERSENSITIVITY

These diseases are summarized in Table 19–2.

ALLERGIC RHINITIS & CONJUNCTIVITIS

Respiratory allergy involving nasal, sinus, and conjunctival tissues represents a hypersensitivity response to primarily airborne allergens. Allergic rhinitis ranks as the most common of allergic diseases, with a prevalence of

Table 19–2. Clinical evaluation of allergic disorders.

Disease	Symptoms/History	Signs	Diagnostic Tests	Treatment
Allergic rhinitis	• Recurrent or chronic pattern of watery rhinorrhea, paroxysmal sneezing, nasal stuffiness, nasal/palatal itching • Seasonal or perennial pattern • Family history of atopy • Personal history of asthma, atopic dermatitis	Allergic shiners Mouth breathing Nasal crease Nasal mucosal edema Conjunctivitis	• Nasal smear for eosinophils (suggestive) • Skin testing to aeroallergens	• Avoidance/environmental control • Antihistamines/decongestants • Nasal cromolyn • Nasal corticosteroids • Allergen immunotherapy
Sinusitis	• Acute—facial pain, headaches, fever, purulent nasal secretions • Chronic—nasal discharge, cough, halitosis, nasal obstruction	Inflamed nasal turbinates Purulent rhinnorrhea "Cobblestone" features Recurrent/chronic otitis	• Waters x-ray (screening) • Sinus CT scan *Frontal view of max sinuses, orbits, nasal structures & zygomas.*	• Antibiotics • Analgesics • Antihistamines/decongestants • Nasal corticosteroids • Surgery
Food allergy (immediate-type)	• Immediate response to food intake (within 2 h) • Mouth/perioral itching, nausea, abdominal cramping, diarrhea; urticaria, angioedema; atopic dermatitis; anaphylaxis; rhinitis/asthma (rare)	Hives Angioedema Eczema	• Skin testing to select foods (screening) • Food elimination/challenge	• Elimination of specific foods • Epinephrine kit prn
Anaphylaxis	• Immediate reaction to inciting agent • Upper/lower airway obstruction, urticaria/angioedema, nausea, abdominal pain, diarrhea, cardiovascular instability/collapse	Pruritus Skin erythema Hives Swelling Stridor/wheeze Hypotension/shock	• Skin, in vitro testing to suspected food, drug, insect venom allergens • Serum/plasma tryptase	• Acute event: epinephrine IV fluids oxygen ± IV/IM antihistamines ± IV aminophylline ± Endotracheal intubation/tracheostomy • Avoidance • Epinephrine prn
Insect sting reaction	• Systemic reaction including upper/lower airway obstruction, cardiovascular instability/collapse	See anaphylaxis (above)	• Skin testing to Hymenoptera venoms or fire ant	• See anaphylaxis (above)
Urticaria/angioedema	• Multiple hives • Lips, tongue, pharyngeal, periorbital, genital swelling • Gastrointestinal symptoms (hereditary angioedema [HAE])	Hives Localized swelling	• Skin, in vitro testing to suspected allergens (food, drug) • Ice cube test (cold urticaria) • ± Complete blood count, erythrocyte sedimentation rate, chem panel, LFTs, CXR, stool O&P (chronic urticaria) • C4 level (screening) • C1 inhibitor/function (HAE)	• Avoidance of offending agent if known; treatment of underlying disease • H_1 antagonists • H_1 + H_2 antagonists • Androgens (HAE)
Drug allergy (immediate hypersensitivity)	• Urticaria/angioedema, upper/lower airway obstruction, cardiovascular instability/collapse, gastrointestinal symptoms	Hives Localized swelling Stridor/wheeze Hypotension/shock	• Skin testing to β-lactams (major and minor determinants) and other selected agents	• Acute event (see anaphylaxis) • Avoidance; use of alternative agent • Desensitization

LFTs = liver function tests: CT = computed tomography; CXR = chest x-ray; O&P = ova and parasites.

10–12%. Although the condition can begin at any age, it most often begins in childhood or adolescence.

Allergic rhinitis and conjunctivitis may be seasonal or perennial, as defined by the predominant pattern of reactivity. Most seasonal allergies are caused by pollens from local tree, grass, or weed species. Perennial allergens include indoor inhalants such as dust mite, cockroach, animal proteins, molds, and occasionally foods.

Respiratory allergy is suggested by nasal symptoms that are more frequent than expected for age, persist without interval between acute episodes, and are not caused by viral infections. Characteristic symptoms are profuse watery rhinorrhea, paroxysmal sneezing, nasal obstruction, nasal and palatal itching, and conjunctivitis, correlated with particular exposures. A family history of atopy is usually present. Allergic shiners, nasal mucosal edema, middle ear effusions, and ocular involvement corroborate historical findings. Allergic rhinitis often coexists with atopic dermatitis and asthma in children.

The differential diagnosis in patients with perennial nasal obstruction should include anatomic obstruction (septal deviation or spurs, polyposis, tonsillar and adenoidal hypertrophy, or foreign body), vasomotor rhinitis, rhinitis medicamentosa, and drug effects. Vasomotor or nonallergic rhinitis is an entity of nasal mucosal hyperirritability, characterized by nasal congestion and postnasal drainage in the absence of skin test reactivity. Pregnancy, as well as the use of oral contraceptive agents and tricyclic antidepressants, may produce nasal congestion. Hypothyroidism, nasal mastocytosis, and nasopharyngeal tumors represent uncommon causes of chronic rhinitis. Persistent rhinitis accompanied by chronic or recurrent purulent secretions, headache, recurrent otitis, and cough may suggest a complicating sinusitis (see below).

Clinical suspicion of allergic rhinitis or conjunctivitis may be supported by the presence of eosinophils in nasal secretions. Identification of responsible antigens is confirmed by immediate skin test reactivity. Evaluation of total serum IgE concentration and peripheral eosinophil counts is rarely helpful.

Treatment should include patient education, avoidance of relevant allergen and irritant triggers, and pharmacotherapy or immunotherapy. Antihistamines and decongestants are helpful in the symptomatic management of seasonal or episodic allergic rhinitis. Treatment of chronic allergic rhinitis or conjunctivitis should focus on anti-inflammatory therapies, such as nasal or ocular cromolyn or nasal steroid aerosols. Immunotherapy is indicated for patients with evidence of clinically relevant skin test reactivity who cannot avoid relevant allergen exposure and have inadequate response to environmental control and pharmacotherapy.

SINUSITIS

Sinusitis should be considered in the presence of protracted symptoms of upper respiratory tract infection, allergic rhinitis, asthma unresponsive to conventional therapy, or chronic cough. Factors contributing to the development of sinusitis include swelling of sinus ostia, mucociliary abnormalities, mucus overproduction, and immune deficiency (especially IgA). The resulting accumulation of secretions in the sinus cavities leads to bacterial proliferation and subsequent infection.

Although acute sinusitis frequently presents with facial pain, headache, fever, and purulent nasal secretions, chronic sinusitis, defined by greater than 6 weeks duration, may have subtler findings, including chronic nasal discharge, persistent cough, halitosis, and recurrent otitis media. Infraorbital edema, inflamed nasal turbinates, with purulent rhinorrhea and pharyngeal lymphoid hyperplasia ("cobblestone" features) may also be suggestive of chronic sinusitis (see Chapter 9, Sinusitis).

ALLERGIC ASTHMA

Asthma is discussed in Chapter 18. It is the most common chronic illness of childhood and seriously affects the quality of life. Despite an increased understanding of the pathophysiology of the disease, as well as the availability of new treatments, the morbidity and mortality of asthma appear to be increasing. This is particularly true in young, poor, urban, and minority populations. Important factors contributing to this trend are underdiagnosis and undertreatment. Acute exacerbations from asthma, resulting in emergency department care and hospitalization, are largely preventable, especially if diagnosis and treatment are comprehensive and ongoing.

There has been increased recognition of the importance of airway inflammation in the patient with even mild asthma. Inflammation induced by exposure to certain airway triggers can lead to airway hyperresponsiveness and bronchial obstruction. Bronchial provocation models suggest that exposure to allergen in a sensitized individual may induce airway inflammation. Allergic triggers are particularly important in pediatric asthma. In children and young adults, asthma is almost always associated with IgE-mediated disease. Prevalence of skin test reactivity to allergen has been correlated with asthma severity. Studies have demonstrated that allergen exposure in early life may influence the age of onset and severity of asthma.

Because of the high prevalence of allergy in childhood asthma, evaluation for environmental triggers and sensitization to allergen is essential. Recognition of allergic triggers and subsequent control of environmental allergens are important in the overall management of many pediatric asthma patients. Patient education, objective monitoring of airway function through peak flow monitoring and spirometry, bronchodilator and anti-inflammatory pharmacotherapy, and continuing care are additional tools in the management of these patients.

ATOPIC DERMATITIS

Atopic dermatitis (allergic eczema) is discussed in Chapter 12. An inflammatory skin condition primarily of early childhood, atopic dermatitis is characterized by a chronic or relapsing pruritic dermatitis with typical morphology and distribution. Although the pathogenesis of this condition is unknown, evidence supports an important role for IgE-mediated hypersensitivity. Approximately two thirds of children with atopic dermatitis have a positive family history for atopy; in 50–80% of children, allergic rhinitis or asthma develops. Both elevated serum total IgE levels and evidence of positive immediate skin test reactivity to dietary and environmental allergens are characteristic of these patients. Recent studies have confirmed an important role for food allergens in 30–40% of patients with moderate or severe atopic dermatitis. Both immediate and late phase reactions have been observed in patients with food-sensitive atopic dermatitis after challenge.

FOOD ALLERGY

Although food allergy represents a broad spectrum of immunologic disease, mechanisms involving type I immediate hypersensitivity are the most common and best understood. Immediate-type food-induced reactions involving IgE-mediated hypersensitivity include atopic dermatitis, urticaria, angioedema, and anaphylaxis. An unusual manifestation of food hypersensitivity in infants is allergic gastroenteropathy (eosinophilic gastroenteropathy), characterized by multiple IgE food sensitivities associated with local gastrointestinal tract pathology. Patients with allergic gastroenteropathy present with acute gastrointestinal symptoms, peripheral eosinophilia, and gut loss of fluid, protein, and blood. Immunologic mechanisms other than type I hypersensitivity reactions are implicated in protein-induced enteropathy, gluten-sensitive enteropathy (celiac disease), and dermatitis herpetiformis. True food allergy should be distinguished from food intolerance to dyes, flavorings, and toxins; gastrointestinal structural abnormalities; enzyme deficiencies; inflammatory bowel disease; ulcer disease; and effects of pharmacologic agents that may mimic food allergy.

Immediate-type food allergy is characterized by IgE-mediated sensitization of intestinal mast cells by food antigens or antigenic fragments. Macromolecules pass through the gastrointestinal epithelium, interact with the mucosal immune system, and access the general circulation. Food allergy is more common in infants and young children. This is thought to reflect an immaturity of the gastrointestinal epithelial barrier and insufficient levels of protective secretory IgA. Immediate-type food allergy often occurs within minutes after specific food ingestion. Mouth and perioral pruritus and urticaria may precede intestinal complaints such as nausea, cramping, abdominal pain and distention, vomiting, and flatulence. Skin reactions include acute urticaria and angioedema (less commonly chronic urticaria) and atopic dermatitis. Rhinitis and asthma occur rarely. Systemic anaphylaxis may be observed, particularly involving selected foods and exercise.

Foods commonly inducing immediate-type food allergy in children younger than 3 years include milk, egg, peanut, soy, fish, and wheat. Allergy to peanut, tree nuts, egg, milk, and soy, as well as fish and other seafood, most commonly affects older children and adolescents.

Food allergy is suggested by the proximity of symptoms to specific food ingestion and by the presence of a family or personal history of atopy. Preparation of the food, amounts consumed, and concurrent medications may influence the expression of food allergy. A suspected food may fail to induce an allergic reaction consistently. A 10-to 14-day diet record may be useful for establishing a cluster of suspected foods. Epicutaneous skin testing of suspected foods offers greater specificity than sensitivity. Negative skin testing is usually more reliable at excluding food hypersensitivity, whereas positive tests have an approximately 40–50% positive predictive value. RAST is less sensitive than skin testing.

A 3- to 4-week trial elimination of suspected allergenic foods, as determined by history and skin testing, may be instituted to look for resolution of symptoms. Elimination diets followed by return of suspect foods to the diet would be applied only in cases in which symptoms are not life-threatening, such as chronic hives, eczema, gastrointestinal symptoms, and rhinitis. If removal of one or several foods from the diet is not successful in eliminating symptoms, a short trial of a restrictive elimination diet may be warranted. If symptoms do not abate with a severe elimination diet, they are not associated with foods. Empiric use of severe elimination diets should be avoided, as malnutrition may result.

Avoidance of foods identified as allergens is the only specific treatment for food allergy. Patients and families must be educated to scrutinize ingredient labels and to recognize technical and scientific names for foods. Epinephrine kits should be prescribed for patients with a history of life-threatening symptoms after food exposure, as inadvertent ingestion is not uncommon. Prophylactic drugs and desensitization therapy have no current role in treating patients with food allergy.

ANAPHYLAXIS

Anaphylaxis defines a generalized, immediate, life-threatening hypersensitivity reaction affecting multiple target organs. IgE-mediated reactivity and subsequent release of bioactive mediators is the predominant mechanism of anaphylaxis. There is no special predilection for atopic individuals. The clinical syndrome is marked by the onset of upper or lower airway obstruction, urticaria (hives), angioedema, gastrointestinal symptoms, and cardiovascular instability or collapse within seconds to minutes after ingestion or injection of an inciting agent. Involvement of some or all of the target organs may occur. Allergens known to elicit human anaphylaxis commonly include foods, drugs, and insect venoms. Any food may induce anaphylaxis, although most frequently incriminated are peanuts, nuts, fish, and egg white. Penicillins and cephalosporins are the most common drugs known to elicit anaphylaxis, although a large array of antimicrobials, chemotherapeutic agents, vaccines, and other medications can produce anaphylaxis. Anaphylaxis to latex has been increasingly recognized as a risk factor for certain high-risk patients, including children with spina bifida and urogenital anomalies, health care workers, rubber industry workers, and patients with prior undiagnosed intraoperative anaphylaxis. Anaphylactic-like reactions (anaphylactoid) to radiographic dyes, aspirin and other nonsteroidal anti-inflammatory drugs, opiate analgesics, intravenous immune globulin, and exercise mimic true anaphylaxis but involve nonimmunologic mechanisms. Recurrent idiopathic anaphylaxis has been described in adults.

Diagnosis is based on the proximal association of clinical symptoms with an inciting event. Measurement of serum or plasma tryptase, a specific marker of mast cell activation, may be useful in the diagnosis of anaphylaxis. Attempts to identify responsible antigens by specific IgE testing may be useful for food, venom, latex, and certain drug exposures several weeks after the initial anaphylactic event. Skin testing to Hymenoptera venoms (see below) or to the major and minor determinants of penicillin (see below) are useful in detecting IgE sensitization. RAST may be helpful in identifying suspected agents.

Effective treatment of anaphylactic or anaphylactoid events requires early recognition of the clinical syndrome. Administration of 0.01 mg/kg of 1:1000 epinephrine subcutaneously should be followed by repeated injections every 15–30 minutes as indicated. Intravenous access is essential for antihistamine and fluid administration and possible use of vasopressors. Oxygen should be given, and endotracheal intubation or emergent tracheostomy may be necessary. Intramuscular or intravenous antihistamines (diphenhydramine, 1–2 mg/kg) should be administered for urticaria, angioedema, and gastrointestinal reactions. Intravenous aminophylline should be administered for bronchial obstruction. Intravenous corticosteroids are not effective in treatment of acute anaphylaxis but may be useful for prevention of late phase anaphylaxis. Patients who have experienced anaphylaxis should carry epinephrine for injection at all times.

INSECT STING REACTIONS

Reactions to the venom of stinging insects of the order Hymenoptera and to fire ants constitute potentially life-threatening allergic responses. In North America, systemic reactions to hymenopteran stings are mostly due to the members of the apidae (honeybee) and the vespidae (include yellow jackets, yellow hornets, bald-faced hornets, and paper wasps). Cross-reactivity of venom proteins is common within the vespid family, although there is little cross-reactivity between the apidae and the vespidae. Use of specific venom antigens has replaced whole body extracts for diagnostic skin testing and desensitization. Whole-body extracts from fire ants contain most relevant allergens and are still used for the diagnosis and treatment of allergic reactions to fire ants.

Sting reactions manifest from a continuum of local to systemic symptoms. Most immediate reactions are attributable to IgE-mediated mechanisms. Systemic reactions may involve cutaneous, vascular, and respiratory symptoms. Cutaneous reactions (hives) occur most frequently and are the sole manifestation of systemic insect sting reaction in more than 60% of children. Respiratory symptoms occur in 50% of patients; hypotension is uncommon. Children with previous systemic skin reactions alone have only a 10–20% risk of anaphylaxis with subsequent sting.

Diagnosis of insect sting hypersensitivity is based on a history, confirmed by evidence of IgE skin test reactivity. Patients with only local reactions or systemic cutaneous reactions exclusively are not candidates for skin testing and subsequent desensitization. A history of systemic respiratory or vascular reaction, however, warrants referral to an allergist for skin testing to a complete set of venoms. RAST is less sensitive and specific than skin testing.

Patients with positive skin test reactions and an appropriate history of systemic reactions have a 50% risk of anaphylaxis with subsequent sting and therefore should be desensitized by venom immunotherapy. Successful immunotherapy, associated with the production of venom-specific IgG, is 97–99% effective in protecting against subsequent sting anaphylaxis. Symptomatic treatment of local reactions includes application of ice packs, rest, use of oral antihistamines, and a brief tapering course of systemic steroids to treat reactions involving the head and throat. Patients with a history of systemic symptoms should be prescribed an epinephrine kit with careful instruction regarding its indications and proper use.

URTICARIA

Urticaria (hives) affects 20% of individuals during their lifetime. **Acute urticaria,** a cutaneous form of anaphylaxis, is caused by foods, drugs, and insect stings. **Chronic urticaria,** extending beyond 6 weeks, is usually nonimmunologic and of unknown cause.

Urticarial lesions are raised areas of erythema and edema involving the superficial dermis. The lesions may be single or multiple, are intensely pruritic, and usually resolve within 24–48 hours. Diagnostic evaluation of urticaria requires a careful medical and environmental history and physical examination addressing factors known to induce the condition. In addition to food, venom, and drug allergens, physical causes have been associated with urticaria. Cold urticaria induced by local skin cooling is diagnosed by applying an ice cube to the forearm for 5 minutes and observing localized urticaria after skin re-warming. Pressure urticaria is a common feature of all forms of urticaria. Cholinergic urticaria is characterized by punctate wheals with prominent flare after exercise, heat, and emotional stress. Rarely, heat, sunlight (solar), vibration, and water (aquagenic) may induce urticaria. Urticaria may be a symptom of vasculitis, chronic infection, or neoplasm. Aspirin and nonsteroidal anti-inflammatory drugs may induce acute or chronic urticaria by non–IgE-mediated mechanisms. Specific diagnostic tests for infection, neoplasm, and connective tissue disease are indicated only if history and examination findings suggest these diagnoses in the absence of urticaria.

Therapy involves avoidance of specific inciting agents when possible. Drug treatments with histamine H_1 receptor antagonists are the primary therapy. The combined use of H_1 and H_2 antagonists is recommended if histamine H_1 blockers are unable to decrease episodes. Epinephrine injections may provide transient relief and should be used when pharyngeal or laryngeal edema is present. Oral corticosteroids are rarely indicated in the management of chronic urticaria because of the risk of systemic adverse effects.

ANGIOEDEMA

Angioedema is often seen in conjunction with urticaria. Angioedema is defined by well-demarcated areas of non-pitting subcutaneous edema involving any area of the body, especially the lips and the periorbital and genital regions. Idiopathic or chronic urticaria and angioedema may involve the tongue and pharynx. Hereditary angioedema (HAE), an autosomal-dominant inherited disorder, involves life-threatening edema of the gastrointestinal and upper respiratory mucosa. Specific IgE mechanisms, such as insect venom hypersensitivity and drug or food reactions, may occasionally cause angioedema.

Two forms of HAE have been described. Most patients (85%) have low levels of normally functioning C1 inhibitor protein, a compound that stabilizes the initial complex in the classic complement pathway. Deficient levels of C1 inhibitor protein promote autoactivation of the complement system. Fifteen percent of patients with HAE have normal or elevated levels of C1 inhibitor, but the existing protein is nonfunctional. C4 levels are decreased between attacks and frequently undetectable during episodes. C2 levels are frequently decreased during attacks as well.

Acquired C1 inhibitor deficiency has been described in association with lymphoproliferative disease or connective tissue diseases such as systemic lupus erythematosus. Acquired states are marked by diminished C1 levels in addition to affected C1 inhibitor, C4, and C2 levels as in HAE.

Treatment of HAE involves prophylactic administration of androgens such as danazol and stanozolol, which probably augment synthesis of C1 inhibitor protein. Treatment of acute episodes is similar to treatment of acute anaphylaxis.

DRUG ALLERGY

Allergy to drugs represents only 5–10% of broadly defined adverse drug events and may involve any of the Gel and Coombs immunologic mechanisms. Large-molecular-weight compounds, such as heteroantisera, can serve as complete antigens and directly induce an immune response, whereas small-molecular-weight compounds, such as penicillin and its metabolites, bind to carrier proteins or cell surfaces and become immunogenic. Drug dose, route of administration, and host reactivity influence expression of drug allergy. Drugs and agents known to cause IgE-mediated events include antibiotics, animal-derived hormones (insulin), enzymes (chymopapain), vaccines, and toxoids. The clinical manifestations of drug allergy may involve single or multiple target organs. The clinical presentation, propensities of certain drugs to induce allergy, and the temporal relationship of the reaction to drug exposure assist in identifying the likely immunopathologic mechanism and therefore have important implications regarding diagnosis, treatment, and prognosis. Immunodiagnostic testing, including immediate or delayed hypersensitivity skin testing, may be useful in confirming a suspected reaction.

Anesthetic Agents

Adverse reactions to general or local anesthetic agents are not uncommon. Type I hypersensitivity reactions have not been clearly demonstrated to cause hypersensitivity to local anesthetics. There is disagreement as to the value of immediate hypersensitivity skin testing to assess the risk of hypersensitivity to local anesthetics. Provocative or challenge testing may be useful for local agents suspected to cause allergy.

β-Lactam Hypersensitivity

β-Lactam–induced immunologic reactions may involve types I, II, or III Gel and Coombs mechanisms. β-Lactam agents, such as penicillin, are the most frequent class of drugs that cause IgE-mediated hypersensitivity. Hypersensitivity reactions occur in up to 10% of treatments with penicillin; anaphylactic reactions occur in 0.01%, and fatal reactions in about 1 per 50,000 treatment courses. Identification of the relevant immunologic metabolites of penicillin have made possible prospective identification of patients at risk for systemic or potentially fatal type 1 immediate (IgE-mediated) hypersensitivity reactions. In vivo, a small portion of administered penicillin is metabolized to biochemically active compounds that can haptenate plasma proteins and elicit immunologic responses. The penicilloyl product is the most abundant metabolite, accounting for 95% of protein-bound drug metabolites, and is thus termed the "major determinant." This determinant is commercially available. Three other penicillin metabolites, the "minor determinants," consist of penicillin, penicilloic acid, and penillic acid. When testing is performed by trained personnel, patients with a history of an adverse reaction to penicillin and negative epicutaneous and intradermal skin tests with major and minor determinants, have less than a 1% risk of a subsequent IgE-mediated systemic reaction. Positive skin test reaction to any of the penicillin determinants carries approximately a 70% chance of systemic reactions when the drug is administered subsequently. The sensitivity of testing with the penicilloyl (major) determinant alone is only 76%, whereas the sensitivity of testing with the penicilloyl and benzylpenicillin determinants is approximately 93%. In vitro tests are unable to detect minor determinants and are less reliable for the detection of IgE reactivity. Patients with prior adverse reactions to β-lactam antibiotics that are consistent with the spectrum of immediate hypersensitivity events should be considered for alternative antibiotics. Skin testing to assess the risk of hypersensitivity should be performed by a trained allergist if there is an immediate absolute indication for the drug and lack of a suitable alternative. Positive skin testing in that setting may indicate the need for acute desensitization if no alternative drug exists.

REFERENCES

MECHANISMS

Frew AJ, Kay AB: Postgraduate course: Eosinophils and T-lymphocytes in late-phase allergic reactions. J Allergy Clin Immunol 1990;85:533.

Kaliner M: Asthma and mast cell activation. J Allergy Clin Immunol 1989;83:510.

Serafin WE, Austen KF: Mediators of immediate hypersensitivity reactions. N Engl J Med 1987;317:30.

Vercelli DV, Geha RS: Regulation of IgE synthesis in humans: A tale of two signals. J Allergy Clin Immunol 1991;88:285.

DISEASE PROCESSES

Bochner BS, Lichtenstein LM: Anaphylaxis. N Engl J Med 1991;324:1785.

Creticos PS: Immunotherapy with allergens. JAMA 1992;268:2834.

Duff AL, Platts-Mills TAE: Allergens and asthma. Pediatr Clin North Am 1992;39:1277.

Kaliner M, Lemanske R: Rhinitis and asthma. JAMA 1992;268:2807.

Patterson R: Diagnosis and treatment of drug allergy. J Allergy Clin Immunol 1988;81:380.

Sampson HA, Metcalfe DD: Food allergies. JAMA 1992;268:2840.

Wald ER: Sinusitis in children. N Engl J Med 1992;326:319.

20

Endocrinology

Stephen M. Rosenthal, MD, & Stephen E. Gitelman, MD

SHORT STATURE

Short stature may be defined as a height that is 2.5 SD or greater below the mean for age, or a height that is 2.5 SD or greater below the expected mean on the basis of the midparental height (using a specialized chart that determines the appropriateness of the height of the child in relation to that of the parents). Suboptimal growth, however, may be present without absolute short stature (eg, an unexplained change in height from 1 SD above to 1 SD below the mean) and becomes apparent on plotting either a linear growth chart or a height velocity chart. Subnormal growth rate is defined as a height velocity less than the third percentile for age, or less than 4 cm/y at any time between 5 years of age and the onset of puberty (Table 20–1). Growth charts for absolute height and height velocity are widely available. Figure 20–1 shows growth charts comparing absolute height with midparental height. It should be remembered that the most commonly available growth charts have been derived from white groups and may not be applicable to all populations.

The differential diagnosis of short stature is extensive. Etiologies include normal variants (which are often familial), virtually any chronic disease, endocrine abnormalities, intrauterine growth retardation, and a large number of genetic syndromes. Worldwide, protein-calorie malnutrition is the most common cause of growth failure.

NORMAL VARIANTS

The most common causes of short stature in the United States—familial short stature (ie, short parents) and constitutional delay in growth and adolescence—are both normal variants. The hallmarks of constitutional delay in growth are summarized in Table 20–2. Such children are of normal size at birth and, during the first 2–3 years, fall below the mean, particularly for height and, to a lesser extent, for weight. Head circumference remains normal. This growth pattern appears to be an exaggeration of the normal shifting along growth curves that may occur during the first 2 years after birth. Subsequently, height velocity is normal, although the timing of adolescence, including the pubertal growth spurt, often is delayed. Such children typically achieve an adult height in the normal to low-normal range for family. With the exception of a delayed bone age, an index for skeletal maturation, laboratory evaluations are unrevealing. The family history often reveals a similar pattern of delayed growth and adolescence in one of the parents.

CHRONIC NONENDOCRINE DISEASE

Chronic nonendocrine disease often is associated with short stature. Occasionally, poor growth may be the first presenting sign. Table 20–3 lists examples of chronic disease associated with suboptimal growth. Abnormal metabolic demands or malnutrition are thought to contribute to growth failure in chronic disease.

HORMONAL CAUSES

Although children with short stature are often referred to an endocrinologist for evaluation, the hormonal causes of growth failure are relatively rare. These include hypothyroidism of any etiology, growth hormone (GH) deficiency, glucocorticoid excess (whether from exogenous or endogenous sources), and poorly controlled diabetes mellitus. Hypothyroidism, hypercortisolism, and diabetes mellitus are discussed in subsequent sections of this chapter.

Growth Hormone Deficiency

The common clinical features of GH deficiency are summarized in Table 20–4. Children with congenital GH deficiency are of normal size at birth. However, after approximately 6 months of life, when linear growth becomes GH dependent, growth failure becomes apparent. Patients

Table 20–1. Definition of subnormal growth.

Height ≥ 2.5 SD below mean for age, *or*
Height ≥ 2.5 SD below mean for that expected based on the midparental height, *or*
Height velocity less than 3rd percentile for age, or < 4 cm/y at any time between 5 y and the onset of puberty

Table 20–2. Clinical features of constitutional delay in growth.

Normal size at birth
Height velocity subnormal during first few years, then normalizes
Delayed adolescence
Delayed skeletal maturation
Final height normal to low-normal range for family
Family history often positive for constitutional delay

with GH deficiency have short stature associated with a pudgy, immature, doll-like appearance. GH also plays a significant role in glucose homeostasis through its effects on fat metabolism (**lipolysis**). GH deficiency therefore may be associated with severe hypoglycemia in addition to short stature, particularly in infancy. Uncomplicated GH deficiency is associated with a normal head circumference and normal intelligence.

The clinical characteristics of GH deficiency result from abnormalities at all levels of the "physiologic growth hormone axis." The secretion of GH from the anterior pituitary gland is regulated principally by the hypothalamic stimulatory factor GH releasing hormone (GH-RH), and by the hypothalamic inhibitory factor somatostatin. GH mediates its growth-promoting effects primarily through local generation, as well as through circulating levels of insulin-like growth factors (IGFs), peptides that play a role in the growth and differentiation of a wide variety of

tissues. GH secretion is normally regulated by a wide range of physiologic and metabolic processes, which are summarized in Table 20–5. In many cases, these processes exert their effects on GH secretion by influencing hypothalamic GH-RH or somatostatin. The biologic effects of IGFs, which are mediated through specific cell-surface receptors, may be modified either positively or negatively by IGF binding proteins.

The differential diagnosis of abnormalities that result in deficiency of the GH physiologic axis is summarized in Table 20–6. Most patients with GH deficiency (80–90%) are GH-RH deficient and are capable of secreting GH in response to exogenous GH-RH. GH deficiency may be isolated or associated with other hypothalamic and pituitary hormone abnormalities; it also may be associated with a wide variety of conditions, including breech delivery, midline developmental defect syndromes, intracranial

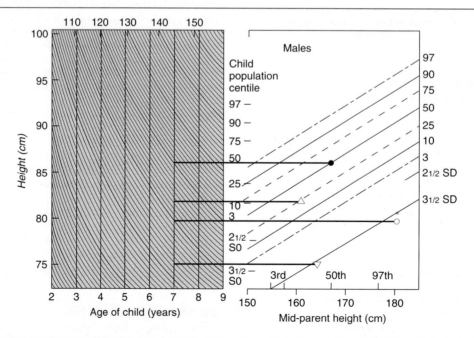

Figure 20–1. Appropriateness of the height of the child to that of the parents (mean midparental height) is indicated on the Tanner-Whitehouse chart. The point of intersection of the height of the child with the median parental height is shown for four children (7-year-old boys). (Reproduced, with permission, from Tanner JM et al: Standards for children's height at ages 2–9 years allowing for heights of parents. Arch Dis Child 1970;45:755.)

Table 20–3. Examples of chronic nonendocrine disease and short stature.

Organ System	Examples
Renal	Renal tubular acidosis, chronic renal failure
Gastrointestinal	Inflammatory bowel disease, malabsorption syndromes, chronic liver disease
Cardiac	Congestive heart failure, cyanotic heart disease
Pulmonary	Severe asthma, cystic fibrosis
Hematologic	Hemoglobinopathies
Skeletal	Rickets, osteochondrodystrophies, pseudohypoparathyroidism, pseudopseudohypoparathyroidism

Table 20–5. Factors that influence growth hormone secretion.

Potentiating Factors	Inhibiting Factors
Exercise	Obesity
Sleep (stage III, IV)	Hyperglycemia
Stress	Hypothyroidism
Hypoglycemia	Glucocorticoid excess
Sex steroids	Increased β-adrenergic tone
Increased α-adrenergic tone	Psychosocial deprivation

tumors, infections, central nervous system (CNS) irradiation, and CNS trauma. Significant emotional deprivation may be associated with transient GH deficiency.

OTHER CAUSES

Other causes of short stature include intrauterine growth retardation, malnutrition, and a large number of dysmorphic syndromes, including those associated with primary skeletal abnormalities. Short stature is seen in virtually all patients with Turner syndrome (**gonadal dysgenesis**), Down syndrome, Russell-Silver syndrome, or Prader-Willi syndrome and in a variety of other conditions with or without associated chromosomal abnormalities. Primary skeletal abnormalities often are associated with abnormal body proportions, which become apparent with measurement of arm span and sitting height.

EVALUATION OF A CHILD WITH SHORT STATURE

An important aspect in the evaluation of a child with short stature is deciding whether to launch an extensive laboratory investigation. A thorough history, physical examination, and plotting of growth charts provide etiologic clues that are as important as the laboratory evaluation. The history should focus particular attention on perinatal events, growth patterns, a history of emotional or family-related problems, and final adult heights of family members. In addition to careful measurements of height (on a wall-mounted device), weight, and head circumference, particular attention should be given to body proportions, the presence or absence of dysmorphic features, and the genital and neurologic examinations.

An algorithm for the evaluation of short stature and/or subnormal height velocity is presented in Figure 20–2. Initially, it is important to determine whether chronic nonendocrine disease, malnutrition, or poorly controlled diabetes—each of which may be associated with suboptimal growth—is present. In the absence of these conditions, the evaluation is based on assessment of body proportions, height velocity, birth weight/gestational age, bone age (as a measurement of skeletal maturation), karyotype, and relative obesity. Abnormal body proportions often are apparent by measurement of the sitting height and arm span (the latter normally closely approximates the standing height) and usually indicate a primary skeletal abnormality or disease and/or irradiation of the spine.

In children with short stature associated with normal body proportions, it is essential to evaluate the height velocity, preferably by serial measurements using the same wall-mounted device over a period of at least 4–6 months. In the absence of a history of intrauterine growth retardation, normal height velocity will usually lead to a diagnosis of idiopathic short stature, familial short stature, or constitutional delay. Of note, height velocity in children with familial short stature or constitutional delay usually is subnormal before 3–4 years of age and normal there-

Table 20–4. Common clinical features of growth hormone (GH) deficiency.

Normal size at birth
Growth failure at or after 6 mo of age, when linear growth becomes GH dependent
Excessive adiposity
Hypoglycemia in 10–20% of patients
Normal head circumference and normal intelligence in uncomplicated GH deficiency

Table 20–6. Differential diagnosis of growth hormone (GH) deficiency.

GH deficiency (80–90% are GH-RH deficient)
  Isolated: idiopathic or genetic
  Multiple hypothalamic and pituitary hormone deficiencies
    Idiopathic, genetic
    Associated with breech delivery or traumatic delivery
    Associated with midline developmental defect syndromes
    Intracranial tumors, infections, infiltrative or hemorrhagic processes
    CNS irradiation, CNS trauma
  Transient GH deficiency
    Emotional deprivation
  Abnormalities in GH signaling, IGF generation, or IGF signaling
  Structurally abnormal GH

CNS = central nervous system; IGF = insulin-like growth factor; RH = releasing hormone.

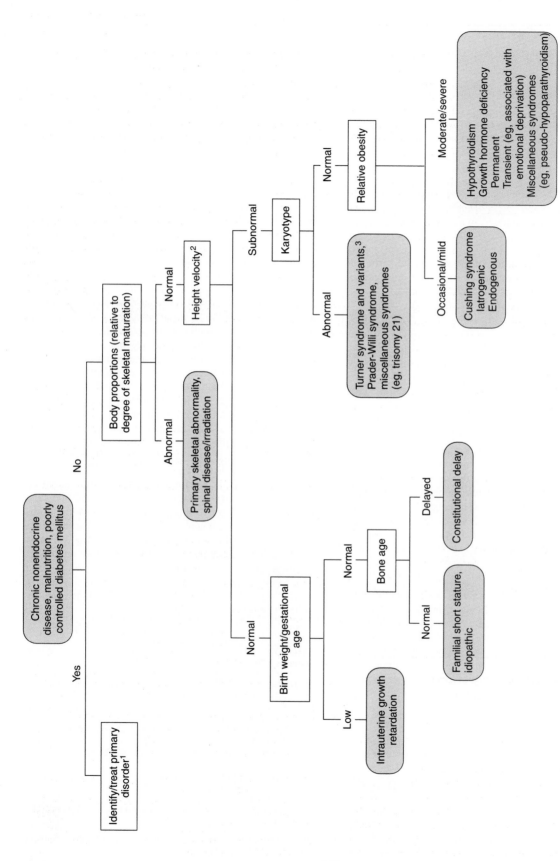

Figure 20–2. Approach to the child with short stature (height ≥ 2.5 SD below the mean for chronologic age). [1]As short stature may be a primary manifestation of chronic nonendocrine disease before other signs or symptoms are apparent (eg, certain gastrointestinal or renal disorders), generalized screening tests (eg, complete blood count, routine serum chemistries) are often considered useful to identify otherwise subtle chronic disease. [2]Height velocity in children with familial short stature is usually normal after 2–3 years of age. Height velocity in children with constitutional delay is usually normal after 3–4 years of age. [3]Girls with Turner syndrome may have some degree of intrauterine growth retardation and, in late childhood, may have abnormally immature body proportions secondary to greater retardation in growth of the legs. Height velocity is usually normal before 3 years of age and decelerates thereafter.

after. A delayed bone age distinguishes constitutional delay from familial or idiopathic short stature, although it is not uncommon for a child to have a combination of familial short stature and constitutional delay.

Subnormal height velocity in children with normally proportioned short stature often will lead to a diagnosis of an endocrine disorder or to a diagnosis of one of a number of syndromes. A karyotype analysis will identify girls with Turner syndrome and its variants and may be useful in the identification of other syndromes associated with short stature. In patients with subnormal height velocity and a normal karyotype, the presence and degree of obesity often are useful diagnostic indicators. Occasional or mild obesity in this context occurs in hypothyroidism, GH deficiency, (permanent and transient forms), and miscellaneous syndromes (eg, pseudohypoparathyroidism).

The diagnosis of GH deficiency is often difficult to make with a single blood test in view of the pulsatile nature of GH secretion. IGF-I and IGF binding protein-3 levels may serve as useful screening tests. If GH deficiency is suspected from the initial evaluation, standard provocative tests of GH secretion should be carried out. Moderate to severe obesity in a patient with subnormal height velocity warrants an investigation for possible Cushing syndrome, including iatrogenic and endogenous causes (see section on Endocrine Causes of Obesity).

TREATMENT

Appropriate treatment of short stature is directed at the cause of the growth failure. Commercial availability of recombinant human GH has led to many studies addressing its potential usefulness in non–GH-deficient short stature in addition to its use in classic GH deficiency. GH may augment final height in girls with Turner syndrome and may be of benefit in other types of non–GH-deficient short stature. The long-term risks and benefits of GH treatment in non–GH-deficient short stature are not yet known.

ABNORMALITIES OF PUBERTY

Puberty, the transitional period between the juvenile state and adulthood, is characterized by the attainment of secondary sex characteristics and, ultimately, reproductive capability. The physical changes that occur during puberty result from a marked increase in plasma gonadal sex steroid concentrations, which in turn result from pulsatile pituitary secretion of gonadotropins, that is, luteinizing hormone (LH) and follicle-stimulating hormone (FSH). Gonadotropin secretion is a consequence of synchro-

nous, pulsatile release of gonadotropin-releasing hormone (GnRH) from neurons in the medial basal hypothalamus.

Puberty is not a sudden event, but rather a developmental milestone in the activity of the hypothalamic-pituitary-gonadal axis (Table 20–7). The hypothalamic-pituitary portal circulation is functional before the end of the first trimester of gestation, and the morphogenesis of the hypothalamic-pituitary gonadotropin unit is complete by midgestation.

Subsequently, a characteristic pattern of activity emerges. Fetal gonadotropin secretion becomes pulsatile by midgestation and is initially unrestrained. At term, gonadotropin secretion is reduced to low levels, presumably secondary to the maturation of sex steroid negative feedback and other mechanisms. Shortly after birth, the GnRH neurosecretory neurons (referred to as a "pulse generator") are again highly active, concurrent with the withdrawal of maternal and placental sex steroids from the fetal environment. Late infancy and childhood are characterized by marked inhibition of pulsatile GnRH secretion. This restraint of the GnRH pulse generator is a consequence of both a highly sensitive sex steroid negative

Table 20–7. Ontogeny of the hypothalamic/pituitary gonadotropin/gonadal unit.

Fetus
- GnRH detected in human fetal brain by 4.5 wk gestation
- Hypothalamic/pituitary portal circulation intact by 11.5 wk gestation
- Morphogenesis of hypothalamic/pituitary gonadotropin unit complete by midgestation
- GnRH/gonadotropin secretion
  Pulsatile at least by midgestation
  Initially unrestrained
  Decreases to low levels at term, presumably secondary to sex steroid negative feedback and other mechanisms

Early infancy
- GnRH pulse generator highly functional by 2 wk
- Transient rise in gonadal sex steroids to midpubertal levels

Late infancy/childhood
- Inhibition of GnRH pulse generator secondary to:
  Highly sensitive sex steroid negative feedback mechanism
- Intrinsic CNS inhibitory mechanism

Late prepubertal/early pubertal period
- Disinhibition of GnRH pulse generator secondary to:
  Decreased sensitivity of sex steroid negative feedback
  Decreased effectiveness or a modification of CNS inhibitory mechanism
- Increased amplitude and frequency of GnRH pulses
- Increased amplitude and frequency of gonadotropin pulses; initially most prominent with sleep
- Increased secretion of gonadal sex steroids

Puberty
- Progressive development of secondary sex characteristics
- Spermatogenesis in males
- Development of estrogen-induced positive feedback mechanism and LH surge in females
- Ovulation in females

CNS = central nervous system; GnRH = gonadotropin-releasing hormone; LH = luteinizing hormone.

feedback mechanism and an as yet poorly defined CNS inhibitory mechanism. After a quiescent period of approximately 10 years, the GnRH pulse generator is disinhibited, ultimately leading to the attainment of clinical puberty. The hypothalamic-pituitary-gonadal axis is functionally intact in the prepubertal child as well as in the fetus; the CNS inhibitory mechanism is considered to be rate limiting in the onset of puberty.

Adrenarche is an independent, although temporally related, developmental process typified by the appearance of pubic hair and acne. Adrenarche represents a poorly understood maturational process in the zona reticularis of the adrenal cortex, which results in enhanced secretion of the androgen dehydroepiandrosterone (DHEA) and its sulfated form (DHEA[S]). An increase in circulating adrenal androgens begins at 6–8 years of age, and approximately 2 years later, clinical adrenarche is manifest.

The normal age of onset of secondary sex characteristics, defined as 2.5 SD on either side of the mean, or where approximately 99% of the population falls, is 8–13 years in girls and 9–14 years in boys. Girls complete secondary sexual development within an average of 4.2 years. In boys, secondary sexual development is completed in 3.5 years.

Clinically, puberty in the boy begins with testicular enlargement ($\geq$ 2.5 cm in maximum diameter) followed by the development of sexual hair and phallic enlargement (see Chapter 2). The growth spurt occurs during midpuberty; growth continues until there is full maturation and fusion of the growth centers in the long bones and spine. Laboratory evidence of puberty includes an increase in circulating testosterone to concentrations of greater than 50 ng/dL associated with evidence of pulsatile gonadotropin secretion and an increase in LH of at least 2 ng/mL above baseline (or approximately 15 mIU/mL) after an intravenous injection of synthetic GnRH.

In approximately 90% of girls, breast enlargement is the initial sign of secondary sexual development. Ten percent of girls demonstrate sexual hair as their initial secondary sexual characteristic. The growth spurt occurs early in puberty, whereas menarche occurs toward the end of puberty and is normally followed within 1–2 years by completion of linear growth. Laboratory evidence of puberty in girls includes a circulating estradiol level of greater than 10 pg/mL associated with pulsatile gonadotropin secretion and a "pubertal" gonadotropin response to synthetic GnRH similar to that described above for boys.

PUBERTAL DELAY

Delayed puberty may be defined, in boys, as lack of an increase of testicular size above prepubertal size by 14 years of age, and in girls, as lack of initiation of breast development by 13 years of age. The differential diagnosis of delayed puberty comprises three major categories: constitutional delay in growth, hypogonadotropic hypogo-

nadism, and hypergonadotropic hypogonadism (Table 20–8).

Constitutional delay in growth, the most common cause of delayed puberty, is a normal variant (see this chapter, Short Stature: Normal Variants). Such patients often have a family history of delayed puberty and have a delayed bone age but do not have evidence of endocrinopathy or other organic disease.

Hypogonadotropic hypogonadism may result from a variety of CNS disorders. A defect at the level of the hypothalamus or pituitary results in deficient GnRH or gonadotropin secretion, as measured by low basal LH and FSH values and the absence of an appropriate LH response to exogenous GnRH. Gonadotropin deficiency can be isolated, as in Kallmann syndrome. This syndrome is associated with anosmia or hyposmia and is transmitted in an X-linked or autosomal-dominant fashion with variable penetrance. In addition to microphallus and undescended testes, Kallmann syndrome may be associated with renal aplasia and with skeletal and ocular anomalies. Hypogonadotropic hypogonadism also may occur in association with multiple hypothalamic and pituitary hormone deficiencies. Etiologies include idiopathic, CNS tumors (primarily third ventricular), CNS infection, trauma, cranial irradiation, and congenital midline defect syndromes. Functional gonadotropin deficiency may occur in association with chronic systemic disease and malnutrition, hypothyroidism, hypercortisolism, hyperprolactinemia, diabetes mellitus, anorexia nervosa, and marijuana use. It also may occur in some female athletes and ballet dancers.

Table 20–8. Causes of delayed puberty.

Constitutional delay in growth—normal variant
Hypogonadotropic hypogonadism—defect at level of hypothalamus/pituitary
• Isolated gonadotropin deficiency
Kallmann syndrome
In association with other syndromes that may include cleft palate, congenital deafness, X-linked form of congenital adrenal hypoplasia (can be associated with glycerol kinase deficiency and muscular dystrophy), Prader-Willi syndrome, Laurence-Moon-Biedl syndrome
• Multiple hypothalamic/pituitary hormone deficiencies
Idiopathic
CNS disorders: tumors (involving primarily third ventricular area), infection, trauma, other invasive disease, irradiation, congenital malformations
• Functional gonadotropin deficiency: chronic systemic disease and malnutrition, hypothyroidism, hypercortisolism, hyperprolactinemia, diabetes mellitus, anorexia nervosa, some female athletes and ballet dancers, marijuana use
Hypergonadotropic hypogonadism—defect at level of the gonads
• Primary testicular failure: Klinefelter syndrome and its variants, anorchia and cryptorchidism, XY gonadal dysgenesis, Noonan syndrome, other causes
• Primary ovarian failure: Turner syndrome and its variants, XX gonadal dysgenesis, other causes

CNS = central nervous system.

In general, weight loss to less than 80% of ideal weight may result in functional gonadotropin deficiency.

Hypergonadotropic hypogonadism indicates a defect at the level of the gonads, with serum concentrations of the gonadotropins, particularly FSH, elevated in children older than 10 years. Primary testicular failure is associated with Klinefelter syndrome (the XXY form of seminiferous tubule dysgenesis), XY gonadal dysgenesis, anorchia (associated with apparent testicular regression after fetal male differentiation), and cryptorchidism; it also may be seen after chemotherapy or local irradiation. Primary ovarian failure is most commonly found in patients with Turner syndrome (45X or in association with structural abnormalities of the X chromosome and mosaicism) and, less commonly, in XX gonadal dysgenesis. Primary ovarian failure also may occur in association with autoimmune disease.

An algorithm for evaluating delayed puberty is presented in Figure 20–3. One should initially measure basal plasma gonadotropins (LH, FSH). If these levels are elevated, such patients have hypergonadotropic hypogonadism (primary ovarian or testicular failure). A karyotype analysis should then be performed to distinguish Turner or Klinefelter syndrome for other causes of primary hypogonadism associated with a normal chromosomal pattern. If basal plasma gonadotropin levels are low or normal, the patient has either constitutional delay or hypogonadotropic hypogonadism. The demonstration of a pubertal LH response to an injection of synthetic GnRH will identify patients with constitutional delay; however, many patients with constitutional delay, when initially examined, will have a prepubertal LH response to GnRH indistinguishable from that seen in patients with hypogonadotropic hypogonadism. Unless other clinical findings point to CNS abnormalities associated with hypogonadotropic hypogonadism or to functional gonadotropic deficiency, only prolonged clinical observation will distinguish constitutional delay from hypogonadotropic hypogonadism. Sexual maturation will become apparent on follow-up examinations in those with constitutional delay. If hypogonadotropic hypogonadism is strongly suspected, an evaluation of possible causes (see Table 20–8) should be carried out. Although the bone age is invariably delayed in all causes of delayed puberty, and therefore is not diagnostically useful, the bone age may nevertheless be useful to determine the severity of the pubertal delay.

Short-term hormonal therapy may be useful in constitutionally delayed adolescents, whereas long-term therapy is indicated in hypergonadotropic or hypogonadotropic hypogonadism. In addition to reassurance and observation, some adolescents with constitutional delay may benefit from a short course of testosterone enanthate (TE) for boys or conjugated estrogen or ethinyl estradiol for girls. Long-term hormonal therapy for boys with hyper- or hypogonadotropic hypogonadism includes monthly injections of TE. Long-term hormonal therapy for girls includes the use of estrogen and progestin cycling in doses that sustain full development of secondary sexual charac-

teristics, result in adequate withdrawal bleeding, and prevent osteoporosis.

SEXUAL PRECOCITY

Sexual precocity usually is defined as the development of secondary sexual characteristics before age 8 years in girls or before 9 years in boys. The differential diagnosis of precocious sexual development is extensive but conceptually straightforward. As sexual precocity results from an increase in circulating sex steroids, etiologic considerations may be divided into exogenous and endogenous sources for these steroids. Exogenous sources include estrogen-containing creams, birth control pills, and anabolic steroids. Endogenous sources include the gonads and the adrenal cortex, either of which may inappropriately secrete sex steroids as the result of a primary process intrinsic to these tissues or secondary to a circulating stimulating factor.

Endogenous Feminizing Sexual Precocity in Girls

The differential diagnosis for endogenous causes of feminizing sexual precocity in girls is summarized in Table 20–9. The most common form of early sexual development in girls is premature thelarche. Premature thelarche is the appearance of unilateral or bilateral breast tissue between infancy and early childhood. This condition is benign and is often associated with single or multiple ovarian follicular cysts. There are no other signs of puberty, such as increased growth velocity, vaginal mucosal thickening, or the appearance of pubic hair. These patients require close follow-up, with observation for other signs of sexual precocity. A pelvic ultrasound study may be considered to evaluate the ovaries, as well as uterine size and contour. No treatment is required.

Other primary ovarian processes include large ovarian cysts, which may be seen with McCune-Albright syndrome, and rare tumors. McCune-Albright syndrome is characterized by a clinical triad of irregularly shaped café-au-lait spots (Coast of Maine lesions), polyostotic fibrous dysplasia of long bones and skull, and sexual precocity (primary ovarian cysts). It also may be associated with other endocrine abnormalities.

Secondary ovarian processes occur in idiopathic true precocious puberty (the most common etiology of precocious puberty, especially in girls), in associated CNS disease or injury, and after late treatment of congenital virilizing adrenal hyperplasia (CVAH). Adrenal neoplasms are rarely the source of precocious feminization. In girls, ectopic secretion of the human chorionic gonadotropin (hCG) will not by itself cause puberty.

Endogenous Virilizing Sexual Precocity in Girls

The endogenous causes of virilization in girls are summarized in Table 20–10. Primary adrenal processes in-

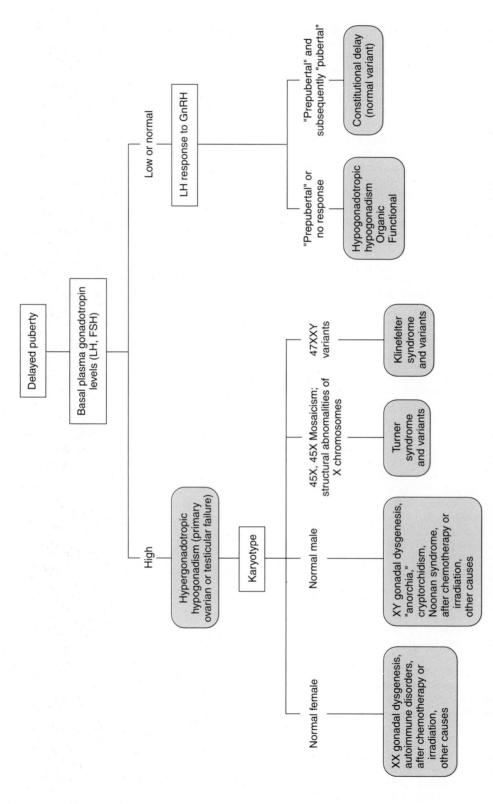

Figure 20–3. Approach to patients with delayed puberty. FSH = follicle-stimulating hormone; GnRH = gonadotropin-releasing hormone; LH = luteinizing hormone.

Table 20–9. Sexual precocity in females: Endogenous causes.

Ovary
- Primary processes
  Premature thelarche/follicular ovarian cyst(s)
  McCune-Albright syndrome: ovarian cysts associated with abnormal skin pigmentation and polyostotic fibrous dysplasia
  Tumors: granulosa or theca cell tumors, gonadoblastoma, lipoid tumors, ovarian carcinomas
- Secondary processes: precocious puberty
  Idiopathic
  CNS disease or injury: hamartoma of the tuber cinereum, tumors, subarachnoid cysts, congenital malformations, other invasive disease, infection, irradiation, severe trauma
  After late treatment of congenital virilizing adrenal hyperplasia

Adrenal neoplasm

CNS = central nervous system.

Table 20–11. Sexual precocity in males: Endogenous causes.

Adrenal cortex
- Primary processes
  Premature adrenarche
  Congenital virilizing adrenal hyperplasia (CVAH)
    21-OH deficiency (P450$_{c21}$)
    11-OH deficiency (P450$_{c11}$)
  Virilizing adrenal neoplasm
- Secondary process
  Cushing disease

Testis
- Primary processes
  Leydig cell tumor
  Familial Leydig cell hyperplasia
  McCune-Albright syndrome
- Secondary process
  Precocious puberty
  Idiopathic
  CNS disease or injury: hamartoma of the tuber cinereum, tumors, subarachnoid cysts, congenital malformations, other invasive disease, infection, irradiation, severe trauma
  After late treatment of CVAH
  Ectopic hCG-secreting tumors

CNS = central nervous system; hCG = human chorionic gonadotropin; OH = hydroxylase.

clude premature adrenarche, CVAH, and virilizing adrenal neoplasms. Premature adrenarche is the most common cause of premature pubic hair development, or pubarche. This is a benign condition without significant growth acceleration; no other signs of pubertal changes are seen. Excessive corticotropin (ACTH) stimulation of the adrenal cortex in Cushing disease may result in virilization in addition to signs of glucocorticoid excess. Virilization may also result from ovarian neoplasms.

Endogenous Sexual Precocity in Boys

The differential diagnosis for endogenous causes of sexual precocity in boys is summarized in Table 20–11. Primary adrenal processes include premature adrenarche, CVAH, and virilizing adrenal neoplasms. As noted previously, Cushing disease may result in virilization from increased adrenal androgens. Primary testicular processes are rare and include Leydig cell tumors, familial Leydig cell hyperplasia, and McCune-Albright syndrome. Secondary testicular processes resulting in sexual precocity include premature reactivation of the hypothalamic-pituitary-gonadal axis (true precocious puberty) and ectopic

Table 20–10. Endogenous causes of virilization in females.

Adrenal cortex
- Primary processes
  Premature adrenarche
  Congenital virilizing adrenal hyperplasia
    21-OH deficiency (P450$_{c21}$)
    11-OH deficiency (P450$_{c11}$)
    3β-Hydroxysteroid dehydrogenase deficiency
  Virilizing adrenal neoplasm
- Secondary process
    Cushing disease

Ovary
  Virilizing ovarian neoplasm

OH = hydroxylase.

hCG-secreting tumors. Endogenous feminization in male adolescents (gynecomastia) is associated with elevated estradiol-testosterone ratios. This form of gynecomastia is common and is discussed further in Chapter 2. Gynecomastia also may be seen in patients with Klinefelter syndrome and in those with partial androgen resistance.

Evaluation of the Child With Sexual Precocity

Evaluation of a Girl With Precocious Feminization. To evaluate precocious feminization in girls (Figure 20–4), one must first consider the possibility of an exogenous source of estrogens. If the source of estrogens is endogenous (from the ovary or, rarely, from the adrenal cortex), it is essential to assess the clinical severity and rate of progression of the sexual precocity. In addition to the physical examination (eg, breast size, vaginal mucosa for evidence of estrogen effect, and growth rate), a bone age examination is useful. If the degree of feminizing sexual precocity is mild and the bone age is not advanced, the patient most likely has premature thelarche, as discussed above, and requires only observation. If the sexual precocity has progressed rapidly and the bone age is advanced, it would then be appropriate to carry out a GnRH stimulation test. A prepubertal response to GnRH indicates a primary ovarian process (eg, large ovarian cyst or tumor) or, rarely, a feminizing adrenal neoplasm; imaging studies can be used for confirmation. A pubertal response to GnRH indicates precocious puberty and should be followed by a cranial magnetic resonance imaging (MRI) study to determine whether there is evidence of CNS disease, injury, or malformation.

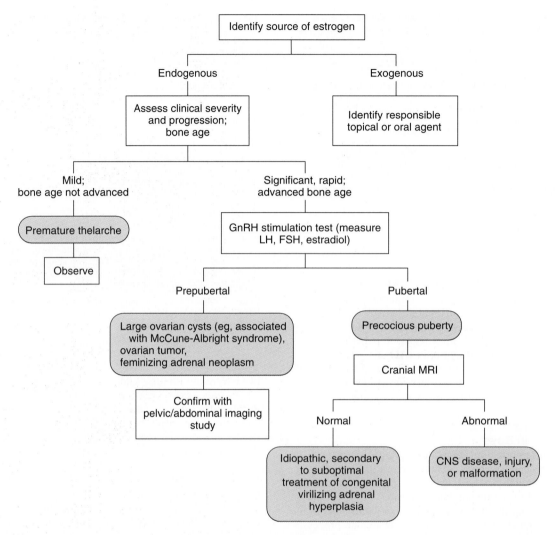

Figure 20–4. Approach to the evaluation of girls with feminizing sexual precocity. CNS = central nervous system; FSH = follicle-stimulating hormone; GnRH = gonadotropin-releasing hormone; LH = luteinizing hormone; MRI = magnetic resonance imaging.

Evaluation of a Girl With Precocious Virilization.
To evaluate precocious virilization in girls (Figure 20–5), it is again important to begin by considering an exogenous source of androgens. In the absence of an exogenous source, the androgens causing precocious or excessive virilization are derived either from the adrenal cortex or from the ovaries. A bone age study should then be obtained. If the bone age is not advanced, the patient most likely has premature adrenarche, a benign condition in which there is early maturation of the adrenocortical zona reticularis, resulting in mild to modest elevations of the principal adrenal androgens, DHEA and DHEA(S). Although a nonadvanced bone age in a girl with virilization usually will lead to a diagnosis of premature adrenarche, this latter condition also may be associated with a bone age that

is significantly advanced. If the bone age is advanced, one should carry out an ACTH stimulation test during which plasma levels of androgens (DHEA, DHEA[S], androstenedione, and testosterone) and cortisol and its precursors (in particular, 17-OH-progesterone and 11-deoxycortisol) are measured just before and 60 minutes after an intravenous injection of ACTH. As indicated in the algorithm, the ACTH test results can be used to diagnose a variety of primary virilizing adrenal disorders. Markedly elevated DHEA(S) or testosterone levels before ACTH stimulation suggest the possibilities of a virilizing adrenal or ovarian neoplasm, respectively.

Evaluation of a Boy With Precocious Virilization.
An algorithm for evaluation of virilizing sexual precocity in boys is presented in Figure 20–6. If an exogenous

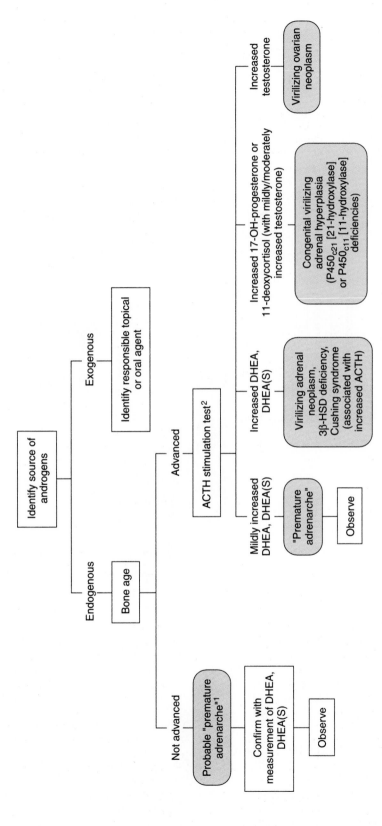

Figure 20–5. Approach to the evaluation of girls with virilizing sexual precocity. [1]Patients with premature adrenarche may have bone ages that range from not advanced to significantly advanced. [2]Adrenocorticotropic hormone (ACTH) test: Measures androgens—dehydroepiandrosterone (DHEA), DHEA sulfate (DHEA[S]), androstenedione, and testosterone—cortisol, and cortisol precursors—17-OH-progesterone and 11-deoxycortisol. 3β-HSD = 3β-hydroxysteroid dehydrogenase deficiency.

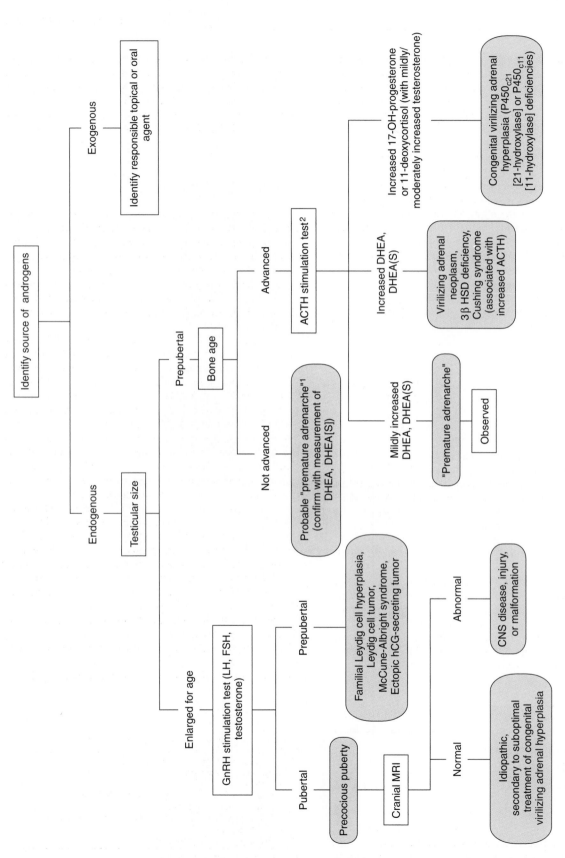

Figure 20–6. Approach to the evaluation of boys with virilizing sexual precocity. [1]Patients with premature adrenarche may have bone ages that range from not advanced to significantly advanced. [2]Adrenocorticotropic hormone (ACTH) test: Measures androgens—dehydroepiandrosterone (DHEA), DHEA sulfate (DHEA[S]), androstenedione, and testosterone—cortisol, and cortisol precursors—17-OH-progesterone and 11-deoxycortisol. CNS = central nervous system; MRI = magnetic resonance imaging; 3β HSD = 3β-hydroxysteroid dehydrogenase deficiency.

source of androgens has been excluded, it would then be appropriate to proceed with an evaluation based on the testicular size. If the testes are enlarged, a GnRH stimulation test should be carried out. A pubertal response to GnRH indicates precocious puberty, and a cranial MRI study should be performed, as noted for girls with precocious puberty. If one or both testes are enlarged but the response to GnRH is prepubertal, the patient either has a primary testicular process (eg, familial Leydig cell hyperplasia, McCune-Albright syndrome, a Leydig cell tumor) or has an ectopic hCG-secreting tumor. If the testes are not enlarged, a bone age study should be obtained. If the bone age is not advanced, the patient most likely has premature adrenarche, which can be confirmed by measurement of DHEA and DHEA(S) levels. This benign condition requires observation only. As noted above, patients with premature adrenarche also may have a bone age that is significantly advanced. If the bone age is advanced, an ACTH stimulation test should be performed, as described above, which will distinguish a variety of primary adrenal disorders.

Treatment

The appropriate therapy for sexual precocity is directed toward the particular cause. Treatment of idiopathic central precocious puberty is aimed at prevention of early epiphyseal fusion and adult short stature, as well as preventing premature menses in girls. The current approach for treatment of true precocious puberty is the use of a long-acting GnRH agonist. GnRH agonists desensitize the pituitary to endogenous GnRH stimulation, resulting in decreased gonadotropin secretion and, ultimately, decreased gonadal sex steroid secretion. These analogues are currently administered daily by subcutaneous or intranasal routes or monthly in a depot form. Recent studies indicate that after such treatment, the normal pubertal process resumes, both hormonally and clinically. Assessment of long-term side effects of these agonists is not yet complete. Medroxyprogesterone acetate, which has direct inhibitory effects on gonadal steroidogenesis, is useful in the rare disorders of familial Leydig cell hyperplasia and McCune-Albright syndrome. Testolactone and ketoconazole, which also inhibit gonadal steroidogenesis, have been used in nontumor primary gonadal causes of sexual precocity.

ENDOCRINE CAUSES OF OBESITY

Obesity in children and adolescents most often is exogenous in nature and usually is associated with a normal or above-average height velocity and stature. In contrast, endocrine causes of obesity, which include Cushing syndrome, hypothyroidism, and GH deficiency, are virtually always associated with subnormal height velocity and often short stature. The clinical presentation, diagnosis, and management of hypothyroidism and GH deficiency are discussed elsewhere in this chapter.

CUSHING SYNDROME

Cushing syndrome results from exogenous or endogenous glucocorticoid excess. The differential diagnosis of Cushing syndrome is summarized in Table 20–12. Exogenous or iatrogenic glucocorticoid excess may occur in patients with adrenal insufficiency who receive overtreatment and in patients with a variety of disorders treated chronically with pharmacologic doses of glucocorticoids. Prolonged use of topical glucocorticoids may also result in Cushing syndrome.

Endogenous hypercortisolism is either ACTH dependent or ACTH independent. Of the ACTH-dependent causes, a pituitary adenoma (usually a microadenoma) is most common. In this condition, referred to as **Cushing disease,** individual ACTH levels may be only minimally or moderately elevated. However, these patients have loss of diurnal variation in ACTH secretion and thus, over the course of 24 hours, have an overall increase in ACTH secretion. A less common ACTH-dependent cause of endogenous hypercortisolism is ectopic ACTH production, associated with oat cell carcinoma, carcinoid tumors, pancreatic islet cell tumors, neuroblastoma, pheochromocytomas, and other neoplasms. ACTH-independent causes result from increased glucocorticoid production in disorders of primary adrenocortical hyperfunction, including adenomas, carcinomas, and primary macronodular hyperplasia. Ectopic ACTH syndrome and ACTH-independent syndromes are less common than Cushing disease. Ectopic production of corticotropin-releasing hormone (CRH) is a rare cause of Cushing syndrome.

The characteristic clinical features of Cushing syndrome of any etiology are summarized in Table 20–13. Marked impairment of linear growth, often with some degree of truncal obesity, is one of the most important clinical signs of Cushing syndrome in the pediatric population

Table 20–12. Differential diagnosis of Cushing syndrome.

Exogenous/iatrogenic glucocorticoid excess
Endogenous hypercortisolism
ACTH-dependent
Pituitary ACTH-secreting adenoma (Cushing disease)
Ectopic ACTH production
Ectopic corticotropin releasing hormone production
ACTH-independent
Primary adrenal hyperfunction

ACTH = adrenocorticotropic hormone.

Table 20–13. Clinical features of Cushing syndrome.

Growth: impaired linear growth; retardation of skeletal maturation
Habitus: "buffalo hump"; truncal obesity
Facies: rounding, plethora
Skin: thin; wide striae
Endocrine: some degree of insulin resistance and hyperglycemia
Other: weakness, fatigue; depression; hypertension

and may be present long before other features commonly associated with this syndrome are noted.

If hypercortisolism is suspected and iatrogenic causes have been excluded, one proceeds with a laboratory evaluation (Table 20–14) to document excessive cortisol levels, establish the cause, and determine the appropriate treatment. Hypercortisolism is first established by obtaining a 24-hour urine collection for 17-hydroxycorticosteroids (17-OHCS) and free cortisol excretion. Urinary creatinine levels and total urinary volume should be measured to determine the adequacy of the collection. Baseline values of 5 mg/m² or greater of 17-OHCS and greater than 100 µg of free cortisol per total volume of urine indicate hypercortisolism. A single, overnight dose of dexamethasone at 11:00 PM with subsequent measurement of plasma cortisol concentration at 8:00 AM has also been useful to distinguish patients with mild hypercortisolism (as may be seen in exogenous obesity, depression, or stress) from patients with true Cushing syndrome. With true Cushing syndrome, plasma cortisol will not suppress to less than 5 µg/dL during this test. The distinction between ACTH-independent and ACTH-dependent Cushing syndrome usually is straightforward, as plasma ACTH levels are low in the former and normal or elevated in the latter.

The principal challenge in the differential diagnosis of Cushing syndrome is the distinction of Cushing disease (pituitary overproduction of ACTH) from ectopic ACTH production. For approximately 20 years, the standard approach has been to carry out a low- and high-dose dexamethasone suppression test. This test begins with a 2-day baseline period during which 24-hour urine collections are

obtained for 17-OHCS, free cortisol, and creatinine; plasma is serially sampled in the morning and afternoon for cortisol and ACTH concentrations to determine whether the normal pattern of diurnal variation is present. Subsequently, low-dose dexamethasone (5 µg/kg every 6 hours for 2 days) and then high-dose dexamethasone (20 µg/kg every 6 hours for 2 days) are administered. Daily urine collection and plasma cortisol and ACTH sampling continue until 6 hours after the last dose of dexamethasone. As with the overnight dexamethasone test, individuals with mild hypercortisolism secondary to exogenous obesity, depression, or stress suppress ACTH and cortisol levels with low-dose dexamethasone. Patients with pituitary adenomas may show some degree of suppression with low-dose dexamethasone and usually suppress significantly (> 50%) with high-dose dexamethasone. In contrast, patients with ectopic ACTH production usually do not suppress with either low or high doses.

Unfortunately, the low- and high-dose dexamethasone suppression test does not always accurately distinguish Cushing disease from ectopic ACTH production. Of note, approximately 20% of patients with Cushing disease do not suppress with high-dose dexamethasone, whereas an equivalent percentage of patients with ectopic ACTH production suppress under similar conditions. Peripheral CRH administration with measurement of plasma ACTH concentration in serial samples may help to distinguish some patients with pituitary adenomas from those with ectopic ACTH production. An MRI of the hypothalamic and pituitary areas should be obtained if Cushing disease is suspected, whereas chest and abdominal imaging studies should be obtained if ectopic ACTH production is a likely consideration.

The treatment of choice for an ACTH-secreting pituitary adenoma is transphenoidal adenomectomy. Occasionally, findings on surgical exploration of the pituitary will be negative even when all laboratory studies indicate pituitary disease. Therapeutic options include repeated pituitary exploration, bilateral adrenalectomy, pituitary irradiation, and use of pharmacologic agents that directly impair cortisol synthesis and secretion.

Table 20–14. Laboratory evaluation of hypercortisolism.

- 24-h urine for 17-OHCS, free cortisol, creatinine
- Baseline AM, PM plasma cortisol, ACTH (multiple samples) concentrations
- Dexamethasone suppression test
- Overnight (limited value), or
- Standard low- and high-dose test (more informative)
- Peripheral CRH stimulation test
- Consider bilateral inferior petrosal sinus sampling, pre-CRH and post-CRH, with simultaneous peripheral ACTH sampling
- MRI of hypothalamic and pituitary areas or of chest and abdomen

ACTH = adrenocorticotropic hormone; CRH = corticotropin-releasing hormone; MRI = magnetic resonance imaging; 17-OHS = 17-hydroxycorticosteroids.

APPROACH TO THE CHILD WITH AMBIGUOUS GENITALIA

SEXUAL DIFFERENTIATION

Although most infants are easily identifiable as male or female, some have ambiguous genitalia. The evaluation of the child with ambiguous genitalia is founded on an understanding of the normal sexual differentiation process. Sexual differentiation occurs at three anatomic levels: gonads, genital ducts, and external genitalia. The fetus has the primordia of both male and female genital ducts; under normal circumstances, the bipotential fetal gonads become either testes or ovaries, and the bipotential external genitalia become those of either a normal male or female infant (Figure 20–7).

Sexual differentiation follows an orderly sequence that begins at approximately the 6th week of fetal life and is completed by the 12th week. The bipotential gonads in the male or female infant are initially indistinguishable. Under the influence of the testis-determining factor (TDF), the gonads begin testicular differentiation by 43–50 days of gestation. TDF recently has been identified as a gene near the pseudoautosomal region of the Y chromosome. (**Pseudoautosomal** refers to a small region of homology between the X and Y chromosomes that allows pairing of the sex chromosomes during meiosis.) This gene, which encodes a DNA-binding protein, has been termed sex-determining region Y (SRY). SRY is thought to function as a switch mechanism, initiating a cascade of events involving genes on the autosomes as well as on the X chromosome that ultimately results in testicular differentiation. Strong evidence that SRY is the TDF comes from studies in which transgenic female mice carrying and expressing the SRY gene develop as male mice. Thus, if SRY is present, the bipotential gonads become testes, with differentiation of Leydig cells, Sertoli cells, and, later, spermatogonia. In the absence of SRY, the bipotential gonads become ovaries.

Differentiation of the genital ducts is a direct consequence of gonadal differentiation. As noted above, the developing fetus has the primordia of both male and female genital ducts. If testes are present, testosterone from Leydig cells cause the male (or wolffian) ducts to develop into the epididymis, vas deferens, seminal vesicles, and ejaculatory ducts. Antimüllerian hormone (AMH), a dimeric glycoprotein secreted by Sertoli cells, prevents differentiation of the ipsilateral female (or müllerian) ducts into the fallopian tubes, uterus, cervix, and the upper third of the vagina. In the absence of testosterone and AMH (ie, if an ovary or a nonfunctional testis is present), the male genital ducts involute, and the female genital ducts continue to develop.

Differentiation of the bipotential external genitalia occurs between the 8th and 12th weeks of gestation. Masculinization of the external genitalia and urogenital sinus results from the action of the androgen dihydrotestosterone (DHT). Testosterone is converted to DHT in the target tissues by the enzyme 5α-reductase. In the complete absence of DHT or of a normally functioning androgen receptor, the bipotential external genitalia feminize. If the DHT concentration or androgen receptor function is partially deficient in an otherwise normal male fetus, the external genitalia appear as intermediate between those of a male and female fetus, and thus ambiguous. Conversely, if inappropriately elevated androgen levels (which can be converted to DHT in the target tissues) are present in the developing female fetus, the external genitalia masculinize to varying degrees. There is, however, a critical period for androgen action on the external genitalia. After approximately the 12th week of gestation, fusion of the labioscrotal folds to form a scrotum does not occur, no matter how intense the androgen stimulation. Phallic growth, however, does continue in response to androgen stimulation after the 12th fetal week. The normal pattern of sexual differentiation is summarized in Table 20–15.

There are three categories of ambiguous external genitalia: female pseudohermaphroditism, male pseudohermaphroditism, and true hermaphroditism.

FEMALE PSEUDOHERMAPHRODITE

A female pseudohermaphrodite is an individual with a 46XX karyotype, normal ovaries, and normal female genital ducts but with ambiguous external genitalia. Ambiguous external genitalia in these individuals is either a consequence of inappropriate androgen stimulation or is associated with non–androgen-induced structural malformations of the intestine and urinary tract. If the pseudohermaphroditism results from excess androgens, the source is either fetal or maternal. Fetal sources are essentially limited to the adrenal cortex and usually ensue from one of three virilizing forms of congenital adrenal hyper-

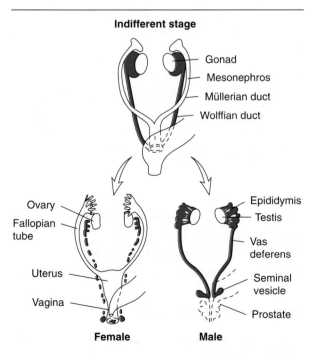

Indifferent stage

Gonad
Mesonephros
Müllerian duct
Wolffian duct

Ovary
Fallopian tube
Uterus
Vagina

Female

Epididymis
Testis
Vas deferens
Seminal vesicle
Prostate

Male

Figure 20–7. The differentiation of the internal genital ducts in the male and female. (Reproduced, with permission, from Wilson JD, Foster DW [editors]: *Williams Textbook of Endocrinology.* Saunders, 1992, p 873.)

Table 20–15. Sexual differentiation.

Gonad
- Bipotential
- Testicular differentiation at 6th–7th wk of fetal life, SRY-dependent
- Ovarian differentiation occurs in the absence of SRY

Genital ducts
- Fetus has primordia of both male and female ducts by 7th wk of gestation
- Male (wolffian) ducts: epididymis, vas deferens, seminal vesicles, ejaculatory ducts; testosterone-dependent
- Female (müllerian) ducts: fallopian tubes, uterus, cervix, upper third of vagina; develop in the absence of AMH

External genitalia
- Bipotential
- Differentiation occurs between 8th–12th wk of fetal life
- Normal masculinization is DHT-dependent
- Inherent tendency to feminize with androgen deficiency or unresponsiveness

AMH = antimüllerian hormone; DHT = dihydrotestosterone; SRY = sex-determining region Y.

plasia (see this chapter, Adrenal Insufficiency); these include, most commonly, deficiency of $P450_{c21}$ (21-hydroxylase [21-OH]) with or without salt loss and, less often, deficiency of $P450_{c11}$ (11-hydroxylase activity) or deficiency of 3β-hydroxysteroid dehydrogenase (3β-HSD or 3β-OL). Rarely, female pseudohermaphroditism results from fetal/placental aromatase deficiency, in which the placenta is unable to aromatize androgens to estrogens. This defect leads to an accumulation of androgens in the fetal and maternal circulations, resulting in virilization of the fetus' external genitalia and temporary virilization in the mother (which regresses after the pregnancy). Potential maternal sources include androgens or synthetic progestins with androgenic activity transferred from the maternal circulation. Unclassified forms of abnormal sexual development also occur in females and are associated with absence or anomalous development of the uterus, fallopian tubes, and vagina. A uterus is present in all other instances of female pseudohermaphroditism noted above.

MALE PSEUDOHERMAPHRODITE

A male pseudohermaphrodite is an individual with a 46XY karyotype (rarely XO/XY mosaicism) whose gonads are testes but who has ambiguous external genitalia. Ambiguity of the external genitalia in these individuals results from deficient DHT or response to androgens. DHT deficiency may arise from several causes, including testicular unresponsiveness to hCG/LH, an inborn error in testosterone biosynthesis, deficient 5α-reductase activity, and various forms of dysgenetic testes. Deficient androgen responsiveness results from androgen receptor or postreceptor defects. In these individuals, male genital duct development is variable.

Additional, unclassified forms of male pseudohermaph-

roditism also exist. Hypospadias occurs as an isolated finding in 1/700 male newborns and usually does not appear to be associated with either androgen deficiency or unresponsiveness. Rarely, ambiguous external genitalia can occur in XY male newborns without obvious explanation in association with multiple congenital anomalies.

TRUE HERMAPHRODITE

True hermaphroditism is a condition in which individuals have both ovarian and testicular tissue and usually have ambiguous external genitalia. Some degree of uterine development is present in all cases. Most true hermaphrodites have a 46XX karyotype, and a minority have either 46XY or sex chromosome mosaicism or chimerism. If all other forms of male and female pseudohermaphroditism have been excluded in the workup of ambiguous genitalia, true hermaphroditism should be evaluated by histologic examination of the gonadal tissue.

EVALUATION OF A CHILD WITH AMBIGUOUS GENITALIA

An approach to the evaluation of ambiguous genitalia is summarized in Figure 20–8. A number of clinical clues assist in the differential diagnosis. The presence of palpable gonads in the external genitalia or inguinal area indicates the presence of testes (or, rarely, an ovotestis) and thus a genotype that most likely will be 46XY. Another useful point is that, with the possible exception of patients with dysgenetic testes, all other patients with male pseudohermaphroditism make antimüllerian hormone and thus will not have a uterus. Therefore, if no gonads are palpated and a pelvic ultrasound study reveals a uterus, the infant probably has female pseudohermaphroditism. While awaiting the results of karyotyping, one can perform the Barr body analysis of cells from the buccal mucosa on the first postnatal day. This will reveal a sex chromatin body corresponding to a partially inactivated X chromosome in 20–30% of the nuclei of 46XX interphase cells (or cells in which two or more X chromosomes are present). In normal 46XY male infants, the sex chromatin body is absent. Using this approach, the clinician can determine relatively quickly, whether the infant is a male or female pseudohermaphrodite. For example, an individual with ambiguous genitalia who has no palpable gonads, has a uterus by ultrasound, and has a positive Barr body analysis most likely is a female pseudohermaphrodite, which is most commonly secondary to deficiency of $P450_{c21}$.

MANAGEMENT

The birth of a child with ambiguous genitalia may not only represent a medical emergency, particularly if there

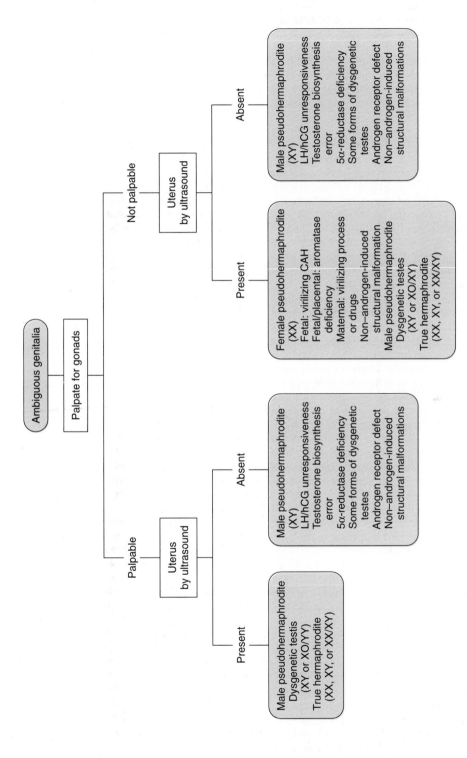

Figure 20–8. An approach to the evaluation of ambiguous genitalia. CAH = congenital adrenal hyperplasia; hCG = human chorionic gonadotropin; LH = luteinizing hormone.

is underlying congenital adrenal hyperplasia with associated adrenal insufficiency, but also is an immediate psychosocial emergency. The usual first question asked by parents and family of a newborn is the child's sex. If the gender is not readily identifiable, this presents immediate difficulties for the family. The family must cope not only with the notion of having a child with a physical malformation, but also with the question of what to tell other relatives and friends. What health care providers communicate to the parents in the first few hours of life can have a crucial effect on the parents' future relationship with the child.

The parents should be allowed to see the infant's genitalia with the physician so that they can understand the problem and ask questions. It is helpful to describe the problem as either "overdevelopment" or "underdevelopment," rather than "something in between." Parents should be reassured that urgent investigations will establish the child to be definitely male or female. They should be advised to postpone giving the child a name and not to complete the birth certificate until a final decision has been made regarding the child's sex of rearing.

If it is established that the infant is a female pseudohermaphrodite, hormonal studies to evaluate whether excess androgens are present can be carried out, with results available often within 1 week. Determining the particular cause of male pseudohermaphroditism often requires a longer period of time, particularly if one embarks on a trial of testosterone treatment to determine androgen responsiveness. Management issues in the infant with ambiguous genitalia are complex, involving not only diagnostic considerations, but also an assessment of which sex for rearing is most compatible with a well-adjusted life and sexual adequacy. Female pseudohermaphrodites who have inborn errors of cortisol and aldosterone biosynthesis can be treated with hormonal replacement and with surgical repair of the external genitalia. Female pseudohermaphrodites usually are fertile. In contrast, virtually all patients with male pseudohermaphroditism are infertile. In such patients, it is recommended that male sex assignment be based on adequacy of phallic size.

THYROID GLAND

The thyroid gland produces the thyroid hormones thyroxine (T_4) and triiodothyronine (T_3), which regulate the rate of metabolism in virtually all tissues. These hormones mediate the rate of growth and development, oxygen consumption and heat production, neural development, erythropoiesis, respiratory drive, skeletal maturation, and many other processes.

The thyroid gland forms as an invagination of endoderm at the base of the tongue during the first trimester of pregnancy and then descends along the midline to its final position anterior to the second to fourth tracheal cartilage rings. Integration of the thyroid axis proceeds during the second to third trimesters and results in a classic negative feedback loop between hypothalamus, pituitary, and thyroid gland (Figure 20–9).

Problems with thyroid gland function may occur at any time of life and may stem from either hypo- or hyperfunctioning. Hypothyroidism is relatively common in the newborn period and usually comes to medical attention after routine neonatal screening, at which time the child may be asymptomatic. Perturbations in thyroid hormone secretion later in life may be detected through clinical symptomatology but often present with enlargement of the entire thyroid gland, termed goiter, or with single isolated masses within the gland. These problems are discussed in the sections below.

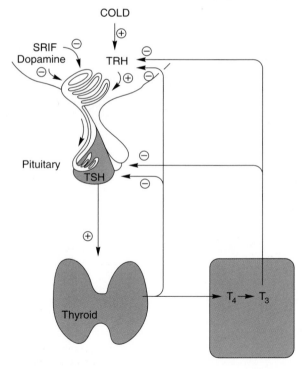

Figure 20–9. Feedback control of the thyroid gland. Plus sign indicates positive feedback, and minus sign indicates negative feedback. SRIF = somatostatin; T_3 = triiodothyronine; T_4 = thyroxine; TRH = thyroid-releasing hormone; TSH = thyroid-stimulating hormone. (Reproduced and adapted, with permission, from Fisher DA: Page 90 in Kaplan SA [editor]: *Clinical Pediatric Endocrinology,* 2nd ed. Saunders, 1990.)

CONGENITAL HYPOTHYROIDISM

A defect in the thyroid axis is one of the most common inborn errors in metabolism, with a frequency of 1/4000. Potential signs and symptoms of thyroid hormone deficiency include lethargy, hypotonia, constipation, poor feeding, prolonged jaundice, umbilical hernia, large fontanelle, macroglossia, and hypothermia. However, even the most astute clinician has trouble detecting an affected infant early in life, as many of the findings are nonspecific and subtle, and the infant may be asymptomatic early in life. Despite mild or even no initial symptoms, the consequence of delayed treatment of congenital hypothyroidism is permanent mental retardation. As a result, most industrialized countries have instituted a neonatal screening program with the goal of detecting problems and initiating thyroid hormone replacement in infants early in life so as to prevent neurologic deficits. Blood is collected on a piece of filter paper at 24 hours of age or later and sent to a central laboratory. In North America, most laboratories first perform a T_4 measurement. If it is in the lowest tenth percentile for the day, a thyroid-stimulating hormone (TSH) assay is subsequently performed. Some laboratories now perform a direct TSH assay. The physician is notified if the TSH level is elevated, and then further diagnostic evaluation is pursued. This approach is designed to detect those infants with a defect in the thyroid gland itself, that is, primary hypothyroidism, but not those with a defect in the pituitary or hypothalamus (secondary and tertiary levels, respectively). These latter defects are much rarer, occurring in about 1 in 100,000 infants. In addition, secondary and tertiary hypothyroidism usually occurs in conjunction with other CNS anomalies or midline defects. Therefore, the physician should already have been alerted to the potential of thyroid hormone deficiency in these children.

Approach to the Infant With an Abnormal Screening Test Result

An approach to the infant with an abnormal newborn thyroid screen is outlined in Figure 20–10. One should see the child as soon as possible to perform a complete history and physical examination and to repeat the T_4 and TSH assays to verify that the child indeed has hypothyroidism. If the screening test was done when the child was younger than 24 hours of age, a false-positive result may occur because of the physiologic neonatal TSH surge. Early hospital discharges of newborns now account for up to five false-positive results for every true case of congenital hypothyroidism.

The history may suggest the etiology of the abnormal

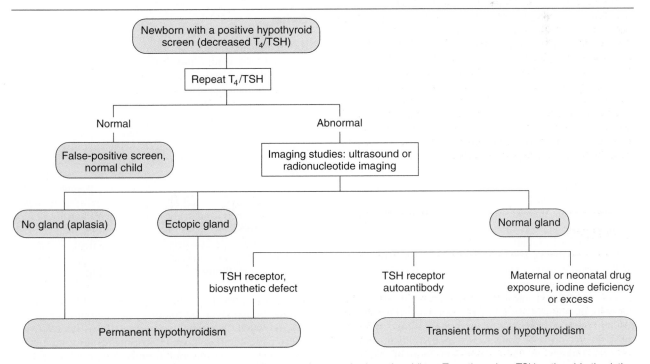

Figure 20–10. Approach to a newborn with a positive screening test for hypothyroidism. T_4 = thyroxine; TSH = thyroid-stimulating hormone.

screening result. If the mother has a history of autoimmune thyroiditis, maternal IgG directed against the thyroid gland could have crossed the placenta and disrupted neonatal thyroid hormone production. In addition, if the mother has Graves disease, thioamide, the medication used to block thyroid hormone synthesis, may cross the placenta and block neonatal thyroid hormone production. Finally, a family history of recurrent hypothyroidism may suggest either an autoantibody-mediated process or an inborn error in thyroid hormone synthesis, transmitted as an autosomal-recessive trait.

All infants with abnormal thyroid function tests on follow-up should undergo an imaging study, if possible, with either ultrasonography or radionucleotide imaging. If no gland is visualized by ultrasonography, or if the gland is ectopic (superior to its expected location), the child will have permanent primary hypothyroidism, and will need to receive therapy for life. A normal-appearing gland in the normal location may indicate either the presence of a TSH receptor defect, a TSH receptor blocking antibody (which may be detectable by an additional serum study and would constitute a transient defect), or a defect in thyroid hormone synthesis, either as a permanent inherited enzymatic defect or as a transient defect from exogenous drugs. Because a reliable ultrasound study is dependent on the experience of the sonographer, many clinicians prefer to use a radionuclide scan for such evaluations. Furthermore, sonography provides only anatomic information about the thyroid gland, whereas a scan with either ^{123}I or technetium may reveal additional insight into gland function.

A bone age obtained from the distal femur and proximal tibia may be helpful in the management of the neonate. The degree of impairment in skeletal maturation has been correlated with severity of congenital hypothyroidism and with eventual neurologic outcome.

Treatment

Thyroid hormone replacement therapy should begin as soon as the diagnosis of hypothyroidism has been confirmed. It has been estimated that if congenital hypothyroidism is untreated, such infants may lose up to 5 IQ points monthly during the first year of life. Thus, their initial evaluation should be completed within a 2–5 day period, and treatment should not be delayed if the ancillary studies, such as thyroid imaging, cannot be immediately obtained. The goal of therapy is to normalize serum T_4 concentrations as rapidly as possible. To ensure adequate replacement, the T_4 level is maintained in the upper half of the normal range. The initial dose is 10–15 μg/kg/d. With such therapy, growth and development of these infants is normalized, and long-term neurologic assessment suggests that aggressive and early thyroxine replacement results in normal outcomes, even in those infants with the most severe forms of congenital hypothyroidism. Infants who are thought to have a transient form of hypothyroidism usually receive treatment for 3–4 years to ensure normal neurologic development. At the end of that time,

the children are given a trial period without thyroid hormone replacement. If their TSH and T_4 levels remain within the normal range, they are considered to have had a transient condition.

THYROID MASS

Up to 5% of school-aged children present with enlargement of their thyroid glands. In the initial evaluation, the principal issue is to determine whether the neck mass is actually part of the thyroid gland or potentially one of the many other neck structures. Possibilities include lymph nodes or branchial cleft cyst if the mass is lateral. Midline masses include an ectopic thyroid gland that failed to migrate far enough inferiorly to its proper location. Another possibility is a thyroglossal duct cyst, a fluid-filled remnant that remains as part of the tract from descent of the thyroid gland from the base of the tongue. Both an ectopic gland and thyroglossal duct cyst will arise on swallowing. With an ectopic gland, a normal thyroid gland will not be detected inferiorly. The distinction between gland and cyst can be made definitively with an imaging study, again by either ultrasonography or a radionuclide scan.

The thyroid mass should be determined to be either symmetric enlargement of the gland, termed goiter, or a separate nodule or nodule(s) within the gland. These possibilities are discussed below.

Goiter

There are several possible causes for a goiter, and the differential diagnosis may be readily constructed after a history is obtained, a physical examination is performed, and the thyroid status of the patient is determined (Figure 20–11). In many instances, the patient presents with clinical euthyroidism. With hyperthyroidism symptoms may include hyperactivity, irritability, temperature intolerance, and weight loss despite hyperphagia. On physical examination, one may note tachycardia, widened pulse pressure, proptosis, lid lag, diaphoresis, and accelerated growth rate. With hypothyroidism, symptoms may include lethargy, weight gain without excessive caloric intake, constipation, and physical findings such as retardation in growth rate, bradycardia, and scaling of skin with hair loss. Thyroid function tests (TSH and free T_4 rather than total T_4 with T_3 resin uptake) should be obtained in all patients with thyroid gland enlargement.

Euthyroid Goiter. Patients presenting with clinical and biochemical evidence of euthyroidism have two primary etiologies for goiter. Hashimoto thyroiditis, or chronic lymphocytic thyroiditis, is an autoimmune disorder in which the gland is infiltrated by lymphocytes. These patients often have autoantibodies directed against thyroglobulin and thyroid hormone peroxidase (previously referred to as antimicrosomal antibody). There is a female to male predominance with autoimmune thyroid

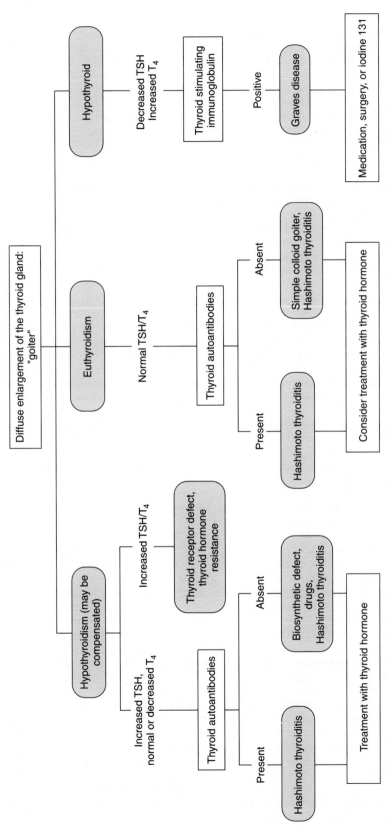

Figure 20–11. Approach to the patient with goiter. Note that serum autoantibodies do not detect all patients with an underlying diagnosis of Hashimoto thyroiditis; therefore, a negative autoantibody study does not rule out this condition. The autoantibodies present with Hashimoto thyroiditis also may be detected in Graves disease, but patients with this disorder frequently have thyroid stimulating immunoglobulin as well. T_4 = thyroxine; TSH = thyroid-stimulating hormone.

disorders, as well as a higher incidence in the Asian population. Patients may present with either euthyroidism or hypothyroidism (see below). The second possibility is simple colloid goiter, also known as nontoxic goiter. It may present in similar fashion to Hashimoto thyroiditis but is always associated with normal thyroid function test results, and there is no evidence for the autoantibodies associated with Hashimoto thyroiditis. Although the thyroid gland usually is symmetrically enlarged in both these conditions, some patients may have solid or cystic nodules (see below).

Goiter With Hypothyroidism. Individuals may present either with compensated primary hypothyroidism, in which T_4 concentration is normal but TSH level is elevated, or with frank hypothyroidism, in which the elevated TSH is unable to maintain T_4 concentration in the normal range. Most of these patients have Hashimoto thyroiditis. Other considerations include mild cases of inborn errors in thyroid hormone biosynthesis, treatment with drugs that block thyroid hormone biosynthesis, or dietary ingestion of substances that also cause such a phenomenon (termed goitrogens). Worldwide, iodine deficiency is one of the most common reasons for such a presentation. However, iodine supplementation makes this consideration extremely rare in the United States. An unusual pattern may also be encountered with thyroid hormone resistance. This constellation results from a defect in the thyroid hormone receptor.

Goiter With Hyperthyroidism. If the patient presents with a goiter and signs and symptoms of hyperthyroidism, then the diagnosis is usually Graves disease. This autoimmune disorder results from autoantibodies directed against the TSH receptor, termed thyroid-stimulating immunoglobulins (TSI), resulting in autonomous production of thyroxine. Thus, T_4 levels are elevated, and TSH is suppressed. These patients may also have a mixture of thyroglobulin and peroxisomal autoantibodies as well, and Hashimoto and Graves disease are thought to represent opposite ends of a spectrum of autoimmune thyroiditis. Rarely, individuals with Hashimoto thyroiditis may present with hyperthyroidism, usually in the early stages of the illness, when autoimmune destruction results in release of pre-formed thyroid hormone into the circulation. The clinical course and autoantibody pattern help to distinguish this entity from Graves disease.

Treatment. Treatment for hypothyroidism and goiter is thyroxine, and the gland will slowly shrink in size over time as TSH is suppressed. Patients with euthyroid goiter may also receive treatment in attempts to shrink the size of the gland, if it is of cosmetic concern to the patient. Individuals with a hyperthyroid goiter should receive agents to suppress thyroid hormone synthesis, such as methimazole. Alternatively, they may elect to have surgical correction with subtotal thyroidectomy or ablation by ingestion of radionuclide (^{131}I).

Painful Thyroid Gland. The above-mentioned conditions are associated with a painless goiter. However, if the patient presents with a painful thyroid gland, the diagnosis may be acute suppurative thyroiditis. The gland may be infected with staphylococci or with mixed aerobic and anaerobic organisms. The white blood cell count and erythrocyte sedimentation rate are elevated, but thyroid function test results often are normal. Treatment includes salicylates, antibiotics, and, occasionally, surgical drainage. Subacute thyroiditis is rare in childhood and is a self-limited illness often associated with an upper respiratory tract infection. Typically, the thyroid gland is enlarged and tender, and the patient initially has hyperthyroidism from leakage of pre-formed thyroid hormone into the circulation from the damaged gland.

Solitary Nodule. Thyroid carcinoma is much more common in adults than in children. Yet, the risk for a malignant solitary nodule is much greater in childhood, necessitating great care in the evaluation of such individuals. Important risk factors from the history include a prior history of radiation exposure to the neck; a family history of thyroid cancer, which may be suggestive of a multiple endocrine neoplasia syndrome; and a rapidly growing neck mass. Physical findings suggestive of malignant disease include a single, hard nodule; compressive symptoms, such as hoarseness or dysphagia; and, as the thyroid cancer metastasizes locally, adenopathy. The differential diagnosis of a solitary thyroid nodule includes thyroid follicular adenoma, cystadenoma, and a functioning adenoma. Multiple follicular nodules often are seen with Hashimoto thyroiditis. These patients often have euthyroid goiter, although an individual may have hypothyroidism or hyperthyroidism and positive autoantibodies from autoimmune thyroiditis rather than from malignant disease. Imaging studies are most helpful in evaluation of these patients. Ultrasonography is useful in defining the number of nodules present, the size of each nodule, and whether the mass is solid or cystic. Cystic lesions generally are considered benign, although they may contain some solid elements from a degenerating carcinoma. Radionuclide scanning with ^{123}I or ^{99m}Tc (pertechnetate) provides additional insight into the nature of the lesion: Functional nodules that demonstrate increased concentration of radionuclide (referred to as "warm" or "hot") usually are benign, whereas cold lesions are more typically malignant. Thus, an individual with a nodule that is solid by ultrasound and hypofunctioning by radionuclide scanning would be at high risk for a malignant disease and would warrant aggressive evaluation. Such patients are referred to a surgeon for open biopsy of the lesion. In some centers, fine-needle aspiration in an outpatient setting is used for the initial evaluation of a thyroid nodule, although the use of such an approach in pediatrics remains controversial. Individuals with a suspicious fine-needle biopsy result proceed to open surgical resection of the nodule. Patients with benign-appearing tissue obtained by fine-needle biopsy may be given a trial of daily thyroid hormone treatment in attempts to suppress nodule growth.

HYPOGLYCEMIA

Hypoglycemia is an endocrine emergency. Although absolute hypoglycemia or a significant and rapid decrease in blood glucose concentration may be associated with clinically evident seizure activity, permanent CNS damage may occur during hypoglycemia even in the absence of overt symptoms. Thus, appropriate evaluation and management of hypoglycemia are of crucial importance.

At any time, the blood glucose concentration is a reflection of glucose production and use. Glucose production depends on three factors: (1) adequate substrate for gluconeogenesis and for glycogen breakdown; (2) enzyme activities for gluconeogenesis, glycogenolysis, and other metabolic processes that enter into these pathways; and (3) normal function of insulin and the counter-insulin hormones, which exert their effects on blood glucose principally by regulating the previously noted enzyme activities. Glycogen stores can provide a child with adequate glucose for 8–12 hours, after which glucose homeostasis becomes dependent on gluconeogenesis. The principal substrates for gluconeogenesis are amino acids (from muscle breakdown or from transamination of amino acid precursors), lactate (from glycolysis), and glycerol and acetyl-CoA (from lipolysis).

The principal hormones that regulate blood glucose concentrations are insulin and the counter-insulin hormones glucagon, epinephrine, cortisol, and GH. The principal mechanisms by which these hormones regulate blood glucose are summarized in Table 20–16. Insulin is an anabolic peptide produced by the pancreatic β cells. The principal target tissues for insulin action are adipose tissue and muscle, where insulin promotes glucose uptake and storage, promotes amino acid uptake and protein synthesis, and decreases use of fat stores for energy. In the liver, insulin inhibits glycogen breakdown and promotes glycogen synthesis by inhibiting adenyl cyclase activity and, therefore, cyclic adenosine monophosphate (cAMP) generation. In addition, insulin recently has been shown to inhibit transcription of phosphoenolpyruvate carboxy-kinase (PEPCK), the rate-limiting enzyme in gluconeogenesis.

Both epinephrine and glucagon increase blood glucose concentrations principally by promoting glycogen breakdown. Epinephrine and glucagon activate adenyl cyclase, leading to an increase in cAMP, which ultimately promotes glycogen breakdown by activating the enzyme phosphorylase and inhibits glycogen synthesis by inactivating the enzyme glycogen synthetase. cAMP also upregulates the rate-limiting enzyme in hepatic gluconeogenesis, PEPCK. In addition, epinephrine and glucagon promote lipolysis, ultimately generating glycerol and acetyl-CoA, which are substrates for gluconeogenesis. Cortisol increases glucose production by increasing the activity of gluconeogenic enzymes and by increasing amino acid substrates for gluconeogenesis through protein breakdown. GH increases glucose production principally by increasing lipolysis.

Although the precise definition of hypoglycemia is somewhat controversial, hypoglycemia is generally agreed to be present when the blood glucose concentration is 40 mg/dL or less. Maintenance of euglycemia in infants normally requires glucose production (derived from dietary intake and metabolic processes) of 5–7 mg/kg/min. In contrast, older children and adults normally require a glucose production rate of 1–2 mg/kg/min.

KETOTIC HYPOGLYCEMIA

The differential diagnosis of hypoglycemia may be divided conceptually into two general classes: ketotic and nonketotic (Table 20–17). Ketosis results from lipolysis, with β-oxidation of free fatty acids and accumulation of acetyl-CoA. Essentially every cause of hypoglycemia is associated with ketosis unless the process of ketone generation is inhibited or the pathway for generating ketones is defective. Ketotic forms of hypoglycemia include decreased substrate (inadequate gluconeogenic substrate and inadequate dietary intake), transient and nontransient abnormalities of gluconeogenesis, some forms of glycogen storage disease, deficiencies of one or more of the

Table 20–16. Hormonal regulation of blood glucose.

Hormone	Action(s)
Insulin	Glucose uptake by cells; glycogen synthesis and storage
Glucagon	Glycogen breakdown; lipolysis and gluconeogenesis
Epinephrine	Glycogen breakdown; lipolysis and gluconeogenesis
Cortisol	Gluconeogenesis
Growth hormone	Lipolysis and gluconeogenesis

Table 20–17. Differential diagnosis of hypoglycemia.

Ketotic
Decreased substrate
Transient and nontransient abnormalities of gluconeogenesis
Some forms of glycogen storage disease (excluding glucose-6-phosphatase deficiency)
Deficiency of counter-insulin hormone(s)
Other abnormalities of amino acid and carbohydrate metabolism (eg, defects in metabolism of branched-chain amino acids, galactose, fructose)
Nonketotic
Hyperinsulinism
Fatty acid oxidation abnormalities, with or without associated carnitine deficiency
Glucose-6-phosphatase deficiency (glycogen storage disease type I)

counter-insulin hormones, and abnormalities in amino acid metabolism or carbohydrate metabolism that limit conversion of metabolites to substrates that can enter the gluconeogenic pathway. All these forms of hypoglycemia may be associated with ketosis, as insulin is suppressed and stress-induced lipolysis occurs.

NONKETOTIC HYPOGLYCEMIA

The principal cause of nonketotic hypoglycemia is hyperinsulinism. The high concentrations of insulin lead to an accelerated rate of glucose use, decreased hepatic glucose production, and general suppression of the ketogenic pathway. Less common causes result from specific defects in the ability to produce ketones, such as abnormalities of fatty acid oxidation. This includes deficiency of carnitine, which plays a role in translocation of free fatty acids from the cytosol to the mitochondria, where β-oxidation occurs.

INFANTS WITH HYPOGLYCEMIA

The frequency of ketotic versus nonketotic forms of hypoglycemia is age related. In infants with transient hypoglycemia, ketotic forms predominate and are associated with prematurity, intrauterine growth retardation, asphyxia, sepsis, starvation, and maternal ingestion of propranolol. Such stressed infants may have depleted glycogen stores and a transient defect in gluconeogenesis but have an intact lipolytic and ketogenic pathway. Transient neonatal hypoglycemia may be nonketotic when associated with transient hyperinsulinism in infants of diabetic mothers or with erythroblastosis fetalis, or in association with maternal ingestion of oral hypoglycemic drugs.

Among the nontransient forms of hypoglycemia from birth to 1 year of age, nonketotic forms predominate. Hyperinsulinism, the most common cause of nonketotic hypoglycemia, appears to result principally from a process often referred to as **nesidioblastosis.** In this condition, hyperinsulinism was initially thought to arise from a diffuse proliferation of endocrine cells budding off from the exocrine ducts. However, a more recent study indicates that the histologic pattern of nesidioblastosis is not a pathologic entity, as it may occur in age-matched infants without hypoglycemia. Whereas some infants with hyperinsulinism may have areas of β-cell hyperplasia (as may be seen in Beckwith-Wiedemann syndrome) or small adenomas, most may have hyperinsulinism secondary to abnormalities in the regulation of insulin secretion. Ingestion of oral hypoglycemic drugs also may result in nonketotic hypoglycemia. Ketotic forms of hypoglycemia in this group include counter-insulin hormone deficiencies, some forms of glycogen storage disease, gluconeogenesis abnormalities, and abnormalities in the metabolism of galactose, fructose, and branched-chain amino acids. Ingestion of ethanol, salicylates, and acetaminophen also may be associated with ketotic hypoglycemia.

CHILDREN WITH HYPOGLYCEMIA

In children from about 18 months of age through midchildhood, hypoglycemia is most often ketotic. Such children usually do not have an obvious abnormality in glycogen breakdown or gluconeogenesis, nor a deficiency of the counter-insulin hormones. Plasma alanine concentrations, however, may be decreased in such children, possibly reflecting decreased efflux of amino acids from skeletal muscle. Hypoglycemia in these children most often occurs when fasting is sustained for 8–16 hours and frequently is associated with an intercurrent illness. This condition often resolves spontaneously as the child approaches the peripubertal years. In late childhood, nonketotic hypoglycemia again predominates, with hyperinsulinism (often associated with multiple endocrine neoplasia) the most common cause.

EVALUATION OF HYPOGLYCEMIA

Useful diagnostic clues in the evaluation of hypoglycemia can be found in the history, physical examination findings, and treatment course. A history of intrauterine growth retardation, prematurity, or maternal drug use, should be sought. Physical examination should include a search for midline defects (cleft lip or palate and optic nerve abnormalities, which may be associated with hypopituitarism), ambiguous genitalia (may be associated with cortisol deficiency), omphalocele, macroglossia, visceromegaly (Beckwith-Wiedemann syndrome), microphallus and undescended testes (which may be associated with multiple hypothalamic/pituitary abnormalities), and hepatomegaly (which may be associated with glycogen storage disease and other metabolic disorders).

Laboratory Evaluation

The initial laboratory evaluation of hypoglycemia is outlined in Table 20–18. It is desirable to obtain both urine and plasma samples before administering glucose (0.5–1 g/kg intravenous bolus as 10 or 25% dextrose in water, followed by a glucose infusion). The urine sample should be analyzed for ketones, organic acids, and reducing substances (eg, galactose, fructose). Ketones may not always be present in the urine during acute hypoglycemia associated with one of the ketotic causes. The plasma sample should be analyzed for glucose, ketones, insulin, GH, cortisol, glucagon, lactate, electrolytes (to determine whether there is an abnormally high anion gap), organic acids, and alanine concentrations. Of crucial importance, the glucose sample must be placed in a tube with sodium fluoride or another inhibitor of enzymes involved in glucose metabolism. Otherwise, if analysis is delayed, the

Table 20–18. Laboratory evaluation of hypoglycemia.

Urine
Ketones
Organic acids
Reducing substances
Plasma: Simultaneous with glucose ≤ 40 mg/dL for measurement of concentrations of
Ketones
Insulin (insulin [μU/mL]:glucose [mg/dL] ratio should not exceed 0.3)
Growth hormone
Cortisol
Glucagon
Lactate
Electrolyte (to measure anion gap)
Organic acids
Alanine

glucose concentration in the sample will decrease at a rate of 5–10 mg/dL/h at room temperature. Moreover, the previously noted blood tests are most useful when the simultaneous blood glucose is 40 mg/dL or less. Therefore, if hypoglycemia is suspected, it may be prudent to determine the blood glucose concentration by Chemstrip at the bedside initially and then to proceed with the evaluation as outlined previously, including a laboratory blood glucose determination, if indicated. An algorithm for the evaluation of hypoglycemia in infants is shown in Figure 20–12.

Of particular diagnostic importance are the glucose requirements to maintain euglycemia and the glucose response to an injection of glucagon (0.1 mg/kg intramuscularly, up to 1 mg). Glucose requirements of 15 mg/kg/min or greater are virtually diagnostic of hyperinsulinism. In addition, a major glycemic response to glucagon during hypoglycemia probably will lead to a diagnosis of hyperinsulinism.

MANAGEMENT

Appropriate long-term management of hypoglycemia requires proper treatment of the underlying disorder. The optimal management of nontransient hyperinsulinism is somewhat controversial. Medical management often includes a low-leucine diet (leucine is an insulin secretogogue in most individuals) and oral diazoxide therapy, which inhibits insulin secretion. Side effects of diazoxide increase when the dose exceeds 15–20 mg/kg/d and include fluid retention, decreased white blood cell count, thrombocytopenia, hyperuricemia, hypertrichosis, and soft tissue facial abnormalities with prolonged use. If medical management is unsuccessful, subtotal pancreatectomy (85–95%) often is undertaken. Hypoglycemia may persist even after 95% pancreatectomy, whereas pancreatic exocrine insufficiency and diabetes may also occur. Somato-

statin analogues, which suppress insulin secretion, have been used with some success in patients with hyperinsulinism.

THE CHILD WITH POLYURIA

Polyuria, which must be distinguished from urinary frequency, is one of the principal presenting signs of two endocrine disorders: diabetes mellitus and diabetes insipidus (DI). In general, polyuria may result from an osmotic agent (eg, hyperglycemia in diabetes mellitus), a deficiency or impaired responsiveness to antidiuretic hormone (ADH), or excessive water intake (primary polydipsia).

An algorithm for evaluating polyuria is presented in Figure 20–13. Initially, one should determine whether an osmotic agent, such as glucose, is present in the urine. The finding of glycosuria suggests the diagnosis of diabetes mellitus, as discussed below, although some medications (eg, pharmacologic doses of glucocorticoids) may cause glucose intolerance and glycosuria. If an osmotic agent is not present in the urine, one would then determine the response to fluid restriction, as discussed below. Decreased urinary output and increased urinary concentration after fluid restriction suggest the diagnosis of primary polydipsia. Continued polyuria without an increase in urinary concentration indicates the diagnosis of DI. An antidiuretic response to exogenous ADH indicates ADH deficiency, or central DI, whereas lack of an antidiuretic response indicates nephrogenic DI.

ANTIDIURETIC HORMONE PHYSIOLOGY

Because deficiency or impaired responsiveness to ADH constitutes the principal components of the differential diagnosis of polyuria, it is important to review the principles of ADH physiology. ADH, in concert with an intact thirst mechanism, maintains plasma osmolality in the normal range of 280–290 mOsm/kg.

Arginine vasopressin (AVP) is the principal ADH in humans. This nonapeptide is produced in the supraoptic and paraventricular nuclei of the hypothalamus. Axons from these neurons terminate in the posterior pituitary gland, where they secrete AVP. The principal action of AVP in regulating water balance is to increase permeability to water in the renal collecting tubules and thus enhance its absorption.

AVP secretion is regulated principally by changes in plasma osmolality and in effective circulating volume. Osmoreceptors in the hypothalamus stimulate the secre-

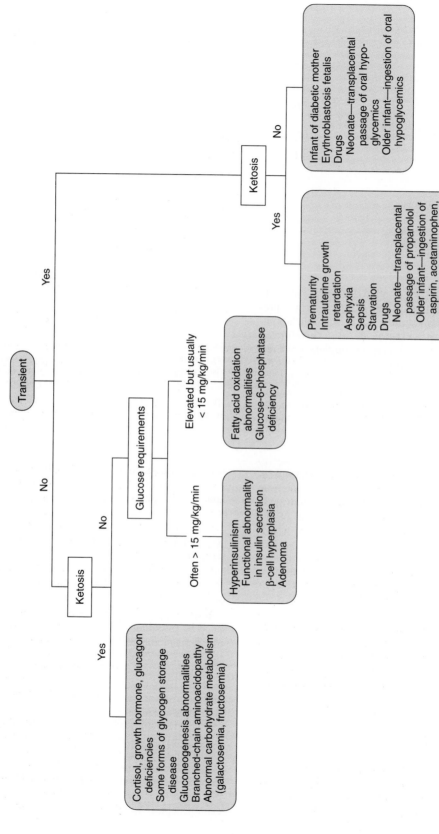

Figure 20–12. An approach to the evaluation of hypoglycemia in infants.

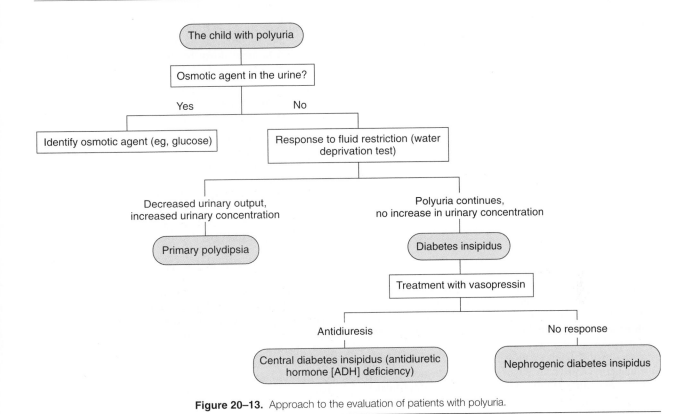

Figure 20–13. Approach to the evaluation of patients with polyuria.

tion of AVP when plasma osmolality increases by as little as 1%. In normal individuals, AVP levels normally are low and do not increase until the plasma osmolality exceeds 280 mOsm/kg. AVP secretion is also regulated by changes in blood volume. Baroreceptors in the systemic venous circulation, right side of the heart, and left atrium ("low pressure"), as well as in the systemic arterial systems of the carotid sinus and aortic arch ("high pressure"), transmit information to the hypothalamus via the vagus and glossopharyngeal nerves, respectively. These baroreceptors become activated when stretched by increases in intravascular volume. Baroreceptor activity leads to inhibition of AVP secretion. In addition, many other factors affect AVP secretion. AVP is stimulated by pain, stress, and drugs such as β-adrenergic agents, morphine, and barbiturates; it is inhibited by α-adrenergic agents, ethanol, and phenytoin.

DIABETES INSIPIDUS

Deficiency of AVP or impaired responsiveness of the kidney to AVP results in DI, characterized by polyuria, polydipsia, and defective urinary concentrating ability. Hypernatremia usually does not occur if the patient has an intact thirst mechanism and adequate access to fluids and does not have additional ongoing fluid losses, such as from diarrhea. Infants with DI, in addition to polyuria and polydipsia, may present with irritability, fever of unknown origin, growth failure secondary to inadequate caloric intake, and hydronephrosis. Older children may also present with nocturia and enuresis. DI may not be apparent in patients with concurrent untreated glucocorticoid deficiency, because cortisol is required to generate a normal free water loss.

DI results from a wide range of abnormalities, as summarized in Table 20–19. AVP deficiency is most commonly acquired but rarely occurs as a familial, autosomal-dominant disorder. Acquired forms of DI may be idiopathic or may occur in association with tumors, trauma, neurosurgery, infection, granulomas, histiocytosis, and vascular and autoimmune diseases of the hypothalamus and pituitary. Impaired AVP responsiveness, also called **nephrogenic DI,** may be familial or acquired. Familial nephrogenic DI (X-linked) may result from either a defect in the ADH receptor or a postreceptor signaling pathway defect. Acquired nephrogenic DI occurs with some forms of primary renal disease, obstructive uropathy, hypokalemia, hypercalcemia, and sickle-cell disease, and may also be induced by drugs such as lithium and

Table 20–19. Etiology of diabetes insipidus.

Arginine vasopressin deficiency: Central diabetes insipidus
- Acquired: CNS disease: tumors, trauma, neurosurgery, infection, granulomas, histocytosis, vascular and autoimmune diseases
- Familial

Impaired arginine vasopressin responsiveness: Nephrogenic diabetes insipidus
- Familial X-linked
- Acquired: Some forms of primary renal disease, obstructive uropathy
- Metabolic: hypokalemia, hypercalcemia, sickle-cell disease
- Drug-induced (eg, lithium, demeclocycline)
- Secondary to prolonged polyuria of any cause

CNS = central nervous system.

demeclocycline. Prolonged polyuria of any cause may result in some degree of nephrogenic DI, secondary to a reduction of tonicity in the renal medullary interstitium and a subsequent decrease in the gradient necessary to concentrate the urine.

A modified 7-hour water deprivation test is useful to distinguish patients with DI from those with normal urinary concentrating ability. After unrestricted fluid intake the night before the test, the patient is given a normal breakfast. The patient urinates (the urine is discarded), and a 7-hour fast is begun. During the first hour, plasma and urine osmolality are measured. After 6 hours, the patient again urinates and discards the urine. After 7 hours, plasma and urine osmolality are measured again. If the initial urine-plasma osmolality ratio is greater than 1.5, normal concentrating ability is demonstrated, and it is unnecessary to continue the test. After 7 hours, normal function is indicated by a urine-plasma osmolality ratio greater than 1.5, an increase from the beginning of the fast in the urine-plasma osmolality ratio of 1 or greater, or a final urine osmolality greater than 450 mOsm/kg. In small children, weight, as well as serum and urine osmolality, should be monitored periodically during the water deprivation test to avoid excessive water loss. If DI is suspected, a baseline plasma sample should be obtained for radioimmunoassay for AVP. AVP or a synthetic analogue should then be administered to distinguish AVP deficiency from AVP unresponsiveness. Aqueous AVP or 1-deamino-8D-arginine vasopressin (DDAVP; subcutaneously or intranasally) may be administered. DDAVP, which has a longer duration of action than AVP, is the drug of choice in most patients with AVP deficiency. Hydrochlorothiazide, alone or in combination with the K$^+$-sparing diuretic amiloride, is the principal treatment for nephrogenic DI.

If DI is associated with significant hypernatremia from free water loss, the free water deficit should be replenished slowly.

Rapid correction can result in swelling of cells, cerebral edema, and seizures. It is recommended that plasma sodium be brought down by 10–12 mmol/L/d. The free water deficit may be calculated by the following formula:

$$(0.6) \times (\text{body wt in kg}) \times \left(1 - \frac{140}{\text{plasma Na}+}\right)$$

If patients have mild hypernatremia, hypotonic NaCl intravenous solutions or oral fluids may be used as initial therapy. If hypernatremia is severe, initial therapy should include normal saline solutions to minimize the risk to iatrogenic cerebral swelling.

DIABETES MELLITUS

One of the most common reasons for polyuria is the presence of a nonresorbable solute, usually glucose. When serum glucose concentration exceeds 180 mg/dL, then the filtered glucose level exceeds the capacity of the renal tubule to reabsorb the solute fully. The result is an obligate diuresis in which water is excreted in conjunction with glucose. Thus, the principal complaint with new onset of diabetes mellitus is polyuria, with concomitant polydipsia. The criteria established for the diagnosis of diabetes mellitus relate to the degree of derangement in carbohydrate metabolism: a random serum glucose concentration more than 200 mg/dL or fasting glucose concentration more than 125 mg/dL with an abnormal oral glucose tolerance test on two occasions (Table 20–20).

Types of Diabetes

Hyperglycemia is caused by a variety of different processes, and diabetes mellitus refers to a heterogeneous group of disorders. As one approaches a patient with newly diagnosed diabetes, it is helpful to consider the possible mechanisms of the patient's carbohydrate metabolism derangement (Figure 20–14). In simplest terms, diabetes may be considered as either a deficiency of insulin, as occurs in type I, or insulin-dependent diabetes mellitus (IDDM), or as a state of insulin resistance, referred to as type II. These two distinct types of diabetes are considered in further detail in the following sections (Table 20–21).

Table 20–20. Criteria for diagnosis of diabetes.

Random plasma glucose > 200, with classic symptoms
Fasting plasma glucose > 125 on two occasions
Oral glucose tolerance test
  1.75 g/kg glucose, to maximum of 75 g
  2 h plasma glucose > 200
  One intervening value > 200
  On two separate occasions

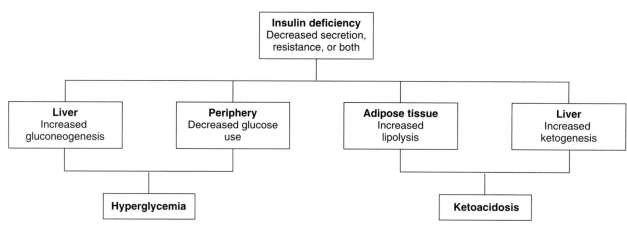

Figure 20–14. Pathophysiologic basis of diabetic ketoacidosis.

Table 20–24. Dia[...]

Maintain airway [...]
Institute insulin t[...]
Correct metaboli[...]
Determine caus[...]
Look out for con[...]

be started whe[...]
tients respond [...]
U/kg of regula[...]
of 0.1 U/kg/h[...]
much less effe[...]
action exagger[...]
poor peripheral[...]
reduce serum [...]
75–100 mg/dL[...]
lality. As the s[...]
mg/dL, intrave[...]
trose to maint[...]
insulin infusio[...]
resolves, whic[...]
the serum gluc[...]

Associated[...]
course of rehy[...]
associated me[...]
Patients with [...]
though they r[...]
urinary loss, t[...]
from the intra[...]
in the face of [...]
perlipemia. S[...]
crease as defic[...]
fusion, and o[...]
serum levels [...]

In addition[...]
deficits, but t[...]
high, normal,[...]
for extracellu[...]
acidosis, but [...]
into the cell. [...]
tration may [...]
DKA procee[...]
sium concent[...]
begin aggres[...]
meq/L. This [...]
or in part w[...]
bonate), or [...]
phosphate re[...]
placement at[...]
pokalemia. [...]
while the pa[...]
monitor. Agg[...]
tate hypocal[...]
such replace[...]

Type I. For most children, the derangement in carbohydrate metabolism is the result of type I, or IDDM. This process follows the autoimmune destruction of the pancreatic β cell, now known to occur over many years. IDDM appears to be a complex, multigenetic process, with greatest risk conferred by genes in the class II region of the HLA locus. Nonetheless, the genetic risk is quite low, as first-degree relatives of an individual with IDDM have approximately a 5% chance of acquiring the disease. There appears to be a synergy between an underlying genetic risk and environmental exposure(s). The actual environmental triggers are unknown but are postulated to include viruses or toxins. Pancreatic destruction can be tracked by detection of autoantibodies directed against the β cell as early as 5–10 years before the clinical presence of disease. As β-cell destruction proceeds, one may detect abnormal metabolic function with an intravenous glucose tolerance test before clinical symptoms become prominent. Overt clinical evidence for diabetes is not apparent until 80–90% of the β-cell mass has been destroyed. As a result of lingering insulin insufficiency, patients often present with polyuria and polydipsia, in addition to a thin body habitus and weight loss despite polyphagia.

Type II. Type II, or non–insulin-dependent diabetes mellitus (NIDDM), also referred to as adult-onset diabetes mellitus, occurs most commonly in adults but is now being detected with increasing frequency in children. The cause of this form of the disease is not well delineated but results from either a defect in insulin secretion or peripheral insulin action. It is considered primarily as a disorder of insulin resistance, rather than insulin deficiency. These patients therefore may have elevated insulin levels and they are expected to have readily measurable C-peptide levels, reflecting processing of pro-insulin to insulin. There is a much stronger risk for genetic transmission of this disorder than with type I diabetes. Maturity-onset diabetes of the young (MODY) is one form of type II diabetes that may present in childhood and is transmitted in autosomal-dominant fashion. In some instances, a mutation in the glucokinase gene is found. The classic patient has obesity and, on physical examination, may have acanthosis nigricans, a velvety hyperpigmented overgrowth of skin noted in the skin folds that is associated with insulin resistance. However, such a body habitus is not always apparent. A number of disease states and pharmacologic agents may induce a type II form of diabetes. Glucocorticoids induce glucose production and cause peripheral insulin resistance; therefore, endogenous overproduction of cortisol (Cushing syndrome or disease) or exogenous steroid treatment for any underlying disorder may induce diabetes. Hyperthyroidism and GH overproduction have also been linked to diabetes. Stress may play a major role in glucose metabolism; production of counter-regulatory hormones leads to insulin resistance and, in some patients, induces diabetes. Drugs (eg, Dilantin, cyclosporin, diuretics, β antagonists, and even oral contraceptives) can in-

Table 20–21. Classification of diabetes mellitus.

Type I (IDDM)	Type II (NIDDM)
Insulin deficient	Insulin resistant
Ketosis prone	Ketosis not present
Usually < 18 y	More frequent in adults
Often thin	Often overweight
90% with no FHx	Strong FHx, may be dominant
1.7 million in United States	13 million in United States
Autoantibodies	No autoantibodies

FHx = family history; IDDM = insulin-dependent diabetes mellitus; NIDDM = non–insulin-dependent diabetes mellitus.

hibit insulir
tribute to th

Clinical Fe

An unde
these patier
to distinguis
abolic ager
glycogen, a
sulin on fat
hydrate me
insulin, ther
further gluc
nesis, and c
nario is obs
tant hyperg
polyuria an
failure to us
with weigh
weakness, v
of muscle p
gluconeoge
lead to leth
and entering

Diabetic K

The con
type II diab
bination of
levels of cc
using fat as
the fatty ac
ketoacidosi
I diabetes f
type II dia
lipolysis bu
olism. The
pH that ma
with serum
increased
(Table 20–:
pirations th
type, reflec
lying metal
The fruity

Table 20–22.

• Hyperosr
• Lipemia,
• Hyponatr
   Na depre
   Artifact fr
• Potassiur
• Blood ure
• Leukocyt

---

sentation has occurred (Table 20–25). It may be the initial diagnosis with type I diabetes. An underlying stress, such as an infection, may have precipitated the episode of DKA. Therefore, one needs to examine the patient carefully for evidence of infection and consider appropriate laboratory tests, such as urinalysis or chest radiograph. The white blood cell count may not be helpful initially in guiding the workup because it is often nonspecifically elevated secondary to the stress of DKA. Noncompliance with insulin therapy should be considered in any patient with known diabetes.

Cerebral Edema. The most worrisome complication encountered in the treatment of DKA is cerebral edema. Although excessive fluid, rapid decrease in serum glucose concentration and osmolality, and use of sodium bicarbonate have all been considered as possible causes, none has been definitively linked with this complication. Although cerebral edema during the treatment of DKA is rare, it does carry a significant risk for morbidity and mortality. Younger patients appear to be at highest risk, particularly those younger than 5 years and those with their initial DKA presentation. The symptoms often develop in the first 24 hours of treatment, as the patient is improving. The patient's status should be evaluated at least hourly for changes in the neurologic examination during treatment of DKA. If cerebral edema is suspected, then one must act quickly and aggressively to prevent central, downward herniation of the brain: Mannitol, fluid restriction, elevation of the head of the bed, intubation with hyperventilation, and immediate consultation with a neurosurgeon may all be indicated.

Hyperglycemia Without Ketoacidosis

Individuals presenting with hyperglycemia but without ketoacidosis may not need intensive treatment with an insulin drip. These patients either may have type I diabetes with early presentation or may represent a type II pattern of diabetes. One will need to consider the features outlined in Table 20–21, determine serum acid-base status, and consider measurement of urinary ketones, serum C-peptide, insulin levels, and autoantibodies to distinguish between the types of diabetes. In those suspected of hav-

Table 20–25. Precipitating factors in diabetic ketoacidosis, hyperosmolar coma.

Too little insulin
Infection (even minor)
Severe stress (physical or ? emotional)
Hypokalemia, usually diuretic induced
Renal failure
Most important: inadequate fluid intake caused by:
   Old age (decreased sensitivity to thirst)
   Infancy (cannot get to or drink water)
   Incapacitation occurring at any age (cannot get to or drink water)

---

ing type I diabetes, or in type II patients with blood glucose concentrations in excess of 600 mg/dL or those receiving glucocorticoids, insulin often is the initial treatment of choice. Patients with lower blood glucose concentrations and a pattern more suggestive of type II diabetes may respond quickly to an oral agent. Two different classes of drugs are now available for such treatment: sulfonylureas such as glyburide, which serve to enhance insulin secretion, and metformin, a biguanide that sensitizes the response to insulin.

Outpatient Management of Diabetes

Insulin Therapy. For the patient whose DKA has been resolved with a continuous intravenous insulin infusion, one must convert the patient to a subcutaneous insulin regimen in preparation for outpatient management. The pharmacokinetics of the most frequently used types of insulin are shown in Table 20–26. Because subcutaneous regular insulin has a delayed onset of action, it must be given 30 minutes before discontinuation of the intravenous insulin, which has an action limited to minutes. Traditionally, patients have been placed on a regimen of sliding scale regular insulin around the clock for one or more days and then converted to a regimen that incorporates a longer-acting insulin, such as neutral protamine Hagedorn (NPH). However, one may directly institute an outpatient regimen using a combination of short- and long-acting insulins, often a combination of regular and NPH insulins. The dose is initially derived empirically, with many children requiring 0.5–1.0 U/kg/d. The simplest initial regimen that approaches physiologic glucose control is administration of regular and NPH insulin before breakfast and before dinner (Figure 20–15). Patients usually require more insulin during the day than at night, primarily to cover the carbohydrate that is ingested during the day. Therefore, two thirds of the total dose is commonly given in the morning. In addition, two thirds of the total insulin dose often is given as the longer-acting NPH. Blood glucose concentrations are monitored with a glucometer before each meal and at bedtime to evaluate the action of insulin at each interval. The fasting blood glucose level reflects the action of the bedtime NPH dose; the pre-lunch glucose concentration documents the morning regular insulin dose effect; the pre-dinner glucose concentration determines the efficacy of the morning NPH dose; and the bedtime reading reflects the dinnertime regular in-

Table 20–26. Current insulin armamentarium.

Type	Onset	Peak	Duration
Regular	0.5 h	2–4 h	6–16 h
NPH	1–2 h	4–8 h	14–24 h
Ultralente	4–6 h	10–14 h	24–36 h

NPH = neutral protamine Hagedorn.

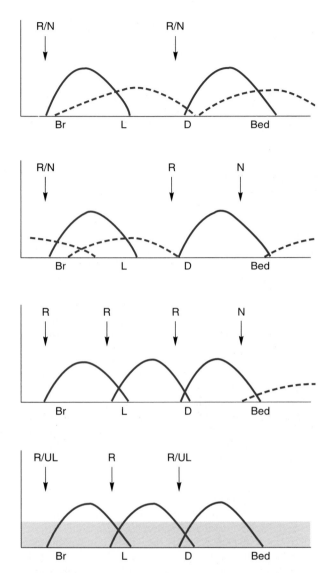

Figure 20–15. Possible insulin regimens. The Y axis denotes the levels of insulin activity, and the X axis refers to times of the day. Arrows indicate the timing of insulin injection, and letters refer to the type of insulin used. The actions of regular insulin are shown in the solid lines; neutral protamine Hagedorn (NPH) action is represented by the dashed line; ultralente is denoted by the shaded box. Bed = bedtime; Br = breakfast; D = dinner; L = lunch; N = NPH; R = regular; UL = ultralente.

sulin effect. A sliding scale is determined for the patient so that higher blood sugar readings can be compensated for with additional insulin and the dose can be reduced by an appropriate amount if the blood sugar reading is low.

Individuals may be initially resistant to insulin for the first several days after recovery from DKA, but their insulin needs may decrease significantly thereafter. This change may reflect increased physical activity or different dietary habits after leaving the hospital. In patients newly diagnosed with diabetes, this may be represent their entrance into a remission or honeymoon phase of diabetes. At the time of initial diagnosis, many patients still have 10–20% of β-cell function; as blood glucose concentrations are reduced with initial insulin therapy, endogenous insulin secretion will resume for a period of time. However, this usually is for no more than 1–2 years. During this period, individuals may find that it is relatively easy to maintain blood sugar control, while exogenous insulin supplements ongoing endogenous insulin secretion.

As the honeymoon period wanes, patients may find that their previous insulin dose does not consistently correct their blood sugar concentrations. Whereas they may have been able to go to bed in the past with an elevated blood sugar level and awaken to find that it had normalized without supplemental exogenous insulin, they now note that their blood sugar levels remain elevated. Their dose of insulin supplementation may need to be increased to compensate for decreased endogenous insulin secretion, with replacement ranging from 0.25 U/kg/d in toddlers up to as much as 1.5 U/kg/d in adolescents. Patients may become limited by the twice daily administration of insulin, particularly with insulin coverage at night. If they eat dinner at 6 PM, then the pre-dinner NPH dose will peak 4–8 hours later, sometime between 10 PM and 2 AM. At this time, the NPH peak is not matched with carbohydrate absorption, and the patient is at risk for nocturnal hypoglycemia. These patients may awaken with elevated blood sugar concentrations in the morning as a result of a Somogyi reaction, in which counter-regulatory hormones have been secreted to compensate for the previous hypoglycemia. Alternatively, blood sugar levels naturally tend to increase between 4 and 8 AM, as cortisol and growth hormone levels increase; this process is known as the dawn phenomenon. In addition, the pre-dinner NPH effect is waning by this time; thus, the individual may simply be running out of insulin. To distinguish between these possibilities for patients with morning hyperglycemia, one may need to check the patient's blood glucose concentration in the early morning hours. Nonetheless, one may need to not only increase the nighttime NPH dose, but also split the pre-dinner injection, giving regular insulin to cover dinner carbohydrate absorption and moving the NPH component to bedtime, at 10–11 PM (Figure 20–15). Many school-aged children are reluctant to administer insulin at school; therefore, one of the most common regimens for these patients is to continue receiving three injections per day, with regular and NPH insulins before breakfast, regular at dinner, and NPH at bedtime.

Some patients can achieve tighter blood glucose control and more dietary flexibility with more frequent injections of regular insulin during the day. Many of these patients will move to an injection of regular insulin before each meal with NPH at bedtime (Figure 20–15). Alternatively, one can use an even longer acting basal insulin, such as ultralente, in combination with regular insulin injection before food ingestion. This regimen has the most dietary flexibility, as the basal insulin coverage allows one to eat meals late, or even skip meals, without having to adjust the insulin regimen. Finally, some individuals may opt to use the insulin pump, a sophisticated insulin delivery device that infuses regular insulin subcutaneously continuously throughout the day. At this time, the pump cannot sense blood glucose concentration and release an appropriate amount of insulin, that is, it is not a closed loop system. The patient instead must pre-set the pump to cover food intake and basal insulin needs between meals and to correct high blood sugar levels.

One newly available tool for the management of diabetes is an insulin that acts significantly faster than regular insulin. This new form is referred to as LysPro, as the last two amino acids of the β chain have been reversed in their position from the native insulin molecule. Regular insulin has a significant delay in its onset of action because it first associates into a larger crystal and must dissociate into a monomeric form to become biologically active. The Lys-Pro modification renders the molecule less likely to remain in a larger aggregate; thus, its onset of action is within minutes, with a peak from 30 to 90 minutes. Hence, this form of insulin is better designed to deal with postprandial carbohydrate absorption, which peaks 1–2 hours after ingestion. This new insulin will become incorporated into some of the insulin regimens referred to above; however, because of its short duration of action, it will need to be used in conjunction with a longer acting insulin, such as NPH or ultralente.

Nutrition & Activity. Blood sugar concentration is affected not only by insulin, but also by food intake and exercise. Consistency in blood sugar readings is related to a reproducible pattern of food intake and exercise each day. Traditionally, individuals with diabetes have been taught to use an exchange system, with monitoring of protein, fat, and carbohydrate intake at each meal. Current recommendations are for patients with diabetes to follow a meal plan similar to that recommended generally for all individuals, with approximately 60% of caloric intake coming from carbohydrate and the remainder derived from an equal distribution between protein and fat. The carbohydrate intake often is divided evenly among the three daily meals but may be altered according to the patient's eating habits. Furthermore, attention is now focused solely on total carbohydrate intake, and there is no attempt to subdivide carbohydrate intake into exchanges of fruit, dairy, and bread, for example. Thus, the patient's diet or meal plan consists of a known total quantity of carbohydrate at each meal, and the specific components of the meal are left to the discretion of the individual. This approach lends more freedom to food selection. The pharmacokinetics of insulin action make it necessary for many patients to have small carbohydrate snacks, often 15–30 g, between meals and at bedtime. With more experience, individuals can alter their insulin dose to compensate for greater or lesser carbohydrate intake and may therefore eat according to

appetite and food availability, rather than be tied to a rigid meal plan.

Activity level will also affect blood sugar levels and often enhances sensitivity to a particular insulin dose. These effects may occur during the exercise itself or may linger for hours after the event. One may compensate for such effects by either decreasing the dose of insulin or increasing carbohydrate intake before or during the activity, or by some combination of the two.

To achieve reasonable blood glucose control, patients and families must make a number of decisions regarding their diabetes management each day, integrating concerns about insulin dose, diet, and exercise. They must understand all aspects of diabetes so as to make these decisions independently; therefore, education is one of the cornerstones for successful long-term management. Such ongoing teaching and management is best provided with a team-based approach, in which the family interacts with an educator, dietitian, psychologist or social worker, and physician.

Long-term Issues. After 10 or more years, individuals with diabetes may have complications resulting from microvascular disease, manifest as retinopathy, neuropathy, and nephropathy, and macrovascular disease, with atherosclerosis. Diabetes is currently the leading cause of blindness in adults in the United States, the leading cause of end-stage renal disease, and a significant risk factor for amputation of a lower extremity, as well as for myocardial infarction or stroke. The Diabetes Control and Complications Trial (DCCT) has confirmed the long-held suspicion that better blood glucose control lessens the risk for development of such complications. Better glucose control reduces the risk of development of microvascular complications in patients who have never had such findings and improves the condition in those with long-standing diabetes in whom complications have already developed. This study was conducted primarily in an adult population; approximately 10% of the study population were adolescents. It remains controversial as to how to apply such findings to younger children because signs of end-organ damage rarely are detected in pre-pubertal individuals, regardless of the duration of their diabetes. However, preliminary studies suggest that pre-pubertal blood glucose control may alter the rate at which complications develop during adult years. Nevertheless, one must exercise caution in how tightly one attempts to control blood sugar levels in children. Children appear to be at greater risk for development of hypoglycemia than adults, perhaps because of less predictable daily schedules, with more variable exercise and diet. Furthermore, children younger than 6 years with diabetes who have experienced recurrent hypoglycemia are at risk for neurocognitive deficits. Therefore, one may need to accept less stringent control of blood sugar levels in the toddler, to avoid the risks of hypoglycemia, but expect tighter control as the child approaches adulthood. Screening for complications should begin when the child has had diabetes for 5 years and has entered puberty. The studies should include a yearly dilated retinal examination to screen for retinopathy and a urine test to screen for microalbuminuria, which is an early sign of nephropathy.

Future Developments

"Cures" for type I diabetes have proved elusive over the years. Transplantation of pancreas tissue or β cells is currently possible but requires ongoing immunosuppression to inhibit graft rejection by the recipient. The resultant side-effects render this approach unacceptable, except in those individuals who require an additional organ transplant, such as in the case of renal failure. Current research efforts are directed at means of bypassing the immune system, such as transplanting β cells in a semi-permeable membrane. With such a system, glucose can diffuse across the membrane to the β cells and secreted insulin can diffuse out into the circulation, but lymphocytes and larger molecules, such as antibodies and cytokines, cannot directly contact and destroy the cells. Development of an "artificial" pancreas has also met numerous roadblocks. Such a device will need to function as a closed loop system, in which it senses blood glucose and delivers an appropriate amount of insulin to maintain glucose levels in a normal range. Although the technology currently exists for insulin delivery, as with insulin pumps, the ability to detect glucose accurately has proved to be a more difficult task. Ongoing efforts are directed at development of invasive sensors that rest within a blood vessel or subcutaneous tissues and noninvasive monitoring, such as transcutaneous infrared devices.

Investigators are also seeking ways to screen for and prevent the development of type I diabetes. Many agents have been used in an attempt to prolong the honeymoon phase, but none have proved reliable, and it appears that too much β-cell damage may have been incurred by that time. The presence of islet cell autoantibodies and an abnormal intravenous glucose tolerance test result are more sensitive indicators for those in whom diabetes will likely develop in the future, and trials are underway to determine whether treatment with insulin will help prevent diabetes in these individuals.

HYPONATREMIA

Hyponatremia may result from a variety of causes. An algorithm for evaluating nonartefactual hyponatremia in the absence of an osmotic agent (eg, glucose or mannitol) is presented in Figure 20–16. This algorithm is based on two principal criteria: an estimation of the degree of hydration and a measurement of the urinary sodium level. Hyponatremia in patients with volume depletion and low urinary sodium levels is a consequence of loss of salt and water with replacement of water only. This combination of events may occur in patients with substantial gastrointestinal salt loss associated with vomiting and diarrhea or in patients with substantial salt loss associated with exces-

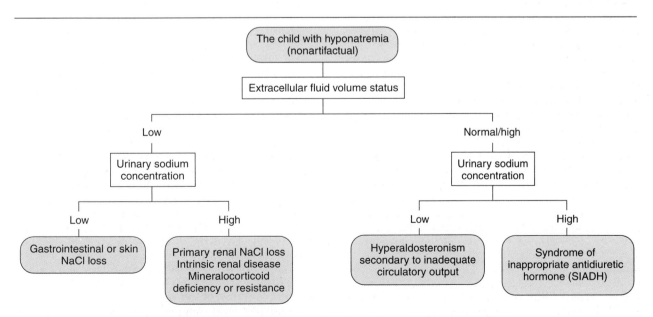

Figure 20–16. Approach to evaluation of children with nonartefactual hyponatremia.

sive sweating. Volume depletion with elevated urinary sodium levels indicates primary renal NaCl loss, which may be a consequence of intrinsic renal disease, use of diuretics, or primary adrenal insufficiency. The latter results in urinary salt loss as a consequence of either mineralocorticoid deficiency or, less commonly, mineralocorticoid resistance. The causes of salt-losing, primary adrenal insufficiency are listed in Table 20–27.

If a patient's hydration status is found to be normal or expanded, an assessment of urinary sodium is again useful to determine the cause of hyponatremia. Patients with normal or expanded extracellular fluid (ECF) volume and low urinary sodium levels may have hyperaldosteronism secondary to inadequate circulating volume (eg, associated with congestive heart failure or cirrhosis). Hyponatremia in patients with normal or expanded ECF in association with elevated urinary sodium levels indicates the syndrome of inappropriate antidiuretic hormone (SIADH).

Artefactual hyponatremia may be caused by excessive accumulation of plasma lipids or proteins.

ADRENAL INSUFFICIENCY

Embryology & Anatomy

The adrenal glands, once referred to as suprarenal glands, are so named for their location just above the kidney. The adrenal gland consists of an outer cortex, in which steroid hormones are produced, and an inner medulla, which produces catecholamines (Figure 20–17). The cells of the adrenal cortex originate from mesoderm, whereas the medulla arises from ectoderm. The cortical cells derive from the gonadal ridge, an enlarge for the steroidogenic cells of both the adrenal cortex and gonad. The adrenocortical cells migrate to their location superior to the kidneys at about the sixth week of gestation. These cells are invaded by sympathetic neural cells between the seventh and eighth week of gestation, giving rise to the medulla. The fetal adrenal gland consists of an outer "definitive" zone, which will persist into adulthood, and a larger inner "fetal" zone, which makes androgenic precursors for placental production of estriol. This latter zone makes the fetal cortex quite large, exceeding the size of the kidney at midgestation and remaining approximately

Table 20–27. Causes of salt-losing primary adrenal insufficiency.

Salt-losing forms of congenital adrenal hyperplasia (includes mineralocorticoid and glucocorticoid deficiencies)
Isolated defects of aldosterone synthesis
Destructive lesions of the adrenal cortex
Autoimmune
Fulminating infection
Hemorrhage
Peroxisomal disorders (including adrenoleukodystrophy)
Tumor metastases

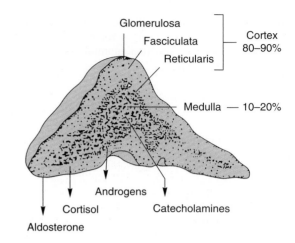

Figure 20–17. Anatomic zones and secretions of the adrenal gland. (Reproduced, with permission, from Guyton AC: *Textbook of Medical Physiology.* Saunders, 1986.)

one third the size of the kidney at birth. The fetal zone begins to involute at birth and disappears by 1 year of age.

Physiology

To understand the mechanism for salt loss with adrenal insufficiency, one must first understand the normal physiology of steroid hormone production within the adrenal cortex. No clinical condition results from absence of the medulla, and it will not be discussed further in this context. The cortex may be further subdivided into three layers histologically, each of which produces a distinct class of steroid hormones; the production of these hormones is mediated by different factors (Table 20–28).

The glomerulosa is the outermost cortical layer in which mineralocorticoids are produced. Aldosterone is the end product of this pathway. Aldosterone acts on the kidney at the distal tubule, where it augments sodium reabsorption and potassium and hydrogen secretion, thereby expanding vascular volume and maintaining blood pressure. The production of aldosterone is mediated principally by the renin-angiotensin system (Figure 20–18). Diminished blood pressure and sodium depletion stimulate release of renin from the juxtaglomerular apparatus in the kidney. Renin then acts enzymatically on angiotensinogen to convert it to angiotensin I. This product is, in turn, converted to angiotensin II by converting enzyme, a protein synthesized in the lungs and vasculature. Angiotensin II subsequently acts at two different levels to maintain blood pressure: First, it acts directly on the vasculature as a potent vasoconstrictor. Second, it stimulates synthesis and secretion of aldosterone, in turn promoting sodium retention and expansion of vascular volume.

The middle layer of the adrenal cortex, the fasciculata, is the site of glucocorticoid production. The end product of this pathway is cortisol. Cortisol influences a number

Table 20–28. Steroid hormone production within the adrenal cortex.

Zone	Type of Steroid	End Product	Regulator of Production
Glomerulosa	Mineralocorticoid	Aldosterone	Renin/angiotensin
Fasciculata	Glucocorticoid	Cortisol	Corticotropin-releasing factor (CRF), Adrenocorticotropic hormone (ACTH)
Reticularis	Androgens	Dehydroepiandrosterone (DHEA), androstenedione	Unknown

of basic physiologic processes essential to survival, including maintenance of vascular tone and integrity, maintenance of serum glucose levels, and clearance of free water. Cortisol production is mediated directly by ACTH release from the pituitary gland, which in turn is stimulated indirectly by corticotropin-releasing factor (CRF) from the hypothalamus (Figure 20–19). The release of CRF and ACTH is modulated by cortisol in a classic negative feedback loop. ACTH and cortisol are produced in a pulsatile manner, with diurnal variation: Peak concentrations are achieved in the early morning, and lower values are noted in the afternoon and evening. The adrenal gland produces 6–9 mg/m^2/d of cortisol; however, under stress this may increase to 3–15 times this amount. Cortisol circulates principally attached to binding proteins, of which transcortin (also known as corticosteroid-binding globulin) is the main such factor.

The innermost layer of the adrenal cortex, the reticularis, is where the adrenal androgens DHEA, DHEA(S), and androstenedione are produced. These are weaker androgens that have only limited clinical effects on virilization. In the peripheral tissues, they are converted to testosterone and dihydrotestosterone, resulting in pubic and axillary hair growth, body odor, and acne. A central factor from the hypothalamus and pituitary gland has been postulated to regulate androgen production, but no such factor has been identified to date.

Disorders of Adrenal Cortical Function

Adrenal insufficiency may result either from a problem in the adrenal gland itself, termed a primary defect, or from a problem in the pituitary gland or hypothalamus (a secondary or tertiary defect, respectively). Possible causes of a primary defect are shown in Table 20–29. The most common cause is congenital adrenal hyperplasia (CAH; see section on Ambiguous Genitalia), which is secondary to an enzymatic defect in the biosynthesis of cortisol (Figure 20–20). These are autosomal-recessive defects and have been described at every possible step of steroid hormone production. The effect on steroidogenesis may be predicted from inspection of the pathway, with some enzymatic defects affecting both glucocorticoid and mineralocorticoid synthesis (such as 21-OH deficiency), some having an isolated effect on glucocorticoid synthesis (such as 11-β hydroxylase deficiency) or mineralocorticoid synthesis (aldosterone synthase deficiency), and some having an effect on neither but affecting androgen production (17-β hydroxysteroid dehydrogenase deficiency). The heterogenous collection of disorders affecting glucocorticoid

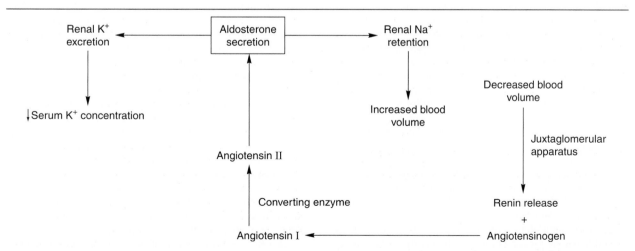

Figure 20–18. Regulation of aldosterone secretion by the renin-angiotensin system and the potassium concentration. (Reproduced, with permission, from Griffin JE: *Manual of Clinical Endocrinology and Metabolism.* McGraw-Hill, 1982.)

Stress and other signals

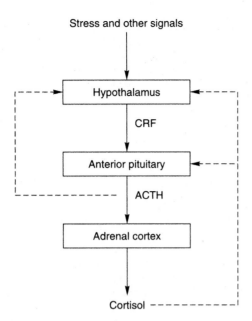

Figure 20–19. Regulation of glucocorticoid secretion. Solid arrows indicate stimulation; dashed arrows indicate inhibition. Glucocorticoids are known to inhibit both pituitary corticotropin (ACTH) and hypothalamic corticotropin-releasing factor (CRF) secretion. ACTH also exerts a short negative feedback effect on CRF release. (Reproduced, with permission, from Griffin JE, Ojeda SR [editors]: *Textbook of Endocrine Physiology.* Oxford, 1988.)

production is referred to as CAH because the defect leads to increased secretion of ACTH, which in turn results in hypertrophy of the adrenal gland.

21-Hydroxylase Deficiency. 21-OH deficiency is the most common form of CAH, accounting for approximately 95% of cases in the United States. The clinical presentation depends on the severity of the enzymatic block. The most severe deficiency, in which no 21-OH activity is present, occurs early in life with salt-wasting crisis. This condition is relatively common, occurring in approximately 1/12,000 individuals. Because 21-OH is involved in both aldosterone and cortisol production, individuals with absence of this enzyme lack the ability to synthesize either hormone. Transfer of maternal steroid hormones across the placenta helps to maintain the neonate for the first 5 days to 2 weeks of life. These patients then manifest their hormone deficiency with nonspecific gastrointestinal symptoms, such as nausea and vomiting, and finally progress to dehydration and shock. Biochemical findings include metabolic acidosis with hyponatremia, hyperkalemia, and hypoglycemia. Another manifestation of this enzymatic defect results from an accumulation of steroid hormone precursors in the glucocorticoid and mineralocorticoid pathways. These precursors are then diverted into the sex steroid pathway and result in overpro-

duction of testosterone. Female infants are virilized, and the condition therefore may be detected before the onset of salt loss by virtue of the physical examination. In male infants, however, the condition may not be detected (unless there is a prior family history of this disorder). A subtle clue on physical examination may be the presence of hyperpigmentation, most notable over the labioscrotal folds and in other skin creases. This finding is the result of overproduction of melanocyte-stimulating hormone, which is secreted in conjunction with ACTH.

The specific diagnosis of CAH is confirmed by measurement of the steroid hormone intermediate immediately preceding the enzymatic block, such as 17-hydroxy progesterone (17-OHP) in the case of 21-OH deficiency. The levels of this steroid intermediate are mildly elevated in normal infants for the first 24 hours after birth and are even more elevated in premature infants. In equivocal cases, an ACTH stimulation test will confirm the diagnosis: One obtains baseline levels of cortisol and steroid hormone precursors, including 17-OHP, then gives an intravenous bolus of ACTH and measures the steroid hormone levels again 60 minutes later. If 21-OH deficiency is present, a hyperresponsiveness of 17-OHP is noted. A nomogram to verify this diagnosis has been established for baseline and ACTH-stimulated 17-OHP values. Initial treatment of CAH requires stress dose glucocorticoid replacement along with dextrose, normal saline, and aldosterone replacement (see section on Treatment). When stable, treatment may be continued with oral glucocorticoid, mineralocorticoid, and sodium chloride.

Most cases of 21-OH deficiency that present in the newborn period are associated with salt loss, at least to some degree. Milder forms of 21-OH deficiency may manifest as ambiguous genitalia without salt loss in the neonatal period or with premature pubarche during childhood; such cases are referred to as simple virilizers. Even milder cases of 21-OH deficiency have been described as presenting later in life with hirsutism and menstrual irregularities; these individuals are considered to have nonclassic CAH. Such variant forms of 21-OH deficiency occur quite commonly, affecting about 1/1000 individuals.

Other Causes of Primary Adrenal Insufficiency

Additional disorders that may cause primary adrenal insufficiency are listed in Table 20–29 and are referred to collectively as Addison disease. In the past, tuberculosis was the most common cause of adrenal insufficiency, but now the most common cause is autoimmune adrenalitis. The inciting antigens appear to be the steroidogenic enzymes themselves. This condition may be associated with other endocrinopathies; when occurring in conjunction with thyroiditis or diabetes mellitus, it is referred to as Schmidt syndrome. More extensive multi-organ involvement may be noted with autoimmune polyglandular syndromes, one of which also involves chronic mucocutaneous candidiasis. There may be an underlying developmental defect in adrenal gland formation, result-

Table 20–29. Causes of adrenal insufficiency

Primary
  Congenital adrenal hyperplasia
  Autoimmune adrenalitis—
    may be component of polyglandular syndromes
  Congenital adrenal hypoplasia or aplasia
  Infection
    Tuberculosis, fungal
    AIDS, opportunistic infections
    Hemorrhage secondary to sepsis (meningococcus, others)
  Trauma
  Adrenoleukodystrophy
  Metastatic disease
  Infiltration
    Sarcoidosis, hemochromatosis
  ACTH unresponsiveness
Secondary
  Withdrawal from glucocorticoid therapy
  Isolated CRF or ACTH deficiency
  Hypothalamic defect or hypopituitarism—
    may be from developmental defect, tumor, infiltrative lesion, radiation.

ACTH = adrenocorticotropic hormone; CRF = corticotropin-releasing factor.

ing in congenital adrenal aplasia or hypoplasia. This is transmitted in autosomal-recessive or X-linked fashion: The latter is associated with a contiguous gene syndrome, in which a gene affecting adrenal development is deleted along with genes causing Duchenne muscular dystrophy and glycerol kinase deficiency. Congenital lipoid adrenal hyperplasia may have a similar clinical presentation but entails grossly enlarged adrenal glands in which cholesterol cannot be shuttled into the mitochondria for subsequent metabolism. The adrenal gland may also be destroyed by massive adrenal hemorrhage during a traumatic delivery and during sepsis with meningococcus (Waterhouse-Friderichsen syndrome), as well as by other organisms. In addition, the adrenal gland may be destroyed by various agents in the stages of AIDS. Adrenoleukodystrophy is an X-linked disorder of very–long-chain fatty acid metabolism characterized by CNS white matter disease in association with adrenal insufficiency. The neurologic disorders may either precede or follow adrenal defects, depending on the nature of the genetic lesion. Finally, infiltration from metastatic cancer, sarcoid, or hemochromatosis can also lead to adrenal insufficiency.

The aforementioned disorders are all associated with defects of both mineralocorticoid and glucocorticoid deficiency. With sudden absence of the steroid hormones, patients may present with adrenal crisis, in similar fashion to the neonate with salt-losing CAH. More insidious onset of hormonal insufficiency will be initially associated with milder symptomatology, including malaise, weakness, dizziness with orthostatic hypotension, nonspecific gastrointestinal complaints, and hyperpigmentation (Table 20–30). A superimposed stressful event, such as an infection, may in turn precipitate an acute adrenal crisis.

An isolated defect in cortisol production, without mineralocorticoid deficiency, may also present with hyponatremia, although this does not result from salt loss. Rather, glucocorticoid deficiency results in an inability of the kidneys to clear free water thought to be secondary to inappropriate secretion of ADH. Isolated cortisol deficiency usually occurs with defects in either CRF or ACTH production. Although an isolated defect in this particular axis may occur, it usually is associated with a lesion that affects other hormonal axes, such as CNS tumor, infiltrative or granulomatous lesion, and destruction radiation therapy. The most common reason for an isolated defect in this axis is chronic treatment with glucocorticoids at supraphysiologic levels. Exposure to more than the equivalent of 20 mg/m²/d of cortisol for more than 10 days may lead to suppression of the adrenal axis at the hypothalamic levels, and it may take 6 months or longer to recover from such suppression. Finally, a rare mutation of the ACTH receptor may be associated with isolated cortisol deficiency and is referred to as ACTH unresponsiveness.

Diagnosis

The diagnosis of adrenal insufficiency may be established by monitoring endogenous secretion of cortisol or by evaluating the response to provocative stimuli. With the diurnal and pulsatile nature of cortisol secretion, it is difficult to establish adrenal insufficiency on the basis of a single blood test result. However, a morning cortisol level of less than 5 μg/dL is very suspicious, especially if coupled with an elevated ACTH value. To evaluate cortisol secretion over time, it often is helpful to measure a 24-hour urine collection for 17-OHCS, with normal being 3 ± 1 mg/m²/d. The ACTH stimulation test (as described in the section on CAH) is often used to evaluate adrenal function, with a stimulated cortisol value greater than 20 μg/dL considered a normal response. Various other provocative stimuli have been used to evaluate the entire CRF-ACTH-adrenal axis, including metyrapone (a compound that block the final enzymatic step in cortisol production), response to insulin-induced hypoglycemia, and the CRF stimulation test.

Treatment

To treat adrenal insufficiency, one must replace the missing steroid hormones at physiologic doses. Cortisol production has been estimated at 6–9 mg/m²/d of cortisol. Such an amount is adequate for parenteral supplementation, but one often needs to use slightly greater amounts (approximately 10–15/m²/d) for enteral replacement. There are a number of different preparations that one can select (Table 20–31). Some agents have combined glucocorticoid and mineralocorticoid actions, whereas others have isolated glucocorticoid effects. These medications have vastly different potencies in their glucocorticoid-like activity. In children, the replacement doses often are so small and require such fine incremental changes that the least potent glucocorticoids (usually hydrocortisone) are used. This enables one to minimize overtreatment, with

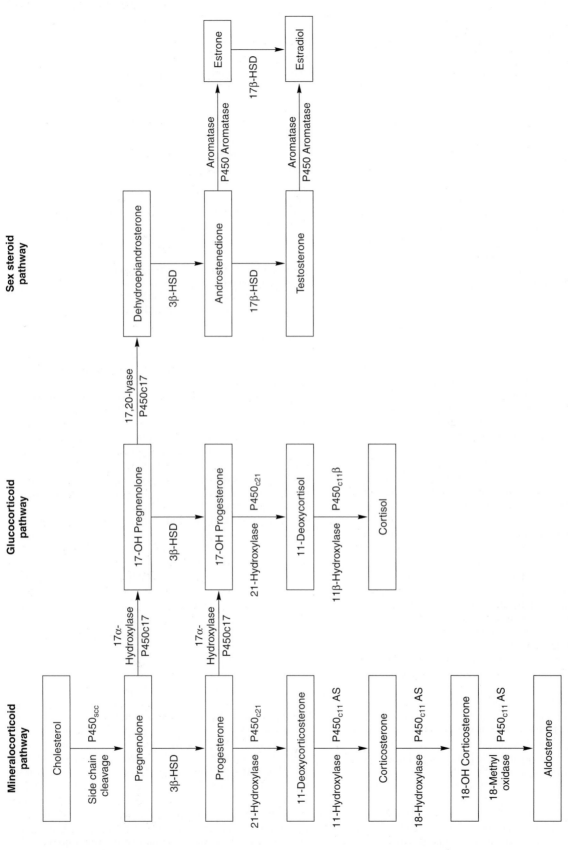

Figure 20–20. Biosynthetic pathways of adrenal steroid production. The diagram is laid out according to the layers of the adrenal cortex, with the outermost layer, glomerulosa, shown on the left (site of aldosterone production); the fasciculata layer (site of cortisol production) is in the middle; and the innermost reticularis layer (site of androgen production) is on the right. These enzymatic reactions occur primarily in the gonads, not in the adrenal cortex. The enzymatic activity is shown on the left or above each arrow, whereas the actual enzyme is shown on the right or below each arrow. Different enzymatic steps are often mediated by a single enzyme. 3β-HSD = 3β-hydroxysteroid dehydrogenase; 17β-HSD = 17β-hydroxysteroid dehydrogenase; $P450_{c11}$ AS = $P450_{c11}$ aldosterone synthetase. (Reproduced and adapted, with permission, from Miller WL: Molecular biology of steroid hormone synthesis. Endocrine Rev 1988;9:295.)

Table 20–30. Signs and symptoms of adrenal insufficiency.

Lethargy, weakness
Anorexia
Nonspecific gastrointestinal complaints; nausea and vomiting
Postural hypotension
Salt craving
Hyperpigmentation (primary)
Dehydration
Hyponatremia, hyperkalemia, hypoglycemia, metabolic acidosis

Table 20–32. Features of syndrome of inappropriate diuretic hormone.

Persistent secretion of ADH despite hypotonic plasma
Inability to maximally dilute the urine in face of hyponatremia
    and volume overload
Laboratory
    Plasma: hyponatremia (dilutional and secondary to natriure-
        sis), hypo-osmolality
    Urine: concentrated relative to plasma, inappropriate and
        persistent sodium excretion

ADH = antidiuretic hormone.

the attendant problems of Cushing syndrome, including growth suppression. During times of stress, such as a febrile illness or a surgical procedure, an individual with a normal adrenal axis will produce 3–15 times the basal amount of cortisol. Patients with adrenal insufficiency must mimic this stress response at such times, administering three times their usual dose of glucocorticoid to avoid adrenal crisis. If the patient is vomiting and unable to take medications enterally, then they must receive parenteral glucocorticoid treatment. Families must be instructed on the use of intramuscular hydrocortisone: The patient receives a single injection of 50 mg/m^2 and then is brought to the emergency department for further management. In the emergency department, the physician must quickly assess the patient's cardiovascular status (blood pressure, heart rate, perfusion) and glucose and electrolyte levels. The patient may require ongoing support with parenteral glucocorticoid treatment (50 mg/m^2/d of hydrocortisone, divided into doses every 6 hours), normal saline, and dextrose intravenous fluids. When the stress has passed, and the patient has been afebrile for 24 hours, the usual maintenance regimen may be quickly reinstated.

For mineralocorticoid replacement, one uses 9α-fluorocortisol at doses of 0.05–0.2 mg/d. Blood pressure, electrolyte levels, and plasma renin activity are monitored to determine whether the dose is adequate. Unlike glucocorticoids, the mineralocorticoid replacement does not need to be altered in the face of stress; aldosterone secretion does not change acutely in such settings. These patients also need additional sodium chloride in their diet. Neonates usually are given a very salt-restricted diet, with limited sodium in their formula, and may need up to 1–3 g of added salt per day. Older children may be able to adjust their salt intake spontaneously, either choosing salty food

items or using additional table salt in their foods to maintain an appropriate balance.

SYNDROME OF INAPPROPRIATE ANTIDIURETIC HORMONE

SIADH is characterized by an inability to dilute urine maximally in the face of hyponatremia and volume overload (Table 20–32). In this condition, secretion of ADH persists despite a hypotonic plasma. This results in water retention and hyponatremia, which is primarily dilutional but also in part is due to a volume expansion-induced natriuresis. The causes of SIADH are outlined in Table 20–33. Most commonly, excessive ADH secretion is associated with CNS diseases, including tumors, trauma, and infection. Less frequently, inflammatory lung disease may cause SIADH, apparently by decreasing the normal baroreceptor-mediated inhibition of ADH secretion. SIADH is also associated with pharmacologic agents that potentiate ADH secretion or action. Ectopic ADH secretion is rare in children and may be associated with carcinoma of the lung and pancreas, thymoma, hepatoma, lymphoma, or carcinoid tumors.

Therapy for SIADH includes treatment of the underlying disorder and fluid restriction. Replacement of lost body sodium also may be necessary but usually can be achieved through normal dietary salt intake. Severe hyponatremia (plasma sodium < 120–125 mmol/L) may be associated with CNS abnormalities, such as seizures, and may require treatment with hypertonic intravenous so-

Table 20–31. Relative potency of various steroids (relative to hydrocortisone).

	Glucocorticoid	Mineralocorticoid
Hydrocortisone	1	1
Prednisone	4	1
Dexamethasone	25	0
Betamethasone	20	0
Aldosterone	0.2	400
9α-fluorocortisol	8	400

Table 20–33. Causes of syndrome of inappropriate diuretic hormone.

ADH from posterior pituitary
• CNS disease (eg, tumors, trauma, infection)
• Lung inflammatory disease
• Drugs that stimulate ADH release

Ectopic ADH production
• Carcinoma of lung and pancreas
• Thymoma
• Hepatoma
• Lymphoma
• Carcinoid tumors

ADH = antidiuretic hormone; CNS = central nervous system.

dium chloride solution (3%). Concurrent use of a diuretic, such as furosemide, may be indicated when volume expansion is severe. The sodium deficit is calculated by the following equation:

Sodium deficit = (0.6) × (body weight in kilograms)
× (normal plasma sodium − observed plasma sodium).

However, the plasma sodium concentration should not be corrected too quickly. Overzealous treatment may re-sult in CNS damage, including central pontine myelinolysis. It is generally recommended that plasma sodium be corrected to a "safe" level of approximately 125 mmol/L at a rate no greater than 0.5–1 mmol/L/h. Thereafter, plasma sodium concentration can be corrected gradually over several days. Chronic SIADH is treated with fluid restriction and may require supplementation with a diuretic or an agent such as demeclocycline, which impairs the responsiveness of the renal tubule to AVP.

REFERENCES

SHORT STATURE

Blizzard RM, Johanson A: Disorders of growth. Page 383 in Kappy MS et al (editors): *Wilkins The Diagnosis and Treatment of Endocrine Disorders in Childhood and Adolescence.* Thomas, 1994.
Hoey HM: Psychosocial aspects of short stature. J Pediatr Endocrinol 1993;6:291.

ABNORMALITIES OF PUBERTY

Ehrhardt AA, Meyer-Bahlburg HF: Psychosocial aspects of precocious puberty. Horm Res 1994;41(Suppl 2):30.
Grumbach MM, Styne DM: Puberty: Ontogeny, neuroendocrinology, physiology, and disorders. In Wilson JD et al (editors): *Williams Textbook of Endocrinology.* Saunders, 1997.
Lee PA: Advances in the management of precocious puberty. Clin Pediatr 1994;33:54.
Rosenfield RL: Normal and almost normal precocious variations in pubertal development: Premature pubarche and premature thelarche revisited. Horm Res 1994;41(Suppl 2):7.
Shankar RR, Pescovitz OH: Precocious puberty. Adv Endocrinol Metab 1995;6:55.

CUSHING SYNDROME

Tsigos C, Chrousos GP: Differential diagnosis and management of Cushing's syndrome. Annu Rev Med 1996;47:443.

SEXUAL DIFFERENTIATION

Federman DD, Donahoe PK: Ambiguous genitalia: Etiology, diagnosis, and therapy. Adv Endocrinol Metab 1995;6:91.
Goodfellow PN, Lovell-Badge R: SRY and sex determination in mammals. Annu Rev Genet 1993;27:71.
Grumbach MM, Conte FA: Disorders of sex differentiation. In Wilson JD et al (editors): *Williams Textbook of Endocrinology.* Saunders, 1997.

THYROID GLAND

Burrow GN et al: Maternal and fetal thyroid function. N Engl J Med 1994;331:1072.

Dayan CM, Daniels GH: Chronic autoimmune thyroiditis. N Engl J Med 1996;335:99.
Fisher DA: Management of congenital hypothyroidism. J Clin Endocrinol Metab 1991;72:523.
Foley TP Jr: Goiter in adolescents. Endocrinol Metab Clin North Am 1993;22:593.
Ridgeway EC: Clinician's evaluation of a solitary thyroid nodule. J Clin Endocrinol Metab 1992;74:231.

HYPOGLYCEMIA

Fernandes J, Berger R: Hypoglycaemia: Principles of diagnosis and treatment in children. Baillieres Clin Endocrinol Metab 1993;7:591.
Hawdon JM et al: Prevention and management of neonatal hypoglycaemia. Arch Dis Child Fetal Neonatal Ed 1994;70: F60.

ANTIDIURETIC PHYSIOLOGY

Frasier SD et al: A water deprivation test for the diagnosis of diabetes insipidus in children. Am J Dis Child 1967;114: 157.
Kovacs L, Robertson GL: Syndrome of inappropriate antidiuresis. Endocrinol Metab Clin North Am 1992;21:859.
Robertson GL: Diabetes insipidus. Endocrinol Metab Clin North Am 1995;24:549.
Robinson AG, Verbalis JG: Diabetes insipidus. Curr Ther Endocrinol Metab 1994;5:1.

DIABETES MELLITUS

Atkinson MA, Maclaren NK: The pathogenesis of insulin-dependent diabetes mellitus. N Engl J Med 1994;331:1428.
Chase HP et al: Diabetic ketoacidosis in children and the role of outpatient management. Pediatr Rev 1990;11:297.
Diabetes Control and Complications Research Group: Diabetes Control and Complications Trial (DCCT): The effect of intensive treatment of diabetes on the development and progression of long-term complications in adolescents with insulin-dependent diabetes mellitus. J Pediatr 1994;125: 177.
Plotnick L: Insulin-dependent diabetes mellitus. Pediatr Rev 1994;15:137.

Santiago JV: Insulin therapy in the last decade. Diabetes Care 1993;16(Suppl 3):143.

Siperstein MD: Diabetic ketoacidosis and hyperosmolar coma. Endocrinol Metab Clin North Am 1992;21:415.

ADRENAL INSUFFICIENCY

Grinspoon SK, Biller BMK: Laboratory assessment of adrenal insufficiency. J Clin Endocrinol Metab 1994;79:923.

Miller WL: Genetics, diagnosis, and management of 21-hydroxylase deficiency. J Clin Endocrinol Metab 1994;78:241.

New MI et al: The adrenal hyperplasias. Page 1881 in Scriver C et al (editors): *The Metabolic Basis of Inherited Disease.* McGraw-Hill, 1989.

Oelkers W: Adrenal insufficiency. N Engl J Med 1996;335:1206.

21

The Nervous System

Donna M. Ferriero, MD, & William Weiss, MD

Clinical Evaluation

Clinical evaluation of infants and children with signs and symptoms referable to the nervous system demands complete and careful attention to all historical details related by the parents or caregivers and particularly the child, if possible. It is important to obtain prenatal, perinatal, and developmental histories, as well as the history of the present illness, to understand completely the nature of the clinical problem; in addition, a complete history of the biologic family should be obtained. The history describes the nature of the pathophysiologic process. A complete general and neurologic examination must then be carried out to determine the part of the nervous system affected by the illness.

Physicians must develop their own methods of performing the neurologic examination, selecting from a variety of available clinical techniques and examining procedures. They must be careful not to overlook assessment of any part of the nervous system. This is sometimes difficult in a young, frightened child, and repeated observations and examinations may be necessary to obtain sufficient information.

The single most important piece of information to ascertain in the evaluation of the child with neurologic problems is whether the problem is new or old, static or progressive. The physician needs to listen to the story of how the child gained (or lost) milestones.

A child may be referred to the neurologist because she or he is "slow." Usually, this term means that the child is slow in acquisition of motor or intellectual milestones. A broad understanding of normal development is necessary to see whether the child's development is delayed. Having obtained information about development, the next step is to look carefully at the child (and parents) for clues to the etiology of the problem.

Skin. Neurocutaneous stigmata, such as café-au-lait spots or hypopigmented macules, can be clues to major diseases (neurofibromatosis or tuberous sclerosis, respectively). Fair complexion can be seen in patients with phenylketonuria; a "tan" in those with adrenoleukodystro-phy and Wilson disease; and telangiectasias in those with ataxia-telangiectasia.

Face. Coarse facial features can be a sign of storage diseases; certain dysmorphisms, such as epicanthal folds, can be a clue to chromosomal disease (eg, Down syndrome).

Hair. Sparse, wiry hair is seen in patients with tricho-poliodystrophy; premature graying in those with ataxia-telangiectasia and homocystinuria; and breakable, dry hair in those with oasthouse urine disease.

The next step is to perform a careful general examination to feel for the following:

Organomegaly. This is seen in some of the storage diseases, for example, big spleen in Gaucher disease and big liver in glycogenesis, Gaucher, and Niemann-Pick diseases.

Cardiac Heaves & Thrusts. These are seen in the storage diseases.

Bony Deformities. These are seen in some storage diseases and in tuberous sclerosis.

Examination of the motor system will determine whether the slow child is weak or clumsy (ataxic). Ataxic children are often mislabeled as weak because they are slow to accomplish a motor task. Conversely, some slowing of movement can be a subtle sign of weakness. Having a child rise from a seated position on the floor without support can test for leg weakness. Children who must use their hands to climb up their legs in order to get up from the floor are performing a **Gower maneuver**—a sign of proximal weakness. Ataxia can be acute, chronic, or intermittent, and its pattern can be a clue to the disease category. Some infectious diseases, for example, varicella-zoster virus, can cause an acute cerebellar ataxia during the infection or afterward. Tumors and structural lesions of the cerebellum can present as a chronic ataxia, and some metabolic diseases, such as the aminoacidurias, can be quite intermittent. When recognized, abnormalities of the control of movement, such as tremor, dystonia, chorea, and myoclonus, can help identify the neurologic problem.

Examination of the eyes, especially the funduscopic examination, is crucial for determining the diagnosis in a progressive neurologic disorder in childhood. Cherry red spots, optic atrophy, cataracts, corneal opacities, and pigmentary degeneration of the retina are all clues to the neurologic syndrome affecting the child. Likewise, eye movement abnormalities may be seen in a number of degenerative diseases of the nervous system; once identified, these abnormalities can provide important diagnostic information.

Perhaps the most difficult part of the history and physical examination of the neurologically impaired child is the ascertainment of cognitive function. Depending on the age of the child, there may be very little information available about intellectual development. The social skills of a developing child are major indicators of intellectual function. Often a child who is dementing will show changes in behavior rather than memory or language.

In the following sections, common neurologic problems of childhood are presented according to the most common symptoms; special attention is given to the evaluation and treatment of a child with such a symptom. Normal development is presented in Chapter 1.

PAROXYSMAL DISORDERS

Paroxysmal disorders can be either epileptic or nonepileptic. **Epileptic** paroxysmal disorders are recurrent seizures that result from generalized or focal electrical discharges arising in the brain. **Nonepileptic** paroxysmal disorders do not involve electrical discharges arising in the brain, although the behavioral motor components may simulate "seizure activity." For example, breath-holding spells are nonepileptic, but the clinical manifestations of loss of consciousness and stiffening can mimic a seizure.

In assessing the child with a new-onset paroxysmal disorder, it is important to be able to observe the event. This can be done by instructing the caregivers to videotape the event so it can be reviewed in the clinic by physician and parents together.

If the paroxysmal spells are believed to be seizures, it is important to determine whether the seizure occurred in the setting of fever and whether the seizure had a focal onset at the start of the episode. A single seizure does not mean that an infant or child has epilepsy, nor does it imply the presence of pathology in the central nervous system (CNS). Recurrent seizures are termed "epilepsy" and are classified according to their mode of onset and accompanying clinical syndromes. An approach to the evaluation of a child with a paroxysmal disorder is shown in Table 21–1.

Table 21–1. Evaluation of the child presenting with a paroxysmal disorder.

Consciousness lost	
Yes	Generalized seizure; focal seizure with secondary generalization; syncope
No	Focal seizure with or without impairment of consciousness; movement disorder; migraine; other paroxysmal nonepileptic disorder
Child febrile	Consider lumbar puncture, especially in young infant
Focal neurologic signs or persistent impairment of sensorium	Complete blood count; glucose, Ca++, electrolytes, toxicology screens; emergent CT *without and with* contrast, *OR* MRI if available on an emergency basis; lumbar puncture (depending on results of CT/MRI); EEG as soon as possible.
Simple, single, afebrile seizure, and normal examination	Observe, consider EEG
Abnormal examination	Proceed as for focal seizure; blood ammonia concentration, screen for inborn errors of metabolism

CT = computed tomography; EEG = electroencephalogram; MRI = magnetic resonance imaging.

CLASSIFICATION OF SEIZURES

Partial or focal seizures are those in which the first clinical changes suggest abnormal activity of the localized anatomic or functional system of neurons located in one hemisphere. Partial seizures can be a manifestation of a variety of lesions, including tumors, traumatic lesions, infection, or ischemia. The body seizure is contralateral to the abnormal hemispheric epileptic discharge, and the symptoms can be motor, sensory, autonomic, or combinations thereof. Focal seizures are characterized by clonic jerking of a limb or of two limbs on the same side of the body. The focal nature of these seizures is evident on electroencephalogram (EEG) and is often caused by focal brain pathology, such as stroke.

Complex partial seizures are characterized by episodic alterations of behavior associated with motor and/or psychosensory symptoms and signs that make the episode appear semi-purposeful in nature. Complex partial seizures can be associated with lesions in the temporal lobe. Simple partial and complex partial seizures can evolve secondarily into generalized seizures with tonic-clonic activity. Therefore, it is important to obtain an accurate history of the beginning of the spell, when possible.

Generalized seizures are those in which there is complete loss of consciousness, followed by clinical features that do not manifest signs or symptoms referable to a single anatomic location. The EEG patterns from the onset of the seizure are bilateral, synchronous, and usually symmetric over both hemispheres. The generalized seizures consist of absence, myoclonic, clonic, tonic, tonic-clonic, and atonic seizure types. Generalized tonic-clonic seizures usually start with an ictal cry followed by a brief tonic seizure, then repeating clonic motor activity. Urinary incontinence is not a consistent hallmark of a seizure and therefore should not be used as a clinical guide to the presence of a seizure.

Myoclonic seizures consist of rapid jerking movements of a limb or group of limbs and suggest diffuse brain damage. The EEG may be normal or may show epileptic or decremental activity. In tonic seizures, the limbs extend and remain rigid, often in association with eye deviation and apnea. Similar limb extensions may also be seen in decerebrate posturing, an often terminal indication of midbrain compromise, and in opisthotonus, an arching of the back indicative of meningeal irritation. Tonic seizures, like myoclonic seizures, are often seen in association with metabolic diseases of the nervous system.

TREATMENT OF CHILDHOOD SEIZURES

Phenobarbital, phenytoin, valproate, and carbamazepine are equally effective for treatment of generalized tonic-clonic seizures (Table 21–2). Phenobarbital may be associated with learning difficulties in childhood, and phenytoin is associated with hirsutism, gingival hyperplasia, and coarse facial features in childhood. Therefore, we usually use carbamazepine for control of generalized and complex partial seizures and valproic acid in cases of mixed seizures. Valproic acid has been associated with fatal hepatic necrosis, primarily in young children (< 2 years) who are receiving multiple medications, and therefore must be used with caution.

In general, a single agent should be used, and plasma concentrations should be increased until control is achieved or side effects become limiting. At that time, alternative monotherapy or polytherapy should be considered. Experience with newer agents, such as gabapentin and lamotrigine, is limited in children; at this time, these agents are used as add-on therapies for children with refractory seizures.

FEBRILE SEIZURES

Fever may provoke epileptic seizures in children with afebrile seizures or may be associated with a familial, benign, and age-limited syndrome of febrile seizures. This syndrome occurs in 4% of children, starting at 3 months and usually remitting by 5–6 years. Seizures are either simple (isolated, generalized, and lasting less than 5 minutes) or complicated (multiple, focal, or lasting more than 5 minutes). Risk of recurrence is greatest for children with young age, low degree and short duration of fever, and positive family history for febrile or afebrile seizures. The risk of afebrile seizures increases with the increased number of complicating features.

The findings of the neurologic examination are normal. EEG usually is not indicated. Lumbar puncture (LP) should be considered in any patient presenting with fever and seizure. This generally is a benign syndrome and does not require treatment. Antipyretics usually are not effective, and the side effects of antiepileptic drugs make them of limited utility for most children. There is no evidence that treatment of febrile seizures reduces the risk of afebrile seizures.

NEONATAL SEIZURES

In the newborn period, it is difficult to determine whether the paroxysmal activities are electrical seizures, because the motor manifestations of the electrical event are often fragmentary and can be dissociated from the electrical recordings obtained by EEG (see discussion below on electroclinical dissociation). In addition, normal neonates may be jittery and often have choreoathetotic movements that can mimic seizures. Babies also may exhibit benign nocturnal myoclonus—jerking movements when falling asleep or awakening. Because many cortical tracts are not myelinated in the newborn infant, the motor manifestations of seizure activity are highly variable. Seizures can manifest as myoclonic jerks, tonic eye deviation, or focal or multifocal tonic or clonic activity (Table 21–3). Therefore, synchronized and generalized tonic-clonic seizures are uncommon in the neonate.

Multifocal clonic seizures are focal seizures in which .

Table 21–2. Pharmacologic data on commonly used anticonvulsants.

Drug	Elimination Half-life (h)	Time to Reach Steady-state (days)	Steady-state Dose (mg/kg)	Therapeutic Range (μg/mL)
Phenobarbital	90	14	5	15–40
Phenytoin[1]	12	~14	5	10–20
Carbamazepine	12	3	25	8–12
Valproic acid	12	2	45	80–140

[1]Does not follow first-order kinetics.

Table 21–3. Types of neonatal seizures.

Apnea
Focal
Multifocal clonic
Myoclonic
Tonic
Subtle

Table 21–4. Etiology of neonatal seizures.

Infectious	Bacterial meningitis or sepsis, herpes or other viral encephalitides
Postinfectious	TORCH infections: *toxoplasmosis, rubella, cytomegalovirus, herpes*
Intoxication	Drug toxicity or withdrawal, kernicterus
Metabolic	Hypoxic-ischemic encephalopathy, hypoparathyroidism-hypocalcemia, hypoglycemia, pyridoxine dependence, urea cycle disorders, maple syrup urine disease, organic acidemias
Mass lesions	Cerebral infarction or hemorrhage, cerebral malformations
Genetic	Familial neonatal seizures, tuberous sclerosis

jerking movements migrate from limb to face or from limb to limb in a random pattern. The EEG shows multifocal epileptiform activity and probably reflects the neonatal equivalent of a generalized tonic-clonic seizure. This is a common manifestation of hypoxic ischemic encephalopathy; it also is seen in infants of addicted mothers in the setting of withdrawal.

Babies exhibiting motor movements that are not clonic, tonic, or myoclonic are said to have "subtle seizures." These events include bicycling movements, lip smacking, blinking, and sucking movements. Many subtle seizures do not have associated epileptiform activity on EEG, and treatment of these disorders with anticonvulsant drugs remains controversial. Conversely, sick neonates undergoing EEG monitoring commonly have electrical seizures without clinical accompaniment (electroclinical dissociation). These seizures should be treated. The EEG therefore is an essential tool in the evaluation of neonatal seizures, and long-term video-EEG monitoring is clearly the most informative technique in this regard. If such monitoring is unavailable, or if the EEG is normal interictally, the infant may be attached to a bedside EEG monitor that can be turned on and off by caretakers during a clinical spell.

Periodic breathing in the absence of vital-sign abnormalities is normal in the premature neonate and reflects immaturity of respiratory centers in the pons. **Apnea** is characterized by breathing pauses associated with decreases in heart rate and may be normal or pathologic in the neonate. Intracranial hemorrhage may present with apnea and is often accompanied by changes in mental status. Isolated apnea rarely is epileptic in origin. Epileptic manifestations of apnea usually are subtle seizures with or without accompanying bradycardia.

Etiology

Many conditions may be associated with seizures in the newborn infant (Table 21–4).

Bacterial meningitis is commonly associated with seizures in neonates and with other signs of sepsis, such as apnea, hypotension, and respiratory distress. Common organisms include group B *Streptococcus, Escherichia coli,* and *Listeria monocytogenes.* Diagnosis requires LP, which usually shows elevated white blood cell count and protein concentration and depressed glucose levels. Gram stain and culture of the cerebrospinal fluid (CSF) usually identify the causative organism. Morbidity and mortality are very high in this age group. **Herpes simplex virus** infections are commonly acquired through birth-canal passage in affected mothers; these infections also may be ac-

quired transplacentally in women who contract primary herpes during pregnancy. The mortality rate may exceed 50%, and long-term sequelae are common. Symptoms may be delayed for 1–2 weeks after birth and commonly include a vesicular rash, conjunctivitis, jaundice, irritability, and seizures. The EEG is diffusely abnormal or may show focal temporal spikes. CSF may be normal or may show increased opening pressure, with pleocytosis, hemorrhage, and decreased glucose concentration. Treatment includes intravenous (IV) acyclovir. Cesarean section should be considered for at-risk mothers.

Opiate withdrawal in the neonatal period is commonly associated with tremor, irritability, a high-pitched cry, and feeding difficulty. Myoclonic jerks are common, but seizures are relatively rare, occurring more commonly with methadone rather than heroin withdrawal. Urine toxicology screens should be performed in all children at risk, and these babies may benefit from replacement and slow withdrawal of the opiate (eg, paregoric). Cocaine intoxication in utero may be associated with intracranial hemorrhage and stroke. Even in the absence of these findings, infants at risk can present with tremulousness, hypertonicity, irritability, and, rarely, seizures.

Kernicterus is a yellow discoloration of the basal ganglia and hippocampus and is associated with high plasma levels (> 20 mg/dL) of unconjugated bilirubin. This disorder is now rare, but it was once commonly seen as a complication of hemolytic disease in the newborn. Patients present with lethargy, followed by hypertonia and opisthotonic posturing 2–3 days after birth. Affected babies then normalize their tone, and athetosis, gaze disturbances, hearing loss, and mental retardation develop. Diagnosis relies on demonstrating high levels of unconjugated bilirubin and may be aided by brainstem auditory evoked response (BAER) and magnetic resonance imaging (MRI) abnormalities. Prevention is aimed at maintaining plasma bilirubin levels in the normal range.

The differential diagnosis of neonatal seizures depends in part on the time of onset. Seizures during the first postnatal day often result from neonatal asphyxia at the time of birth. **Hypoxic-ischemic encephalopathy (HIE)** results from both hypoxemia (decreased blood oxygen content) and ischemia (decreased organ perfusion). Neonatal brains are quite resistant to hypoxic ischemic insults; with prolonged injury, however, brain damage may occur. In the term infant, HIE is the clinical manifestation of neonatal asphyxia and may first present as lethargy after birth. When stimulated, the baby becomes jittery and hyperalert. Tone is normal or decreased, and power may be decreased proximally, consistent with watershed injury to parasagittal brain areas. In more severe cases, lethargy is pronounced, and seizures occur. Sucking and swallowing reflexes may be absent, and primitive reflexes are diminished.

Severely affected infants may remain obtunded for prolonged periods, gradually becoming more alert and hypertonic. Such infants tend to have long-term neurologic sequelae. The EEG may help delineate the degree of brain injury, and computed tomography (CT) and MRI can show brain edema and evolving stroke. Treatment is supportive only. Seizures are usually managed with phenobarbital; in rare cases, phenytoin may be added.

Pyridoxine dependency is a rare autosomal-recessive disorder characterized by intractable multifocal clonic seizures or status epilepticus (SE) shortly after birth. Late-onset disease may also be seen. Seizures are characteristically refractory to all antiepileptic drugs but cease in response to 100 mg IV pyridoxine, which is best given during the EEG recording. Long-term treatment with pyridoxine prevents further seizures. Developmental handicaps are common.

Hypoglycemia and hypocalcemia are common in neonates. The serum glucose concentration commonly decreases during the first hours and is usually asymptomatic. Pathologic hypoglycemia is associated with glucose levels of less than 20 mg/dL in preterm and less than 40 mg/dL in term infants and includes such disorders as maternal or neonatal diabetes, malnutrition, prematurity, asphyxia, sepsis, aminoacidurias, hypopituitarism, or defects in carbohydrate metabolism. These patients may have seizures and coma or may be jittery, irritable, and hypotonic. Treatment is aimed at restoring glucose homeostasis. Calcium levels less than 7 mg/dL are an uncommon cause of seizures but may contribute to the morbidity of at-risk children. Causes of hypocalcemia include prematurity, hypoparathyroidism, DiGeorge syndrome, vitamin D deficiency, pseudohypoparathyroidism, and renal disease. Treatment is aimed at restoring calcium homeostasis. (See Chapter 16.)

Six recognized enzymatic deficiencies lead to **urea cycle disorders** (see Chapter 6). Ornithine transcarbamoylase deficiency is X-linked, and all others are autosomal recessive. In the newborn period, these typically present with hyperammonemia, which is associated with seizures, lethargy, vomiting, and hypotonia. Ammonia is produced as a by-product of amino acid breakdown; therefore, levels increase when protein is introduced in the diet. Diagnosis requires measurement of serum ammonia levels, and therapy is aimed initially at reducing the ammonia level. This can be achieved with dialysis or, in less severe cases, by reducing nitrogen intake and augmenting alternative pathways for nitrogen excretion with the use of arginine, sodium benzoate, and sodium phenylacetate.

Maple syrup urine disease is an autosomal-recessive disorder in which there is a defect in branched-chain amino acid metabolism (leucine, valine, and isoleucine) characterized by sweet-smelling urine and buildup of branched-chain ketoacids. Infants appear healthy at birth, but lethargy develops after feeding; ultimately, seizures and cerebral edema develop. Diagnosis is suspected with the occurrence of sweet-smelling urine and a positive urine dinitrophenylhydrazine test result. Definitive diagnosis is established by urine organic acid analysis. Treatment is aimed initially at removing branched-chain ketoacids with dialysis. Later, dietary restriction of branched-chain amino acids prevents recurrence of lethargy and seizures.

Nonketotic hyperglycinemia is a relatively uncommon autosomal-recessive disorder associated with hypotonia, intractable seizures, apnea, and obtundation. Most infants die in the neonatal period. Of those who survive, many are severely handicapped. In rare cases, however, the infant remits spontaneously. EEG characteristically shows a burst suppression or hypsarrhythmic pattern. Urine examination shows an elevated glycine concentration in the absence of ketones or other organic acids, and CSF analysis shows elevation of glycine levels out of proportion to that seen in serum.

Organic acidemias are characterized by a baby who is normal at birth but becomes lethargic after feeding and experiences vomiting, dehydration, seizures, and failure to thrive. Diagnosis requires demonstration of acidosis and analysis of urine organic acids. Treatment of these disorders is mainly dietary.

Full-term babies commonly have **subarachnoid hemorrhage** secondary to passage through the birth canal. In most cases, this is not associated with long-term neurologic problems. **Subdural hemorrhage** usually results from a more traumatic birth injury and may cause brainstem compression. This serious condition has a high degree of neurologic morbidity and mortality. Subdural hemorrhage is readily visualized with CT. **Intraventricular hemorrhage (IVH)** may result from mechanical trauma but more commonly is a sequela of HIE that manifests shortly after birth. In preterm infants, IVH is associated with bleeding in the germinal matrix, a periventricular region that is the site of neuronal origin and migration to the cortical layers. The germinal matrix involutes at term, and the choroid plexus then becomes the primary site of IVH. Asphyxiated preterm infants typically present with IVH 1–2 days after birth. IVH may be associated with periventricular hemorrhagic infarction, hydrocephalus, or brain parenchymal injury (intracranial hemorrhage). In general, both short- and long-term outcomes are a function of the degree of hemorrhage. IVH in the preterm infant may be clinically silent or may be associated with acute respiratory compromise, bulging fontanelle, and a decreasing hematocrit. In the term baby, deterioration may be rapid in association with a large hemorrhage or may be much more gradual (saltatory syndrome) or clinically silent. Hypotension associated with HIE and IVH may lead to cerebral infarction; the periventricular white matter is especially at risk in the premature infant. Cystic lesions in the periventricular white matter, termed **periventricular leukomalacia,** are associated with static encephalopathy, more commonly involving motor abnormalities than cognitive problems. Prevention is largely aimed at delaying preterm delivery and ensuring that high-risk deliveries are performed at experienced centers. Seizures are managed with appropriate antiepileptic drugs (usually phenobarbital). Hydrocephalus may require ventriculoperitoneal shunting after resolution of the hemorrhage. In evolving hydrocephalus, some centers use diuretic therapies (acetazolamide or furosemide) and serial LPs before shunt placement.

Benign neonatal seizures are a transient syndrome of multifocal clonic seizures that begin in the neonatal period and remit spontaneously after 3 weeks. This disorder is commonly not associated with other neurologic abnormalities, and there is often a positive family history. Some cases show linkage to chromosome 20q.

Treatment

Phenobarbital remains the drug of choice in neonatal seizures, although inpatient therapy with lorazepam is becoming increasingly popular. Initial blood phenobarbital levels of 20 µg/mL should be sought; however, these levels may be insufficient in a minority of patients. Learning difficulties may be associated with long-term use of phenobarbital, and patients usually are given alternative therapies after 1–2 years of age. Phenytoin is commonly used in addition as a second-line drug in children whose condition is refractory to phenobarbital. Oral therapy is difficult with this medication, because absorption is erratic, and it is available only in suspension form. Phenytoin levels of 15–20 µg/mL are adequate for antiepileptic therapy. Lorazepam is a long-acting benzodiazepine anticonvulsant with less respiratory depression and hypotension than other benzodiazepine drugs. This drug may be used as monotherapy or may be added to phenobarbital or phenytoin treatment. Most infants require lorazepam at dosages of 0.05–0.10 mg/kg for antiepileptic effects.

Duration of therapy is a function of the cause of the seizure and the results of the neurologic examination. In patients with metabolic abnormalities that have subsequently normalized, and in whom the examination results also normalize, it is reasonable to discontinue therapy after 2 weeks. If the cause of seizures is structural, and the clinical examination and EEG findings are abnormal, it is reasonable to continue treatment at discharge and reevaluate after 1 month.

EPILEPTIC SYNDROMES

Infantile Spasms

Infantile spasms are an age-dependent form of myoclonic epilepsy. In some children, these spasms are caused by congenital malformations and metabolic disorders (symptomatic infantile spasms), whereas in others they are caused by unknown mechanisms (cryptogenic infantile spasms). Onset is before 1 year of age, and seizures consist of clusters of flexor or extensor spasms involving the head, trunk, and limbs. Diagnosis requires EEG, which usually is abnormal. A characteristic pattern of chaotic, high-amplitude, and random spike-and-wave activity is called **hypsarrhythmia,** and the combination of this pattern, infantile spasms, and mental retardation is called **West syndrome.**

Diagnosis relies on characteristic seizures and abnormal EEG results. Causes of infantile spasms must be sought, although approximately 15% of cases are idiopathic or cryptogenic. A small percentage of patients have normal EEG and examination findings, and their seizures ultimately are called "benign neonatal myoclonus." Despite the generalized nature of these seizures, some children have focal abnormalities on functional imaging studies and may benefit from focal cortical resection. Medical therapy usually is initiated with adrenocorticotrophic hormone (ACTH), which stops seizures in most cases. However, most children have new seizures after the first few years, even if their spasms are controlled. Mental retardation is very common.

Lennox-Gastaut Syndrome

The Lennox-Gastaut syndrome occurs between 3 and 5 years and consists of multiple types of generalized seizures (myoclonic, atonic, or atypical absence), spike-and-wave EEG, and mental retardation. This is a label rather than a diagnosis and, like infantile spasms, requires a workup for etiology. Twenty percent of these patients have a history of infantile spasms. More than half have structural brain damage or other metabolic disorders. Treatment of myoclonic and atonic seizures is difficult; most children are given valproic acid in combination with clonazepam or other long-acting benzodiazepines.

Benign Rolandic Epilepsy of Childhood

Benign rolandic epilepsy of childhood is a self-limited autosomal-dominant disease of childhood; onset usually occurs between 5 and 10 years. Typically, the seizures awaken the child and/or parents, who notice twitching of the face, which sometimes spreads to the limbs, and associated drooling and inability to speak. Examination is normal and EEG may be characteristic, showing discharges in the rolandic (centrotemporal) region. Therapy is not required for rare nocturnal seizures. Seizures usually remit by 14 years.

Juvenile Absence Epilepsy

Absence seizures are a form of primary generalized epilepsy transmitted as an autosomal-dominant trait. Onset is between 4 and 8 years and always before age 20. Seizures typically occur up to 100 times a day and are less than 1 minute in duration. The child may stare into space, and there may be fluttering of the eyelids. In contrast to complex partial seizures, there is no aura or postictal drowsiness. The examination is normal, but seizures may be provoked by cerebral vasoconstriction associated with hyperventilation. A paper towel is held in front of the child's mouth, and the child is instructed to blow on it repeatedly for 2 minutes. EEG is pathognomonic and shows 3 per second spike-and-wave activity in all leads. In a child with normal development and examination, the characteristic seizures and EEG establish the diagnosis, and no further testing is necessary. Treatment is with ethosuximide. If generalized tonic-clonic seizures develop, valproic acid should be used, because ethosuximide does not treat the generalized tonic-clonic component adequately.

Juvenile Myoclonic Epilepsy

Juvenile myoclonic epilepsy of Janz (JME) is a common autosomal-recessive disorder with onset typically in adolescence. A characteristic history is that of a child with frequent myoclonic seizures who has a first grand mal seizure and is taken to the emergency department. When asked, parents offer the history that the child frequently flings or drops objects, usually in the morning, and therefore is labeled "clumsy" or "rude." Patients usually have absence epilepsy as well and often have 4- to 6-Hz generalized spike-and-wave activity seen on EEG. A characteristic history and EEG, along with a normal neurologic examination, establish the diagnosis. Therapy involves valproic acid and may be needed throughout the patient's life.

Progressive Myoclonic Epilepsies

These rare, progressive disorders are of infectious or metabolic origin. They are differentiated from JME on the basis of the progressive nature of seizures and of abnormalities on the neurologic examination.

STATUS EPILEPTICUS (SE)

Unlike SE in adults, SE in children does not usually portend devastating neurologic disease. In fact, of the children who present with SE:

* 25% have febrile convulsions that usually do not progress to epilepsy

* 25% have remote neurologic disorders, such as old trauma or infarct

* 25% have new acute CNS problems, such as infection or toxin exposure

* 20% have no obvious reasons for the seizures

* only 5% have progressive neurologic disease.

Over the past two decades, morbidity and mortality from SE have decreased substantially, so that only children with serious underlying neurologic disease die (< 4%). The morbidity of SE is more often a result of the anticonvulsant therapy (oversedation requiring intubation and admission to intensive care units) than of the precipitating cause. Again, children with progressive neurologic disease rarely present with SE. Those children who present with afebrile SE as their first seizure have the same risk of recurrence for epilepsy as those who present with a brief generalized tonic-clonic seizure.

Treatment

IV access should be achieved, and, if necessary, the airway should be controlled. The serum glucose concentration should be measured and supplemented if necessary. Lorazepam (0.1 mg/kg) should be administered and may be repeated after 10 minutes if indicated. If seizures are still occurring, 20 mg/kg of phenobarbital (in neonates) or phenytoin is given next; an additional 10 mg/kg may be given if needed. Phenytoin is not as effective for SE that is associated with fever. In the case of febrile SE, it is best to use benzodiazepines and barbiturates to their maximal tolerated doses. If seizures still recur, a neurologist should be consulted, and midazolam or pentobarbital coma considered. It is unusual for children to require multiple drugs if SE is treated promptly. Prehospital treatment of SE in children with rectal diazepam appears to decrease morbidity (Table 21–5).

Therapy is aimed at recognizing the cause of SE, but the general guidelines for drug therapy are as follows:

* Febrile SE: Use sedative-hypnotic drugs (benzodiazepines such as lorazepam and midazolam).

* Afebrile SE: Use phenytoin.

After seizures are controlled, a full physical and neurologic examination must be performed, and LP considered.

Table 21–5. Barbiturate anesthesia: Protocol for refractory status epilepticus.

1. Intubation and ventilation, admission to intensive care unit, arterial line (central venous pressure line and/or Swan-Ganz if preexisting cardiopulmonary disease).
2. Electroencephalogram (EEG) for monitoring control of seizures and level of anesthesia (check q 15–30 min during induction, then q 1–2 h once burst-suppression pattern is attained).
3. Pentobarbital—loading dose of 15 mg/kg over 1 h, maintenance infusion of 1–2 mg/kg/h, additional loading doses (5 mg/kg to maximum of 30 mg/kg in first 12 h) as needed to control seizures or attain burst-suppression.[1]
4. Low-dose dopamine (followed by dobutamine, if necessary) for hypotension.
5. Continue maintenance phenytoin and phenobarbital with monitoring of blood levels.
6. Stop pentobarbital at 12 h and observe. If seizures recur, reinstate infusion and continue for 24 h before withdrawal. Repeat as needed.

[1]The initial maintenance infusion we now recommend is 0.5 mg/kg/h, with adjustment to higher doses on the basis of clinical and EEG responses.

Laboratory analysis should include a complete blood count (CBC), liver function tests, a toxicology screen, and measurement of electrolyte, dextrose, calcium, and magnesium levels. An electrocardiogram (ECG) should be considered, as seizures may be a secondary manifestation in children with primary heart disease.

Remember that convulsive SE can degenerate into nonconvulsive SE; therefore, it is imperative to obtain an EEG after convulsions cease to determine whether the electrical seizures have ceased as well. Nonconvulsive SE also can be seen when either absence seizures or complex partial seizures are continuous. In these cases, the child may just seem unaware of the environment ("out of it"), with little else except a change in behavior or language function. Again, an EEG will determine whether there are continuous electrical discharges. Benzodiazepine is given during the test to make the diagnosis.

NONEPILEPTIC PAROXYSMAL DISORDERS

These disorders are listed in Table 21–6. Migraine, syncope, night terrors, and hyperventilation are all paroxysmal disorders in childhood. Narcolepsy may start in early childhood and consists of daytime sleepiness, cataplexy (loss of muscle tone induced by startle or laughter), and vivid (hypnagogic) hallucinations. Myotonic dystrophy also can present with so-called sleep attacks and is more common than narcolepsy in this age group.

Breath-holding Spells
Breath-holding spells occur in 5% of children, may start in infancy, and tend to be familial. Children hold their breath in response to anger, frustration, or other external stimuli. In cyanotic breath-holding, children hold their breath, become cyanotic, and may lose consciousness in association with tonic or clonic movements. These children then recover and seem normal. Diagnosis rests on the history, and no treatment is required.

Table 21–6. Nonepileptic paroxysmal disorder in infancy and childhood.

Infants
Breath-holding spells
Infantile masturbation
Movement disorders
Infantile shuddering
Sandifer syndrome
Children
Night terrors
Migraine, migraine variants, migraine equivalents
Movement disorders
Chorea
Dystonia
Syncope
Pseudoseizures

In pallid breath-holding, the child becomes pale and loses consciousness, possibly also with associated tonic-clonic movements. Treatment may not be necessary in this spell; however, with longer durations of pallor and unconsciousness, atropine may be beneficial.

Migraine Equivalents
Migraine equivalents in childhood include leg cramps, cyclic vomiting, vertigo, and torticollis, all of which may be paroxysmal. Diagnosis rests on history, family history, and demonstration of a normal examination. Treatment usually is not indicated in infancy. Treatment of childhood migraine is discussed below.

Migraine Variants
Children with **benign paroxysmal vertigo** typically present between 2 and 6 years of age. These children have sudden, brief episodes of fright, with difficulty maintaining equilibrium but without loss of consciousness. Full recovery is seen after minutes. If the neurologic examination is normal and the story is characteristic, no further workup is needed. Paroxysmal torticollis may present similarly and may also be a migraine variant.

Children with cyclic vomiting have episodes of unexplained abdominal pain, nausea, and vomiting, sometimes leading to obtundation with or without headache. Patients characteristically are free of abdominal pain between complaints. Vomiting may be severe enough to require IV hydration. The results of gastrointestinal evaluation and neuroimaging are characteristically negative.

HEADACHE

Evaluation of the Child With Headache
Headache is a common childhood illness. The overall incidence of significant headache during childhood is 40% by age 7 years and 75% by 15 years. In one study, 12% of adolescents missed a day of school in the preceding month secondary to headache. Patients with headache often do not seek medical help. The patient's history often is provided by the parents, but every attempt should be made to ask the child about the nature and duration of head pain. It is important to appreciate that migraine episodes may occur without head pain. They are, however, still classified as headaches. The single most important question regarding headache is, "Does the head pain wake you up from sleep?" Other important information includes school absences, as well as frequency, duration, quality, timing, location, and precipitating and relieving factors (Table 21–7). Specific questions should be asked about changes in vision and accompanying weakness or

Table 21–7. Important aspects of history in evaluation of headache.

Location:	Where is the pain (eyes, neck, face)
Frequency:	Daily, weekly, monthly
Severity:	Wakening from sleep, stopping play
Duration:	Seconds, minutes, hours, days
Auras:	These are uncommon in children, but there may be a history of macropsia, micropsia, or visual obscurations
Triggers:	Foods, stresses
Maneuvers that increase or decrease pain	
Presence of associated weakness or numbness	
Medications used to relieve pain	

Table 21–8. Classification of headaches in children, based on site of origin.

Extracranial structures
  Paranasal sinuses—acute or chronic sinusitis
  Middle or external ear—acute or chronic otitis
  Teeth—dental infections or trauma
  Neck and scalp muscles—muscle contraction ("tension")
  Orbit—orbital infection
  Eyes—refractive errors

Dura & venous sinuses
  Traction—distortion by space-occupying lesions: tumor, abscess, hematoma, pseudotumor cerebri, hydrocephalus
  Inflammation—acute or chronic meningitis

Vascular structures
  Nonmigrainous—hypertension, fever, convulsive disorders
  Migraine—classic, common, complicated

Psychogenic
  Depression
  Hypochondriasis

numbness. The history should include a discussion of headache triggers. A minority of patients have headaches bought on by ingestion of specific foods, including chocolate, preserved meats, monosodium glutamate, and food rich in tyramine (strong cheese and red wine). Many patients are not aware that certain foods trigger headache. By paying attention to the association of food and headache, avoidance of triggers may help reduce headache frequency.

One goal of the physical examination is to rule out systemic abnormalities, because headache can be a nonspecific accompaniment to a number of systemic disorders. Blood pressure should be measured to evaluate for hypertension. The skin should be examined for café-au-lait spots, petechiae, or striae. Head circumference must be recorded, and the head should be palpated for areas of focal tenderness or signs of trauma. Auscultation of the skull for bruits, which are common in children, should be performed for all new-onset headaches. The neurologic examination should include assessment of meningeal signs, visual fields, and eye movements. A careful funduscopic examination must be performed, and the pupils should be dilated if the full fundus is not visualized. A detailed motor examination will help rule out focal abnormalities.

Worrisome headaches are new, progressive, severe at onset, or consistently localized. These headaches feature pain that awakens the patient, occurs in the early morning, or is associated with straining or with neurologic signs or symptoms. However, there are no absolute indicators of ominous headache, and one should probably err on the side of caution. CT and LP are useful in the acute management of headache, but MRI generally is a better test to rule out a brain tumor. Contrast should be used in evaluating any potential inflammatory lesion and should be administered after a noncontrast scan is obtained.

Classification

The anatomic sites from which headaches originate, as well as the conditions associated with headache, are shown in Table 21–8.

Even though the site of head pain is usually nonlocalizing, pain-sensitive structures do exist within the skull and consist mainly of blood vessels, which react to vasodilatation, inflammation, and traction displacement. The brain and its membranous coverings are insensitive to pain. Vascular pain originating in structures above the tentorium is transmitted mainly via the trigeminal nerve, whereas infratentorial vascular pain is transmitted by spinal nerves C1–C3. Dural pain is transmitted via the ophthalmic division of the trigeminal nerve (V1) to the eye and forehead, whereas posterior fossa pain is referred to the neck. Extracranial structures sensitive to pain include skin, subcutaneous tissues, muscles, mucous membranes, teeth, and large vessels.

Acute Headaches. The patient presenting with an acute generalized headache must be evaluated for infection, trauma, and hypertension. LP should be considered in all such patients after careful exclusion of a space-occupying lesion (lack of papilledema, CT scan). Post-LP headache is seen mainly in older children and adults; it is caused by dural tears and CSF leaks resulting from the spinal needle. This is a postural headache that occurs in 10–30% of patients, starting minutes to days after the LP attempt and persisting up to 2 weeks. Headaches usually are frontal and throbbing but may be occipital. Treatment is symptomatic for mild headaches, but more severe headaches will respond to IV caffeine or to an autologous blood patch. Another cause of acute generalized headache is severe postexertional (eg, weight-lifting) headache, which may be responsive to indomethacin.

Sinusitis is a common cause of acute localized headache, with pain provoked by palpation of the sinuses. Diagnosis requires demonstration of sinus opacification by CT or MRI. Treatment with antibiotics usually is curative; symptomatic pain is relieved with analgesics. Otitis media can cause headache and is readily diagnosed by otoscopy and pneumatoscopy. Uncorrected refractive errors are a rare cause of headache. Malocclusion of the teeth, dental abscesses, caries, and temporomandibular joint swelling are all causes of focal pain in the jaw, mouth, or ear. Head trauma may be associated with localized headache, and pain onset may be delayed relative to the timing of head trauma.

Chronic Headaches

Common Migraine. Migraine accounts for most cases of recurrent headache in childhood. This is an autosomal-dominant condition with increasing prevalence with age, affecting 2–10% of children. Triggers commonly include stress, exercise, head trauma, certain foods, and the premenstrual decline in circulating estrogen. Many adults with migraines experienced paroxysmal recurrent abdominal pain, leg cramps, or car sickness when they were children, generating some debate about whether these represent pediatric migraine equivalents.

Clinical characteristics include abdominal pain and nausea or vomiting, in association with a cranial throbbing, pulsatile pain. Complete relief occurs after a brief period of rest. Although migraine may be associated with visual, sensory, or motor auras, these are uncommon in childhood. Auras may be secondary to regional changes in blood flow. Characteristic auras include blurred vision, brightly colored lights, scotomata, and moving lights and zigzag lines said to look like the battlements of a castle (fortification spectra). Somatosensory auras include speech, motor, or sensory disturbances. Auras attributable to basilar artery symptoms cause the so-called Alice-in-Wonderland syndrome (distortions of vision, space, and time) and may also cause transient blindness. After the aura (or in the absence of aura), the headache usually occurs. Pain is characteristically pounding and usually is not maximal at onset. Anorexia, photophobia, and hyperacusis are common migraine accompaniments.

Focal motor deficits accompanying migraine (usually hemiplegia or ophthalmoplegia) are called **complicated migraine** and usually abate within hours. Although the condition usually is benign, patients with such syndromes may warrant imaging studies (MRI and magnetic resonance angiography [MRA]) even in the absence of localizing features on examination. Epilepsy and migraine commonly coexist, and headache may be an ictal or postictal symptom. EEG should be considered in all such patients, especially those with a history of postictal confusion during or after their headache.

Regional changes in blood flow and characteristic throbbing support a vascular contribution to migraine headaches. Numerous studies have suggested that serotonin plays a role in migraine, and serotonergic drugs (acting at 5 HT-1 receptors, sumatriptan), antiserotonergic drugs (acting at 5 HT-2 receptors, methysergide), and other drugs that alter serotonin metabolism appear to have some efficacy. Models for migraine suggest that external influences and serotonergic influences (both central and possibly peripheral from platelets) contribute to the brain and vascular changes seen in this disorder.

Cluster Headache. This is rare in childhood. Hemicranial pain usually begins around one eye and then spreads.

The headache is associated with tearing, conjunctival irritation, and other signs of autonomic dysfunction. Attacks usually are short but may recur daily for a number of weeks. Treatment includes oxygen, prednisone, lithium, or various anticonvulsant drugs.

Tension Headache. This is a diagnosis of exclusion and may account for chronic nonprogressive diffuse headaches that have a pounding quality. Some practitioners believe that daily headache is nonmigrainous and that such patients (at least those who have progressive headache) should undergo imaging studies to rule out increased intracranial pressure (ICP) as a cause of headache. Depression is not an uncommon accompaniment, and the findings of physical examination are normal. Therapy is similar to that for migraine headache.

Benign Intracranial Hypertension

Increased ICP in the absence of an intracranial lesion, infection, or hydrocephalus is called pseudotumor cerebri or **benign intracranial hypertension (BIH)** (Table 21–9). This syndrome may be seen in children of either sex, despite the fact that it occurs more frequently in women in the second and third decades during adulthood. The major morbidity of BIH is visual loss. Presenting signs usually are headache and visual change; diplopia secondary to sixth-nerve palsies occurs in 20% of patients. Nausea is common, and tinnitus has been described. BIH may be associated with numerous conditions, including otitic hydrocephalus (an intracranial venous sinus thrombosis secondary to acute and chronic otitis media); pregnancy; endocrinopathies; vitamin A toxicity; use of oral contraceptives, tetracycline, or nalidixic acid; iron deficiency anemia; and systemic lupus erythematosus.

Diagnosis and therapy are determined according to the results of LP. Opening and closing pressure must be recorded and used to guide how much CSF should be removed. Large-volume taps may be needed, and the closing pressure measurement should be less than 100 cm H_2O. Diuretic agents (such as acetazolamide) and corticosteroids have been used as adjuvant therapy. Severe cases unresponsive to medical therapy occasionally require lumboperitoneal shunting. Retinal sheath fenestra-

Table 21–9. Differential diagnosis of benign intracranial hypertension (BIH).

Symptomatic intracranial hypertension without localizing signs simulating BIH
Infection adjacent to cranial cavity—otitis media
Intracranial venous sinus thromboses
Endocrine and metabolic disorders (steroid administration)
Drugs and toxins
Systemic illness
Increased cerebrospinal fluid protein concentration
"Meningism" with systemic bacterial or viral infections
Idiopathic BIH

tion probably is not effective in preserving optic nerve function in these patients.

Treatment

The pharmacologic treatment of headache is divided into two components, abortive and prophylactic (Table 21–10). **Abortive** therapies are aimed at individuals with rare headaches, fewer than two per week. These therapies include acetaminophen or nonsteroidal anti-inflammatory agents. Newer therapies include dihydroergotamine and sumatriptan, although experience is limited with these agents in children. In particular, sumatriptan should be avoided in children with basilar artery symptoms (eg, vertigo), as this drug theoretically may worsen existing vasospasm in such patients.

In children with more frequent headaches, **prophylactic** therapy is initiated on a daily basis to decrease headache frequency. Commonly used abortive medications included β-blockers (acting through central mechanisms), cyproheptadine, other tricyclic antidepressants, and valproic acid. These drugs usually take a number of days before an effect is seen, and dosages must be increased steadily until an effect is realized. Propranolol is the drug used most commonly, but its use is limited in patients with asthma or heart disease. It is given initially at 2 mg/kg in divided doses but also may be given once daily in much higher doses. Cyproheptadine is given in a split dose of 0.2–0.4 mg/kg; the dose is increased as needed. Valproic acid is used in the dose and frequency ranges required for anticonvulsant activity. Biofeedback also may be effective in treating headaches.

Most patients with headache respond to treatment but often require a number of different therapies before one becomes successful. Treatment usually is continued for 6 months. At that time, if the patient is free of headaches while receiving treatment, therapy may be discontinued. The natural history of migraine is poorly documented, but a number of children can be expected to "outgrow" their headaches. Many children will have headaches that recur while they are not receiving therapy, and the migraine may require treatment for longer periods of time.

COMA

Pathophysiology

Coma, which refers to a deep state of unconsciousness from which the patient cannot be aroused, may accompany an array of neurologic conditions. Speech is absent, the eyes are closed, and there is no purposeful movement of the limbs. This is in contrast to **stupor,** in which the patient can be aroused during periods of vigorous stimulation; **obtundation,** in which the patient can be aroused during and after periods of vigorous stimulation; and **lethargy,** which is a state of sleepiness.

Coma requires a disorganization of both awareness and arousal. **Awareness** is the ability to recognize the external world and requires input from both hemispheres. **Arousal** is equivalent to wakefulness, which is evidenced by the ability to open both eyes spontaneously or in response to external stimuli. Arousal requires activation of the reticular activating system, which is a brainstem structure in the midbrain and the pons. Arousal can exist without awareness, as is seen in patients with bi-hemispheric injury, and is characterized by a persistent vegetative state. Disturbances of arousal and awareness may be the result of structural lesions, diffuse encephalopathies, and SE (Table 21–11). Structural lesions are neoplastic, infectious, or traumatic in origin. They can cause altered consciousness by impinging directly on brain structures and by causing downward or uncal herniation. Diffuse encephalopathies can be caused by metabolic abnormalities or toxic ingestions, usually are symmetric, and feature preservation of pupillary light reflexes. Seizures may occur in the absence of motor accompaniments and can be followed by a deep postictal period, especially in patients with preexisting brain damage.

Mass Lesions. Expanding supratentorial masses can be associated with somnolence from compression of the contralateral hemisphere or the inferior diencephalon (Figure 21–1). Somnolence progresses to stupor and

Table 21–10. Treatment of headache.

Prophylaxis Agent	Dose (mg/kg)
Propranolol	2.0
Cyproheptadine	0.2–0.1
Valproic acid	25
Tricyclic antidepressants	15 mg every night to start

Abortive Agent	Comment
Oxygen	Best for cluster headahces
Sumatriptan	Not indicated for basilar migraine
Cafergot	Use only at onset
Dihydroergotamine (DHE 45)	Best for intractable migraine

Table 21–11. Causes of coma.

Structural	Mass lesions
Metabolic	Anoxic-ischemic coma
	Hypoglycemia
	Hyperglycemia
	Hyponatremia and SIADH
	Hepatic dysfunction
	Renal failure
Toxins	Lead
	Sedative and hypnotic drugs
Trauma	Head injuries
Infection	Meningitis, encephalitis, severe generalized infection
Nonconvulsive status epilepticus	

SIADH = syndrome of inappropriate antidiuretic hormone.

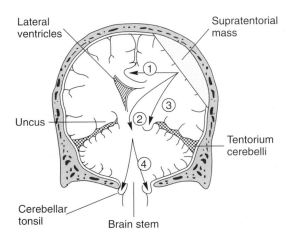

Lateral ventricles

Uncus

Cerebellar tonsil

Supratentorial mass

Tentorium cerebelli

Brain stem

Figure 21–1. Anatomic basis of herniation syndromes. An expanding supratentorial mass lesion may cause brain tissue to be displaced into an adjacent intracranial compartment, resulting in *(1)* cingulate herniation under the falx, *(2)* downward transtentorial (central) herniation, *(3)* uncal herniation over the edge of the tentorium, or *(4)* cerebellar tonsillar herniation into the foramen magnum. Coma and ultimately death result when *(2)*, *(3)*, or *(4)* produces brainstem compression. (Reproduced, with permission, from: Greenberg DA et al: *Clinical Neurology,* 2nd ed. Appleton & Lange, 1993.)

coma, and such progressive downward transtentorial herniation is usually fatal once the pons is affected. Supratentorial masses also can cause herniation of the uncus across the tentorium cerebelli, causing compression of the midbrain and oculomotor nerve. Subtentorial herniation is usually of sudden onset and features focal brainstem signs.

Anoxic & Ischemic Coma. Acute anoxia causes coma rapidly, whereas ischemia leads to a more gradual depression of consciousness. Causes include failure of the heart, lungs, and neuromuscular systems. Acute ischemia or anoxia is seen after blood pressure falls accompanying cardiac arrest and in suffocation. Consciousness is lost quickly, followed by seizures and decerebrate rigidity. Cerebral edema may build up over 72 hours after arrest and can be associated with herniation. Physical examination and EEG evaluation can be used to prognosticate. Patients with no pupillary responses immediately after arrest usually do poorly, as do patients lacking pupillary and motor responses at 24 hours. Burst suppression or flat-line patterns on EEG also are associated with bad outcomes.

Infection. Bacterial, viral, and fungal agents all can cause meningoencephalitis associated with coma. Infants may have fever, irritability, and a full fontanelle; meningeal irritation can be assessed in the older child by neck stiffness, knee flexion during neck flexion (Kernig sign), or inability to extend the leg completely when the thigh is flexed on the trunk of a supine patient (Brudzinski sign).

The organisms causing meningoencephalitis are discussed in Chapter 9.

Hypoglycemia. Hypoglycemia usually is a complication of insulin excess but may occur in newborn infants with metabolic disorders (see Chapter 6). Symptoms usually appear with blood glucose levels less than 50 mg/dL. Symptoms initially include dizziness and restlessness and progress to depressed consciousness and coma. Seizures may occur, as may focal neurologic signs that can alternate from side to side. Treatment involves administration of glucose, and outcome is a function of the duration of hypoglycemia. Most children fully recover.

Hyperglycemia. Diabetic ketoacidosis may be the presenting feature of insulin-dependent diabetes mellitus; it also may occur in patients with known diabetes. Children have a metabolic acidosis with a compensatory respiratory alkalosis. Fatigue may progress rapidly to coma, and mortality approaches 10%. Cerebral edema usually accompanies this disorder and is caused largely by parenteral administration of hypotonic fluid. This disorder is discussed in Chapter 20.

Hypernatremia. Dehydration may be associated with water loss in excess of sodium and may be aggravated by administering hypertonic fluids to such patients. A rapid decrease in serum sodium levels also contributes to encephalopathy in these patients. Venous sinus thrombosis is a further complication of dehydration and may cause focal neurologic signs in these patients. Treatment involves a slow but steady restoration of fluid losses.

Hyponatremia & Syndrome of Inappropriate Antidiuretic Hormone Secretion (SIADH). Hyponatremia may accompany dehydration in which sodium is lost in excess of solute (as seen in vomiting and diarrhea); it also may be caused by SIADH. Hyponatremia results in swelling of cells in the brain and may be accompanied by vomiting, lethargy and coma, and seizures. Serum sodium concentration in such patients usually is less than 125 meq/L, but the rate of sodium decrease is also a factor in the clinical presentation. Rapid overcorrection of serum sodium levels may be associated with central pontine myelinolysis; therefore, sodium deficits should be replaced over 1–2 days. SIADH is seen primarily in patients with meningitis, head trauma, and pulmonary disease. These patients inappropriately dilute their urine in spite of serum hyponatremia and may progress to seizures and coma if they do not receive treatment. Diagnosis is determined by simultaneous measurement of serum and urine osmolality. The disorder usually is transient and responds to fluid restriction. (See discussion in Chapter 20.)

Hepatic Dysfunction. Hepatic failure can lead to coma, as seen in hepatitis, acute acetaminophen overdosage, or other toxic exposures. A number of inborn errors of metabolism feature hepatic dysfunction and can result in coma. A once-frequent cause of hepatic dysfunction and coma is Reye syndrome. This mitochondrial disorder may accompany viral infection and subsequent salicylate ingestion. The disorder progresses from vomiting to progressive confusion, delirium, and coma with decorticate and then decerebrate posturing. The final stage features flaccidity, apnea, and fixed, dilated pupils. Laboratory examination demonstrates hypoglycemia, hyperammonemia, and elevated serum transaminase levels. Liver biopsy is diagnostic. Differential diagnosis includes primary carnitine deficiency, ornithine transcarbamylase deficiency, and valproic acid hepatotoxicity. Children with Reye syndrome should undergo a full examination for inborn errors of metabolism. Treatment is supportive and aimed mainly at controlling ICP.

Renal Failure. Coma is rarely seen as a complication of uremia, but confusion and lethargy are common, and myoclonus, tetany, and frank seizures may follow. Asterixis (a flapping tremor of extended hands or feet) is an early sign. Renal failure causes depression of consciousness through a number of mechanisms, including increases in blood urea nitrogen concentration, hyperammonemia, and other ion disturbances. Hypertensive encephalopathy may accompany renal failure and contributes to alterations in consciousness. Treatment involves dialysis, which usually reverses the encephalopathy.

Toxic Ingestions. Toxic ingestions commonly cause depression of consciousness. In general, smaller children ingest household products, whereas older children ingest sedative or hypnotic drugs. Coma caused by many such drugs characteristically features preservation of the pupillary responses and loss of extraocular movements. Diagnosis usually requires urine and serum toxicology screens. Treatment depends on the ingested substance but usually is supportive. Gastric cleansing and specific antidotes may be helpful.

Head Trauma. Dural hematomas may cause alteration in consciousness, often occurring hours after the initial injury. Subdural hematomas may result from relatively minor head injury and usually are venous in origin. Epidural hematomas usually are associated with skull fractures and with tearing of the middle meningeal artery and vein. Complications include focal neurologic deficits, cerebral edema, and herniation. Diagnosis usually requires imaging by head CT. Surgical evacuation may be lifesaving.

Nonaccidental trauma is an all too common form of child abuse in young children. Typically, an infant is shaken, resulting in tearing of bridging cerebral and retinal veins, and optic sheath hemorrhages occur. The child usually is unconscious and seizing, with a bulging fontanelle. Diagnostic evaluation includes a dilated funduscopic examination, head CT, and skeletal survey. Treatment is supportive and may require hematoma evacuation. Outcome depends on the degree of injury but usually is poor because of **diffuse axonal injury.**

Diagnosis & Management

Airway, breathing, and circulation should be assessed initially, as discussed in Chapter 10. Dextrose should be given parenterally, as hypoglycemic coma is a common metabolic encephalopathy and is easily treated. The goal of management is to identify and treat acute life-threatening abnormalities quickly. A systematic examination is performed to determine whether anatomic abnormalities exist. The results of the examination dictate the course of therapy. The physical examination should focus on traumatic injury, specifically for CSF leaks; the existence of tympanic hematomas, Battle sign (ecchymoses over the mastoids), and raccoon eyes (indicating basilar fracture) should be carefully excluded. Blood pressure should be recorded, because an increase can result from intracranial hypertension (Cushing triad—hypertension, bradycardia, and respiratory abnormalities). A stiff neck or other meningeal signs might indicate infection, subarachnoid blood, or herniation, although these signs are unreliable before the age of 2 years.

The neurologic examination should be done in its entirety but rests principally on findings in three areas: pupillary response, eye movements, and motor examination (Figure 21–2).

Pupils usually are reactive in metabolic disorders. The absence of a pupillary light reaction implies structural abnormalities or administration of mydriatic drugs. Small, reactive pupils may be associated with a bilateral Horner syndrome (ptosis, meiosis, anhydrosis) and can be seen with thalamic damage with early herniation, involving the descending sympathetic chain. Midbrain lesions are associated with midline, fixed, dilated pupils from compression of the parasympathetic fibers in the third nerve. Pinpoint pupils are associated with pontine lesions (or opiate toxicity).

Extraocular movements can be tested by oculocephalic (doll's eye) or oculovestibular (cold water caloric) maneuvers. In the doll's eye test, the head is rotated by the examiner, and eye movements are observed. In the absence of a response, cold water is instilled into one ear, causing tonic deviation of the eye toward the stimulated side. A normal response bilaterally indicates intact brainstem function, whereas a unilateral abnormality may result from structural damage.

The **motor response** to pain is assessed by sternal rub. The best response is purposeful withdrawal, which can be distinguished from reflexive withdrawal by testing a movement that requires limb abduction. Abnormal posturing can be decorticate (elbow flexion, shoulder adduction, leg extension) and decerebrate (elbow extension, internal shoulder rotation, and leg extension). Decorticate posturing indicates a lesion of the thalamus, often from compression. Decerebrate posturing implies midbrain or diffuse brain damage. Lesions of the pons and medulla are often associated with no response to pain.

Laboratory investigations should be individualized but must address structural, infectious, and metabolic causes of coma. CT or MRI should be performed if mass lesions are suspected. An LP (with opening pressure measurement) must be done if the differential diagnosis includes meningitis or encephalitis. LP may be associated with herniation if an intracranial mass lesion is present; imaging before LP may be helpful in this regard. Laboratory stud-

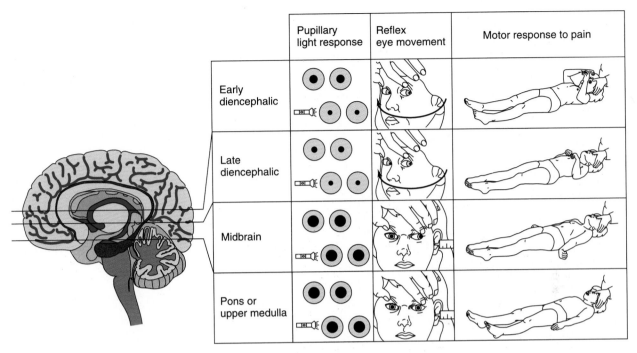

Figure 21–2. Neurologic signs in coma with downward transtentorial herniation. In the early diencephalic phase, the pupils are small (approximately 2 mm in diameter) and reactive, reflex eye movements are intact, and the motor response to pain is purposeful or semi-purposeful (localizing) and often asymmetric. The late diencephalic phase is associated with similar findings, except that painful stimulation results in decorticate (flexor) posturing, which also may be asymmetric. With midbrain involvement, the pupils are fixed and midsized (approximately 5 mm in diameter), reflex adduction of the eyes is impaired, and pain elicits decerebrate (extensor) posturing. Progression to involve the pons or medulla also produces fixed, midsized pupils, but these are accompanied by loss of reflex abduction, as well as adduction, of the eyes, and by no motor response or only leg flexion on painful stimulation. Note that although a lesion restricted to the pons produces pinpoint pupils as a result of the destruction of descending sympathetic (pupillodilator) pathways, downward herniation to the pontine level is associated with midsized pupils. This happens because herniation also interrupts parasympathetic (pupilloconstrictor) fibers in the oculomotor (III) nerve. (Reproduced, with permission, from: Greenberg DA et al: *Clinical Neurology,* 2nd ed. Appleton & Lange, 1993.)

ies to consider include CBC, erythrocyte sedimentation rate, blood glucose and electrolyte concentrations, liver function tests, ammonia level, and blood and urine toxicology screen and osmolality. An EEG may be indicated if seizures are a suspected etiology of coma.

BRAIN DEATH & PERSISTENT VEGETATIVE STATE

Brain death in adults and children requires irreversible cessation of all cortical and brainstem function. Hypoglycemia, sedative medication, hypothermia, neuromuscular blockade, and shock must be excluded before an individual can be pronounced brain dead. The criteria for brain death are summarized in Table 21–12. A diagnostic approach is presented in Figure 21–3.

The persistent vegetative state refers to a state of arousal without awareness seen in some patients after recovery from coma. The patient may have physiologic sleep-wake cycles, spontaneous eye opening, and intact brainstem functions. Diagnosis requires that the patient is at no time aware of self or environment. Patients in a persistent vegetative state may survive for years, and discontinuation of therapy, nutrition, and hydration may be considered in some cases.

INCREASED INTRACRANIAL PRESSURE

After closure of the fontanelles and sutures, the skull contents are fixed into a rigid space. The pressure in that space is derived from the components of the intracranial space, ie, the brain, blood, and CSF. Altering cerebral blood flow, increasing CSF resorption, and compression

Table 21–12. Guidelines for determination
of brain death in children.[1]

A. History: Determine the cause of coma to eliminate remediable or reversible conditions.
B. Physical examination criteria
 1. Coma and apnea
 2. Absence of brainstem function
  a. Midposition or fully dilated pupils
  b. Absence of spontaneous oculocephalic (doll's eyes) and caloric-induced eye movements
  c. Absence of movement of bulbar musculature and corneal, gag, cough, sucking, and rooting reflexes
  d. Absence of respiratory effort with standardized testing for apnea
 3. Patient must not be hypothermic or hypotensive.
 4. Flaccid tone and absence of spontaneous or induced movements excluding activity mediated at the spinal cord level
 5. Examination should remain consistent for brain death throughout predetermined period of observation.
C. Observation period according to age
 1. 7 d to 2 mo: two examinations and EEGs 48 h apart
 2. 2 mo to 1 y: two examinations and EEGs 24 h apart or one examination and an initial EEG showing ECS combined with a radionuclide angiogram showing no CBF, or both
 3. > 1 y: two examinations 12–24 h apart; EEG and isotope angiography optional

[1]Reproduced, with permission, from Berg: *Clinical Neurology. A Clinical Manual,* 2nd ed. Lippincott, 1994.
CBF = cerebral blood flow; ECS = electrocerebral silence.

of brain parenchyma are the main mechanisms available to relieve pressure. Spreading of unfused cranial bones is another adaptive mechanism seen in infancy.

Cerebrospinal Fluid

Normal CSF is clear and colorless. Clouding occurs when there are approximately 400 cells/mm^3. Xanthochromia is cell-free yellow fluid. Pigments causing xanthochromia include oxyhemoglobin, bilirubin, and methemoglobin. A protein concentration greater than 150 mg/dL will result in binding to bilirubin and cause a yellow hue. Normal infants have yellow CSF from high protein and bilirubin levels. Neonates have up to 32 cells/mm^3 (mean, 6–7) and have protein concentrations of 20–170 mg/dL (mean, 73). CSF glucose level is usually two thirds of plasma values but can also be closer to plasma levels. Protein concentrations decrease during the first few months of life: 20–100 mg/dL at 1–3 months, 15–50 mg/dL at 3–6 months, and 15–20 mg/dL at 6 months to 10 years.

CSF is absorbed via arachnoid villi and granulations found in the intracranial venous sinuses and along emerging spinal nerve roots. CSF production is approximately 0.35 mL/min, and ventricular volume in adults is 150 mL. Carbonic anhydrase in the choroid plexus is important for CSF formation, and the carbonic anhydrase inhibitor ac-

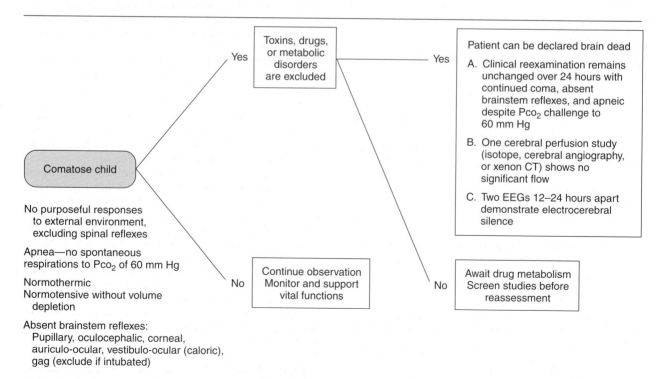

Figure 21–3. Sequential decisions in determining brain death. CT = computed tomography; EEG = electroencephalogram; Pco$_2$ = partial pressure of carbon dioxide. (Reproduced, with permission, from: Swaimann KF: *Pediatric Neurology. Principles and Practice,* 2nd ed. Mosby-Year Book, 1994.)

etazolamide (Diamox) has been shown to reduce CSF flow and formation.

General Clinical Features

CSF pressure in children younger than 8 years usually is less than 100 cm H_2O. In older children and adults, CSF pressure is less than 200 cm H_2O. The presenting features of a child with increased ICP are a function of age. In infancy, the fontanelle may be bulging, cranial sutures may separate, and head circumference may increase. With continued increases in ICP, infants vomit, fail to thrive, and, sometimes, have impaired upgaze (sun-setting sign) from pressure on the midbrain tectum. The Cushing triad (hypertension, bradycardia, and respiratory irregularities) may be present. In older children and adults, headache, sometimes associated with vomiting, is the usual presenting symptom of increased ICP. This headache probably results from stretching of intracranial vessels and may be focal or generalized. The headache may have a postural component; it decreases when the patient rises to a standing position. The sixth nerve may also be involved, as evidenced by abducens palsy or diplopia.

With prolonged increases in ICP, venous return from the retina may be compromised, leading to loss of venous pulsations and papilledema. Flame hemorrhages and nerve fiber infarcts (cotton-wool spots) may be present. Papilledema must be distinguished from drusen, a normal variant in which the disk is congenitally elevated.

General Therapeutic Considerations

The child with increased ICP requires emergent diagnostic evaluation. Given the risk of herniation, LP is contraindicated until obstructive mass lesions are ruled out. Treatment of elevated ICP depends on the cause, but palliative measures include head elevation to 30 degrees, hyperventilation (to constrict arterial inflow), and osmotic diuresis. Vasogenic edema induced by mass lesions may respond to corticosteroids. The efficacy of barbiturate coma for management of increased ICP is controversial.

Causes of Increased Intracranial Pressure

The conditions causing increased ICP are presented in Table 21–13.

Cerebral Edema. Brain swelling due to cerebral edema is an important cause of increased ICP. Such swelling results in increased CNS water content and can

Table 21–13. Causes of increased intracranial pressure.

Cerebral edema
Tumors
Epidural hematoma and subdural hematoma
Hydrocephalus
Subarachnoid hemorrhage
Central nervous system infections
Toxins

be divided into three principal forms: vasogenic, cytotoxic, and interstitial (Table 21–14).

Hydrocephalus. This is caused by obstruction to CSF outflow, which leads to ventricular dilatation. The white matter is affected preferentially because oligodendroglial cells and astrocytes appear to be especially vulnerable to pressure-induced injury. Cranial ultrasound will reveal the ventricular dilatation before actual head enlargement occurs. This progressive subclinical dilatation probably has associated morbidity: Studies have shown impaired blood velocity in cerebral arteries and abnormal visual evoked potentials in these babies, which are correctable after shunting. It is unclear whether irreversible injury occurs during the period of ventricular dilatation before overt head enlargement.

In approaching an infant at risk for hydrocephalus, certain physical findings are helpful. Head circumference should be measured in all children; in babies, a head circumference above the 90th percentile has a high correlation with ventricular enlargement. Only 15% of babies with hydrocephalus will have evidence of increased ICP. The anterior fontanelle and cranial sutures should be examined carefully. With rapidly progressive hydrocephalus, apnea, decreased alertness, and oculomotor abnormalities can occur. Management of rapidly evolving hydrocephalus requires neurosurgical intervention. Mortality may be as high as 60% in untreated cases. Management for more indolent cases is directed at controlling hydrocephalus, but treatment options toward this end remain controversial. Serial LP may be performed, but this procedure has no proven efficacy for preventing hydrocephalus. External drains and diuretic drugs may be considered.

Subarachnoid Hemorrhage. This may result from trauma or may reflect an underlying vascular abnormality such as aneurysm or arteriovenous malformation (AVM). Bleeding may be dramatic, with sudden loss of consciousness and increased ICP. More commonly, the lesions bleed indolently, causing headache and occasionally focal neurologic signs. In traumatic subarachnoid hemorrhage, blood products may accumulate slowly, and children become difficult to arouse hours after the head injury. Diagnosis is determined by imaging or LP, but angiography may be required. If subarachnoid hemorrhage is suspected, CSF should be spun immediately after LP, and supernatant fluid should be examined for xanthochromia. A useful pearl is that xanthochromia is first seen in half a day, peaks in half a week, and resolves in half a month. Because large aneurysmal subarachnoid hemorrhages usually are lethal, diagnosis of sentinel bleeds is imperative. Aneurysms are contained by neurosurgical clipping, whereas AVMs may be more difficult to access. AVMs may require initial treatment by interventional neuroradiology to reduce arterial inflow before neurosurgical excision.

Brain Tumors. The most common solid tumor of childhood, brain tumor, frequently presents with increased ICP from both localized edema and obstruction of CSF outflow. Most tumors are supratentorial in children younger

Table 21–14. Types of cerebral edema.

	Vasogenic	Cytotoxic	Interstitial
Pathogenesis	Increased capillary permeability	Cellular swelling	Blocked CSF absorption
Location of edema	White matter	Grey and white matter	Periventricular white matter
Clinical disorders	Tumors/abscess, infarction, trauma, ischemia, meningitis	Hypoxia, ischemia, meningitis	Obstructive hydrocephalus, meningitis
Steroids indicated	Yes	No	Uncertain

CSF = cerebrospinal fluid.

than 2 years and infratentorial in later childhood. Brain tumors in children and adults usually are glial in origin, although posterior fossa neuronal tumors (medulloblastomas), ependymal tumors, and choroid plexus tumors also occur (Tables 21–15 and 21–16). Tumors usually cause breakdown of the blood-brain barrier and therefore are best seen with contrast enhanced imaging. Most childhood tumors arise in the posterior fossa, an area prone to CT scatter artifact. Therefore, MRI is the imaging modality of choice. Treatment and outcome depend on location and on tumor type. Surgical removal and postoperative radiation therapy are the usual treatment modalities. Therapeutic advances in this area have been disappointing.

Epidural & Subdural Hematomas. Epidural and subdural hematomas resulting from head trauma are discussed above (see section on Coma). IVH is commonly seen in premature infants and may cause an acute or indolent ventricular dilatation. In acute cases, clotted blood may obstruct CSF absorption through obstruction of arachnoid villi. In chronic cases, hemorrhage leads to an obliterative arachnoiditis with blockade of CSF flow. Rarely, aqueductal obstruction occurs from debris and gliosis in that area.

Infections. Infections of the brain and meninges are commonly associated with increased ICP. Infections cause edema secondary to inflammation and may impair venous outflow and CSF resorption. Common infections of the brain and meninges in childhood are discussed in Chapter 9.

Toxins. Toxins may cause increased ICP; lead is the most common toxin. Exposure of children to lead-based paint continues to be a major environmental hazard, although most of these cases are chronic ingestions that lead to long-term intellectual disabilities but not to acute toxicity. Severe lead encephalopathy may start insidiously, with gastrointestinal disturbances and irritability, and then progress to decreased level of consciousness and seizures. Diagnosis is determined by ascertaining serum lead levels, by basophilic stippling on blood smear, and by the presence of lead lines on bone radiographs. Treatment is aimed at reducing ICP and chelating lead from blood, as well as removing unabsorbed lead from the gastrointestinal tract. Mortality may be as high as 50%, and many survivors have residual seizures and other residua of brain injury.

Increased ICP in the absence of an intracranial lesion, infection, or hydrocephalus is called benign intracranial hypertension or pseudotumor cerebri. This condition is discussed above.

WEAKNESS

Evaluation

In assessing a child with weakness, it is important to distinguish static from evolving lesions and to determine whether the pattern of weakness reflects a central or pe-

Table 21–15. Types of brain tumors in childhood.

Tumor Type	Incidence (%)
Glial origin	
Astrocytoma	
Cystic, solid cerebellar astrocytoma	20–30
Brainstem glioma	10–20
Optic nerve, chiasm, hypothalamic glioma	5
Cerebellar hemispheric astrocytoma	8
Medulloblastoma	18
Ependymoma	8
Nonglial origin	
Craniopharyngioma	5
Choroid plexus papilloma	< 0.5
Pineal region tumors	1
Meningioma	1
Metastatic tumors	Unknown

Table 21–16. Clinical manifestations of brain tumors in childhood.

Increased intracranial pressure
  Headache, stiff neck
  Vomiting
  Impaired vision
    Papilledema
    Cranial nerve dysfunction
  Head enlargement

Focal neurologic signs
  Cranial nerve dysfunction
  Corticospinal tract dysfunction
  Cerebellar dysfunction
  Endocrine abnormalities
  Visual loss (optic nerve or craniopharyngioma)
  Seizures

ripheral lesion. Lower motor neuron weakness usually reflects a disordered motor unit. The differential diagnosis of lower motor neuron weakness is narrowed further by identifying the site of pathology within the motor unit (Table 21–17).

In older children, upper motor neuron lesions present with spasticity, hyperreflexia, and a Babinski sign, whereas lower motor neuron abnormalities feature hypotonia and hyporeflexia. In infancy, however, the motor examination may be similar in upper and lower motor neuron diseases. CNS dysfunction usually does not present with isolated weakness but with hypotonia and increased stretch reflexes. Other signs of CNS involvement, such as encephalopathy, spasticity, cortical thumbing, and exaggerated or persistent primitive reflexes (tonic neck, Moro), usually are present and aid in localizing the site of pathology. A few disorders present with both upper and lower motor neuron disease. In diseases such as mitochondrial encephalomyelopathies and metachromatic leukodystrophy, the upper motor neuron injury is profound. Other lower motor neuron diseases, such as myotonic and Duchenne dystrophy, may have more subtle signs of upper motor neuron dysfunction. These are discussed later in this section.

Clinical Assessment

Weakness in infancy may present as motor delay, whereas weakness in childhood is often manifest by difficulty in keeping up with peers. In assessing the infant with weakness, power is measured on a three-point scale: movement against gravity, movement insufficient to overcome gravity, and lack of movement. Appendicular tone in infants is measured as in adults, whereas central or postural tone should be assessed by analyzing head lag and horizontal and vertical suspension. In older children, power is measured on a five-point scale, as in the adult.

The distinction between neuropathic and myopathic weakness can be difficult. The distribution of weakness may reflect the distribution of a particular root or peripheral nerve. Fasciculations are specific for disease of the anterior horn cell. Reflexes in myopathy are said to reflect the degree of weakness, whereas in neuropathy, the reflexes may be markedly diminished in the presence of minor degrees of weakness. In many cases, electromyography (EMG) with nerve conduction can help localize and classify neuropathy versus myopathy. Muscle and or

nerve biopsy also may be indicated in selected individuals.

The physical examination of a weak ambulatory child should include observation of the child's ability to rise from a sitting position without using the hands to push or pull off the floor. In the presence of pelvic girdle muscle weakness, a child will use the hands to climb up the body; this is referred to as the Gower maneuver (Figure 21–4).

Power in large leg muscles may be assessed by having the patient hop on either foot and perform a deep knee bend. Heel and toe walking should be observed. In testing power, the examiner should also palpate tested muscles for texture and signs of muscle atrophy. In particular, minor degrees of weakness may be best seen in small distal muscles, where weakness and wasting are most evident.

Table 21–17. Anatomic location of weakness.

Upper motor neuron	Static encephalopathy (cerebral palsy), spasticity, rigidity
Anterior horn cell	Spinal muscular atrophy, poliomyelitis
Peripheral nerve	Demyelinating and axonal neuropathies
Neuromuscular junction	Myasthenia, neonatal botulism
Muscle	Muscular dystrophy and congenital and acquired myopathies

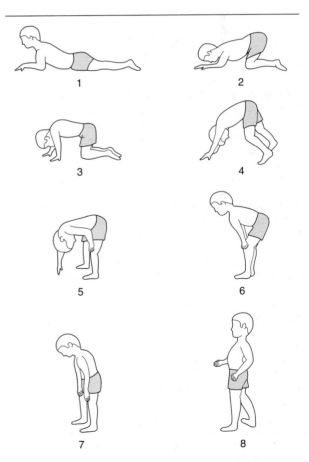

Figure 21–4. The Gower maneuver showing sequence of postures used in getting up from the ground: *1,* lying prone; *2, 3,* getting onto hands and knees; *4,* legs and arms extended and legs brought as close as possible to arms; *5,* hand placed on knee; *6,* both hands on knees, knees extended; *7,* hands move alternately up thighs ("climbing up himself"); *8,* erect posture. (Reproduced, with permission, from: Dubowitz V: *Muscle Disorders in Childhood,* 2nd ed. Saunders, 1995.)

Cerebral Palsy

Cerebral palsy is not a disease, but rather a constellation of physical signs. In 1990, at an international conference in Brioni, Yugoslavia, a definition was developed stating that cerebral palsy is a "term covering a group of nonprogressive, but often changing, motor impairment syndromes secondary to lesions or anomalies of the brain arising in the early stages of development." It is a diagnosis that cannot be made until after the age of 2 years. Some pediatric neurologists prefer to call this category of diseases "static encephalopathy." In addition to these motor impairments, children with cerebral palsy often have other disabilities, such as epilepsy, visual and motor handicaps, and learning difficulties. Recent epidemiologic studies have associated risk of development of cerebral palsy with such conditions as preterm delivery, twin pregnancies, fetal growth retardation, and perinatal asphyxia. Children at risk should be identified early in life so that appropriate interventions can be instituted.

Diseases of the Spinal Cord

Myelitis. Transverse myelitis is a demyelinating disorder of the spinal cord that evolves rapidly and may involve other areas of the brain (acute disseminated encephalomyelitis) or the optic nerve (Devic disease). These disorders may be post- or para-infectious, although there is no clear evidence of an infectious or postinfectious etiology. Patients usually have both central and peripheral patterns of weakness.

Transverse myelitis occurs mainly in school-aged children, with maximal deficit within days of onset. Most children recover with no or minimal residua, but 10% may not recover. Diagnosis is determined by MRI, and corticosteroids (prednisone) are used in most patients on the basis of efficacy noted in case reports. A sensory level should be determined (using sweat level or temperature localization) and followed through the course of disease. Many children with bladder dysfunction will not be aware of this, and postvoid residuals must be measured.

Myelomeningocele. Abnormalities of neural tube closure that involve the spinal cord are called myelomeningocele. The neural tube starts as a flat plate of cells and forms a tube by 6 weeks' gestation. Prevention of neural tube defects, therefore, must be aimed at women planning their pregnancies, as the tube usually closes before most women know they are pregnant. Most of these lesions occur in the thoracolumbar cord, and many occur in conjunction with a Chiari II abnormality. The Chiari malformation consists of inferior displacement of the medulla, fourth ventricle, and lower cerebellum into the upper cervical cord; elongation and thinning of the medulla and pons with persistence of the embryonic "S"-shaped flexure of these structures; and bony abnormalities of the foramen magnum, occiput, and upper cervical vertebrae. This malformation causes hydrocephalus secondary to the hindbrain malformation with concomitant blockade of CSF outflow from aqueductal stenosis, which occurs in more than 50% of cases as an associated malformation.

In approaching the child with myelomeningocele or suspected myelomeningocele, the skin defect should be kept clean and free of infectious agents. A sensory and motor level should be assessed, and postvoid residuals measured. The skin defect should not be probed. Diagnosis usually is made by physical examination, but all children should undergo a head ultrasound study to exclude hydrocephalus. Early surgical intervention ensures the best outcome and probably is indicated in all cases. The most effective treatment is prevention; supplemental folate given to the mother in early pregnancy reduces the incidence of neural tube defects.

Tethered Cord. Children with midline cord defects may have an underlying abnormality that tethers the spinal cord and causes it to stretch during linear growth. A child with tethered cord may present with gait disorders, asymmetric reflexes in the lower extremities, or incontinence. In children with no known midline defect, MRI is the study of choice. In a child with a known midline defect, imaging studies have limited utility, as the cords of most such children appear tethered on MRI. Diagnosis in such children relies on the history and physical examination. Neurosurgical intervention is indicated to prevent progression. Surgery may not reverse existing deficits, however, so early diagnosis of these disorders is essential.

Diseases of the Anterior Horn Cell

Spinal Muscular Atrophy. The spinal muscular atrophies are characterized by progressive loss of anterior horn cells with subsequent loss of the peripheral nerves and muscles provided by those nerves. Although these disorders are named on the basis of age of onset and may follow characteristic courses (Table 21–18), most cases in all pediatric age groups are linked to the same genetic locus on chromosome $5q$. The biology of anterior horn cell death in these disorders is poorly understood.

Clinically, the spinal muscular atrophies are characterized by weakness, hypotonia, and hyporeflexia. Muscle bulk is diminished, and fasciculations may be present. Infants may show paradoxical breathing. The diaphragm, which is spared early in the disease, descends in inspiration, with consequent abdominal distention and intercostal retraction (Figure 21–5). Intellect is characteristically

Table 21–18. Clinical classification of progressive spinal muscular atrophies (PSMA).

Type	Onset	Course	Life Expectancy
Werdnig-Hoffmann disease (PSMA type I)	Birth to 6 mo	Never sits	< 2 y
Werdnig-Hoffmann disease, intermediate type (PSMA type II)	6–18 mo	Never stands	Variable
Kugelberg-Welander disease, chronic form (PSMA type III)	> 18 mo	Stands	Variable

spared in the spinal muscular atrophies, and the image of an alert and expressive infant who is unable to oppose gravity is a particularly sad and striking feature.

Poliomyelitis. Poliomyelitis is an infection of the anterior horn cell (see Chapter 9). The course differs from that of spinal muscular atrophy in that weakness follows a febrile illness featuring CSF pleocytosis and is usually asymmetric.

Diseases of the Peripheral Nerve

Bell Palsy. The seventh nerve may become compressed and demyelinated in response to inflammation within the facial canal or the stylomastoid foramen. Children with idiopathic facial nerve dysfunction (Bell palsy) present with paralysis of one side of the face over a period of hours. Diagnosis is based on clinical examination, the results of which should be otherwise normal, and should include examination of the ipsilateral ear for herpetic lesions. Herpes infection of the geniculate ganglion (Ramsay Hunt syndrome) can mimic Bell palsy and may be treated with antiviral agents, such as acyclovir. Treatment of Bell palsy in children usually is not indicated, as full recovery in the absence of treatment is the rule. Although

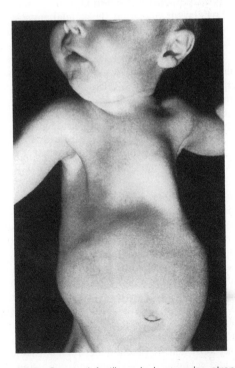

Figure 21–5. Severe infantile spinal muscular atrophy in a 3-month-old infant showing marked respiratory deficit with intercostal paralysis and reduction in chest size and marked costal recession, with normal diaphragmatic function. (Note alert, expressive face.) (Reproduced, with permission, from: Dubowitz V: *Muscle Disorders in Childhood,* 2nd ed. Saunders, 1995.)

prednisone is widely used early in the disease in adults, it is rarely used in children.

Recurrent facial nerve palsy (Melkersson-Rosenthal syndrome) is thought to be a genetic disorder because there is often a family history. The triad for diagnosis is facial swelling, facial nerve palsy, and fissured tongue.

Acute & Chronic Inflammatory Demyelinating Polyneuropathy. Acute inflammatory demyelinating polyneuropathy (the Guillain-Barré syndrome) is an acute monophasic illness characterized by demyelination of peripheral nerves. A symmetric ascending weakness may progress rapidly, and involvement of respiratory musculature can be life-threatening. Involvement of the facial musculature, autonomic insufficiency, and sensory involvement may accompany the muscular weakness. Diagnosis is by nerve conduction studies showing demyelination and by LP showing elevation of protein concentration in the absence of a pleocytosis in the CSF. Treatment involves plasmapheresis or γ-globulin infusion, suggesting an immune-mediated etiology. Full recovery is the rule, although a minority of children have lasting residual weakness.

Chronic inflammatory demyelinating polyneuropathy presents similarly to the Guillain-Barré syndrome. The onset may be more gradual, and relapses may occur over subsequent months. This disorder, unlike the Guillain-Barré syndrome, is responsive to steroids.

Hereditary Polyneuropathies. The hereditary motor and sensory neuropathies (HMSN) are a group of genetic disorders of the peripheral nerve. **Charcot-Marie-Tooth disease (HMSN type I)** is a demyelinating disorder featuring pes cavus, hammer toes, peroneal weakness, and decreased ankle jerk. The disorder is inherited as a dominant trait with genes identified to chromosomes 1 and 17. One subtype is X-linked dominant. Life expectancy is normal, and disease progression may be very slow. The **neuronal type of Charcot-Marie-Tooth disease (HMSN type II)** is milder than HMSN type I and features an axonal neuropathy. Linkage is to chromosome 1, but this type is distinct from HMSN-I. The **hypertrophic neuropathy of infancy (HMSN-III [Dejerine-Sottas disease])** is a demyelinating disorder linked to the same chromosomal 1 and 17 genes found mutated in HMSN I. This disorder usually occurs sporadically, although the mutations involved are dominant. Onset occurs in infancy, with prominent motor delay. This disorder may progress in later life, leading to loss of the ability to walk. **HMSN IV (Refsum disease)** is an inborn error of phytanic acid metabolism with onset in childhood or adulthood. Ataxia and retinitis pigmentosa accompany the neuropathy, and slow progression is noted.

Diseases of the Neuromuscular Junction

Myasthenia. Myasthenia is **fatigable weakness** that improves after rest. Congenital myasthenia gravis is a rare, often familial, group of diseases that arise from structural abnormalities of the neuromuscular junction.

Immune-mediated myasthenia gravis is a chronic disorder characterized by antibodies to the acetylcholine receptor. The disease occurs at any age and is more common in females. Myasthenia gravis usually affects the ocular muscles, but other muscles may be involved as well. Fatigue may manifest as diplopia after reading or as ptosis that worsens after wakening. Respiratory involvement in myasthenia may be life-threatening, and the status of forced vital capacities should be followed carefully.

Diagnosis is by clinical examination demonstrating fatigable weakness. Edrophonium chloride (Tensilon), a short-acting anticholinesterase inhibitor, may restore power to weak muscles briefly and may be useful diagnostically. A characteristic decremental response is seen after repetitive nerve stimulation, and antibody against the acetylcholine receptor is present in most patients. Treatment involves anticholinesterase therapy. Steroids, cytotoxic drugs, plasmapheresis, and thymectomy may be indicated in severe cases.

Newborn infants of women with immune-mediated myasthenia gravis may have a **transient myasthenic syndrome** from passive transfer of antibody from the mother. Babies present with hypotonia and feeding difficulties starting from birth to the third day and progress for a few days before their condition improves. Duration of symptoms is from days to weeks, and recovery usually is complete.

Botulism. Infantile botulism is an age-limited disorder that results from growth in the infant gut of ingested *Clostridium botulinum*. The *C botulinum* exotoxin blocks presynaptic acetylcholine release, resulting in cholinergic blockade of skeletal muscle and autonomic nerves. Patients present with constipation, feeding difficulties, and hypotonia, which may progress to respiratory failure. Cranial nerve involvement is common. This disorder may resemble hypoxic-ischemic encephalopathy or spinal muscular atrophy. Sluggish pupillary reaction in botulism is an important distinguishing characteristic. Diagnosis is by clinical examination, toxin identification from stool, and characteristic EMG findings. Treatment is supportive and may be required for months, but recovery usually is complete.

Diseases of Muscle

Muscular Dystrophy. The muscular dystrophies are genetically determined primary diseases of muscle that feature progressive muscle fiber degeneration in the absence of other nervous system abnormalities. This definition is not wholly accurate, because we now know that both Duchenne and myotonic dystrophy can affect the CNS, and, rarely, Becker dystrophy may be relatively nonprogressive. The most common muscular dystrophy is the Duchenne-Becker type, an X-linked disease resulting from nearly complete (Duchenne) or partial (Becker) loss of function mutations in the dystrophin gene product. The conventional wisdom is that dystrophin serves as a link between the cytoskeleton and the extracellular matrix; in its absence, this linkage is lost, and muscle contraction it-

self may damage the cell membrane, leading to muscle-cell death.

Duchenne muscular dystrophy has an incidence of 1:3000 children. Two thirds acquire dystrophin mutation from their mother, and one third have spontaneous mutations. The disease usually develops before the age of 5 years. Weakness is prominent in proximal muscles, and children often present with toe-walking and difficulty climbing stairs. The gait is waddling, and patients fall frequently. A Gower sign is eventually present. Pseudohypertrophy of the calves and deltoids is a prominent feature, in which the calves are large and feel firm. Strength declines steadily, and most children are nonambulatory in their teens. Mean intelligence quotient is in the low-normal range. Death usually is from respiratory failure.

Becker muscular dystrophy is similar to Duchenne but has a milder course. Weakness may present later in life, and ambulation is preserved into the third decade. Intelligence may be normal. Laboratory analysis shows elevated creatine phosphokinase (CPK) levels, which decrease over time. Muscle biopsy specimens show degeneration of muscle fibers with progressive fibrosis. Dystrophin protein levels are low to absent in muscle biopsy specimens from these patients, and this finding can be used for diagnosis. Carrier detection by DNA testing is being developed.

Myotonic Dystrophy. **Myotonia** is the sustained contraction or delayed relaxation of skeletal muscle. Myotonic dystrophy is an autosomal-dominant condition with prevalence of 5:100,000 and features muscle weakness, wasting, and myotonia. Onset usually occurs in adolescence, although a congenital form may present in the newborn period. Patients have a characteristic facies with a hollowing of the temporal fossae, ptosis, and a swan-shaped neck. Cataracts may be present, and the testes may be atrophic in boys. There is often a history of excessive daytime sleepiness.

Strength testing reveals weakness in the face and distal limbs. Percussion of the thenar eminence demonstrates abduction of the thumb and contraction of the thenar eminence, which is maintained for several seconds. In shaking hands, patients may have difficulty relaxing the grip. Myotonia may develop late in children with this disorder.

The gene for myotonic dystrophy encodes a protein kinase called myotonin and maps to chromosome 19. Mutations leading to myotonic dystrophy are dynamic in nature and result from expansion of a CTG DNA repeat in the 3′ untranslated region of the gene. Whether this mutation affects the activity of myotonin protein kinase is unclear at this time. However, the presence of the expanded repeat can be used as a diagnostic aid in this disorder.

Myopathies. The distinction between muscular dystrophies and myopathies is vague and confusing. Many congenital and metabolic myopathies exist, some of which feature systemic involvement and are nonprogressive. In general, the myopathies are a rarer group of disorders than the muscular dystrophies and are not discussed in this volume.

Inflammatory Diseases of Muscle. Dermatomyositis and **polymyositis** are inflammatory disorders of muscle seen in childhood. Dermatomyositis, which is more common, is the result of an underlying angiopathy with vascular occlusion. The disease presents as a triad of muscle weakness, skin lesions, and malaise. There is no underlying malignant disease predisposing to this disorder. Diagnosis is mainly clinical, although a muscle biopsy specimen showing inflammatory changes may be helpful. Steroids and other immunosuppressive agents are useful therapies. Polymyositis may be considered as part of the spectrum of dermatomyositis.

STROKE

Stroke occurs in children much less frequently than in adults. The incidence ranges from 2.5/100,000 to as high as 13/100,000, depending on study inclusion criteria. As in the adult, localization of the lesion helps to identify possible mechanisms of disease; therefore, complete general and neurologic examinations are essential. Because the pathophysiology and evaluation of stroke in the newborn period differ from those in older children, perinatal stroke is discussed separately at the end of this section.

Etiology

Stroke can be embolic or thrombotic, from an arterial or venous source. An important mechanism for thrombotic or thromboembolic stroke is dissection of one of the great vessels (carotid or vertebral). Vascular events usually are ischemic (55%) but can be hemorrhagic or convert later into hemorrhagic stroke. Thrombosis of the dural venous sinuses in infancy and childhood can lead to cortical infarction, which may be unilateral or bilateral. Often, seizures are the presenting sign, but headache and change in mental status are also frequent complaints. This disorder is seen more commonly in the younger child who is at risk for dehydration in the setting of infection. Meningitis and mastoiditis are common precipitating infectious sites. MRI with venogram is essential for making the diagnosis.

The great mimickers of cerebrovascular disease are tumor, infection, and trauma. A brain tumor can present acutely as unilateral weakness when a tumor outgrows its blood supply and undergoes necrosis with subsequent edema and hemorrhage into the necrotic areas. Brain abscess from any infectious cause, tuberculoma, or cerebritis from herpes simplex encephalitis can cause sudden changes in mental status and hemiparesis. With both accidental and nonaccidental trauma, closed head injury can present as a mass lesion with acute or subacute onset of unilateral weakness with or without change in mental status.

Risk Factors

Risk factors for stroke in children differ substantially from those in adults (Table 21–19). Congenital heart disease is the leading identifiable cause of stroke, but acquired heart disease from endocarditis, cardiomyopathies, Kawasaki disease, or rheumatic fever also may result in stroke. Any systemic disorder that leads to a hypercoagulable state or produces volume depletion can cause stroke. Any disease that affects the development or integrity of the vasculature can lead to stroke. Such conditions as ho-

Table 21–19. Risk factors for stroke in children.

Congenital or acquired heart disease—congenital heart defects
Cardiac surgery—cardiomyopathies
Endocarditis
Kawasaki disease
Rheumatic fever
Immunoproliferative disorders
Leukemia
Lymphoma
Vasculopathies
Homocystinuria
Systemic lupus erythematosus
Marfan syndrome
Moyamoya disease
Fibromuscular dysplasia
Fabry disease
Hematologic disorders
Sickle-cell disease
Antiphospholipid antibodies
Hemolytic-uremic syndrome
Protein C, S deficiencies
Antithrombin III deficiency
Intracranial infection
Meningitis
Meningoencephalitis
Syphilis
Mycoplasma
Trauma
Subdural hematoma
Epidural hematoma
Shaken baby syndrome
Fat embolism
Vascular malformations
Arteriovenous malformations
Aneurysms
Drugs
Cocaine
Methamphetamine
Oral contraceptives
L-asparaginase
Organ transplantation
HIV infection (AIDS)
Migraine
Mitochondrial disorders
MELAS
Leigh disease
Dehydration
Neurocutaneous syndromes
Neurofibromatosis
Tuberous sclerosis
Sturge-Weber syndrome
von Hippel-Lindau disease
Klippel-Trenaunay-Weber syndrome

MELAS = myopathy, encephalopathy, lactic acidosis, and stroke-like episodes.

mocystinuria, fibromuscular dysplasia, moyamoya disease, AVM, Ehlers-Danlos syndrome, Marfan syndrome, polycystic kidney disease, systemic lupus erythematosus, and Fabry disease are important examples. Several hematologic disorders, such as sickle-cell disease, and hypercoagulable states, including protein C or S deficiency, antithrombin III deficiency, and Factor V Leiden mutation, also can result in stroke. Acquired hypercoagulable states include antiphospholipid syndrome, myeloproliferative disorders, and systemic neoplastic conditions. In fact, any coagulation factor deficiency puts a person at higher risk for hemorrhagic stroke.

Clinical Features

The child with a stroke usually presents with an acute or abrupt onset of unilateral weakness (Table 21–20). This is especially true in cases of embolic stroke. At times, the weakness has a stuttering or slower onset when a larger vessel is undergoing thrombosis. If the weakness is predominantly in the face and arm, a cortical lesion should be suspected. The weakness usually is more pronounced distally, so that the extensors of the arm and flexors of the leg are the weakest groups (pyramidal tract signs). Stretch reflexes are increased on the side of the weakness, and the plantar response usually is extensor. In subtle cases, the only sign that might be present is a pronator drift (pronation of the supinated outstretched arm after prolonged extension at 90 degrees from the body) or inability to heel-walk. With cortical strokes, there can be evidence of speech dysfunction (receptive or expressive aphasia) or visual problems (homonymous hemianopsia). When the face, arm, and leg are equally involved with weakness, the lesion is smaller in size and subcortical in location, usually in the internal capsule or basal ganglia. Children, like adults, may have small "lacunar" subcortical infarctions, but hypertension is not a cause of this type of stroke in children. In fact, the pathogenesis of lacunar infarcts in children is unknown, but they have been associated with vasculitis from a variety of causes (eg, infection, chemotherapy).

It is important to consider great-vessel dissection, because diagnosis can be missed by conventional angiographic techniques; a special fat-saturated MRI therefore must be performed. A history of trauma is not necessary for dissection; however, this problem is being observed with increasing frequency in young children who "head the ball" in soccer. There is often a history of neck pain extending to the head on the side of the dissection. Systemic conditions, such as Marfan syndrome or fibromuscular dysplasia, also can predispose a child to this type of stroke.

Large hemorrhagic strokes are often associated with change in mental status (lethargy) and sudden acute head pain ("the worst headache of my life"—subarachnoid hemorrhage). Focal motor seizures can herald a hemorrhagic event or an ischemic embolic stroke. In one series, 49% of patients with stroke had at least one seizure. Most seizures occurred within 1 day of the onset of weakness. When unilateral weakness follows a focal motor seizure and resolves over the course of hours, it most probably is not a stroke and is then referred to as a Todd hemiparesis. If the weakness lasts longer than 24 hours, stroke becomes much more likely.

Patients with alteration of consciousness and paralysis of upward gaze associated with the hemiparesis have "disturbance of vigilance," a clinical symptom complex seen after thalamic stroke. If there are crossed findings, for example, involvement of the face on one side of the body and weakness of the arms and legs on the other side of the body, the lesion is located in the brainstem and can be localized best by evaluating the cranial nerves. Unilateral ataxia usually is caused by a vascular lesion in the ipsilateral cerebellum.

Headaches, seizures, or both are frequent accompanying clinical signs in pediatric stroke and are discussed below.

Evaluation

Stroke is a medical emergency. Conditions that may mimic stroke should be carefully excluded. On the basis of the risk factors, history, and examination, a stepwise

Table 21–20. Presenting signs in childhood stroke.

Hemiplegia and hemiparesis
Seizures
Fever
Speech or language abnormality
Headache
Depressed level of consciousness

Table 21–21. Studies to be performed for evaluation of stroke.

Blood studies:	Complete blood count with differential, platelet count, ESR, prothrombin time, and partial thromboplastin time; blood culture if febrile; blood sample saved for special studies (hemoglobin electrophoresis, coagulation factors, antiphospholipid antibodies, HIV)
Urine studies:	Toxicology screen (methamphetamine, cocaine); urine nitroprusside (homocystinuria); urinalysis and specific gravity
CT scan without contrast; if no blood noted, do contrast study	
MRI with fat saturation (for vessel dissection) followed by MRA, if indicated	
If no mass effect on CT:	
Lumbar puncture:	Check for xanthochromia, infection (CSF lactate if mitochondrial disorders are suspected)
Cardiac evaluation:	ECG, chest radiograph, and echocardiogram if heart murmur noted (especially if lesion is embolic)

CSF = cerebrospinal fluid; CT = computed tomography; ECG = electrocardiogram; MRA = magnetic resonance angiography; MRI = magnetic resonance imaging.

evaluation can be planned (Table 21–21). The most urgent are intra- and extracerebral mass lesions. Intracerebral mass lesions, such as abscess or tumor, may present suddenly when there is rapid expansion from hemorrhage or edema. A head CT scan without and with contrast (in that order to determine first whether blood is present and then to look for blood-brain barrier problems with contrast enhancement) will determine the nature and extent of the lesion. Extracerebral mass lesions, such as epidural and subdural hematoma, may present with an abrupt onset of unilateral hemiparesis. With epidural hematoma, there is sometimes a lucid interval between onset of hemorrhage and frank decompensation. In an infant with apnea or seizures, nonaccidental head trauma may cause expanding subdural hematoma. Emergent CT scan with subdural windows is indicated. The presence of retinal hemorrhages is the sine qua non for diagnosis of "shaken baby syndrome."

Occasionally, a child or teen may present with a psychogenic cause of unilateral weakness. The weakness is usually present on the nondominant side (opposite the side of handedness). Physical or sexual abuse must be considered in these cases.

Treatment

Prevention of further morbidity from stroke requires astute early management. Systolic blood pressure is often elevated during acute stroke, and blood pressure should not be lowered by antihypertensive agents. The increase in blood pressure assists in providing adequate cerebral perfusion to nondamaged areas.

In documented arterial dissection, intraluminal thrombus may break up and cause embolic injury distally. In this type of stroke, as well as in stroke in evolution and stroke secondary to atrial fibrillation, treatment with heparin is indicated. The pharmacokinetics of heparin are poorly understood. The dose response is not linear; the half-time ($t_{1/2}$) of a 100-U/kg dose is 56 minutes, and the $t_{1/2}$ of a 400-U/kg dose is 152 minutes. The volume of distribution is 40–60 mL/kg. The therapeutic range should be reached within 48 hours maximum. The ratio of the patient's activated partial thromboplastin time (APTT) over the mean control APTT should be 1.5–2.5. Heparinization also should be considered if the patient is thought to have subacute bacterial endocarditis or a documented intramural cardiac thrombus or valvar vegetations. If an intracranial hemorrhage has resulted from a hypercoagulable state, heparin also may be useful. The role of thrombolysis in childhood stroke has not been clarified, although drugs like streptokinase, urokinase, and tissue plasminogen activator (TPA) are being used with increasing frequency in adults. With subarachnoid hemorrhage, rebleeding and vasospasm can lead to further morbidity. Vasospasm can be reduced by the administration of the calcium-channel blocker nimodipine (0.7 mg/kg initially, followed by 0.35 mg/kg every 4 hours). Aneurysm clipping is done as soon as possible. If there has been an intracerebral hemorrhage, therapy should be aimed at restoring clotting function (eg, platelet transfusions, fresh-frozen plasma, vitamin K).

Chronic Management. Most neurologic diseases require support from a pediatric rehabilitation team. This is most important in the case of a child recovering from a stroke. The approach to the patient is based on age and the developmental capacity of the child before the illness or event. It is very important to set realistic goals for restoration of function. The primary goals are to restore mobility, age-appropriate self-care skills, and functional communication. Speech and language specialists, physical and occupational therapists, skilled nurses, physician specialists, medical social workers, and clinical psychologists are involved in an interdisciplinary approach. Discharge planning is done through the combined efforts of the team, and community resources are contacted before discharge from hospital so that patients who live in remote areas will be assured of continued outpatient therapy.

Outcome

Most strokes occur as single episodes without recurrence in childhood. However, recurrent seizures may occur after stroke in childhood, especially if seizures occur more than 2 weeks after the stroke episode. Cortical involvement increases the likelihood of recurrent seizures. Younger patients tend to have less motor and language deficit because of the plasticity of the developing nervous system. Usually children regain ambulation, although clinically evident hemiparetic gait may be present. An unfortunate residual effect of subcortical infarctions, especially involving the basal ganglia, is dystonia of the involved limb. This movement disorder is often refractory to medical management.

Perinatal Stroke

There are no consistent intrauterine or perinatal events that explain the occurrence of stroke in newborns. However, when stroke occurs in the setting of perinatal asphyxia, outcome is uniformly poor, and strokes involve more than one vascular territory, for example, bilateral watershed infarctions. Seizures usually accompany stroke and may be the only clinical sign of the event, as it is often difficult to demonstrate unilateral weakness in a newborn infant because of the poor representation of motor function in the cortex. Apnea is also a frequent clinical sign of the event and may accompany seizures. Cranial ultrasound study is insensitive to even large cortical infarctions; if the diagnosis is suspected, CT or, preferably, MRI, should be performed. EEG usually correctly identifies the lesion in all babies who have seizures, either by the appearance of focal slowing or by focal spike-wave activity. Metabolic causes of stroke should be ruled out, especially inborn errors such as homocystinuria, sulfite oxidase deficiency, and NADH-coenzyme Q reductase deficiency. If the lesion is hemorrhagic, hematologic disorders, such as coagulation factor deficiency, vitamin K deficiency, and vascular malformations associated with neurocutaneous syndromes, should be investigated if the clinical picture is suggestive (Table 21–22).

The etiology of the underlying disorder usually helps to predict outcome. Outcome after stroke from perinatal asphyxia or infection depends on the size and extent of the lesions. If the etiology is not determined and the stroke is a unilateral cortical ischemic event of the newborn, the outcome is uniformly favorable.

ATAXIA

Ataxia is the breakdown of coordinated movement, which causes disturbance of posture, station, and gait. There is also an associated loss of fine motor control of the limbs, depending on the location of the lesion in the cerebellar pathways. Common terms used to describe cerebellar movement abnormalities include the following:

- Dysmetria: a disturbance of the placement of a body part during movement

- Dysdiadochokinesis: inability to perform rapid alternating movements

- Titubation: tremor of the head or trunk

- Opsoclonus: bouncing eyes

- Nystagmus: rhythmic to-and-fro movement of eyes, usually gaze-provoked.

Lesions in midline structures of the cerebellum (vermis, flocculonodular lobe, fastigial nucleus) cause truncal ataxia, titubation, head tilt, lower limb ataxia, and eye movement problems, such as dysmetria and nystagmus.

Table 21–22. Studies to be performed in newborn infants with stroke.

Blood studies:	Complete blood count with differential, platelet count; prothrombin time and partial thromboplastin time—if abnormal, clotting factors; blood culture; plasma amino acid levels; ammonia, lactate, and pyruvate concentrations
Urine studies:	Toxicology screen (methamphetamine, cocaine); urine nitroprusside (homocystinuria); urinalysis and specific gravity; urine for organic acids

CT scan without contrast; if no blood, contrast scan
MRI with MR venogram
Lumbar puncture (especially to measure lactate)
Cardiac evaluation: ECG, echocardiogram, chest radiograph
EEG: Continuous if paralyzed

CT = computed tomography; ECG = electrocardiogram; EEG = electroencephalogram; MRI = magnetic resonance imaging.

When lateral structures (cerebellar hemispheres) are involved, the resulting clinical picture can include ipsilateral limb ataxia, tremor, scanning speech, or eye movement problems, including opsoclonus, ocular bobbing, flutter, dysmetria, or nystagmus.

The course of the illness can be acute, intermittent, or chronic. The causes of ataxia are listed in Table 21–23.

Acute Cerebellar Ataxia

Acute cerebellar ataxia may develop after a variety of illnesses, most commonly viral (varicella). In a recent series, 26% of children had chickenpox, 52% had other presumed viral illnesses, 3% had an immunization-related onset, and 19% had no definite prodrome. This disorder affects the young child (2–4 years) but has been reported in children of all ages. Fever is an uncommon sign. The latency of the prodromal illness to development of ataxia can range from 1 to 43 days but is usually 10 days. The ataxia is truncal and manifests as a gait ataxia. Dysmetria is also common. Nystagmus is not common, and cranial nerve palsies and corticospinal tract signs are infrequent. Laboratory evaluation of this condition is presented in Table 21–24. The white blood cell count usually is increased to 15,000/mm^3 or more, with a lymphocytic predominance. However, the pleocytosis in the CSF is usually low, in the range of 20 cells/mm^3 with both granulocytes and lymphocytes. A minority of patients have elevated protein concentrations in the CSF, but more than half have an elevated CSF IgG relative to the level in serum (IgG index). MRI may reveal T2 signal abnormalities in the cerebellum. Although these patients do not have seizures, the EEG can be abnormal, showing diffuse slowing or epileptiform activity. Fortunately, the outcome usually is excellent; most children recover completely. Cognitive abnormalities are seen in the acute setting, manifesting as behavioral changes (irritability, hyperactivity, withdrawal). These behaviors are not permanent, but learning disabilities have been noted in a minority of children.

Of the other etiologies for acute cerebellar ataxia, ingestions and Guillain-Barré syndrome are the most common discharge diagnoses. When ingestion is the cause, the patient usually has a change in mental status, such as lethargy.

The management of acute cerebellar ataxia depends on the underlying condition. For the most part, treatment is symptomatic. Steroids are essential if there is a tumor exerting mass effect. Otherwise, steroids may be beneficial in the setting of acute disseminated encephalomyelitis if the ataxia is severe enough to prevent ambulation.

Inpatient rehabilitation is important in providing patients with the skills necessary to recover balance and function.

Opsoclonus-Myoclonus-Ataxia Syndrome

The syndrome of opsoclonus, myoclonus, and ataxia is associated with occult neuroblastoma. These signs usually

Table 21–23. Causes of cerebellar ataxia in children.

Acute ataxia
   Toxins and drugs
      Heavy metals (lead, mercury)
      Phenytoin, ethanol
   Infections
      Viral meningitis
      Cerebellitis
      Encephalitis
      Labyrinthitis
   Posterior fossa tumors
      Cerebellar astrocytoma
      Ependymoma
      Medulloblastoma
      Cerebellar hemangioblastoma
      von Hippel-Lindau disease (occult neuroblastoma)
   Head injury
      Concussion
      Hematoma
   Metabolic disturbances
      Hypoglycemia
      Hyperammonemia
      Hyponatremia
      Acute cerebellar stroke
   Acute obstructive hydrocephalus syndrome associated with neuroblastoma
   Peripheral demyelinating disease
      Guillain-Barré syndrome (Miller-Fisher variant)
   Central demyelinating disease
      Multiple sclerosis
      Acute disseminated encephalomyelitis
Chronic-static ataxia
   Developmental anomalies
      Arnold-Chiari syndrome
      Dandy-Walker syndrome
      Basilar impression
      Cerebral palsy
Chronic-progressive ataxia
   Toxins and drugs
      Heavy metals (lead, mercury)
      Ethanol
   Metabolic disorders
      Hypothyroidism
      Vitamin E deficiency
      Vitamin B_6 excess
      Refsum disease (phytanic acid deficiency)
      A-betalipoproteinemia
   Genetic disorders
      Ataxis-telangiectasia
      Olivopontocerebellar atrophy
      Hypomyelination
      Friedreich ataxia
      Ramsay Hunt syndrome
      Hereditary neuropathies
      Charcot-Marie-Tooth disease
      Roussy-Lévy syndrome
      Childhood ataxia with diffuse central nervous system hypomyelination
   Acquired neuropathies
Intermittent ataxias
   Metabolic
      Hartnup disease
      Pyruvated decarboxylase deficiency
      Carnitine acetyltransferase deficiency
      Maple syrup urine disease
   Migraine
      Benign paroxysmal vertigo
      Basilar migraine
   Genetic
      Dominant recurrent ataxia
      Paroxysmal ataxia and myokymia

Table 21–24. Studies to be performed in the evaluation of acute ataxia.

Blood	White blood cell count, ammonia, glucose and electrolyte concentrations
	Save for special studies (eg, thyroid, serum amino acids, Pb)
Urine	Toxicology screen
	Save for special studies (eg, organic acids, heavy metals, homovanillic acid/vanillylmandelic acid)
MRI	If mass noted: neurosurgical consultation
	If no mass noted: lumbar puncture for cells, protein, IgG index, cultures)

MRI = magnetic resonance imaging.

precede the diagnosis of tumor, which is found in the thorax or abdomen. Children with tumor have a better prognosis with regard to their cancer, but major cognitive disabilities are associated with the movement disorder. The syndrome has been said to be immune-mediated, although data are lacking to support this concept. This syndrome also can be seen after infection, anoxia, intracranial hemorrhage, and cocaine or thallium poisoning (Table 21–25). It has also been described in adults with tumors of the breast, uterus, and thyroid, as well as those with small cell carcinoma. In addition to the standard evaluation for ataxia, studies should include urinalysis for catecholamine products and chest and abdominal MRI. To treat the movement disorder, most patients receive ACTH, and 80% show a good response. Patients tend to relapse when the medication is withdrawn. High-dose immunoglobulin therapy has been reported to diminish the symptoms.

Chronic Ataxias

Chronic ataxias tend to be progressive, but some disorders are relatively static (see Table 21–23). When ataxia is a chronic condition, generalized hypotonia usually is associated. The ataxia is truncal and involves gait, and often there is a history of delayed motor milestones. The most frequent causes are communicating hydrocephalus, developmental anomalies of the cerebellum, and a history of perinatal problems, such as asphyxia. Many degenerative diseases of the CNS present with ataxia, but other neurologic signs usually are present (Table 21–23).

Perhaps the best known degenerative ataxia is ataxia-

Table 21–25. Etiology of opsoclonus-myoclonus-ataxia syndrome.

Parainfectious	Coxsackie B2, B3; parainfluenza 3; immunization
Drugs	Cocaine
Metabolic	Nonketotic hyperosmolar coma; biotin-responsive multiple carboxylase deficiency
Neoplasms	Neuroblastoma; hepatoblastoma; adult cancers (uterine, breast, thyroid, small cell carcinoma)

telangiectasia. The gene identified for this autosomal-recessive condition, *ATM,* recently has been identified by positional cloning on chromosome 11q22–23. The protein product is similar to phosphatidylinositol-3′ kinase involved in signal transduction. The cellular phenotype of this disease is characteristic. In addition to chromosomal instability, cells have reduced life span, defects in the cytoskeleton, increased sensitivity to ionizing radiation, and increased requirements for growth factors. Serum levels of α-fetoprotein are elevated in these patients, and this finding serves as a diagnostic marker.

The disease is characterized by progressive cerebellar ataxia, oculocutaneous telangiectasias, premature aging, growth retardation, choreoathetosis, frequent sinopulmonary infections due to immunodeficiency, and a predisposition to lymphoreticular neoplasia. Affected patients have a particular oculomotor apraxia, wherein a defect of voluntary and involuntary saccadic eye movements is associated with eye blinking or head thrusts. Patients require careful immunologic investigation and support, including frequent immunoglobulin therapy and prophylaxis against common infections.

The telangiectasias usually are noted around 4 years of age on the bulbar conjunctivae and exposed areas of skin, such as the nasal bridge, antecubital and popliteal fossae, and ears. Vitiligo, café-au-lait spots, and scleroderma are frequent accompaniments. Choreoathetosis gradually becomes as disabling a condition as the ataxia, and these patients become wheelchair-bound by the end of the first decade. Death is secondary to overwhelming infection, respiratory failure, or cancer.

A progressive syndrome of childhood ataxia with diffuse CNS hypomyelination has been described recently. These patients have been girls presenting with ataxic diplegia. Initially, growth and development are normal, but these patients lose the ability to walk early in the first decade. MRI reveals diffuse hypodensity of the white matter of the cerebral hemispheres and cerebellum with no atrophy. Cognition is relatively preserved, and some patients have seizures. Eye movements remain normal. Metabolic investigations have been unrevealing.

Friedreich ataxia is another chronic progressive ataxia with onset in early childhood. Most patients manifest an autosomal-recessive mode of inheritance, and the main presenting symptom is abnormal gait. Ataxia of gait and limbs with depressed or absent deep tendon reflexes should suggest the diagnosis. Sensory nerve conduction studies are helpful to confirm the diagnosis. Cardiac involvement is appreciated by ECG changes, even in the absence of symptoms. Diabetes mellitus is a late complication of the disease.

A number of acquired and hereditary neuropathies may cause a sensory ataxia. The cornerstone of the evaluation is neurophysiologic testing of the involved limbs. In some cases, genetic testing is available (Charcot-Marie-Tooth disease), whereas in others the diagnosis can be made by looking for the appropriate abnormality in blood or urine (eg, Refsum disease).

MOVEMENT DISORDERS

Many pathologic movements that appear later in life are physiologic during early development. For example, every infant has frequent choreoathetotic movements and dystonic postures. These movements are slowly dampened as the brain myelinates and matures during the first year of life. Mirror movements are involuntary, symmetric movements of the arm or hand performed by the corresponding part on the opposite side. They are common during childhood, usually abating after the first decade. Persistence of mirror movements is seen in Klippel-Feil deformity, in which there is absent decussation of the pyramidal tracts associated with skeletal abnormalities in the cervical region.

Movement disorders usually are apparent at rest but become more obvious when the patient is anxious. Except in some patients with severe dystonia and myoclonus, the abnormal movements disappear during sleep. Although they are considered separately, these movement disorders often blend into one another.

Athetosis & Chorea

Athetosis describes slow, irregular, writhing or twisting movements that are primarily distal and can affect the trunk or limbs. There is usually alternating flexion, extension, or hyperextension of the wrists and digits, often one digit at a time. Facial grimacing and incoordination of oropharyngeal muscles may be present, resulting in dysarthria and drooling. The causes of athetosis and chorea are presented in Table 21–26.

Chorea is characterized by quick, uncoordinated muscle movement from place to place without semblance of regularity. Initially, one may believe that the patient is fidgety or restless. Commonly, the face, neck, and distal muscles are affected; however, any skeletal muscle can be involved. Volitional movements often are exaggerated because choreic movement usually is superimposed on them. Usually, chorea and athetosis are seen together, except in the case of athetosis from perinatal asphyxia or kernicterus. Chorea and athetosis can be caused by toxic, metabolic, infectious, or inflammatory disease of the CNS (see Table 21–26).

Sydenham chorea occurs after group A *Streptococcus* infection and is one of the major Jones criteria for rheumatic fever. It appears after the late phase of the infection, although a history of sore throat is noted only in 50% of children. Cardiac manifestations are present in 33%, and joint manifestations at some stage in 25%. There is often emotional instability and restlessness. The movements are random and irregular in time and space but are predominantly seen in the face and upper limbs. Movements are greatest distally in the limbs and interfere with function. Although the neuropathology is not well es-

Table 21–26. Causes of athetosis and chorea.

Drugs	Anticonvulsants, oral contraceptives, tricyclic antidepressants (especially phenothiazines), stimulants, sedative-hypnotics
Infectious	Sydenham chorea, bacterial meningitis, viral infections
Inflammatory	Systemic lupus erythematosus
Metabolic	Kernicterus, hyperthyroidism, hypoparathyroidism, pregnancy, Addison disease, hypernatremia, hypocalcemia, vitamin B_{12} deficiency
Structural	Moyamoya disease, neoplasms
Genetic	Wilson disease, Huntington chorea, Hallervorden-Spatz syndrome, familial paroxysmal choreoathetosis, ataxia-telangiectasia
Postasphyxial	Perinatal stroke, post-perfusion (cardiopulmonary bypass)

tablished, there have been reports of antineuronal antibodies in the caudate and subthalamic nuclei. The treatment for Sydenham chorea begins with penicillin. Children with this syndrome should have a full course of penicillin at diagnosis and penicillin prophylaxis for life because of the risk of cardiac involvement with recurrent streptococcal infection.

Post-pump chorea is seen within 2 weeks after cardiopulmonary bypass in 1–2% children with congenital heart disease. Young infants (< 8 months) seem to recover completely, whereas older infants and children often have severe persistent chorea. Risk factors for persistence include rapid cooling period, prolonged hypothermia, prolonged pump time with circulatory arrest, severe cyanotic heart disease, and young age. The disorder is presumed to be caused by asphyxial damage to the basal ganglia, but predisposing factors are unclear.

Dystonia

Dystonia is the result of contractions of agonist and antagonist muscle groups, which cause a disturbance of posture with irregular, somewhat slow twisting or torsion of limb or trunk muscles. It can be generalized or confined to a specific region, such as the face, tongue, hand, or neck, and can be present during sleep. Focal dystonias include **blepharospasm, writer's cramp,** and **torticollis.** A peculiar cervical dystonia syndrome in infancy associated with gastroesophageal reflux is called **Sandifer syndrome.**

The most common presentation of dystonia in childhood is the acute idiosyncratic reaction caused by drugs, especially phenothiazines. Reactions include **opisthotonos, torticollis, oculogyric crisis,** and **trismus.** There usually is a quick resolution after IV administration of diphenhydramine.

Torticollis is a focal dystonia commonly seen in young children. When associated with head tilt, fourth-nerve palsy should be ruled out. If torticollis presents acutely and is associated with pain and hyperreflexia of the lower limbs, abnormalities of the cervicomedullary junction should be sought carefully. Benign paroxysmal torticollis

is a migraine variant occurring in infants and young children. Attacks can last for hours to days, and some are associated with vomiting. With time, the episodes may evolve into benign paroxysmal vertigo or migraine.

Generalized dystonias can be idiopathic or associated with a number of genetic neurologic conditions, such as mitochondrial disorders. A dopa-responsive dystonia called **Segawa disease** presents with gait problems early in the first decade. There is often a particular diurnal variation to the dystonia, with worsening as the day progresses. Immediate, but temporary, administration of levodopa eliminates the dystonia.

Idiopathic torsion dystonia usually is an autosomal-dominant disorder with childhood onset in the second decade. Most children present with abnormalities of gait caused by dystonia of the legs or feet. Patients progress relentlessly, and 50% are bedridden within a decade. An autosomal-recessive form is seen in Ashkenazi Jews, with a uniform course and less involvement of axial muscles.

The evaluation of dystonia is similar to that for choreoathetosis (Table 21–27). Trihexyphenidyl is the drug of first choice for progressive dystonias. Diazepam and tetrabenazine also have been used in difficult cases. Often patients seek surgical ablative therapy. Although phenothiazines are effective, long-term use causes tardive dyskinesias.

Tics

Tics, the most common movement disorder in childhood, can be motor, vocal, or sensory. Children with vocal tics, such as throat clearing, coughing, or sniffing, often are thought to have allergies before the tic disorder is recognized. Sensory tics are peculiar sensations. Motor tics can be dystonic or myoclonic, but in both cases these movements are quick. Most tics are more easily suppressed by voluntary movements than any of the other types of movement disorders.

When pathologic, tics are complex, stereotyped movements or verbal expressions that are intrusive and purposeless. Tics disappear with sleep and are exacerbated by stress. **Tourette syndrome** is part of a spectrum that includes obsessive-compulsive behavior and attention deficit disorder. Laboratory tests, such as EEG, neu-

Table 21–27. Etiology of dystonias.

Inflammatory	Syphilis, tuberculous meningitis, encephalitis
Drug intoxication	Phenothiazines, cocaine
Tumors	
Perinatal brain injury	Asphyxia, postinfectious, post-stroke
Genetic	Wilson disease, Huntington chorea, Parkinson disease, Hallervorden-Spatz syndrome, dopa-responsive dystonia, dystonia musculorum deformans, familial paroxysmal dystonia
Trauma	

with lines. Most children prefer to look at a card with lines. As progressively thinner and closer lines are presented to children, their ability to resolve these lines is measured. This test requires time and considerable cooperation on the part of the child.

Vision-evoked potential testing has not found much use clinically for the measurement of visual acuity, but it is used for research investigations. The child's vision can be estimated by measuring the electrical potential with leads over the visual cortex, after presenting the child with a visual target (usually a checkerboard).

OCULAR ALIGNMENT

The examination should then proceed to an assessment of ocular alignment. The Hirschberg test identifies whether a light shined at the eyes projects a reflex off the center of each cornea. If the reflex is deviated inward in one eye, that eye may actually be turned out, implying **exotropia.** On the other hand, a light reflex that projects on the outside of one cornea may indicate that an eye has **esotropia.** Even seasoned clinicians occasionally mistake prominent epicanthal folds for true esotropia. The value of the Hirschberg test is increased in children who have these prominent skin folds over the bridge of their nose.

The cover test is even more accurate than the Hirschberg test. A clinician who can successfully induce the child to regard a visual target, by covering one eye and then the other, can look for movement of the uncovered eye, which would indicate the possible presence of a strabismus problem. For example, in the case of exotropia of the left eye, the child fixates on a visual target with the right eye. Covering the right eye would then cause the left eye to shift in to take up visual fixation on the object of interest. On the other hand, covering the left eye causes no shifting of the right eye, because it was and is already the preferred fixing eye. It is therefore important to cover each eye separately.

THE RED REFLEX

Next the clinician should determine the quality of the red reflex. This part of the examination requires a direct ophthalmoscope and a view through the pupil of each eye from a distance of 2–4 ft. The red reflex actually should appear orange and approximately the same color in each eye. If the reflex is obscured by any opacification, this is cause for concern. Whitening of the cornea, cataract, or, even more ominously, retinoblastoma, are potential causes of so-called leukocoria. On the other hand, if the red reflex is somewhat asymmetric, that is, darker in one eye than in the other, this may indicate that there is an asymmetric or refractive error. This asymmetry of red reflex forms the basis of the Bruchner reflex test, which is admittedly unreliable unless the observer has considerable experience in judging the red reflex.

OTHER OCULAR STRUCTURES

Inspection of the ocular adnexal structures is germane when symptoms related to eyelids or tear function exist. Excess discharge or tearing can be evaluated by looking closely at the conjunctiva or surface of the eye.

Finally, the clinician should attempt to examine the ocular fundus. The optic nerve is located slightly nasal to center; evaluation with a direct ophthalmoscope should be performed with this in mind. In children who have significant myopia (nearsightedness), the optic nerve will appear large. Hyperopia (farsightedness) causes an optical distortion of the optic nerve in which the nerve appears smaller.

The macula can be examined simply by asking the child to look directly at the light. It may be helpful to dim the light somewhat because of sensitivity in some children. The center of the macula, termed the fovea, looks like a small pit. The macula should appear slightly orange and is framed by retinal blood vessels.

APPROACH TO VISION ABNORMALITIES IN CHILDREN

The approach to vision abnormalities in children should focus on several aspects of the history and physical examination (Figure 22–1). Clinicians should pay serious attention to how well the child appears to function from a visual standpoint. In other words, the preverbal child may have a normal physical examination, but the family may complain that the child does not use his or her vision. Visual acuity should be determined or estimated as described above. The child's ability to see in different lighted conditions is also an important determination.

Normal visual acuity is 20/20 in each eye. If there is more than one line difference in vision between each eye, a careful investigation should be undertaken for possible pathology. In addition, if one or both eyes has vision that is worse than 20/30, then further investigation is warranted to determine the cause and nature of the reduced vision. Clinicians should use their judgment regarding children who test 20/30 in each eye. If there are other complaints about vision, then further investigation is warranted.

Refractive errors are the usual cause of reduction in vision in children. The pinhole test can be used to screen for refractive errors in children who can cooperate with this examination. A tiny hole placed in front of the eye screens extraneous light rays and allows only light rays that are directed perpendicular to the macula to enter the eye. Thus, children with low vision due to a refractive error will be able to see much more clearly when a pinhole is placed in front of their eye.

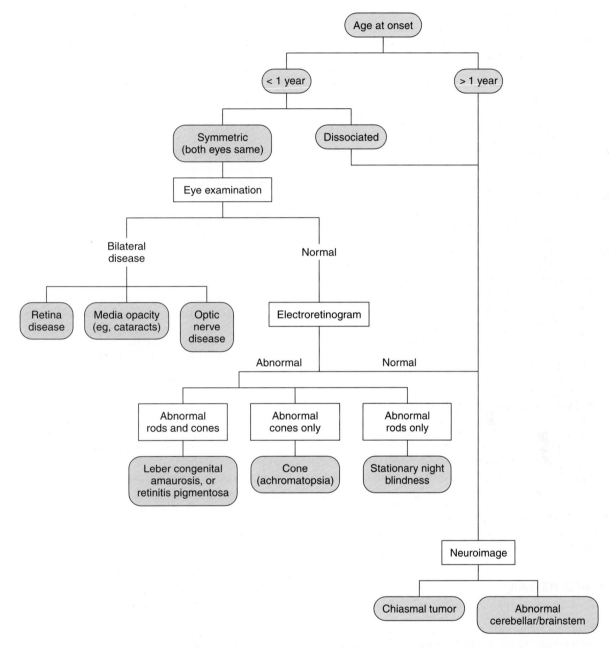

Figure 22–1. Evaluation of the young child with no or poor vision.

Clinicians should look carefully for the presence of nystagmus. **Nystagmus** is defined as rhythmic oscillations of the eye, usually horizontal, but of varying amplitudes and speed, depending on the condition causing the nystagmus and also on the child. Nystagmus in childhood usually indicates bilateral anterior afferent visual pathway disease and implies vision worse than 20/60 in both eyes. Nystagmus has myriad causes in the first year, but most of these occur in severely neurologically damaged children.

In the outpatient setting, the emphasis in the evaluation of children with nystagmus should be on the visual system. Examples of conditions that can cause nystagmus include bilateral optic nerve hypoplasia, untreated congenital cataracts, retinal disease, and corneal opacities. Unilateral lesions usually do not cause nystagmus. Lesions in the posterior visual pathways (ie, visual cortex) also do not produce nystagmus. Neuroimaging studies probably should be reserved for children with an entirely normal eye evaluation who otherwise show signs suggesting central nervous system (CNS) or optic chiasm disease.

Good ocular alignment is usually a prerequisite to good vision in each eye. If a child prefers visual fixation with one eye, and allows the other eye to drift either in (esotropia) or out (exotropia), this implies some degree of amblyopia (loss of vision) in the nonfixing eye. On the other hand, if the child is content to fixate with either eye, this implies that both eyes have equal vision.

Some children see well in the light but poorly in the dark, and vice versa. Rod photoreceptor cells are responsible for good vision in the dark. Cone photoreceptor cells allow for good color vision and also light-adapted vision. Differences in dark versus light vision can provide important clues to the possible etiology of vision problems. Retinitis pigmentosa, for example, will often present initially as trouble seeing in the dark (**nyctalopia).** Children with cone cell abnormalities, also termed **cone dystrophies** or **achromatopsia,** may show photophobia and difficulty seeing under lighted conditions. An **electroretinogram** can often be helpful in sorting out whether a child has one or another of these retinal diseases. The electroretinogram measures electrical activity of the retina (in response to a flash of light).

AMBLYOPIA

Amblyopia is defined as loss of vision in one or both eyes with an otherwise normal eye examination. Amblyopia is divided into three categories: form deprivation, strabismus, and anisometropic.

Form deprivation amblyopia occurs when one or both eyes are occluded early in life. Possible etiologies would include congenital cataracts, severe ptosis, and corneal opacifications. The sensitive period for amblyopia to occur (and be reversed) is short in this type of amblyopia—usually 3–4 months. For that reason, the determination of the red reflex in the nursery is critically important to exclude corneal and lens opacities. The child should have this reflex tested during the first several well-baby visits because lens and corneal opacities can occur postnatally as well. If the cause of form deprivation can be reversed promptly, the prognosis is good.

Strabismic amblyopia occurs when one eye is preferentially used for visual fixation, while the other, strabismic, eye is allowed to deviate. The critical period for this type of amblyopia is approximately ages 4–5 years. Treatment with patching or penalization (eg, pharmacologically causing an eye to see more poorly than the other eye) can be very effective.

Anisometropic amblyopia occurs when one eye has a refractive error closer to normal than the other eye. Usually, either one eye shows no refractive error and the other eye demonstrates high hyperopia, or one eye shows no refractive error and the other eye demonstrates high myopia. In this setting, the eyes may maintain their ocular alignment and there may be no other clue to the diagnosis other than the measurement of visual acuity. Fortunately, the critical or sensitive period for the development of (and also treatment of) this type of amblyopia is about 9 years; in addition, some recent evidence has suggested an even longer sensitive period. The etiology of this type of amblyopia is unknown, but treatment is similar to that for other types of amblyopia. Patching may be useful, and optical correction of the abnormal eye is also indicated.

Treatment is most often restricted to a patching regimen in almost all types of amblyopia. Although deprivation amblyopia can be corrected by surgery in some cases, patching the fellow normal eye will help to augment vision in the amblyopic eye.

CORTICAL VISUAL IMPAIRMENT

Some children have impaired vision due to CNS disease. In adults, the term **cortical blindness** is often used to describe this condition. In children, **cortical visual impairment (CVI)** is the preferred terminology, because most children with cortical abnormalities have some residual vision, albeit very little. The diagnosis of CVI is based on altered visual acuity, abnormal responses to the environment, and neurobehavioral abnormalities.

Children with CVI often show a constellation of behavioral abnormalities that can be clues to the diagnosis. They may stare at bright lights and, paradoxically, also be photophobic. They often wave their fingers between their eyes and a light source, as though stimulating their vision. They prefer colored objects over black and white contrasted objects. They may have variable visual performance, presumably because of other neurologic disease that accompanies CVI.

The usual etiology of CVI is perinatal or postnatal hypoxic ischemia; however, myriad other causes have been noted. If this condition is suspected, a careful investigation is warranted, usually including a neuroimaging study.

Management of such children is complicated and problematic. There usually is no specific treatment for the disorder, but efforts at rehabilitation can be helpful.

THE CHILD WITH THE RED EYE

The most common ocular complaint in children is that of a red eye. In this section the diagnosis and management of the red eye is reviewed. Clinicians who use a logical and systematic approach to red eyes are unlikely to miss serious or occult disease (Figure 22–2).

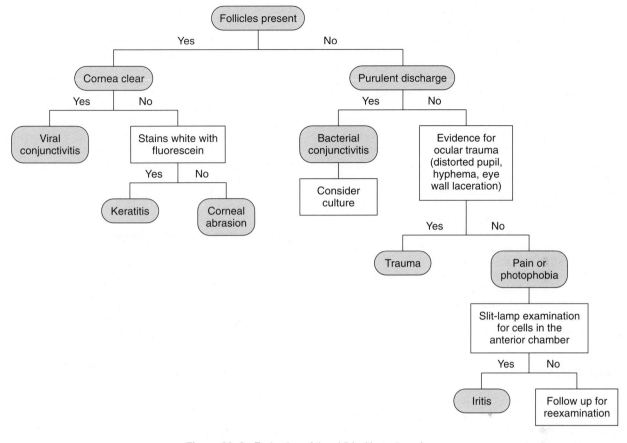

Figure 22–2. Evaluation of the child with acute red eye.

INFECTIOUS DISEASES

Viral conjunctivitis represents the most common cause of red eyes. The usual cause is an adenovirus, and many children have preexisting or simultaneous upper respiratory infections. Certain strains of adenovirus can cause viral conjunctivitis without causing an upper respiratory infection. In these situations, a mild and superficial keratitis often accompanies the conjunctivitis.

The physical findings in viral conjunctivitis consist of mild to moderate mucinous discharge, redness, and chemosis (swelling) of the conjunctiva. Follicles of the palpebral conjunctiva are probably the most reliable physical finding and are fairly specific to viral and chlamydial infection. Furthermore, the presence of a preauricular lymph node helps substantiate a diagnosis either of viral or chlamydial infection.

Viral conjunctivitis usually is a self-limited condition. The duration of symptoms is 7–10 days. If the condition is thought to be viral in nature, no specific antibiotic treatment is indicated. Because the disease is infectious and contagious for 2 weeks after the onset of symptoms, care

should be taken regarding the child's return to preschool or classroom settings. Health care providers should also take precautions.

Bacterial conjunctivitis usually does not cause follicles. Symptoms consist of a papillary conjunctivitis with more purulent discharge and usually more swelling of the conjunctiva. The onset is usually acute, but preauricular lymph nodes are seldom noted, except with gonococcal conjunctivitis.

Cultures are usually not necessary in suspected bacterial conjunctivitis, except when gonococcal, meningococcal, or chlamydial infections are suspected. Empiric treatment with an antibiotic, such as sulfacetamide or erythromycin, for 7–10 days is usually effective. Typically, bacterial conjunctivitis resolves within 2–3 days with antibiotic treatment.

Allergic conjunctivitis is also often acute. The most specific and important sign is itching. The eyelids are swollen and accompanied by chemosis, but children rub their eyes and complain of itching. Treatment is often symptomatic and includes cold washcloths and compresses and the occasional use of topical vasoconstrictors and antihistamines. In refractory cases, cromolyn sodium can be used, but long-term therapy usually is required to achieve success. Topical steroids should not be used except under careful guidance by an ophthalmologist, because misdiagnosis can lead to severe exacerbation of an infectious conjunctivitis and because topical steroids carry the potential for significant side effects, including cataract and glaucoma.

With chronic conjunctivitis, chlamydial infection should be considered. This infection typically causes a chronic follicular conjunctival reaction. Treatment should be systemic (erythromycin) as well as topical (erythromycin ointment). In sexually active patients, a careful investigation for sexually transmitted disease, of both the patient and consorts, is imperative. In neonates, a diagnosis of chlamydial conjunctivitis should always be accompanied by a careful investigation into possible systemic signs of chlamydial disease (eg, pneumonia). Systemic treatment with erythromycin is indicated.

Another cause of chronic follicular conjunctivitis is molluscum contagiosum. Molluscum bodies should be searched for in cases of chronic unilateral follicular conjunctivitis. Ablation of the molluscum lesion will result in prompt resolution of the eye irritation and follicular conjunctivitis.

UVEITIS

A triad of symptoms—pain, redness, and photophobia—indicate the possibility of uveitis. Uveitis is categorized according to the part of the eye affected. **Anterior uveitis,** often designated as iritis, consists of inflammatory cells occurring in the anterior chamber of the eye. The distribution of redness is often in the so-called ciliary region; however, diffuse redness can also occur. The palpebral conjunctiva should be spared. Anterior uveitis occurs in the setting of juvenile rheumatoid arthritis, HLA-B27 diseases (Reiter syndrome, psoriasis, and ankylosing spondylitis), and other rare conditions.

Posterior uveitis indicates inflammatory cells occurring in the posterior aspects (vitreous) of the eye. Redness may be present, but the usual symptoms are complaints of seeing spots or diminished vision. Inflammatory cells in the posterior aspect of the eye occur with sarcoidosis, multiple sclerosis, and pars planitis.

A search for the possible cause of posterior uveitis should be instituted, and appropriate treatment provided. Treatment for anterior uveitis usually consists of topical steroids and cycloplegic agents. Posterior uveitis may require steroid injections of the posterior subtenons fascia, a tissue layer located behind the eye. This treatment carries the risk of causing glaucoma but also offers considerable improvement in the posterior uveitis.

Scleritis is rare in children. Causes include rheumatoid arthritis and Behçet disease; some are idiopathic. The diagnosis is based on redness of the sclera with relative sparing of the overlying conjunctiva. Treatment should be aimed at the underlying disease. Topical steroids and subconjunctival injections pose a risk of causing scleral melting and should be administered very carefully.

EYE TRAUMA

Traumatic injuries to the eye represent the most common cause of vision loss in children. With an estimated 300,000 eye injuries per year in the United States, physicians must be aware of signs and symptoms of traumatic injuries to the eye. In particular, it should be recognized that some children may have eye trauma without a good history. Eye trauma may be a presenting feature of child abuse.

Corneal abrasions, the most common type of eye trauma, are associated with denudation of the corneal epithelium, with considerable pain and diffuse redness of the eye. The diagnosis is based on fluorescein staining, which highlights the area of absent corneal epithelium. An investigation for corneal infiltration is indicated (ie, whiteness of the cornea) because this would indicate a superimposed keratitis. Usually there is no keratitis, and treatment consists of topical cycloplegic agents to control pain and topical antibiotics (ointments), with patching of the eye. The patient with corneal abrasion should be examined on a daily basis until the entire corneal epithelial defect has healed.

Blunt trauma to the eye can cause iritis. Pain, redness, and photophobia occur. Treatment may consist of topical steroids if symptoms are prominent.

Lacerations of the eyelid margin require special investigation and management. Apposition of the lid margins, with careful suturing techniques, is important because lid margin injuries can cause cosmetically deforming notches if handled improperly. Lacerations of lid margins in a medial distribution could include the superior or inferior canaliculus. In such cases, children require surgical intervention to place stents in the canaliculi to ensure future drainage in the lacrimal system.

Eye wall laceration represents the most serious form of eye injury. Anterior lacerations occur on the cornea, no more than 5–6 mm from the corneoscleral limbus. Posterior lacerations are posterior to this zone and carry a much poorer prognosis because the retina underlies this region of the eye wall and is very vulnerable to injury.

The diagnosis of an eye laceration is based on findings of decreased vision, distorted ocular anatomy, and, usually, an obvious laceration. When laceration is suspected, an examination under anesthesia may be warranted. Emergent surgical intervention is indicated for lacerations; they should be closed, and concurrent eye injuries managed as needed (eg, retinal detachment and cataract).

Traumatic cataracts can also occur with blunt trauma. The diagnosis is based on an abnormal red reflex. In the first 5 years of life, amblyopia is a risk and prompt cataract removal is indicated. After the age of 5 or 6 years, cataracts should also be removed if they are restricting vision to a significant degree. However, cataract surgery can be more elective, and the surgeon has the option of considering the use of an intraocular lens implant to manage the aphakia created by cataract surgery.

Retinal injuries can also occur with blunt trauma to the eye. Macular holes often reduce vision to 20/200 or 20/400, and there is no specific treatment. Retinal dialysis occurs with severe blunt trauma and must be managed with retinal detachment-reattachment surgery.

Traumatic optic neuropathy can occur with blunt trauma to the forehead or face. Diagnosis is based on diminished vision in one eye with an otherwise normal eye examination. An afferent pupil defect is usually seen (the involved pupil reacts less briskly to light than the fellow pupil). When the diagnosis is suspected, an emergency computerized tomography (CT) scan with coronal reformats of the optic canal should be obtained. If a canal fracture is suspected, emergency surgery may be indicated to try to decompress the optic canal. Indications for surgery are very low vision, prompt diagnosis, and failure to improve spontaneously (within several days) or with systemic steroids. An optic nerve contusion in the absence of a fracture is also possible and can be managed, depending on the clinical situation, with high-dose intravenous steroids.

It is important to recognize that eye injuries seldom occur alone, and a careful assessment for the presence of other injuries should be instituted.

FOREIGN BODY

A foreign body trapped on the surface of the eye, or having penetrated the eye, may cause redness. The most common foreign body is a small piece of stone or other particle blown onto the eye. Hammering metal on metal (eg, hammering a nail into a metallic sheet) can create a rapidly moving projectile that has the potential to penetrate the eye.

Any unilateral red eye should be scrutinized carefully for a possible foreign body. The conjunctival fornices (the area between the eyelid and eyeball, upper and lower) should be searched for particulate matter. A small foreign body embedded on the cornea will usually create a positive test on fluorescein staining. Otherwise, the foreign bodies may be so small that they must be evaluated using magnification, as with a slit lamp.

A foreign body penetrating the eye can be suspected on the basis of redness and evidence of anatomic distortion inside the eye. For example, the pupil may be irregular, the iris may have a perceptible hole in it, or eye discomfort may be out of proportion to a slight amount of redness. Nevertheless, intraocular foreign bodies can be missed easily; therefore, the clinician should refer suspected cases to an ophthalmologist for a full, prompt, careful evaluation.

Management of foreign bodies is removal. A nonembedded foreign body can be irrigated and removed. Corneal foreign bodies must be removed, either with irrigation or with a small, sharp instrument that can dislodge

them. Intraocular foreign bodies require urgent attention and surgical intervention.

EVALUATION OF EYE PAIN

Pain receptors exist throughout the eye and surrounding structures, and the evaluation of pain around the eye proceeds as for pain anywhere else in the body. One exception is an unusual reflex that can cause intense photophobia (light sensitivity; see below). The complaint of pain should elicit a search for potential lacerations, foreign bodies, and blunt trauma. The cornea is one of the most sensitive organs in the body, and even relatively minor injuries, such as a slight debridement of corneal epithelium, can cause substantial pain. The diagnosis of corneal irritation is based on direct inspection and on fluorescein staining, which will cause an area of denuded epithelium to turn bright green when exposed with a blue light.

A reflex exists between sensory nerve endings to the eye and efferent or motor nerve fibers to the pupil. Irritation to the surface of the eye and internal structures will usually cause an intense pupillary spasm and ensuing deep, significant intraocular pain. The etiology of this pain serves as the basis for treating corneal abrasions with topical anticholinergic drops. These drops paralyze the pupil and reduce discomfort.

In anterior uveitis, patients also complain of deep ocular pain that is particularly aggravated by light. Light sensitivity is experienced as a type of pain by most patients but is not limited to uveitis. For example, irritation of the cornea, cataract, and even optic neuritis (inflammation of the optic nerve) can cause photophobia.

STRABISMUS FUNDAMENTALS

Strabismus is divided into several categories: esotropia, exotropia, and vertical deviations. Although it is beyond the scope of this chapter to explore the etiologies and treatment ramifications of each of these conditions, we will direct our attention to important fundamentals in the diagnosis and management of each of them.

CONGENITAL ESOTROPIA

In congenital esotropia, the child's eyes are deviated toward the nose. Typically, the onset of congenital esotropia occurs in the first 2–3 months after birth. The risk for amblyopia in congenital esotropia is less than in other types of esotropia. Nevertheless, efforts to exclude the possibility of amblyopia should be made so that equal vision can be ensured as best as possible. Congenital eso-tropia is also frequently accompanied by nystagmus, over-action of oblique muscles, and a tendency for one eye to drift up under binocular conditions (divergent vertical de-viation).

The management of congenital esotropia is usually surgi-cal. Nevertheless, children should undergo a careful refrac-tion study, and any significant hyperopia should be treated. Ideally, surgery should be performed after amblyopia has been managed successfully. Most children with congenital esotropia should undergo an operation by 1 year of age. Ap-proximately two thirds of children with congenital esotropia achieve ocular alignment with one operation; however, two or more operations may be required. Surgical alignment does not imply that ophthalmic management is unnecessary. The risk for amblyopia and refractive errors persists even though the eyes are aligned; thus, children in whom congen-ital esotropia is diagnosed should be observed at least to 5 or 6 years of age, regardless of alignment outcome.

ACCOMMODATIVE ESOTROPIA

Accommodative esotropia usually occurs between 18 and 36 months of age. Children with accommodative eso-tropia usually have hyperopia in the 2–4 diopter range. Although the etiology of accommodative esotropia is un-known, the pathogenesis involves too much convergence per unit of accommodation. Thus, hyperopic children who must accommodate to see clearly experience esotropia as a result.

The risk of amblyopia in this type of esotropia is quite high. The majority of such children require patching or some other form of antiamblyopic management.

Treatment is aimed at managing the hyperopia and ac-commodation. The use of spectacles with full correction of hyperopia is warranted. If the condition is diagnosed promptly and spectacle therapy instituted within a few months, the prognosis for alignment is good with specta-cles alone. Delays in diagnosis and management, how-ever, often result in failure and the need for surgical re-alignment. Ultimately, most children with accommodative esotropia can be weaned off their glasses. However, a pe-riod of several years is usually required to control the ac-commodative esotropia before tapering therapy.

When the onset of esotropia occurs after the age of 4 years, the possibility of a brainstem tumor should be considered. There may be other ocular or neurologic find-ings to support brainstem pathology, for example, nystag-mus, long tract signs, or the inability to use the eyes to-gether (fuse). Prompt referral to an ophthalmologist familiar with this presentation is indicated.

EXOTROPIA

Exotropia occurs either as a constant or intermittent phenomenon. Constant exotropia in the first year of life is uncommon and usually indicates a craniofacial anomaly or CNS disease (eg, static encephalopathy). Intermittent exotropia surpasses esotropia as the most common type of strabismus by the age of 5 years.

The management of all forms of strabismus begins with a careful search for amblyopia and diagnosis of refractive errors. Both of these abnormalities should be treated be-fore any specific treatment for the strabismus is under-taken. In congenital and constant exotropia, assuming that the child's neurologic status permits, prompt surgical re-alignment is indicated.

On the other hand, management of intermittent exo-tropia varies. If the exotropia occurs only occasionally, no treatment may be indicated. When the eyes are exotropic more than one third of the time, alternative forms of treat-ment should be considered.

One approach consists of deliberately oversubtracting the patient's prescription to induce accommodation. Con-vergence accompanies accommodation, and the eyes can be forced to turn into a more normal position with this maneuver. About 50% of children with intermittent exo-tropia can be managed successfully by this approach. Be-cause initial conservative management does no harm, the use of spectacles and optical interventions is appropriate.

If the child rejects the optical treatment, or if it fails, sur-gical management may be indicated. This can be accom-plished with considerable success, but there is a tendency for the exotropia to relapse within 5–10 years after surgery.

VERTICAL STRABISMUS PROBLEMS

A number of important conditions result in vertical mis-alignment of the eyes.

Fourth Cranial Nerve Palsies

Fourth nerve palsies may be congenital or acquired. Children can compensate for these palsies by developing an ability to move their eyes together (large, vertical fu-sion amplitudes). However, the compensatory phase of this condition also usually includes a head tilt. Children will tilt their head away from the side of the fourth nerve palsy (eg, to the right in a left fourth nerve palsy). A child with a head tilt, at any age, should have a careful eye ex-amination to exclude the possibility of fourth nerve palsy. Management often includes surgery, depending on the de-gree of head tilt and the amount of vertical deviation.

Brown Syndrome

Brown syndrome is the inability to elevate one eye when it is adducted. Although this diagnosis may be sub-tle, children usually compensate for the problem by ele-vating their chin somewhat and maintaining the eyes in a downward gaze.

The possible causes of Brown syndrome are numerous, but many are idiopathic. If the diagnosis is known, no par-ticular investigation is warranted. If primary gaze is affected, prism therapy and glasses or surgical intervention are warranted.

Double Elevator Palsy

When a child cannot elevate an eye adequately in any field of gaze, double elevator palsy is diagnosed. The usual cause is tightness of the inferior rectus muscle, which then fails to allow the eye to rotate up efficiently. Rare causes include paralysis of the superior rectus muscle (usually accompanied by ptosis) and CNS (midbrain) conditions.

Children compensate for this inability to elevate one eye by tilting their head so that they can use both eyes together, but in a downward gaze. Surgical management is often indicated. Prism therapy may be useful if the amount of deviation in primary gaze is small.

Blowout Fractures

The cause of blowout fracture is blunt trauma to the eye. It is assumed that the floor of the orbit has the weakest bony structure and therefore is most vulnerable to fracture. Orbit contents can prolapse into the maxillary sinus through the floor fracture. As a result, children with blowout fractures may demonstrate enophthalmos and strabismus. Because the inferior rectus muscle is usually trapped, difficulty may occur in rotating the eye either down or up.

The child with vertical strabismus should undergo a careful investigation for the possibility of a fracture. When a fracture is diagnosed, its cause should be clearly delineated. Child abuse is of major concern. There is no need to manage the fracture per se. Only in the setting of cosmetically significant enophthalmos or strabismus should clinicians be concerned about correcting the fracture itself.

Surgical management may have to be performed in several stages. Often the floor fracture needs to be closed primarily to reduce the degree of enophthalmos. If strabismus persists after this primary procedure, it may have to be treated.

PITFALLS IN THE DIAGNOSIS & MANAGEMENT OF STRABISMUS: A PEDIATRICIAN'S PERSPECTIVE

In the office management of strabismus, pediatricians should be aware of certain strabismus presentations that may indicate serious CNS disease. The first of these is cranial nerve palsy. Fourth nerve palsies seldom imply CNS disease. On the other hand, an acquired sixth nerve palsy may indicate posterior fossa or brainstem tumor. Unless there is an obvious antecedent history of trauma (and even when there is trauma!), a CNS scan is indicated. Similarly, third nerve palsies, when acquired, and with no obvious antecedent cause (eg, trauma, congenital), should be managed by obtaining a neuroimaging scan. The risk of a brain tumor in this setting is small, but it could be harmful to the child to delay this diagnosis.

A constant exotropia in the first year of life may indicate either craniofacial defect or significant neurologic disease. A more focused neurologic examination and skull examination is warranted with this type of strabismus.

Esotropia that presents after 4 years of age may also indicate brainstem tumor. Once again, neuroimaging investigations are occasionally warranted, depending on other clinical circumstances.

When nystagmus occurs simultaneously with strabismus, a more detailed investigation is indicated, usually with neuroimaging studies.

The vast majority of cases of strabismus in childhood have no underlying CNS disease. In most cases, children can be managed by an ophthalmologist familiar with strabismus without concern about more ominous CNS pathology.

OPHTHALMOLOGY IN THE NURSERY

RETINOPATHY OF PREMATURITY

Retinopathy of prematurity (ROP) is a disease of retinal vascularization. The migration of retinal blood vessels normally runs from posterior (optic nerve) to anterior (peripheral aspects of retina). The nasal retina is entirely vascularized earlier than the temporal retina because there is less retinal area on the nasal side. Complete vascularization usually occurs by 33–34 weeks' gestation. In very low birth weight infants, an arrest in this vascularization process can occur. A demarcation line develops between vascularized and nonvascularized retina; neovascularization may occur along this line, and this can cause scarring and subsequent retinal detachment.

The exact etiology of ROP is unknown. A national study done in the 1950s documented that high concentrations of oxygen delivered to low-birth-weight infants increased the likelihood of ROP. However, because of advances in neonatal care, combined with better ability to monitor arterial oxygen saturation in newborn and premature babies, other factors have become more important.

Very low birth weight infants are at particularly high risk. The incidence of ROP is negligible in infants with birth weights greater than 1500 g. Below this weight, the risk of ROP increases as birth weight decreases. At 500 g birth weight, the risk of ROP is 90–95%.

In addition to gestational age, risk factors include sepsis, blood transfusions, and pulmonary disease. Increased bilirubin levels appear to offer protection against ROP, perhaps because bilirubin is a scavenger for oxygen free radicals, a putative causative factor.

ROP usually appears 4–10 weeks after birth, regardless of gestational age. In most infants, it progresses to a certain point then regresses spontaneously, causing no damage to the retina. In approximately 20% of babies, ROP progresses to cause visual damage.

ROP is categorized according to the zone of the retina in which it occurs and its severity in that particular zone (stage). **Zone 1** refers to ROP that exists within twice the distance between the optic nerve and the fovea. Zone 1 disease carries a particularly bad prognosis. In **zone 2 ROP,** a demarcation line exists 360 degrees around the retina. In **zone 3 ROP,** the area of affected retina occurs only on the temporal side.

Stage 1 indicates a line that exists between vascularized and nonvascularized retina. In **stage 2,** the line is elevated. In **stage 3,** neovascularization has occurred in this demarcation region. **Stage 4** indicates local retinal detachment. **Stage 5** indicates a complete retinal detachment. The pathogenesis of retinal detachment includes neovascularization in the demarcation region followed by regression of neovascularization with cicatrization (scarring), pulling on the retina, and retinal detachment.

Vision loss occurs from retinal detachment. However, the pulling forces can also occur tangentially along the retina, leading to traction and warping of the macular region without an actual retinal detachment. This "dragging" of the retina virtually always causes vision to be worse than 20/400.

Treatment of ROP is multifaceted. Efforts have been aimed at attempting to prevent the condition. Careful monitoring of oxygen saturation remains important. Vitamin E as a preventive treatment is debated. Further studies are required to clarify its role in helping retard or prevent ROP.

Babies who weigh less than 1500 g should be monitored closely by an ophthalmologist familiar with ROP. In certain cases, when the ROP progression is severe, cryotherapy or laser therapy to the retina may help accelerate the regression of the ROP and prevent complications. Most ophthalmologists choose to treat babies who have reached a minimum of zone 2. If stage 3 disease is particularly bad in one sector of the eye, local or complete treatment may be advisable. Babies who have severe zone 1 disease should have both eyes treated. When the disease is in the zone 2 distribution bilaterally, the ophthalmologist should discuss with the family the option of treating one or both eyes, and proceed accordingly. Because long-term effects of cryosurgery are unknown (eg, whether it could cause late complications heretofore unknown), the family may choose treatment for only one eye.

If retinal detachment recurs, the prognosis is poor. Scleral buckling procedures may be helpful in reattaching the retina. Intraoperative techniques include vitrectomy and endolaser. Sadly, although anatomic success in reattaching the retina may be achieved, most of these children have no useful vision.

CONDITIONS OF INTEREST TO THE OPHTHALMOLOGIST

The list of conditions that can affect the eyes together with other organ systems is long. Some of the more common conditions are discussed below.

Some drugs used by mothers are teratogenic and may cause ocular complications. Alcohol can cause fetal alcohol syndrome, the most prominent feature of which is poor prenatal and postnatal growth. Mental retardation is common. Midfacial abnormalities (flat philtrum) and cardiac defects are also noted. The ocular findings can include ptosis, strabismus, and optic nerve hypoplasia, but the eyes may be normal.

Recently, cocaine has been implicated as an in utero cause of fetal abnormality. Cocaine can cause genitourinary abnormalities and neurobehavioral disruption in the first 6 months after birth. Ocular findings include optic nerve abnormalities, eyelid edema, and delayed visual maturation. Of these, delayed visual maturation is probably the most common eye abnormality seen in "crack babies" and consists of poor visual attentiveness, despite a normal eye and normal neurologic (including scan) examination. The prognosis in delayed visual maturation is good; however, many of these children may go on to have other minor but troubling neurologic abnormalities, such as attention-deficit disorder and learning disabilities.

Craniofacial abnormalities are not infrequent and are of importance to the ophthalmologist. Strabismus occurs commonly in children with craniofacial defects. Children with strabismus should have at least one careful eye examination. Hydrocephalus can cause damage to the optic nerves or cortical visual impairment. Children with hydrocephalus should be monitored closely with regular eye examinations.

The ophthalmologist is often asked to help diagnose one of the congenital *tox*oplasmosis, *r*ubella, *c*ytomegalovirus, *h*erpes simplex (TORCH) infections (see Chapters 4 and 5). The lesions in congenital toxoplasmosis are characteristic, usually consisting of unilateral or bilateral macular scars. Congenital rubella frequently causes impaired vision in children. Microphthalmia, as well as congenital cataracts, may occur. Glaucoma may also occur but usually does not accompany congenital cataracts. Pigmentary retinopathy occurs with later gestational infection. Herpes infections can cause dermatitis and keratitis. With CNS involvement, retinitis can also occur. Cataracts occasionally accompany the retinitis. Cytomegalovirus also may cause congenital eye abnormalities. Colobomas of the eye have been reported, and cataracts occur occasionally. Retinitis can also accompany congenital cytomegalovirus infections.

Congenital syphilis usually does not cause congenital eye lesions. However, interstitial keratitis can present later in childhood.

Certain eye abnormalities may be an indication that a baby has a particular syndrome. For example, the ophthalmologist may be asked to look for ocular colobomas. Their presence may indicate simple autosomal-dominant transmission or a more ominous and serious syndrome. The CHARGE syndrome includes colobomas, heart defects, choanal atresia, retardation, genitourinary abnormalities, and ear anomalies, with hearing problems. Aicardi syndrome consists of severe CNS defects with delays in development, infantile spasms, and colobomas. Trisomy 13 can also cause colobomas of the eyes.

Congenital cataracts are discussed below. Their presence may be an indication of any of a number of syndromes or diseases, although the usual cause is autosomal-dominant transmission or sporadic occurrence.

Optic nerve abnormalities also accompany certain syndromes and genetic defects. Septo-optic dysplasia syndrome includes absence of the septum pellucidum, optic nerve hypoplasia, and pituitary gland insufficiency. Children with this syndrome who present with optic nerve hypoplasia (and nystagmus) are at risk for pituitary insufficiency and midline CNS abnormalities. They should be evaluated by an endocrinologist, and neuroimaging is indicated. Optic nerve hypoplasia also occurs in fetal alcohol syndrome, in infants of young mothers, and in infants of diabetic mothers.

Retinal abnormalities are a feature of a number of syndromes. In tuberous sclerosis, astrocytic hamartomas may be found. In neurofibromatosis type 1, optic nerve abnormalities (hypoplasia and atrophy) and Lisch nodules (hamartomatous bumps on the anterior surface of the iris) can occur. In neurofibromatosis type 2, retinal hamartomas and posterior subcapsular cataracts can occur.

Pigmentary retinopathy can occur as an isolated finding associated with impaired vision and can be a sign of more severe and occasionally degenerative neurologic disease. Because pigmentary retinopathies occur with a variety of organ system abnormalities, children should be examined carefully for the possibility of other disease.

Cherry-red spots occur in the macula when ganglion cells become engorged with metabolic by-products. Tay-Sachs disease is an example of a condition with this feature.

THE CHILD WITH AN ABNORMAL RED REFLEX

From the ophthalmologist's perspective, an investigation for the presence of a normal red reflex is an important part of the neonatal eye examination. An abnormal reflex, or frank leukocoria, usually is a sign of serious eye, or even systemic, disease. The most common abnormality causing a poor red reflex is congenital cataracts. These may occur unilaterally or bilaterally. Their diagnosis is crucial, because failure to treat congenital cataracts can lead to irreversible monocular or bilateral amblyopia. The approach to the child with abnormal red reflex is outlined in Figure 22–3.

problem z central vision, images from z eyes often so diff they cannot be fused

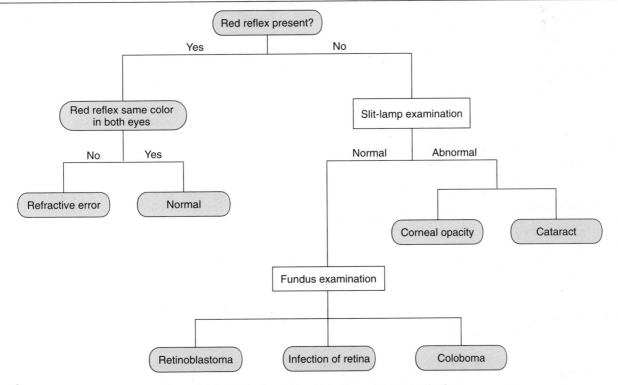

Figure 22–3. Evaluation of the child with an abnormal red reflex.

CATARACTS = *Loss of transparency of the lens of the eye.*

The causes of cataracts are myriad. The evaluation of the child with congenital cataracts should begin with a careful history and physical examination. If the findings are normal, with no organ system abnormalities, further investigation is seldom warranted. On the other hand, a search for a systemic cause of congenital cataracts is indicated if there are neurologic or systemic problems.

The treatment for congenital cataracts is usually surgical removal of the lens. Occasionally small cataracts can be observed if they do not take up the entire visual axis.

RETINOBLASTOMA

The most ominous cause of an absent red reflex is retinoblastoma. Retinoblastoma usually presents with leukocoria. Occasionally children with retinoblastoma present with strabismus or hyphema. *→ blood in the anterior chamber of the eye.* Retinoblastoma is the most common eye tumor in children. It can occur unilaterally or bilaterally. It can occur as a sporadic tumor, or it can be inherited in an autosomal-dominant fashion.

When the tumor occurs unilaterally with no family history and with a relatively late onset (after age 18 months), it is usually sporadic, with little chance of the occurrence of additional tumors in the same or other eye. On the other hand, bilateral onset, positive family history, and early onset (younger than 1 year) all indicate the possibility of inherited tumor, and genetic counseling and very close surveillance of the patient become even more important.

Treatment of retinoblastoma consists of local treatment for small tumors (irradiation or thermal ablation). Large tumors need to be removed by enucleating the eye. Any investigation for metastatic disease should include lumbar puncture and bone marrow aspiration. Children with the hereditary form of retinoblastoma are at significant risk for the development of second tumors (especially osteosarcoma).

CORNEAL OPACITIES

Although uncommon, corneal opacities also pose a formidable challenge to visual development. The Peter anomaly consists of central corneal scars, often in conjunction with cataracts. Congenital corneal infections occur occasionally and can cause whitening of the central part of the cornea. Rare congenital dystrophies also present with whitening or haziness of the cornea. Congenital glaucoma is notorious for causing corneal haziness, large eyes, tearing, and photophobia. The differential diagnosis of the cloudy cornea at birth is presented in Table 22–1.

CONCLUSION

A systematic approach to eye problems in children is advised. Monitoring visual acuity is paramount. Most eye problems can be diagnosed by direct observation with an ophthalmoscope.

Table 22–1. Differential diagnosis of cloudy cornea at birth.

Forceps injury (linear tear across cornea)
Mucopolysaccharidosis
Keratitis — *inflammation of the cornea*
Congenital corneal dystrophy
Peters anomaly (central opacity)
Glaucoma (symptoms of tearing and photophobia)

REFERENCES

Good WV: Behaviors of visually impaired children. Semin Ophthalmol 1991;6:158.
Hoyt CS et al: Disorders of the eye. In Taeusch HW et al (editors): *Schaffer and Avery's Diseases of the Newborn,* 6th ed. Saunders, 1991.

Isenberg SJ (editor): *The Eye in Infancy.* Year Book, 1989.
Taylor DSI (editor): *Pediatric Ophthalmology.* Blackwell, 1990.

Orthopedic Problems

John T. Smith, MD

Orthopedic problems in children are common. Most problems are straightforward and require a basic understanding of the growth and development of the musculoskeletal system to be managed properly. Form, structure, and function are closely interrelated.

Initial orthopedic assessment begins with observation of the child. Abnormalities of gait and limb function are easily detected when the child is unaware of the examiner, such as during play or walking in a relaxed setting. The child should be examined in a parent's lap when appropriate and should be undressed to allow inspection of the limbs and trunk.

MUSCULOSKELETAL TRAUMA

Musculoskeletal injuries in children account for 10–15% of all childhood injuries. The presence of open cartilaginous growth plates, greater elasticity of the bones, small size and blood volume, and the potential for growth disturbance are unique considerations in pediatric injuries and fractures.

FRACTURES

Evaluation

The initial evaluation of a suspected fracture begins with a thorough physical examination. Deformity, neurocirculatory status, and skin integrity should be documented. Any suspected fracture, regardless of how minor the trauma, must be assessed with radiographs in two planes. The joint above and below the fracture should be visualized. Comparison views of the opposite normal extremity may be helpful if the injury involves a growth plate. Splinting the extremity during the evaluation provides comfort and reassurance for the child.

Children's fractures demand accurate description to facilitate communication between the primary care physician and the consulting physician. Fractures should be described by anatomic location, location in the bone, fracture pattern, alignment, and status of the surrounding soft tissues.

Management Principles

Treatment of a given fracture must be individualized. The need for fracture reduction, splinting, and a plan for follow-up should be determined in conjunction with the consulting orthopedist. Most children's fractures heal rapidly with nonoperative care. Children tolerate prolonged immobilization physically and emotionally better than do adults. Growth and remodeling of long bone fractures will correct minor inaccuracies of alignment in many instances, especially when residual deformity is in the plane of motion of the adjacent joint. Growth plate injury can produce prolonged growth disturbance and residual deformity. Figure 23–1 depicts an algorithm for the management of a patient with a fracture.

Growth Plate Injury

Longitudinal growth of the axial skeleton occurs at the growth plate (physis). Normal growth-plate function is controlled by mechanical, local, and systemic factors. Physeal growth begins with the orderly multiplication of germinal cells on the epiphyseal side of the growth plate. These cells progress through a process of multiplication, hypertrophy, and vascular invasion, followed by ossification of physeal cartilage into metaphyseal bone. The epiphysis "grows away" from the metaphysis. The normal growth process results in limbs of symmetrical length and alignment. Injuries to this mechanism can produce significant growth disturbance and angular deformity.

The cartilaginous growth plate is vulnerable to injury because it is mechanically weaker than the surrounding bone and supporting ligaments. Fractures involving the growth plate may produce mechanical or vascular injury to the germinal cells of the physis, disrupting normal longitudinal growth. The Salter-Harris classification of

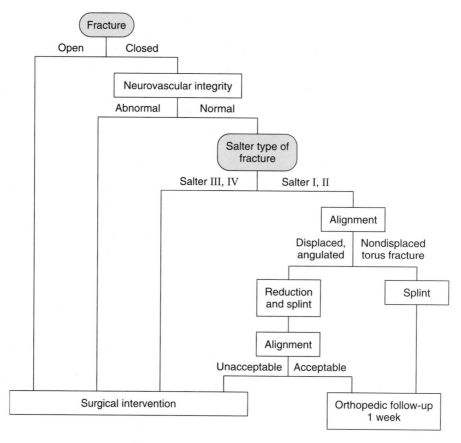

Figure 23–1. Algorithm for fracture care.

growth-plate injuries correlates closely with the risk of subsequent growth disturbance (Figure 23–2). In type I injury, the fracture traverses the physis through the zone of hypertrophy and does not involve the germinal physeal fragment. Type I and II injuries have a low incidence of subsequent growth disturbance and often can be managed with closed reduction and casting. Fractures of the distal femoral physis, however, are a major exception. Type III and IV injuries cross the germinal layer of the physis. Most of these injuries require surgical reduction and stabilization. Injury to this layer or an imperfect reduction can result in the formation of a bridge of bone across the physis, which functions as a tether to future growth. Angular deformity or limb-length inequality can result. Type V injury results from a crush injury to the germinal physeal cells; this diagnosis is made retrospectively.

A common pitfall when treating pediatric injuries is to confuse a physeal separation with a "torn ligament," which is relatively rare in children. For example, an ankle injury in a skeletally immature patient is as likely to produce an injury to the distal fibular physis as is a simple ligamentous ankle sprain. A suspected physeal injury should be referred to an orthopedist.

Fracture Remodeling

Children's fractures, unlike their adult counterparts, have a considerable capacity to remodel with growth. This ability is dependent on the age of the child, the location of the fracture, the degree of deformity, and the proximity of the fracture to the growth plate. Deformity in the plane of motion of a joint remodels readily. Angular deformity is slower to remodel, and rotational deformity has no capacity to correct with growth.

The process of fracture healing also may produce stimulation of growth. Fracture healing begins with an inflammatory response facilitated by increased local blood flow. It is common to see 1 cm of "overgrowth" after healing of a femoral-shaft fracture. This must be accounted for at the time of treatment, or unequal limb lengths will result. Metaphyseal fractures of the medial aspect of the tibia can produce asymmetrical growth simulation, resulting in angular deformity (*genu valgum*).

Common Fractures in Children

Forearm Fractures. Forearm fractures are common in children, typically resulting from a fall on the outstretched arm. These fractures vary from a minimal buckle

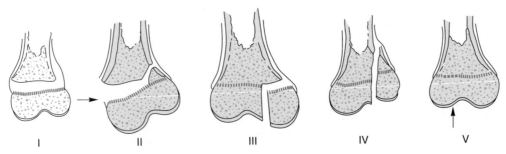

Figure 23–2. The Salter-Harris classification of growth-plate injuries. Type I physeal fractures occur through the region of provisional calcification. The proliferating portion of the physis remains attached to the epiphysis and is not damaged. Type II fractures extend through a segment of the metaphysis. Again, the proliferative portions of the physis are intact. Type III fractures extend through a segment of the provisional calcification zone and then cross through the epiphysis to the articular surface. Type IV fractures extend obliquely from the metaphysis across the physis and into the epiphysis. They, too, are regular fractures. Type V fractures are crush injuries of all or a portion of the physis. The proliferative zones of the physis sustain irreversible damage. (Reproduced, with permission, from Salter RB, Harris WR: Injuries involving the epiphyseal plate. J Bone Joint Surg [Am] 1963;45:587.)

or torus fracture to an obviously displaced fracture of the radius and ulna requiring manipulation and reduction. These fractures may involve the physis.

All suspected forearm fractures should be evaluated radiographically. When a fracture is present, a decision regarding reduction is made depending on the severity and degree of deformity. Torus fractures have little associated deformity and require only splinting or a below-elbow cast for protection; healing is rapid. Fractures with displacement, gross deformity, or angulation require manipulative reduction followed by splinting. A "sugartong" splint is preferred initially because it allows for swelling and provides sufficient ability to maintain fracture alignment. After swelling is reduced, a carefully molded cast is applied until radiographic union is achieved.

Elbow Fractures. Elbow fractures are common in children and may be difficult to recognize. The ossification centers of the distal humeral epiphysis appear sequentially beginning at age 2 years and are all present by age 10. A large portion of the elbow is cartilaginous, making fractures difficult to visualize radiographically. Subtle physeal injuries are easily missed, resulting in adverse long-term outcomes. The normal development of the ossification centers of the elbow and their relationships to each other are well established. An alteration in these normal relationships or the presence of a joint effusion should lead to a strong suspicion that a fracture is present. Comparison views of the contralateral elbow, oblique views, or arthrography are often useful adjuncts to confirm the diagnosis.

Treatment of elbow fractures in children must be individualized. A major portion of these fractures appears relatively benign radiographically yet is inherently unstable and requires operative treatment. Good examples of this include **supracondylar fractures** and **lateral condylar fractures.** The consequences of failure to recognize these injuries are angular deformity or non-union. Early referral

and operative care, when appropriate, produce the best long-term outcome.

Nursemaid's elbow, a common injury unique to children, is not actually a fracture. The usual mechanism of injury is forced hyperextension and supination of the forearm producing subluxation of the annular ligament around the radial neck at the elbow. Injured children typically stop using their elbows and avoid motion because of pain. Radiographs of the injury usually are normal. Nursemaid's elbow is easily reduced by rapidly taking the elbow through a full flexion, with pronation and supination of the wrist, and then into full extension. A palpable or audible "pop" may be felt, followed shortly by relief of pain, full range of motion, and return of normal function.

Femur Fractures. Fractures of the femur are frequently the result of high-energy trauma and may be associated with major multisystem trauma. In infants younger than 12 months, these injuries have a high association with nonaccidental trauma. These fractures are best treated by rapid stabilization to facilitate mobilization of the child or care of associated injuries. There are a variety of methods to treat these injuries, including immediate hip casting, prolonged skeletal traction, external fixation, and internal fixation. Treatment decision are individualized on the basis of the age of the patient, associated injuries, and other factors.

Fractures of the femoral neck and proximal femur are surgical emergencies. These injuries are frequently unstable. The blood supply of the proximal femoral epiphysis is at risk in these injuries, a risk minimized by early operative stabilization of the hip. Casting is successful in only a small percentage of stable fractures in this region.

Fractures of the distal femur often involve the distal femoral epiphysis. These injuries are easily mistaken for "knee sprains." Stress views of the distal femoral epiphysis readily distinguish these injuries. The distal femoral epiphysis tolerates injury poorly, with the incidence of subsequent growth disturbance as high as 30%. Most physeal injuries of the distal femur require anatomic reduction and pinning.

Tibia Fractures. Fractures of the tibia are relatively common in children and may occur with seemingly minimal trauma. One common example is the so-called **toddler's fracture,** an oblique minimally displaced fracture of the tibial shaft without an associated fibular fracture. This injury usually results from a minor fall with a twisting component, followed by refusal to walk. The oblique nature of the fracture often makes it difficult to visualize on initial radiographs. Most of these injuries are stable, requiring only cast immobilization.

Fractures of the distal epiphysis of the tibia and fibula should be considered when evaluating any ankle injury. Until skeletal maturity, the yield strength of the physis is lower than that of the surrounding ligaments. Therefore, ankle sprains are easily confused with these fractures by physical examination but should be easily distinguished radiographically.

Compartment Syndrome

The development of compartment syndrome after an injury to an extremity can have serious consequences. Compartment syndrome develops when there is bleeding into a closed fascial compartment, producing progressive swelling and an increase in intracompartmental pressure. As the pressure increases, venous blood flow is impaired, followed by ischemia, which if prolonged will result in cell death of the surrounding muscle and nerves.

Compartment syndrome is characterized by the "five P's": pain, pallor, paresthesia, pulselessness, and paralysis. The earliest sign of compartment syndrome is pain. A child with a splinted fracture should be comfortable with minimal analgesia. If not, then compartment syndrome should be suspected. The remaining "P's" are late findings. Compartment syndrome is confirmed by direct measurement of compartment pressures. If compartment syndrome is found, it is treated by immediate surgical fasciotomy. Without treatment, irreversible damage to the compartment structures occurs within 6 hours after onset.

CHILD ABUSE

Nonaccidental trauma (NAT), or **battered child syndrome,** must be recognized and reported by primary care physicians treating pediatric injuries. The diagnosis of NAT is rarely straightforward (see Chapter 10). About 75% of abused children are younger than 3 years. The consequences of failure to diagnose NAT are significant, with a 35% risk of repeat injury and risk of death up to 10%.

Child abuse covers a broad spectrum, from emotional neglect to physical injury. Several historical features and patterns of fracture strongly suggest the diagnosis of NAT, which should prompt further investigation (Table 23–1). Fractures highly suggestive of NAT include multi-

Table 23–1. Radiographic signs suggesting child abuse.[1]

High specificity
  Metaphyseal lesions
  Posterior rib fractures
  Scapular fractures
  Spinous process fractures
  Sternal fractures

Moderate specificity
  Multiple fractures, bilateral
  Fractures of different ages
  Epiphyseal separations
  Vertebral body fractures
  Digital fractures
  Complex skull fractures

Common but low specificity
  Clavicular fractures
  Long bone fractures

[1]Reproduced, with permission, from Kleinman PK (editor): *Diagnostic Imaging of Child Abuse.* Williams & Wilkins, 1987.

ple fractures in differing stages of radiographic healing, metaphyseal corner fractures, spinous process fractures, posterior rib fractures, complex skull fractures, and epiphyseal separations. Spiral fractures involving the femoral diaphysis in a child younger than 12 months should prompt suspicion of NAT.

These physical findings must be correlated with the history of the injury. No single historical feature or behavior is consistently present in NAT. Abusive parents rarely offer accurate information. Step-parents or boyfriends are frequent abusers. If the history is inconsistent with the physical findings, it is best to ensure the safety of the child and initiate further investigation into the circumstances of the injury.

SPORTS MEDICINE IN CHILDREN

Organized sports for children are increasing in the United States. Both children and their parents are driven by the tangible rewards for exceptional performance. This has resulted in a major increase in injuries associated with organized sports. Sports injuries in children are divided into two groups: overuse syndromes and sports trauma.

OVERUSE SYNDROMES

Overuse syndromes result from placing a highly repetitive stress on a given structure until injury occurs. This can produce several patterns of injury unique to the growing skeleton.

Shin Pain

This is a nonspecific symptom complex characterized by pain along the anterior aspect of the leg with activity. Persistent shin pain requires investigation to look for an underlying cause. The differential diagnosis includes stress fractures, shin splints, periostitis, nerve entrapment, muscle strain, infection, tumors, and exercise-induced compartment syndrome.

Stress Fractures

Repetitive application of loads to a bone can produce a stress fracture. It presents with the gradual onset of pain with activity. The tibia and metatarsals are the most common sites. Initial radiographs may be normal, whereas a bone scan will demonstrate early increased uptake. These early findings must be interpreted carefully, because stress fractures can easily imitate infection, osteoid osteomas, and malignant neoplasms. Treatment is directed at avoidance of the offending activity, casting, or bone grafting if spontaneous healing fails.

Sever Disease

Sever disease presents as activity-related heel pain. Radiographs may show increased density and fragmentation of the calcaneal apophysis but are nonspecific. Treatment involves rest and activity modification. Symptoms resolve at the completion of growth.

Throwing Syndromes

Most throwing syndromes result from repetitive valgus stress at the elbow. Osteochondrosis of the capitellum, or so-called **Little League elbow,** is commonly seen in baseball pitchers and gymnasts. Patients complain of pain, grinding, and reduced range of motion of the elbow. Radiographs show fragmentation of the capitellum with or without a loose body. Treatment involves activity modification or avoidance, strengthening, and surgery if a loose body is present.

Other throwing syndromes seen less frequently include epiphysiolysis of the proximal humerus, osteochondritis of the radial head, and stress injury or fracture to the medial epicondyle.

SPORTS TRAUMA

Ligamentous injuries and fractures of the ankle, knee, and shoulder often occur in association with participation in organized sports. Each injury requires careful evaluation to avoid confusing "simple" sprains with more complex physeal injuries or osteochondral fractures. Major swelling, hemarthrosis, or inability to bear weight should prompt x-ray evaluation.

Ankle Sprains

These are a common sports injury. The usual mechanism is inversion of the ankle, producing a varying degree of disruption of the lateral stabilizing ligaments or the an-terior ankle capsule. Treatment is based on the severity of the injury and follows the basic principles of rest, ice, compression, and elevation ("RICE") and some degree of immobilization. For most sprains, rehabilitation exercises, taping, or a compressive ankle brace are adequate. More severe injuries may require casting or, rarely, surgical reconstruction of the ligaments.

Acute Knee Injuries

Acute knee injuries, especially those associated with hemarthrosis or inability to walk, require careful assessment. In the younger child, ligamentous injury is decidedly rare, with avulsions of bone at ligamentous insertions, osteochondral fractures, or physeal injury more common. In the adolescent, pure ligamentous disruption is similar to the adult pattern of injury. A clinical history of a forceful twisting injury to the knee, associated with a "pop," pain, and rapid onset of swelling, suggests a major injury. Examination of the knee after acute injury is often compromised by pain and swelling. Radiographs, including standard, oblique, and stress views, are helpful. In some instances, examination under anesthesia is necessary.

Treatment is age and diagnosis specific. Many problems, such as acute patellar dislocation, anterior cruciate ligament tears, and collateral ligament injuries, are initially managed with bracing and an aggressive rehabilitation program. In children, ligamentous reconstruction is delayed until skeletal maturity.

Acute Shoulder Dislocation

Dislocation of the shoulder is rare in children but may occur in adolescence. The most common mechanism is that of forced abduction and external rotation of the shoulder producing an anterior dislocation. Immediate reduction under sedation is recommended. The incidence of chronic instability and recurrence is higher when the initial dislocation occurs before 20 years of age.

CHRONIC KNEE PROBLEMS

Evaluation of the Painful Knee

A variety of unique, painful conditions affect the growing skeleton. Although most problems are self-limited and resolve at the completion of growth, each requires careful evaluation. Any knee pain associated with limping, swelling, or restriction of function should be evaluated radiographically. The clinician should bear in mind that the most common pitfall is to miss significant pathology of the hip that presents as referred pain to the knee.

Osgood-Schlatter Disease

Osgood-Schlatter disease is characterized by swelling and pain over the apophysis of the proximal tibia at the insertion of the patellar ligament. It presents as activity-related pain and swelling over the tibial tubercle and is often bilateral. It is more common in active boys. Radiographs show fragmentation of the tibial tubercle and soft-tissue swelling. Treatment involves rest, activity restriction, and anti-inflammatory medications. The symptoms resolve at the completion of growth.

Peripatellar Pain

Anterior peripatellar knee pain is common in children, especially adolescents. Overuse is a common etiology; patellar tendinitis, recurrent subluxation, and dislocation of the patella should also be considered. Radiographs, including patellar views, should be obtained but rarely confirm the diagnosis. Treatment is directed toward strengthening the quadriceps mechanism to restore proper patellar tracking and balance. Physical therapy often accelerates recovery.

Osteochondritis Dissecans

This is a process in which a small segment of subchondral bone becomes avascular. The etiology is uncertain, but trauma and endocrine problems have been suggested. Children often present with an aching pain in the knee. The segment may become necrotic and then detached from the adjacent bone, producing catching or locking of the knee. Radiographs of the knee, especially a "tunnel or notch" view, are diagnostic. The lesion typically involves the lateral surface of the medial femoral condyle. In situ lesions are treated with rest and activity restriction, whereas detached fragments require surgical repair.

Popliteal Cysts (Baker Cysts)

These frequently occur in the popliteal fossa under the medial head of the gastrocnemius muscle. They are an out-pouching of the synovium of the capsule enclosing the knee joint. They are usually asymptomatic, and their size fluctuates. Spontaneous regression is to be expected. Indications for surgical excision include persistent pain, rapid change in size, uncertain diagnosis, and parental concern despite reassurance. The recurrence rate is 30% or greater after surgical excision.

SCOLIOSIS & SPINE DEFORMITY

Scoliosis is defined as a curvature of the spine of greater than 10 degrees in the coronal plane. Scoliosis is a physical finding, not a diagnosis. The etiology of scoliosis is varied, and the specific course must be sought before initiating treatment.

Evaluation

Scoliosis is usually detected during a routine physical examination. A complete history and developmental as-sessment should be obtained. Idiopathic scoliosis is usually painless, and a history of back pain suggests other causes. Because scoliosis can be the result of lesions to the spinal cord, a history of changes of bowel or bladder function or neuromuscular changes should be sought. The child must be undressed and examined in both the sitting and standing positions. Scoliosis that resolves in the sitting position may indicate a leg-length inequality. The forward bending test is performed by having the patient bend 90 degrees with the hands joined in the midline. This test will identify asymmetry of the ribs and spinous processes, which suggest an underlying curve. Cutaneous abnormalities, such as dimpling or tufts of hair over the spine may indicate spinal dysraphism. A careful neurologic examination may reveal weakness or altered reflexes, which suggest a neuromuscular etiology.

Radiographs should be obtained if a spinal curvature is detected. An upright 3-foot posteroanterior view of the spine is adequate as a screening exam. Spinal curvature is measured by the Cobb method (Figure 23–3).

Classification

Once a curve is detected, it should be classified, which helps to determine etiology, natural history, and prognosis (Table 23–2).

IDIOPATHIC SCOLIOSIS

This is the most common form of scoliosis in North America. It occurs primarily during the adolescent growth

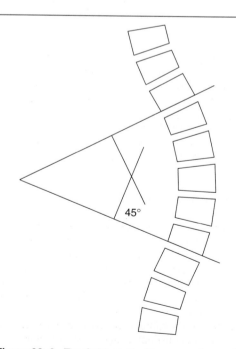

Figure 23–3. The Cobb method for measuring scoliosis.

Table 23–2. Classification of scoliosis.

Idiopathic
  Infantile (0–3 years)
  Juvenile (4 years to puberty)
  Adolescent (puberty to epiphyseal closure)

Neuromuscular
  Cerebral palsy
  Myelomeningitis
  Spinal muscular atrophy
  Syringomyelia
  Friedreich ataxia
  Spinal cord tumor
  Spinal cord trauma

Myopathic
  Arthrogryposis
  Muscular dystrophy

Congenital
  Failures of formation (hemivertebrae)
  Failures of segmentation (unilateral unsegmented bar)
  Mixed

Mesenchymal
  Marfan syndrome
  Ehlers-Danlos syndrome

Other Causes
  Limb length inequality
  Hysterical
  Metabolic
  Soft tissue contractures
  Osteochondrodystrophies

spurt and is much more common in females. "Idiopathic" is a diagnosis of exclusion, and other causes should be sought before treatment is initiated.

Treatment decisions are based on the risk for further curvature progression. The likelihood of progression increases with female sex, onset before menses, skeletal immaturity, and greater magnitude of curvature. Children with curvature less than 25 degrees should be observed for further progression. Children with curvature between 25 and 40 degrees who are still growing warrant bracing. Most curvature of greater than 50 degrees, regardless of skeletal maturity, will progress slowly even after growth is completed. These children therefore require surgery to prevent further progression and to restore structural balance to the spine (Figure 23–4).

CONGENITAL SCOLIOSIS

Congenital scoliosis is caused by the failure of formation or segmentation of the vertebrae during embryonic development. Cardiac, visceral, and renal anomalies are frequently associated with congenital curves. Anomalies of the spinal cord may be present and must be investigated before any treatment is initiated. Management can involve either observation for small, nonprogressive curves or surgical stabilization for larger, progressive curves. Bracing is ineffective in controlling progression in congenital scoliosis.

PARALYTIC SCOLIOSIS

A variety of neuromuscular problems are associated with scoliosis. Paralytic curves tend to be progressive and respond poorly to bracing. Treatment decisions must be individualized depending on the patient, the goals of treatment, and the prognosis of the disease.

KYPHOSIS

Kyphosis is normally present in the thoracic spine. Two types of excessive kyphosis may occur in adolescents. Scheuermann kyphosis is a painful, progressive kyphosis in teenage boys. Examination shows a sharp, well-demarcated kyphosis in the thoracic spine. Radiographs demonstrate irregularity and anterior wedging of the involved vertebral endplates. Treatment is directed at pain control and prevention of progressive deformity and neurologic injury. Bracing is usually appropriate. Postural roundback is an exaggerated kyphosis seen in adolescents because of poor posture; it resolves spontaneously and no treatment is needed.

SPONDYLOLYSIS & SPONDYLOLISTHESIS

Spondylolysis is a defect in the lamina of the vertebrae in the pars interarticularis, usually in the lumbar spine. This defect may allow the adjacent superior vertebrae to slip forward, producing spondylolisthesis. Rest and analgesics may be effective initially. Progressive spondylolisthesis eventually may require treatment.

BACK PAIN

In contrast to adults, back pain is unusual in children and should be investigated completely. A careful history and physical examination are mandatory, and spine radiographs should be obtained. For persistent symptoms, a bone scan and, in some instances, a magnetic resonance imaging scan (MRI) should be obtained to determine the cause.

TORTICOLLIS

Congenital wryneck, or **torticollis,** is characterized by tilting of the neck in infants. It is most often caused by a contracture of the sternocleidomastoid muscle on the side toward which the head is tilted. The etiology of congenital muscular torticollis is unknown; intrauterine positioning and trauma to the sternocleidomastoid muscle have been implicated. There is a high association with developmental dysplasia of the hip (20%), and this should always be

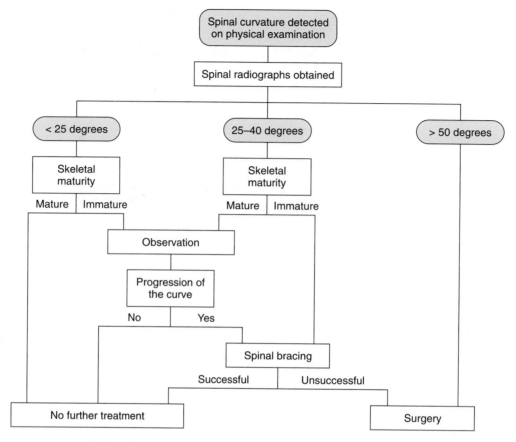

Figure 23–4. Algorithm for treatment of idiopathic adolescent scoliosis.

carefully investigated. Radiographs can detect abnormalities of the cervical spine that may cause torticollis.

Treatment for congenital torticollis begins with passive stretching. In 90% of patients, torticollis resolves with stretching alone. Surgery may be necessary for persistent deformity.

LOWER-EXTREMITY DEFORMITIES

TORSIONAL & ANGULAR DEFORMITIES

Concern regarding the torsional and angular development of the lower extremities in children is ubiquitous. These "deformities" usually represent variations of normal lower extremity development in children and have a favorable natural history. Most torsional deformities correct with growth.

Intoeing

Intoeing is defined as the turning in of the feet toward the midline during walking. Intoeing may result from three anatomic areas: the foot, the tibia, and the femur. These anatomic areas are clearly defined by physical examination (Figure 23–5).

Metatarsus adductus (MA) is defined by the presence of forefoot varus with a normal ankle and hindfoot. The lateral border of the foot is curved like a "kidney bean." MA probably results from intrauterine positioning. Treatment depends on the flexibility of the foot. Flexible, mild deformities usually resolve spontaneously or with passive stretching. Rigid deformities may require serial stretching casts or, rarely, surgery for correction.

Inward tibial torsion is defined as an excessive inward twisting of the tibiofibular unit. It is a variation of normal limb development. Intrauterine positioning may contribute. Inward tibial torsion is the most common cause of

Cause	Appearance	Age	Examination	Treatment
Metatarsus adductus	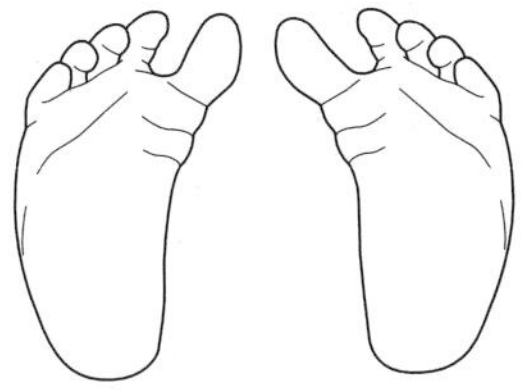	0–2 years	Curved lateral border of foot Heel bisector 4th–5th toe Flexibile versus rigid?	Flexible: stretch Rigid: cast
Inward tibial torsion	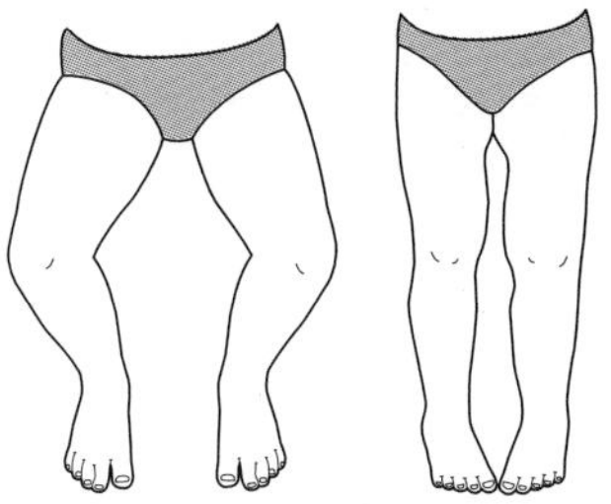	1–3 years	Inward thigh-foot angle Neutral transmalleolar axis	None
Inward femoral torsion	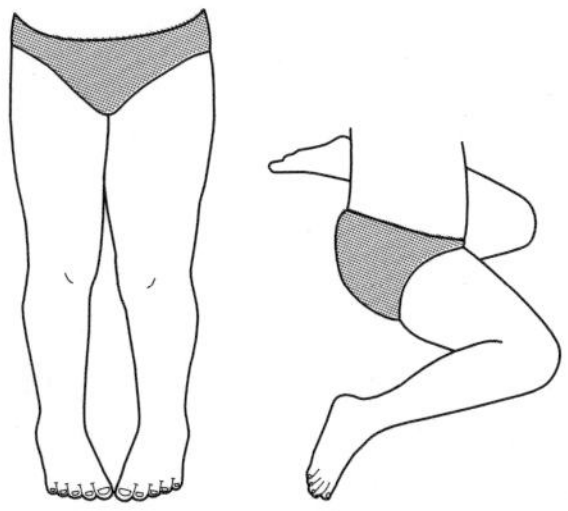	> 3 years	Increased inward hip rotation (prone)	None Surgery (rare)

Figure 23–5. Intoeing and its causes.

intoeing in children younger than 3 years and corrects spontaneously with growth. Torsional bracing, despite its popularity, is rarely indicated and has never been proved efficacious.

Inward femoral torsion, the most common cause of intoeing after age 3 years, is caused by increased anteversion of the femoral neck relative to the knee. Sitting and sleeping habits are often implicated but are probably not etiologic factors. Inward femoral torsion corrects with growth by 10 years of age. Again, bracing has not been demonstrated to be of any benefit and is not indicated. About 1% of children require surgical correction for residual cosmetic or functional problems.

Out-toeing

Out-toeing is rarely a functional problem. Causes include outward rotation contracture of the hip, torsional variations in femoral and tibial development, and flexible flatfeet. Toddlers learning to walk often have a wide-based gait for stability, which looks like out-toeing. Out-toeing rarely requires treatment, and parents should be assured that spontaneous correction is the rule.

Genu Varum & Genu Valgum (Bowlegs & Knock Knees)

Bowlegs and knock knees usually represent normal variations in limb development in children. Most deformities resolve spontaneously with growth. Bowlegs that have not resolved by age 2½ years and knock knees after age 7 years require referral to an orthopedist. Pathologic forms of bowlegs such as rickets, Blount disease, and skeletal dysplasia must be sought when deformities persist.

HIP PROBLEMS

Developmental Dysplasia of the Hip

Developmental dysplasia of the hip (DDH) represents a spectrum of hip problems ranging from mild instability of the hip in the acetabulum to frank dislocation. The inaccurate term **congenital dislocation of the hip** is no longer used, as some dislocations occur after birth.

About 1:100 children have dislocatable hips in the newborn nursery, and complete dislocation of the hip develops in 1:1000. Several factors are associated with the development of hip dysplasia. Mechanical, environmental, hormonal, and genetic factors are thought to increase the incidence of DDH (Table 23–3). The diagnosis of DDH is made primarily by physical examination and confirmed by radiographic and ultrasound studies. Several clues in the physical examination can point to the diagnosis. Asymmetry in the fat folds of the thigh can reflect the relative shortening of the leg because of the proximal dislocation of the femoral head out of the acetabulum. Similarly, the Galiazzi test (Figure 23–6) compares the level of the knees after the baby is carefully placed flat on the examination table with the hips and knees flexed. If one knee is higher than another, this may indicate a dislocatable hip. The Ortolani maneuver (Figure 23–7) is the sensation of a "clunk" when the hips are abducted with hips and knees flexed. The thighs should be able to abduct until they are flat against the examination table. The clunk represents the passive reduction of the femoral head back into the acetabulum. The Barlow maneuver (Figure 23–8) attempts to dislocate the femur that tends to rest in the acetabulum. Gentle but firm pressure directed posteriorly on the proximal medial thigh by the thumb while the hip is adducted elicits a clunk with subluxation or dislocation of the hip. The physical findings change depending on the age of the child. The Ortolani and Barlow maneuvers are reliable only until the child reaches 3 months of age, after which limited abduction becomes the most prominent physical finding (Table 23–4).

Treatment of confirmed DDH is age dependent. The principles are to obtain a reduction of the hip into the acetabulum, maintain a reduction, and allow adaptive changes in the hip to resolve residual abnormalities until the hip is normal (Figure 23–9). Early diagnosis is essential and simplifies management.

Legg-Calvé-Perthes Disease

Legg-Calvé-Perthes (LCP) disease is an idiopathic

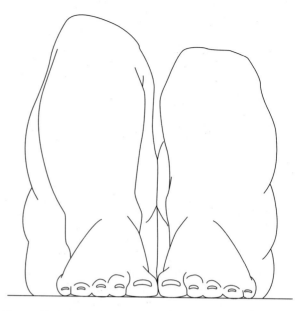

Figure 23–6. The Galiazzi test. (Reproduced, with permission, from Skinner SR: Orthopedic problems in childhood. Page 2136 in: Rudolph AM et al [editors]: *Rudolph's Pediatrics*, 20th ed. Appleton & Lange, 1996.)

process in which the capital femoral epiphysis becomes avascular, is resorbed, and then is revascularized. The etiology of LCP is uncertain, but hormonal, genetic, infectious, and traumatic factors may be involved. LCP is more common in boys aged 4–10 years who are short in stature. Skeletal age is usually delayed.

LCP typically presents with a limp of insidious onset, associated with groin and knee pain. Examination suggests an irritable hip with restricted range of movement, especially abduction and inward rotation. The diagnosis is confirmed with plain radiographs of the pelvis. Bone scans and MRI may be helpful in early diagnosis but are usually unnecessary. The prognosis is dependent on age at onset, extent of femoral head involvement, and the stage of healing at the time treatment is initiated.

During the resorption and revascularization phase of LCP, the femoral head demonstrates "biologic plasticity" and responds to the forces placed on it. Therefore, the principle of treatment is to maintain containment of the femoral head in the acetabulum during the healing and remodeling process. This is achieved by either abduction bracing or surgery. Revascularization and healing of the femoral head usually takes 18–36 months.

Slipped Capital Femoral Epiphysis

In slipped capital femoral epiphysis (SCFE) disorder, the capital femoral epiphysis slips off the metaphysis through the growth plate, producing deformity of the proximal femur. The etiology is uncertain; mechanical

Table 23–3. Etiologic factors associated with developmental dysplasia of the hip.

Mechanical
Breech presentation
First born
Oligohydramnios
Hormonal
Estrogens
Relaxin
Genetic
Environmental
Infant swaddling

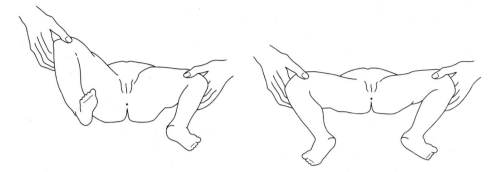

Figure 23–7. The Ortolani test. (See text for description.) (Reproduced, with permission, from Skinner SR: Orthopedic problems in childhood. Page 2137 in Rudolph AM et al [editors]: *Rudolph's Pediatrics,* 20th ed. Appleton & Lange, 1996.)

and hormonal factors have been implicated. SCFE typically affects obese adolescents during the adolescent growth spurt.

Most children present with an insidious onset of limping and pain that suddenly increase in severity. The pain may localize to the knee, thigh, or groin, and the clinician may miss this diagnosis if only the joint presenting with pain is examined. During examination of the hip, flexion produces marked outward rotation and reproduces symptoms.

Radiographs confirm the diagnosis of SCFE. Anterior-posterior and frog lateral views of the pelvis are obtained for initial assessment of the hips. Early radiographic signs of SCFE, including widening of the physis, a metaphyseal blanche, or varus position of the epiphysis relative to the metaphysis, may be subtle. As the slippage becomes more chronic, the deformity becomes more obvious. In chronic

SCFE, there is evidence of remodeling of the femoral neck.

On recognition, SCFE requires immediate surgical treatment to prevent further slipping of the femoral epiphysis. This is accomplished by epiphysiodesis of the capital femoral growth plate by percutaneous insertion of one or two cannulated screws.

FOOT PROBLEMS

Foot deformities are a source of considerable concern to parents and grandparents. Treatment myths abound but rarely have a scientific basis. Most problems are minor and have a favorable prognosis. However, some seemingly minor foot deformities may be the first sign of a significant neurologic problem; each must receive careful

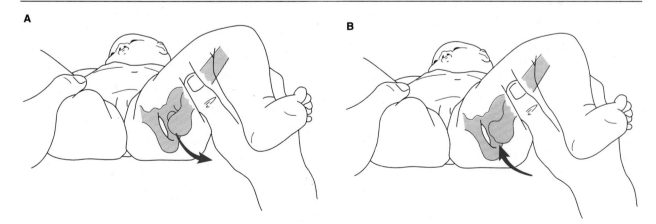

Figure 23–8. The Barlow maneuver. **A:** Gentle pressure by the thumb is first placed in the infant's groin in a posterior and lateral direction to dislocate the hip. **B:** The fingers then push the greater trochanter of the femur anteriorly and medially to return the femoral head to the acetabulum. (Reproduced, with permission, from Skinner SR: Orthopedic problems in childhood. Page 2137 in: Rudolph AM et al [editors]: *Rudolph's Pediatrics,* 20th ed. Appleton & Lange, 1996.)

Table 23–4. Clinical signs of developmental dysplasia of the hip.

Test	Age		
	0–1 mo	1–3 mo	3–6 mo
Ortolani (%)	100	29	15
Limited abduction (%)	7	67	86

consideration. Evaluation of the foot begins with a thorough physical examination. Position, alignment, and flexibility of the foot should be documented. Management depends on the diagnosis, severity, and expected natural history (Figure 23–10).

Clubfoot

A clubfoot has three components: extreme plantar flexion of the ankle (equinus), medial angulation of the hindfoot (varus), and adduction and supination of the forefoot. Clubfeet can be divided into three categories. **Postural** clubfeet result from intrauterine molding and correct rapidly after birth with stretching or several serial casts. **Congenital** clubfeet, the most common form, probably represent a true limb dysplasia. Congenital clubfeet rarely correct with casting alone. **Teratologic** clubfeet are asso-

ciated with other problems, such as myelomeningocele, and usually require surgery for correction.

Treatment begins with application of stretching casts, preferably in the newborn nursery. Serial casts are continued until either the foot is completely corrected or a plateau is reached. This plateau typically occurs at about 3 months of age. Clubfeet resistant to serial casting require surgery, which is best accomplished by a pediatric orthopedist when the child reaches about ages 4–6 months.

Calcaneovalgus Foot

Calcaneovalgus foot deformity is apparent at the time of birth and is the result of in utero positioning. The dorsum of the foot is positioned along the anterior aspect of the tibia. This deformity resolves spontaneously with simple stretching and time. Residual deformity is unusual.

Congenital Vertical Talus

Congenital vertical talus (CVT) is a rare deformity in which the talus is positioned in marked plantar flexion; the talonavicular joint is dislocated with the navicular positioned dorsally on the talus. Diagnosis is frequently delayed because CVT is often confused with a calcaneovalgus foot or a flexible flatfoot. CVT is distinguished by a

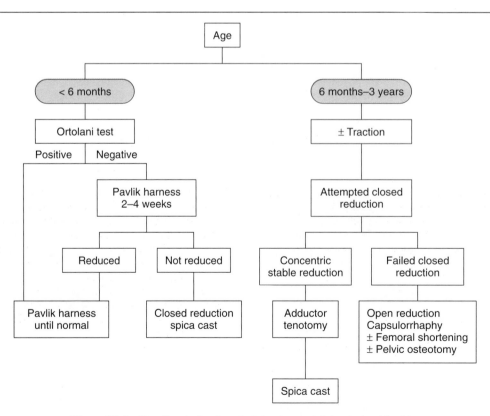

Figure 23–9. Algorithm for treatment of developmental dysplasia of the hip.

Condition	Age at presentation	Appearance	Main feature	Treatment
Clubfeet	Birth	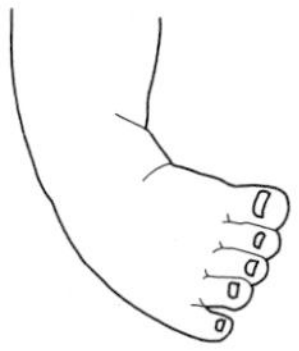	Fixed equinovarus	Serial casts; surgery in 80%
Calcaneovalgus feet	Birth	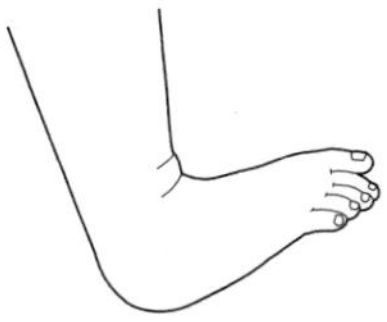	Dorsum of foot rests on shin	Reassurance, stretching
Metatarsus adductus	Birth	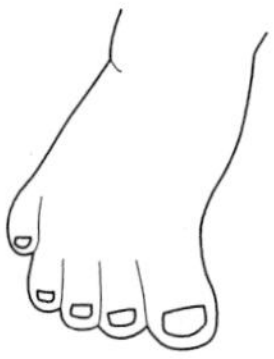	Forefoot adduction	Stretching, casting
Vertical talus	Birth	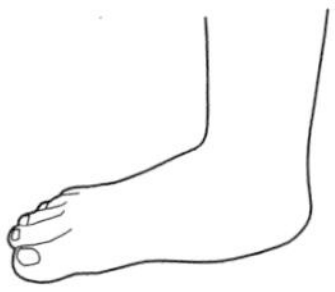	Rocker-bottom foot	Surgery
Flexible flatfoot	2 years plus	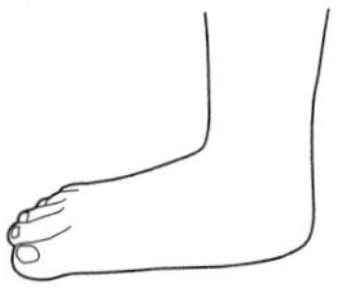	Flexible flatfeet	None

Figure 23–10. Common foot deformities in children and their management.

rigid **rocker-bottom deformity** and equinus of the hindfoot. The etiology of CVT often has a neurologic basis.

Nonoperative treatment consisting of stretching casts may improve flexibility of the foot but does not achieve full correction. Surgical correction of the foot is usually required.

Pes Planus (Flatfeet)

Flatfeet occur when there is loss of the longitudinal arch of the foot. Most flatfeet are flexible and may be associated with generalized ligamentous laxity. Most chil-

dren with flatfeet can wear normal shoes and rarely have problems such as pain, excessive shoe wear, or functional difficulties. The use of arch supports, "orthopedic" shoes, and other treatment modalities to attempt to recreate a "normal" arch have no scientific basis. If a child has problems with excessive shoe wear and positioning problems, orthotics may be appropriate.

A rigid flatfoot must be distinguished from a flexible flatfoot. A rigid foot may be associated with neurologic disorders, tarsal coalition, trauma, infection, tumors, and other problems.

REFERENCES

Engle MG, Staheli LT: The natural history of the angle of gait, tibial torsion, knee angle, hip rotation, and development of the arch in normal children. Clin Orthop 1974;99:12.

Hensinger RN: Congenital dislocation of the hip. Treatment from infancy to walking age. Orthop Clin North Am 1987;18:597.

Kling TF: Angular deformities of the lower limbs in children. Orthop Clin North Am 1987;18:513.

Salenius P, Vankka E: The development of the tibiofemoral angle in children. J Bone Joint Surg [Am] 1975;57-A:259.

Staheli LT et al: Lower extremity rotational problems in children: Normal values to guide management. J Bone Joint Surg [Am] 1985;67-A:39.

Wenger DR et al: Corrective shoes and inserts as treatment for flexible flatfoot in infants and children. J Bone Joint Surg [Am] 1989;71-A:800.

24

Ethical Issues in Pediatrics

Bernard Lo, MD, & Ann Alpers, JD

Physicians and medical students often confront ethical issues in their clinical work. Some pediatric cases can present dramatic dilemmas, such as whether to discontinue mechanical ventilation in a 400-g, 22-week-old infant who has respiratory failure and intracerebral hemorrhage. Typically, however, ethical issues are more subtle. For example, a pediatrician may have nagging doubts about whether to inform a child of a grave diagnosis or whether to tell the parents of an adolescent that their child has sought care for a sexually transmitted disease.

In this chapter, we offer suggestions on how to approach common ethical problems and analyze the reasons for and against conflicting courses of action. We first address two fundamental questions:

1. Which standards should be used in making decisions about the health care of children?
2. Who should make medical decisions for children?

We then discuss decisions about life-sustaining interventions, the relationship between the pediatrician and the parents and children, conflicts of interest, clinical research, and the role of the pediatrician and medical student.

WHICH STANDARDS SHOULD BE USED IN MAKING MEDICAL DECISIONS?

Although acting in the best interests of the child is the fundamental ethical guideline in pediatrics, other factors may need to be considered.

BEST INTERESTS OF THE CHILD

The expected benefits of a medical intervention should outweigh the possible risks. The **best interests** of the child are often vague and difficult to interpret. Individuals may disagree over how to determine which factors constitute a child's best interests and which outcomes are desirable and how to weigh the benefits and burdens of interventions. By promoting some of a child's interests, one may set back other interests.

A child's best interests include both **duration** and **quality of life.** For example, in deciding about the use of chemotherapy for a child who has cancer, parents usually consider not only the projected survival but also the likely side effects of treatment and the child's expected level of functioning. Although judgments about quality of life seem unavoidable, they may be problematic ethically, because it is difficult to predict the quality of life of a child. Healthy persons tend to underestimate the quality of life of persons who have chronic illness. The determination of quality of life should not be confounded by burdens to third parties or the costs to society. Despite these shortcomings, the concept of best interests is important because children deserve respect as individuals separate from their parents, with their own interests and rights.

PREFERENCES OF THE CHILD

To the extent that children have the capacity to make informed decisions about their medical care, their self-determination and choices should be respected. When children cannot give informed consent, their assent to interventions is still ethically important. It is disturbing to force a therapeutic intervention on a child who is actively resisting it. Although a child's objections are not necessarily decisive (eg, a child who objects to receiving shots should still receive immunizations), the child's lack of assent should take on more weight as the child becomes more capable of making informed decisions. The child's refusal to assent also becomes important when the benefits of treatment are unclear because they are balanced by serious burdens or because the possible benefits are speculative.

FUTILE INTERVENTIONS

Some parents may insist on an intervention that physicians regard as futile in the strict sense that it has no pathophysiologic rationale, it has already failed in the patient, maximal treatment is failing, or the goals of care cannot be achieved. Under these circumstances, physicians have no ethical obligation to provide such care, and parents are not entitled to demand whatever care they desire.

In some cases, physicians use the term "futile" in a looser sense when they believe that the parents' goals for care are not worth pursing, the likelihood of success is small, the child's quality of life is unacceptable, or the costs are prohibitive. In these circumstances, unilateral decisions by physicians to withhold interventions could be arbitrary and inconsistent. Such decisions are inappropriate unless authorized by society. For example, it would be problematic to withhold ventilatory support from a child with cerebral palsy who has chronic lung disease as a result of premature delivery on the basis of futility when that child, although developmentally disabled, is alert and capable of some interaction with his or her parents.

INTERESTS OF PARENTS & FAMILY MEMBERS

The interests of parents and other family members must also be considered. The time and expense of caring for a sick child may compromise the rearing of other children or jeopardize the family home or business. Although parents and families should be expected to make some sacrifices, they should not be expected to devote their entire lives to a sick child. Pediatricians should help provide parents with emotional and social support so that families do not feel overwhelmed by the burdens of care.

PREVENTION OF HARM TO OTHERS

Society has an interest in maintaining the public health and preventing the spread of infectious disease. For example, public health officials have the legal power to compel vaccination. They can also require directly observed therapy (watching a child swallow pills) of children with tuberculosis to ensure adherence to treatment until cure. In addition, sexually transmitted diseases, such as gonorrhea, are reported to the public health department, which does contact tracing.

JUST ALLOCATION OF RESOURCES

Physicians should allocate limited health care resources in a fair manner. Pediatricians whose patients lack prenatal care and immunizations may be outraged when large amounts of money are spent on intensive care for neonates who have a very small likelihood of survival. However, the allocation of resources on a public policy level needs to be distinguished from rationing decisions at the bedside or in the office. Pediatricians can advocate for universal access to health care and more equitable allocation of resources, but they should not limit beneficial care for one child in an effort to save money for other health care priorities, unless society or the parents have authorized them to do so. Furthermore, attempts at bedside rationing are usually ineffective gestures because money saved on one patient cannot be redirected to more worthwhile social goals. In exceptional situations, if the provision of scarce resources (such as a bed in the intensive care unit or extracorporeal membrane oxygenation) to one child would deny care to another child who would obtain much greater medical benefit, it would be appropriate to limit the care of the former child.

WHO SHOULD MAKE MEDICAL DECISIONS FOR CHILDREN?

Children usually cannot make informed decisions about their medical care or protect themselves from harm. Hence, adults must make decisions for them and look after their welfare.

PRESUMPTION OF PARENTAL DECISION-MAKING

Parents are presumed to be the appropriate decision-makers for children because, in most cases, love motivates them to act in the best interests of their children. The culture of the United States prizes parental responsibility, the integrity of the family, and strong parent-child relationships. Society therefore grants parents considerable power and discretion to raise children according to their own values. The parents' view of what is best for the child should usually be respected. In most circumstances, parents give pediatricians permission to carry out recommended care. Parents are permitted to decline interventions when they believe the risks outweigh the benefits.

Exceptions to Parental Decision-Making

In some cases, the presumption of parental decision-making may be invalid. Some parents may be estranged from their children or unwilling to be involved in decisions about their care. Other parents lack the capacity to make informed decisions; they may be severely impaired by such factors as alcohol or substance abuse, developmental disability, or immaturity. Nevertheless, it is expected that parents make decisions for their children unless a court has appointed someone else as guardian. The judicial process, however, may be too slow for medical decisions to be made in a timely manner. In practice, physicians often make informal arrangements with other family members when the parents are absent or incapable of making decisions.

In exceptional situations, the parents' assessment of the child's best interests may be overridden. For example, as discussed later, parents are not permitted to refuse highly effective life-saving therapy that is associated with few side effects, such as antibiotics for bacterial meningitis, for a previously healthy child.

Emergencies

In emergency situations, when a parent or guardian is not available and delay in treatment would jeopardize the child's health or life, the physician should provide appropriate treatment without parental permission. The rationale is that delaying treatment until approval is obtained would violate the child's best interests.

ADOLESCENT PATIENTS

As children mature, they develop the capacity to make informed decisions about their health care. By statute, adolescents older than 18 years can consent to or refuse medical care without parental involvement. In certain situations, the law may also allow younger minors to make their own decisions about health care. Because statutes vary from state to state, pediatricians need to be familiar with the laws in their jurisdiction.

Mature Minors

Mature minors are those who are capable of giving informed consent. Mature minors should be allowed to consent to or refuse medical treatment, just like adults. Pediatricians need to assess an adolescent's capacity to give informed consent and to help him or her obtain appropriate support from parents or other adults. Physicians need to ask directly about the adolescent's understanding of the proposed intervention, the alternatives, the risks and benefits of each, and the likely consequences. In general, adolescents older than 14 or 15 years can be shown to have such decision-making capacity, whereas younger children often have difficulty entertaining different alternatives, appreciating the consequences of decisions, and appraising their future realistically.

Emancipated Minors

Adolescents who are living apart from parents and managing their own finances, are married, have children, or have served in the armed forces are considered **emancipated minors.** Most states regard them as de facto adults, capable of consenting to their own medical care. Some states require a judicial hearing and declaration of emancipation.

Treatment of Specified Conditions

Most states allow minors to consent to treatment for such sensitive conditions as sexually transmitted diseases, contraception, pregnancy, substance abuse, and psychiatric illness—without parental consent. Requiring parental permission would deter many adolescents from seeking treatment for important public health problems.

Parental Requests for Treatment

Parents may ask the physician to test an adolescent for illicit drug use or pregnancy without telling the child. Although such requests are usually motivated by concern, surreptitious testing is unacceptable because it undermines the child's trust in the physician and compromises future care.

INSTITUTIONAL ETHICS COMMITTEES

Interdisciplinary institutional ethics committees can provide a supportive forum to discuss difficult ethical issues, allow health care workers and parents to develop a better understanding of each other's views, and suggest ways to resolve disagreements. These committees should serve an advisory role and should not relieve pediatricians of their responsibility for decision-making.

COURTS

The courts have the power to intervene in health care decisions to protect the well-being of vulnerable children. Physicians may need to initiate legal proceedings to override parental decisions that severely violate the best interests of the child. This step should be a last resort because the adversarial legal process may polarize parents and health care workers, thereby complicating subsequent care.

DECISIONS ABOUT LIFE-SUSTAINING INTERVENTIONS

Dilemmas may occur when parents refuse life-sustaining interventions.

REFUSAL OF MEDICAL INTERVENTIONS

Parents may refuse interventions that have limited effectiveness, impose serious side effects, are controversial, or require long-term treatment. In such situations, the parents' informed refusals should ordinarily be decisive. Pediatricians need to keep in mind the importance of parental discretion, family integrity, and ongoing care by parents. Refusal of life-sustaining interventions may be ethically appropriate even if the patient's life may be shortened.

Extraordinary & Ordinary Care

The commonly used terms "heroic," "extraordinary," and "ordinary," although intuitively plausible, are confusing and should be abandoned. Interventions such as mechanical ventilation are sometimes categorized as extraordinary because they are invasive, expensive, and highly technological. The crucial ethical issue is not whether a medical technology can be labeled as inherently heroic or ordinary, but how the benefits of the intervention compare with the risks. Any medical intervention may be withheld if the risks outweigh the benefits for the particular patient.

Withholding Versus Withdrawing Interventions

There are no ethical or legal differences between withdrawing and withholding interventions, although there may be a great emotional difference. For example, many physicians or nurses are reluctant to discontinue mechanical ventilation in a child who has severe cystic fibrosis, even though they would not have started the procedure if they had known that the child could not be weaned. This distinction, however, is not tenable. The reasons that justify not starting the intervention—refusal by parents or a mature child in the face of a poor prognosis—would also justify withdrawing the ventilator. Indeed, the reasons to withdraw an intervention are often stronger because the prognosis is clearer after a trial of ventilatory support. Furthermore, if one were not permitted to stop the ventilator, parents and pediatricians might forego at the onset a trial of intensive care, which would determine whether additional treatment, such as antibiotics, would increase the chance of survival.

Do Not Resuscitate Orders

When a child is in cardiopulmonary arrest, cardiopulmonary resuscitation (CPR) needs to be started immediately to have any prospect of success. Therefore, CPR is attempted unless a do not resuscitate (DNR) order has been written. Pediatricians caring for children who have terminal or chronic illness need to raise the issue of DNR orders with parents or mature minors. DNR orders are appropriate if the parents or an informed, competent adolescent refuses CPR or if the child would not survive the hospitalization even if CPR were administered.

DNR orders should be written in the medical record, together with a progress note explaining the decision and plans for further care. "Slow" or shadow codes, in which CPR is perfunctorily administered in a manner known to be ineffective, are unethical because families are deceived into believing that maximal care is being provided. A DNR order means only that CPR will not be administered and does not preclude other interventions. Everyone needs to understand that DNR does not mean withdrawal of all care or abandonment of the patient.

Relief of Distress

After a decision is made to withhold or withdraw life-sustaining interventions from a child who has a terminal illness, the pediatrician should provide adequate relief of distressful symptoms, such as pain or shortness of breath. No predetermined ceiling on the dose of narcotics or sedatives should be set. If lower doses have not adequately controlled symptoms, the dose should be increased to the level necessary to achieve this goal. In rare cases, the dose that provides adequate relief of distress may also depress respiration or even shorten life. In these circumstances, the appropriate goal of care is to relieve distress, not to prolong life.

The Decision-Making Process

Decisions to withhold or withdraw interventions should be discussed with all health care workers who are involved with the patient, including house staff, students, nurses, and social workers. This approach allows them to understand the rationale for the decision; to voice their questions, concerns, and objections; and to make suggestions. This reasoning should also be clearly presented in the medical record.

HANDICAPPED INFANTS

The Federal **Baby Doe Regulations** apply to decisions to withhold medical treatment from disabled infants younger than 1 year of age. The intent of these regulations is to ensure that such interventions as surgery for duodenal atresia or tracheoesophageal fistula in disabled infants (eg, those with Down syndrome) are performed. This particular surgery can cure swallowing problems and allow these children to lead lives that they and their families generally find meaningful. Under the Baby Doe Regulations, treatment other than "appropriate nutrition, hydration, or medication" need not be provided in several situations:

1. when the infant is irreversibly comatose
2. when treatment would merely prolong dying
3. when treatment would not be effective in ameliorating or correcting all life-threatening conditions
4. when treatment would be futile in terms of survival
5. when treatment would be virtually futile and inhumane under such circumstances.

The implication is that medically appropriate nutrition, hydration, or medication must be provided in all cases.

The pediatrician's reasonable medical judgment presumably determines what is medically appropriate. Physicians are not required to provide treatment that, in their judgment, is inappropriate. Decisions to withhold medically indicated treatment may not be based on subjective opinions about the child's future quality of life.

The Baby Doe Regulations have been sharply criticized. Many terms used in the regulations, such as "appropriate" and "futile," are subject to conflicting interpretations. In addition, parents are not mentioned in the decision-making process, despite their customary role as surrogates. Commentators have pointed out that the regulations often are neither literally followed nor strictly enforced.

REFUSAL OF EFFECTIVE LIFE-SAVING THERAPY ASSOCIATED WITH FEW SIDE EFFECTS

Parents sometimes refuse treatments that cure life-threatening conditions and are associated with few medical side effects. For example, Jehovah's Witnesses commonly refuse blood transfusions for children who sustain acute trauma. Christian Scientist parents often refuse antibiotics even for curable life-threatening infections, such as bacterial meningitis. Physicians who are unable to persuade parents to accept such interventions should seek a court order to administer treatment. As one court declared, although "parents may be free to become martyrs themselves," they are not free to "make martyrs of their children."

RELATIONSHIP BETWEEN THE PEDIATRICIAN & THE CHILD & PARENTS

Physicians may face ethical conflicts concerning the disclosure of information, confidentiality, and truth-telling. Appropriate actions are important because they show respect for the child, lead to beneficial consequences, foster trust in the medical profession, and facilitate future care.

DISCLOSURE OF INFORMATION

For parents to make informed decisions, pediatricians must inform them of their child's prognosis, the alternatives for care, and the benefits, risks, and likely consequences of each alternative. Furthermore, to obtain assent from children, pediatricians need to inform them of their

condition and the plan of care, in terms that children can comprehend. Even when children cannot understand medical details, they still want to know what will be done to them.

Some parents do not want their children to know about serious diagnoses, such as cancer. Pediatricians should elicit the parents' concerns and fears. Parents may believe that the child will not be able to handle bad news or that peers will reject the child. Physicians can explain how it is beneficial for children to understand their diagnosis and the proposed therapy. Children may already suspect that something is seriously wrong and may cope better if they can discuss the situation with adults and receive support. Adherence to medical regimens may be enhanced if the child understands the rationale. Physicians can usually persuade parents to disclose information to the child and help the family cope with the bad news.

Parental requests for secrecy are particularly difficult when adolescents are capable of making health care decisions. Pediatricians should ask adolescents whether they want to know what is wrong with them.

Physicians should not promise parents that the child will never learn the diagnosis. Other members of the health care team may disclose it. In addition, pediatricians should not deceive children who ask directly about their condition.

CONFIDENTIALITY

Medical information should be kept confidential because the privacy of children and their parents should be respected. Moreover, the patients and their families might be less willing to seek care if sensitive information were disseminated inappropriately. Confidentiality is not absolute, however, and may be overridden when disclosure has been authorized by parents or adolescents, when the statutes or courts require it, or when it is necessary to protect the public health or to prevent harm to identified third parties. In such instances, physicians should disclose only information that is truly needed. For example, a school needs to know only that the child's absence was medically indicated, not the diagnosis.

Child Abuse & Neglect

Physicians and other health care workers are obligated by law to inform child protective services agencies about cases of suspected child abuse or neglect. Definitive proof of abuse and neglect is not required. The privacy of the parents is overridden to protect vulnerable children from the possibility of serious harm. Intervention may enable parents to obtain enough assistance and support to prevent further abuse. In extreme cases, the child may be removed from parental custody. In evaluating possible cases of child abuse, pediatricians should treat parents with respect, keeping in mind that most parents are trying their best to deal with a difficult situation.

Adolescents' Requests for Confidentiality

Adolescents may wish to keep certain information confidential from their parents. For instance, they may not want parents to know that they are receiving care for a psychiatric condition, a sexually transmitted disease, pregnancy, or substance abuse. State laws generally protect confidentiality in such situations. Physicians should routinely offer adolescents an opportunity to talk privately, apart from their parents. In most cases, however, pediatricians should encourage adolescents to discuss medical decisions with their parents, who can often provide support and advice. Physicians can also help patients disclose information to their parents. In some situations, however, such disclosure may be counterproductive or even dangerous to an adolescent, as when abuse has occurred.

Parental notification regarding abortion is a particularly controversial issue. Several states require that minors who seek an abortion must either have parental permission or obtain a judicial waiver.

TRUTH-TELLING

Some parents may ask physicians to misrepresent the child's diagnosis. For example, a parent may want to have the child excused from school requirements or they may want to obtain insurance coverage. Pediatricians understandably believe that children should receive needed care. Nonetheless, deception undermines trust in physicians. If physicians are willing to use deception to benefit patients, they might also be deceptive in other circumstances that could harm patients.

CONFLICTS OF INTEREST

As professionals, pediatricians and medical students should act in the best interests of their patients even if their own self-interest may be compromised. **Conflicts of interest** occur when advancing the interests of the child would harm the self-interest of the physician or the interests of third parties, such as hospitals or insurers.

FINANCIAL CONFLICTS OF INTEREST

These conflicts may occur under any reimbursement system. Fee-for-service reimbursement and physician investment in health care facilities to which they refer patients create incentives for physicians to order services of little or no clinical utility. On the other hand, prospective payment and capitated reimbursement offer physicians incentives to withhold expensive interventions that may benefit patients. Regardless of the reimbursement system, pediatricians should order tests and treatments that are in the child's best interests and to which parents agree, no more and no less.

MEDICAL TRAINING & THE CARE OF CHILDREN & YOUTH

Medical students and house officers need to assume clinical responsibility and to learn invasive procedures to benefit future patients. This need to learn may sometimes conflict with the needs of current patients. The attending pediatrician and trainee need to inform parents and children of the roles of members of the medical team and the identity of the health care professionals who are performing the procedures. Requests to exclude trainees from the case or from procedures should be honored when possible. Trainees should be adequately supervised and be willing to ask for help if they encounter difficulties during a procedure.

RESPONSES TO MISTAKES

Many physicians and medical students feel uncomfortable calling attention to mistakes because their reputations and careers may suffer. Pediatricians also may be reluctant to tell parents or patients about mistakes, even those that clearly caused serious harm. They may fear that the family will worry needlessly, get angry, or sue. There are cogent reasons, however, to disclose mistakes. Families and patients often benefit from knowing what happened and what is being done to mitigate the mistake, particularly if changes in care are necessary. In teaching hospitals, discussing mistakes candidly in rounds and conferences enables others to learn from them.

IMPAIRED OR INCOMPETENT COLLEAGUES

Physicians and medical students may observe that a colleague is impaired because of such factors as alcohol abuse or depression. A physician may be reluctant to report the problem to appropriate authorities, fearing that colleagues will regard him or her as a "snitch," or that the other physician will retaliate. Students and residents may be particularly reluctant to raise such issues because they fear their grades and recommendations will suffer. In such situations, the ethical ideal is clear: The well-being of patients should be paramount. Patients may be gravely harmed if an impaired or incompetent physician is allowed to continue to practice. Trainees can usually find ways to raise their concerns in a constructive manner; for example, they can ask the chief resident to review the case.

RESEARCH ON CHILDREN

Traditionally, society has sought to protect children from the potential harms of clinical research. Because children cannot give their own consent, their participation in research has been limited. Clinical research is essential, however, to improve the care of pediatric patients. The scientific basis for pediatric practice is compromised if therapies are not adequately tested in children. Increasingly, the public is viewing research not as exploitation of vulnerable children, but rather as access to promising new therapies for such grave conditions as HIV infection, cystic fibrosis, and cancer.

According to Federal guidelines, several categories of pediatric research may be permitted:

1. research that presents no greater than minimal risk to children
2. research that offers the prospect of direct benefit for participants, provided that the benefit-risk ratio is acceptable
3. research that is likely to yield vitally important knowledge about the patient's disorder or condition, provided that the risk is only slightly more than minimal.

Minimal risks are defined as risks similar to those encountered in ordinary life and in routine physical examinations or tests. Parents or guardians must give their permission for the child to participate in the research. In addition, children must assent to the study if they are capable of doing so.

THE PEDIATRICIAN'S ROLE IN DECISION-MAKING

When ethical issues are complex, reasonable and well-meaning individuals may disagree. Pediatricians and medical students can play a key role in ensuring that difficult decisions are made as wisely as possible.

PROMOTE INFORMED DECISION-MAKING BY PARENTS & CHILDREN

In addition to informing parents and older children of pertinent medical information, physicians help families to deliberate by eliciting their concerns and questions, pointing out overlooked considerations, and recommending what they believe is best for the child. When possible, one pediatrician should have primary, ongoing responsibility for care.

ACT AS THE CHILD'S ADVOCATE

Pediatricians can remind everyone that the goal is to do what is best for the child. They need to try to persuade parents to accept highly effective interventions that have few side effects. In addition, physicians, together with social workers and nurses, can often mobilize emotional support and social resources. For example, the parents and child might benefit from meeting another child who has undergone the same recommended treatment.

OVERRIDE PARENTS ONLY AS A LAST RESORT

Pediatricians are understandably distressed when a child's care at home is suboptimal. They may consider asking the courts to remove the child from parental custody on the basis of neglect. However, lifestyles that physicians may find objectionable, such as alcohol abuse or an untidy home, do not in themselves constitute neglect. Although judicial intervention may be useful for limited interventions, such as a single blood transfusion, it is usually impractical in cases of chronic illness that require ongoing care. Even if a child with asthma or diabetes is not receiving medications, disruption of the parent-child bond causes emotional distress for the child. Foster placement or institutionalization may be worse for the child than are the attempts of well-meaning parents to cope with difficult circumstances. In general, the best response is for pediatricians to try to mobilize more support and resources so that the parents can provide better care.

In summary, it is not enough simply to be a good person or to follow one's personal beliefs when responding to ethical dilemmas. Pediatricians also need to justify their plans to persuade others of their approach. Ethical guidelines help ensure that decisions in similar cases are consistent and fair. Yet, guidelines cannot be applied by rote in difficult cases. Part of the art of clinical medicine is to act with discretion, compassion, and respect for each individual child and family.

REFERENCES

American Academy of Pediatrics Committee on Bioethics: Informed consent, parental permission, and assent in pediatric practice. Pediatrics 1995;95:314.

Clark FI: Intensive care treatment decisions: The roots of our confusion. Pediatrics 1994;94:98.

Council of Ethical and Judicial Affairs of the American Medical Association: Mandatory parental consent to abortion. JAMA 1993;269:82.

Holder AR: Minors' rights to consent to medical care. JAMA 1987;257:3400.

Kopelman LM et al: Neonatologists judge the "Baby Doe" regulations. N Engl J Med 1988;318:677.

Susman EJ et al: Participation in biomedical research: The consent process as viewed by children, adolescents, young adults, and physicians. J Pediatr 1992;121:547.

Index

Page numbers in **boldface** indicate major discussions; those followed by *i* or *t* indicate illustrations or tables.

℘ TITLES OF RELATED INTEREST ℘

Hay, Groothuis, Hayward & Levin
CURRENT Pediatric Diagnosis & Treatment
Thirteenth Edition
a LANGE medical book
1997, 1217 pp., illus., Paperback, ISBN 0-8385-1400-6, A1400-9

Merenstein, Kaplan & Rosenberg
Handbook of Pediatrics
Eighteenth Edition
a LANGE medical book
1997, 1029 pp., illus., Paperback, ISBN 0-8385-3625-5, A3625-9

Hoffman & Greydanus
Adolescent Medicine
Third Edition
1998, 936 pp., illus., Case, ISBN 0-8385-0067-6, A0067-7

Gomella, Cunningham, Eyal & Zenk
Neonatology
Management, Procedures, On-Call Problems, Diseases, and Drugs
Third Edition
a LANGE clinical manual
1994, 620 pp., illus., Spiral, ISBN 0-8385-1331-X, A1331-6

Rudolph, Hoffman & Rudolph
Rudolph's Pediatrics
Twentieth Edition
1996, 2337 pp., illus., Case, ISBN 0-8385-8492-6, A8492-9

Appleton & Lange books are available through your local

health science bookstore or by calling

1-800-423-1359

Appleton & Lange P.O. Box 120041 Stamford, CT 06912-0041